SURGERY

A Monthly Journal Devoted to the Art and Science of Surgery

VOLUME 23

JANUARY—JUNE, 1948

ST. LOUIS
THE C. V. MOSBY COMPANY
1948

Printed in the
United States of America

Press of
The C. V. Mosby Company
St. Louis

SURGERY

Vol. 23 | January, 1948 | No. 1

Original Communications

THE ARTERIAL BLOOD SUPPLY OF THE COMMON AND HEPATIC BILE DUCTS WITH REFERENCE TO THE PROBLEMS OF COMMON DUCT INJURY AND REPAIR

Based on a Series of Twenty-Three Dissections

Alfred L. Shapiro, M.D., and Gregory L. Robillard, M.D., Brooklyn, N. Y.

(From the Surgical and Pathological Services of the Brooklyn Cancer Institute, Beth El, and Norwegian Hospitals)

In the course of a study, appearing elsewhere, on the morphology and variations of the duodenal blood vasculature in relation to the problem of postgastrectomy duodenal stump leakage, we[80] had frequent occasion to trace the small blood vessels supplying the ductus choledochus. In attempting to compare our findings with previous anatomic descriptions, review of some thirty treatises, atlases, dissection manuals, and applied texts[1-30] failed to disclose any definitive consideration of the blood supply of the biliary passages proper, although considerable detail on the variational anatomy of the hepatic arteries was generally incorporated. Painstaking search of the literature revealed no reasonably complete study of the topic; however, a few writers[32, 34, 40, 48, 49, 66, 76] briefly referred to one or more small arteries actually or presumably supplying the bile ducts. Contrary to our observations, these vessels were generally indicated as arising primarily from the hepatic arteries.[16, 32, 34, 42, 48] A single fairly recent foreign paper, comprehensive and well executed, dealing with the venous circulation of the extrahepatic ductal system, but without reference to its arteries, was encountered.[54] No articles in the English language journals were found, and with few exceptions the meager depications appear to be relatively at variance with our findings.

The greatly increased clinical importance of bile duct surgery in recent decades warrants, in our opinion, this somewhat detailed re-presentation of its blood supply. The voluminous literature and discussions of common duct injury incident to surgery and the numerous operative descriptions of reparative, reconstructive, or the newer radically resective procedures apparently omit all consideration of the intrinsic blood supply of this tube.[38, 41, 67-71, 74, 75, 77, 88]

Received for publication, April 29, 1946.

Accurate knowledge of the origins and distribution of these delicate vasa propria may be of great significance if the bile ducts are correctly considered as analogous to gut from the surgical point of view.[79] It is well established that the viability of enteric segments involved in various surgical technical procedures is primarily dependent on maintenance of an adequate circulation. Carter and Maraffins,[67] Allen[70] and Cole,[71] among others, stress the advisability of securing mucosal lined rather than fistulous channels in hepatic or common duct plastic procedures without, however, emphasizing the need to safeguard the blood supply of structures utilized.

The hepatic and common ducts in rudimentary fashion resemble small intestine in structure.[85-88] The mucosal lining, tunica muscularis, and serosa or tunica propria of the 7.0 cm. to 8.5 cm. long ductus would appear to require an adequate circulation for viability no less than similar endodermally derived tissue elsewhere. The possible role that devascularization and consequent ischemic necrosis (secondary to stripping a large cuff or surface of these ducts), might play in the formation of strictures and fistulas, or in the failure of duct reconstructions and choledochoenteroanastomoses, does not appear to have been given suitable consideration. As cited in greater detail in our papers on duodenal and colonic arterial supply, Welsh and Mall, as quoted by Eisberg,[46] Rothschild[57] and other investigators reported that mesenteric ligations of the intestinal vasa recta effectively devascularizing segments as little as 3 to 5 cm. in length produce gangrene of the loop. The intestinal vasa recta are considerably larger and relatively more abundant than the vessels demonstrably supplying the biliary ducts. Anastomotic marginal arteries running the entire length of the common duct and insuring sufficient circulation with relatively complete stripping appear to be infrequent. More often than not small blood vessels approaching almost at right angles to the ducts appear to serve as end arteries for segments several centimeters long and are so arranged that widespread separation of the structures in the hepatoduodenal ligament might lacerate these relatively fine trunks. To what extent such manipulation might result in localized ischemic necrosis and later unexpected stricture formation, so-called spontaneous postoperative rupture, fistulas, or failure of anastomatic procedures, is a problem for the solution of which experimental surgery is indicated. At present we are investigating the effect of such devascularization in animal surgery, utilizing fluorescein and ultraviolet light as an adjuvant method, as advocated by Lange[97] and others, to determine circulatory adequacy. On completion of these studies a detailed report is contemplated. However, it is our present impression that minimal stripping for surface exposures, particularly along the medial border, is probably advisable under most circumstances in order to reduce the danger of devascularization and ischemic necrosis in common duct surgery. As a rule, the cystic and hepatic arteries can be suitably identified without denuding too great a segment of bile duct. It should be noted that in dilatation of the common duct its tiny blood vessels often hypertrophy to a size readily discernible in nonfatty hepatic pedicles.

ARTERIAL DISTRIBUTION TO THE BILE DUCTS

The following survey of the arterial circulation of the extrahepatic biliary passages is drawn in the main from our own investigations and to some extent from the several sources quoted. Dissections were made of twenty-three bodies, all refrigerated, of individuals who had died less than two days before. The anatomic studies were made in the course of complete necropsy and no cases were included where pathology or extreme obesity existed of such a nature as to obscure the structure of the celiac and superior mesenteric trunks or branches. India ink injected[44] in the ligated hepatic, gastroduodenal, and superior mesenteric arteries was utilized for contrast filling of small arteries. For demonstration of the detailed distribution of the ductal vasa propria they were often cannulated by blunted hypodermic needles of small size and injected with India ink from a 1 c.c. tuberculin syringe. Unless otherwise specified, figures given are derived from this series of cases. Corroborative or explanatory reference citations are often indicated by number alone. In studies of this nature no claim for originality of observations can very well be made. Our intent is rather to collate and amplify the meager, widely scattered, and hitherto somewhat inaccessible information available on this somewhat neglected topic. In all probability prior descriptions exist but are difficult to trace.

In our material the small branches supplying the common and hepatic ducts showed great variation in distribution. It would appear possible, as pointed out by us with reference to the arterial supply of the duodenum[80] and transverse colon,[81] that in certain cases a scanty configuration of supplying twigs may render the individuals concerned especially prone to operative ischemic injuries to the bile ducts with resultant fibrosis or fistula formation. Certainly the subject with only two or three demonstrable vessels runs a greater risk of devascularization with one or two small trunks injured than does a person with biliary passages completely ringed by the elaborately ramifying branches of a half-dozen or more proximate arteries. In a fairly thoroughly review of the literature on the possible causes of bile duct injury, a brief statement by Dragstedt and associates[72] that the blood supply of the biliary passages themselves might be involved was the only consideration given to this obvious etiologic factor.

The usual explanations[67, 69, 70, 71, 77, 89-96] given for so-called benign strictures of the common bile duct concur in attributing them, in by far the majority of instances, to cholecystectomy. Occasionally a local stricture at the junction of cystic and choledochal ducts is found, possibly secondary to inflammation, abscess, or choledochostomy. Most writers[67, 70, 89, 91-93, 96] stress the etiologic rule of inadvertent clamping, ligation, section, or excision of a segment of nonvisualized duct. Cattell[96] and Lahey[92] pointed out the danger of injury to the intrapancreatic termination of the duct in duodenal mobilization secondary to subtotal gastrectomy. Calculus ulceration, chronic sclerosing pancreatitis,[94] necrotization by activated pancreatic reflux into the biliary passages,[89] and obliterative cholangitis[93] have been proposed as nontraumatic causative factors.

However, known cholangitis and cholelithiasis are conditions often escaping surgery without the recorded development of stricture formation, whereas the obliteration of the ducts in several hundred reported cases in the literature has almost invariably followed surgery. The premise that factors other than traumatic are frequently responsible would, therefore, in our opinion, be unsubstantiated.

Inasmuch as benign postsurgical fibrotic obliteration of the common bile duct is, in the majority of cases, observed to be extensive or even complete, the possibility of devascularizing injury (followed by similar fibrotic degeneration in ischemic gut) deserves consideration. Since often only the uppermost hepatic or the lowermost intrapancreatic segments are spared, that part of the duct supplied as a rule by twigs from the cystic arteries or less usually by the right hepatic artery appears to be most commonly involved.

The retroduodenal portion of the common duct usually receives three to five twigs from the superior posterior pancreatic duodenal artery as it loops around the common duct.[40, 53, 66] The existence of a posterior pancreaticoduodenal arcade as a constant structure, as discussed in our paper on the duodenal vasculature, is mentioned in only three[2a, 5, 88] of some thirty standard anatomy treatises, texts, and atlases. Pierson,[53] Petren,[55] Ramodnowskaja,[58] Wilmer,[62] and Ziegler,[64] among other recent writers,[31, 43, 45, 50, 63] confirm the presence of both an anterior and a posterior pancreaticoduodenal arcade in from 75 to 80 per cent of human bodies. Quoting our own previously published findings,[80] "the posterior superior pancreaticoduodenal artery generally originates independently from the right dorsal side of the gastroduodenal and in 75 per cent of cases as it descends crossed anteriorly to the right of the retroduodenal common bile duct, curves round it, and, crossing it dorsal to its intrapancreatic portion, descends toward the left thus usually forming an arterial hook around the duct, contributing to it several small branches at the same time. One or more of these twigs extends along the common duct and may form an accessory cystic."

Since it is noted[37, 40, 53] that the most important twigs to the lower ductus choledochus as a rule stem from a sizable vessel, the posterosuperior pancreaticoduodenal artery, which itself has received insufficient anatomic or surgical recognition, it is small wonder that the intrinsic blood supply of the duct proper has been accorded even less attention as a primary subject.

In two of our cases the supraduodenal artery,[61, 62] in both instances larger than usual, gave a discernible branch to about the junction of the lower and middle thirds of the common duct. Here the unusually prominent supraduodenal artery notably overlapped the region of duodenum usually supplied by the superior pancreaticoduodenals. The right hepatic artery, as described many years ago by Haller,[34] may contribute several small branches to the central and upper secetions of the ductus choledochus. We have found such branches with relative constancy, but disagree with Rouviere,[16] Soulsloff,[36] and Faure[48] as to their importance. In accordance with Branco[40] our impression is that these hepatic artery twigs are generally so fine and minute as to contribute only a minor part of the choledochal blood supply in most instances. However, in two of our cases, with a low or common trunk origin of the posterosuperior pancreaticoduodenal the apparently replacing branches came primarily from the right hepatic artery. In another two cases the posterosuperior pancreaticoduodenal arose from the hepatic, and in both of these instances the gastroduodenal and common hepatic arteries gave definite twigs to the common bile duct, which in one example ascended as an accessory cystic, a finding noted also by Branco[40] and Michels[66] and apparently illustrated by Belou[28] in a single figure. Flint,[49] Haller,[34] and Descomps[37] in picturing a fair-sized branch of the gastroduodenal or hepatic artery passing directly to the lower anterior surface of the common bile duct appear to have described the exceptional rather than the regular modes of supply. Descomps,[37] however, noted that the precholedochal ascendant branch might arise from the pancreaticoduodenal arcades.

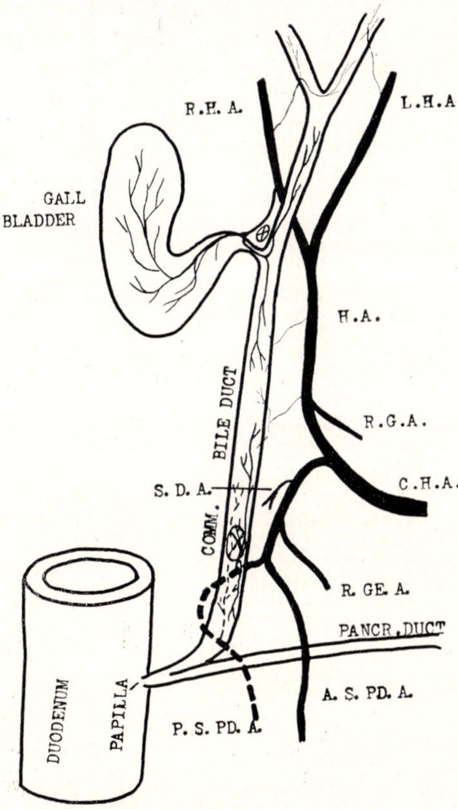

Fig. 1.

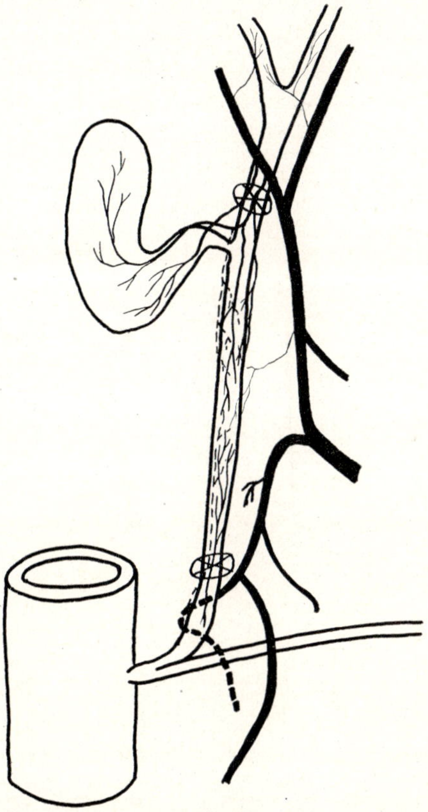

Fig. 2.

Fig. 1.—Usual supply. Note looping of posterosuperior pancreaticoduodenal artery around retroduodenal portion of common duct and origin of ascending and postcholedochal twigs from loop. The right hepatic artery may pass anterior or posterior to the duct. Cystic arterial branch to the duct is of fair size; rami from hepatic arteries are minute and fine. *R.H.A.*, right hepatic artery; *L.H.A.*, left hepatic artery; *C.H.A.*, common hepatic artery; *R.G.A.*, right gastric artery; *S.D.A.*, supraduodenal artery; *A.S.PD.A.*, anterospuperior pancreaticoduodenal artery; *P.S.PD.A.*, posterosuperior pancreaticoduodenal arteries; *R.GE.A.*, right gastroepiploic artery; *H.A.*, hepatic artery.

Fig. 2.—Double cystic artery supplying increased number of descending twigs (four cases). Devascularization would ensue if twigs were lacerated at sites marked by crossed ellipses.

The cystic arteries likewise, as stated also by Faure,[48] send small arterial channels to the upper part of the common duct and, where the bifurcation is low, to the right hepatic duct. Both right and left hepatic arteries may send fine almost hairlike vessels to the extrahepatic segment of the hepatic ducts. Occasionally (two cases) when the ascending branches along the retroperitoneal and posterior segment of the choledochal tube are not strongly developed, the

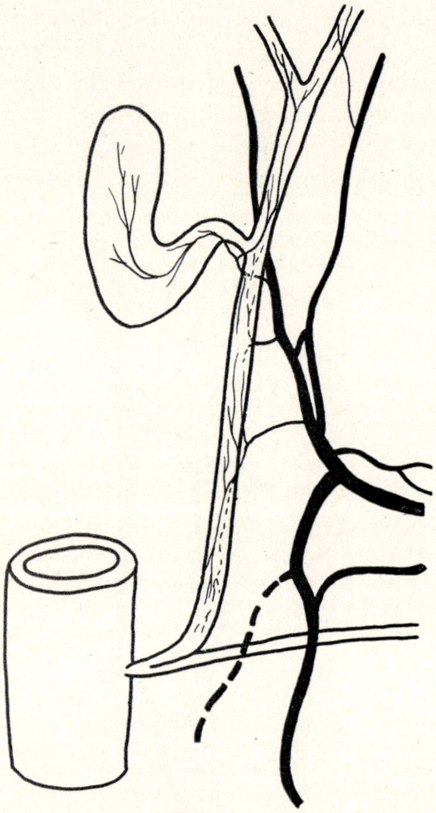

Fig. 3.

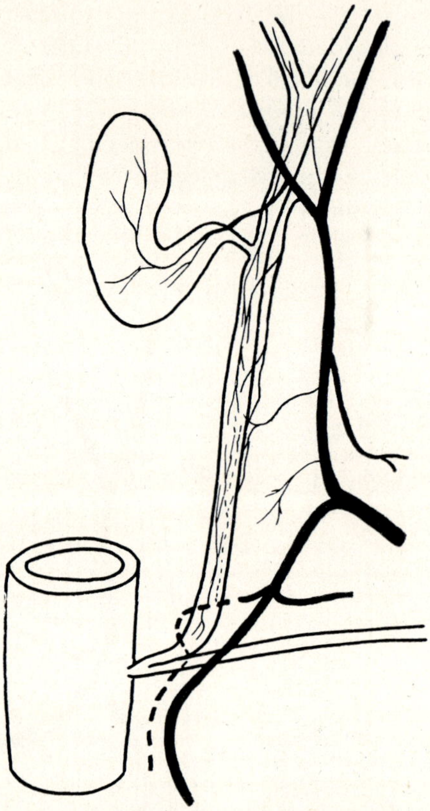

Fig. 4.

Fig. 3.—Replacing arteries from right hepatic; low origin (common trunk) of antero- and posterosuperior pancreaticoduodenal vessels without looping or ascending ductal branches (two cases).

Fig. 4.—Composite supply; several fairly well developed twigs from cystic, hepatic, and posterosuperior pancreaticoduodenal arteries (one case).

cystic or right hepatic artery may provide a usually well-defined descending twig or two which may be traced anteromedially particularly, to almost the lower third of the common duct. Calot, as cited by Branco,[40] appears to have considered this, contrary to our experience, as a typical finding.

Several diagrammatic sketches of the arterial branches to the common bile duct that we have encountered are illustrated in Figs. 1 to 6 to depict the more usual sources of supply as well as the hooking of the posterosuperior pancreaticoduodenal artery around the retroduodenal portion of the common bile duct. At the points indicated by the crossed ellipses, laceration during operation of the arterial branches to the duct proper, or vasa propria, which seem to be functional end-arteries, would apparently devascularize a segment several centimeters long. The dotted lines indicating twigs along the posterior aspect of the common bile duct and hepatic ducts should be borne in mind. As has occurred with the concept of the pancreaticoduodenal circulation, surgeons and anatomists are prone to visualize only the anterior blood supply of these organs. However, as in the case of the small intestine,[44, 46, 47, 56] it is likely that neither

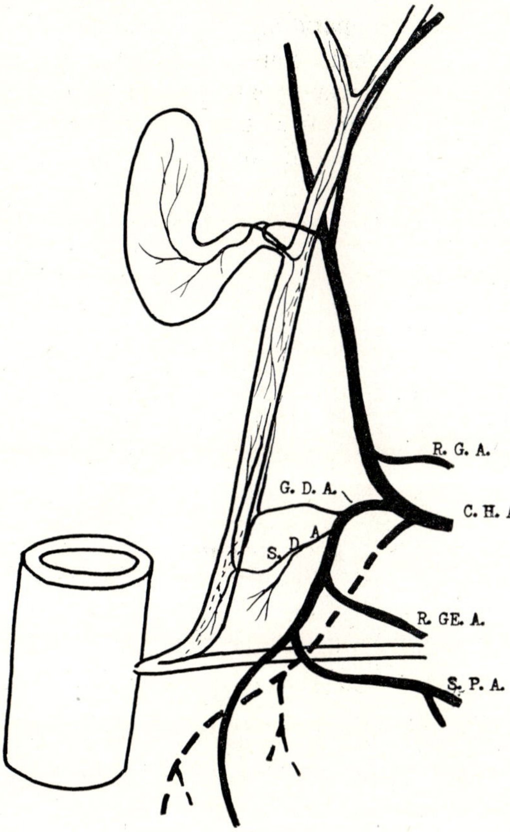

Fig. 5.

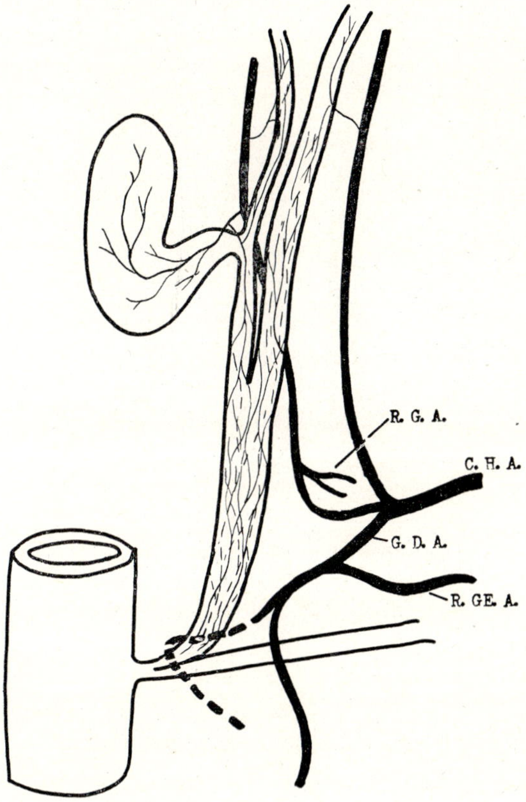

Fig. 6.

Fig. 5.—Origin of superoposterior pancreaticoduodenal artery from common hepatic, superior pancreatic from gastroduodenal; replacing ascending choledochal arteries from gastroduodenal and supraduodenal vessels (one case). *R.G.A.*, right gastric artery; *G.D.A.*, gastroduodenal artery; *C.H.A.*, common hepatic artery; *S.D.A.*, supraduodenal artery; *R.GE.A.*, right gastroepiploic artery; *S.P.A.*, superior pancreatic artery.

Fig. 6.—Ringing of ducts by multiple ascending and descending twigs with elaborate pericholedochal anastomosing arterial plexus. Incidental low bifurcation of hepatic ducts and arteries illustrated (three cases). *R.G.A.*, right gastric artery; *C.H.A.*, common hepatic artery; *G.D.A.*, gastroduodenal artery; *R.GE.A.*, right gastroepiploic artery.

anterior nor posterior twigs provide a completely circumferential anastomosis and that both sets of vessels are necessary to secure adequate blood supply. Histologic studies to determine this point are in progress.

An accessory cystic artery, reported by Flint[49] and other authors[51, 59] as present in about one-sixth of bodies dissected, occurred in three cases, arising in two from the hepatic and one from the gastroduodenal. Only in the latter instance did it provide rami of any size to the bile duct. In none of the cases studied in detail for this report was any remarkable anomaly of the hepatic arteries encountered, therefore we are unable to describe what variations occur in the choledochal blood supply in these cases.[41, 52, 73] Similarly, no accessory or anomalous hepatic or cyst ducts were noted. A retroductal position or low bifurcation of the hepatic vessels, or low division of the common duct, either occurring in about one-quarter and likely to coexist, is not considered abnormal for purposes of this paper.

In the dissection of the hepatic pedicle tiny arteriolar branches from the hepatic arteries, noted also by Branco,[40] were observed to course to the larger lymph nodes and ganglia of both the pedicle and porta hepatis. As a rule the arteries to the biliary passages ran lengthwise for variable distances. In only three instances could a noteworthy pericholedochal network of arterial loops be demonstrated, a finding referred to by Wiart,[32] and Guillaume[35] as a cause of hemorrhage in denuding or incising the hepatocholedochal canal. Friend[76] stated that a plexus of veins and arteries covers the common duct, but reference to his accompanying illustration reveals nonanastomosing ramifying branching of an anterior descending arterial twig from the cystic artery and an ascending anterior vessel from the gastroduodenal in the occasionally encountered prolific pattern referred to previously.

In three bodies, from six to nine branches, ascending and descending, were found to encircle the common duct, the upper coming from the cystic and right hepatic arteries, the lower from the gastroduodenal and superior pancreaticoduodenal. Some of these vessels, however, seemed to form a pericholedochal anastomotic plexus between the cystic and hepatic arteries and the pancreaticoduodenal vessels which did not afford tributaries to the bile ducts proper since they could be easily lifted away intact without lacerating any demonstrable vasa propria. This was, however, not a typical arrangement. No vessels of significance appeared to enter the biliary passages from any of the retroperitoneal structures or the gastric or gastroepiploic arteries.

For purposes of completeness a brief description of the veins of the extrahepatic biliary passages is included in this paper. In our material the upper veins ascended to the porta hepatis. According to Petren[54] they then enter the hepatic vein radicles directly. As a rule, the lower veins drain only the lowermost portion of the common duct and empty into the portal vein. Rouviere,[16] Faure,[48] and Branco[40] portrayed a venous anastomosis between hepatic and portal systems along the common bile duct and indicated that the major venous drainage of the bile ducts is downward and into the portal vein via the superior pancreaticoduodenal or gastroduodenal veins. In several bodies, however, we found that injection of the portal vein filled only the lowermost venules primarily of the retroduodenal portion of the common duct, an apparent substantiation of Petren's[54] contention that the venous drainage of both gall bladder and biliary ducts is into the hepatic vein radicles directly, without major anastomoses between the portal and hepatic venous systems. For this reason, he claimed,[54] there is no dilation of veins along the common bile duct in hepatic cirrhosis.

SUMMARY

The proximate and intrinsic circulation of the ductus choledochus and the hepatic ducts is described as present in twenty-three bodies dissected. The possible etiologic significance of ischemic necrosis in common bile duct and hepatic injury, as obliterative fibrosis, rupture, or fistula formation, or failure of reconstructive ductal anastomoses is considered. The important arterial branches to the common and hepatic ducts are demonstrated as arising primarily from the cystic and posterosuperior pancreaticoduodenal arteries rather than the hepatic artery, as usually represented in the few prior descriptions available in the literature. The venous drainage of the extrahepatic biliary passages ascends in the main to empty directly into the hepatic vein radicles without demonstrable major anastomoses with the portal system.

REFERENCES

1. Callander, C. L.: Surgical Anatomy, ed. 2, Philadelphia, 1942, W. B. Saunders Company.
2a. Cunningham, D. J.: Manual of Practical Anatomy, ed. 8, New York, 1927, Oxford University Press.
2b. Cunningham, D. J.: Textbook of Anatomy, ed. 8, New York, 1943, Oxford University Press.
3. Deaver, J. B.: Surgical Anatomy of the Human Body, ed. 2, Philadelphia, 1927, The Blakiston Company.
4. Grant, J. C. B.: Atlas of Anatomy, Baltimore, 1943, Williams & Wilkins Company.
5. Grant, J. C. B.: Method of Anatomy, ed. 3, Baltimore, 1945, Williams & Wilkins Company.
6. Herzler, J. C.: Practical Anatomy, Philadelphia, 1912, J. B. Lippincott Company.
7. Jamieson, E. C.: Companion to Manuals of Practical Anatomy, ed. 2, Baltimore, 1928, William Wood & Company.
8. Jamieson, E. C.: Illustrations of Regional Anatomy, Baltimore, 1942, Williams & Wilkins Company.
9. Lewis, W. H.: Gray's Anatomy, ed. 24, Philadelphia, 1942, Lea & Febiger.
10. Mainland, D.: Anatomy, New York, 1945, Paul B. Haeber, Inc.
11. Massie, A.: Surgical Anatomy, ed. 3, Philadelphia, 1937, Lea & Febiger.
12. McGregor, A. L.: Synopsis of Surgical Anatomy, ed. 5, Baltimore, 1943, Williams & Wilkins Company.
13. Morris, H.: Human Anatomy, ed. 9, Philadelphia, 1942, The Blakiston Company.
14. Piersol, G. A.: Human Anatomy, ed. 9, Philadelphia, 1930, J. B. Lippincott Company.
15. Quain, J.: Elements of Anatomy, London, 1914, Longmans, Green & Co.
16. Rouviere, H.: Anatomie Humaine, Paris, 1924, Masson & Cie.
17. Testut, L.: Traite d'Anatomie Humaine, ed. 7, Paris, 1926, Gaston Doin & Cie.
18. Shearer, E. M.: Manual of Human Dissection, Philadelphia, 1937, The Blakiston Company.
19. Sobotta, J.: Atlas of Human Anatomy, New York, 1928, G. E. Stechert & Company.
20. Spalteholtz, W.: Hand Atlas of Human Anatomy, ed. 7, Philadelphia, 1940, J. B. Lippincott Company.
21. Treves, F.: Surgical Applied Anatomy, ed. 8, Philadelphia, 1926, Lea & Febiger.
22. Toldt: Atlas of Human Anatomy, reprinted in 1944.
23. Warren, J.: Handbook of Anatomy, Cambridge, 1942, Harvard, University Press.
24. Wilson, E.: A System of Human Anatomy, Philadelphia, 1858, Blanchard and Lea.
25. Jones, J., and Shepard, E.: Manual of Surgical Anatomy, Philadelphia, 1945, The Blakiston Company.
26. Pauchet, V., and Dupret, S.: L'Anatomie en Poche, Paris, 1926, Doin & Cie.
27. Adachi, B.: Dis Arteriensystem der Japanner, Kyoto, 1933.
28. Belou, P.: Revision Anatomica del Sistema Arterial, Buenos Aires, 1934.
29. Hovaloque, A.: Les Arteres Mesenteriques, Paris. 1936, Doin & Cie.
30. Testut, L., and Jacob, O.: Traite d'Anatomie, Topographique avec Applications Medico-Chirurgicales, ed. 4, Paris, 1925, Doin & Cie.
31. Del Campo, J. C.: Circulacion del duodeno, An. Fac. de med. de Montevideo 12: 404, 1927.
32. Wiart, J.: Recherches sur la forme et les rapport du pancreas, J. de l'anat et physiol. 1: 104, 1899.
33. Bergmann, Bruns, and Mickulicz, W.: Handb. d. prakt. Chir. ed. 3, Stuttgart, 1907.

34. Haller, A.: Disputationum Anatomicarum Selectarun, Vandenhoeck Gottingen, 1748.
35. Guillaume, E.: De la Choledocotomie, These de Paris, 1906.
36. Sousloff, H.: Document pour l'anatomie chirurgie des voies biliaries, Arch. Russes de Chir., 1907.
37. Descomps, W.: Le Tronc Coeliaque, These de Paris, 1910.
38. Budde, A.: Beitrage Zur Kenntnis der Topographie der normal Art Hepatica, Deutsche Ztschr. f. Chir. **86**: 18, 1906.
39. Descomps, W., and Siraul: Note sur l'anast de la vesicule biliaire, Lyon med., 1895.
40. Branco, D. R.: Tronc Coeliaque et ses Branches de l'artere Hepatique, Paris, 1912, Steinheil.
41. Browne, E.: Variations in Origin and Course of the Hepatic Artery, SURGERY **8**: 424, 1940.
42. Brewer, G. E.: Some Observations Upon the Surgical Anatomy of the Gall Bladder, Baltimore, 1900, Johns Hopkins Press.
43. Brunschwig, A.: Surgery of Pancreatic Tumors, St. Louis, 1942, The C. V. Mosby Company.
44. Cokkinis, A. J.: Observations on the Mesenteric Circulation, J. Anat. **64**: 200, 1930.
45. Edwards, L. F.: The Retroduodenal Artery, Anat. Rec. **81**: 351, 1941.
46. Eisberg, H. B.: Intestinal Arteries, Anat. Rec. **28**: 227, 1924.
47. Eisberg, H. B.: On the Viability of the Intestine, Ann Surg. **81**: 926, 1928.
48. Faure, J. L.: Quelques Points de L'Anatomie des Vois Biliaires, Paris, 1898.
49. Flint, E. R.: Abnormalities of the Right Hepatic, Cystic and Gastroduodenal Arteries, Brit. J. Surg. **10**: 509, 1922.
50. Kellog, E. L.: The Duodenum, New York, 1933, Paul B. Hoeber, Inc.
51. Lindner, H., and others: Structures in the Hepatic Pedicle, Quart. Bull., Northwestern Univ. M. School **15**: 103, 1941.
52. Lipschitz, B.: A Composite Study of the Coeliac Axis, Ann. Surg. **65**: 213, 1917.
53. Pierson, J. M.: The Arterial Blood Supply of the Pancreas, Surg., Gynec. & Obst. **77**: 426, 1943.
54. Petren, T.: Veins of the Extrahepatic Biliary System, Verhandl. d. anat Gesellsch. **41**: 139, 1932.
55. Petren, T.: Die Arteren und Venen des Duodenums und des Pancreaskopfes beim Menschen, Ztschr. f. Anat. u. Entwchlngsgesch. **90**: 234, 1929.
56. Reeves, T. B.: Study of Arteries Supplying Stomach and Duodenum, Surg., Gynec. & Obst. **30**: 374, 1920.
57. Rothschild, N. S.: Safety Factors in Mesenteric Ligatures, Ann. Surg. **89**: 878, 1929.
58. Ramodnowskaja, Z.: Die Arterien der Bauchspeicheldruse, Ztschr. f. Anat. u. Entwcklngsgesch. **79**: 506, 1926.
59. Thompson, J. M.: Arteries in Hepatic Pedicle, Univ. California Publ., Anat. **1**: 55, 1933.
60. Wharton, G. K.: Blood Supply of the Pancreas, Anat. Rec. **53**: 55, 1932.
61. Wilkie, O. P. D.: Blood Supply of the Duodenum, Surg., Gynec. & Obst. **70**: 662, 1940.
62. Wilmer, H. A.: The Blood Supply of the First Part of the Duodenum, SURGERY **9**: 679, 1941.
63. Yule, E.: The Arterial Supply to the Duodenum, J. Anat. **61**: 345, 1927.
64. Ziegler, H. P.: Excision of the Head of the Pancreas for Carcinoma, Surg., Gynec. & Obst. **74**: 137, 1942.
65. Cavalie, M.: La vesicule biliare et l'artere Cystique, Compt. rend. Congr. de. Med. (Sect. d'anat.), Paris, 1900.
66. Michels, N. A.: Variations in Blood Supply of Liver, Gallbladder, Stomach, Duodenum, and Pancreas, J. Internat. Coll. Surgeons **6**: 502, 1945.
67. Carter, R. F., and Maraffino, B.: Hepato-cholecystenterostomy for Relief of Jaundice in Obliteration of the Hepatic Ducts, Am. J. Surg. **44**: 217, 1944.
68. Eisendrath, D. N.: Operative Injury of the Common and Hepatic Bile Ducts, Surg., Gynec. & Obst. **31**: 1, 1920.
69. Judd, E. S.: Sequelae and Accidents of Biliary Surgery, New England J. Med. **199**: 712, 1928.
70. Allen, A. W.: A Method of Re-establishing Continuity Between the Bile Ducts and the Gastro-Intestinal Tract, Ann. Surg. **121**: 412, 1945.
71. Cole, W. H., Ireneus, C., Jr., and Reynolds, J. T.: Use of Vitallium Tubes in Strictures and Absence of the Common Bile Duct, Ann. Surg. **122**: 490, 1945.
72. Dragstedt, L. R.: Implantation of the Hepatic Duct Into the Duodenum or Stomach, Surg., Gynec. & Obst. **77**: 126, 1943.
73. Perez, G. E.: Arteries Mesentericos, Rev. de med. y cir. Habana **49**: 116, 1944.
74. McWhorter, G. L.: New Method of Gall Bladder Dissection, Surg., Gynec. & Obst. **36**: 256, 1923.
75. Hackett, W. L.: Surgical Anatomy of the Gall Bladder Region, J. Michigan M. Soc. **26**: 26, 1927.
76. Friend, E.: Abnormalities of the Bile Ducts and Their Blood Vessels, Illinois M. J. **56**: 169, 1929.

77. Colp, R., and Ginzburg, L.: Mortality in Surgical Diseases of the Biliary Tract, **105**: 9, 1937.
78. Lurje, A.: Topography of the Extrahepatic Biliary Passages, Ann. Surg. **105**: 161, 1937.
79. Halpert, B.: Note on Distribution of Blood Vessels in Wall of Gall Bladder, Am. Ass. Anat. **35**: 1927.
80. Shapiro, A. L., and Robillard, G. L.: Morphology and Variations of the Duodenal Blood Vasculature, Arch. Surg. **52**: 571, 1946.
81. Shapiro, A. L., and Robillard, G. L.: Variational Anatomy of the Middle Colic Artery, J. Internat. Coll. Surgeons **10**: 157, 1947.
82. Herrlin, J. O., Glasser, S. T., and Lange, K.: New Methods for Determining the Viability of Bowel, Arch. Surg. **45**: 785, 1942.
83. Kopoch, F.: Anatomie des Menschen, Thiene Leipzig, 1911, Georg Thieme.
84. Osler, G. F., and Dow, R. S.: Variations and Anomalies of the Biliary Duct System and Its Associated Blood Supply, West. J. Surg. **53**: 316, 1945.
85. Bremer, J. L.: Textbook of Histology, ed. 6, Philadelphia, 1944, The Blakiston Company.
86. Smith, P. E.: Bailey's Textbook of Histology, ed. 11, Baltimore, 1944, William & Wilkins Company.
87. Sobotta, J.: Textbook and Atlas of Histology, New York, 1928, G. E. Stechert & Company.
88. Poierier, P., and Charpy, A.: Traite d'Anatomie Humaine, ed. 4, Paris, 1901, Masson & Cie.
89. Colp, R.: Repair of Strictures of the Common and Hepatic Bile Ducts, Bull. New York Acad. Med. **22**: 306, 1946.
90. Judd, E. S.: Strictures of the Common Bile Duct, Ann. Surg. **84**: 404, 1926.
91. Cole, W. H.: Strictures of the Common Duct (editorial), Surg., Gynec. & Obst. **82**: 104, 1946.
92. Lahey, F. H.: Strictures of the Common and Hepatic Bile Ducts (editorial), Surg., Gynec. & Obst. **80**: 555, 1945.
93. Flickinger, E. M., and Masson, J. C.: Reconstructive Operations for Benign Stricture of the Bile Ducts, Surg., Gynec. & Obst. **83**: 24, 1946.
94. Peterson, L. W., and Cole, W. H.: Chronic Sclerosing Pancreatitis Causing Complete Stenosis of the Common Bile Duct, Arch. Surg. **51**: 15, 1945.
95. Walters, W., and Heim, D. J.: Stricture of the Common and Hepatic Ducts, Proc. Staff Meet., Mayo Clin. **21**: 377, 1946.
96. Cattell, R. B.: Benign Strictures of the Bile Ducts, Causes and Methods of Repair, S. Clin. North America **23**: 701, 1943.
97. Herrlin, J. O., Glasser, S. T., and Lange, K.: Two New Methods to Determine Viability of Blood, Arch. Surg. **45**: 785, 1942.

UNUSUAL INNERVATION OF THE INTRINSIC MUSCLES OF THE HAND BY MEDIAN AND ULNAR NERVE

EUGENE E. CLIFFTON, M.D., NEW HAVEN, CONN.

IN THE course of examining a large number of peripheral nerve injuries, in a neurosurgical and hand surgery center, it was surprising to find cases in which the innervation of the small hand muscles, apparently, was through unusual channels. Reports of several of these cases were first presented at the Hand Conference at Wakeman General Hospital late in 1945.

The usual innervation of the small hand muscles as described in standard anatomic and peripheral nerve texts is as follows:

MEDIAN	ULNAR
Flexor pollicis brevis	Adductor pollicis
Opponens pollicis	Lumbricales, 3 and 4
Abductor pollicis brevis	Dorsal and palmar interossei
Lumbricales, 1 and 2	Abductor digiti quinti
	Opponens digiti quinti
	Palmaris brevis
	Flexor digiti quinti brevis

It is considered common for the flexor pollicis brevis to have dual innervation, the medial head by the ulnar and the lateral head by the median.

In the cases to be reported, partial function of these muscles remained despite complete section of the nerve involved, either median or ulnar. This same observation has undoubtedly been made by others and five cases with partial function were reported by Murphy and associates.[1] It has not been common knowledge, however, even among neurosurgeons and hand surgeons. Brief mention of the condition has been made in the excellent books on peripheral nerves by Pollack and Davis[2] and Haymaker and Woodhall,[3] and in the report of the Medical Department in World War I.[4] A very complete discussion of the entire problem may be found in the text by Stookey.[5]

In discussing any of these unusual innervations it is well recognized that certain false, trick, or anomalous movements may lead one astray unless great care is taken in the muscle test. It is also well recognized that the only absolute proof of muscle function is palpation of the muscle in its actual contraction, or else palpation of motion of the tendon. However, where this is impossible, one can with a fair degree of accuracy rule out false motions, if strict adherence to the type of motion is insisted upon. Furthermore, one can practically rule out false motion by observations of other muscles and tendons which must take over the function of the muscles being tested. For instance, in testing for the interosseus by motion, the contraction of the extensors of the fingers can be easily visualized and palpated if they are taking over the indicated function.

Received for publication, April 12, 1947.

Although false motion cannot be completely and absolutely ruled out, it was felt that the careful check system used in these cases made the findings fairly definite. Other observations are also important in confirming an opinion that incomplete paralysis is present where a complete paralysis is expected. These include lack of the usual atrophy and, in the case of an ulnar nerve lesion, the absence of an ulnar Griffe. In all the cases to be reported atrophy was absent or minimal and ulnar Griffe was absent or minimal. All nerve checks were made in the nerve laboratory, the staff of which consisted of at least one specially trained medical officer and one specially trained physiotherapist whose sole work was a disinterested testing of each peripheral nerve case by voluntary and electrical tests. Each case was then rechecked by at least one other member of the neurosurgical staff. These tests were performed at least one time preoperatively, one month postoperatively, and at three-month intervals until the patient was discharged. Standard methods of examination were used, especially as outlined in the standard texts on peripheral nerves (Pollack and Davis,[2] Haymaker & Woodhall[3]).

The cases to be described were drawn from a total group of over 3,000 cases of nerve injuries, all of which were carefully observed and followed as outlined. Of this total group we have accurate and complete records on 250 ulnar nerve, 150 median nerve, and 151 combined median and ulnar nerve injuries. Of this group neurorrhaphies were performed on 143 ulnar nerves, 81 median nerves, and on both nerves in 36 cases.

All photographs were produced in the routine manner to show function of the involved muscles, with the usual precautions to prevent false motions. The charts are reproduced exactly as they were found in our files.

The voluntary tests are marked on the approximate basis of 0, no function; 1, just perceptible contraction, 2, 25 to 50 per cent of normal; 3, 50 to 75 per cent of normal; and 4, normal.

In the electrical tests F indicates response to faradic current, but with an asterisk it indicates only sluggish response. G_3 indicates a brisk response to galvanic current. Only a faradic response is considered evidence of normal innervation by this test.

CASE REPORTS

Attention was first drawn to this interesting condition on Dec. 29, 1944, shortly after the admission of the first patient (Case 1).

CASE 1.—This soldier received a severe penetrating wound of the posteromedial forearm 8 cm. below the condyles of the humerus, Sept. 24, 1944. Thirty-one hours later at the Fifteenth Evacuation Hospital a débridement with removal of the shell fragment from the anteromedial forearm and suture of the ulnar nerve with closure of the wound was performed. It is of particular interest that the approximation was by a single sling suture of silk and that the nerve ends were still separated by 1 cm. at closure, despite great tension. On the first examination at the nerve laboratory, Wakeman General Hospital, he was found to have voluntary function of all but the palmar interosseous 3, and faradic response on all ulnar nerve muscles, but with anesthesia in the ulnar distribution. Atrophy was minimal. At operation, Feb. 8, 1945, a branch of the medial antibrachial cutaneous nerve was found divided but unsutured and the ulnar nerve was found to contain a neuroma with the silk suture imbedded in its center. Stimulation of the nerve above the neuroma resulted in very slight contraction of the small hand muscles. As the dissection was extended, however, a nerve fiber was found to enter the ulnar nerve below the neuroma. This fiber extended upward and medially and was found to originate from the median nerve. A small fiber left the ulnar nerve just above the neuroma and joined this cross fiber (Fig. 1, *C*). Stimulation of the cross fiber resulted in contraction of all the ulnar small hand muscles. A secondary

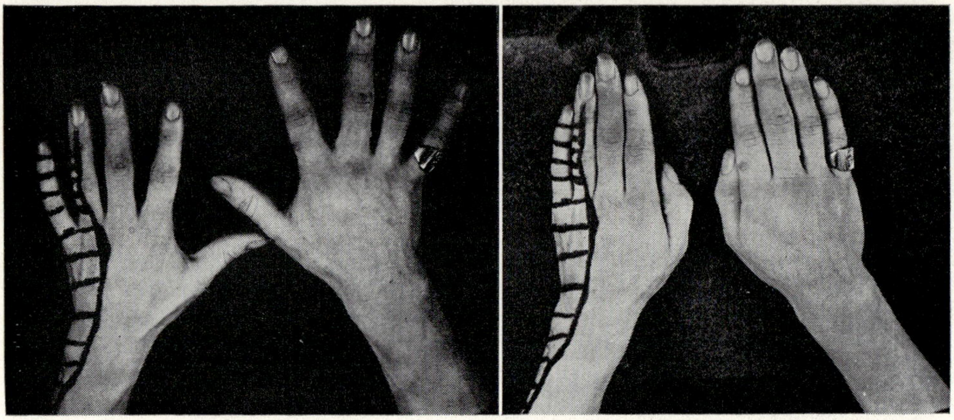

A. *B.*

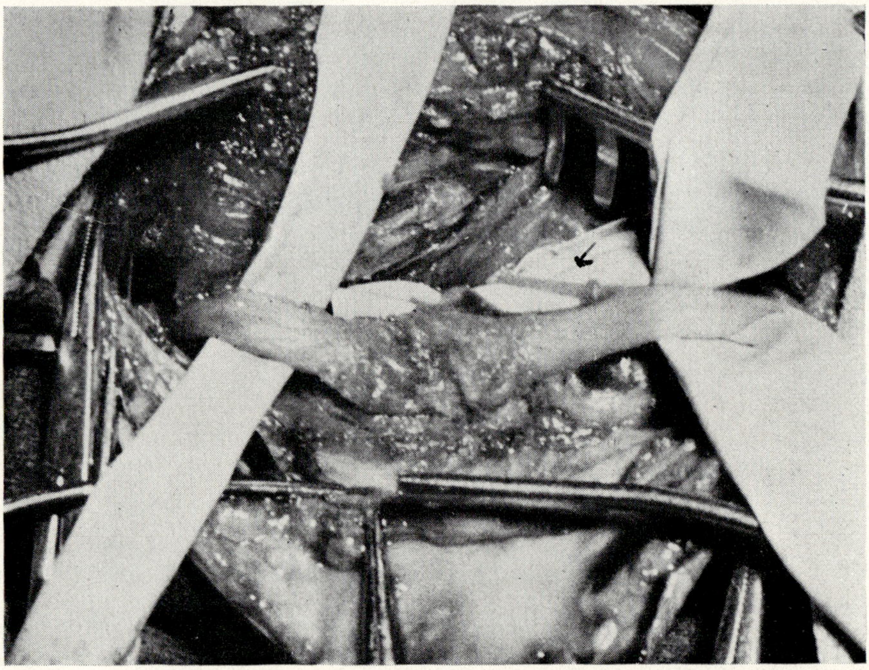

C.

Fig. 1.—*A* and *B*, Note ability to spread and approximate fingers and lack of atrophy. Anesthesia area is outlined. *C*, Operative photograph showing scarring and neuroma formation. The arrow points to the communicating branch from the median nerve entering the ulnar below the neuroma. The branch leaving the ulnar nerve to join this communicating branch can just be seen as it passes over the cottonoid at the neuroma level.

partial neurorrhaphy was performed leaving the cross fiber intact. The nerve chart of this patient (Table I) shows his further course graphically (Fig. 1, *A*, *B*, and *C*, Table I).

During the remaining fifteen months covered by this study an additional three cases with complete division of the ulnar nerve in the elbow region or above and with good function of the small muscles of the hand were found. Cases 1, 2, and 3 were secondary to war wounds. Case 4 was of different etiology.

TABLE I (CASE 1). VOLUNTARY AND FARADIC RESPONSE RECORDED ON ALL MUSCLES*

DATE	1/3/45		4/12/45		5/9/45		8/10/45		11/13/45	
	PREOP.		POSTOP.		POSTOP.		POSTOP.		POSTOP.	
ULNAR NERVE	VOL	EL	VOL	EL	VOL	EL	VOL	EL	VOL	EL
Flexor carpi ulnaris	3	F	3	F	3	F	3	F	4	F
Flexor digitorum profundus 4	2	F	1	F	2	F	2	F	3	F
Flexor digitorum profundus 5	2	F	1	F	2	F	2	F	3	F
Abductor digiti quinti	2	F	2	F	3	F	3	F	3	F
Opponens digiti quinti	2	F	2	F	3	F	3	F	3	F
Dorsal interosseous 1	2	F	2	F	3	F	3	F	3	F
Dorsal interosseous 2	1	F	2	F	3	F	3	F	3	F
Dorsal interosseous 3	1	F	2	F	3	F	3	F	3	F
Dorsal interosseous 4	1	F	2	F	3	F	3	F	3	F
Palmar interosseous 1	2	F	2	F	3	F	3	F	3	F
Palmar interosseous 2	1	F	2	F	3	F	3	F	3	F
Palmar interosseous 3	1	F	2	F	2	F	3	F	3	F
Adductor pollicis	2	F	2	F	3	F	3	F	3	F
Sensory	A		A		A		A		H & A	

*Note the moderate improvement in function postoperatively. Sensation beginning to return only on last test.

CASE 2.—This soldier received a severe penetrating shell fragment wound, Oct. 7, 1944. The fragment entered the medial part of the arm 7 cm. above the condyle and lodged in the anterior part of the forearm 8 cm. above the wrist joint. He was first examined in the nerve laboratory, Wakeman General Hospital, Feb. 15, 1945. Because of a trigger point in the wound, anesthesia in the ulnar distribution, and failure of the Tinel sign to advance, exploration was carried out March 14, 1945. The nerve was found completely divided except

TABLE II (CASE 2). SLUGGISH RESPONSE TO FARADIC CURRENT*

DATE	21/15/45		4/9/45		6/7/45		8/11/45	
	PREOP.		POSTOP.		POSTOP.		POSTOP.	
ULNAR NERVE	VOL	EL	VOL	EL	VOL	EL	VOL	EL
Flexor carpi ulnaris	3	F	3	F	3	F	3	F
Flexor digitorum profundus 4	2	F*	2	F	3	F	3	F
Flexor digitorum profundus 5	1	F*	2	F	2	F	3	F
							3	F
Abductor digiti quinti	2	F*	2	F	2	F		
Opponens digiti quinti	1	F*	2	F	2	F	3	F
Dorsal interosseous 1	2	F	2	F	3	F	3	F
Dorsal interosseous 2	2	F	2	F	3	F	3	F
Dorsal interosseous 3	2	F	2	F	3	F	3	F
Dorsal interosseous 4	2	F	2	F	3	F	3	F
Palmar interosseous 1	2	F	2	F	3	F	3	F
Palmar interosseous 2	2	F	2	F	3	F	3	F
Palmar interosseous 3	2	F	2	F	3	F	3	F
Adductor pollicis	3	F	3	F	3	F	3	F
Sensory	A		A		A		A	

*Note the good voluntary function throughout. Sluggish response to Faradic current on the first examination is indicated by the asterisks. Anesthesia throughout.

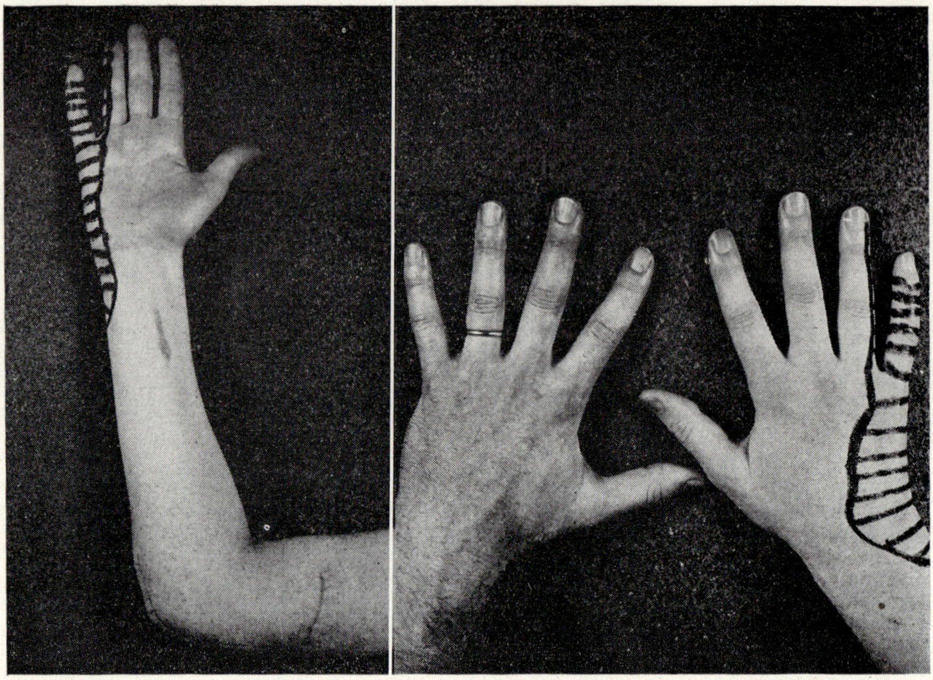

A. B.

Fig. 2.—*A*, Area of anesthesia outlined. Note the scar of the recent operation, three weeks postoperatively. Also note the scar of exit of the shell fragment. Note lack of ulnar Griffe. *B*, Note lack of atrophy, ability to spread fingers and area of anesthesia, postoperatively.

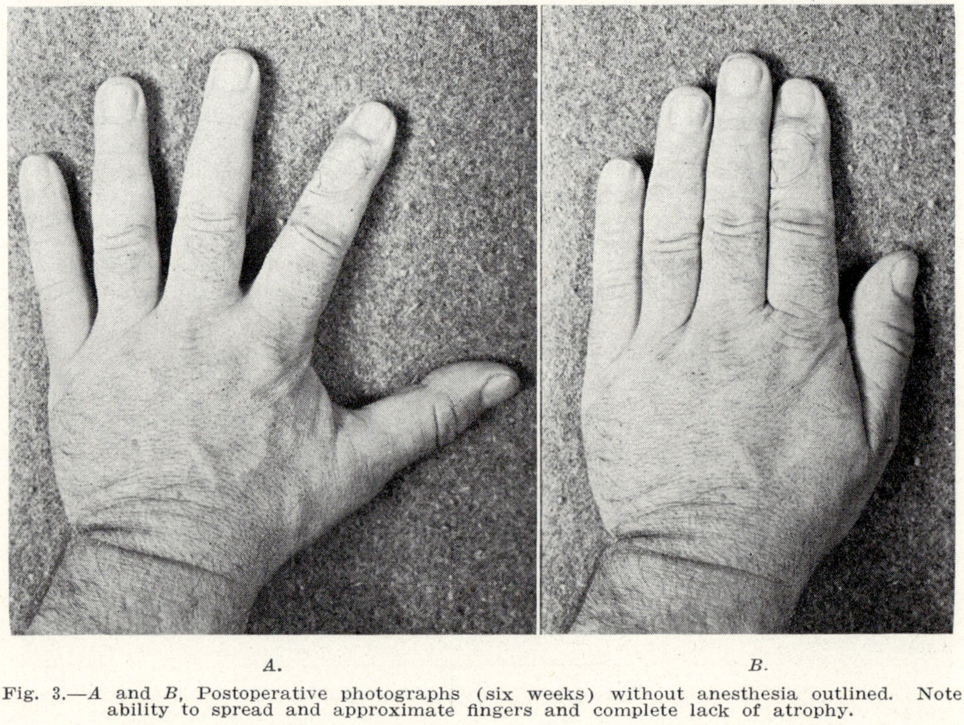

A. B.

Fig. 3.—*A* and *B*, Postoperative photographs (six weeks) without anesthesia outlined. Note ability to spread and approximate fingers and complete lack of atrophy.

for a band of scar tissue. Stimulation of the median nerve gave contraction of some of the small hand muscles of the ulnar nerve. Stimulation of the ulnar nerve above and below the neuroma failed to give any contraction of these muscles. Neurorrhaphy was performed after resection of the neuromas. Function remained after operation. Improvement gradually ensued and the final note, Sept. 5, 1945, stated, "Practically normal motor function. Sensory loss limited to distal two phalanges of 5th finger. Patient has been recommended for C.D.D." (J. R. R.) (Fig. 2, *A* and *B*, Table II.)

CASE 3.—This soldier received a perforating wound, the entrance in the posterolateral part of the arm 6 cm. above the condyles, the exit in the medial part of the arm 8 cm. above the condyles, with associated fracture of the humerus, caused by a rifle bullet on Nov. 3, 1944. At débridement fourteen hours after injury it was noted that the ulnar nerve was lacerated. When seen first in the nerve laboratory at Wakeman General Hospital, April 8, 1945, he was found to have questionable function of the small muscles of the hand, with definite function of the first interossei, palmar and dorsal, and definite function of the adductor of the thumb. In view of the statement that the ulnar nerve was completely divided, it was felt most certain that this function was due to innervation through the median nerve. A recheck on April 23 gave the result shown in Table III. At operation, April 25, 1945, the nerve was found to be completely divided, the tips of the neuromas being separated by 4 cm. Three centimeters of neuroma were excised and a neurorrhaphy was performed with silk technique after transplanting the nerve. The patient had such good function three months after operation that the chief of section without knowledge of his status asserted, "The paralysis of the ulnar nerve has shown satisfactory recovery and all muscles show gross response and the area of the hypesthesia has diminished." He was separated from the service at this time (Table III).

TABLE III (CASE 3). MINIMAL FUNCTION OF SEVERAL MUSCLES TO VOLUNTARY TESTS*

DATE	4/23/45		5/28/45		7/23/45	
	PREOP.		POSTOP.		POSTOP.	
ULNAR NERVE	VOL	EL	VOL	EL	VOL	EL
Flexor carpi ulnaris	2	F	2	F	2	F
Flexor digitorum profundus 4	2	F	2	F	2	F
Flexor digitorum profundus 5	2	F	2	F	2	F
Abductor digiti quinti	0	F	?	F	1	F
Opponens digiti quinti	0	F	1	F	1	F
Dorsal interosseous 1	2	F	3	F	3	F
Dorsal interosseous 2	2	F	2	F	2	F
Dorsal interosseous 3	1	F	1	F	2	F
Dorsal interosseous 4	0	F	1	F	1	F
Palmar interosseous 1	1	F	2	F	2	F
Palmar interosseous 2	1	F	1	F	1	F
Palmar interosseous 3	1	F	1	F	1	F
Adductor pollicis	2	F	2	F	2	F
Sensory	A		A		H	T35

*However all respond to Faradic current.

CASE 4.—A 40-year-old Staff Sergeant was admitted on the General Surgery Section, Wakeman General Hospital, for treatment of a mass in the axilla. At operation, June 2, 1945, the tumor mass (6 by 3 cm.) was found to arise from the ulnar nerve and a neurosurgeon was called. He excised the tumor and did a neurorrhaphy. Twenty-eight days after operation, at examination in the nerve laboratory, the patient was found to have anesthesia in an ulnar distribution smaller than usual, but fair to good function of all ulnar muscles. Strangely enough, the flexor profundus 4 and 5 along with the abductor digiti quinti and the opponens digiti quinti were relatively the weakest (see Table IV). There were no other sensory changes. He was discharged Oct. 5, 1945, with function still present. The Tinel sign had advanced only 30 cm., or to the elbow (Fig. 3, *A* and *B*, Table IV).

All four of these patients with complete division of the ulnar nerve showed fair to good function of most of the ulnar nerve hand muscles, with little atrophy

TABLE IV (CASE 4). POSTOPERATIVE EXAMINATION*

DATE	6/30/45		9/30/45	
	POSTOP.		POSTOP.	
ULNAR NERVE	VOL	EL	VOL	EL
Flexor carpi ulnaris	3	F	4	F
Flexor digitorum profundus 4	2	F	1	F
Flexor digitorum profundus 5	2	F	2	F
Abductor digiti quinti	1	F	3	F
Opponens digiti quinti	2	F	3	F
Dorsal interosseous 1	3	F	3	F
Dorsal interosseous 2	2	F	3	F
Dorsal interosseous 3	2	F	3	F
Dorsal interosseous 4	2	F	3	F
Palmar interosseous 1	3	F	3	F
Palmar interosseous 2	2	F	3	F
Palmar interosseous 3	2	F	3	F
Adductor pollicis	3	F	3	F
Sensory	A		A	

*No preoperative tests because lesion not suspected. Note anesthesia.

and the usual anesthetic area. This is significant in Case 4 since it might be considered that one of the sensory nerves was involved rather than the ulnar, as we first suspected in Case 1. This condition remained postoperatively despite known complete division of the nerve. In one patient, Case 1, a branch from the median nerve was proved to carry at least some of this function. In another patient, Case 2, stimulation of the median nerve in the upper arm gave contraction of some of the ulnar muscles, showing that the functioning elements were carried in this nerve in the area of operation.

At least three other cases of severance of the ulnar nerve without intrinsic muscle paralysis have been reported. All of these were cases of tumor similar to our Case 4. In Goldman's[6] case, a tumor and 5 cm. of the ulnar nerve were removed from above the elbow without any disturbance in motility of the hand or fingers. Auerbach and Brodnitz[7] found no paralysis in the ulnar distribution after complete section of the ulnar nerve above the elbow, for excision of a nerve tumor. Halipré[8] also found no motor loss after complete severance of the ulnar nerve in his case. In addition, at the time of operation he stimulated both cut ends of the nerve without any motor response. However, stimulation lower on the ulnar nerve did give contraction of the small hand muscles. During transfer procedures from Wakeman General Hospital the records of one other case were lost. This man was one of the original cases presented at the Wakeman General Hospital conference.

The first case reported here of function of median nerve muscles despite complete section of the nerve was also found purely by chance.

CASE 5.—This soldier suffered a guttering wound of the anticubital space and the adjacent arm on Aug. 10, 1944. The wound was covered by a pedicle graft measuring 11 by 6 cm. which had been applied on Sept. 1 and Oct. 6, 1944. He was sent to neurosurgery from the orthopedic section for consultation, Feb. 16, 1945, because of severe pain with use of an extension cast to correct the flexion deformity of the elbow. The patient was checked in the nerve laboratory and on examination he was found to have function of all the median nerve muscles except the flexor digitorum profundus of the index finger and the flexor pollicis longus. There was normal sensation in the median nerve distribution. There was a trigger point, marked, over the median nerve in the elbow region at the lower edge of the graft. Pressure on this trigger area or extension at the elbow, beyond 120 degrees, resulted in severe pain and paresthesia along the course of the median nerve and in its sensory area. There was, in addition, marked tissue loss in the wound area and the biceps muscle tendon had been completely divided with much loss of substance. Flexion at the elbow was carried out by the brachioradialis muscle. At operation, March 7, 1945, the nerve was found to be divided except for a thin scar tissue bridge with the neuromas separated by 3.5 cm. The

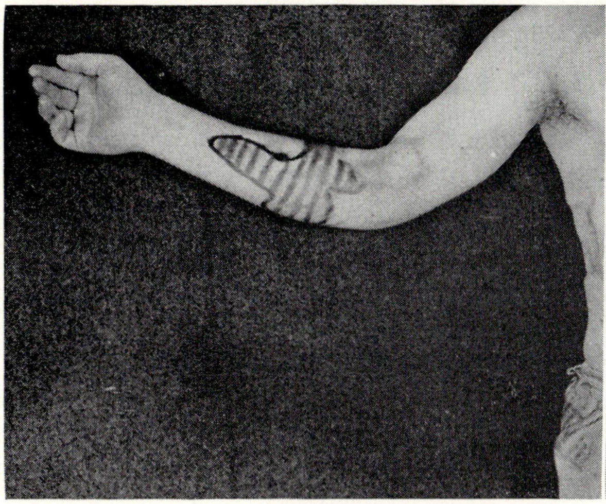

A.

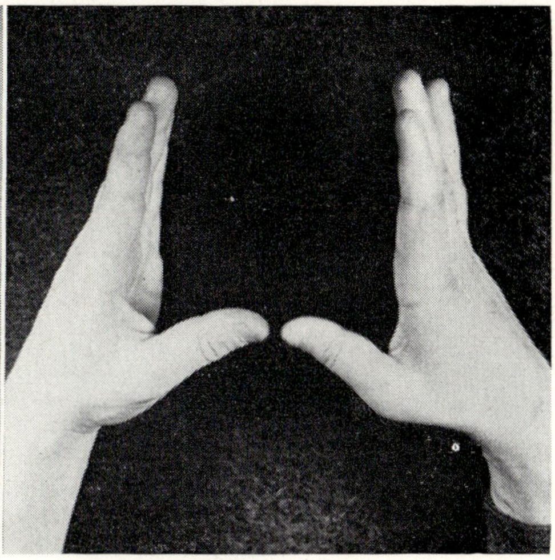

B.

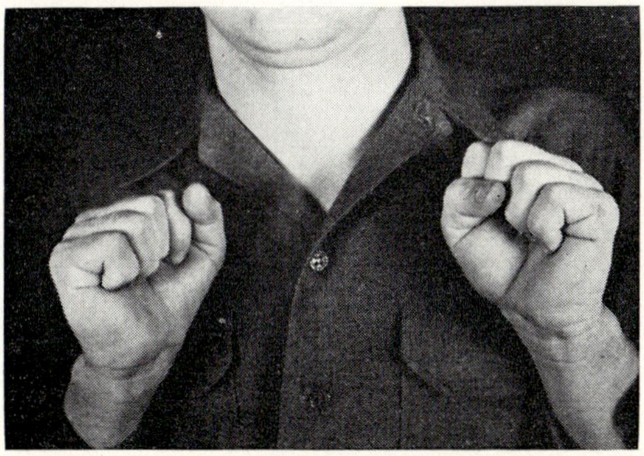

C.

Fig. 4.—*A*, Note large wound covered by skin graft and area of anesthesia. *B*, Postoperative action photograph to show function abductor pollicis brevis. Note moderate atrophy of right thenar eminence. *C*, Postoperative photograph to show function of median muscles.

proximal neuroma was exquisitely tender. An additional 4 cm. of neuroma were removed and neurorrhaphy was performed using silk. One month postoperative he had the same function as before operation. By three months after operation there was return of function of the flexor profundus to the index finger. Hypesthesia of the distal two phalanges of the second and third fingers was noted at this time. The patient was discharged on Dec. 11, 1945, with function of all median muscles although the small thumb muscles were weak and the function of the flexor pollicis longus was questionable. He also had normal extension of the elbow without pain or paresthesia (Fig. 4, *A*, *B*, and *C*).

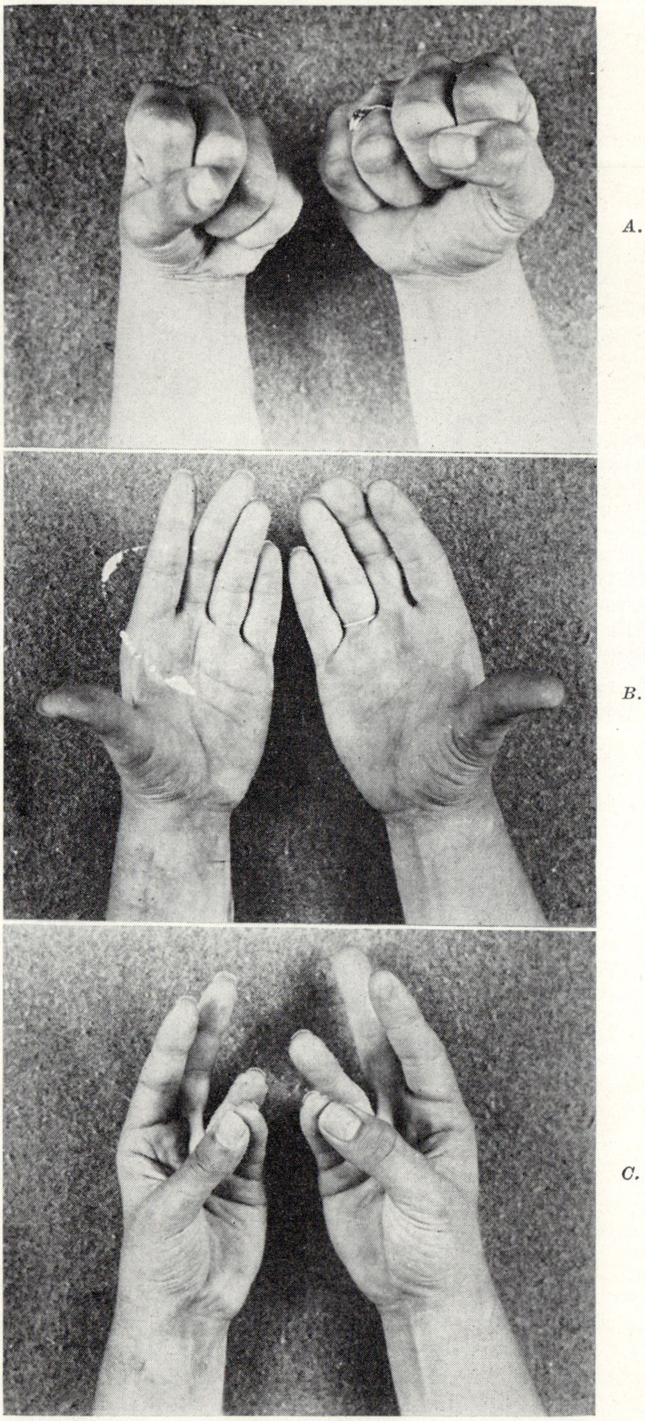

Fig. 5.—*A*, Photograph to show function of median muscles. Note poor function of flexor pollicis longus. *B*, Photograph to show function of abductor pollicis brevis. This is imperfect in that there is too much associated extension of thumb. *C*, Photograph to show function of opponens pollicis. Note lack of atrophy.

TABLE V (CASE 6). DECREASE IN FUNCTION OF THE FLEXOR POLLICIS LONGUS, FLEXOR DIGITORUM PROFUNDUS 2, AND FLEXOR POLLICIS BREVIS*

DATE	7/10/45		8/17/45		9/27/45		11/27/45		12/20/45	
	PREOP.		POSTOP. 1 PREOP. 2		POSTOP. 2		POSTOP. 2		POSTOP. 2	
MEDIAN NERVE	VOL	EL	VOL	EL	VOL	EL	VOL	EL	VOL	EL
Pronator teres	3	F	3	F	4	F	4	F	4	F
Flexor carpi radialis	3	F	3	F	4	F	4	F	4	F
Flexor digitorum sublimus	3	F	4	F	4	F	4	F	4	F
Flexor digitorum profundus 2	3	F	1	F	2	F	3	F	3	F
Flexor digitorum profundus 3	3	F	3	F	3	F	4	F	4	F
Flexor pollicis longus	3	F	1	F	2	G3	3	F	3	F
Opponens pollicis	3	F	4	F*	4	F	4	F	4	F
Abductor pollicis brevis	3	F	3	F	3	F	4	F	4	F
Flexor pollicis brevis	3	F	3	F*	3	F	4	F	4	F
Sensory	A		A		A		A fingers H palm		A index and thumb H remainder	

*After the first operation; note rapid return postoperatively.

CASE 6.—This soldier received a moderate guttering wound of the palmar surface of the right forearm 9 cm. above the tip of the radius, Dec. 19, 1944. There was an associated severe laceration of the radial artery. Débridement and ligation of the radial artery and repair of a sensory branch of the radial nerve were performed seven hours after injury. A secondary closure and skin graft were performed, Jan. 27, 1945. The soldier was examined first in the nerve laboratory, March 28, 1945, two days after admission to Wakeman General Hospital. He was found to have anesthesia in the radial distribution. There was also anesthesia in the median distribution but no motor dysfunction. Because of a persistent trigger point in the wound over the median nerve, and the anesthesia, exploration was considered justified. It was our feeling that a neuroma would be found and that a neurolysis would be indicated. Much to our surprise at operation, July 17, 1945, the median nerve was found to be completely divided with a gap of 6 cm. and a large neuroma and glioma. One centimeter was removed from each end and a first stage neurorrhaphy performed with 000 silk sutures in the sheath. A secondary neurorrhaphy was performed, Aug. 27, 1945, by another operator. There was decreased function of the flexor profundus 2 and the flexor pollicis longus after the first operation, as indicated in the photograph of the fist (Fig. 5, *A*), but this function returned rapidly after the second operation. The patient was discharged, Dec. 29, 1945, still with good motor function and a decrease in the area of anesthesia, which now included only the index finger and thumb (Fig. 5, *A*, *B*, and *C*, Table V).

TABLE VI (CASE 7). LOSS OF FARADIC RESPONSE AFTER SECOND OPERATION

DATE	6/7/45		7/24/45		8/25/45		10/12/45		12/17/45		1/12/45	
	PREOP.		PREOP.		POSTOP. 1 PREOP. 2		POSTOP. 2		POSTOP. 2		POSTOP. 2	
MEDIAN NERVE	VOL	EL	VOL	EL	VOL	EL	VOL	EL	VOL	EL	VOL	EL
Pronator teres	3	F	3	F	3	F	–	F	3	F	3	F
Flexor carpi radialis	3	F	3	F	3	F	2	F	2-3	F	3	F
Flexor digitorum sublimus	3	F	3	F	3	F	2-3	F	3	F	3	F
Flexor digitorum profundus 2	3	F	3	F	3	F	2	F	3	F	3	F
Flexor digitorum profundus 3	3	F	3	F	3	F	3	F	3	F	3	F
Flexor pollicis longus	3	F	3	F	3	F	1	G3	3	G3	3	F
Opponens pollicis	3	F	3	F	3	G3	2	G3	3	F	3	F
Abductor pollicis brevis	3	F	3	F	3	G3	1-2	G3	2-3	G3	2-3	F
Flexor pollicis brevis	3	F	3	F	2	G3	0-1	G3	2-3	G3	2-3	F
Sensory												

Case 7.—On New Guinea in early 1944, this soldier developed symptoms of a painful tumor of the hand. On April 26, 1944, at the 116th Station Hospital, it was excised and found to be a neuroma of the median nerve. He was first examined in the nerve laboratory at Wakeman General Hospital, June 7, 1945, at which time it was noted that he had anesthesia in most of the median nerve distribution, but almost normal motor function. A

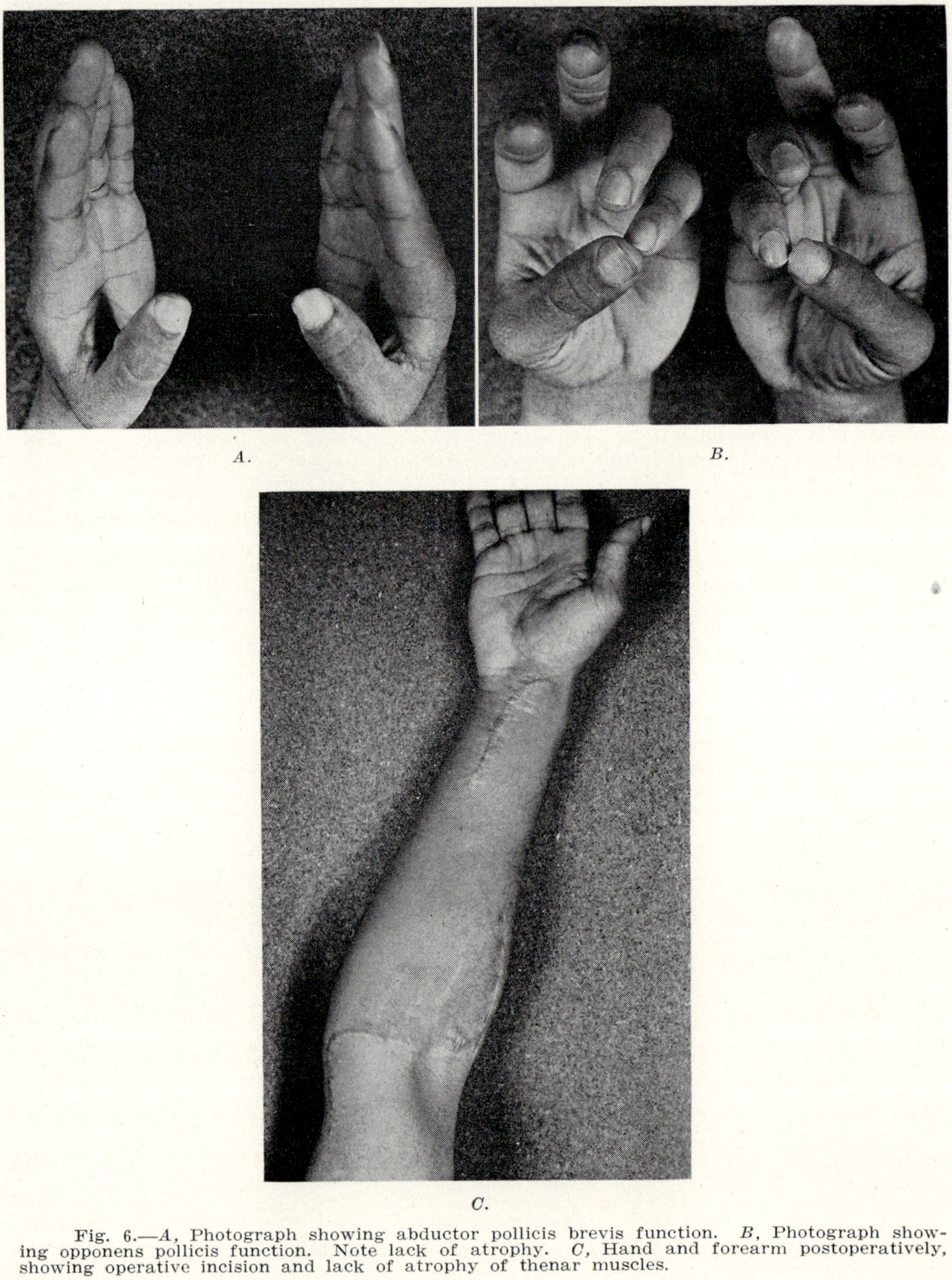

A. *B.* *C.*

Fig. 6.—*A*, Photograph showing abductor pollicis brevis function. *B*, Photograph showing opponens pollicis function. Note lack of atrophy. *C*, Hand and forearm postoperatively, showing operative incision and lack of atrophy of thenar muscles.

tender mass was palpable just above the wrist, palpation of which caused paresthesia in the second and third fingers. At exploration, Aug. 1, 1945, the median nerve was found to be completely divided and the proximal end had retracted to above the wrist. After excision, for biopsy, the nerve was drawn down to the transverse carpal ligament by tension sutures. The pathologic report was benign neuroma. There was temporary decrease in function of the thumb muscles three weeks postoperatively, as recorded (Table VI). This was evidently due to the operative trauma in the region of the thenar eminence. At a third operation, Sept. 17, 1945, a neurorrhaphy was performed with marked tension despite transplantation anterior to the pronator muscle. Function was poor four weeks after this operation, but rapidly returned to the preoperative level three and four months after operation. There was, by this time, return of sensation except for the distal phalanges of fingers 2 and 3. He was discharged on Jan. 12, 1946 (Fig. 6, *A, B,* and *C,* Table VI).

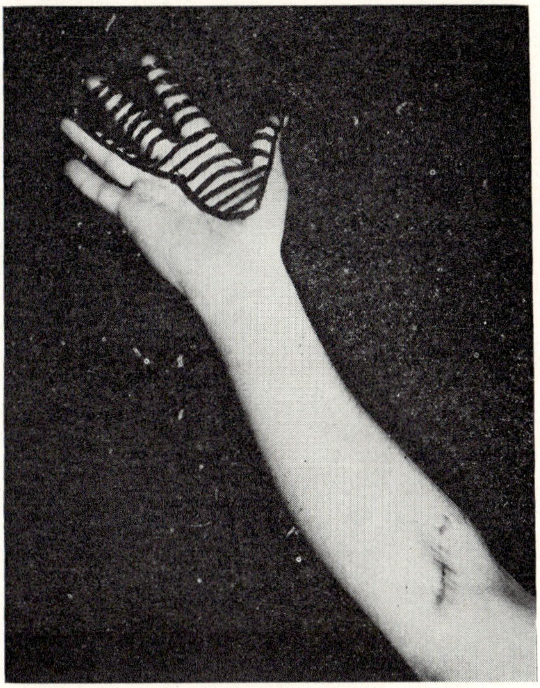

Fig. 7.—Photograph to show scar of wound and area of anesthesia. Note minimal thenar atrophy.

Case 8.—This soldier received a moderate perforating wound, from the posterolateral to the anterior part of the forearm, 4 cm. below the condyles, June 14, 1944. This was associated with complete, comminuted fracture of the radius. When first examined in the nerve laboratory, April 2, 1945, he had function of all median muscles, although several failed to respond to faradic current. There was anesthesia in the median distribution, plus a trigger point in the scar, for which operation was considered necessary. A neuroma was expected. At operation, May 7, 1945, a large neuroma 9 by 3 cm. was found, excised, and neurorrhaphy performed. The postoperative nerve laboratory examination showed function of all median muscles which persisted except for the flexor pollicis longus, function of which was lost after three months. There was gradual return of sensation until discharge, Feb. 1, 1946, when, only the fingers were still anesthetic (Fig. 7).

Case 9.—This soldier received a perforating wound through the forearm from the posterior to the anterior part, 5 cm. above the wrist on July 3, 1944. Débridement was done thirty hours later. A preoperative examination was not made in the nerve laboratory, but the preoperative test by the operating neurosurgeon revealed function of all median muscles, with anesthesia in the median distribution and a trigger point in the wound. At operation, Dec. 7, 1944, a hard neuroma was found. Stimulation above and below the neuroma gave no contraction of the thumb muscles. Excision of the neuroma and neurorrhaphy were carried out. At the first examination in the nerve laboratory, one month postoperatively, there was decrease in function of the abductor pollicis brevis, but no other change in motor function or sensation. Through the postoperative course there was gradual, slow improvement in function until nine months postoperative, when all muscles functioned well and there was return of sensation except for the tip of the index finger (Table VII).

TABLE VII (CASE 9). LACK OF FARADIC RESPONSE OF OPPONENS AT SIX AND NINE MONTHS*

DATE			3/8/45		6/2/45		9/10/45	
	PREOP.		POSTOP.		POSTOP.		POSTOP.	
MEDIAN NERVE	VOL	EL	VOL	EL	VOL	EL	VOL	EL
Pronator teres	4		4		4	F	4	F
Flexor carpi radialis	4		4		4	F	4	F
Flexor digitorum sublimus	4		4		4	F	4	F
Flexor digitorum profundus 2	4		4		4	F	4	F
Flexor digitorum profundus 3	4		4		4	F	4	F
Flexor pollicis longus	4		4	G3	4	F	4	F
Opponens pollicis	3		3	F	3	G3	4	G3
Abductor pollicis brevis	2		1	F	3	F	3	F
Flexor pollicis brevis	4		3	F	3	F	4	F
Sensory	A		A		A fingers		A fingertips	

*Otherwise, function throughout. No electrical tests preoperatively as this examination was not done in nerve laboratory.

CASE 10.—This soldier received two penetrating wounds of the right upper extremity, Dec. 14, 1944. He was first seen in the nerve laboratory, Wakeman General Hospital, on March 2, 1945. It was noted at that time that he had marked limitation of motion of the elbow. With extension to 110 degrees he had severe pain in the wound area with radiation through the course of the median nerve into the median nerve distribution of the hand. There had been return of function of all median muscles except the flexor pollicis longus, but anesthesia was present throughout the median distribution. It was thought that perhaps a foreign body pressed on the nerve, causing the symptoms and signs indicated. The patient was continued on physiotherapy without improvement and operation was performed on July 4, 1945. The branches to the forearm muscles were scarred, but the main trunk was almost completely divided. No stimulator was available for tests. A neurorrhaphy was performed on the main trunk. At examination, one month postoperatively, he was found to have the same function as before operation and in addition the Tinel sign also remained at 20+ cm. as before operation. Six months postoperatively, there was beginning return of function of the flexor pollicis longus and by the time of discharge, one year postoperatively, there was sensation, although far from normal, present throughout the median distribution. The foreign body was removed, Feb. 21, 1946, because of a persistent draining sinus through the wound.

These six patients with median nerve injury examined pre- and postoperatively all showed function of the thumb muscles, according to the usual criteria. Unfortunately, neither the ulnar nor the musculocutaneous nerves were stimulated in any of these cases.

The cases to follow show the possibility of considering good function as an operative result rather than realizing that the function was present before operation. Some of these cases are from the Wakeman General Hospital and we have definite proof from the records. Others are from other hospitals, about which there may be some question. However, no case had been considered without definitely recorded objective tests, usually the physiotherapists, from other institutions.

CASE 11.—This soldier received a penetrating, severe wound of the axilla and shoulder region on July 3, 1944. Diagnosis was severe brachial plexus injury with complete musculocutaneous and ulnar nerve paralysis and partial radial and median nerve paralysis. At operation on Nov. 16, 1944, the ulnar nerve was found to be completely separated by 5 cm., and a neurorrhaphy under tension was performed using tantalum wire stay and epineural sutures. The radial nerve was partially divided and a partial neurorrhaphy was performed. Neurolysis was done on the median and musculocutaneous nerves, because there was contraction of the muscles when the median and musculocutaneous nerves were stimulated. There was no function with ulnar or radial nerve stimulation. It was a complete surprise to find voluntary function of some, and faradic response of all, ulnar small hand muscles six weeks after operation. Three months postoperatively, there was function of all ulnar muscles, but still complete ulnar anesthesia. It was at this point that the entire record was carefully re-examined and we found that the last examiner, one week before operation, had observed beginning function of some of the ulnar muscles. These records are not available for reproduction.

If this return of function had been delayed longer there is little question that this return would have been claimed as an operative result.

CASE 12.—This soldier was wounded on Dec. 31, 1944. On March 29, 1945, a neurorrhaphy of the median nerve, 5 inches above the wrist, was performed in an overseas hospital. On examination in the nerve laboratory, July 17, 1945, he was found to have some function of all median muscles except the abductor pollicis brevis. This was considered a possible return of function until his overseas records were checked and it was found that he had had good to normal function of median muscles sixteen days before operation. Two months after operation another observer had noted that he showed return of function of all median muscles, but still had complete anesthesia. By failure to check the preoperative records this would have been considered a return of function through regrowth of the nerve (Table VIII).

TABLE VIII (CASE 12). PREOPERATIVE RECORDINGS COPIED FROM THE RECORDS OF 67TH GENERAL HOSPITAL*

DATE	3/13/45		7/17/45		9/19/45	
	PREOP.		POSTOP.		POSTOP.	
MEDIAN NERVE	VOL	EL	VOL	EL	VOL	EL
Pronator teres	N	F	2	F	4	F
Flexor carpi radialis	G	F	2	F	2	F
Flexor digitorum sublimus	N	F	2	F	2	F
Flexor digitorum profundus 2	N	F	1	G3	0-1	G3
Flexor digitorum profundus 3	N	F	2	G3	0-1	F
Flexor pollicis longus	N	F	2	F	2	F
Opponens pollicis	N	F	1	F	2	F
Abductor pollicis brevis	N	F	2	G3	3	F
Flexor pollicis brevis	G	F	0	G3	1	G3
Sensory	A		A		A	

*Recordings are shown as N, normal and G, good, rather than 1, 2, 3, and 4. Postoperative function was not so good as preoperative function if this is accurate.

CASE 13.—This soldier was wounded in action on Aug. 6, 1944. Operation was performed on March 13, 1945, at another general hospital, when the median nerve was found to be completely separated and a neurorrhaphy was performed. The patient was transferred to Wakeman Convalescent Hospital with a report (on Surgeon General form 941) of returning function of the median nerve. However, this would be virtually impossible since the lesion was in the mid-upper arm, 50 cm. from the hand. On careful examination of the previous records it was noted that he had had definite function before operation.

Case 14.—This soldier who was wounded Sept. 24, 1944, had a neurorrhaphy of the median nerve performed at another general hospital on Jan. 25, 1945. When he was found to have function four months after operation, he was considered to be showing return of function. However, on careful examination of the records, a physiotherapy record at one month postoperatively was found, which showed function of all median nerve muscles. Since this would be too early for return of function after operation, one must consider that he also had function before operation.

The last patient (Case 15), although possibly belonging with Cases 5 to 10, is considered separately because he was returned to duty without operation from another neurosurgical hospital.

Case 15.—This soldier received a lacerating wound of the volar aspect of the wrist on Dec. 12, 1944. After healing of the wound he was returned to duty from a general hospital with a neurosurgical service and did full duty until he was returned to the Zone of Interior for separation. He was seen in consultation from the separation center on March 12, 1946. He had anesthesia in the median distribution, but good motor function. Admission and exploration were advised. At exploration, March 20, 1946, the nerve was found to be completely divided with a gap of 1½ cm. between the tips of the neuroma and glioma. Stimulation of the median nerve before and after dissection gave no contraction of the opponens pollicis, flexor pollicis brevis, or abductor pollicis brevis. Stimulation of the ulnar nerve gave good contraction of the thumb muscles. After the dissection, however, as the glioma was excised from the distal end of the median nerve, the patient complained of pain in the exact median nerve distribution and electrical stimulation of the distal end of the nerve gave the same reaction, that is, pain in the median distribution. Postoperatively, excellent function remained. He had very slow return of sensation in the median distribution and by Oct. 24, 1946, he had return of pain and touch sensation except in the distal two phalanges of the second and third fingers (Table IX).

Table IX (Case 15). Excellent Function of All Muscles With Anesthesia

DATE	3/12/46		4/11/46		6/24/46		8/27/46		10/24/46	
	PREOP.		POSTOP.		POSTOP.		POSTOP.		POSTOP.	
MEDIAN NERVE	VOL	EL	VOL	EL	VOL	EL	VOL	EL	VOL	EL
Pronator teres	4	F	4	F	4	F	4	F	4	F
Flexor carpi radialis	4	F	4	F	4	F	4	F	4	F
Flexor digitorum sublimus	4	F	3-4	F	3	F	3	F	3	F
Flexor digitorum profundus 2	4	F	3	F	3	F	3	F	3	F
Flexor digitorum profundus 3	4	F	3-4	F	3	F	3	F	3	F
Flexor pollicis longus	4	F	3-4	F	3	F	3	F	3	F
Opponens pollicis	4	F	4	F	3	F	3	F	3	F
Abductor pollicis brevis	4	F	3-4	F	3	F	3	F	3	F
Flexor pollicis brevis	4	F	4	F	3	F	3	F	3	F
Sensory	A		A		A		H palm A fingers		H all but distal 2 & 3 fingers	

This last case (Case 15) revealed another interesting phenomenon which was found on at least five median nerve cases during operation with local anesthesia. Stimulation either by grasping or by the stimulator current, of the distal end of the completely divided nerve gave a painful sensation in the area of distribution of the median nerve. All of these injuries were in the lower forearm. We failed to make the obvious test of blocking the ulnar and radial nerves to determine which carried the pain impulses to the central nervous system. One other possibility would seem to be the periarterial sympathetics. As far as is known this phenomenon did not occur on any nerves other than the median.

DISCUSSION

If one can confirm function of muscles which are usually innervated through an already divided or seriously damaged nerve, as in these cases, an anomalous innervation must be considered. Further proof can sometimes be produced by stimulation or block of the nerve which is supposed to carry the anomalous or unusual nerve fibers. These unusual innervations are of great importance in primary diagnosis and planned treatment of nerve injuries and of especial importance in judging the recovery following repair of nerves. If care is not taken in determining preoperative function of these muscles by careful tests, one may be led to claim a good result from nerve repair on the basis of the usual innervation when the unusual innervation is the true cause of the good function. This would be more likely to occur in cases with temporary paralysis of the second nerve and return of function between examinations. Several of the cases reported show clearly these pitfalls in determining return of motor function.

As far as the original diagnosis is concerned one may be led to accept a partial function of muscles to mean only slight damage to the nerve and thus to procrastinate, expecting further return of motor function and sensation. Such is Case 15. In many cases undoubtedly these patients have been discharged with the assurance that there would be rapid continued return of function. Certainly this was almost done in several of these cases and it was done in one shortly after operation (Case 3).

If we are going to accept this unusual condition, even as a possibility, we must first establish the fact that there are nerve pathways other than the so-called normal pathways over which the stimuli may be carried. Fortunately several of the older anatomists have by their evident tedious and careful work furnished us with the proof of the presence of several such variations in the nerve pathways to the hand.

The explanation for the variations in these particular nerves lies in their embryology. In the human being there are three nerves, median, ulnar, and musculocutaneous, serving one basic muscle group, the primitive ventral musculature of the arm. For the primitive dorsal musculature in contradistinction, there is just one nerve, the radial. Communicating fasciculi between the median and ulnar nerves and between the median and musculocutaneous nerves are not uncommon. A communication between the median and ulnar nerves was found in 38 of 125 cadavers by Gruber[9] and in 15 per cent of 406 cadavers by Thompson.[10] According to Piersol[11] such a communication is found in 20 to 25 per cent of cases.

The communications occur most frequently in the forearm as in Case 1, in a second case of the Wakeman General Hospital group not reported in this series, and in one of the cases reported by Murphy and co-workers.[1] Thompson[10] described four specific types of communication:

(1) A communication arising from the anterior interosseous nerve about 5 cm. below its origin from the median which joined the ulnar nerve in its middle one-third passing below the ulnar artery upon the flexor digitorum profundus

(2) A branch from the main trunk of the median nerve joining the ulnar in the same manner as in (1)

(3) A sling communication occurring over the flexor digitorum profundus formed by both median and ulnar nerves, with branches from the sling supplying the flexor digitorum profundus to the fourth and fifth fingers

(4) A branch arising from the median nerve in the elbow region passing superficial to the flexor muscles and joining the ulnar nerve in its middle one-third

Borchardt and Wjasmenski[12] traced some of these communications more thoroughly and found that frequently the communicating branch divided into sensory and motor fibers. The sensory branch joined fibers in the ulnar nerve which supplied the skin on the inner part of the palm, over the palmaris brevis muscle, and the fourth and fifth fingers. The muscular branch joined that part of the ulnar nerve which supplied the intrinsic muscles of the hand.

Less commonly, communications between the median and ulnar nerves occur in the arm as high as the axilla. I visualized such communications in two cases.

Within the hand itself there are two communications of some importance. One is sensory for the adjacent surfaces of the third and fourth fingers. The other, described and illustrated best by Fröhse and Frankel,[13] is motor between the deep branch of the ulnar and the motor branch of the median, passing through the abductor pollicis brevis and along the flexor pollicis brevis. In Piersol's[11] text it was stated that the communications in the forearm are usually from median to ulnar, while in the hand they may be in either direction. Turner[14] went further and stated that the communication in the hand is usually from ulnar to median.

These facts would fit in with the finding that in no instance of division of the ulnar nerve below the upper forearm was definite function found of the ulnar intrinsics, except of the first interosseous in a few cases, whereas in the median nerve, function was found even with division at the wrist. As far as the first interosseous is concerned, it evidently occasionally receives twigs from the median nerve, as shown by Turner[14] and Mackenzie.[15] Communications between median and ulnar nerves have also been described in textbooks of anatomy by Cunningham,[16] McClellan,[17] Quain,[18] Toldt,[19] Verchere,[20] and Villar.[21]

The anatomic variations which might explain the residual function of the median nerve thumb muscles are even more varied than those of the ulnar nerve. In addition to the possible communications in the arm, forearm, and primarily in the hand between the ulnar and median nerves, there are variations in formation of the median nerve and its relations to the musculocutaneous nerve. The two or more heads of the median nerve may unite as low as the elbow (Piersol[11]).

Communications between the median and musculocutaneous nerves are very common. In fact in some vertebrates, such as the ruminants, the median and musculocutaneous nerves are united in a single trunk. Some early anatomists including Hyrtl[22] considered the musculocutaneous to be a branch of the median nerve. Such an origin does occur but is unusual. The median nerve may take over some or even all of the musculocutaneous function. Much more rarely the musculocutaneous nerve may take over partly or completely the motor and sensory distribution of the median nerve (Gegenbauer,[23] Gruber,[24] and Krause[25]). According to Gegenbauer,[23] some form of communication may be found in 70 per cent of cases. The extent of communication between these two nerves may also vary somewhat according to the type of plexus. The passage is more commonly from the musculocutaneous to the median in the post-fixed plexus, and the reverse in the prefixed plexus. In the post-fixed plexus this communication from musculocutaneous to median is most likely to contain fibers from the fifth cervical root.

By finer dissection three general types of musculocutaneous to median fibers have been shown. In some instances all three types may be present in one communicating branch. Type 1 passes to the median nerve, runs in it for a short distance, and then returns to the musculocutaneous nerve. Type 2 enters the funiculus of the median nerve which is destined for the pronator teres and flexor carpi radialis and has been traced as far as the humeral head of the pronator teres. Type 3 divides into two branches, one entering a sensory path in the dorsal aspect of the nerve trunk; the other branch has been followed through the median nerve into the forearm where it communicates with the funiculus supplying the thenar muscles.

Variations in the median and musculocutaneous nerves have also been described by Piersol,[11] Borchardt and Wjasmenski,[12] Fröhse and Frankel,[13] Cunningham,[16] Quain,[18] Villar,[21] Testut,[26] and Cruveilhier.[27]

These variations in origin or communication with the musculocutaneous by the median nerve might well explain the result in Cases 5, 10, and 13, where the division of the median nerve was above the elbow. This is especially true of Case 10 where a Tinel sign to 20+ cm. below the point of division was present both pre- and postoperatively. Other possibilities in this case (Case 10) would be that fibers were carried through the branches to the forearm muscles rejoining the main trunk below the elbow or even a junction of heads of the median nerve below the elbow. Those patients with division in the forearm (Cases 8, 9, and 12) could have their innervation through branches in the forearm from the ulnar or from the anterior interosseous, or in the hand from the deep ulnar, as must have occurred in those with division at the wrist (Cases 7 and 15).

Those patients with pain on stimulation of the distal stumps of the median nerve can be explained only on the basis of communication with the central nervous system through some other nerve in the hand. This could be through the ulnar (Piersol,[11] Borchardt and Wjasmenski,[12] Fröhse and Frankel,[13] and McClellan,[17] the musculocutaneous, or the radial (Piersol,[11] Fröhse and

Frankel,[13] and Toldt[19]). Another possibility might be a communication through the periarterial sympathetics. The fact that the median nerve is the only nerve in which this phenomenon was noted and is the nerve in which causalgia is most common might make one consider this remote possibility.

The question may be asked, how do such small communicating branches produce such great function? It must be reiterated that function in these cases was not entirely normal, but ranged from fair to good. It is well known that there are intraneural plexuses with branches between the individual funiculi, in all nerves (Langley and Hashimoto[28]). It is not too difficult to suppose that these branching fibers may communicate with several funiculi by intraneural plexuses and, in fact, this has been shown by careful anatomic dissections. That two or three funiculi may carry some function to all muscles served by a given nerve was adequately proved by another patient treated at Wakeman General Hospital. This soldier, who had a thigh wound, had causalgia in the tibial distribution, but weak function of all tibial and peroneal muscles and some sensation throughout. At operation two intact funiculi of approximately eight present in the peroneal nerve were saved and three of the eight in the tibial nerve were saved. Stimulation above the area of injury after division of all but these intact funiculi gave some contraction of all muscles, and stimulation below gave not only the same motor function but also some pain sense. Dissection of these intact funiculi down into the distal nerve revealed several small fibrils passing from them into other funiculi which were divided proximally. These were evidently part of the intraneural plexus. A partial neurorrhaphy was performed leaving the intact funiculi. Some function was lost immediately postoperatively, but function had returned to almost the preoperative level by three months after operation.

The greater actual and relative number of median nerve cases is undoubtedly on the basis of the fact that it is so difficult to be sure of function of the small hand muscles served by the ulnar. Two questionable cases of the ulnar nerve were considered, but ruled out on the basis of uncertainty, and one certain case was lost. Function of the first interosseous has occurred in approximately 10 per cent of the cases of ulnar nerve division.

It was also observed in several of these cases that the relative size of the nerves was changed. Thus, in at least two of the median nerve cases the nerve looked much smaller than the normal median nerve, both proximally and distally, while the ulnar seemed larger than usual. The same relative change held true we believe in the reversed cases. No objective measurements were made.

CONCLUSIONS

1. Several cases of residual function of the small hand muscles, despite complete section of the nerve which usually supplies them, are reported.

2. Anatomic pathways (communications between the median and ulnar and median and musculocutaneous) for nerve impulses to these muscles are described.

3. These unusual cases are of importance in judging cases of peripheral nerve injury preoperatively and in evaluating return of function postoperatively.

REFERENCES

1. Murphy, Francis, Kirklin, John W., and Finlayson, A. I.: Anomalous Innervation of the Intrinsic Muscles of the Hand, Surg., Gynec. & Obst. 83: 15, 1946.
2. Pollock, L. J., and Davis, Loyal: Peripheral Nerve Injuries, New York, 1932, Paul B. Hoeber, Inc., pp. 21, 22.
3. Haymaker, W., and Woodhall, B.: Peripheral Nerve Injuries, Philadelphia, 1945, W. B. Saunders Company.
4. Medical Department of the United States Army in the World War, Vol. II, War Department, Washington, D. C., 1927, Government Printing Office, p. 872.
5. Stookey, Byron, P.: Surgical and Mechanical Treatment of Peripheral Nerves, Philadelphia, 1922, W. B. Saunders Company.
6. Goldman, E.: Beiträge zu der Lehre von den Neuromen, Beitr. z. klin. Chir. 10: 13, 1893.
Idem: Ueber das Fehlen Von Funktions Stoerungen nach der Resektion von peripheren nerven, Beitr. z. klin. Chir. 51: 183, 1906.
7. Auerbach, S., and Brodnitz: Neurofibrom des Nervus Ulnaris Oberarm: Extirpation Herlung, Mitt. a.d. Grenzgeb. d. Med. u. Chir. 21: 589, 1910.
8. Halipré, A.: D'une cause d'erreur dans l'appreciation de l'importance des lesions du nerf Cubital au bras, Rev. neurol. 24: 236, 1917.
9. Gruber, W.: Ueber die Verbindung des Nervus Medianus mit dem Nervus Ulnaris am Unterarme des Menschen und der Saugethiere, Arch. f. Anat., Physiol. u. wissensch. Med., Leipzig 37: 501-522, 1870.
10. Thompson, A.: Third Annual Report of the Committee of Collective Investigation of the Anatomical Society of Great Britain and Ireland for the year 1891-1892, J. Anat. & Physiol. 27: 183, 1893.
Idem: Frequency and Arrangement of Communications Between the Median (or Anterior Interosseous) and Ulnar Nerves in the Forearm, J. Anat. & Physiol. 27: 192-194, 1893.
11. Piersol, G.: Human Anatomy, Philadelphia, 1923, J. B. Lippincott Company.
12. Borchardt, M., and Wjasmenski: Der Nervus Medianus, Beitr. z. klin. Chir. 107: 553, 1917.
13. Fröhse, F., and Frankel, M.: Die Muskeln des Menschen Armes, Jena, 1908, Gustav Fischer.
Idem: Bardeleben Handbuch d'Anat. d. Menschen, Vol. 2, Sect. 2, Part 2, Jena, 1913, Gustav Fischer.
14. Turner, W.: Further Examples of Variations in the Arrangement of the Nerves of the Human Body, J. Anat. & Physiol. 8: 297, 1873.
15. Mackenzie, I.: Reactions of the Ulnar Nerve in Disease, Edinburgh M. J. 31: 413, 1924
16. Cunningham, G.: Textbook of Anatomy, ed. 5, revised, New York, 1917, William Wood & Company, pp. 735-736.
17. McClellan, G.: Regional Anatomy, Vol. I, Philadelphia, 1893, J. B. Lippincott Company, p. 393.
18. Quain, S.: Anatomy. Vol. III, Part II, London, 1909, Longmans, Green & Co., pp. 75-83.
19. Toldt, C.: Anatomy. Part VI, New York, 1904, Rebman Co., p. 832.
20. Verchère, F.: Note sur l'innervation des Muscles Flechisseurs Communs des doigts, Anastomose du Nerf Median et du Nerf Cubital, Union méd. 35: 205, 1883.
21. Villar, F.: Quelques Recherches sur les Anastomoses des Nerfs du Membre Superieur, Bull. Soc. anat. de Par. 2: 613, 1888.
22. Hyrtl, J.: Ueber das Vorkommen eines dritten Kopfes des Biceps Brachii, Oesterr. Ztschr. f. prakt. Heilk. 5: 479, 1859.
23. Gegenbauer, C.: Ueber das Verhältnis des Nervus Musculocutaneous zum nervus Medianus, Jenaische Ztschr. f. Naturw. 3: 258, 1867.
24. Gruber, W.: Neue Anomalien als Beiträge zur Physiologischen Chirurgischen und Pathologischen Anatomie, Berlin, 1849, Verlag von Albert Forstner.
25. Krause, W.: Beiträge zur Systematischen Neurologie des Menschlichen Armes, Arch. f. Anat., Physiol. u. wissensch. Med. 31: 349, 1864.
26. Testut, J. L.: Recherches Anatomiques sur l'Anastomose du Nerf Musculocutané avec Le Nerf Median, J. Anat. & Physiol. 19: 103-108, 1883.
27. Cruveilhier, J.: Traité d'Anatomie Descriptive, ed. 1, vol. IV, Paris, 1836, Felix Lòquin, p. 800.
28. Langley, J. N., and Hashimoto, M.: On the Suture of Separate Nerve Bundles in a Nerve Trunk and on Internal Nerve Plexuses, J. Physiol. 51: 318, 1917.

TANTALUM GAUZE IN THE REPAIR OF HERNIAS COMPLICATED BY TISSUE DEFICIENCY

A Preliminary Report

Tom Dercum Throckmorton, M.D., Des Moines, Iowa

THERE are many admirable methods of repairing the various hernial apertures of the body. Necessarily some of these procedures are better than others and, depending upon the situation which confronts the surgeon, one or the other of them may be the "best." The choice of herniorrhaphy must have basis: sound knowledge of the anatomy and physiologic requirements of the region; a recognition of the fundamental factors concerned in wound healing and tissue repair; and a certain ingenuity which allows an occasional disregard of "routine procedures." The skillful application of these factors to the requirements of the individual operation is of far more importance than certain technical knickknacks which are dignified by the term "modifications." In conformance with surgical principles, the operation must be made to fit the patient. Many unsatisfactory results are occasioned when standard procedures are attempted in unusual surgical situations.

Nowhere is this more apparent than in difficult herniorrhaphy. If the surgeon finds his repertoire exhausted, he must extemporize to meet the problem. The defect to be covered may be enormous; the structures may be attenuated and friable, and the whole inguinal canal may present such a wreck that the possibility of cure seems remote. It may seem quite impossible for *usual* methods to succeed. Thus, the surgeon is confronted with three possibilities: (1) as is commonly the case, he may resort to a policy of masterly inaction; (2) he may employ some hypertrophied variety of the primeval truss, with all its discomforts, uncleanliness, perennial adjustments, and eventual failure; (3) he may improvise some operative method which goes beyond the mere autoplastic aims of usual surgical repair. It is in this latter instance that the employment of tantalum gauze offers a useful adjunct to the performance of a difficult herniorrhaphy.

Tantalum gauze is a finely woven mesh of monofilament tantalum wire, 2 to 5 mils in diameter.* The finest weave, 100 by 100, resembles heavy sheer cloth. The weave more commonly used, 50 by 50, is a light pliable screen.† This material was first developed as a dressing for burns. Brief experience soon made it evident that it offered no advantages, and that it did make for certain disadvantages as compared to other materials available for that purpose. This has been confirmed by Lam.[4] However, the innate properties of tantalum, enhanced by

The materials for this work were furnished through the courtesy of the Ethicon Suture Laboratories, New Brunswick, N. J. It is a pleasure to acknowledge the aid of Mr. I. R. McCall in developing a tantalum gauze suitable for herniorrhaphy, and his help in metallurgical problems.

Received for publication, April 16, 1947.

*A mil is 0.001 of an inch, used as a measure of wire diameter. For example, 10 mil wire is B. and S. gauge 30, or 000 U.S.P. catgut size.

†Tantalum gauze is now available only as a 50 by 50 weave of 3 mil wire.

its employment as a fine mesh, prompted its use in the repair of large abdominal defects and particularly in difficult herniorrhaphy when the size or location of the defect seemed otherwise an almost insurmountable obstacle.

The relation of tantalum sutures and appliances to tissue repair is well known. Its position is that of a biologically inert foreign body. Tissue repair progresses rapidly and unimpeded in its presence, allowing nature to proceed in an orderly fashion and with a minimum of interference.

The use of metallic filigrees, grids, plates, and mesh is not new to the field of herniorrhaphy. Such appliances had some vogue at the turn of the century. Phelps[7] (1894) treated many inguinal hernias by placing coiled silver wire on the floor of the inguinal canal and approximating the layers of the abdominal wall over it. Witzel[8] (1900) constructed, in the tissues, a rude network of crossed silver wires and suggested to the surgical world the idea of embedding a ready-made filigree. Goepel[3] (1900) was the first to make use of such a ready-made filigree. Meyer[6] (1902) reported the use of a silver wire netting made up after the fashion of ordinary mosquito bar. Bartlett[1] (1903) introduced a filigree of wire loops, usually held in position by a central strand. These appliances were made of heavy silver wire. Many of them were so rigid that the discomfort of the patient dictated their subsequent removal. The sutures employed were also of silver wire, which frequently broke on the knot and became fugitive in the tissues. Wound infections occasionally developed and, with metallic implants in place, drainage was often prolonged—probably in many instances by the vigorous therapy directed toward the sinus tracts. However, eventual healing was the rule. Accurate statistics as to the operative results are not available; but it is evident that many hernias, otherwise considered inoperable, were cured. The practice gradually fell into disuse for three reasons: (1) Occasional discomfort experienced by the patient. McGavin[5] (1907) reporting on silver filigree herniorrhaphy, stated: "The greatest difficulty has been with rigidity. Pliability is necessary so that the implant shall at all times and in all positions yield to bodily movements. Most rigid gridirons, having a stout framework supporting a heavy wire trellis, were so uncomfortable that they had to be removed." (2) The fact that silver wire and appliances are ill-suited for tissue implantation, because they are not inert and because they rapidly work-harden. (3) A sentimental distrust of a foreign body in the tissues.

The tantalum mesh now in use, from the standpoint of both its innate properties and its physical fabrication, has little resemblance to the earlier filigrees except in its ultimate purpose (Fig. 1). It is strong, pliable, biologically inert in the tissues, and forms a scaffold for the ingrowth of sturdy white fibrous tissue which firmly closes the hernial defect. Its use is relatively simple when compared to many autoplastic procedures, and its adaptability to the various situations which arise during a difficult herniorrhaphy is satisfactory.

A hernia frequently is associated with a deficiency in fascial structures. When the proportions of the defect are such that the approximation of its edges is difficult or impossible, the logical mind searches for a suitable patch. The autoplastic procedures have run the gamut from the simple fascial flap or fascial suture to periosteal flaps, free or pedicled fascial transplants, and dermis grafts. Certain of these methods, as the Gallie fascial suture, have enjoyed well-earned popularity; but when such a herniorrhaphy must be performed under tension, a recurrence follows. The extent to which various relaxing incisions or maneuvers may be helpful, each surgeon may readily determine for himself. Autoplastic procedures are valuable; they are often difficult, and they are far from uniformly successful under adverse conditions.

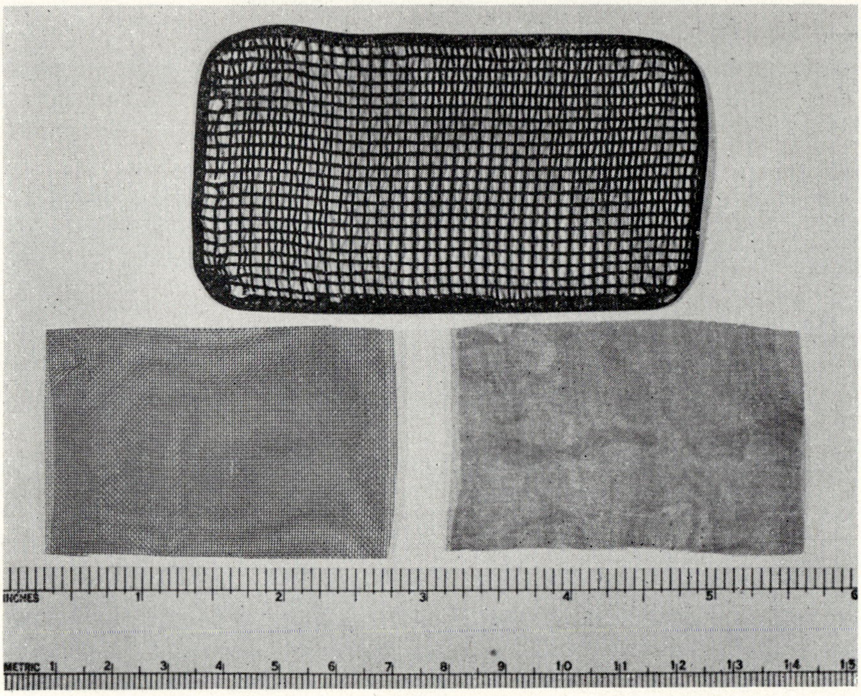

Fig. 1.—The difference in the silver wire screens used *circa* 1900 and the tantalum gauze used in this series of cases is shown. *Above* is a silver screen implanted by the late Dr. David S. Fairchild, Sr. of Clinton, Iowa, and which was subseuently removed because of ulceration and subjective discomfort. *Lower left* is the heaviest tantalum gauze used—a 50 by 50 weave of 5 mil wire. *Lower right* is the finest tantalum gauze used—a 100 by 100 weave of 2 mil wire.

THE TECHNIQUE OF TANTALUM GAUZE HERNIORRHAPHY

The technique of tantalum gauze herniorrhaphy is capable of almost unlimited modification to fit the individual situation. Such a mesh, together with its ensheathing white fibrous tissue, forms an impervious patch wherever the surgeon places it. In the continued use of this material, certain features have assumed increasing significance:

1. The cut edges of the implant should be folded under for approximately 1 cm. This serves the double purpose of creating a smooth, atraumatic edge, and also making it possible, when suturing the mesh in place, to pass all sutures through a tough, double thickness of material.

2. All sutures holding the implant in position should be placed in strong white fascia or periosteum and the dissection must expose these structures adequately. The dimensions of the implant are limited not by the size of the actual defect to be covered, but by the position of *reliable* supporting structures.
3. The implant must be of such generous proportions that it can be sutured in place *without tension.* More herniorrhaphies have been defeated by tension than by choice of suture material.

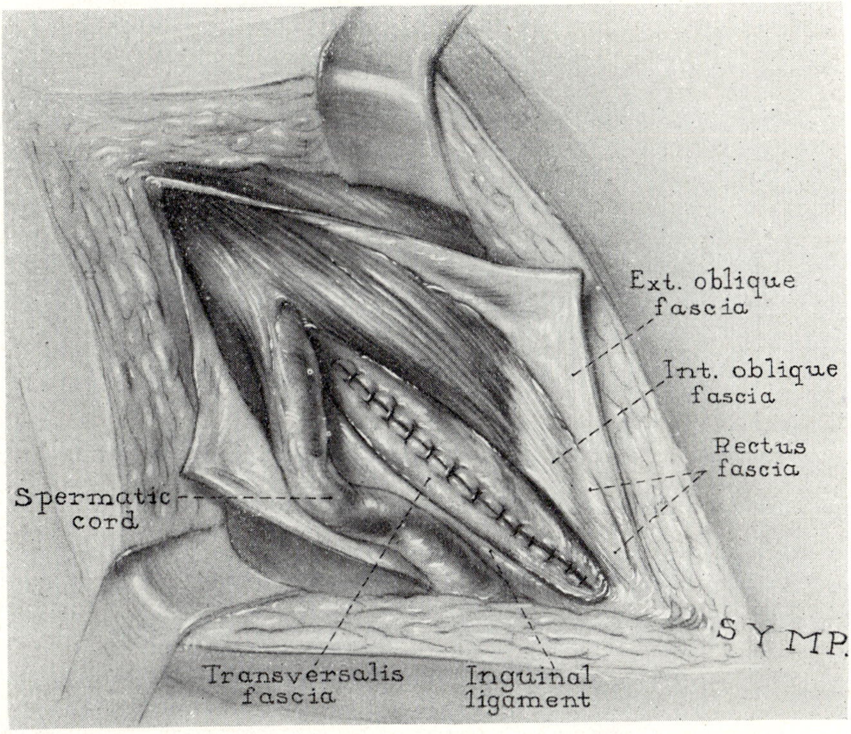

Fig. 2.—The inguinal canal is open; the direct hernial sac has been excised and the peritoneum closed. The rent in the transversalis fascia has been repaired with a row of interrupted sutures of 10 mil tantalum wire.

4. The suture material used to hold the tantalum gauze in place should be monofilament tantalum wire. The 10 mil size has seemed best suited to this purpose. The braided tantalum wire, although slightly easier to tie, was discarded because its finely serrated surface produced a notable "drag" when drawn through the screen. Other types of wire sutures were not used because of a difference in electrolytic potential between them and the gauze implant.
5. The wire sutures should be cut "on the knot." If unaccustomed to the use of metallic sutures, the surgeon may experience some initial difficulty with tantalum wire. A continuous type of suture should not be used. One-handed knots are not satisfactory. A simple

square knot should be tied, with only sufficient tension on the first throw to co-apt the structures being sutured. The second throw must lie flat and should be set snugly. The ends of the suture are then crossed to form a V, with the apex just above the knot. The suture is then cut at this apex, leaving no irritating ends.

The Tantalum Gauze Inguinal Herniorrhaphy.—The tantalum gauze herniorrhaphy performed for the cure of direct inguinal hernia associated with tissue deficiency is as follows: The usual inguinal incision is made; the inguinal canal is opened by incising the fascia of the external oblique, and the structures of

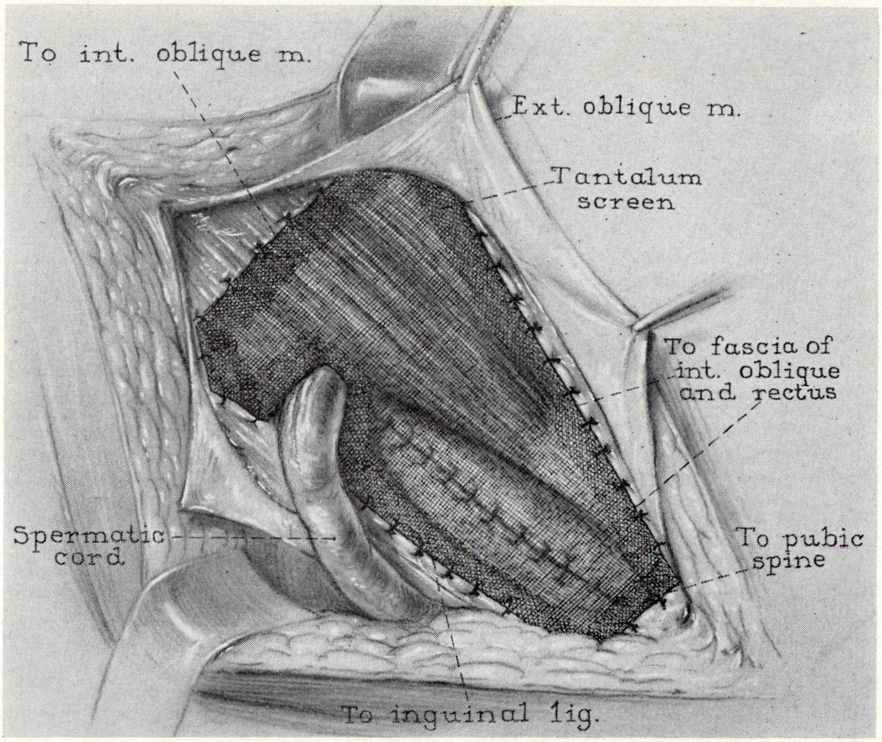

Fig. 3.—The hernial defect is covered by an implant of tantalum gauze. This is sutured medially to the periosteum of the pubis, the rectus fascia, and the fascia of the internal oblique. Laterally the implant is sutured to the shelving edge of the inguinal ligament. Superiorly, the sutures are taken in the internal oblique muscle and fascia. The spermatic cord is led through a defect in the lateral border of the implant.

the cord are isolated. These are carefully examined for an indirect sac, and retracted with a strip of Penrose rubber tubing. The direct weakness is identified and the sac treated as the situation requires, either by excision or inversion. If the rent in the transversalis fascia can be repaired, this is done (Fig. 2). No effort is made to suture a friable, attenuated, conjoined tendon to the inguinal ligament. Instead, the defect is covered with a patch of tantalum gauze. This is cut to size at the operating table, the edges doubled under, and it is sutured in place (Fig. 3). All suture material in this repair, save purse strings and ligatures, is 10 mil tantalum wire. The usual tantalum implant is sutured medially to the periosteum of the pubic bone, the edge of the rectus sheath, and the sturdy white fascia of the internal oblique muscle. Laterally, the sutures are usually placed in the shelving edge of the inguinal ligament. On occasion, when this latter structure has been deficient, the inferior-lateral sutures have been placed in Cooper's ligament after the fashion of the McVay herniorrhaphy. The structures of the cord are brought out through a small triangular opening made high on the lateral border of the implant. The cord is then placed in the subcutaneous position by closing the fascia of the external

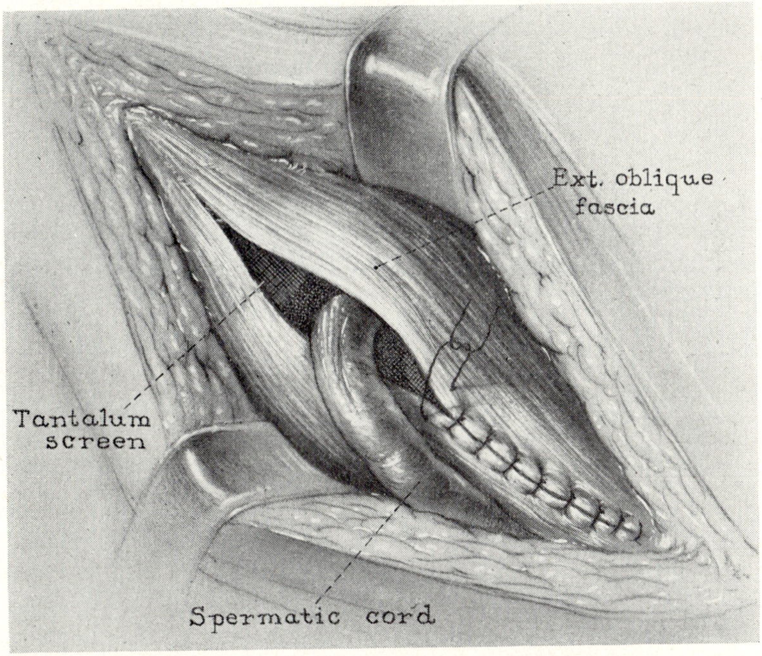

Fig. 4.—The fascia of the external oblique is sutured above the implant, placing the spermatic cord in a subcutaneous position.

oblique beneath it and over the implant (Fig. 4). The superficial fascia and skin are closed as usual. This method is equally applicable, when indicated, to indirect hernias with a large defect in the floor of the canal (as in certain sliding hernias), and to recurrent inguinal hernias. In this latter condition, since the hernia is usually direct and the inguinal region presents such a chaos, it occasionally has been necessary to use Cooper's ligament in lieu of the deficient or absent inguinal ligament. On several occasions, the lateral margin of the implant has extended from the pubic spine to the anterior-superior spine of the ilium, thus reinforcing the entire inguinal ligament.

The Tantalum Gauze Ventral Herniorrhaphy.—The problem of ventral hernia, particularly of a recurrent nature, arises periodically to perplex the surgeon. The moderate-sized ventral hernia, with good adjacent tissues, is satisfactorily repaired by one of several operative techniques. The large ventral defect, in

Table I

Sex and age (yr.)	Type of hernia	Type of repair	Period of follow-up (mo.)	Result
Female, 29	Ventral—P.O. hernia through low midline incision for drainage of pelvic abscess; patient weighed 255 pounds and was 5 feet 3 in. tall	Bilateral salpingectomy and abdominal total hysterectomy, with tantalum gauze repair of large ventral hernia	26	No recurrence
Female, 63	Low midline ventral P.O. hernia; two previous repairs, the last with fascial strips and alloy steel wire; draining sinuses and skin ulceration present	Usual type of tantalum gauze implant	24	No recurrence
Male, 75	Right indirect sliding inguinal hernia, scrotal in type and incarcerated	Usual tantalum gauze repair; the trimmed edges of the sac were sutured together behind the cecum, utilizing a separate laparotomy incision	18	No recurrence
Male, 62	Huge right indirect sliding inguinal hernia, scrotal in type and incarcerated, obese and incapacitated; the inguinal defect was larger than a closed fist	Ochiectomy; tantalum gauze implant from pubic spine to anterior superior iliac spine; sac treated by laparotomy as above	10	No recurrence
Male, 34	Large bilateral direct hernias with absence of the "conjoined tendon"	Usual tantalum gauze implants; the left side was done 2 weeks after the right	6	This patient was operated 26 mo. ago; has not responded to follow-up efforts after 6 mo.
Male, 50	Right inguinal indirect and direct (saddlebag) hernia; poor fascial endowment	Usual tantalum gauze implant	25	No recurrence
Male, 68	Large right direct inguinal hernia, uncontrolled by a truss, in a patient with arrested tabes dorsalis	Usual tantalum gauze implant	19	No recurrence
Male, 75	Large left direct inguinal hernia, uncontrolled by a truss; very poor fascia	Usual tantalum gauze implant	14	No recurrence
Male, 72	Large indirect right scrotal hernia; reducible but not controlled by a truss; associated with complete destruction of the floor of the inguinal canal	Usual tantalum gauze implant	12	No recurrence; patient died of coronary heart disease 1 yr. P.O.
Male, 70	Right recurrent direct inguinal hernia; two previous herniorrhaphies; destruction lower one-third of the inguinal ligament	Tantalum gauze implant utilizing Cooper's ligament	18	No recurrence

TABLE I—CONT'D

SEX AND AGE (YR.)	TYPE OF HERNIA	TYPE OF REPAIR	PERIOD OF FOLLOW-UP (MO.)	RESULT
Male, 58	Right recurrent hernia after Halsted repair with alloy steel wire; marked tissue deficiency	Usual tantalum gauze implant	15	No recurrence
Male, 47	Left recurrent inguinal hernia; three previous repairs, the last being a Torek operation with separation of the spermatic cord and resultant hernial sacs at both inguinal rings so constructed	Excision both sacs; tantalum gauze implant utilizing Cooper's ligament and extending to the anterior-superior iliac spine	16	No recurrence
Male, 64	Bilateral recurrent direct inguinal hernias; poor fascial development and almost complete destruction of the floor of the left inguinal canal	Right Halsted herniorrhaphy with tantalum wire; left inguinal tantalum gauze implant placed in the usual manner	10	No recurrence
Male, 62	Large left direct inguinal hernia, not controlled by a truss; marked obesity and fascial inadequacy	Usual tantalum gauze implant	6	No recurrence
Male, 48	Large left recurrent inguinal hernia; three previous repairs; complete destruction of inguinal supporting structures and absence of the inguinal ligament	Tantalum gauze implant utilizing Cooper's ligament and extending to the anterior-superior iliac spine	3	No recurrence
Male, 69	Right obturator hernia with intermittent intestinal colic and a positive Howship-Romberg sign	Laparotomy; excision of sac; tantalum gauze implant over the internal obturator foramen	19	No recurrence

an obese patient whose flabby abdominal musculature is a covering rather than a support, presents a situation that demands a radical effort if a cure is to be anticipated. The use of a tantalum gauze patch over such an abdominal defect is logical and offers a simple operative procedure in lieu of a difficult one. The operation is carried out as usual to the stage of the actual repair. The peritoneum is closed and the attentuated tissues about the defect are excised back to normal structures. If it is possible to approximate the wound edges by imbrication and without tension, this is usually satisfactory and the use of tantalum mesh is not indicated. However, if imbrication cannot be accomplished without

TABLE II

WIRE DIAMETER (MIL.)	NUMBER OF BENDS (AVERAGE OF 5 DETERMINATIONS)	
	STAINLESS STEEL	TANTALUM
3	762	1,475
8	197	451
10	181	208

tension, the fascia is simply approximated over the peritoneum with interrupted sutures of tantalum wire, and a rectangular tantalum gauze implant is sutured over the repair. All sutures are taken in the fascia and without tension. In case the fascia cannot be approximated over the whole of the defect, the edges can be drawn into proximity with wire sutures and the tantalum mesh implanted directly over the peritoneum as it bulges into the hiatus. The subcutaneous tissues and skin are closed over the implant.

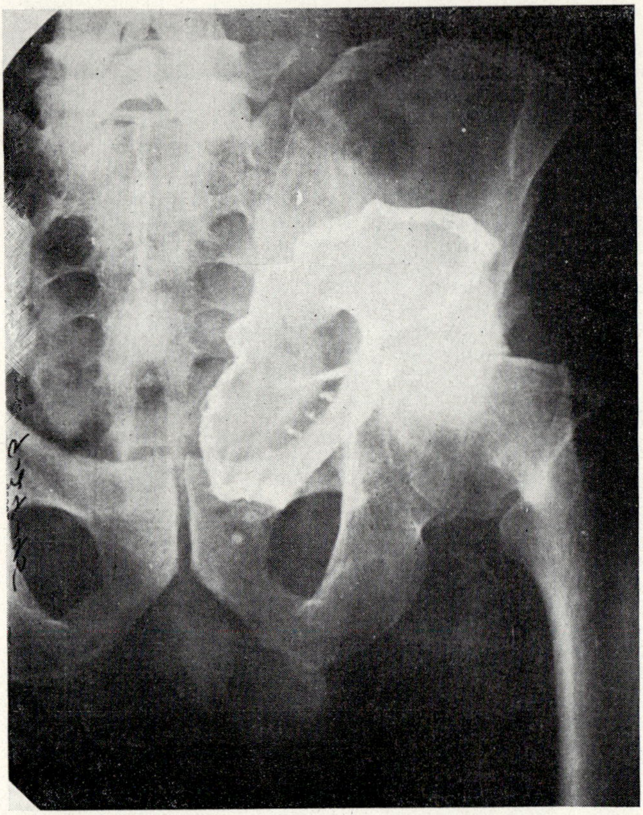

Fig. 5.—Typical x-ray view of the usual inguinal tantalum gauze herniorrhaphy.

In this connection, it is of interest to mention the tantalum gauze ventral herniorrhaphy done by Ferris[2] in October, 1945. The patient had a malfunctioning gastroenterostomy and a huge postoperative ventral hernia. This latter had occurred through an upper midline incision and extended from the xiphoid process to just below the umbilicus. The gastroenterostomy was disconnected, the opening in the jejunum closed, and partial gastrectomy with cholecystectomy was performed. The repair of the ventral hernia was then undertaken and a piece of tantalum gauze 12 by 24 cm. in size was sutured to the fascia at the edge of the defect. Underlying this tantalum screen there was nothing except the abdominal viscera, and overlying it there was only subcutaneous tissue and skin. The patient returned in May, 1946, complaining of a small ulcerated area in the skin where it overlay a wrinkle in the tantalum gauze implant. The tantalum mesh was removed on June 3, 1946. It was dissected free from a thick layer of underlying scar tissue, which of itself was adequate to close and buttress the hernial defect, save for two small areas, 4 to 5 cm. in diameter, which were weak. These were covered by another piece of tantalum gauze of finer weave than that previously employed, and the skin incision was repaired. The result to date has been very satisfactory.

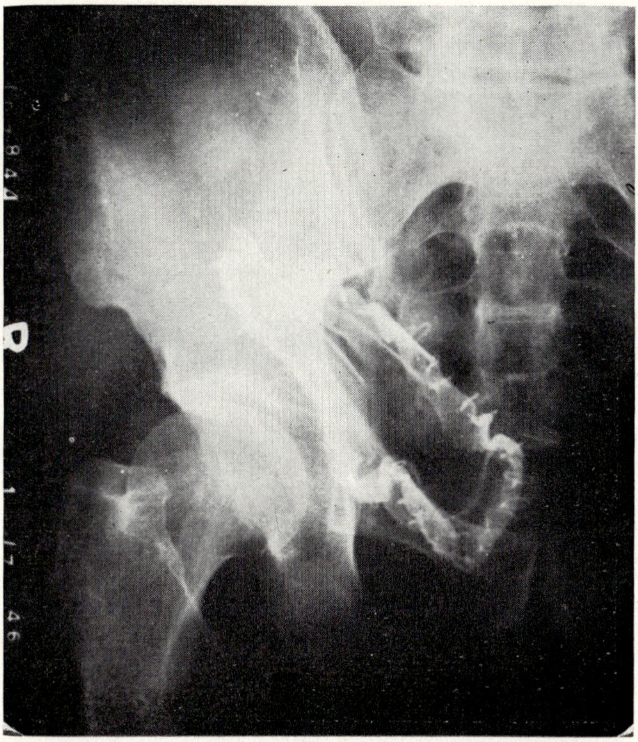

Fig. 6.—Postoperative x-ray view of a patient in whom Cooper's ligament was utilized in the repair.

The Tantalum Gauze Femoral Herniorrhaphy.—No patients have been seen with femoral hernias of such magnitude or tissue deficiency as to require a tantalum mesh implant. The inguinal approach to femoral herniorrhaphy usually is most satisfactory. If the inguinal ligament were deficient, it would be a simple matter to utilize Cooper's ligament in a tantalum gauze herniorrhaphy, as is sometimes done in certain inguinal hernias. Such an implant would completely block the internal femoral ring and should prove as satisfactory in the treatment of difficult femoral hernia as it has in the repair of inguinal hernias with associate tissue deficiency.

The Tantalum Gauze Obturator Herniorrhaphy.—One patient with obturator hernia has been treated with a tantalum gauze implant. This is the subject of a separate report. The procedure was carried out as an intraperitoneal operation. A small rectangular tantalum mesh implant was fastened over the defect with a single suture in each corner, utilizing the periosteum in the superior sutures and the obturator membrane in the inferior ones. The obturator vessels and nerve ran beneath the lateral edge of the implant without compression.

CASE REPORTS

That a larger number of cases has not been submitted to tantalum gauze herniorrhaphy is due to the fact that, although I have been impressed by the practical utility of the operation, I believe it inadvisable to elevate the procedure to the dignity of routine treatment and employ it in all cases of hernia. The

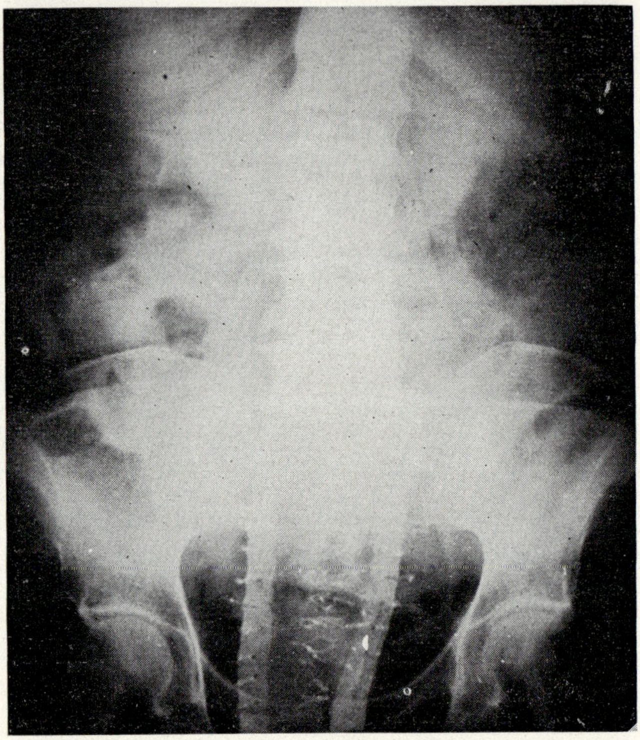

Fig. 7.—Postoperative x-ray view demonstrating the tantalum gauze implant in a ventral herniorrhaphy.

hernias so treated were of the type wherein the application of ''standard operations'' offered little assurance of a satisfactory result. Tissue deficiency, with or without congenital anatomic weakness, was the principal etiologic factor in every hernia in this series.

The information for this study was derived from seventeen herniorrhaphies in which tantalum gauze was implanted, with the purpose of closing and buttressing the defect present. Of these operations, two were done for postoperative ventral hernia, six were done for direct inguinal hernia, five were done for recurrent inguinal hernia, one was done for indirect hernia, two for indirect sliding hernia, and one for obturator hernia. These cases have been followed, except one patient with a bilateral operation, at frequent intervals both by physical examination and roentgenography of the tantalum gauze implants. (Figs. 5 and 6.)

POSSIBLE COMPLICATIONS OF TANTALUM GAUZE HERNIORRHAPHY

Work-hardening.—Metal fatigue or "work-hardening" is a property of all metals and must be considered in their application to surgery. Tantalum is no exception. Repeated bending of a wire ultimately leads to fracture at the site of angulation. Tantalum is not immune to work-hardening, although it is more resistant to fatigue than many other metals commonly used for tissue implantation.

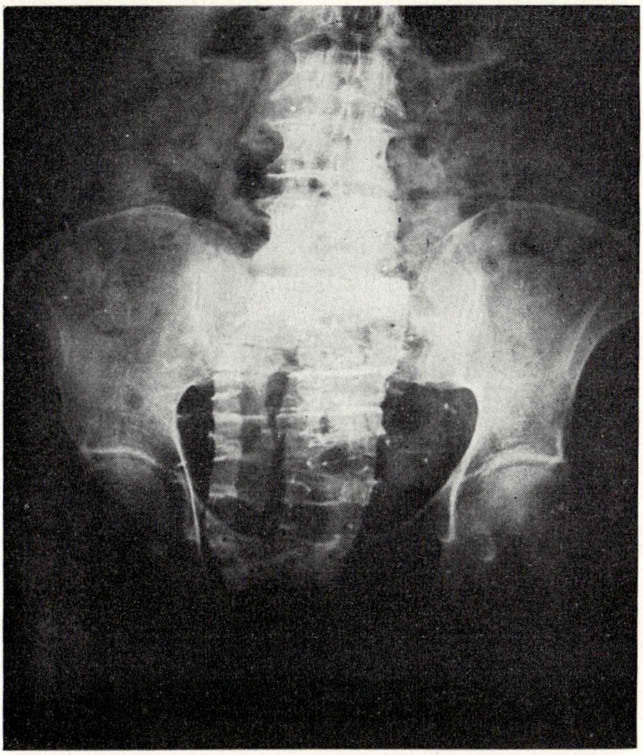

Fig. 8.—X-ray finding in the same patient 17 months postoperatively. The fracture of the implant is evident, but the clinical result remains quite satisfactory after 24 months. This implant was of the 50 by 50, 5 mil tantalum gauze. It is prone to early "work-hardening" and its use has been discontinued.

Tantalum wire resists work-hardening and fracture approximately twice as well as stainless steel alloy wires of comparable sizes. A few bending tests were done using 4 mm. lengths of wire held between clamps and bent through ninety degrees until fractured. The results of these tests are shown in Table II.

It is thus apparent that the larger and more rigid the wire, the more it is subject to metal fatigue. Although there have been no hernial recurrences as yet following the tantalum gauze herniorrhaphies in this series, there is x-ray evidence that some of the implanted mesh has fractured (Figs. 7 and 8). This has become apparent after about twelve months in some patients. The 100 by 100 mesh gauze and the gauze woven of 5 mil wire is more prone to fatigue and fracture than the 50 by 50 mesh gauze woven of 3 mil wire. This was the source of considerable apprehension to me until I persuaded one of the patients to allow the exploration of a previously performed tantalum gauze herniorrhaphy at the time of operation for hernia on the other side. A small secondary incision through the old scar revealed a firm inguinal region. It was impossible to dissect the fascia of the external oblique from the underlying tantalum gauze implant, so firmly were the two united in dense white fibrous tissue. When the upper margin of the implant was freed, a finger could be slipped beneath the entire piece of tantalum mesh with ease. Although the implant was completely ensheathed in dense collagenous tissue, there were no adhesions to the underlying structures. It appeared as if a supplementary sturdy fibrous tissue sheet had been added to this region without the incorporation of underlying contiguous structures. A small corner of this implant was removed for study. The wire gauze was found embedded in dense fibrous tissue, extending approximately 3 to 4 mm. on either side of the mesh. The individual wires of the gauze were clothed by this fibrous sheath much as the steel rods in reinforced concrete. It appeared impossible for the implant, or any fragment thereof, to become fugitive in the tissues. The entire inguinal region was buttressed by a sheath of dense fibrous tissue, reinforced by a fine wire screen. There was no involvement of underlying tissues by this reaction which, microscopically, was the encapsulating reaction seen in response to the presence of a biologically inert foreign body. The work of Ferris[2] would seem to confirm these findings. With these examples in mind, it seems unlikely that a hernia could recur through an abdominal wall so reinforced. Furthermore, the factor of work-hardening would seem to assume more academic than practical importance.

The Strength of the Initial Tantalum Gauze Implant.—The ultimate strength of the tantalum gauze herniorrhaphy is dependent upon the production of a fibrous tissue patch, secondarily reinforced by the ensheathed mesh implant. However, it seems reasonable that the formation of this sheath must require several months. The question then arises as to the strength of this implant during the period of healing. Pull tests, using a Tinius Olsen testing machine, were done on ½ inch strips of 50 by 50 mesh 3 mil wire tantalum gauze. Using a ⅜ inch pull speed per minute, the average stress at the breaking point was 17.5 pounds. A wire mesh of this type, even initially, would seem to have more strength on lateral pull than the tissues to which it is anchored.

Wound Healing.—In this small series of cases, there were three wound complications. One patient, on whom a tantalum gauze herniorrhaphy had been done for direct inguinal hernia, developed a simple accumulation of serous fluid in the subcutaneous tissues. This was aspirated, a pressure dressing applied, and healing progressed without further measures. Another patient had a large recurrent ventral hernia. The overlying skin was ulcerated and two sinus tracts were present from the previous operation. Tantalum mesh was implanted in the process of the repair, and penicillin used postoperatively. There was a slight amount of serous drainage from one angle of the incision for two weeks. The third instance of wound complication followed the repair of an enormus scrotal sliding hernia. A motion picture was taken of this procedure, during which skin towels and drapes were changed several times. The patient subsequently became febrile and several ounces of pus were evacuated from the incision. Healing progressed satisfactorily and all drainage had ceased in four weeks. From these experiences it would seem that the tantalum implant has no deleterious influence on the course of minor wound complications. The remainder of the wounds healed by first intention, without induration and with less discomfort than is usually experienced in catgut or fascial transplant herniorrhaphies.

Subjective Discomfort.—No patient in whom tantalum gauze was implanted had subjective complaint referrable to the implant. In one patient, an extremely slim, elderly man, a corner of the mesh was palpable subcutaneously, but without discomfort. Another patient was operated upon for bilateral recurrent inguinal hernias. Tissue deficiency was so marked on one side that a tantalum gauze implant was used. He knew the implant was used, but remained unable to tell in which side it was inserted. These patients were subjectively unaware of the tantalum gauze, and several of them later did hard physical work.

Testicular Complications.—There were no testicular complications in this small series of tantalum gauze inguinal herniorrhaphies. In the fourteen men operated upon, orchiectomy was done once to effect the complete closure of a huge sliding hernia. In the remaining thirteen cases, the spermatic cord was led from the abdomen through a small triangular defect in the lateral or superior border of the implant and placed in the subcutaneous position. A pressure scrotal dressing was applied at the time of operation, and these dressings were replaced by a conventional scrotal support on the fourth or fifth postoperative day. There were no instances of testicular swelling or subsequent atrophy.

DISCUSSION

The surgeons of forty years ago were much more optimistic in their discussion of herniorrhaphy than their present-day descendants. The terms "radical cure" and "ideal operation" were used carelessly. Most of these surgeons and their special operations are long since forgotten. It is not the purpose of this paper to advocate a new type of herniorrhaphy. It is the purpose of this paper to relate the experiences acquired in the use of a new material as an adjunct to the repair and closure of hernial defects where tissue deficiency plays the principal role. The use of tantalum gauze is not advocated as a routine procedure in the repair of hernias. This material is but another string to the bow of the ingenious surgeon. The application of tantalum gauze and its fibrous tissue envelope as a buttress to an inguinal canal that has failed is rational and, in my experience, satisfactory. Admittedly, the implantation of large pieces of this material is an offense to one's finer surgical sensibilities; but if the results justify the means, the pricks of ingrained convictions are soon assuaged. Serious disorders frequently demand radical measures. The use of tantalum gauze in the repair of an incapacitating incarcerated scrotal hernia is less drastic than the 75 per cent subtotal gastrectomy we so blithely perform for intractable duodenal ulcer.

The series of cases reported is small, limited as it has been by the number of patients in whom this type of repair has seemed indicated. Nevertheless, certain inferences may be drawn. Tantalum gauze implants are well tolerated by the tissues. They are not the source of subjective complaint on the part of the patient. They have not interfered with healing in those cases where wound complications have existed or supervened. The factor of work-hardening has not proved to be a real deterrent in the use of this material, as judged by results in the present group of cases to date. Each patient operated upon in this series was a likely candidate for a hernial recurrence. That there have been no recurrences to date is gratifying, but does not imply the infallibility of this procedure. However, the feasibility of the method is apparent and its further application to hernias associated with tissue deficiency is indicated.

SUMMARY

Tantalum gauze, a woven mesh of fine tantalum wire, is ensheathed by a sturdy envelope of dense collagenous tissue when implanted in the abdominal wall. This sheath, together with its reinforcing implant, may be used advantageously to buttress a hernial defect when local tissue deficiency makes the usual types of autoplastic repair impractical. The implantation of this material is not difficult. In this small series of cases, there have been no wound complications nor subjective discomfort attributable to its use. Tantalum gauze work-hardens, as do other metals, but this factor seems to be of more academic than practical importance. Its routine use in herniorrhaphy is not advocated, but a further trial of this material as an adjunct in the repair of hernias in which tissue deficiency plays a dominant role would seem justified.

REFERENCES

1. Bartlett, Willard: An Improved Filigree for the Repair of Large Defects in the Abdominal Wall, Ann. Surg. 38: 47-62, 1903.
2. Ferris, D. O.: Personal communication.
3. Goepel, R.: Ueber die Verschliessung von Bruchpforten durch Einheilung geflochtener, fertiger Silberdrahtnetze (Silberdrahtpelotten), Verhandl. d. deutsch. Gesellsch. f. Chir., Berl. 29: 4-177, 1900; Centralbl. f. Chir., Leipz. 27: 458-461, 1900.
4. Lam, Conrad: Personal communication.
5. McGavin, Lawrie: The Use of Filigrees of Silver Wire in the Cure of Herniae Usually Considered Inoperable, Brit. M. J. 2: 1395-1398, 1907.
6. Meyer, Willy: The Implantation of Silver Filigree for the Closure of Large Hernial Apertures, Ann. Surg. 36: 767-778, 1902.
7. Phelps, A. M.: A New Operation for Hernia, New York M. J. 60: 291-296, 1894.
8. Witzel, O.: Ueber den Verschluss von Bauchwunden und Bruchpforten durch versenkte Silberdrahtnetze (Einheilung von Filigranpelotten), Centralbl. f. Chir., Leipz. 27: 257-260, 1900.

Ibid.: Nachtrag zur Mittheilung: Ueber den Verschluss von Bauchwunden und Bruchpforten durch versenkte Silberdrahtnetze, Centralbl. f. Chir., Leipz. 27: 457, 1900.

PULMONARY EMBOLISM

A Correlation of Clinical and Autopsy Studies

Richard R. Crutcher, M.D., and Rollin A. Daniel, Jr., M.D.,
Nashville, Tenn.

(From the Department of Surgery, Vanderbilt University School of Medicine)

An analysis of clinical and autopsy records in the Vanderbilt University Hospital has been undertaken in an effort to aid in the clarification of the problem of pulmonary embolism as a cause of death.

Particular attention has been paid to the certainty of diagnosis and the clinical course in patients who died as a result of an embolus to the pulmonary arteries. The records were carefully examined in an attempt to determine the source of the fatal embolus.

Early in the study of these cases it became apparent that a diagnosis of pulmonary embolism was made very frequently in this hospital in both fatal and nonfatal cases. Often the diagnosis was unconfirmed and the data in retrospect seemed insufficient to justify such a diagnosis.

We believe, therefore, that a careful analysis of the data in a group of patients in whom massive pulmonary embolism was noted at autopsy may be of more value than would be any attempt to organize data on a larger group in whom pulmonary embolism might or might not have occurred.

ANALYSIS OF CASES

The Frequency of Pulmonary Embolism as a Cause of Death.—The study reported here is based upon a fifteen-year period, from 1930 to 1944, inclusive. During this period 83,984 patients were admitted to the hospital (Table I) and 35,540 operations were performed. This number includes such minor procedures as skin grafts, tonsillectomies, adenoidectomies, operations upon the eye, and the drainage of soft tissue abscesses. Bronchoscopic and esophagoscopic examinations and surgical procedures performed in the emergency room or outpatient clinic are not included.

There were 4,182 deaths in the hospital during this period and 2,580 autopsies were performed. These figures do not include stillborn infants. Death was caused by pulmonary embolism in 55 of the 2,580 patients upon whom autopsies were performed. Twenty-five of these patients had been operated upon and thirty had not. The incidence of fatal pulmonary embolism in these groups is shown in Table I.

Analysis of Autopsy Cases.—A detailed analysis of the records of the fifty-five patients examined at autopsy in whom pulmonary embolism is thought to have been the primary or immediate cause of death is presented in the accompanying tables.

Table II shows data pertaining to the seasonal, age, and postoperative occurrence of fatal pulmonary embolism.

Received for publication, April 26, 1947.

TABLE I. INCIDENCE OF FATAL PULMONARY EMBOLUS IN FIFTEEN-YEAR PERIOD, 1930-1944

Number of hospital admissions		83,984
Number of deaths in hospital (excluding stillbirths)		4,182
Number of autopsies performed (63% of deaths)		2,580
Number of operations (including ear, eye, nose and throat)		35,540
Number of fatal pulmonary emboli confirmed by autopsy		55
Expected number of fatal pulmonary emboli calculated on basis of 100% autopsies		89
Number of postoperative fatal pulmonary emboli		25
Expected number of postoperative fatal pulmonary emboli calculated on basis of 100% autopsies		39
Expected occurrence of fatal pulmonary embolism for total hospital admissions	0.11%	or 1 in 943
Expected occurrence of fatal pulmonary embolism in postoperative patients	0.109%	or 1 in 911
Occurrence of fatal pulmonary embolism in all patients examined at autopsy	2.14%	or 1 in 47

One-third of the fatal pulmonary emboli occurred in patients less than 40 years old. One patient was a 1-year-old infant with chronic bacillary dysentery.

The seasonal variation was not striking in these cases, approximately an equal number occurring in winter and summer.

Twenty-five patients had been operated upon and in fourteen of these fatal pulmonary embolism occurred within ten days after operation. Seventeen patients had abdominal operations. The types of operations are listed in Table III.

Table IV shows veins in which thrombi were found at autopsy. Twenty-eight (51 per cent) presumably came from the veins of the lower extremities. In twenty-seven (49 per cent) venous thrombi were found above the level of the superficial femoral vein. These veins include the common iliac, hypogastric, uterine, vesicle, periprostatic, ovarian, renal, adrenal, inferior vena cava, and mural thrombi in the right heart which could have been the source of the fatal embolus.

The location of the fatal pulmonary emboli is shown in Table V. Some patients who were critically ill succumbed to emboli which occluded small branches of a pulmonary artery whereas in patients whose general physical condition was good, massive emboli, which occluded the pulmonary conus or the main arteries, were always found.

Many of the fatalities from pulmonary embolism occurred among patients who had diseases which were incurable or in whom the disease was severe and the patient's prognosis grave. On the other hand, pulmonary embolism also occurred in a few patients whose prognosis otherwise seemed excellent.

The patients were, therefore, divided into three groups based upon an evaluation of the severity of the illness. Brief summaries of the entire fifty-five cases are presented in Tables VI, VII, and VIII.

Group I (Table VI) is composed of those patients who were not seriously ill prior to the occurrence of pulmonary embolism.

Group 2 (Table VII) includes patients who were seriously ill and in whom the outcome was uncertain. Many were debilitated. It is believed, however, that these patients might have recovered if pulmonary embolism had not occurred.

TABLE II. OCCURRENCE OF FATAL PULMONARY EMBOLISM

Age (in years)		
0-9	1	
10-19	2	
20-29	4	
30-39	11	
Total	18	(32.7%)
40-49	8	
50-59	14	
60-69	10	
70-79	5	
Total	37	(67.3%)
Grand Total	55	
Sex		
Male	31	
Female	24	
Total	55	
Month		
Winter		
Dec.	6	
Jan.	8	
Feb.	4	
Total	18	
Spring		
March	5	
April	3	
May	5	
Total	13	
Summer		
June	7	
July	5	
Aug.	4	
Total	16	
Fall		
Sept.	4	
Oct.	1	
Nov.	3	
Total	8	
Grand Total	55	
Operation		
Yes	25	
No	30	
Total	55	
Postoperative day fatal embolus occurred		
0-4	4	
5-9	10	
10-14	2	
15-19	2	
20-24	1	
25-29	0	
30-39	1	
Over 40	1	
More than one operation	4	
Total	25	

TABLE III. TYPE OF OPERATION

17 Abdominal Operations	
Cholecystectomy	4
Exploratory laparotomy	3
Abdominal hysterectomy	3
Exploratory laparotomy; Appendectomy	1
Abdominoperineal resection, rectum	1
Incarcerated inguinal hernia	1
Repair of ventral hernia	1
Suprapubic cystotomy	1
Gastrostomy for esophageal stricture; Drainage of lung abscess	1
Entercolostomy for carcinoma of cecum; Laparotomy for peritoneal abscess	1
8 Other Operations	
Craniotomy	2
Incision and drainage hematoma of neurofibroma sacral region	1
Iridectomy	1
Amputation of thigh	1
Extraction of cataract	1
Radical mastectomy	1
Open reduction dislocation of hip; Drainage of soft tissue abscess	1
Total	25

TABLE IV. THE LOCATION OF VENOUS THROMBI FOUND AT AUTOPSY

Unknown	25
Lower extremity below profunda femoral	3
Common femoral and iliac (One extended into vena cava; no thrombi in pelvic vessels)	4
Pelvic vessels only (prostatic, vesicle, uterine, hypogastric; two with extension into common iliac)	6
Combined pelvic and femoral veins (One had ovarian vein thrombus also)	6
Inferior vena cava, ovarian, adrenal, and renal	6
Mural thrombus of right heart	3
Mural thrombus of right heart and periprostatic	1
Mural thrombus of right auricle, left adrenal, and left popliteal	1
Total	55

TABLE V. ANATOMIC LOCATION OF FATAL EMBOLUS

Right and left main pulmonary artery	14
Conus and right and left pulmonary artery	11
Right lower lobe artery	6
Pulmonary conus only	5
Multiple small, right and left	4
Right main pulmonary artery	3
Left lower lobe artery	3
Right and left lower lobe artery	2
Right main pulmonary and left smaller arteries	2
Left main pulmonary artery	1
Right upper and lower lobe arteries	1
Right upper and lower and left lower lobe arteries	1
Left main pulmonary artery and right lower lobe artery	1
Right middle and lower and left lower lobe arteries	1
Total	55

Group 3 (Table VIII) is composed of patients who could not have recovered if pulmonary embolism had not occurred. Life expectancy was short in each case.

Table IX presents a summary of data included in Tables VI, VII, and VIII.

Fourteen patients, or one-fourth of the total number, are included in Group 1. There are twenty patients in Group 2 and twenty-one in Group 3.

The highest proportion of postoperative deaths occurred among the patients in Group 1, the lowest in Group 3.

In only eleven patients was clinical evidence of phlebitis in the lower extremities noted. The tables show that two of these cases were in Group 1, four were in Group 2, and five in Group 3. A total of fifteen patients, all in Groups 2 and 3, had bilateral edema of the lower extremities due to malnutrition, cardiac insufficiency, or renal disease which might have masked evidences of venous clotting. Examination of Tables VI, VII, and VIII shows that eight of the eleven patients in whom evidences of phlebitis were noted had infarcts in the lungs at autopsy. One of these was a patient in Group 1, four were in Group 2, and three in Group 3. Furthermore, in eight of the fifteen patients who had bilateral edema, infarcts were found in the lungs at autopsy.

There were ten patients with recorded episodes suggestive of pulmonary embolism prior to the fatal accident (Table IX). In three of these patients, one in each of the three groups, clinical signs of phlebitis were present. In all of these patients pulmonary infarction was found at autopsy.

Table IX reveals that pulmonary infarcts were found in twenty-six patients at autopsy. Only four of these were in patients in Group 1, in two of whom there was clinical evidence of previous pulmonary infarction. Phlebitis was noted in only one of the four. Thirteen (65 per cent) of the patients in Group 2 exhibited pulmonary infarcts at autopsy. In three of these signs of phlebitis were present before death and in four there was clinical evidence of previous pulmonary embolism; one other patient exhibited signs of both phlebitis and pulmonary embolism prior to the fatal accident. Among the remaining five patients, four had bilateral edema thought to be due to nutritional deficiencies or cardiac decompensation.

In Group 3 pulmonary infarcts were found in nine patients (43 per cent) at autopsy. Three of these had clinical signs suggestive of pulmonary embolism and one of these patients also had bilateral thrombophlebitis. Two other patients of the nine had evidence of phlebitis. In three patients there was massive edema which was due to cardiac insufficiency in two and cystic disease of the kidney in one. It should be recalled that this group is composed of patients with far-advanced incurable diseases.

It is noteworthy that of the twenty-five patients upon whom operation was performed, evidence of pulmonary emboli prior to death was found at autopsy in only nine. Thus, sixteen died as a result of a single pulmonary embolus. Emboli which occluded smaller arteries caused death only in severely ill or debilitated patients.

Table VI.—Group 1, Unexpected Sudden Death Due to Pulmonary Embolus, Patient in Good General Condition

Patient, race, sex, age	Clinical data: Diagnosis	Clinical data: Operation	Clinical data: Remarks	Clinical data: Phlebitis pul. infarct	Autopsy data: Veins involved	Autopsy data: Pul. infarct	Autopsy data: Embolus
W. S., W, M, 48	Duodenal ulcer, hemorrhage		Profuse hemorrhages, Hb. 7 Gm.	None	Rt. auricle and periprostatic	None	Massive rt., lt., and conus
H. L., W, M, 59	Cholecystitis	Cholecystectomy	Uncomplicated P.O. course, died 8th P.O. day, Hb. 13 Gm.	None	Unattached thrombus in inferior vena cava	None	Massive rt., lt., and conus
E. B., N, F, 31	Fibromyoma uterus	Hysterectomy	Uncomplicated P.O. course, died 11th P.O. day, Hb. 13 Gm.	No phlebitis, slight elevation of temp., pulse and resp. 8th P.O. day	Rt. uterine into int. iliac, also lt. ovarian	None	Massive rt., it., and conus
C. A., W, M, 37	Acute cholecystitis	Cholecystectomy	Uncomplicated P.O. course, died 7th P.O. day, Hb. 14 Gm.	None	Unknown	Recent	Massive rt., lt., and conus
S. S., W, M, 30	Rt. hydronephrosis, perinephric abscess	Exploratory laparotomy, appendectomy	Fever 100-104° F., died 15th P.O. day, Hb. 14 Gm.	None	Lt. renal into inf. vena cava loosely attached	Infarcts present	Massive conus
E. R., W, F, 55	Chronic cholecystitis, diabetes mellitus	Cholecystectomy	Temp. 100-100.6° F. P.O., died 5th P.O. day, Hb. 13 Gm.	Thrombosed (old) varicose veins of lt. calf	Unknown	None	Massive conus
M. C., W, F, 56	Intertrochanteric fracture, lt. femur		Temp. 100-100.8° F., Hb. 13 Gm.	None	Mural thrombus in rt. auricle	None	Massive rt. and lt.

M. L., W, F, 42	Varicose veins and ulcers, cholecystitis, chronic	Skin grafts, cholecystectomy	Temp. to 101° F., died 17th P.O. day, Hb. 11 gm.	None	Unknown	None	Massive rt., lt., and conus
T. L., W, M, 62	Cellulitis of face, benign prostatic hypertrophy	Suprapubic cystostomy	Uncomplicated P.O. course except phlebitis, died 6th P.O. day, Hb. 13 Gm.	Thrombophlebitis lt. calf, first noted 10 min. before death	Lt. pudendal and int. iliac into common iliac, femoral not involved	None	Massive rt. and lt.
J. E., W, M, 64	Cataract, bilateral	Extraction cataract rt. eye	Spontaneous pneumothorax 7th P.O. day, died 14th P.O. day, Hb. 15 Gm.	None	Int. and ext. iliac into common iliac and vena cava, loosely attached	None	Rt. pul. artery
V. S., N, F, 44	Fibromyoma of uterus, tubo-ovarian abscess, rt.	Hysterectomy	Uncomplicated P.O. course, died 9th P.O. day, Hb. 9.5 Gm.	None	Rt. hypogastric	None	Rt. main pul. artery and lt. smaller artery
E. S., W, F, 65	Carcinoma of breast, acute mastitis, biliary calculi	Radical mastectomy	Uncomplicated P.O. course, died 5th P.O. day, Hb. 13.5 Gm.	None	Unknown	None	Massive rt., lt., and conus
A. H., W, M, 48	Chronic sinusitis, pul. infarction, multiple		Temp. 99-102° F., Hb. 13 Gm.	No phlebitis, signs of pul. infarct	Unknown	Yes, multiple	Massive rt. and lt.
N. H., W, M, 17	Furunculosis, thrombophlebitis, popliteal and jugular		Lymphangitis, rt. leg, furunculosis of lower extremities, multiple emboli, R.B.C. 4.8 mil., died day of admission	Rt. popliteal, lt. external jugular; signs of pul infarct	Fixed thrombus in rt. int. iliac, unattached in ext. and common iliac, neck veins not examined	Yes, multiple	Massive rt. and lt.

TABLE VII, GROUP 2, SEVERE ILLNESS BUT RECOVERY LIKELY WITHOUT EMBOLUS

	Clinical Data				Autopsy Data		
Patient, Race, Sex, Age	Diagnosis	Operation	Remarks	Phlebitis Pul. Infarct	Veins Involved	Pul. Infarct	Embolus
W. G., W, M, 20	Convulsions, post-traumatic	Craniotomy	Stormy P.O. course, temp. 101-105° F., died 8th P.O. day, Hb. 10 Gm., transfusions	No phlebitis, signs of pul. infarct	Periprostatic	Yes, rt. lung	Massive rt., lt., and conus
C. T., W, F, 36	Puerperal sepsis, septicemia, hemolytic str.		Septic course, positive blood culture, also aspiration vomitus, Hb. 6-10 Gm., 11 transfusions	No phlebitis, signs of pul. infarct	Rt. ovarian, lt. renal and adrenal inf. vena cava organizing thrombus fixed to vein wall	Yes, septic staph. aureus	Lt. lower lobe artery
W. W., N, M, 63	Diabetes mellitus, general arteriosclerosis, gangrene of lt. foot	Amputation lt. mid-thigh (emergency)	Died 2nd P.O. day, N.P.N. 120, sec. anemia, Hb. 11 Gm.	None	Lt. superficial femoral (amputation stump)	No	Massive rt. and lt.
B. M., W, F, 52	Esoph. varicosities with hemorrhage, cirrhosis of liver		Repeated massive hemorrhage, Hb. 4-6 Gm., ascites, pneumonia, multiple transfusions	Lt. femoral, no signs pul. infarction	Lt. int. and ext. iliac into common iliac, unattached thrombi in inf. vena cava	Yes, multiple	Rt. and lt. multiple smaller vessels
W. S., W, M, 49	Infected polypi of rectum and colon, anemia, secondary, wound disruption	Exp. laparotomy, secondary wound closure	Fever 100-101° F., diarrhea for weeks, increasing weakness, Hb. 6-8 Gm., malnutrition	None, bilateral edema of feet and legs	Lt. external iliac, femoral and popliteal, loosely, attached	Yes, multiple	Multiple small vessels
P. B., N, M, 31	Stricture of esophagus, abscess of rt. lung	Gastrostomy, drainage of lung abscess	4 operations, last 4 days before death, Hb. 8 Gm.	None	Unknown	Yes	Rt. main pul. artery
J. S., W, M, 24	Gliosis lt. frontal, post-traumatic, decubiti, buttocks	Craniotomy, excision of motor cortex	Stormy P.O. course, temp. 102-105° F., died 15th P.O. day, Hb. 9-10 Gm.	Edema of lt. leg and thigh	Lt. common iliac, ext. and int. iliac vesicle, prostatic, gluteal and rt. hypogastric, loosely attached	Yes	Massive rt. and lt.

W. D., W, M, 72	Sliding inguinal hernia, strangulated, bronchopneumonia, bilat., paroxysmal auricular fibrillation	Emergency herniorrhaphy	Stormy P.O. course, temp. 102-105° F., died 6th P.O. day, Hb. 12 Gm.	None	Rt. auricle	No	Massive rt., lt., and conus
R. G., W, M, 53	Ventral hernia, coronary thrombosis, recent (autopsy)	Repair of hernia	Bronchopneumonia, bilat., improving at death on 23rd P.O. day, Hb. 14 Gm.	No phlebitis, signs of pul. infarct	Unknown	Yes	Massive rt. and lt.
M. D., W, M, 48	Glomerulonephritis (nephrotic stage), passive congestion of abdominal viscera		General anasarca, N.P.N. 80, T.S.P. 4.2, slow downhill course, Hb. 10 Gm.	Bilateral edema	Unknown	No	Massive rt. and lt.
C. S., W, F, 36	Chronic ulcerative enterocolitis		Temp. 100-101° F. for 3 weeks; diarrhea, malnutrition, increasing weakness, Hb. 11.5 Gm.	Slight edema of both legs	Unknown	No	Lt. lower lobe
D. A., W, M 34	Typhoid fever		Temp. 103-105° F. for 3½ weeks, abdominal distention, malnutrition, Hb. 10 Gm., positive blood culture	Thrombophlebitis of lt. lower extremity, signs of pul. infarct	Lt. femoral common iliac and hypogastric and int. saphenous unattached in common iliac	Yes, septic	Lt. lower lobe
C. B., W, F, 55	Fibromyoma of uterus, pelvic peritonitis, perforation of cecum, operative	Abdominal hysterectomy	Temp. 104° F., P.O. subsiding to normal in six days, abdominal distention, died 8th P.O. day, Hb. 9 Gm.	None	Unknown	No	Massive rt. and lt.
L. Q., W, F, 39	Cardiac decompensation, 3 mo. post partum		Malnourished, marked edema all extremities, died 3rd hosp. day, Hb. 7 Gm., T.S.P. 5.3	Massive edema	Ovarian, uterine veins, bilateral	Yes, multiple	Rt. main multiple small
M. W., W, F, 29	Tube, ovarian abscess, ruptured; genal peritonitis, incomplete abortion		Temp. 100-101° F., rigid abdomen, Hb. 4.6 Gm.; given 4 transfusions but course progressively down hill, died 10th hosp. day	Bilateral edema	Lt. ovarian and both renal veins	Yes, bilateral multiple	Lt. main rt. lower lobe

TABLE VII—CONT'D

PATIENT, RACE, SEX, AGE	DIAGNOSIS	CLINICAL DATA: OPERATION	CLINICAL DATA: REMARKS	CLINICAL DATA: PHLEBITIS PUL. INFARCT	AUTOPSY DATA: VEINS INVOLVED	AUTOPSY DATA: PUL. INFARCT	AUTOPSY DATA: EMBOLUS
W. H., W, M, 1	Chronic bacillary dysentery, marasmus, sec. anemia		Marked malnutrition, temp. 103° F. for several weeks, normal 1 mo. before death, Hb. 10 Gm.	None	Unknown	No	Massive conus
C. H., W, F, 79	Fracture of neck of femur, old left hemiplegia (abscess of epicardium found at autopsy)		Temp. 102-104° F. 9 days before death, Hb. 10 Gm.	Bilateral edema	Unknown	Yes	Lt. main artery, infarct. lt. lower lobe
M. A., W, M, 14	Staph. bacteremia and empyema, staph. pericarditis		Temp. 102-105° F. daily, also multiple lung abscesses, abscess kidney, subgluteal and thyroid gland, Hb. 15 Gm.	No phlebitis, signs of pul. infarct	Unknown	Yes, septic	Massive rt. heart and conus
H. H., W, M, 57	Tuberculous pericarditis, arteriosclerotic heart disease		Decubitus ulcers and cellulitis, temp. 101-102° F. daily, Hb. 12 Gm.	Bilateral edema	Unknown	No	Rt. lower lobe
S. H., N, F, 54	Carcinoma of rectum, acute P.O. intestinal obstruction	Abdominoperineal resection of rectum, laparotomy for intestinal obstruction	Intestinal obstruction following resection, died 8th day after resection, Hb. 10 Gm.	Edema of rt. lower extremity	Rt. and lt. hypogastric into rt. ext. iliac	Yes	Massive rt. and lt.

TABLE VIII, GROUP 3, PATIENTS WITH FAR-ADVANCED DISEASE AND SHORT LIFE EXPECTANCY REGARDLESS OF EMBOLUS

		CLINICAL DATA			AUTOPSY DATA		
PATIENT, RACE, SEX, AGE	DIAGNOSIS	OPERATION	REMARKS	PHLEBITIS PUL. INFARCT	VEINS INVOLVED	PUL. INFARCT	EMBOLUS
H. H., W, M, 41	Neurofibroma (massive) of sacrum, hematoma massive infection and sec. hemorrhage	Incision and drainage of hematoma	Cl. welchii infection of back, temp. 102° F. daily, frequent hemorrhages, expired 30th P.O. day	None	Unknown	None	Rt. main pul. artery
D. A., W, M, 65	Fibrosarcoma, abdominal, extensive; lung abscess		Died few hours after admission, suddenly	Lt. leg	Attached thrombus, rt. common iliac extending into femoral and vena cava	None	Rt. and lt. secondary pulmonary arteries
J. B., W, F, 57	Multiple fractures of ribs; metastatic carcinoma of lungs, ribs, axilla from breast; injury of eye	Iridectomy for eye injury	Temp. 99-102° F. daily, marked malnutrition	None	Lt. popliteal not attached	None	Massive conus, rt. and lt. pulmonary arteries
A. W., W, M, 47	Tetanus, general paresis		Convulsions, coma, temp. 99-104° F. daily, died 6 days after admission	None	Prostaticovesicle plexus	None	Massive rt. and lt.
T. M., W, F, 31	Carcinoma of cecum with necrosis of bowel; metastases to mesenteric and aortic nodes	Enterocolostomy; laparotomy for peritonitis	Temp. 100-102° F., progressive downhill course	Edema of rt. lower extremity	Rt. common iliac	Yes, recent	Rt. lower lobe
H. W., N, M, 55	Carcinoma of stomach with metastases to liver and pleura		Arteriosclerotic heart disease, benign prostatic obstruction, marked malnutrition	None	Unknown	None	Massive conus, rt. and lt. pul. arteries

TABLE VIII.—CONT'D

PATIENT, RACE, SEX, AGE	CLINICAL DATA				AUTOPSY DATA		
	DIAGNOSIS	OPERATION	REMARKS	PHLEBITIS PUL. INFARCT	VEINS INVOLVED	PUL. INFARCT	EMBOLUS
J. D., W, M, 61	Carcinoma of gall bladder; metastases to liver, pancreas, and duodenum	Exploratory laparatomy	Temp. 99-100° F., died 14 hr. after operation	None	Periprostatic	None	Massive conus
H. T., W, F, 25	Arteriosclerotic heart disease; cardiac decompensation		Cardiac insufficiency despite digitalization, increasing fever to 105° F.	Rt. leg	Lt. adrenal, lt. popliteal; mural thrombus rt. auricle	Yes, recent	Rt. and lt. lower lobe arteries
I. E., W, F, 55	Hypertensive cardiovascular disease, cardiac decompensation		Cardiac insufficiency despite digitalization, temp. 100-103° F. daily	Bilateral edema of lower extremities	Unknown	Yes	Rt. lower lobe, lt. lower lobe
J. M., W, M, 71	Rheumatic heart disease, cardiac decompensation		Cardiac insufficiency despite digitalization, temp. 101° F.	Bilateral edema	Mural thrombus in rt. auricle	None	Massive rt. and lt.
N. H., W, M, 65	Pyelonephritis, hypertensive cardiovascular disease, cardiac decompensation, ulcer of lt. foot		Temp. 98-106° F., cardiac insufficiency despite digitalization	Edema of lt. leg	Unknown	None	Rt. upper and rt. lower lobes
P. P., W, M, 70	Arteriosclerotic heart disease with failure		Cardiac insufficiency despite digitalization	Brawny edema of both feet and legs	Unknown	Yes, recent	Rt. lower lobe
J. C., W, M, 72	Fracture of neck of femur, hypertensive heart disease with failure		Cardiac insufficiency despite digitalization, temp. increasing to 105° F., increasing stupor to coma	Edema of both lower extremities, signs of pul. infarct	Unknown	Yes	Rt. lower lobe

R. E., W, M, 63	Arteriosclerotic heart disease with failure, broncho-pneumonia bilateral		Cardiac insufficiency despite digitalization, temp. 102-104° F. for two weeks, gradual decline	Generalized edema	Unknown	None	Rt. lower lobe
J. D., W, M, 53	Arteriosclerotic heart disease with failure		Cardiac insufficiency despite digitalization, temp. 101-102° F. daily	Edema of all extremities	Unknown	None	Rt. middle and lower and lt. lower lobe arteries
A. G., W, F, 62	Arteriosclerotic heart disease with failure, acute cholecystitis, toxic nodular goiter	Anesthesia (general) only, operation abandoned because of poor condition	Cardiac insufficiency despite digitalization, temp. 101° F., died 11th P.O. day	Edema of both lower extremities, signs of pul. infarcts	Unknown	Multiple	Massive rt. and lt.
C. J., W, M, 30	Fracture of pelvis, rupture of bladder and urethra, dislocated hip	Open reduction of disloc. hip; drainage of abscess	Peri-urethral abscess, septicemia, broncho-pneumonia, bilateral; temp. 101-104° F. daily, died 16th P.O. day	None	Unknown	None	Rt. lower lobe
S. E., W, F, 57	Papillary carcinoma of bladder, vegetative endocarditis, rt. hemiplegia		Cerebral accident, temp. 100-103° F. daily, patient comatose after cerebral accident	None	Rt. femoral and ext. iliac with puriform softening	Multiple small	Multiple rt. and lt. small secondary vessels
A. D., W, F, 38	Congenital cystic kidney, bilateral; pyelonephritis, perforation of gastric ulcer with abscess of lt. upper abdomen		Temp. 101-102° F., gradual downhill course, coma, death	Edema of both lower extremities	Renal, bilateral into inferior vena cava	Yes, recent	Rt. upper and lt. lower
J. G., W, F, 62	Abdominal carcinomatosis generalized	Exploratory laparotomy	Temp. 101-102° F. for two weeks, gradual downhill course, died 2nd P.O. day	None	Unknown	None	Massive rt. and lt.
A. J., W, F, 42	Adenocarcinoma of pancreas (head) and liver		Temp. 101-102° F. for six weeks	Thrombophlebitis of rt. and lt. legs, signs of pul. infarct	Rt. ovarian into inf. vena cava	Multiple	Massive rt. and lt.

TABLE IX

	GROUP 1	GROUP 2	GROUP 3	TOTAL
Number of cases in each group	14	20	21	55
Average age	47	40	53	
Postoperative	10 (71%)	9 (45%)	6 (28%)	25
Clinical evidence of phlebitis (lower extremities	2 (14%)	4 (20%)	5 (24%)	11
Edema bilateral (lower extremities)	0	7 (35%)	8 (38%)	15
Clinical signs suggesting pulmonary infarction prior to fatal accident	2 (14%)	5 (25%)	3 (14%)	10
Pulmonary infarction prior to fatal embolus (found at autopsy)	4 (28%)	13 (65%)	9 (43%)	26
Location of thrombus found at autopsy				
Unknown or below profunda femoris	6 (43%)	10 (50%)	12 (58%)	28
Above profunda and below bifurcation of vena cava (including pelvic vessels)	5 (36%)	6 (30%)	5 (24%)	16
Above bifurcation of vena cava	3 (21%)	4 (20%)	4 (18%)	11
Location of fatal embolus in pulmonary vessels				
Massive bilateral embolus	12 (86%)	10 (50%)	8 (38%)	30
Main artery on one side	2 (14%)	4 (20%)	1 (5%)	7
Smaller emboli	0	6 (30%)	12 (58%)	18

Table IX shows that all of the patients in Group 1 (fourteen) died of massive emboli to large pulmonary arteries while twelve patients (58 per cent) in Group 3 died of emboli to small pulmonary arteries.

Origin of Embolus.—The autopsy records were studied in an attempt to determine the source of the embolus. The veins in which thrombi were demonstrated are listed in Table IV. A summary of these findings is included in Table IX. The veins were carefully examined at autopsy down to the thigh. In some cases the popliteal and superficial femoral veins were examined but this was not done routinely. The calf and plantar vessels were not examined.

There were twenty-five cases in which no thrombus was found. In three cases thrombi were demonstrated in the popliteal or the superficial femoral veins. If we assume that all pulmonary emboli in which the source was not found came from the lower extremities, a total of twenty-eight (51 per cent) of the fatal pulmonary emboli originated in the veins of the lower extremities below the opening of the profunda femoris.

There were four cases in which thrombi were found in the common femoral or common iliac veins and were not demonstrated elsewhere. In one of these cases the thrombus was fixed to the walls of the iliac vessel and appeared to have originated there. The other three may have originated in vessels lower in the leg or thigh and extended to the femoral or iliac.

Thrombosis of the pelvic veins or a combination of the pelvic and femoral veins was demonstrated in twelve patients. These pelvic vessels included the uterine, prostatic, vesicle, pudendal, and hypogastric veins. There were eleven cases in which venous thrombosis was found in vessels above the bifurcation of the vena cava. These include the ovarian, renal, adrenal, and mural thrombi in the right auricle. Many of these thrombi extended into the inferior vena cava.

Thus, in twenty-seven (49 per cent) of the fifty-five patients, the fatal pulmonary emboli could have originated from thrombi in veins superior to the level of the profunda femoris vein. Since there were twenty-eight patients in whom no thrombus was found above the level of the profunda femoris vein it was assumed that the fatal pulmonary embolus originated from the veins of the lower extremities. It seems important, therefore, to determine whether there were indications in these cases for ligation of the superficial femoral vein. Twelve of the twenty-eight patients had far-advanced disease and short life expectancy even if pulmonary embolus had not occurred. Venous ligation in those patients would have been difficult to justify even in the presence of signs of venous thrombosis. In only four of the remaining sixteen patients were there any signs to indicate venous thrombosis.

There were six patients in Groups 1 and 2 not included among the sixteen discussed previously who gave evidence of venous thrombosis prior to the fatal embolis. All of these had thrombi, demonstrated at autopsy, in veins above the profunda femoris and would, therefore, probably not have benefited by ligation of the superficial femoral vein.

CONCLUSIONS

Fatal pulmonary embolism occurs at all ages but is more frequent in the advanced groups. Of more importance is the fact that its occurrence increases with the degree of severity of illness of the patient.

Trauma did not appear to have a significant influence upon the frequency of occurrence of pulmonary embolism in this group of patients.

Homans,[1] Rössle,[2] Hunter, Sneeden, Robertson, and Snyder,[3] and others, have demonstrated that clots are frequently found, at autopsy, in the small veins of the legs. We believe it to be of importance to emphasize the fact that in twenty-three of the fifty-five autopsy records reviewed in this study, thrombi were found in veins of the pelvis or the upper abdomen. These vessels include the renal and adrenal veins, the ovarian and spermatic veins, and, in three cases, thrombi in the right side of the heart. If the fatal embolus originated in these pelvic and abdominal veins, a few of the patients might have been saved by ligation of the inferior vena cava.

Clinical evidence of phlebitis was found in only eleven patients among the fifty-five who died of pulmonary embolism, and in five of these patients life expectancy was short because of incurable disease. In all of the remaining six patients thrombi were found at autopsy in the internal iliac vein or its branches. Ligation of the femoral veins could not have prevented pulmonary embolism if the embolus originated in the pelvic veins but ligation of the inferior vena cava might have done so. Furthermore, the presence of swelling or tenderness in the lower extremities does not exclude the presence of additional thrombi in other veins.

The restriction of activity or the fixation of patients in bed is probably of importance in causing thrombosis in veins. During the fifteen-year period from 1930 to 1944 inclusive there were 2,107 admissions to the Vanderbilt University Hospital for pulmonary tuberculosis. Most of these patients were confined to bed before admission and all were kept in bed during hospitalization. These patients, with rare exceptions, were permitted to move about in bed without restriction. Very few were critically ill during the period of hospitalization. Fatal pulmonary embolism did not occur in any of these patients. The importance of the absence of fixation and of prolonged muscular relaxation should be stressed instead of ambulation as a means of preventing venous stasis.

REFERENCES

1. Homans, J.: Thrombosis of Deep Veins of Lower Leg Causing Pulmonary Embolism, New England J. Med. **211**: 993-997, 1934.
2. Rössle, R.: Ueber die Bedeutung und die Entstehung der Wadenvenenthrombosen, Virchows Arch. f. path. Anat. **300**: 180-189, 1937.
3. Hunter, W. E., Sneeden, V. D., Robertson, T. D., and Snyder, G. A. C: Thrombosis of the Deep Veins of the Leg; Its Clinical Significance as Exemplified in 351 Autopsies, Arch. Int. Med. **68**: 1-17, 1941.

TATTOOING WITH MERCURY SULFIDE FOR INTRACTABLE ANAL PRURITUS

With Brief Reference to Vulval Pruritus and Evaluation of Results

Robert Turell, M.D., New York, N. Y.

IN THIS article there is presented an analysis of 93 of a total of 106 patients suffering from intractable anal pruritus who had been treated by tattooing with mercury sulfide[1] during the period between October, 1938, and November, 1942, and who had been followed personally and adequately for from six months to four years.* At some time prior to tattooing, all of these patients had received various forms of treatment without lasting benefit. The antecedent therapeutic procedures included topical medicines, endocrine drugs, irradiation, psychotherapy, subcutaneous injection of oil-soluble, long-acting "anesthetic solutions" or alcohol, anorectal operative procedures, or combinations of these forms of therapy (Table I).

MATERIAL AND RESULTS

The pertinent data concerning this group of patients are depicted in the accompanying tables. Table II shows that fifty-three patients of this series had had regional itching for ten years or longer. Table III shows that these patients had had moderate to severe degrees of characteristic local cutaneous changes which are encountered in advanced chronic anal pruritus.[2] Their circumanal skin was discolored grayish-white, moist, superficially fissured or otherwise ulcerated, indurated, thickened, and folded; in a few patients the skin was reddish, smooth, and glistening. In forty of these unselected cases the histologic studies showed various degrees of edema and inflammatory reaction in the upper portion of the skin. Occasional erosion and excoriation were also observed. It is realized that previous therapy, especially irradiation, influenced the gross and microscopic cutaneous appearance. Leucoplakic perianal and anal lesions resembling those seen in moderately advanced kraurosis vulvae were observed in seven patients.

All of these fifty-three patients, as illustrated in Table IV, were, in varying degrees, relieved of the troublesome itching. Thirty-eight patients graded their therapeutic response as good, while fifteen graded theirs as satisfactory. The itching usually ceased immediately after tattooing and the texture of the skin returned to normal or near normal in three to four weeks.

Ten of the thirty-eight patients who regarded their therapeutic results as good had had anal pruritus for over twenty-five years and had the most advanced cutaneous changes I have ever seen. Significantly, their therapeutic

---

Presented in part, with cinematographic illustration, at a meeting of the Philadelphia Proctologic Society, Dec. 18, 1946.

Received for publication, Jan. 31, 1947.

*This study was completed in October, 1942, just prior to my entry into the Army, but its publication was postponed for obvious reasons.

TABLE I. IMPORTANT THERAPY EMPLOYED PRIOR TO TATTOOING*

THERAPY	NUMBER OF PATIENTS
Topical medication (ointments and lotions)	All
Irradiation	65
Subcutaneous injection of oil-soluble "anesthetics"	85
Subcutaneous injection of alcohol	8
Anorectal operations (hospital or office procedures)	42
Endocrine	14
Psychotherapy	9
Various combinations of the foregoing procedures	All

*This information was obtained from the patients and not always from their physicians or hospitals.

TABLE II. DURATION OF PRURITUS

GROUP	YEARS	NUMBER OF CASES
I	15 or longer	24
II	10 or longer	29
III	5 or longer	33
IV	1 or longer	7
	Total number of cases	93

response was the most gratifying. Although advanced in years, these patients underwent a drastic change in disposition; by their statement and definition, they attained "a new lease on life."

The fifteen of the fifty-three patients in whom "satisfactory" results were obtained have occasionally experienced short-lived episodes of mild pruritus for which further treatment is neither indicated nor desired as they are satisfied with the therapeutic outcome. Some of these patients had a light cutaneous deposit of mercury sulfide as well as external and internal hemorrhoids, associated with recurrent stasis and congestion. For experimental reasons, these hemorrhoids were deliberately left undisturbed. It should be pointed out that external hemorrhoids, tabs, or redundant perianal skin are technically difficult to tattoo properly.

Interestingly, Tables III and IV also show that in sixteen patients of Group III who had had pruritus for five years or longer, but who had also exhibited moderate to advanced cutaneous local manifestations, good therapeutic results had also been obtained.

TABLE III. GROSS CUTANEOUS MANIFESTATIONS CONSISTENT WITH PRURITUS

GROUP	PRESENT (MODERATE TO SEVERE) NUMBER OF CASES	ABSENT OR MINIMAL NUMBER OF CASES
I	24	0
II	29	0
III	16	17
IV	1	6

TABLE IV. RESULTS OF TATTOOING WITH MERCURY SULFIDE

GROUP	GOOD (NUMBER OF CASES)	SATISFACTORY (NUMBER OF CASES)	POOR (NUMBER OF CASES)
I	20	4	0
II	18	11	0
III	16	4	13
IV	1	2	4

Of the twenty-three patients who exhibited either minimal or no cutaneous changes, only six responded satisfactorily to tattooing with mercury sulfide, while the remaining seventeen patients failed to improve.

COMMENT

From the foregoing analysis and study, it is apparent that tattooing with mercury sulfide is effective for chronic recalcitrant anal pruritus that is associated with characteristic cutaneous changes. Confirmation of these results has indirectly been elicited in an experimental study of a small series of cases of intractable vulval pruritus. Those patients who manifested cutaneous changes, especially the hypertrophic manifestations, have responded well to tattooing with mercury sulfide.[3] In four of these women contemplated radical vulvectomy became unnecessary following tattooing. In contrast, fifteen women with vulval pruritus who showed no cutaneous changes have uniformly failed to respond to tattooing with mercury sulfide.*

Most of the patients who had not exhibited characteristic cutaneous manifestations, except for scratch marks, were highly nervous and frustrated individuals. Four of them had received prolonged psychotherapy by recognized experts prior to tattooing without apparent benefit. The psychic factors of these individuals were extremely difficult to evaluate as one could not always be sure of what was cause or what was effect. In some of these individuals the mental status was not apparent before tattooing, while others I treated for experimental reasons because I realized that the continuance of anal itching was conducive to a variety of psychotic manifestations in these neurotic patients. This policy was motivated in 1939 by the satisfactory results obtained in some "psychoneurotic" patients.[4]

The satisfactory results obtained in the six patients of Groups III and IV who had had either minimal or no cutaneous perianal skin changes may to a degree be ascribed to psychotherapeutic influences. This interpretation was recognized in the early course of my studies[4] as I then stated, "It is realized that in some instances tattooing with mercury sulfide, like other therapeutic procedures, may in addition to the pharmacodynamic action exert a psychotherapeutic effect although in normal (nonneurotic) patients our control studies of tattooing with mercury sulfide indicated that the psychic effect is of no therapeutic value in relieving pruritus."

Although individuals with anal pruritus who have minimal or no cutaneous changes are poor candidates for tattooing with mercury sulfide, these patients may nevertheless be given a trial of tattoing only before other drastic therapeutic procedures, such as the subcutaneous injection of ethyl alcohol[5] or the radical resection of the anoperianal skin,[6] are contemplated.

ANOGENITAL PRURITUS

In two men with severe concomitant anal and scrotal pruritus, some amelioration of scrotal itching occurred after the cessation of anal pruritus follow-

*Most of the gynecologic aspects of this study were conducted with the cooperation of the late Dr. S. H. Geist, Mount Sinai Hospital, New York, N. Y.

ing tattooing with mercury sulfide. Subsequent tattooing of the scrotal skin was ineffective in completely eliminating the itching of the scrotum.

To date I have successfully treated twelve women with pruritus ani and pruritus vulvae by tattooing of the anal and perianal regions only. In five of these patients tattooing of the vulva had also been contemplated, and the anoperineal region was tattooed as a preliminary procedure. Following this maneuver there occurred sufficient subjective and objective improvement of the vulval itching so that further treatment became unnecessary.

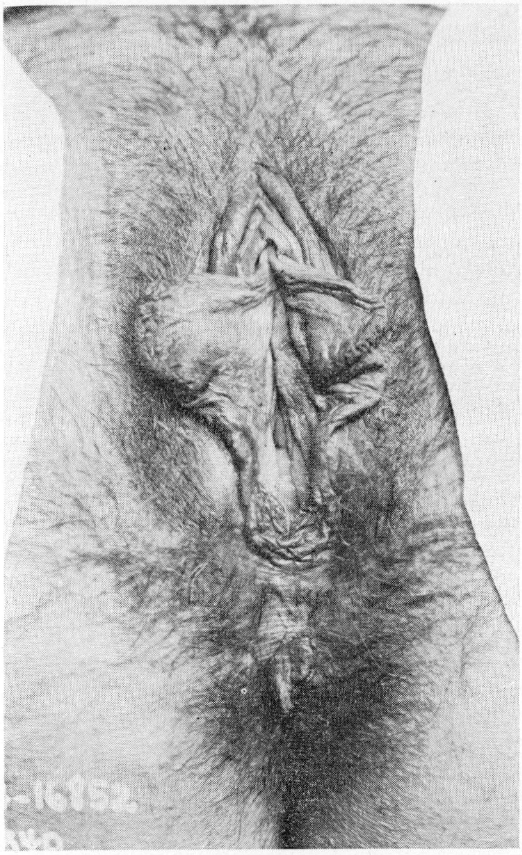

Fig. 1.

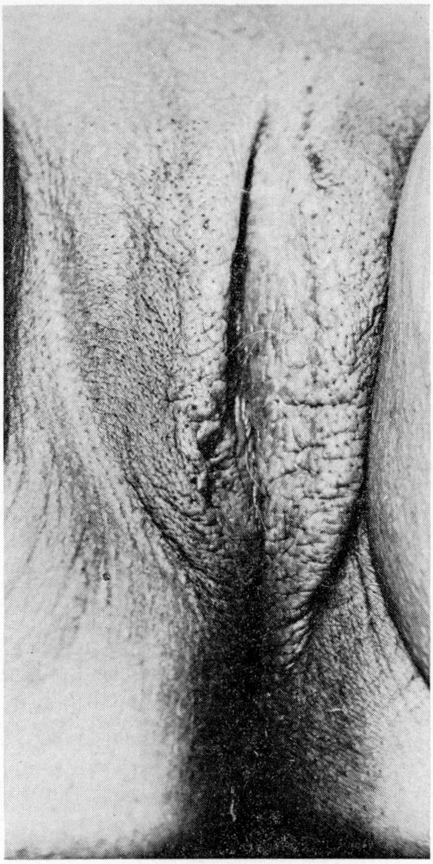

Fig. 2.

Fig. 1.—Pretattoo appearance of anogenital pruritus (see Figs. F and G).

Fig. 2.—Pretattoo appearance of "hypertrophic" vulvitis with areas of leucoplakia (see Fig. H).

GENERAL PROCEDURE

The following procedures are now carried out prior to tattooing with mercury sulfide: (1) A general survey including a patch test for sensitivity to mercury using 2 per cent ammoniated mercury ointment; positive reactors should never be tattooed with mercury or its derivatives. (2) The eradication of anorectal or colonic lesions as well as excision of redundant perianal skin.

(3) The administration of estrogenic therapy to women who develop anal pruritus at or after menopause. Usually about 150,000 to 250,000 R.U. of estradiol benzoate* are administered in biweekly intramuscular doses of from 6,000 to 10,000 R.U. If the localized pruritus is unrelieved by hormonal therapy, tattooing is carried out.

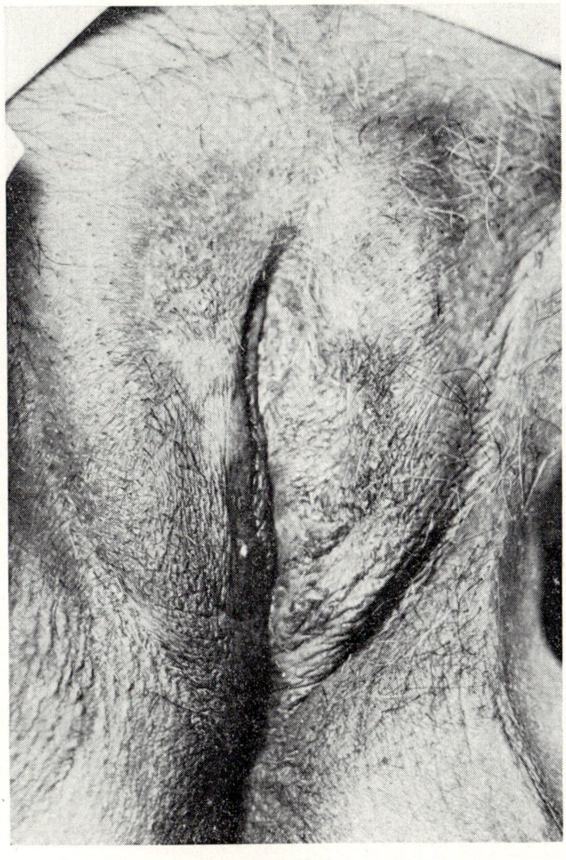

Fig. 3.

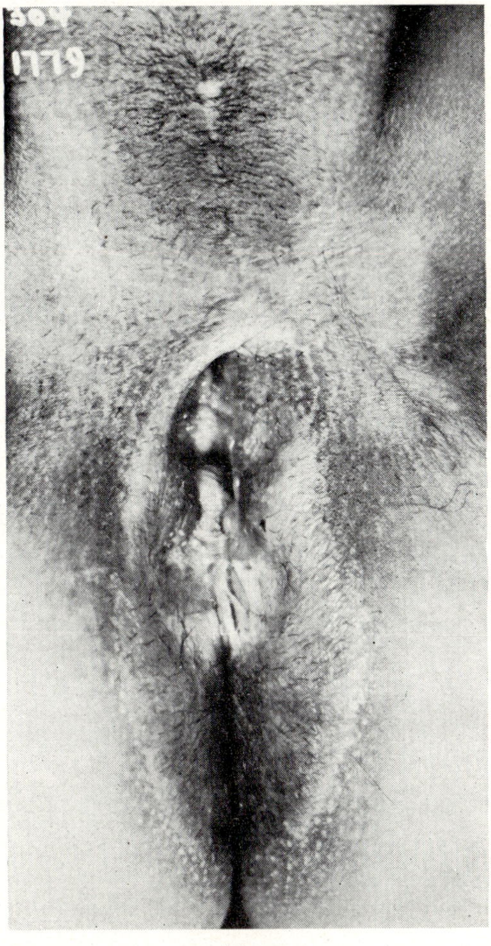

Fig. 4.

Fig. 3.—Same patient as shown in Fig. 2, six months after tattooing (see Fig. I).

Fig. 4.—Pretattoo appearance of anogenital area after four vulval operations for recurrent kraurosis vulvae with pernicious pruritus (see Figs. J and K).

Systemic and general dematologic lesions having anoperianal representation are always appropriately treated and, if possible, eliminated prior to tattooing.

The presence of inflammatory or infectious disease of the anorectum or colon contraindicates tattooing. Lesions, such as anal ulcers, suppuration, fistulas, and hemorrhoids, which apparently are caused by inflammation or

---

*Progynon B supplied for research purposes by the Schering Corporation, Bloomfield, N. J., through Dr. W. H. Stoner.

infection of the anal glands, the pre-formed anal ducts, and the anal crypts should be eradicated surgically prior to tattooing. A contracted anal outlet is etiologically important and should be eliminated.

It has been my policy to perform radical operations on these individuals with respect to excision of perianal skin, especially when redundant folded perianal skin is present. Large, elliptically shaped blocks of skin are removed, but enough integument between wounds is left to prevent postoperative anal stenosis.

Operation and tattooing should never be carried out at one sitting because the primary operation may be adequate for the control of pruritus in many cases, and also because in the presence of open wounds the mercury sulfide may get into the subcutaneous tissues and form mercury proteinate which is soluble and toxic.

TECHNIQUE

Since the details of the technique of tattooing have already been described,[7] only the essential points will be discussed here.* It is important to deposit the mercury sulfide in the corium and to tattoo the anal canal to the mucocutaneous junction along with the circumanal skin for 1 cm. beyond the visible line of demarcation. In the absence of a naturally demarcated zone, the extent of the pruritic involvement should be delineated before the anesthetic is administered. A regional relaxing anesthetic that will last for one hour is satisfactory. The skin to be tattooed is prepared with ether and alcohol as for any anorectal operation and a thin film of petrolatum is applied. The skin should be held taut to obliterate the cutaneous folds and to facilitate

*The technique is well illustrated in a colored motion picture which is suitable for teaching purposes.

Fig. A.—Pretattoo appearance of advanced circumanal cutaneous changes in a patient with intractable anogenital pruritus of over twenty years' duration. Tattooing is effective for this type of lesion.

Fig. B.—Same patient as shown in Fig. A., fifteen months after tattooing of circumanal area which resulted in the disappearance of the anal and vulval pruritus. Note the permanent post-tattoo red stain produced by the mercury sulfide.

Fig. C.—Same patient as shown in Figs. A and B, six years after successful tattooing. (Photograph made July 17, 1947, when patient was almost 80 years old.)

Fig. D.—Pretattoo appearance of anogenital region of patient with pruritus of about five years' duration, but with only minimal skin changes. This type of lesion is as a rule not suitable for tattooing with mercury sulfide (see discussion in the text).

Fig. E.—Same patient as shown in Fig. D., twelve months after experimental tattooing.

Fig. F.—Anogenital pruritus; tattooing of vulva only, failed to relieve the itching. (See Fig. 1 for pretattoo appearance of anogenital region.)

Fig. G.—Same patient as shown in Fig. F., twenty months after extension of tattooing to perianal area which resulted in the disappearance of anogenital pruritus.

Fig. H.—Pretattoo appearance of "hypertrophic" vulvitis with pernicious and intractable pruritus. Note the advanced cutaneous changes with areas of leucoplakia.

Fig. I.—Same patient as shown in Fig. H, eighteen months after successful tattooing. (See Figs. 2 and 3.)

Fig. J.—Appearance of anogenital area three weeks after tattooing of vulva and five days after tattooing of circumanal and perineal regions for recurring kraurosis with intractable pruritus. (See Fig. 4 for pretattoo appearance of anogenital area of this patient.)

Fig. K.—Same patient as shown in Fig. J., appearance of anogenital region fifteen months after successful tattooing. Note the scarred perineum which is but lightly or inadequately tattooed.

Fig. L.—Appearance of unilateral incomplete tattooing (light color and skipped areas) with unilateral recurrent pruritus. The opposite side is well tattooed and nonpruritic.

Fig. M.—Shows superficial perineal fissures which may cause temporary recurrence of pruritus. Note acute dermatitis of vulva which stopped sharply at the line of tattooed perineum.

Note the inadvertent misplacement of Figs. C and L.

SURGERY
VOL. 23, NO. 1, JANUARY, 1948

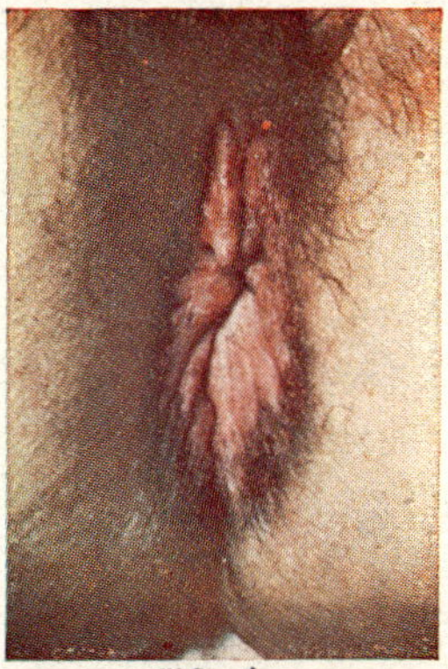
FIG. A

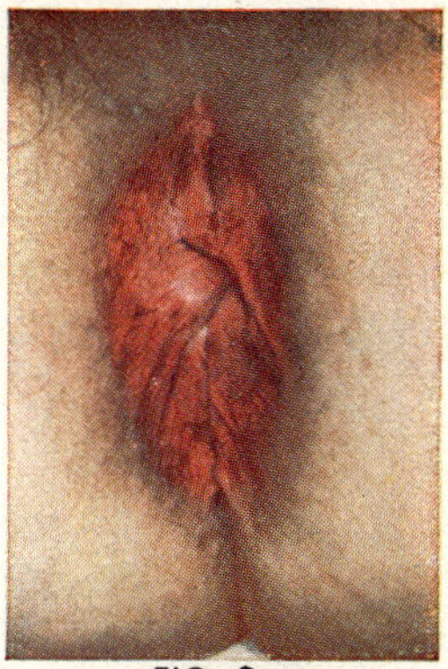
FIG. B

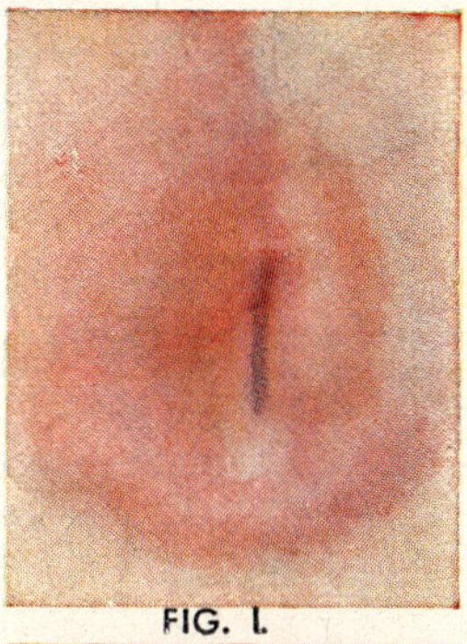
FIG. L

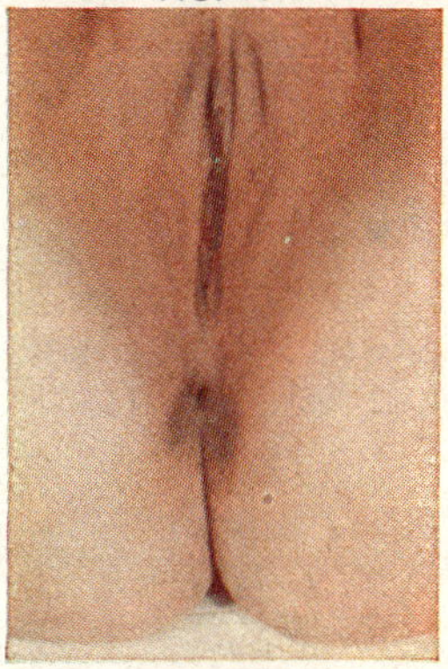
FIG. D

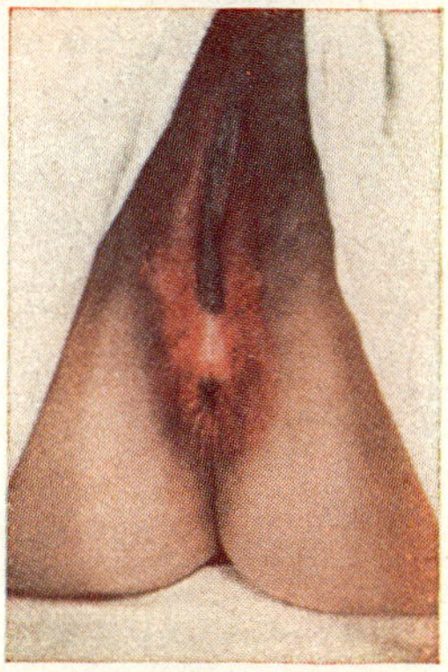
FIG. E

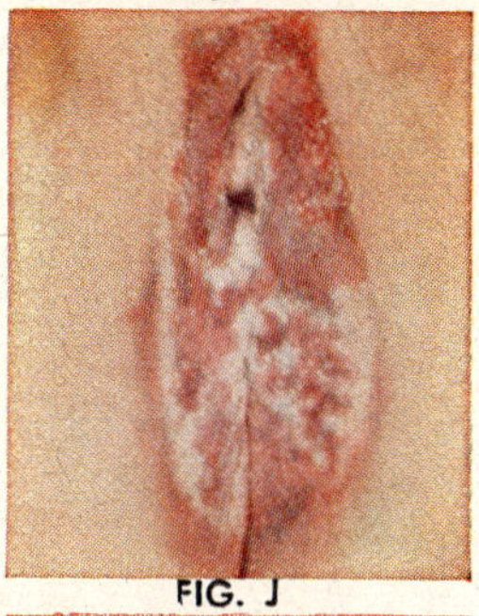
FIG. J

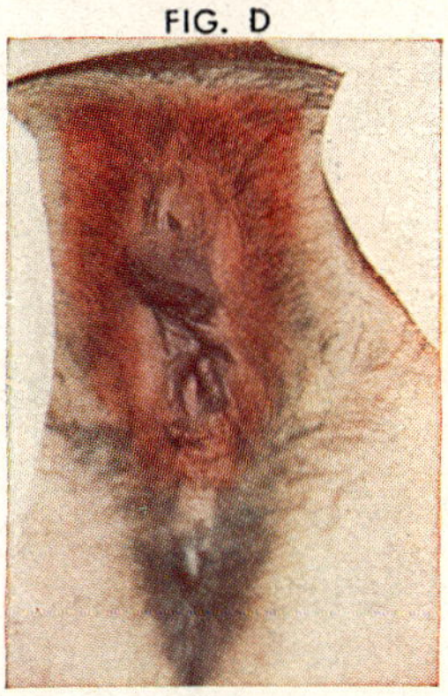
FIG. F

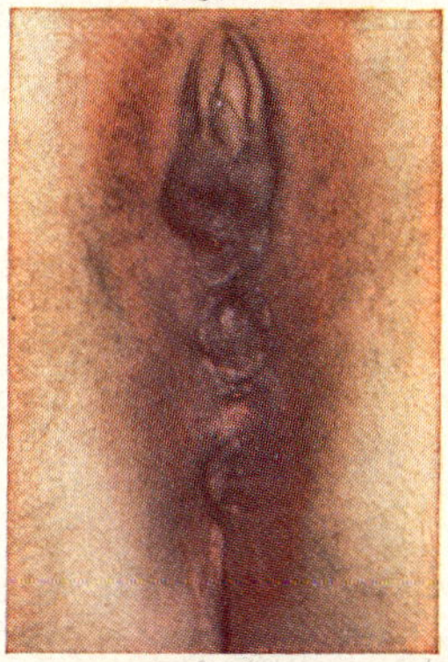
FIG. G

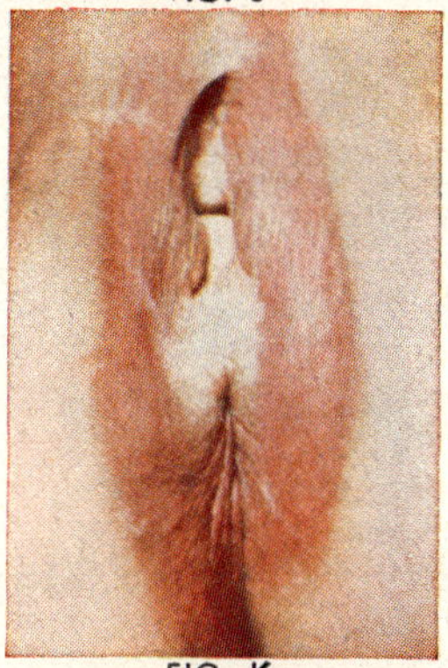
FIG K

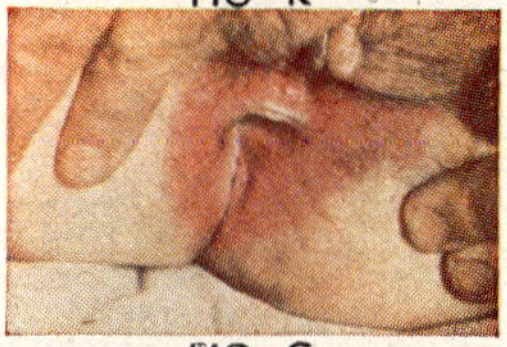
FIG. C

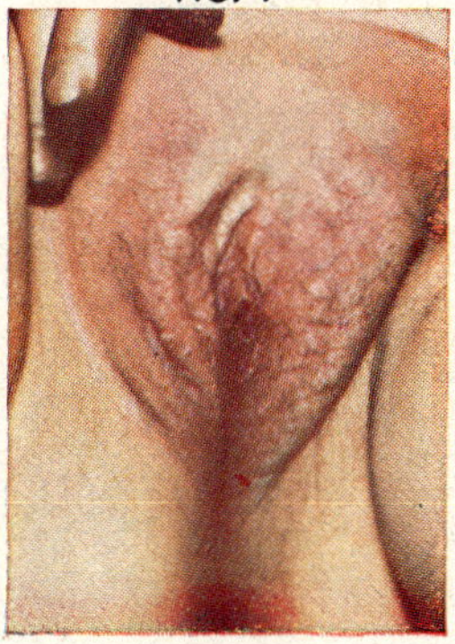
FIG. H

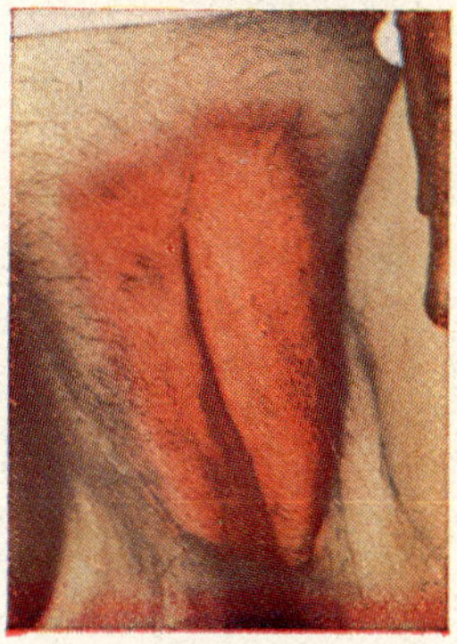
FIG. I

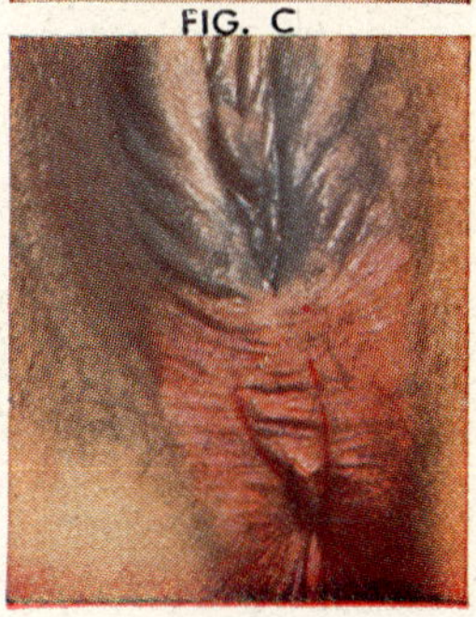
FIG M

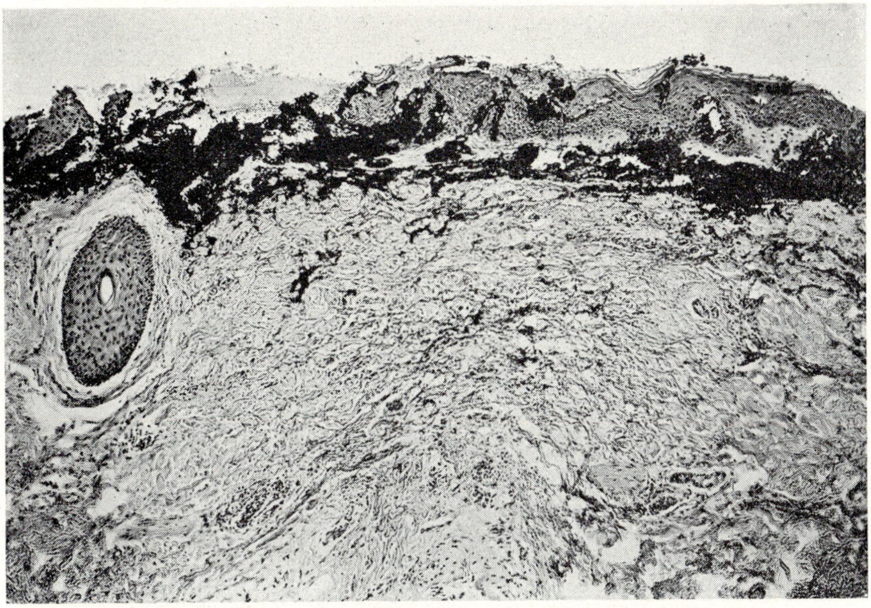

Fig. 5.—Photomicrograph of specimen of tattooed skin obtained immediately after completion of tattooing shows perforations and deposits of mercury sulfide in the epithelium and massive deposition in the upper corium.

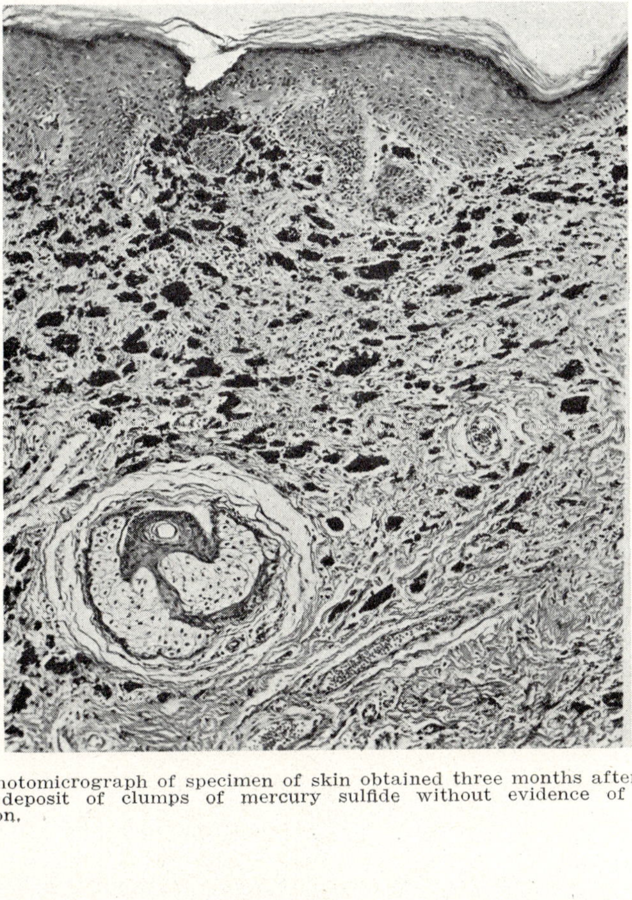

Fig. 6.—Photomicrograph of specimen of skin obtained three months after tattooing shows a subepithelial deposit of clumps of mercury sulfide without evidence of a foreign body giant-cell reaction.

the penetration of the needles and the mercury sulfide into the corium. A paste of mercury sulfide, prepared by mixing the powder with sterile distilled water, is placed on the skin, or the tip of the instrument may be dipped into the paste as often as necessary. The shaft of the instrument should be held at a 45 degree angle or at a right angle to the skin and is advanced slowly, exerting light pressure against the skin; these maneuvers are repeated several times in the same area until the skin shows a uniform and permanent red

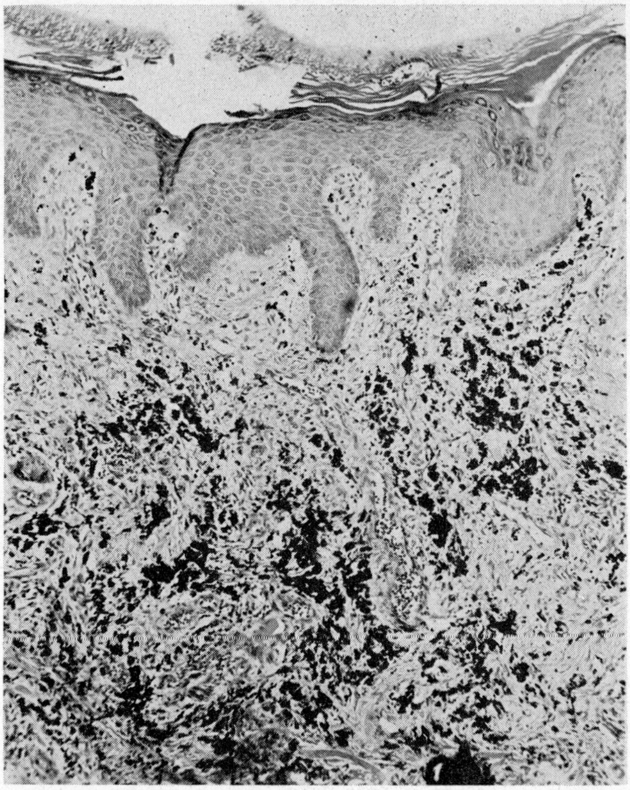

Fig. 7.—Photomicropgraph of a skin specimen obtained eight months after tattooing shows a histologic picture similar to that of Fig. 6.

stain. The speed of tattooing will depend on the type of tattooing instrument employed. The ordinary instrument used by the tattoo artist is satisfactory but makes the procedure extremely tedious and time-consuming. To overcome these objections I have devised a reciprocating (2,000 strokes per minute), pneumatic tattooing pistol utilizing 20 needles in a single row with an adjustable mechanism so that the needles have the necessary protruding travel which varies from 2 to 4 mm. (Fig. 11). With this instrument I am able to do the tattooing for the average case in one sitting in about one hour.

Since the introduction of this instrument the incidence of incomplete tattooing or skipped areas (where localized pruritus may persist and which has erroneously been regarded as a recurrence) has been greatly diminished. Recently I

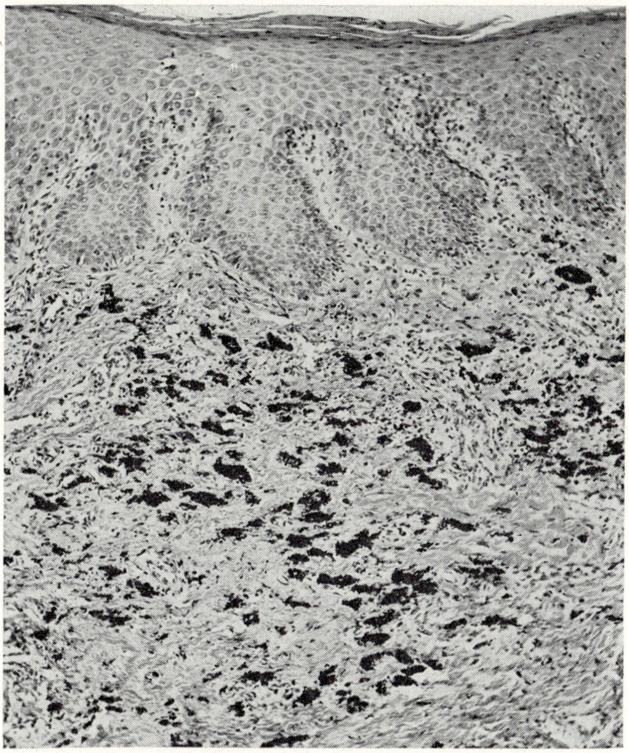

Fig. 8.—Photomicrograph of skin obtained thirty-six months after tattooing shows a histologic picture similar to that observed in Figs. 6 and 7. Again note the absence of a foreign body gaint-cell reaction.

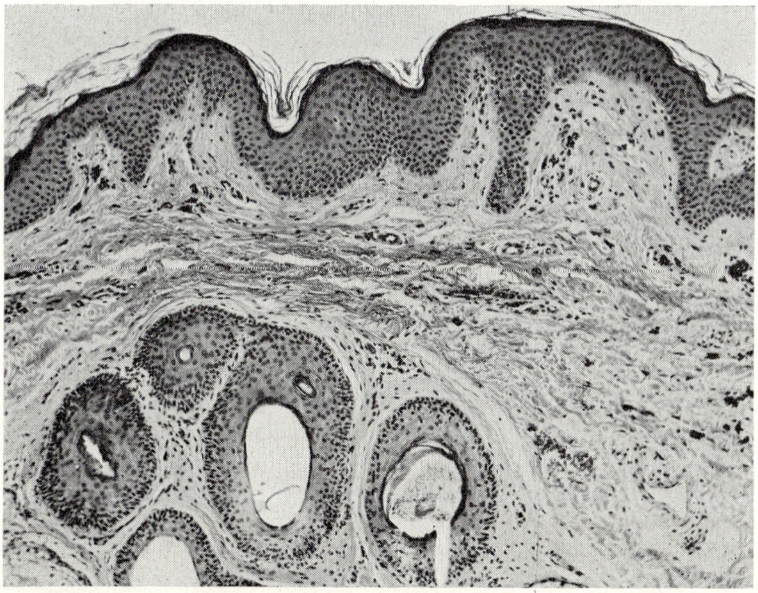

Fig. 9.—Photomicrograph showing a skipped cutaneous area with no or very scant subepithelial deposit of mercury sulfide (see Fig. L.)

have been experimenting with a new effective electric tattooing instrument (Vibro-tool,* Fig. 12). (This instrument is also suitable for tattooing of grafted skin and other phases of plastic surgery.) Following the completion of tattooing, petrolatum gauze is applied. To reduce post-tattoo edema, moist compresses are utilized. Tenderness and moderate pain may persist for about ten to fourteen days and are relieved by moist compresses or sedatives. Desquamation of the tattooed epithelium occurs within a few days after tattooing and re-epithelization ensues in a few weeks.

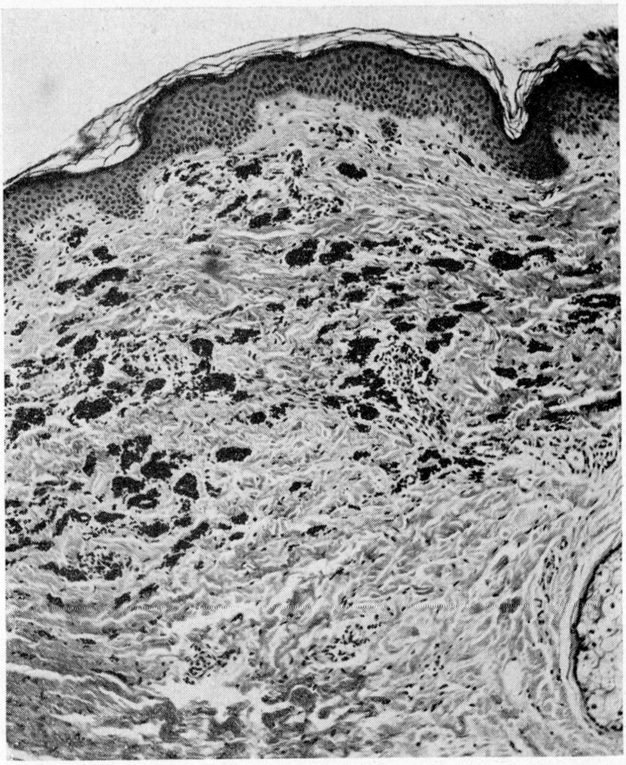

Fig. 10.—Photomicrograph of an adequately tattooed area of skin of the same patient, showing, in contrast, a uniform and abundant subepithelial deposit of mercury sulfide (see Fig. L).

RECURRENCE

Recurrences of anal pruritus in the patient who was considered ideal for this form of therapy have usually been due to inadequate or incomplete tattooing (skipped areas) as shown by gross and histologic studies.[8] This recurrent pruritus promptly disappears following retattooing. Occasionally a pseudo-recurrence may be produced by superficial anal or perineal fissures or suppuration of an anal crypt.

PHYSIOLOGIC PATHOLOGY

The rationale of the tattooing procedure is still undetermined. Personal studies[4] on the mechanism of the action of mercury sulfide deposited in the

*Manufactured by Burgess Battery Co., Chicago, Ill.

corium by tattooing suggest that a functional impairment of the cutaneous sensory terminals is produced which reduces their capacity to respond to adequate stimuli. A change in the cutaneous modalities is produced which apparently is proportional to the quantitative intracutaneous deposit of mercury sulfide.[8] Improvement of the blood supply of the tattooed skin may also play a beneficial role.[9]

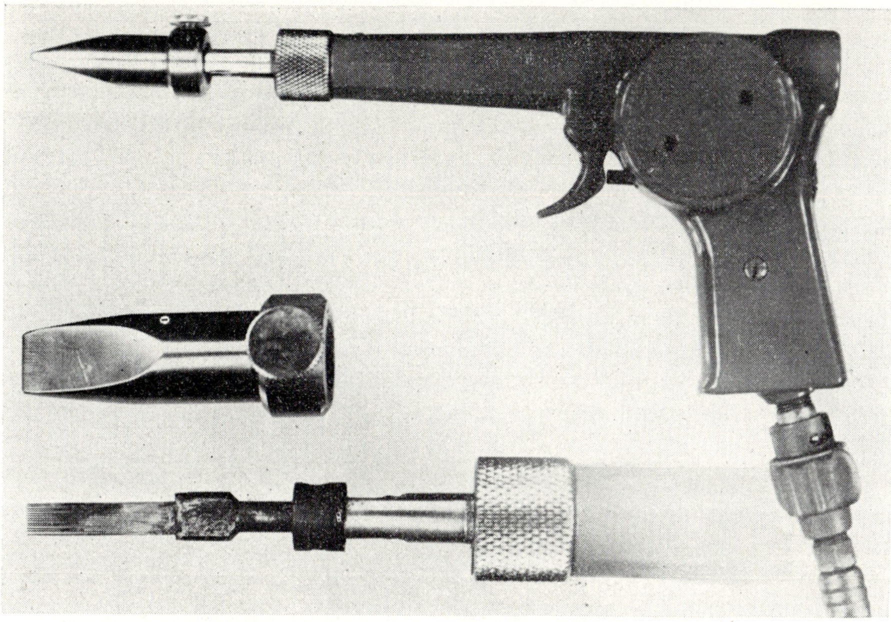

Fig. 11.—Newly developed pneumatic tattooing pistol, assembled and disassembled.

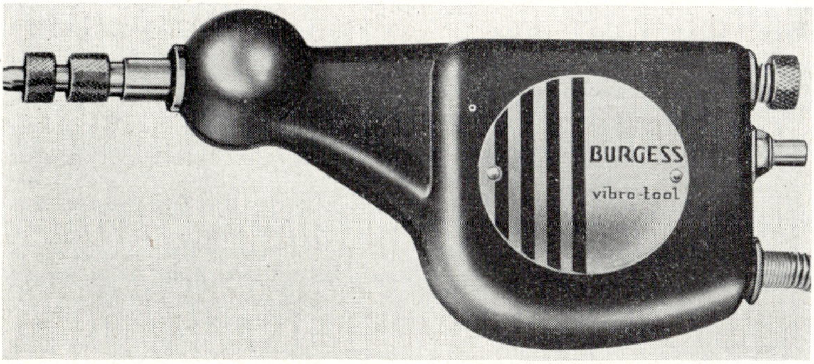

Fig. 12.—The electric Vibro-tool (Burgess) is suitable for tattooing by the addition of a needle holder and an adjusting mechanism as shown in Fig. 11. An even better electric tattooing machine is now in the process of development (Golz).

Mechanical trauma alone as produced by the tattooing instrument without the deposition of mercury sulfide or other chemicals is ineffective in relieving anal pruritus.[4]

Histologic studies of specimens of tattooed skin removed at the conclusion of the tattooing and subsequently at three-month intervals for a period of over three years have shown no evidence of irritation or of a foreign body giant-cell reaction in the skin similar to that observed after the intracutaneous introduction of other foreign substances. Massive deposition in the epidermis and upper corium is seen immediately after tattooing. Subsequently the mercury sulfide is localized in the corium in various sized clumps which have a slight but definite tendency to reach the deeper portion of the corium (Figs. 5, 6, 7, and 8).[8]

SUMMARY AND CONCLUSIONS

Fifty-five of a group of seventy patients who had had chronic and recalcitrant anal pruritus that was associated with definite characteristic cutaneous changes have responded well to tattooing with mercury sulfide; the remaining fifteen patients obtained "satisfactory" results. Confirmation of this has been obtained in the treatment of vulval pruritus with cutaneous changes. Of twenty-three patients with similar complaints but who had no cutaneous changes consistent with chronic anal pruritus, only six obtained "satisfactory" results while seventeen showed no improvement. This too finds confirmation in the unsuccessful treatment by tattooing with mercury sulfide of vulval pruritus without cutaneous changes.

It appears that tattooing with mercury sulfide is an effective form of treatment for intractable anal pruritus which is associated with definite characteristic cutaneous changes in the absence of anorectocolonic lesions. The patient who complains of severe anal pruritus but who has no cutaneous changes consistent with localized pruritus is, in the majority of cases, an unfavorable candidate for this form of therapy. However, since no deleterious effects have, to date, been observed following tattooing with mercury sulfide this form of therapy may be given a trial in all cases of localized pruritus when more radical procedures, such as the subcutaneous injection of ethyl alcohol or the radical excision of perianal or vulval skin, are contemplated.

Acknowledgment is made of the cooperation of Dr. William Leifer in the dermatologic appraisal of many of these patients.

REFERENCES

1. Hollander, E.: Treatment of Pruritus Ani by Tattoo With Mercuric Sulfide, Arch. Dermat. & Syph. **38**: 337-339, 1938.
2. Turell, R.: Pruritus Ani With Special Reference to Therapeutic Tattooing With Mercury Sulfide, New York State J. Med. 42: 1335-1340, 1942.
3. Turell, R.: Tattooing With Mercury Sulfide for Intractable Anogenital Pruritus, With Special Reference to Leukoplakia—Kraurosis, J. Mt. Sinai Hosp. **9**: 147-153, 1942.
4. Turell, R.: Tattooing (Puncturation) With Mercury Sulfide and Other Chemicals for Treatment of Pruritus Ani and Perinei; Further Investigations, J. Invest. Dermat. **3**: 289-297, 1940.
5. Brust, J. C. M.: In discussion of Turell.[2]
6. Young, F., and Scott, W. J. M.: Radical Operation for Intractable Pruritus Ani, SURGERY **13**: 911-915, 1943.
7. Turell, R., and Marino, A. W. M.: Technic of Tattooing With Mercury Sulfide for Pruritus Ani, Ann. Surg. **115**: 126-130, 1942.
8. Turell, R.: Tattooing With Mercuric Sulfide for Treatment of Intractable Pruritus Vulvae and Ani: Anatomical Study, Am. J. Obst. & Gynec. **42**: 290-296, 1941.
9. Ewing, James: Personal Communication.

CEREBRAL HEMORRHAGE FOLLOWING REPAIR OF A COMMON CAROTID-INTERNAL JUGULAR ARTERIOVENOUS FISTULA

A. O. Singleton, M.D., and A. O. Singleton, Jr., M.D., Galveston, Texas

A REVIEW of the literature, in 1939, by Quattlebaum revealed forty-six cases of common carotid-internal jugular fistulas. When the figures on arterial injuries of World War II are published this number will be greatly augmented. We have been able to find published reports of eighteen other more recent cases, although there are undoubtedly many more we have failed to find. (We have also found reports of some seventeen internal carotid-internal jugular arteriovenous fistulas.)

Quadruple ligation has been the general method of attack in these lesions but more recently there has been an increasing effort to restore the continuity of the artery despite the greater technical difficulties, in an endeavor to prevent cerebral anemia which so frequently occurs following ligation.

Interruption of the common, and especially of the internal carotid has long been known to be hazardous. In Zimmerman's series of 70 ligations of the common carotid there were 26 per cent with cerebral symptoms; in Pitz' series of 600 cases there were 32 per cent.[10] It is generally believed that in older people the danger from this procedure is greater, although Reid and others contended that it is equally dangerous in the young. (We have had the experience of a hemiplegia in a boy 9 years of age following common carotid ligation.)

In fifty cases of common carotid-internal jugular fistula found in the literature there were thirty-three cases where the arterial flow was interrupted by ligation of the artery and vein and seventeen cases in which the artery was restored. In the latter there was a cure of the lesion with no complications except in one patient who died of pneumonia on the eleventh postoperative day. Seven of the successful cases were patients over 40 years of age. Two had evidence of peripheral vessel damage, and two had positive serology. Six had evidence of cardiac damage. Three had evidence of cerebral anemia before operation, including one case of eleven months' duration. The duration of the lesions ranged from ten hours to thirty-seven years. The methods of repair included ligation of the fistula and suture of the opening in the artery from the outside. In most cases the vein was not restored.

In the cases where the artery was not restored but ligated there were two deaths and three recurrences. (In these cases only the artery was ligated.) There was also one death six days postoperative from coronary occlusion. One of the deaths occurred in a 20-year-old individual only eight days after the appearance of the fistula. The other was of eighth months' duration in a 59-year-old person. Both deaths resulted from cerebral anemia. The other patients were cured. They were mainly young individuals, although there were patients 37 and 45 years of age. Most of these were of at least several months' duration. One case showed evidence of cardiac decompensation. One boy of

Received for publication, April 17, 1947.

19 years had a quadruple ligation of the artery and vein only nine days after the appearance of the fistula but he had several frontal headaches for ten days postoperatively. There was one case of hemiplegia in an early ligation of the carotid.

Quadruple ligation was the usual procedure in this series. Although there was a high incidence of success in these cases where the arterial flow was interrupted, most of them had been cases which had responded well to testing before operation by occlusion of the involved vessels by pressure or had compressive exercises before ligation was attempted. One patient with quadruple ligation complained of headaches postoperatively.

TABLE I. COMMON CAROTID-INTERNAL JUGULAR ARTERIOVENOUS FISTULAS—RESTORATION OF ARTERIAL FLOW

LOCATION	REF. NO.	AGE (YR.)	DURATION	TYPE OF REPAIR	RESULTS	REMARKS
1. Rt.	2	N. S.	30 days	Lig. of fistula	Cure	Had cerebral symptoms before op.; no evidence of cardiac involvement
2. Lt.	2	N. S.	3 mo.	Lig. of fistula and vein	Cure	No cardiac involvement
3.	2	N. S.	N. S.	Transvenous suture of arterial opening of fistula; lig. of vein	Died of pneumonia 11th day	Sensory aphasia before op.
4. Lt.	2	58	11 mo.	Lig. of fistula and vein	Cure; palpable temporal artery	Cerebral symptoms preop.; cardiac enlargement
5.	3	58	23 mo.	Restoration of artery	Cure; artery patent after 10½ yr.	
6.	3	55	37 yr.	Vein lig. proximal and distal; transvenous suture of artery	Cure for 2 yr. then arterial aneurysm developed	Short of breath and vessels calcified (before op.)
7.	2	25	1 mo.	Lig. vein transvenous suture of artery	Cure	
8. Rt.	14	46	30 yr.	Lig. of fistula	Cure	Preop. cardiac enlargement
9. Rt.	14	21	6 yr.	Lig. of fistula	Cure	Preop. cardiac enlargement
10. Lt.	7	28	22 days	Restoration of artery and vein	Cure	No cardiac envolvement
11. Rt.	7	40	2 mo.	Restoration of artery and vein	Cure	Slight cardiac enlargement; neg. B. W.
12. Rt.	7	41	30 days	Restoration of artery and vein	Cure	Pos., B. W., preop. cardiac enlargement
13. Rt.	16	33	1½ mo.	Restoration of artery and vein	Good pulse in artery	No cardiac involvement; syphilis
14.	8		N. S.	Lig. of vein; suture of fistula	Cure	Damage peripheral vessels
15. Rt.	9	23	5½ mo.	Lig. of vein; suture of fistula	Cure; good temporal pulse	
16. Rt.	9	24	4 mo.	Lig. of vein; suture of fistula	Cure; good temporal pulse	Fistula 1 cm. in diameter
17. Rt.	9	19	7 mo.	Lig. of vein; suture of fistula	Cure; good temporal pulse	Fistula 1 cm. in diameter

TABLE II. COMMON CAROTID-INTERNAL JUGULAR ARTERIOVENOUS FISTULAS—INTERRUPTION OF ARTERIAL FLOW

LOCATION		REF. NO.	AGE (YR.)	DURATION	TYPE OF REPAIR	RESULT	REMARKS
1.	Rt.	4	59	8 mo.	Lig. of artery	Death	Shortness of breath before op.
2.	Lt.	4	20	8 days	Lig. of artery	Hemiplegia and death	Shortness of breath before op.
3.		4	30	N.S.	Erosion of aneurysm	Cure	
4.	Lt.	4	25	1 yr., 8 mo.	Lig. of artery	Recurrence	
5.	Rt.	4	16	3½ mo.	Quad. lig. of artery and vein	Cure	
6.		4	N.S.	N.S.	Quad. lig. of artery and vein	Cure	
7.	Rt.	4	25	N.S.	Excision of aneurysm	Cure	
8.		4	N.S.	N.S.	Lig. of artery above and below fistula	Cure	
9.	Lt.	4	22	N.S.	Lig. of artery above and below fistula	Failure; aneurysm still present	
10.	Lt.	4	37	7 yr.	Quad. lig. of artery and vein	Cure	
11.		4	45	N.S.	Lig. of artery distal to fistula	Cure	
12.		4	N.S.	N.S.	Lig. of artery distal to fistula	Recurred	
13.		4	29	N.S.	Partial excision of aneurysm	Cure	
14.	Rt.	4	N.S.	N.S.	Excision of anuerysm	Cure	
15.		4	N.S.	N.S.	Excision of anuerysm	Cure	
16.	Lt.	4	25	N.S.	Quad. lig. of artery and vein	Cure	
17.	Lt.	4	N.S.	2 mo.	Excision of aneurysm	Cure	
18.	Lt.	4	21	1 mo.	Partial lig. of artery; suture of opening in sac	Cure	
19.	Lt.	4	25	2 days	Lig. of common, external and internal carotid	N.S., presume cure	
20.		2	N.S.	N.S.	Quad. lig. of artery and vein	Cured	Headaches pre-op.
21.	NS	3	10	14 mo.	Occlusion of common carotid distal to lesion with fascia; lig. of vein proximal and distal	Cured; observed 3 yr. and 8 mo. postoperatively	
22.	Lt.	10	22	1½ yr.	Quad. lig. of artery and vein	Cure; no cerebral symptoms	Preop. shortness of breath
23.	Lt.	18 (7 cases)	young	N.S.	Main. quad. lig. of artery and vein	Cure	
24.	Rt.	1	19	9 days	Quad. lig. of artery and vein		
25.		15	N.S.	3 mo.	Excision of aneurysm	Cure	Compression exercises
26.	Lt.	12	40	15 yr.	1st stage clearance of veins and applications of bands on vein and artery; 2nd stage transvenous suture of arterial opening	Improved Died 6 days later of coronary occlusion	Cardiac enlargement; syphilis

TABLE III. ARTERIOVENOUS FISTULA BETWEEN INTERNAL CAROTID AND INTERNAL JUGULAR VEIN—INTERRUPTION OF ARTERIAL FLOW

LOCATION	REF. NO.	AGE (YR.)	DURATION	TYPE OF REPAIR	RESULTS	REMARKS
51. Lt.	4	25	3 mo.	Lig. of external carotid, internal carotid, and internal jugular	Cure	
52.	4	21	N.S.	Quad. lig. of artery and vein	Cure	
53. Rt.	4	28	N.S.	Lig. of internal carotid	Improved	
54. Lt.	4	27	N.S.	Quad. lig.	Cure	Weakness in right side
55. Rt.	4	N.S.	N.S.	Lig. of external, internal, and common carotid and internal jugular vein	Cure	
56. Rt.	4	29	8 mo.	Lig. of internal and common carotid and internal jugular vein.	Cure	
57. Lt.	4	N.S.	1½ mo.	Lig. common carotid	Cure	
58. Rt.	18	Young	N.S.	Quad. lig.		

In the repair of carotid-jugular arteriovenous fistula certain complications have been noted. As has been mentioned when the artery has been ligated, cerebral anemia with hemiplegia and death may occur. When the artery is restored, bleeding at the suture line or thrombosis of the vessel may result. We wish to report a case illustrating a complication of arterial restoration which we hitherto have not seen reported in the literature, a case of cerebral hemorrhage following repair of the artery.

TABLE IV. ARTERIOVENOUS FISTULA BETWEEN INTERNAL CAROTID AND INTERNAL JUGULAR VEIN—RESTORATION OF ARTERIAL FLOW

LOCATION	REF. NO.	AGE (YR.)	DURATION	TYPE OF REPAIR	RESULTS	REMARKS
61.	12	Young	N.S.	Transvenous repair of artery; lig. of vein	Cure	
62.	17	53 yr.	3 mo.	Occlusion of fistula tract	Cure	Minimal evidence of cardiac damage

REPORT OF CASE

C. B. B., a 49-year-old white man, a stock farmer, was admitted to the John Sealy Hospital on July 16, 1946, with the chief complaint of a "thumping" in the neck. When he was 12 years old he had fallen and struck the neck on a rock; since that time he had been conscious of a "whirling" sound in the head. It seemed to be accentuated by exercise or excitement. About three years before admission a swelling appeared in the left side of the neck. Beginning three months before, the patient noticed increasing shortness of

TABLE V

	NUMBER OF CASES	RESTORATION OF ARTERIAL FLOW	RESULTS	INTERRUPTION OF ARTERIAL FLOW	RESULTS
Common carotid-internal jugular	50	17	Cure in all cases except 1 death from pneumonia on 11th P.O. day	33	2 deaths hemiplegia; 3 recurrences; 1 death from coronary occlusion
Common carotid-internal jugular	13	2	All cured	11	All cured

breath on exertion, after meals, and on awakening from exciting dreams at night. There was palpitation of the heart at times and a mild cough. In recent weeks he had noticed some swelling of the ankles during the day. History was otherwise noncontributory.

Physical examination revealed a large man, 6 feet 2 inches tall, weighing 162 pounds. There was a fullness of the neck extending from the clavicle to the angle of the jaw. About two inches above the clavicle in line with the great vessels of the neck there was a small indefinite pulsating tumor. A palpable thrill accentuated during systole was noted over the area. On ausculation a harsh continuous murmur with a louder systolic element could be heard. This was transmitted up into the neck and down into the chest, the greater volume being found in the latter. On reclining, the veins of the neck and forehead were quite distended but this was not seen in the erect position. The retinal veins as seen by the ophthalmoscope were thought to be distended. The patient exhibited a Corrigan type of pulse with a rate of 81. Blood pressure was 140/68. Respirations were about 20. The heart appeared to be enlarged by percussion; the apical beat was noted in the sixth left interspace at the midclavicular line. There was a positive Duroziez' sign. There was an aortic diastolic and systolic murmur. The liver was slightly enlarged. Blood pressure changes were still present. Fluoroscopic examination showed a slowing of the heart with increased dilatation on pressure over the fistula. Venous pressure in the left arm was 18.75 cm. of saline solution and 16.25 cm. in the right arm. Vital capacity was 2,750 c.c.

Roentgenograms of the chest for cardiac size showed an enormous enlargement of the cardiac silhouette. The transverse diameter of the heart was 20 cm. as compared to the transverse thoracic diameter of 31 cm. The heart was globular in shape and dilated in all diameters. The lung fields showed marked increase in the vascular markings and pulmonary artery trunks compatible with left-sided heart failure. Skull films were normal except for a suggestion of some decalcification of the dorsum sellae. Electrocardiograms showed evidence of definite myocardial damage.

Laboratory studies showed a negative blood Wassermann test. Urinalysis revealed specific gravity 1,024, acid reaction, protein 1 plus, sugar negative. Microscopic examination showed 10 white blood cells per high power field and rare hyaline cast. Hematology revealed red blood cells, 5,040,000; hemoglobin, 13.9 Gm., or 90 per cent leucocytes per cubic millimeter. Polymorphonuclear leucocytes, segmenters 58 per cent, stags 3 per cent, lymphocytes 30 per cent, monocytes 7 per cent, and eosinophiles 2 per cent.

A diagnosis of arteriovenous fistula between the left common carotid and internal jugular was made. Aug 14, 1946, the patient was operated upon. Before going to the operating room he got up, shaved himself, and said he was feeling fine. He talked very intelligently and rationally in the operating room and moved himself from the stretcher carriage onto the operating table. He was given a local infiltration anesthetic of ¼ per cent procaine with epinephrine. A vertical incision was made along the anterior border of the left sternomastoid, and an arteriovenous fistula between the second portion of the left common carotid and the internal jugular vein was easily exposed. The veins of the neck were greatly distended and the jugular sacculated at the level of the fistula. The artery had been cut transversely through one-half of its width at the original injury. The opening into the sacculation was large. The jugular vein was ligated proximally and distally to the fistula with plain catgut and the carotid artery was temporarily occluded with rubber-shod bulldog clamps. When the artery was freed, the patient complained of pain and was very apprehensive. He was given cyclopropane and oxygen. The vein was then opened and a fresh blood clot removed from the sac. The fistulous opening was then closed through the vein opening. The borders of the arterial opening were brought together from above downward in an end-to-end manner using interrupted fine chromic catgut sutures. The sac was trimmed off close to the first row of sutures, and a second layer of similar sutures was placed in the area. A segment of vein was then closed over this. The clamps were removed and a pulse was immediately felt in the carotid distal to the fistula and in the corresponding temporal artery. The patient did not require any anesthetic for the last thirty-five minutes of the operation and was thought to be in good condition at the end of the procedure. He was returned to the ward at 10:30 A.M. About 3:00 P.M. the patient was seen in the ward by one of us and was

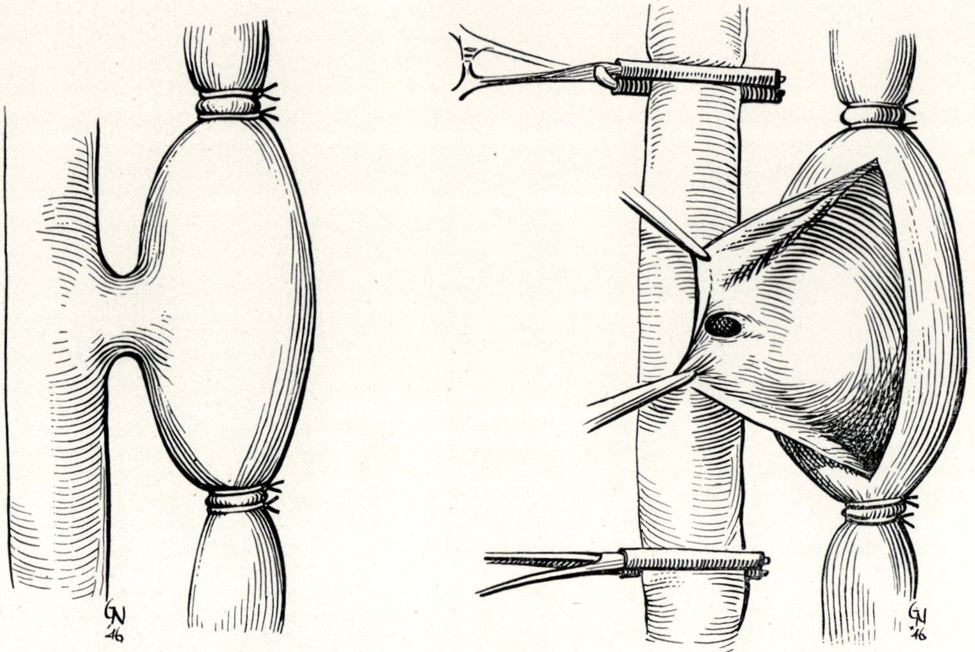

Fig. 1.—Illustrating arteriovenous fistula between carotid artery and jugular vein.

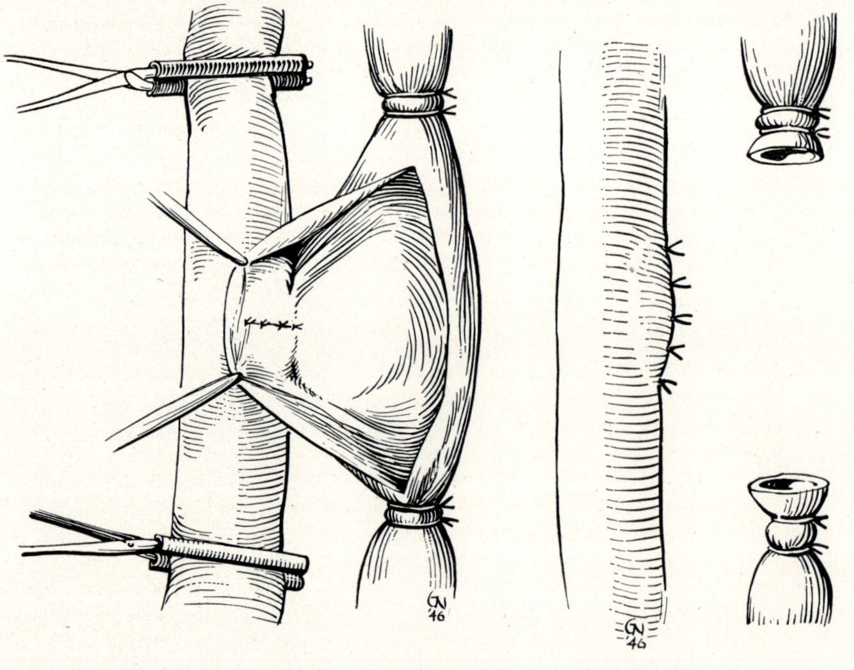

Fig. 2.—Illustrating repair with reconstruction of the artery.

found still sleeping soundly. Blood pressure, pulse, and respirations were normal. All attempts to arouse him were futile. Reflexes were normal but the muscles flaccid. It was felt that he had had a cerebrovascular accident. Thirty cubic centimeters of heparin in 1000 c.c. of 5 per cent glucose was started but within thirty minutes and before 100 c.c. of this solution had been given the respirations ceased and all attempts to resuscitate him failed. He was pronounced dead at 4:45 P.M. and it was felt that a thrombus was the most likely cause of this situation.

Autopsy Findings.—At autopsy it was found that the arterial repair in the neck was intact without thrombosis and that the patient had had a hemorrhage from the left ventriculostriate artery with a large intracerebral blood clot, 6 cm. in diameter in the left temporoparietal region with fresh clots in the entire ventricular system and subarachnoid space, and that the cause of death was evidently the cerebrovascular hemorrhage. On examination of the brain it was found that it weighed 1,520 Gm. The heart weighed 550 Gm. and showed marked hypertrophy and dilatation.

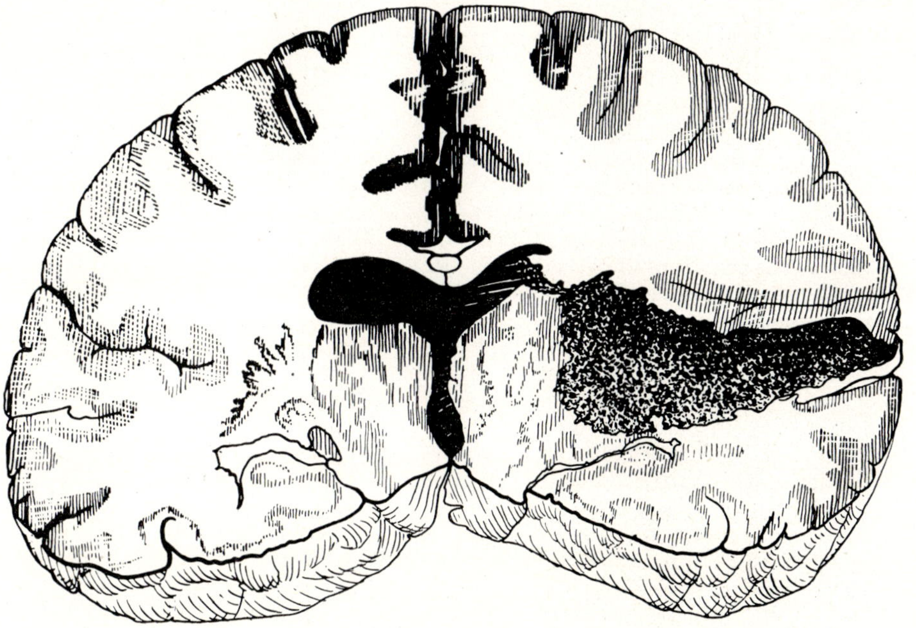

Fig. 3.—Drawing of cross section of the brain showing intracranial hemorrhage which immediately followed reconstruction of the carotid artery.

DISCUSSION

This case showed the classical picture of arteriovenous fistula with the typical thrill and murmer, the slowing of the pulse on occluding the fistula, and the cardiac decompensation that comes on as the lesion persists over a period of time.[11] The points made by Holman recently in regard to the physiologic changes involved in closing the fistula were well illustrated here. When the increased blood volume which was formed to compensate for the leak of the arterial blood through the fistula was suddenly all forced into the arterial system by the closure of the shunt, the blood pressure rose with dilatation of the heart and aortic arch as was observed fluoroscopically. This acting on the end organs of the depressor nerve caused a reflex slowing of the heart with a reduction in blood pressure.

The administration of atrophine by blocking the vagus pathway abolished the slowing of the pulse usually resulting from occulusion of the fistula and the blood pressure did not fall. It was of interest to note here that pressure over the fistula caused the patient to have a headache. This represented an occlusion of the carotid artery rather than the fistula alone. There was no evidence of arteriosclerosis in this patient. The blood Wassermann was negative.

We have assumed that a blood vessel which was formerly carrying a smaller blood volume under a lower pressure was unable to stand the increased load upon it with restoring the carotid artery, resulting in the rupture of the artery in the brain. We were unable to demonstrate any pathology in the artery itself which would predispose to the fatal hemorrhage.

In our zeal to prevent anemia of the brain we restored the artery rather than occluding it by ligation. The procedure was correctly carried out but the fatal outcome was the opposite to what was anticipated.

COMMENT

(Personal communication from Dr. Rudolph Matas)

Your case of arteriovenous aneurysm is indeed very interesting, rare and possibly unique in the literature, at least in the way it terminated. It is possible that other cases of apoplexy following extirpation of the fistula or quadruple ligature may have been recorded in which death was attributed to cerebral ischemia from insufficiency of the Circle of Willis, as is common enough in dealing with pure arterial aneurysms.

But that death should follow the restoration of the cerebral circulation by conservative repair of the artery must indeed be rare, since the cure of an arteriovenous fistula by the transvenous route, or any other procedure that closed the fistula without obliterating the artery, is too new and relatively rare a procedure to have furnished many examples of this unfortunate accident.

I believe your explanation of the hemorrhage is correct. The only question is regarding a predisposing cause. Was there a miliary aneurysm of the Circle of Willis or any other evidence of arterial disease in the finer arteries of the apoplectic zone of Charcot and Bouchard?

If the ruptured artery and its branches have been preserved for careful histologic changes it is more than probable that a weak spot of atheroma or arterial degeneration is found to be responsible for the hemorrhage. Your case is another example of the fact that the cure of an aneurysm sometimes kills the patient, as happens when an aneurysm of the caeliac axis of the aorta is spontaneously obliterated by coagulation, owing to the necrosis of the liver and duodenum by ischemia; likewise, when an aortic aneurysm is obliterated at the renal origin.

REFERENCES

1. Albright, H. L., and Van Hale, L. A.: Traumatic Aneurysms, SURGERY 20: 452, 1946.
2. Bigger, I. A., and Lippert, K. M.: Arteriovenous Fistula Involving the Common Carotid and Internal Jugular Vein, SURGERY 2: 555, 1937.
3. Bigger, I. A.: Treatment of Traumatic Aneurysms and Arteriovenous Fistulas, Arch. Surg. 49: 170, 1944.
4. Callander, C. L.: Study of Arteriovenous Fistulae, Bull. Johns Hopkins Hosp. 19: 259, 1920.
5. Callander, C. L.: Study of Arteriovenous Fistula With an Analysis of 447, Cases, Ann. Surg. 71: 428, 1920.

6. Conway, H., and Plain, G.: Pulsating Hematoma, False Aneurysm, and Arteriovenous Fistula Due to War Injuries, SURGERY **19**: 383, 1946.
7. Elkin, D. C., and Campbell, J. L.: Aneurysm, Am. J. Surg. **24**: 611, 1934.
8. Elkin, D. C.: Vascular Injuries of Warfare, Ann. Surg. **120**: 284, 1944.
9. Freeman, N. E.: Arterial Repair in the Treatment of Aneurysms and Arteriovenous Fistulae, Ann. Surg. **124**: 888, 1946.
10. Holman, E.: Arteriovenous Aneurysm, New York, 1937, The Macmillan Company.
11. Holman, E.: Roentgenologic Kymographic Studies of the Heart in the Presence of Arteriovenous Fistula and Their Interpretation, Ann. Surg. **124**: 920, 1946.
12. Matas, R.: Some Experiences and Observations in the Treatment of Arteriovenous Aneurisms by the Intrasaccular Method of Suture With Special Reference to Transvenous Route, Ann. Surg. **71**: 403, 1920.
13. Mustard, W. T.: The Technique of Immediate Restoration of Vascular Continuity After Arterial Wounds, Ann. Surg. **124**: 46, 1946.
14. Pemberton, J. deJ.: Arteriovenous Aneurysm, Arch. Surg. **16**: 469, 1928.
15. Preston, A. P.: Arterial Injuries of Warfare, SURGERY **20**: 786, 1946.
16. Quattlebaum, J. K.: Carotid-Jugular Arteriovenous Aneurysm, J. M. A. Georgia **28**: 433, 1939.
17. Reid, M. R., and McGuire, J.: Arteriovenous Aneurysms, Ann. Surg. **108**: 643, 1938.
18. Shumacker, H. B., Jr., and Carter, K. L.: Arteriovenous Fistulas and Arterial Aneurysms in Military Personnel, SURGERY **20**: 9, 1946.
19. Matas, R.: Personal Communication, Feb. 14, 1947.

LOBECTOMY FOR PULMONARY CYSTS IN A FIFTEEN-DAY-OLD INFANT WITH RECOVERY

W. Emory Burnett, M.D., and H. Taylor Caswell, M.D., Philadelphia, Pa.
(From Temple University Medical School)

PRIOR to December, 1946, the youngest patients with pulmonary resection were reported by Fischer, Tropea, and Bailey[1] and by Gross.[2] The patient described by Fischer and his associates was 30 days old and the lesion was a large thin-walled pulmonary cyst with bronchiolar mucosa and musculature. The cyst involved the right upper and middle lobes. The follow-up for one year after lobectomy showed normal growth and development with a most satisfactory x-ray appearance of the chest. Gross's recent report was of an infant 23 days old. In this case the congenital cyst involved the upper lobe and extended into the hilar region which necessitated pneumonectomy rather than lobectomy. Follow-up in this case was for six months and the child's progress was excellent.

The case which we are reporting describes a 15-day-old infant with a similar clinical and pathologic picture; this is the youngest patient on record in whom a pulmonary resection was performed. We feel that these cases are of particular interest in that they show the feasibility of major pulmonary surgery in infants suffering with congenital pulmonary air cysts which often indicate a very poor prognosis.

CASE REPORT

Baby U. B. W., female, was born May 4, 1945. She was admitted to Temple University Hospital May 18, 1945, and discharged June 2, 1945.

History.—The chief complaint was of marked dyspnea. The mother stated that the child was apparently normal from birth until five days before admission when dyspnea began and persisted. Four days later this became quite severe, and cyanosis appeared. A physician was consulted who admitted the child to a local hospital. Roentgenograms were made which revealed multiple loculations of air in the left side of the chest which appeared to involve the entire hemithorax and displace the heart and mediastinum markedly to the right. The multiple loculations of the air in the left side of the chest were interpreted as representing stomach and intestinal contents and an area of density in the lower portion of the chest was interpreted as spleen, so that a diagnosis of diaphragmatic hernia was erroneously made. This same evening the patient was transferred to Temple University Hospital.

Physical Examination.—The child was markedly dyspneic and cyanotic, and the respirations were extremely shallow, excessively rapid, and grunting in character. There was retraction of the supraclavicular spaces on inspiration. The left side of the chest was tympanitic with absence of voice and breath sounds. Breath sounds could be heard only in the right axilla and in this region some alveolar râles were also noted on inspiration. The heart was completely displaced into the right side of the chest, and there was a pulse rate of 160 per minute with a suggestion of quadruple rhythm. The abdomen revealed no masses, the liver was normally palpable, and one observer thought that the spleen could be palpated. Peristalsis was present in the abdomen but not in the chest. The umbilicus was recently

Received for publication, March 6, 1947.

healed with no evidence of infection. The extremities were negative, reflexes were normal, and the skin showed a normal turgor. The temperature was normal, and the blood showed 15 Gm. of hemoglobin, 5,300,000 erythrocytes, and 17,800 leucocytes with 70 per cent polymorphonuclears, 47 per cent of which were nonfilamented.

Hospital Course.—The admitting diagnosis of "hernia, diaphragmatic, left, congenital" was accepted on the basis of the symptoms and the x-ray films showing the multiple loculi of air, which were interpreted as intestine, in the left side of the thorax. Because the child's condition had grown rapidly worse in the first few hours after admission and she was unable to take feedings, it was felt there was no time for further study and at 11:00 P.M. on the day of admission, May 18, 1945, laparotomy was performed. Although a thoracic approach was considered, it was discarded in favor of the less shocking left upper rectus approach under local anesthesia with oxygen inhalation. However, at operation it was found that both diaphragms were intact that it was then realized that the pathology was that of a

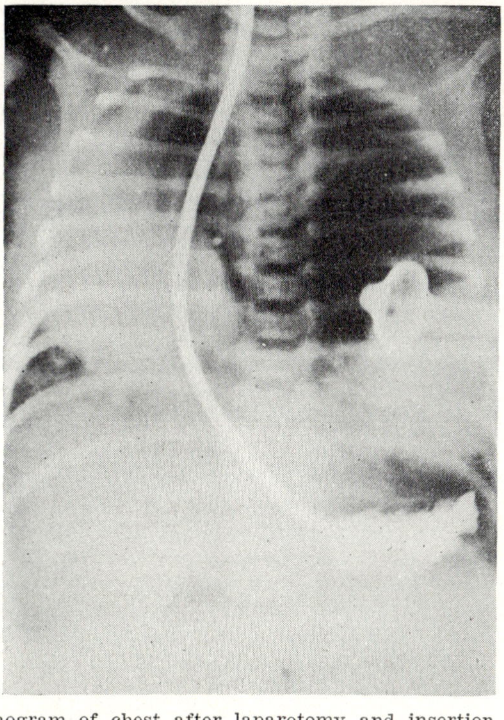

Fig. 1.—Roentgenogram of chest after laparotomy and insertion of mushroom catheter in left side of chest. (Note marked displacement of heart and mediastinal structures and compression of right lung; stomach situated in normal position.)

congenital pulmonary cyst on the left. The abdominal incision was closed. Fearing further major surgery at this time, a needle was inserted into the left side of the chest. Pressure readings varied from plus 5: plus 30 to plus 4: plus 6. After removal of 100 c.c. of gas, there was a temporary decrease in positive pressure and corresponding slight improvement in respiration. In an effort to avoid the return of positive pressure, a stab wound was made deeply into the sixth left interspace and a catheter inserted into the cyst for constant gentle suction. Checking the pressure readings through the catheter revealed the same oscillations as before.

On the following morning, May 19, 1945, there was no appreciable improvement (Fig. 1), and it appeared that the only hope of survival for this infant lay in resection of the involved portion of lung or possibly in the removal of the cyst only, which had been successfully accomplished on several adults previously.

At 2:00 P.M. on this, the day after admission, under field block anesthesia with 1/4 per cent metycaine and positive pressure oxygen by mask, the catheter was removed and an incision was made along the left fifth interspace. The interspace was opened, and the ribs spread with a thyroid retractor. The left upper lobe seemed normal, but the lower lobe was completely diseased, consisting of multiple air cysts in its cephalic half and of firm induration at its base. The lobe was freed from soft adhesions, and dissection was begun on the hilus, but was discontinued because of the patient's poor condition, and a No. 1 chromic ligature was tied about the hilus. Distal to this a transfixion suture of No. 00 chromic catgut was applied, and the lobe was amputated just beyond this point. A flap of pleura was then developed from the posterior chest wall and hinged over the stump. The upper lobe was re-expanded by positive pressure, indicating that the upper lobe bronchus was not obstructed, and 25,000 units of penicillin and a few crystals of sulfanilamide were placed in the pleura. The ribs were approximated with pericostal sutures of No. 1 chromic catgut, each of the two layers of overlying muscle with No. 00 chromic, and the skin and subcutaneous fascia with a continuous lock stitch of No. 35 alloy steel wire. A stab wound was then made in the seventh interspace and a No. 18 French mushroom catheter inserted. By means of positive pressure on the mask and slight suction on the tube, the intrapleural pressure was brought to within normal limits so that there was immediate improvement in the baby's respiratory function. The tube was clamped off and not attached to suction for twenty-four hours to allow the sulfonamides and penicillin to decontaminate the area. There was possible contamination, since one of the thin-walled cysts had ruptured during dissection, and a small amount of mucopurulent material exuded in the field.

Pathology.—Grossly, the apical portion of the lobe appeared to be quite cystic, while in the basilar portion there was considerable induration (Fig. 2). On section it was found that the apical portion contained one large, one medium-sized, and many small air cysts. The indurated basilar portion appeared to be mainly atelectatic with a rather considerable amount of trapped puriform secretions. This material could be expressed from the solid basilar portion into the larger air cysts, indicating their communication. The interior of the cysts showed the fibrillar structure usually visible in pulmonary air cysts.

Pathologic description was as follows: Slides from the consolidated portion of the specimen (Fig. 3, *A*) displayed a maize of channels lined by tall columnar epithelium. Occasionally smaller spaces were found in between which were lined by smaller cuboidal cells. The larger bronchi showed the usual ciliated pseudostratified columnar epithelium. All of the spaces were filled with leucocytes, many undergoing degeneration, giving the exudate a suppurative aspect. Included were many macrophages. Some of these were unusually large, almost giant sized. These were vacuolated, multinucleated, and contained engulfed particles. Inflammatory cells also were found infiltrating the larger bronchial walls, and among these eosinophiles were prominent. There was no fibrosis or any other tissue alteration which would indicate a long-standing process.

Sections of the cystic portion (Fig. 3, *B*) showed a pleura considerably thicker than normal as a result of hemorrhage and edema accompanied by pigment-laden macrophages. The underlying parenchyma contained a slightly greater number of alveoli than seen in the other sections, but dilated bronchioles were still conspicuous. A few macrophages were within the alveolar spaces and bronchial lumens. The inner cyst lining was irregular as a result of papillary projections lined by tall columnar epithelium which were part of bronchioles. The changes observed affecting the bronchial elements were quantitative as well as qualitative. Not only were the bronchioles dilated and filled with exudate, but they exceeded by far the number of alveoli. The paucity of alveoli could not be attributed to obliteration by expanding bronchioles or inflammation since neither atelectasis nor replacement fibrosis were apparent. The bronchiolar increase appeared to be both an absolute and a relative quantity which seemed best explained on a congenital basis. The suppurative exudate was ample proof of an inflammatory reaction. Its nature was nonspecific although the giant cells were unusual and forced the mentioning of the possibility of the so-called "giant-cell pneumonia" seen in infants and thought to be associated with the virus of dis-

Surgery
Vol. 23, No. 1, January, 1948

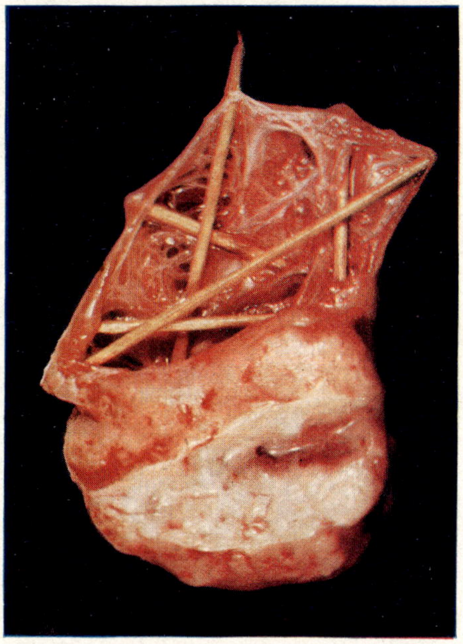

Fig. 2.—Gross specimen, showing the apical cystic portion and also the indurated basilar portion. (Note homogeneous appearance of sectioned basilar portion of this lobe and its resemblance to atelectasis with consolidation.)

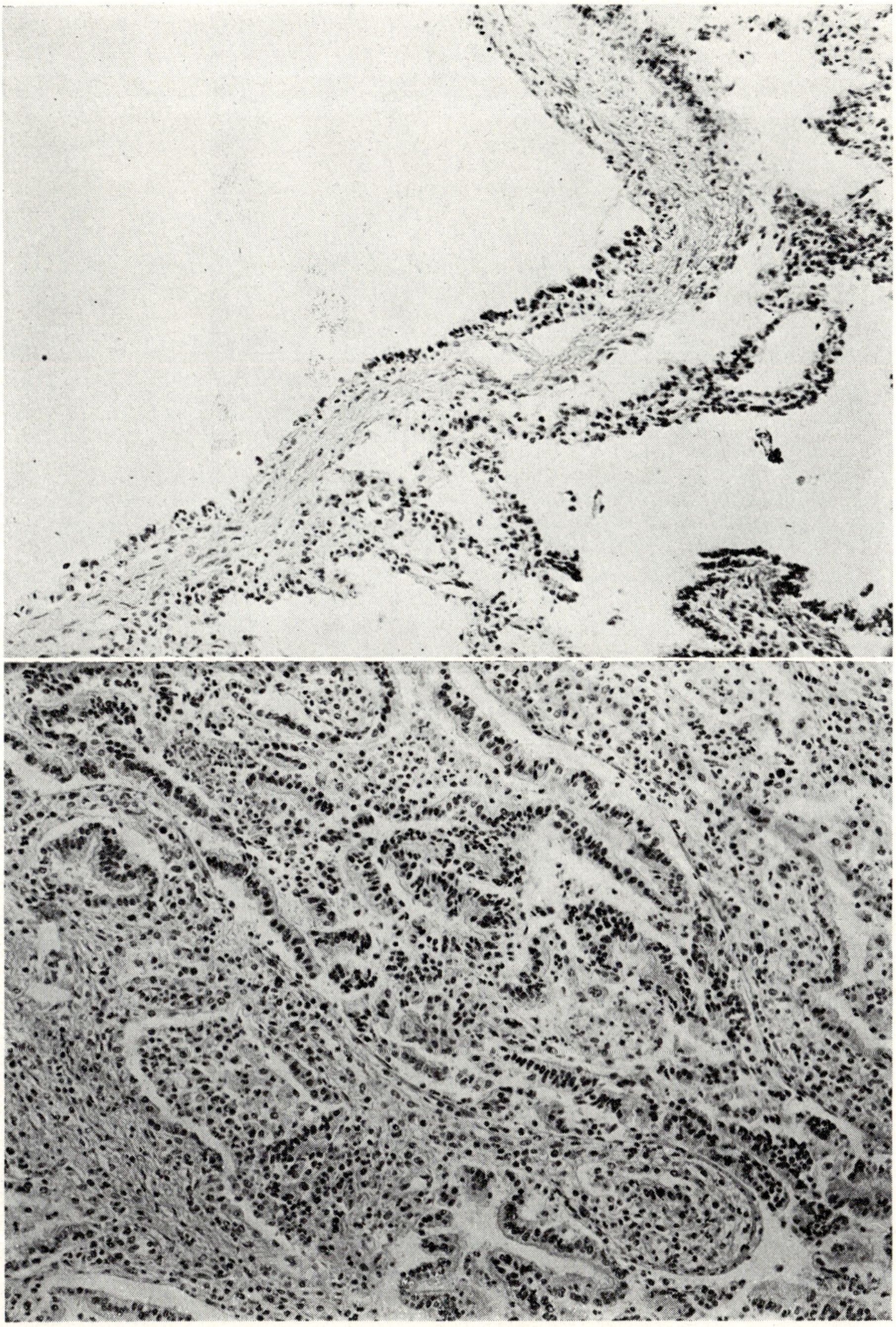

A. B.

Fig. 3.—*A*, Histology of solid portion showing preponderance of bronchial elements with infection causing inflammatory exudate. *B*, Section of cyst wall showing bronchial epithelium lining the cavity.

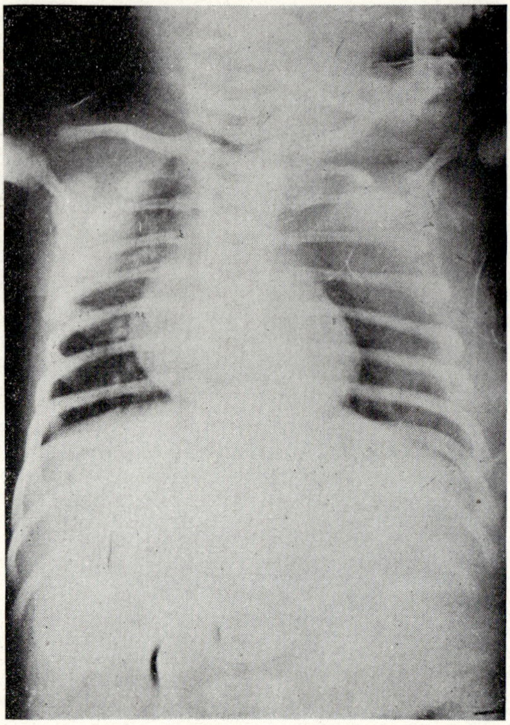

Fig. 4.—Roentgenogram of chest two days postoperatively showing restoration of the mediastinum of the midline and relatively normal expansion of both lung fields.

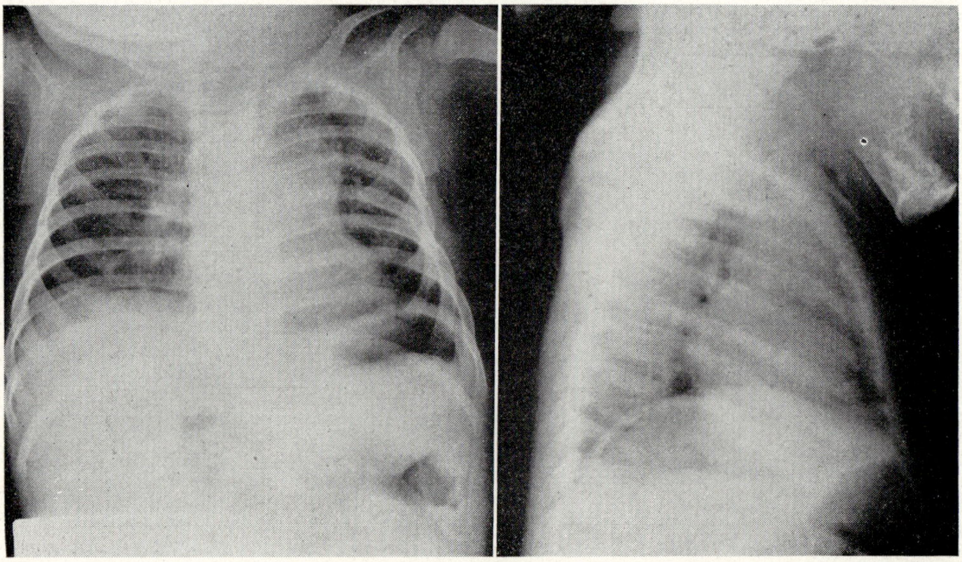

Fig. 5.—Roentgenogram of chest eight months postoperatively showing a normal infant's chest.

temper. Our experience with this particular lesion is admittedly minimal. Breakdown of tissue lipoids can also cause a reaction in which there is the appearance of giant cells.

Obviously the pathogenesis of this lesion was the matter of primary importance and interest. It was felt that there had been abnormal pulmonary parenchymal development, to which had been superimposed a suppurative reaction giving the lesion a dual nature.

Bacteriology.—Cultures from the bronchial stump at the time of operation revealed no growth in five days. Those taken from the puriform material in the congenital cyst were reported as showing an occasional anaerobic *Staphylococcus albus* and a few anaerobic nonhemolytic streptococci.

Postoperative Course.—The postoperative course was most satisfactory. Immediately after operation the patient's condition improved considerably and all dyspnea and cyanosis disappeared within a few hours. On the first two postoperative days the temperature rose to 102.1° F. by rectum from which point it receded gradually until the seventh postoperative day, at which time it became normal and remained so until discharge. The child was given 4,000 units of penicillin intramuscularly at two-hour intervals. Intravenous fluid and blood were continued as indicated through the cannula in the saphenous vein.

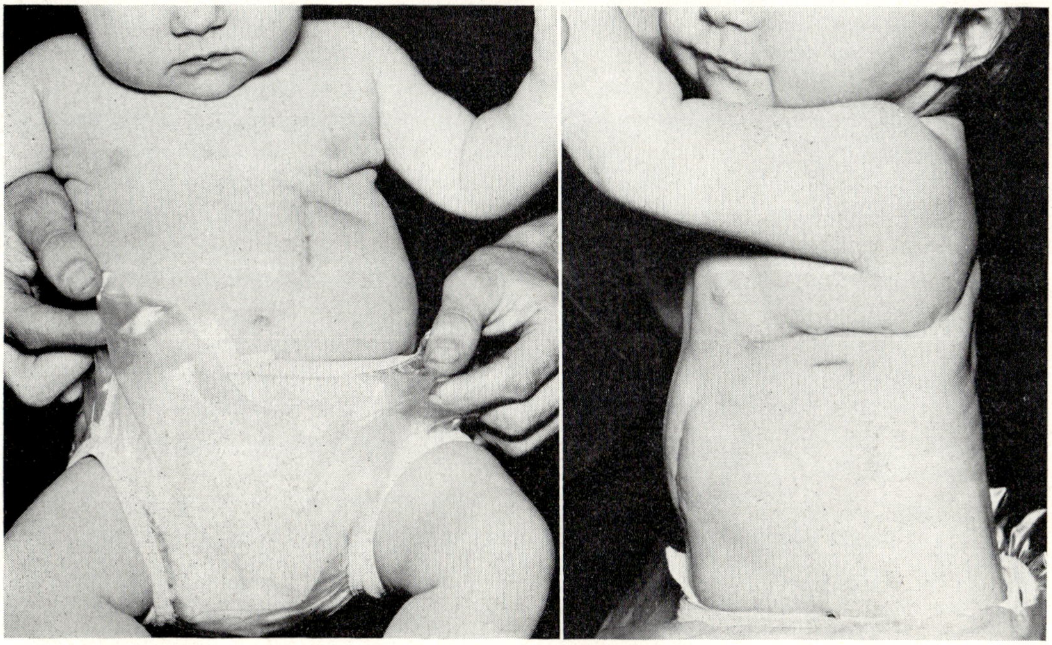

Fig. 6.—Infant six months postoperatively showing normal development.

On the third postoperative day a suppurative thrombophlebitis, involving the area of saphenous canalization, was noted, and culture of this revealed a coagulase positive hemolytic staphylococcus. This responded well to local wet dressings and probably also to the systemic penicillin therapy which was continued for fourteen days postoperatively.

X-ray check-ups, beginning two days following lobectomy (Fig. 4), showed the mediastinal structures to be in the midline, the right lung expanded to normal volume, and aeration of the left upper lobe to be satisfactory. The leaves of the diaphragm moved in phase, and the right was sharply outlined, while that on the left was slightly less sharp and normally situated. The axillary portion of the left side of the chest was obscured by hazy density, representing pleural reaction to the surgical procedure, but by June 1, 1945, the fourteenth postoperative day, the aerated portion of the left lung was more clearly seen, although some pleural thickening was noted about the left base and axillary region with some obscuring of the costophrenic sulcus. However, the aeration of both lungs appeared satisfactory, and the cardiac silhouette remained normally situated.

The child was discharged from the hospital on June 2, 1945, which was the fifteenth postoperative day, in excellent condition. Both the abdominal exploratory wound and the thoracotomy wound had healed by primary intention. There was no dyspnea nor cyanosis, and the baby was gaining weight in a satisfactory fashion on normal feedings.

Re-examination up to and including sixteen months after surgery revealed a child of normal development without respiratory symptoms or loss of energy. The incisions remained well healed, and x-ray check-ups of the chest showed only slight mediastinal displacement to the side operated upon (Fig. 5).

DISCUSSION

The diagnosis of pulmonary air cyst is not difficult if one is suspicious of such a possibility. As pointed out by Anspach and Wolman,[3] the ease of confusion with diaphragmatic hernia or eventration of the diaphragm can be easily overcome by ingestion of small amounts of barium, demonstrating abdominal viscera in their normal or abnormal position (Fig. 1). Single large cysts may be confused with pneumothorax, but the lowered position of the hilus and the persistence, in spite of aspiration, as well as the x-ray and thoracoscopic views of the fibrillar structures inside the cysts, help to differentiate. Multiple cysts may contain fluid or air as described by the previously mentioned authors. This may confuse one with the possibility of infection, and abscess may be thought present. Infection may confuse the picture as in the cases reported by Rosemond and Caswell[4] of pressure pyopneumothorax in the first month of life.

The urgent symptoms and extremely poor condition of some of these infants militate against prolonged study. However, the ingestion of barium is a simple maneuver and was discussed in this case but erroneously omitted. In retrospect, the gastric bubble could easily be seen below the diaphragm of this patient, and very little time would have been consumed in giving a few swallows of barium. We think this error is unjustifiable and should not be repeated. As in some others, this child progressed normally from birth for several days to become increasingly dyspneic. The explanation is probably that the bronchial communication with the cystic areas is oblique or distorted to form a valvular opening which traps increasing amounts of air to balloon the cavity to greater and greater degree, displacing effective parenchyma until pulmonary decompensation occurs. Further evidence for this is found in the positive pressure within the cysts, the temporary improvement from aspiration or drainage, and the disproportion between the size apparent on x-ray views and that of the removed specimen.

The remarkable ease with which lobectomy can be done in infants was noted in this patient and was described by Fischer and his co-workers and by Gross. The hilus forms a small pedicle, as occurs in dogs, making hilar ligation simple and easy and shortening the operation greatly. It has been possible in several of our patients, both adults and children, to excise cysts or large bullae and conserve the remainder of the lung; while in others, particularly with infection, lobectomy has been required.

Field block anesthesia contributes greatly to avoiding shock in these tiny patients and is extremely satisfactory if combined with slight positive pressure oxygen inhalation. We were unwilling to intubate the trachea of this small child but have done so in children of a few months of age.

The pathologic description is interesting in that the indurated basilar portion of the removed lobe, which grossly had appeared to be atelectatic lung, was shown on histologic section to display a maize of channels lined by tall columnar epithelium. These channels were no doubt bronchial in origin and represented a similar histologic but a different morphologic picture than was seen in the larger cystic areas in the upper lobe. The presence of the definite inflammatory change is also of interest and brings up the possibility of pulmonary infection, adding to the already severe situation caused by the marked increase in intrapulmonary pressure.

CONCLUSIONS

1. Pulmonary resection for the treatment of congenital pulmonary air cysts in infants is a feasible and lifesaving procedure.
2. The case of the youngest patient with lobectomy on record is described.

REFERENCES

1. Fischer, C. C., Tropea, F., Jr., and Bailey, C. P.: Congenital Pulmonary Cysts: Report of Infant Treated by Lobectomy With Recovery, J. Pediat. **23**: 219-223, 1943.
2. Gross, R. E.: Congenital Cystic Lung, Ann. Surg. **123**: 229-237, 1946.
3. Anspach, W. E., and Wolman, I. J.: Large Pulmonary Air Cysts of Infancy, Surg. Gynec. & Obst. **56**: 635-645, 1933.
4. Rosemond, G. P., and Caswell, H. T.: Pyopneumothorax in the First Month of Life With Recovery, Am. J. Surg. **68**: 383-387, 1945.

Recent Advances in Surgery

CONDUCTED BY ALFRED BLALOCK, M.D.

THE PROBLEM OF PARENTERAL NITROGEN ADMINISTRATION IN SURGICAL PATIENTS*

WITH SPECIAL CONSIDERATION OF PREOPERATIVE PREPARATION AND OF THE MEANS OF EFFECTING FAVORABLE NITROGEN BALANCE

ARNOLD J. KREMEN, M.D., MINNEAPOLIS, MINN.

(From the Department of Surgery, University of Minnesota Medical School)

INTRODUCTION AND STATEMENT OF THE PROBLEM

THE steady decline of surgical mortality rates concomitant with an ever broadening surgical horizon and a more aggressive surgical attack on well-recognized pathologic states has been one of the outstanding achievements of the past ten years. Many factors each contributing their increment of improvement, have played a part in this accomplishment. Better and safer anesthesia, coupled with judicious and adequate replacement therapy during surgery, has allowed the surgeon to do an unhurried and deliberate operation, leaving nothing to chance. Chemotherapy and antibiotics have been invaluable tools in combating infections. But often the issue is decided before the patient goes to the operating room by the type of preoperative preparation he receives. To this end, a broader understanding, on the part of surgeons, of the general problem of protein metabolism and of the necessity of rebuilding the depleted protein stores of the malnourished patient is of real importance.

It is readily conceded that the oral route when it is available to the patient is to be preferred for this type of preparation. However, in not a small group of patients, particularly those with benign or malignant obstruction of the esophagus or gastric outlet, in chronic or subacute bowel obstructions, in external or internal intestinal fistulas, and in the emaciated state of ulcerative colitis, this avenue of alimentation is not available. It is in this poor-risk group where the ravages of malnutrition and starvation are most marked, and where the need for food is most desperate, that one must avail himself of other means of supplying vitally needed protein and calories. In addition there is a large group of patients in whom, for one reason or another, only a substandard amount of food can be assilmilated orally and in whom protein and caloric needs must be augmented by parenteral means.

The researches presented here were supported by the Augustus L. Searle Fund for Experimental Surgical Research, the Berenice Moriarity and Robert Cooper Funds for Surgical Research.

In partial fulfillment of the requirements for the degree of Doctor of Philosophy in Surgery, May, 1947.

It is proposed in this thesis to present the problem of protein metabolism and protein depletion as it relates to surgical patients. The means of supplying to the poor-risk patient by the intravenous route the protein he so desperately needs have been studied. It will be shown that these patients can be maintained in positive nitrogen balance by parenteral feedings alone, and that, if adequately prepared in this fashion, they can withstand operations of major magnitude with risks comparable to the uncomplicated case.

GENERAL CONSIDERATIONS OF PROTEIN METABOLISM AND A REVIEW OF PERTINENT LITERATURE

Historical Development of Concepts of Protein Metabolism.—In recent years there has been accomplished a fulfillment of the original meaning of the word protein, that is, of first importance. This added emphasis has developed slowly, for originally it was assumed that the proteins of the body were in a very stable state and were regarded more as inert structural elements rather than active dynamic participants in the chain of metabolism.

According to the classical theory of Folin[69-71] protein metabolism consists of two phases, one an endogenous phase which is in progress continuously. This corresponds to the amount of nitrogen excreted on a nitrogen-free diet and its marking end product in the urine is creatinine, neutral sulfur, and to a lesser extent uric acid. The excretion of these end products Folin found to be constant for each individual, regardless of the nitrogen intake or the nitrogen output. The other, an exogenous phase, and variable in character, is related to the amount of nitrogen foodstuff ingested and yields as its end product chiefly urea and inorganic sulfur. It was felt that protein synthesis in the adult organism in nitrogen equilibrium is restricted to replacement of the endogenous quota and when more than this minimal quantity of protein is ingested, it is quickly catabolized and appears in the urine chiefly as urea. Earlier Voit[206] postulated that protein of food passed through the blood stream to the tissues where it was catabolized under the influence of living protoplasm without first becoming an integral part of that protoplasm. Pflüger,[158] on the other hand, felt that all protein catabolized must first be transformed into an integral part of living tissues and as such undergoes oxidation.

McCullum,[132] Osborne and Mendel,[153] and Mitchell[144] questioned whether "wear and tear" or endogenous metabolism really involved the destruction of any intracellular protein. The latter felt that Folin's figures prove only that the excretion of creatinine is constant. Endogenous metabolism may be largely suppressed with protein feedings either because, by virtue of the mass action law, retardation of tissue hydrolysis by amino acids being set free by digestion of protein may occur, or from dietary protein catabolism certain nitrogenous substances become available which otherwise might have had to come from tissue protein. Nevertheless, the concept of the protein tissues of the body being in a more or less static and relatively inert state, that nitrogen ingested in excess of that necessary to replace the "wear and tear" of endogenous metabolism could not be stored and was excreted promptly in the urine as urea was generally believed.

In 1935 Borsook and Keighley[20] first proposed their theory of continuing metabolism of protein which is completely in the opposite direction of previous modifications of Folin's theory. They stated that, in an animal in nitrogen equilibrium, the breakdown of intracellular protein is continuously in progress even when abundant quantities of amino acids are obtained from the diet. This breakdown bears no "wear and tear" connotation and is directly proportional to the level at which nitrogen balance has been set by the previous dietary history. As a consequence, in nitrogen balance a corresponding quantity of amino acids is synthesized into tissue protein and peptides. When protein is ingested in the course of the next twenty-four hour period some of its amino acids contribute toward maintaining constant the concentration of free amino acids in the blood and tissues. A large fraction is synthesized into protein and peptides while the remainder is catabolized; this latter appears in the urine. The evidence for this hypothesis is that when nitrogen balance was maintained for one day with nonsulfur-containing amino acids, the sulfur excretion was considerably in excess of the endogenous sulfur excretion. In view of the fact that nitrogen balance was maintained, an increased endogenous metabolism could not be invoked to account for a sulfur excretion in excess of the endogenous level.

In a series of important contributions from Whipple's[53, 99, 103, 128, 159] laboratory, the concept of a "dynamic equilibrium" between the various stores and depots of body protein was developed. Holman and associates[99] first showed that dogs could be kept in nitrogen equilibrium by administering dog plasma intravenously as the sole source of nitrogen intake. The idea was developed that plasma proteins, without being broken up into amino acids, could leave the circulation and be available for the body needs. This concept was extended and confirmed by Pommerenke and co-workers[159] and by Daft and associates.[53] In 1938 Howland and Harkins,[103] in a well-conceived experiment, showed that when a phlorhizinized dog is fed plasma protein orally, the protein is readily digested to amino acids with conversion of 58 per cent of the protein into sugar, and with excretion in the urine of increased amounts of nitrogen and sugar. When the same plasma protein is given intravenously to phlorhizinized dogs, there is no increased urinary nitrogen excretion and no conversion of protein to sugar. This points to a different metabolic mechanism on the part of the body. It was suggested by Howland and Harkins that there is no need for intravenously injected protein to be broken up into amino acids for utilization, but rather that a partial catabolism of the injected protein occurs, with reassembly of the large aggregates performed by the cells to conform to the needs of their own peculiar type of protein. From plasmophoresis experiments[128] it was shown that there is a fairly large store of body protein which, when plasma protein is withdrawn producing hypoprotenemia, can readily be converted into new plasma protein. This reserve store of plasma protein-producing material is part of the general stores of the body. It is a bulwark against infections and toxemia. In its absence little new plasma protein is formed.

Further evidence that larger aggregates than amino acids are utilized by the body is offered by Reineke and associates[164] who showed, in lactating goats, that glycoprotein is used directly as the precursor of the protein of milk.

It was demonstrated for the first time in 1940 by Wangensteen and coworkers[207] and Kremen and associates[113] that, similarly, man could be maintained in positive nitrogen balance by administering human plasma intravenously as the sole source of nitrogen intake.

Schmidt, Allen, and Tarver[183] in 1940 postulated that a synthesis of proteins can take place in the body by transformation of existing proteins into others without being broken down into amino acids first.

The work of Schoenheimer and his associates,[179, 180] using isotopes of hydrogen, carbon, and nitrogen have demonstrated that every protein in the body is continuously changing and renewing its structure. Rapid amino shifts among the amino acids of the proteins of the body were observed. Amino acids of the body other than those administered were found to contain a considerable quantity of isotopic nitrogen. By measuring the concentration of isotopic nitrogen in a tissue at a certain time, an index of the chemical activity of its proteins could be obtained. Serum proteins always contained the highest concentration of isotopic nitrogen, and then in order of magnitude came viscera, muscles, and skin.

To quote Schoenheimer and Rittenberg:[179]

> Results of experiments with feeding isotopic physiological compounds to animals can scarcely be reconciled with the concept of endogenous and exogenous varieties of metabolism. Body constituents are involved in continuous chemical processes and there exists a close correlation between food materials and body components. Peptide, ester, and probably other linkages of the complex body materials open and close continuously. The amino acids, fatty acids, and other units temporarily liberated mix with others of the same species of whatever source, diet or tissue. By this mixing process they become indistinguishable as to their origin. Nitrogen excreted in urine may be regarded as part of the metabolic pool originating from the interaction of dietary nitrogen with the relatively large amounts of reactive body nitrogen, and the same applies to the other groupings of dietary and tissue substances.

In feeding isotopic nitrogen to rats,[181] an equal amount was rapidly recovered from all the fractions of plasma proteins. The proteins of the red blood cell, however, were found to have considerably less isotopic nitrogen, while the heme fraction of the red blood cells contained the least amounts of isotopic nitrogen. This seems to indicate that the protein of the red blood cell in circulation is involved in a slower cycle of synthesis and destruction than the other proteins of the body. By administering[182] isotopic nitrogen in amino acids to actively immune rats and rabbits, antibody like other serum and body proteins was found to participate in metabolic reactions involving the uptake of dietary nitrogen. The rate of replacement of marked nitrogen by ordinary nitrogen was followed. This indicated the half life of the antibody molecule to be about two weeks, approximately the same as the average serum protein. In a rabbit made passively immune to an antigen by injection of antibody,[93] the absence of uptake of dietary isotopic nitrogen by the passive antibodies is in marked contrast to the appearance of tagged nitrogen in the active antibodies. Shemin and Rittenberg[186] reported that half of the nitrogen in liver proteins is replaced by nitrogen from other sources in seven days. Apparently the most active proteins take up the tagged nitrogen first, then gradually let it go to other proteins until eventually there is an equilibrium of all the protein of the body. Muscle apparently is composed of heterogenous proteins, some reacting slowly with dietary nitrogen and others reacting very rapidly.

Burroughs and associates[26] felt that the discrepancy between the two views, that of Folin and that of Schoenheimer may not be so great if one considers the reactivity of various proteins from a quantitative rather than a qualitative viewpoint. While all organ proteins may be involved, they may react at different rates. Borsook and Dubonoff[21] suggested that the labile or reserve protein may be distinguished not primarily by its difference in composition, but rather by its location. Some organs, the liver,[86] intestine, and kidney,[5] change in size and protein content quickly with fasting and with changes in level of body protein. The labile protein may therefore arise in the course of a fast at first from the substance of the more labile organs.

Causes of Protein Deficiency in Surgical Patients.—

Starvation: Probably the most common cause of protein deficiency in surgical patients is simple starvation. Often this is due to a disease process that prevents the oral ingestion of food. Carcinoma about the oral cavity, esophageal lesions, both neoplastic and inflammatory, and obstruction to the gastric outlet, due either to carcinoma or benign stricture, are among the common offenders. All too frequently, however, because a disease process has precluded the use of solid food, the patient or his advisors have been at fault by the injudicious choice of a liquid diet. Varco[204] has very ably shown what can be accomplished with liquid diets containing large quantities of protein.

Himsworth,[97] Cuthbertson,[48] Elman,[60] and others[146] have pointed out that protein starvation leads to anorexia and asthenia, and thus a vicious cycle may well be established. With resumption of positive nitrogen balance, either by oral or parenteral protein feeding, a return of appetite and a feeling of well-being have been noted time and again by the author.

Altered absorption: Altered absorption of nutritiously adequate protein may be equally at fault in producing a picture of malnutrition and protein depletion. Inadequate absorption often will occur in diarrhea, ulcerative colitis, gastrojejunal colic fistula, and in fistulas of the small intestine. Increased oral intake of protein in this group often will pyramid the loss and recourse must be had to parenteral administration of carbohydrate and protein to replace the marked losses.

Changes in the gastrointestinal mucosa after starvation have been noted by Jackson.[107] Sun,[196] in a histologic study of the small intestinal mucosa after starvation, noted atrophy and sloughing of the tips of the mucosal villi. Most noticeable changes were in the duodenum and upper jejunum. Regeneration of the villi could be demonstrated ten hours after refeeding. If the villus did not regenerate, the animal would not eat and death ensued. Laycock,[119] writing of mass starvation in China, noted marked loss of appetite with diarrhea and a tendency to pass food unaltered in the stool. Cori and Cori[39] found glucose and fructose to be absorbed more slowly in rats after a forty-eight hour fast than after a twenty-four hour fast. At a meeting of the Royal Society of Medicine in 1945, Magee[131] stated that, in the terminal stages of starvation in man a copious and persistent diarrhea with dehydration occurs. The onset of these symptoms invariably presaged a fatal end in spite of treatment. He felt that there is a progressive decline in efficiency of absorption as the process of fasting is increased. At the same meeting, Cuthbertson[131] stated that there is reason to believe that in starvation the alimentary enzymes may share in the general protein depletion and that the power to digest will therefore become affected. In contrast to the impression that there might be real interference with intestinal absorption in extreme starvation, it was the impression of Vaughan,[205] writing of her experience in the treatment of starvation and malnutrition at Belsen, that best results were obtained using large doses of skim milk orally. Similarly Berger and associates[15] after the liberation of Holland noted that protein digests given orally caused no diarrhea but best results in rehabilitation obtained from a high caloric, high protein (300 Gm.), bland diet given orally.

Altered protein synthesis: In the presence of hepatic disease, protein synthesis may be impaired. This is especially true in regard to albumin formation, reversal of the albumin globulin ratio being a common finding in hepatitis and in portal cirrhosis.[140] In addition, there may be large losses of protein in ascitic fluid. Davis and Blalock[54] returned ascitic fluid intravenously to patients in order to replace protein losses. Davis and Getzoff[55] proposed a new classification of hypoproteinemias, a prehepatic state where there is insufficient intake or poor absorption, a hepatic state where hypoproteinemia is due to decreased hepatic synthesis of protein, and a posthepatic state due to excess protein losses. Barnett and associates[11] reported a case of cirrhosis of the liver with a daily loss of 10 Gm. of protein into ascitic fluid over a seven-month period without any lowering of plasma proteins. Madden and associates[125] found that sterile abscesses produced by turpentine in hypoproteinemic dogs have a retarding effect on protein synthesis.

Excessive protein loss: Serious loss of protein may occur in nephritis where large amounts of albumin leave the circulation, producing, if severe enough, a marked hypoproteinemia. Local losses of protein from burns, blood and plasma loss from open wounds, internal bleeding, and suppuration such as empyema or peritonitis, may be of major magnitude and constitute a real drain on a patient's protein stores.

After trauma, mainly fractures, Cuthbertson[43-46] first pointed out that there is a marked increased urinary nitrogen excretion. Disuse atrophy, although it produced an undoubted but small loss of nitrogen, could not wholly account for these changes, as the loss of substance was not wholly confined to the area of trauma. This traumatic catabolism in man reached its maximum toward the end of the first week after injury and then slowly declined. With severe injuries, the ingestion of a diet rich in protein and in calories did not maintain nitrogen equilibrium at the height of the catabolic process, although it did decrease the extent of the nitrogen losses. After trauma there appears to be a general increase of catabolism of protein in particular to meet the enhanced metabolism of the repair process.[47]

Lucido[122] reported increased urinary nitrogen excretion after burns. Cope and co-workers,[38] studying the causes of increased urinary nitrogen excretion after burns, found it was not associated with an increased potassium excretion and concluded that the excess nitrogen excreted did not come from cellular breakdown. They found the loss of nitrogen in the urine to be no greater in the severely burned than in the mildly burned. Croft and Peters[41] reported the urinary nitrogen loss after burns to be substantially reduced by inclusion of 1 per cent methionine in the diet, supplying confirmatory evidence to an earlier suggestion by Cuthbertson[45] that the increased urinary catabolism of protein after trauma was in response to a demand by the body for certain key amino acids for repair purposes, and so renders the healing process independent of dietary nitrogen. Brunschwig and associates[24] found that postoperative nitrogen loss bore no relation to the type of disease but rather was related only to the length of time the patient was deprived of food. Similarly Co Tui and associates[40, 148] felt that the principal cause of nitrogen loss in postoperative patients is starvation. Using a high nitrogen intake of protein digest given by indwelling intestinal tube they reported positive nitrogen balance can be obtained during the postoperative period. Rasmussen and associates[163] reported that by preoperative ingestion of considerable amounts of protein in patients with gastric cancer, serious degrees of hypoproteinemia can be prevented during the postoperative period of negative nitrogen balance.

Howard and associates[102] have reported augmented urinary nitrogen losses after simple fractures reaching a peak in 5.6 days and lasting up to 35 days. Peters[155] and Browne and co-workers[23] felt that a healthy man after injury or an acute infection suffers protein depletion which cannot be prevented. On the other hand, a malnourished and protein depleted individual can summon certain conservative processes that permit him to utilize protein for reconstruction of tissues.

Effects of Protein Deficiency in Surgical Patients.—

Hypoproteinemia: In the protein-deficient animal and in man this deficiency is mirrored in the blood proteins by a fall in the albumin fraction. This was well demonstrated by Weech[211] and has been confirmed by other investigators.[136, 177, 185, 200, 224] Sachar and associates[177] felt that hypoalbuminemia can be used as a quantitative measure of tissue protein depletion, postulating that for every gram of change in total serum albumin, there has been a concomitant change in the same direction of 30 Gm. of tissue protein. Madden and Whipple[128] have shown that, while the reserve stores of protein exist, a hypoproteinemic dog will produce plasma protein on a protein-free diet. Weech[211] found that on refeeding a protein deficient dog there was a slow return of plasma proteins to normal, suggesting that replenishment of the organ responsible for formation of albumin must take place before a rise of circulating plasma albumin occurs. This mechanism is apparently at play with intravenous plasma infusions also, for the rise of plasma proteins following such multiple transfusions is very gradual and slow.[185, 213] In contrast to the fall in the albumin fraction, the serum globulins remain relatively unchanged in protein depletion.[211] Zeldis and associates[224] felt the serum globulins enjoy prior demands on the total available pool of body proteins under such emergency conditions.

Blood volume: Single or even multiple determinations of plasma protein levels may be misleading without data on total plasma and blood volume.[2] That there is a fall in blood volume with protein depletion was first pointed out by Chang,[34] who felt that the plasma proteins had a regulatory effect on blood volume. Melnick and Cowgill[135] similarly felt that the plasma proteins had a regulatory effect on the plasma volume, but only in so far as the red blood cell volume remained constant. Others[2, 123, 155, 185, 211, 217] have pointed out the existence of a contracted plasma volume in starvation and deficiency states. Abbott and associates,[1] on the other hand, have demonstrated a rise in plasma volume in the postburn shock phase that persisted from forty to ninety days. This however, is not comparable to the starvation state mentioned previously. There appears to be a reciprocal arrangement between red cell volume and plasma volume for increases in red cell mass will tend to decrease the plasma volume to keep the total blood volume relatively constant.[17, 133] In anemias, on the other hand, there may be a real as well as an apparent increase in plasma volume.[1]

Edema: Starling[192] first stressed the significance of the osmotic pressure of the plasma proteins in drawing tissue fluid into the capillaries. Present-day theories of edema formation are still explained on the basis of his theory. The major osmotic effect of the plasma proteins[76, 77] was found to reside with the albumin fraction, which, because of its smaller molecular weight, is four times as active osmotically as the globulin fraction. Moore and Van Slyke[145] postulated a critical level of total protein of 5.5 Gm. per cent, or of albumin of 2.5 Gm. per cent or a plasma specific gravity of 1.023, below which edema will occur. By varying the level of sodium chloride intake, exception to the rule occurred. Weech and associates[214] similarly showed hypoproteinemia to be associated with edema. However, they noted that a lower level of plasma protein was necessary to produce edema after plasmaphoresis than after nutritional deficiency. Clinically the effect of large salt and fluid intake as well as hypoproteinemia in producing postoperative edema was first stressed by Jones and Eaton.[108] Also they postulated that edema may be a cause of stomal obstruction in gastroenterostomy during the early postoperative phase. Ravdin[160] later pointed out the same condition and in addition felt that hypoproteinemia reduced the gastric emptying time probably because of edema of the gut wall.[134] This later finding could not be confirmed by Beams and associates,[13] who could not demonstrate any roentgenologic change in gastric motility with edema.

Liver function: In 1914, Opie and Alford,[150, 151] studying the effect of chloroform on the liver, noted that the incidence of hepatic necrosis could be reduced after a high carbohydrate diet while a high fat diet materially increased the susceptibility of the animal to develop liver necrosis. Later Davis and associates[56, 57] noted regeneration of liver tissue on a carbohydrate diet alone. Also they observed that after chloroform anesthesia, when sugar was given, there was much less urinary nitrogen loss than when sugar was witheld. They postulated that the beneficial effect observed from sugar was due to its "protein sparing" effect. A similar effect was reported in 1936 by Daft and co-workers.[52]

In 1939 Goldschmidt, Vars, and Ravdin,[75] working with rats, demonstrated that the major protection afforded the liver to injury by chloroform was related to its protein content. They demonstrated a progressive increase of liver necrosis after chloroform anesthesia as the liver fat content increased. A high concentration of hepatic glycogen per se failed to confer any discernible protection. The liver damage increased with the lipid content independent of the glycogen content. Whatever benefit derived from glycogen was obtained by virtue of its replacing fat.[160] Protein, on the other hand, produced real protection. A high protein intake prior to chloroform anesthesia markedly reduced the incidence of liver necrosis even in those livers with a high lipid content. The injurious effect of fasting was believed to be due to its depletion of the protein stores.

Miller and associates[142, 143] demonstrated in protein depleted dogs that a single protein feeding by mouth, plasma protein intravenously or methionine and cystine may be the effective agent in this action. Brunschwig and associates[25] and others[96, 201] have reached similar conclusions. Harrison and Long[86] have shown in rats that the liver weight rapidly decreases during short periods of fasting, with the major loss being protein. Casein and lactalbumin feedings were effective in replacing this loss. However, from the time necessary to do this they felt that liver protein was not restored to its original level until after the lost body protein had been replaced. Tsan Wen Li[202, 203] stressed the effect of cholesterol which uniformly caused a higher total liver lipid content than ordinary fat. This effect could not be prevented entirely by high protein intake.

Resistance to infection and trauma: In Madden and Whipple's[128] experiments of producing protein depletion it was early appreciated that hypoproteinemic dogs were much less resistant to infection and to toxic agents. Sako[178] working with white rats concluded that animals on a high protein diet were more resistant to pneumococcus infection than a control group of animals; whereas animals on a lower protein diet were less resistant to the same organism. Further evidence of malnutrition reducing resistance to infection can be noted from the increased incidence of active tuberculosis in European countries after World War I and again at the present time. Cannon and his co-workers in a series of papers[29-32] stressed the importance of good protein reserves for formation of globulin and antibodies. In hypoproteinemic rabbits, he demonstrated a deficiency of antibodies.[31] That dietary nitrogen participates in formation of antibodies has been shown with isotopic nitrogen by Schoenheimer and associates.[182] In the foregoing discussion, it was shown there is good evidence to believe that protein depletion is associated with a decreased blood volume. In hypoproteinemic dogs, Ravdin and associates[161] demonstrated a 67 per cent increase in susceptibility to hemorrhagic shock.

Wound healing: In 1919 Clark,[36] working on dogs, showed that the lag phase in wound healing was markedly shortened with a high protein diet.

Harvey and Howes,[89] working on stomach wounds in rats, found no change in the lag period, but did note that once growth had started its rate was noticeably increased by a high protein diet. Thompson and associates,[198, 199] Hartzell and associates[87] and A. O. Whipple[216] wrote of the importance of adequate protein stores for wound healing, and of the high incidence of wound disruption in hypoproteinemic patients. Thompson and co-workers[199] noted an accelerated decline in tensile strength of catgut in hypoproteinemic dogs and recommended that silk be used in its place. A decreased formation of callus in hypoproteinemic dogs was reported by Rhoads and Kasinskas.[165]

In summary, it can be said that the effects of protein deprivation are legion. In the past, related clinical conditions such as pulmonary edema, failure of wounds and anastomoses to heal, sepsis, hepatorenal syndrome, and a poor response to operative trauma and anesthesia may have been dismissed as unavoidable complications. Such conditions, however, are not distantly related to the effects of protein deprivation. It has been only in recent years, when surgeons have concerned themselves with phases of the patient's care in addition to good operative technique, that operative mortalities have declined. It is not the operation per se, but one of its complications which prolongs convalescence and often ends fatally. In uncomplicated major operative cases the patients are ready for dismissal from the hospital in four to five days. A smooth uncomplicated convalescence should be the goal toward which the surgeon embarks on each case. In attaining that goal, attention to many details is necessary, one of which should be an effort to correct the protein-deficient state in poorly nourished patients.

THE RELATIONSHIP OF HEMOGLOBIN METABOLISM TO BODY PROTEIN METABOLISM

In normal man there is a continuous destruction of erythrocytes and a continuous replenishment of new red blood cells from the hematopoietic tissue.[210] An equilibrium between these processes in health maintains the hemoglobin level at around 15 Gm. per cent. Many studies of the average life of the red blood cell have been made. By selective agglutination of donor red blood cells in a recipient's circulation and from the rate of their disappearance, Ashby[9] and others[50, 105, 221] concluded that the survival time of transfused erythrocytes may vary from 50 to 120 days. From a study of bilirubin and urobilinogen excretion, Hawkins and Whipple[91] and others[208] found similar results. Shemin and Rittenberg[187] fed glycine containing isotopic nitrogen, thus incorporating it into the heme fraction of hemoglobin. They concluded that the average life of the red blood cell was 125 days. Other studies[82] using radioactive iron incorporated into the red blood cell were nonconclusive in determining the life of the erythrocyte, for no change in the amount of radioactive iron in the circulating red blood cells could be noted after 120 days. It was felt that the iron liberated by the breakdown of red blood cells was promptly reutilized in the formation of new red blood cells. Hence, no change could be detected in the circulating level of radioactive iron.

The actual site of destruction of red blood cells is not clear. Three possibilities exist, hemolysis, phagocytosis, and fragmentation. Rous and Robertson[170, 175, 176] state that phagocytosis of red blood cells while frequent in the dog, rat, and guinea pig is slight in man, rhesus monkey, and rabbit. They find no support for the thesis of hemolytic destruction of erythrocytes and feel that the principal means of red blood cell destruction is by fragmentation of erythrocytes in the circulation due to aging of the cells and to the stress and strain they are subjected to in their passage through the blood vessels and capillaries. Fragments of various portions of red blood cells can be observed in the circulation and these in turn are removed by the reticuloendothelial system. In summarizing the prevailing views on the fate of the liberated hemoglobin, Rous in 1923[175] stated that the hemoglobin was broken up into globin, the fate of which was unknown, into bilirubin, which was excreted in the bile; and into an iron-containing substance which was retained by the body and possibly utilized. Isaacs[105] in 1937 stated that the concepts of red blood cell destruction were unchanged since the papers of Rous.

Apparently the hemoglobin[181] of the intact red blood cell does not participate in the rapid interchange of amide groups as do the proteins of the remainder of the body. It seems to have a separate and slower cycle of synthesis and destruction than the other body proteins. Hahn and associates[81] and Whipple[218] and Shemin and Rittenberg[187] have shown that the hemoglobin of the red blood cell apparently remains intact as long as the cell exists, and similarly its component iron is not subject to physiochemical change for the life span of the erythrocyte. When the red blood cell is destroyed, the iron is retained by the body and reutilized for new hemoglobin formation,[91] possibly more promptly than iron in storage[42, 82] and certainly in preference to dietary iron.[80]

Itami in 1908[106] postulated that experimental plethora may have a depressing effect on hematopoiesis. Boycott and Douglas[22] in 1910 found that just as anemia can be a stimulus to red blood cell formation, excess circulating red blood cells can be a stimulus to red blood cell destruction in an effort by the body to adjust to a normal status. This problem was again studied by Robertson and Rous[170] in 1917, who gave daily transfusions of whole blood to rabbits. They were not able to produce plethora uniformly, but in some animals hemoglobin levels up to 150 per cent of normal occurred. Concomitant with the production of plethora a decrease of reticulocytes in the circulating blood occurred and often they completely disappeared, to reappear again only when the hemoglobin returned to normal levels. Bone marrow biopsies similarly showed a marked decrease in the number of reticulocytes.

In 1936 Melnick and associates[137] stated that the slow continuous breakdown of injected red blood cells after plasmaphoresis experiments liberated globin which is completely metabolized similar to dietary protein, and in so doing it erased the amino acid deficiency of gliadin.

In a series of papers recently published by Strumia and associates[193, 194] the claim was made that globin prepared by extracorporeal hemolysis of erythrocytes can be given parenterally with good utilization. They felt that it could be converted to plasma protein, citing a 90 Gm. increase of plasma protein after administering 260 Gm. of globin, or a three to one conversion ratio.

In 1935 Pommerenke and associates,[159] working in Whipple's laboratory, reported that hemoglobin and globin could not be utilized by the body. They administered dog hemoglobin intravenously to dogs and noted increased urinary nitrogen excretion equivalent to the amount of hemoglobin nitrogen administered. Similarly Madden and co-workers[127] stated that laked red blood cells afforded little if any material for plasma protein formation when given intravenously. They found no increased plasma protein formation when red blood cells were given intravenously in addition to a basal diet. In later papers[126, 141, 168, 169, 218, 219] from the same laboratory, however, it is reported that hemoglobin and hemoglobin digests given intravenously and parenterally will support nitrogen balance and produce new plasma protein.

Whipple writing in 1942[218] stated:

> Hemoglobin in its production may draw on the plasma protein, but hemoglobin stands apart in the protein economy and does not contribute freely to the protein pool. On the other hand, the body guards jealously the fabrication of hemoglobin and given a real need for both plasma protein and hemoglobin the protein flow favors hemoglobin which under these circumstances is always produced in more abundance than plasma proteins.

In 1944 Whipple and Madden[219] wrote:

> Hemoglobin cannot be contributed to the body protein pool except when the red blood cell is broken up. Hemoglobin is then saved, supplemented, and recast into new protein depending upon the body needs, and much of the rescued hemoglobin or globin may contribute to the building of plasma protein.

In 1933 Daft[51, 52] demonstrated that under conditions of protein starvation the anemic dog can fabricate new hemoglobin from its own body proteins. This is associated with a decrease urinary nitrogen excretion over similar nonanemic periods. Later Hahn and Whipple[85] pointed out that limitation of protein intake eventually will limit the formation of globin and thus cut down the formation of hemoglobin. Since the body can manufacture unlimited quantities of porphyrin pigment, the limiting factors in hemoglobin formation are iron and protein. Similarly Orten and Orten[152] and others [215] showed that a low protein diet produced anemia, whereas an isocaloric diet high in protein resulted in normal hemoglobin levels. They felt that protein building blocks are not available for hemoglobin synthesis under conditions of protein starvation. Taylor and Lytle[197] found that in patients, both hypoproteinemic and anemic, infusions of red blood cells resulted in a definite rise of plasma proteins. This they attributed to a sparing effect on protein which otherwise would have been used for hemoglobin formation. In 1946 Robscheit-Robbins and associates[169] stressed the point that in doubly depleted dogs (hypoproteinemic and anemic) hemoglobin is always produced more abundantly than and often at the expense of plasma proteins.

From the foregoing discussion it may be surmised that hemoglobin formation constitutes a real drain on the protein stores of the body, and will continue even in the fasting state and at the expense of plasma proteins. Also as red blood cells are being destroyed, the proteins of the liberated hemoglobin are made available to the general body pool of proteins for whatever use is most urgent at the moment. From a nutritional viewpoint the administration of whole blood transfusions offers several avenues of benefit to the over-all protein economy of the body. First, protein from the body stores which would have, by priority, been used for building hemoglobin may now become available for other purposes. Second, the plasma proteins contained in the whole blood are available for use in the body economy and, third, as the total circulating hemoglobin or red cell mass is increased, more red blood cells will be destroyed daily liberating their contained hemoglobin, the protein of which also becomes available for general body utilization.

CONSIDERATIONS IN PROTEIN REPLACEMENT THERAPY AND REAFFIRMATION OF THE PROBLEM

The average adult in health when fed adequate quantities of carbohydrate and on a protein-free diet will excrete from 4 to 6 Gm. of nitrogen per day in the urine.[59, 113] This amount is equivalent to 25 to 37.5 Gm. of protein. In addition, if oral feedings are being taken, up to 10 per cent of the ingested nitrogen may normally be excreted in the stools without diarrhea.[144] Chittenden[35] proposed 0.65 Gm. of protein per kilogram body weight as an adequate protein intake for a healthy man. To create an adequate margin of safety most recommendations are placed on a higher level of protein intake. The League of Nations[58] recommendation was set at 1 Gm. of protein per kilogram of body weight per day. A similar figure was reported by Cuthbertson[48] and by the National Research Council[149] with the added recommendation that one-third to one-half of the protein intake be of animal origin and the remainder of vegetable origin. This is in recognition of the fact that proteins of animal origin are more complete in essential amino acids. For replacement therapy when the protein stores of the body are depleted, amounts of protein in the order of magnitude of two to four times this figure may be beneficial[61, 204] and utilized.

The sparing effect of carbohydrate on the body's consumption of its own protein or on ingested protein has been attested to by many authors. Landergen[114] in 1903 showed that urinary nitrogen excretion is markedly reduced on a rich carbohydrate diet. Similarly Cathart[33] showed that urinary nitrogen excretion is less when carbohydrate is consumed than under conditions of total fasting. Shaffer and Coleman[184] reported a decreased nitrogen loss with typhoid fever when a high carbohydrate intake is assured. Writing on the protein sparing action of carbohydrate in 1919, Davis, Hall and Whipple[57] postulated two possible mechanisms for its action: one by conserving the end products of protein catabolism and the other by sparing the autolysis of protein. They felt that both actions may occur. When sufficient carbohydrate is available for energy requirements, protein catabolism is reduced to a minimum. In the absence of sufficient carbohydrate, protein can be used for energy purposes and 58 per cent of it may be converted to carbohydrate, the so-called D/N ratio.[166] More recently others[7, 49, 104, 117, 162] have attested to the protein sparing action of carbohydrate, and to the attainment of increased nitrogen retention when protein is given in conjunction with a high sugar intake, preferably at the same time. Daft and associates[53] suggested that possibly protein intoxication can occur. They noted excessive urinary nitrogen excretion when large doses of protein alone were administered. It was possible to prevent this excess loss of nitrogen by feeding adequate carbohydrate and fat with the protein. Elman and co-workers[63] recently stated that nitrogen retention can occur with a sufficiently high nitrogen intake and an inadequate caloric intake, with the caloric deficit being made up by body fat. This is in contradistinction to reports by Landergen[114] and Cathart,[33] early in this century, who noted much poorer nitrogen retention when fat was substituted for carbohydrate in the diet.

In 1935 Kochakion and Murlin[112] demonstrated that male sex hormones, extracted from urine, constantly led to nitrogen retention when administered to castrated dogs. Kenyon and associates[109, 110] noted that testosterone led to increased nitrogen retention and decreased urinary nitrogen excretion in normal men as well as in eunuchoids, although to a lesser extent in the former. One normal young woman responded in a similar fashion. They feel the effect is related to the stimulus to growth associated with puberty. Similar results are reported by Abels and co-workers.[4] Albright[8] has postulated that the adrenal gland produces an ''N'' or protein anabolic hormone and an ''S'' or sugar or antianabolic hormone and that normally these are balanced. After injury there may be a decreased excretion of ''N'' and an increased excretion of ''S'' hormone producing the increased catabolism of protein described earlier.

The exact amount of protein replacement necessary, prior to embarking on a major operative procedure, cannot be stated categorically. Studley[195] in 1936 reported that the percentage of weight loss by the patient was a good indicator of the surgical risk of that patient. He reported on forty-seven patients with complicated peptic ulcer who were operated upon. In twenty-nine patients who had lost less than 20 per cent of their body weight there was one death, a mortality of 3 per cent, whereas in eighteen patients who had lost over 20 per cent of their body weight there were six deaths, a mortality of 33 per cent. Varco[204] on similar considerations postulated progressively increasing periods of preoperative dietary preparation, the length of preparation being in direct proportion to the weight loss of the patient. In extreme cases, periods of preoperative preparation up to one month are suggested.

However, if the weight loss has been chiefly from the fatty depots no harm will result. In evaluating weight loss one should consider the past dietary history as well as the status of the patient's nitrogen balance. Similarly, the state of hydration can effect weight figures by as much as 10 per cent. Complete replacement of the total protein loss is often impossible and not very practical. Certainly, however, positive nitrogen balance should be established, hypoproteinemia and hemoglobin deficits corrected, and the contracted blood volume that may accompany malnutrition restored to normal by the most propitious means. With a cooperative patient, in whom no obstruction to the esophagus, stomach, or bowel exists, or in whom no avenues of increased food loss such as ulcerative colitis, external intestinal or gastrojejunocolic fistula exists, oral feeding of a high protein, high carbohydrate, and low fat diet is undoubtedly the best avenue of supplying vitally needed protein. For the group of patients, as just mentioned, in whom the oral route is not available, parenteral feeding is necessary.

It is possible to supply parenterally all the essential food elements: water, minerals, vitamins, carbohydrates, and protein. Possibly fat should be included in this group[28] and its parenteral administration has been accomplished,[37, 100] but as yet this method has not reached the stage of clinical trial. Gastrostomy or jejunostomy performed for feeding purposes and preliminary to a major surgical procedure may have rare instances of usefulness, but this should not be necessary often. It subjects a patient to the risk and discomfort of an additional operation, with its subsequent period of increased protein catabolism. In neoplastic diseases of the intestinal tract it is not an uncommon occurrence to return to the peritoneal cavity three to four weeks after having done a jejunostomy for feeding purposes to find what was previously a well-localized carcinoma has spread beyond its original site. The best time to cure cancer is at the initial operation.

In the following sections it will be shown that the positive nitrogen balance can be achieved by parenteral administration of plasma proteins, whole blood, and protein digests. Also it will be shown that these poor-risk patients who cannot be prepared by oral means can be prepared parenterally and will withstand operations of major proportions with risks not greater than similar uncomplicated cases.

CONSIDERATIONS OF PARENTERAL THERAPY

The history of parenteral therapy dates from 1628 when William Harvey[90] discovered the circulation. Dr. Wren (later Sir Christopher)[111] in 1657 first injected medicinals into the veins of animals and reported his findings at one of the early meetings of the Royal Society which had been started in London in 1661. To Richard Lower, also a member of the Royal Society, and stimulated by the work of Harvey and Wren, belongs the credit for giving the first blood transfusion from dog to dog in February, 1666. One year later Jean Denys of Montpellier, and physician to Louis XIV, pursued similar experiments and on June 15, 1667, he transfused into a boy of 15 years, 9 ounces of lamb's blood with no untoward effect. As might have been expected, when these attempts of transfusing animal blood into man continued, fatalities occurred and in 1670 a writ appeared specifically prohibiting the operation of transfusion in France. Similarly in 1678 an edict of Parliament appeared specifically prohibiting the operation of transfusion in England. On Dec. 22, 1818, James Blundell[19] gave the first blood transfusion from man to man. Out of ten transfusions given by Blundell, four were successful. Before blood transfusions could be rendered safe and be performed with relative ease and dispatch, it remained for the work of Landsteiner[116] to demonstrate the four blood groups in man, and for Lewisohn[120, 121] to offer an efficient, practical means of avoiding coagulation of blood by the use of sodium citrate solution.

The first intravenous injection of saline solution was made by Thomas Latta[118] in 1831 for treatment of the dehydration of cholera. To Claude Bernard[16] in 1843 belongs credit for first injecting carbohydrate intravenously. He showed that sucrose, when injected intravenously, soon appeared in the urine, but, if it had been previously acted upon by gastric juice and converted to glucose, it was apparently utilized. Woodyatt and associates[223] first postulated that intravenous nutrition in man might be accomplished by intravenous injection of glucose when he showed that normal man can utilize from 0.8 to 0.9 Gm. of glucose per kilogram per hour. If this rate were exceeded, glycosuria and diuresis would occur. He also warned that death could occur from dehydration from the diuretic effect of extremely large doses of hypertonic intravenous glucose given too rapidly over prolonged periods.

In 1912 Austin and Eisenbrey[10] expressed the belief that dogs could utilize dog and horse serum administered intravenously as a source of tissue nitrogen. They determined the urinary nitrogen excretion on a nitrogen-free diet, following which they administered dog and horse serum intravenously to dogs. This was not associated with any increased urinary nitrogen excretion over the control period. Although their figures do not show positive nitrogen balance, they did find that the protein so administered was retained and used by the body. From the laboratory of Whipple and associates[99] in 1934 and in numerous subsequent reports,[128, 159] it was demonstrated that positive nitrogen balance in animals and man[113, 207] could be obtained using homologous plasma intravenously as the sole source of protein intake.

Plasma protein given intravenously soon disappears from the circulation, apparently going into the general body protein stores. Shearburn[185] using blood volume studies, found an initial rise of circulating plasma protein following massive plasma transfusion. In three days he noted that all the injected plasma proteins had apparently left the circulation. Using protein tagged with radioactive sulfur, Fine and Seligman[66] observed the rate of disappearance of tagged plasma protein from the circulation of normal dogs. At five hours, 90 per cent of the protein remained in the circulation; at fifteen hours, 70 per cent was present; by forty-eight hours, 55 per cent of the tagged plasma protein had left the circulation. They observed similar disappearance curves of plasma protein in shocked animals. Fink and associates[67] in a similar study, but using heavy nitrogen in the lysine fraction of the plasma proteins, reported the same findings. These studies confirm the clinical findings that hypoproteinemia is not readily corrected by plasma transfusions. Apparently depleted protein stores must first be restored or at least must concomitantly be restored as was first suggested by Weech[211] in the case of oral feedings. Sachar and co-workers[177] have computed that plasma proteins are restored in a ratio of one to thirty with body protein stores.

In 1905, Abderholden and Rona[3] demonstrated that nitrogen equilibrium in a dog could be maintained by feeding a pancreatic digestion product of casein containing amino cleavage products equal to 2 Gm. of nitrogen. When the same protein was hydrolysed with acid and an equivalent amount of nitrogen was administered, negative nitrogen balance resulted. The nitrogen loss was equal to that on a nitrogen-free diet. Henriques[94] showed that in the absence of the single amino acid, tryptophane, nitrogen equilibrium cannot be attained. Henriques and Anderson,[95] in 1913, first demonstrated that nitrogen equilibrium could be obtained in the goat by intravenous injection of amino acids (meat digested with trypsin and erypsin plus tryptophane) as the sole source of nitrogen for eighteen days. It is of interest that they chose the goat as their experimental animal so that they could utilize its horns for fixing their intravenous apparatus which they maintained in the jugular vein for long periods. Through the work of Osborne and Mendel[153, 154] and later Rose and associates[171, 172] the nutritutive significance of amino acids for growth was established. Ten amino acids: lysine, leucine, isoleucine, threonine, methionine, phenylalanine, tryptophane, valine, histidine, and arginine, were found to be essential to the body for growth. They cannot be synthesized or substituted for by the body and must be supplied in the food. Burroughs and co-workers[27] postulated a difference between growth where total protein synthesis must occur, and for maintenance of nitrogen equilibrium in an adult where only particular requirements must be met. For such a state lysine, histidine, and arginine may possibly be dispensed with. Elman and Weiner,[64] in 1939, first reported the use of an acid hydrolysate of casein with added tryptophane and cystine for intravenous alimentation and reported positive nitrogen balance with its use. The first clinical use of an enzymatic hydrolysate of casein in which all the essential amino acids are present was reported by Shohl, Butler, and Blackfan[188] and Farr and MacFadyen.[65] Shohl and Blackfan,[189] in 1940, reported a crystalline amino acid solution to be equally effective as an enzymatic hydrolysate of casein in achieving positive nitrogen balance when given intravenously to children. However, their observation periods were only for twelve to twenty-four hours.

In 1940, it was shown that growth of rats was the same when fed casein, or the casein enzymatic digest, amigen, as the sole source of protein.[147] Later, Horwitz and associates[101] claimed growth in rats using amigen as the sole source of protein, subcutaneously. Shohl[190] found nitrogen retention to be equally good when amigen was given either orally or intravenously. From his data it is noted that nitrogen retention was greater both in amount and in proportion to intake when blood transfusions were given in addition to amigen. Madden and co-workers[130] reported that a papain casein digest was found to be equally as effective in producing plasma protein when given either orally or intravenously. However, a greater urinary nitrogen excretion was noted after intravenous administration than after oral feeding of the digest. Others[193, 194] have noted a pyramiding of urinary nitrogen excretion when protein digests are given intravenously. Mixtures of the ten essential amino acids, as described by Rose, were found to rate with the best food proteins in producing new plasma protein.[124, 129] Positive nitrogen balance could be achieved equally well with either oral or intravenous administration.

The mixtures of pure amino acids could be given several times faster than the fastest tolerable rate for protein digest without producing clinical disturbance. Glutamic acid[126] was suggested as being the causative agent in producing nausea and vomiting. Hoffman and associates[98] noted nausea and vomiting occurring in human beings after amigen injection when the blood amino acid level rose above 10 mg. per cent.

EXPERIMENTAL: NITROGEN BALANCE STUDIES

Method.—In order to assay the effectiveness of a given material for parenteral feeding purposes, nitrogen balance studies were performed on selected patients using bovine plasma, human plasma, whole human blood, and casein digests* given intravenously as the sole source of nitrogen intake. These materials were tested individually and in combinations. It was felt that the ability of a nitrogenous material to sustain positive nitrogen balance when given intravenously as the sole source of nitrogen intake would constitute a critical test of that material's ability to sustain protein metabolism and to replenish depleted protein stores.

Subjects were chosen who had lost considerable weight, usually because a carcinoma of the esophagus or stomach had precluded their taking an adequate diet by mouth. All patients were afebrile and were allowed out of bed ad libitum while fluids were not running.

The selection of a proper subject for such a study requires the fulfillment of several considerations. First, the patient's disease must be such to justify and require a prolonged period of parenteral feeding. Second, the cooperation of the patient must be secured so that specimens will not be lost, will be passed on time, and will be passed into the proper receptacle. Third, there must be an adequate number of patent peripheral veins on the arms, hands, and legs, for in the course of such a study many of the vessels will become thrombosed. As the studies progressed, it was appreciated that as a rule men made better subjects for study. They had less difficulty in passing urine and feces separately, whereas even with repeated warning, women would on occasion pass urine at the time of bowel movements. During the period of study the patients were on a protein-free oral intake of sweetened fruit juice and tea. Usually 3000 c.c. of 10 per cent glucose solution, supplying 1,200 calories, was given intravenously daily along with 4.5 Gm. of sodium chloride and therapeutic doses of vitamins B, C, and K. Total urinary output was collected daily, preserved with toluene, and quantitatively analyzed for total nitrogen by the macro Kjeldahl technique,[156] urea nitrogen,[73] amino acid nitrogen,[74] ammonia,[72] creatinine,[157] and sugar.[88] Although all urine specimens were collected and analyzed daily, some of the earlier data were accumulated by periods and are so reported. After an initial test period, during which time there was no nitrogen intake, the urinary nitrogen excretion reached a basal level of around 5 Gm. per day. The test protein or protein digest solution was then given

*Two casein digests were used. One, amigen, an enzymatic hydrolysate of casein, was supplied by the Mead Johnson & Co., Evansville, Ind. The other, parenamine, an acid hydrolysate of casein fortified with tryptophane, was supplied by Fredrick Stearns & Company, Detroit, Mich.

intravenously, in addition to the dextrose solution, daily for four to six days followed by another basal period to determine any delayed nitrogen spillage, if such occured. In some cases the stools were collected by periods and preserved with glacial acetic acid. Total fecal nitrogen excretion was then determined by macro Kjeldahl technique.[156] In Tables VIII and IX, quantitative fecal urobilinogen[209] was determined. The low values of urobilinogen obtained were felt to be due to the fact that there was no oral intake of food during the time and the amount of stool passed was quite meager.

At the beginning and end of each study period, and once during a study period, hemoglobin determinations by the oxyhemoglobin method using a Leitz photoelectric colorimeter, red blood cell counts, hematocrit,[222] total and fractional plasma protein,[78] urea nitrogen,[73] plasma chloride,[220] uric acid,[73] and amino acid levels[74] were determined in the patient's blood. Total nitrogen content of donor plasma and whole blood was determined by macro Kjeldahl technique on an aliquot of each specimen. Blood volume determination, when performed, was done by the technique recommended by Gregerson,[79] using an Evelyn photoelectric colorimeter.

Results of Nitrogen Balance Studies.—From 1939 through 1941, an investigation of the possibility and potentialities of using whole bovine plasma as a blood substitute in man was carried out. These results were published in two papers, in 1940[207] and 1942.[113] It was shown that large doses of bovine plasma or serum could be given to man, but its use was attended by a large (66.6 per cent) incidence of reactions. The incidence of these reactions could be reduced, but could not be abolished by preliminary adsorption of bovine plasma with human red blood cells which partially removed a hemolysin contained in the plasma. Using such a procedure, the incidence of reactions was reduced to 24.5 per cent.

In the course of these investigations, nitrogen balance studies using bovine serum, given intravenously, as the sole source of protein intake were carried out. The results of one such study are shown in Table I and Fig. 1. The patient, O. W. (U. H. No. 702623), was a 48-year-old man with an inoperable carcinoma of the sigmoid colon. Before admission to the hospital the patient had experienced a weight loss of forty pounds, amounting to 34 per cent of his normal body weight. Beginning twelve days after an exploratory laparotomy and transverse colostomy, the patient was started on a nitrogen balance study. During the preliminary period, when there was no protein intake, the total urinary nitrogen excretion was 47.32 Gm. with an average daily nitrogen excretion of 7.88 Gm. This is a somewhat higher figure than most of our studies have shown during the basal period of protein starvation, with a caloric intake maintained at around 1,500 daily. From Jan. 9, 1941 through Jan. 13, 1941, 500 c.c. daily and a total of 2,500 c.c. of whole bovine serum, containing a total of 30.75 Gm. of nitrogen, were administrated intravenously. The remainder of the conditions were identical with the basal period. It is noted there was no increased urinary nitrogen excretion during this period, but rather a slight decrease as shown by an average daily nitrogen excretion of 6.91 Gm. as compared to 7.88 Gm. excreted during the basal period. Although positive nitrogen balance was not achieved, nitrogen equilibrium was almost reached as compare 6.15, the average daily nitrogen intake, against 6.91, the average daily nitrogen excretion. During the subsequent period, Jan. 14, 1941 through Jan. 17, 1941, when again there was no protein intake, it is noted there was no augmented urinary nitrogen excretion over the preliminary basal period, indicating that no delayed catabolism of the ingested protein occurred. At no time was any protein noted in the urine. Also, there did not appear to be any shift in the urine urea nitrogen to total urine nitrogen ratio which might indicate an abnormal catabolism of protein. The circulating plasma proteins appear to have risen slightly from a level of 5.62 Gm. per cent at the beginning of the experiment to 6.19 Gm. per cent at the completion of the injection period. However, without blood volume determination one cannot definitely substantiate that impression. Nevertheless, from these studies it would appear that bovine plasma protein given intravenously to man, although not capable, in the amounts used, to produce positive nitrogen balance, is retained by the body for nitrogen metabolism or for replenishment of protein stores.

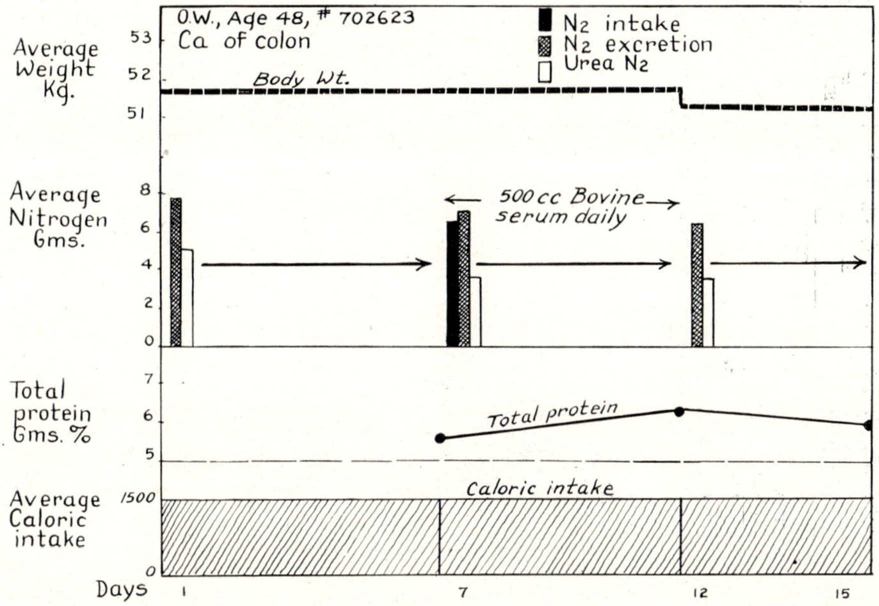

Fig. 1.—Nitrogen balance study attending intravenous administration of bovine serum.

In Table II and Fig. 2 are shown the results of a similar study of nitrogen balance attending the intravenous administration of equivalent amounts of nitrogen in the form of the casein digest, amigen, and whole human plasma. The patient, J. O. (U. H. No. 695929), a man, had a carcinoma of the hepatic flexure of the colon. He had complained of weakness, anorexia, and a weight loss of twenty-five pounds, amounting to 20 per cent of his normal body weight. He was operated upon Aug. 16, 1940, at which time exploratory laparotomy revealed the lesion to be unresectable and nothing further was done. On the

Table I. Nitrogen Balance Studies Attending Intravenous Administration of Bovine Serum

O. W., U. H. No. 702623, aged 48 years, carcinoma of colon

		Urine		Blood					
Period	Date	Total N_2 (Gm.)	Urea N_2 (Gm.)	Total protein (Gm.)	N.P.N. (mg. %)	B.U.N. (mg. %)	Daily caloric intake	Nitrogen intake as bovine serum intravenously (c.c.)	Weight (Kg.)
1	1/3/41 through 1/8/41	47.32	28.54	5.62	23	10.5	1500	0	51.8
	Av. daily	7.88	4.91						
2	1/9/41 through 1 13/41	34.55	17.28	6.19	23.3	15	1500	2500 Total N 30.75 Gm. Av. daily 6.15 Gm.	51.8
	Av. daily	6.91	3.46						
3	1/14/41 through* 1/17/41	25.80	13.73	5.95	32		1500	0	51.3
	Av. daily	6.45	3.43						

*Patient developed general urticaria and edema lasting 2 days, from 1/15/41 to 1/17/41.

Table II. Nitrogen Balance Attending Intravenous Administration of Amigen and of Human Plasma

J. O., U. H. No. 695929, aged 51 years, carcinoma of colon

		Urine		Blood					
Period	Date	Total N_2 (Gm.)	Urea N_2 (Gm.)	Total protein (Gm.)	N.P.N. (mg. %)	B.U.N. (mg. %)	Average daily caloric intake	Nitrogen intake	Weight (Kg.)
1	8/29/40 through 9/2/40	15.06	9.37	5.73	29.75	9.4	660	0	46.8
	Av. daily	3.01	1.87					1000 c.c. 5 % amigen I.V. daily	
2	9/3/40 through 9/8/40	51.59	34.14	5.88	27.8	17.2	1350	Total N 36.0	46.5
	Av. daily	8.59	5.83					Av. daily 6.0	
3	9/9/40 through 9/12/40	25.04	17.17	6.03	28.2	14.7	600	0	45
	Av. daily	6.26	4.29					500 c.c. whole human plasma daily IV	
4	9/13/40 through 9/17/40	21.88	13.80	6.09	26	14.7	600	Total N_2 28.0	44.2
	Av. daily	4.37	2.76					Av. daily 5.6	
5	9/18/40 through 9/22/40	16.95	9.53	6.38	30.3	11.2	1000	0	44.3
	Av. daily	3.39	1.90						

tenth postoperative day, the present study was started. During Period 1, when there was no protein intake, the urine nitrogen excretion averaged 3.01 Gm. per day. In Period 2 the patient received, in addition to the same fluids given during Period 1, 1000 c.c. of 5 per cent amigen solution containing 6 Gm. of nitrogen intravenously daily. This was associated with a prompt rise of urinary nitrogen excretion so that the patient remained in negative nitrogen balance of 2.59 Gm. of nitrogen per day. Again in Period 3, there was no nitrogen intake and the urinary nitrogen excretion declined, there being noted an average urinary nitrogen loss of 6.26 Gm. per day. This was due to an augmented urinary nitrogen spillage during the early part of the period, a delayed effect from the amigen period, while during the latter days of the period the urinary nitrogen excretion more closely approached the original

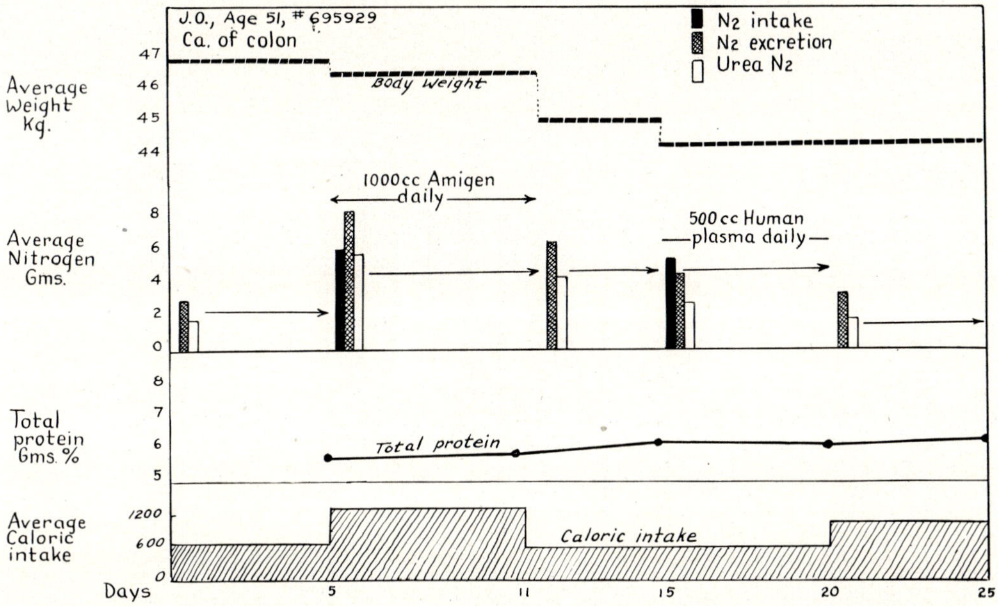

Fig. 2.—Nitrogen balance study attending the intravenous administration of amigen and whole human plasma.

basal level. During the five days of Period 4, the patient received intravenously daily as the sole protein intake 500 c.c. of human plasma, containing an equivalent amount of nitrogen, 5.6 Gm. per day as determined by Kjeldahl analysis. In contradistinction to Period 2 there was no rise of urinary nitrogen excretion noted, and definite positive nitrogen balance, a daily intake of 5.6 Gm. against a daily urinary excretion of 4.37 Gm., was obtained. In Period 5 no delayed excess nitrogen spillage over the basal period was noted, indicating that the plasma protein given was apparently retained by the body. No significant change in total circulating plasma protein was noted during the experiment. During the twenty-five day span of this study, in a patient with far advanced inoperable carcinoma of the colon, and while the metabolic requirements were met by parenteral feedings, there was a weight loss of 2.5 kg.

In Table III and Fig. 3 are recorded the results of another nitrogen balance study attending the use of intravenous amigen. This patient, C. S. (U. H. No. 698650), a 62-year-old man, had about three months earlier, a gastric resection for carcinoma of the stomach. At the time of the study he had developed almost complete obstruction at the gastrojejunal anastomosis, presumably from recurrent carcinoma. He was unable to sustain himself by oral feeding, and there had been a thirty-five pound weight loss experienced in eight months, amounting to 26 per cent loss of his normal body weight. In Period 2, when

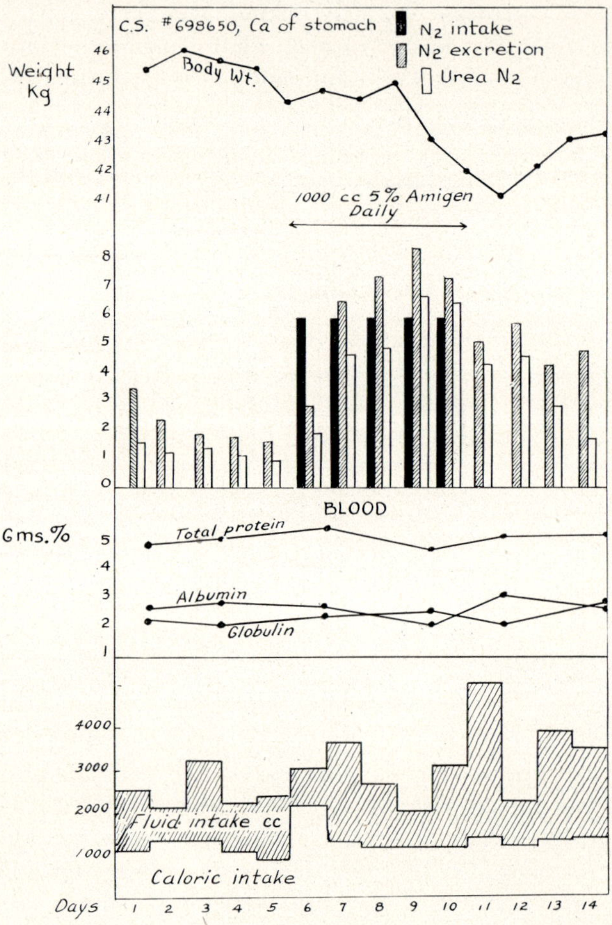

Fig. 3.—Nitrogen balance study attending the intravenous administration of amigen.

6 Gm. of nitrogen contained in 1000 c.c. of 5 per cent amigen solution was given intravenously daily as the sole source of nitrogen intake, a pyramiding of nitrogen excretion over the basal figure occurred and positive nitrogen balance could not be achieved. Again during the follow-up period (Period 3) the urinary nitrogen excretion gradually fell until it approached the basal figure. Similar results are shown in another study, on J. B., summarized in Table IV and Fig.

TABLE III. NITROGEN BALANCE STUDY ATTENDING INTRAVENOUS ADMINISTRATION OF AMIGEN

C. S., U. H. No. 698650, carcinoma of stomach

		URINE				BLOOD									
PERIOD	DATE	VOL. (C.C.)	TOTAL N_2 (GM.)	UREA N_2 (GM.)	AMINO ACID N_2 (GM.)	TOTAL PROTEIN (GM. %)	ALBUMIN (GM. %)	GLOBULIN (GM. %)	N.P.N. (MG. %)	B.U.N. (MG. %)	AMINO ACID (MG. %)	CAL. INTAKE	N_2 INTAKE (GM.)	WEIGHT (KG.)	FLUID INTAKE (C.C.)
1	12/18/40	1230	3.49	1.68	.096	5.0	2.77	2.23	24.3	20.2	5.3	1108	0	45.6	2600
	12/19/40	880	2.39	1.22	.097							1400	0	46.1	2215
	12/20/40	545	1.82	1.42	.056	5.16	2.99	2.17	23.3	10.3	7.5	1400	0	45.8	3300
	12/21/40	330	1.78	1.01	.060							1060	0	45.6	2325
	12/22/40	455	1.64	.79	.046							900	0	44.4	2400
	Total N_2		11.12									5% Amigen			
	Av. daily		2.56									1000 c.c.			
												I.V. daily			
2	12/23/40	755	2.75	1.98	.147	5.53	2.97	2.56	31.3	17.3	6.8	2200	6	44.7	3050
	12/24/40	1215	6.62	4.64	.279							1400	6	44.5	3600
	12/25/40	1195	7.52	4.97	.478							1200	6	45	2600
	12/26/40	880	8.43	6.72	.475	4.92	2.29	2.63	53	24	8.0	1200	6	43	2000
	12/27/40	820	7.43	6.54	.308							1200	6	42	3100
	Total N_2		32.75									Total N_2 30			
	Av. daily		6.55									Av. daily 6.0			
3	12/28/40	1010	5.13	4.38	.252	5.38	3.14	2.24	73	54	9.3				
	12/29/40	1030	5.77	4.69	.224							1400	0	41.2	5000
	12/30/40	1125	4.39	2.80	.127							1200	0	42.2	2200
	12/31/40	1320	4.09	2.69	.093	5.45	2.72	2.93	56	33	8.7	1300	0	43.0	3950
	Total N_2		19.38									1335	0	43.3	3500
	Av. daily		4.84												

TABLE IV. NITROGEN BALANCE STUDY ATTENDING THE INTRAVENOUS ADMINISTRATION OF PARENAMINE

J. B., U. H. No. 703888, appendicitis

		URINE				BLOOD									
PERIOD	DATE	VOL. (C.C.)	TOTAL N_2 (GM.)	UREA N_2 (GM.)	AMINO ACID N_2 (GM.)	TOTAL PROTEIN (GM. %)	ALBUMIN (GM. %)	GLOBULIN (GM. %)	UREA N_2 (MG. %)	N.P.N. (MG. %)	AMINO ACID (MG. %)	CAL. INTAKE	N_2 INTAKE (GM.)	WEIGHT (KG.)	FLUID INTAKE (C.C.)
1	3/18/41	3785	4.16	3.94	.246							1460	0	60.8	4650
	3/19/41	3030	3.18	.939	.276	7.13	3.97	3.16	4.7	21.6	5.7	1448	0	60.1	4400
	3/20/41	3430	3.18	.892	.261							1436	0	60.0	3650
	Total N_2		10.52									Parenamine I.V. daily			
	Av. daily		3.51												
2	3/21/41	3915	5.44	3.33	.458	6.85	4.04	2.81	5.0	24.3	7.7	1840	6.15	59.8	5600
	3/22/41	3055	6.32	3.48	.379							1578	6.15	60.4	5100
	3/23/41	3845	7.92	4.69	.400							1600	6.15	61.0	5400
	3/24/41	3715	9.99	6.59	.473	6.25	3.72	2.53	9.3	30	7.8	1700	6.15	60.5	5300
	3/25/41	3885	9.29	4.34	.415							1800	6.15	60.3	5100
	Total N_2		38.96								Total N_2		30.75		
	Av. daily		7.79								Av. daily		6.15		
3	3/26/41	3355	7.72	3.93	.309	5.84	2.41	3.43	13.5	30	6.0	1426	0	60.6	3950
	3/27/41	3425	4.72	2.81	.315							1446	0	59.3	4350
	3/28/41	2685	4.00	2.90	.234	6.01	3.80	2.21	12.0	29.0	6.25	1460	0	58.8	3450
	3/29/41	955	3.05	2.09	.115								0	57.3	2200
	3/30/41	1695	3.85	2.31	.188								0	57.8	2475
	Total N_2		23.34												
	Av. daily		4.67												

4. This patient, J. B. (U. H. No. 703888), a 68-year-old man, developed a small bowel obstruction subsequent to peritonitis from a ruptured appendix. This necessitated a decompressive enterostomy. The obstruction would recur when the enterostomy tube was clamped, or when oral feedings were allowed. For this reason, a period of parenteral feedings was elected. During the illness, the patient had lost twenty-eight pounds amounting to 18 per cent of his normal body weight. In this study 6.15 Gm. of nitrogen daily, in the casein digest

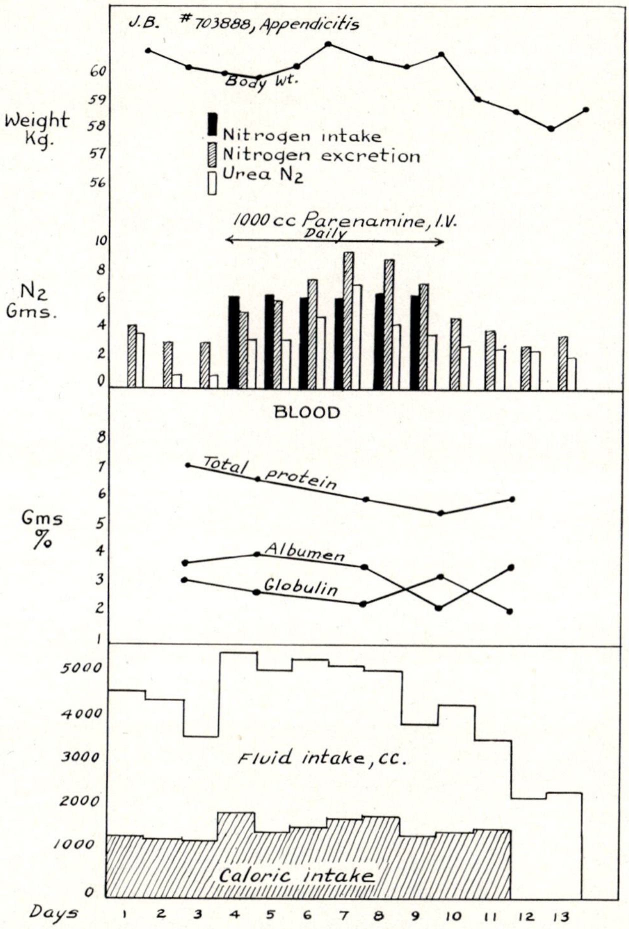

Fig. 4.—Nitrogen balance study attending intravenous administration of parenamine.

parenamine, given intravenously during Period 2, failed to produce positive nitrogen balance. It was noted (Tables III and IV) that the major portion of increased urinary nitrogen during the injection period was not amino acid nitrogen, although a slight increase of urine amino acid nitrogen did occur. This was more noticeable in Table III. The blood amino acid levels remained within normal limits throughout both studies. These determinations were done, however, from eight to twelve hours after injection of the casein digest and do not reflect the amino acid level during administration of the material. In

TABLE V. NITROGEN BALANCE STUDIES ATTEND
W. J., U. H. No. 773121, a

PERIOD	DATE (1947)	URINE: VOL. (C.C.)	SP. GR.	TOTAL N_2 (GM.)	UREA N_2 (GM.)	AMINO ACID N_2 (GM.)	AMMONIA N_2 (GM.)	CREATININE (GM.)	SUGAR (GM.)	INTAKE: VENOUS PR. CM. H_2O	NITROGEN INTAKE (GM.) / I.V. WHOLE BLOOD C.C.	GM. N_2	AGE (DAYS)	CAL. INTAKE	FL I TA (C
1	1/14	2180	1.005	11.70	7.02	.227	.366	1.09	2.79	8		0		2000	4
	1/15	5295	1.001	7.25	6.00	.290	.344	1.27	7.70			0		2000	5
	1/16	4425	1.003	7.66	6.62	.244	.176	1.64	3.63			0		1840	5
2	1/17	5130	1.002	8.98	6.83	.447	.246	1.39	5.08		490	13.2	2	1850	4
	1/18	3420	1.003	5.13	4.04	.220	.054	1.27	12.65		425	10.1	2	1600	4
	1/19 }*	9940	1.003	12.98	9.43	.710	.458	3.08	16.47		490	12.15	3	1840	4
	1/20 }										490	10.78	3	1850	4
	1/21	6150	1.001	6.33	5.78	.185	.369	1.38	2.02	5½	425	10.62	3	1600	4
	1/22	5230	1.007	5.60	4.18	.262	.424	1.41	6.22		380	7.18	3	1440	3
	1/23	4900	1.003	5.29	4.00	.131	.261	1.21	4.10		425	8.50	3	1800	4
			Total N_2	44.31							Total N_2	72.53			
			Av. daily	6.33							Av. daily	10.36			
3	1/24	2900	1.002	5.22	4.85	.218	.211	1.45	5.70	7		0		1720	4
	1/25	3540	1.005	5.80	4.77	.071	.265	1.27	4.07			0		1680	4
	1/26	4500	1.003	4.73	3.16	.113	.405	1.44	3.06			0		1680	4
	1/27	4280	1.003	4.84	4.07	.598	.212	1.07	2.19	6.0		0		1600	4

*Urine specimens over two days collected together.

Table III some azotemia apparently resulted during Period 2 which abated at the completion of the study. This effect was not noted in other studies with amigen.

In Table V and Fig. 5 are recorded the results of a nitrogen balance study on a patient in whom the sole source of protein intake consisted of whole blood transfusions. This patient, W. J. (U. H. No. 773121), a 65-year-old man, was admitted to the University Hospital with a diagnosis of carcinoma of the stomach. He had lost thirty pounds in weight, amounting to 20 per cent of his normal body weight, in the preceding six months. At the completion of this study, and without further preparation, the patient was operated upon (see Case 7, Chart 7), at which time a segment of lower ileum about 30 inches in length was resected because of obstructing metastatic carcinoma in that area.

During Period 1 the patient received no protein intake, the caloric intake being maintained by intravenous glucose solution. In Period 2 the patient received daily, in addition to the intravenous glucose, one bottle of whole blood preserved with citric acid dextrose mixture. All the blood given was three days old or less. Its total nitrogen content as determined on each specimen by macro Kjeldahl analysis is listed as the nitrogen intake. As noted during Period 2, this was associated with no increase in urinary nitrogen excretion.

E INTRAVENOUS ADMINISTRATION OF WHOLE BLOOD
years, carcinoma of stomach

	BLOOD											STOOL		
IGHT (KG.)	HB. (GM. %)	HE-MAT-OCRIT	R.B.C.	TOTAL PROT. (GM. %)	AL-BU-MIN (GM. %)	GLOB-ULIN (GM. %)	UREA N_2 (MG. %)	PLASMA CL. (MG. %)	URIC ACID (MG. %)	PLASMA VOL. (L.)	BLOOD VOL. (L.)	RETIC-ULO-CYTES (%)	N_2 (GM.)	URO-BIL-INOGEN (MG.)
5.9	13.3	42.5	4.07									0.7		
3.4														
5.6														
													Av. daily 0.5	31
5.0	12.8	41	4.2	6.50	4.12	2.36	16.8	590	2.5					
5.0														
5.4														
5.3	13.7	44	4.5	7.2	5.10	2.00	12.8	581	2.7	2.85	5.09			
3.2														
.4														
5												1.0		
													Av. daily 0.11	7.1
4.5	16.8	53.5	5.8	7.6	4.70	1.57	12.0	510	2.6	2.86	6.15			
5.8														
5.0														
.6	16.3	54.0	5.8	7.2	4.24	2.10	11.6	617	2.8	2.50	5.42			
													Av. daily 0.19	49.0

The slightly downward trend of urinary nitrogen excretion started on the first day of Period 1 is continued throughout the experiment until the end of Period 3. By the criteria of total nitrogen intake plotted against output, the patient was in marked positive nitrogen balance during the six-day period when whole blood transfusions constituted the sole source of protein intake.

No clinical ill effects due to the mild plethora produced by transfusion were noted either subjectively by the patient or objectively by physical examination. The venous pressure remained within normal limits throughout the experiment. Subjectively the patient felt stronger and his mental outlook was much more cheerful following the blood transfusions.

Unfortunately the specimens for blood volume determination on Jan. 17, 1947, were lost, and blood volume changes are known for only the last four days of Period 2. However, the changes here were quite definite. The blood volume increased entirely by virtue of increased red cell mass, with the plasma volume remaining constant and then falling somewhat after the transfusions were stopped. Also in Period 3 there was a fall in total circulating hemoglobin, although the hemoglobin and hematocrit levels remained fairly constant. From these data it appears that most of the injected plasma proteins contained in the whole blood soon leave the circulation, whereas all of the hemoglobin or red blood cells injected can be accounted for by an increase in the blood volume and, more particularly, its red blood cell component. Studies of the urobilinogen content of the stool, in an effort to demonstrate increased red blood cell destruction, were inconclusive. Although a definite increase was shown in Period 3, the total amounts are so small as to cast doubt as to their validity. Because the oral intake was restricted to only clear liquids, the amount of stool passed was quite meager. This may have been a factor in the results obtained.

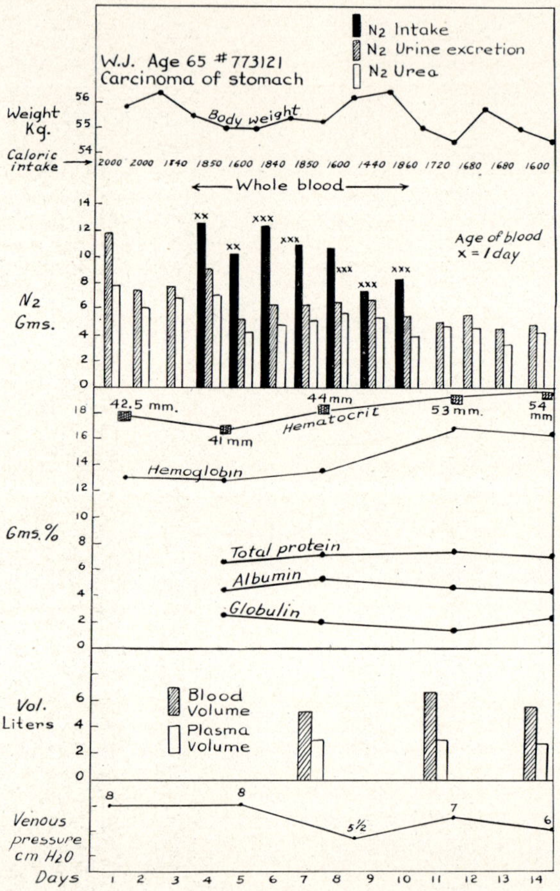

Fig. 5.—Nitrogen balance study attending the intravenous administration of whole blood.

Since it has been shown by Flink and Skubi,[68] Ross and Chapin,[174] and others[14] that there is an increased destruction of stored citrated blood following its transfusion, as compared to fresh blood, a study as tabulated in Table VI and Fig. 6 was carried out. This patient, J. T. (U. H. No. 775120), a 66-year-old man, was admitted to the University Hospital with a diagnosis of carcinoma of the esophageal gastric junction. He had lost forty-five pounds, amounting to 30 per cent of his normal body weight, and was unable to maintain his nutrition by oral means. At the completion of this study the patient was operated upon (Case 9, Chart 9).

Results quite similar to those in W. J., Table V, Fig. 5, were obtained. Whereas in W. J., blood three days old or less was used for transfusion, in J. T., all transfused blood was seven days old or more. During Period 2 no augmentation of urinary nitrogen excretion over Period 1, when only glucose was given, was noted. Also in the succeeding days, Period 3, there was no increased urinary nitrogen excretion over the preliminary basal period. On the contrary, the nitrogen conservation in Period 3 is considerably more efficient than

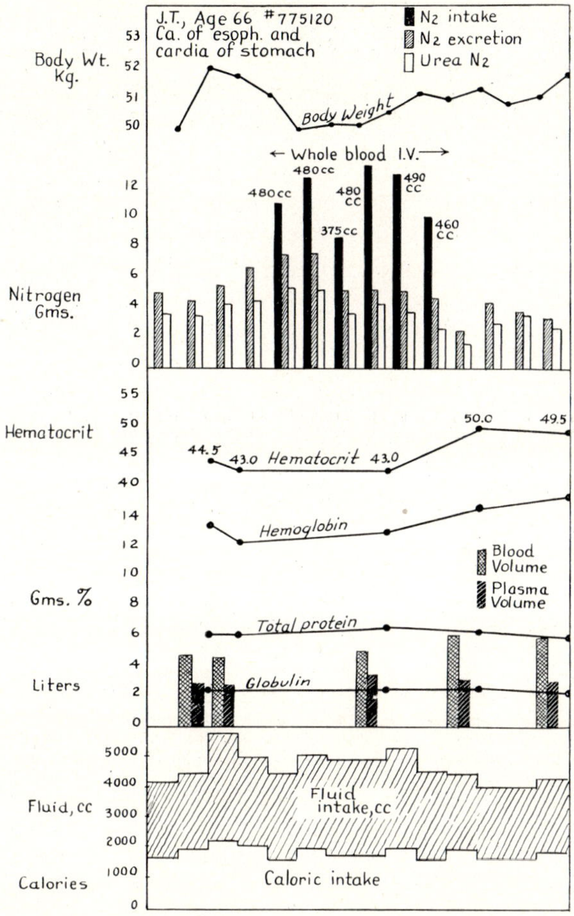

Fig. 6.—Nitrogen balance study attending the intravenous administration of whole blood.

during Period 1, as noted by respective figures of 14.53 as the total nitrogen excretion in the four days of Period 3 as against 22.15 for the four days of Period 1. Again during Period 2, if one considers only total nitrogen intake, marked positive nitrogen balance resulted.

The effect of the transfusions was quite closely mirrored by changes in the patient's blood. Ninety per cent of the transfused red blood cells can be accounted for by the increased blood volume and total red cell mass. Plasma volume changes were less marked, with about 50 per cent of the total plasma

TABLE VI. NITROGEN BALANCE STUDY ATTEND[illegible]
J. T., U. H. No. 775120, aged 66 yea[illegible]

				URINE						INTAKE				
PERIOD	DATE (1947)	VOL. (C.C.)	SP. GR.	TOTAL N_2 (GM.)	UREA N_2 (GM.)	AMINO ACID N_2 (GM.)	AMMONIA N_2 (GM.)	CREATININE (GM.)	SUGAR (GM.)		NITROGEN INTAKE (GM.)		CAL. INTAKE	FLU[illegible] IN[illegible] TA[illegible] (C.[illegible]
1	1/29	1950	1.002	5.29	3.83	0.247	0.380	0.917	1.13		0		1680	42[illegible]
	1/30	4300	1.005	4.47	3.71	0.245	0.593	0.774	36.1		0		1820	45[illegible]
	1/31	3140	1.006	5.53	4.29	0.298	0.226	1.162	30.8		0		2280	57[illegible]
	2/1	3500	1.007	6.86	4.61	0.409	0.466	1.400	24		0		2000	50[illegible]
		Total N_2		22.15										
		Av. daily		5.54										
										I.V. WHOLE BLOOD C.C.	GM. N_2	AGE (DAYS)		
	2/2 } 2/3 }*	6680	1.007	15.49	10.79	1.358	1.358	2.406	71	480	11.28	8	1632	44[illegible]
										480	12.62	9	1850	50[illegible]
2	2/4	2300	1.010	5.15	3.87	0.287	0.127	0.759	23.8	375	8.81	8	1700	50[illegible]
	2/5	3000	1.010	5.22	4.39	0.120	0.261	0.990	37.5	480	13.68	7	1700	50[illegible]
	2/6	3650	1.008	5.00	3.82	0.438	0.467	1.200	50.9	490	13.08	7	1900	54[illegible]
	2/7	3100	1.002	4.71	2.63	0.583	0.930	0.992	14.6	460	10.02	7	1600	46[illegible]
		Total N_2		35.57							69.49			
		Av. daily		5.93							11.58			
3	2/8	2960	1.006	2.55	1.83	0.207	0.530	0.829	26.1		0		1800	45[illegible]
	2/9	3400	1.003	4.21	3.06	0.340	0.340	1.258	12.8		0		1600	40[illegible]
	2/10	3800	1.005	3.99	3.83	0.342	0.247	1.102	30.4		0		1600	40[illegible]
	2/11	2250	1.012	3.78	2.78	0.203	0.339				0		1760	44[illegible]
		Total N_2		14.53							0			
		Av. daily		3.63							0			

*Urine collected over two days as one specimen.

protein contained in the donor blood or their equivalent having left the circulation. Again the stool urobilinogen studies were inconclusive probably for the same reasons as in the study of W. J., although there was an increase noted in Periods 2 and 3 over the control, Period 1. During this fourteen-day period, while nutrition was maintained by parenteral means, the patient's weight remained constant. Subjectively and objectively the patient felt better and stronger than he had before the study was started. From data on Mrs. C. N. (Case 6, Chart 6, U. H. No. 775502), a similar retention of transfused hemoglobin occurred. On Feb. 5, 1947, the following findings were noted. Hemoglobin was 5.6 Gm. per cent, hematocrit was 23.5, plasma volume was 2.18 L., and blood volume 2.84 L. The total circulating hemoglobin (5.6 by 2.84 by 10) was 159 Gm. In the next five days, she received 4,500 c.c. of whole blood by transfusion. On Feb. 10, 1947, the patient's hemoglobin was 16.5 Gm. per cent, hematocrit was 58.5, the plasma volume was unchanged at 2.18 L. The total blood volume was 5.29 L. The total circulating hemoglobin (16.5 by 5.29 by 10) was 872 Gm. Assuming the donor blood to contain 15 Gm. of hemoglobin per 100 c.c., 675 Gm. of hemoglobin were administered. Allowing for errors in technique this constitutes complete retention of transfused red blood cells in the circulation.

e INTRAVENOUS ADMINISTRATION OF WHOLE BLOOD
cinoma of esophagus and cardia of stomach

	BLOOD												STOOL	
IGHT KG.)	HB. (GM. %)	HE-MAT-OCRIT	R.B.C.	TOTAL PROT. (GM. %)	AL-BU-MIN (GM. %)	GLOB-ULIN (GM. %)	UREA N_2 (MG. %)	PLASMA CL. (MG. %)	URIC ACID (MG. %)	PLASMA VOL. (L.)	BLOOD VOL. (L.)	RETIC-ULO-CYTES (%)	N (GM.)	URO-BILO-GEN (MG.)
0												1.4		
2	13.7	44.5	4.72	6.2	3.74	2.50	10.0	564	2.5	2.77	4.99			
1.8	12.6	43.0	4.56	6.2						2.49	4.37			
1.2												1.1		
													0.893	21.6
													0.223	5.4
0.0														
0.2														
0.2														
0.6	13.15	43.0	4.5	6.6	3.52	2.54	14.1	598	2.5	3.14	5.50			
1.2														
1.0												0.6		
													3.82	106.8
													.64	17.8
1.4	14.7	50	5.32	6.4	3.28	2.70	9.0	600	3.0	3.11	6.22			
0.9														
1.0														
0.8	15.5	49.5	5.26	6.0	3.4	2.36	11.4	550	3.0	3.14	6.21			
													1.05	84.4
													.26	21.1

Table VII and Fig. 7 show the results of a nitrogen balance study attending the intravenous administration of whole blood and amigen separately. The patient, T. A. (U. H. No. 773207), was a 53-year-old woman admitted to the University Hospital with a carcinoma at the outlet of the stomach producing complete obstruction. The patient had been unable to take and retain any food by mouth. She had lost thirty-five pounds in weight, amounting to 25 per cent loss of her normal body weight. The study was terminated on the third postoperative day after a gastric resection when it became possible for the patient to take food by mouth again (see Case 4, Chart 4).

During Period 1, while the patient was receiving no protein, the urinary nitrogen excretion averaged 4.8 Gm. per day. When the patient received 500 c.c. of whole blood daily, in addition to 3,000 c.c. of 10 per cent glucose intravenously, the urinary nitrogen excretion remained close to the basal level. In Period 3 when the patient received 24 Gm. of nitrogen daily as 4,000 c.c. of 5 per cent amigen in 5 per cent glucose solution, a marked rise of urinary nitrogen excretion resulted. However, there still occurred a fairly strong positive nitrogen balance with the amigen, an average daily urinary nitrogen excretion of 18.98 Gm. against an average daily nitrogen intake of 24 Gm. associated with the administration of intravenous amigen. In Period 3, there was a weight gain of three kilograms. This is not a true weight gain, but a retention of water by the body. Such an effect has been noted in other instances when large amounts of amigen have been given intravenously. It does not appear to be due to sodium chloride effect alone for the sodium chloride content of amigen as given by the manufacturer is 3 per cent of the dried powder. For 200 Gm. of amigen, the amount given in this experiment, this would make a sodium chloride intake of 6 Gm. per day, an amount hardly enough to produce edema in a patient with apparently normal renal function.

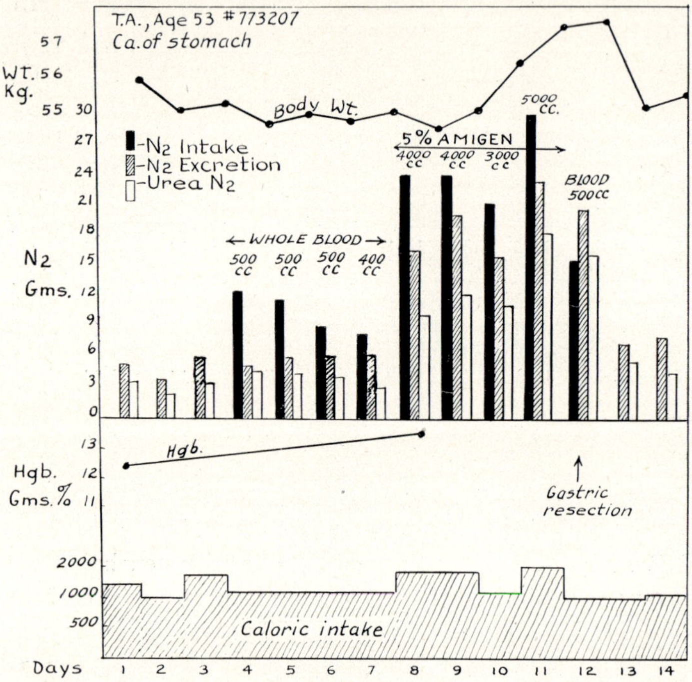

Fig. 7.—Nitrogen balance study attending the intravenous administration of whole blood and amigen.

Tables VIII and IX, Figs. 8 and 9, show the results of two similar studies. E. E. (U. H. No. 764398) was a 59-year-old white man who in the preceding eight months had noticed marked asthenia, loss of appetite, and a weight loss of one hundred pounds, amounting to thirty-five per cent of his normal body weight. On admission to the hospital, x-ray examination revealed a large carcinoma of the stomach producing a high-grade obstruction at the gastric outlet. C. A. (U. H. No. 768842) was a 64-year-old white man with a carcinoma involving the upper third of the esophagus. The patient had been unable to take any food other than small amounts of clear liquids by mouth for the preceding two weeks. Symptoms in all were of about six months' duration. During this time, the patient had lost fifty pounds, amounting to 30 per cent of his usual body weight. After a preliminary period of zero nitrogen intake, 3,000 c.c. of 5 per cent amigen in 5 per cent glucose solution containing 18 Gm.

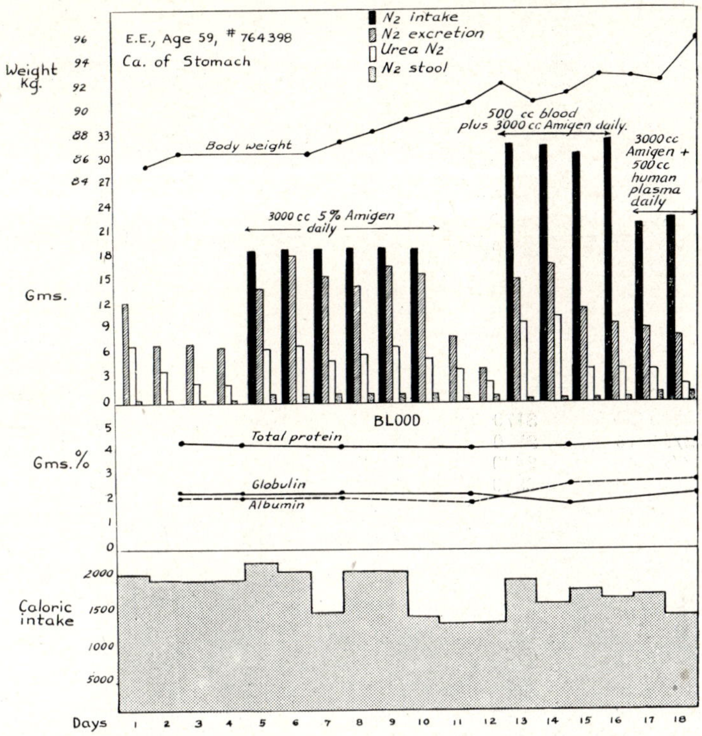

Fig. 8.—Nitrogen balance study attending the intravenous use of amigen, human plasma, and whole blood.

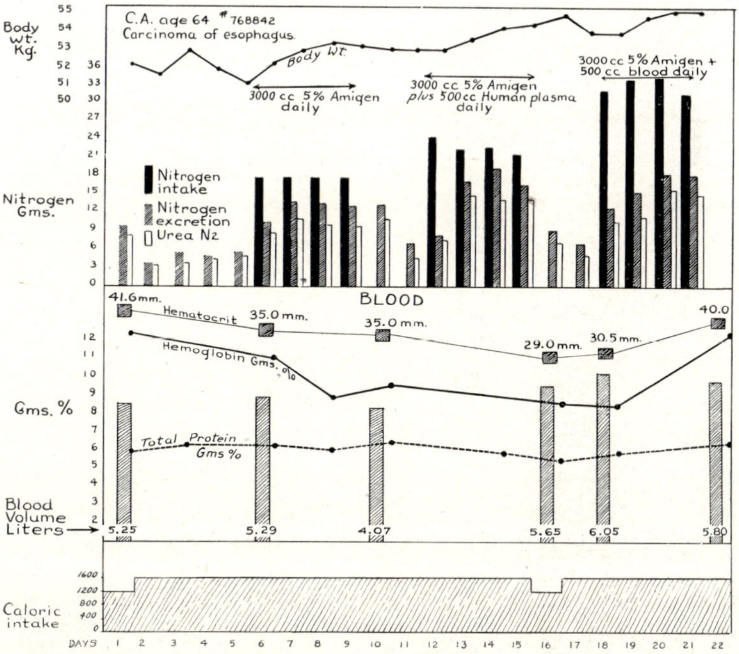

Fig. 9.—Nitrogen balance study attending the intravenous administration of amigen, human plasma, and whole blood.

TABLE VII. NITROGEN BALANCE STUDY ATTENDING T
T. A., U. H. No. 773207, ag

		OUTPUT					
PERIOD	DATE	VOLUME (C.C.)	SPECIFIC GRAVITY	TOTAL N_2 (GM.)	UREA N_2 (GM.)	AMINO ACID (GM.)	CREATINI (GM.)
1	12/ 7/46	1490	1.012	5.16	3.39	0.450	1.340
	12/ 8/46	1620	1.005	3.67	2.61	0.98	0.810
	12/ 9/46	4690	1.011	5.47	3.75	1.20	1.870
			Total	14.30			
			Av. daily	4.86			
	12/10/46	3170	1.012	4.82	3.85	0.190	1.080
2	12/11/46	2550	1.005	5.92	4.19	0.630	0.765
	12/12/46	2690	1.005	5.98	3.79	1.23	0.646
	12/13/46	2890	1.006	5.95	2.97	1.67	0.434
			Total	22.67			
			Av. daily	5.53			
3	12/14/46	2430	1.012	16.67	10.64	3.600	1.940
	12/15/46	2300	1.017	19.96	12.18	2.980	1.47
	12/16/46	2230	1.012	15.97	11.09	2.39	1.27
	12/17/46	3160	1.012	23.31	18.07	2.27	1.07
			Total	75.91			
			Av. daily	18.98			
4	12/18/46*	3115	1.021	20.87	15.78	3.19	1.31
	12/19/46	2140	1.008	7.48	5.47	0.77	0.984
	12/20/46	1540	1.006	7.99	4.54	1.35	1.108

*Day of operation, gastric resection.

of nitrogen were given intravenously daily (Period 2). In both studies positive nitrogen balance was obtained, although it was more marked in C. A., Table IX. As happens uniformly when giving casein digests parenterally, there is a pyramiding of urinary nitrogen excretion. When using smaller amounts of the digest (see Tables II, III, and IV), this increased nitrogen excretion was so marked that positive nitrogen balance could not be obtained. However, when the amount of digest is increased, although the urinary nitrogen excretion is also increased, a stage is reached where positive nitrogen balance can uniformly be obtained. This had been achieved without fail in five instances where 18 Gm. of nitrogen contained in amigen were given daily. From Tables VIII and IX, it can be noted that most of the increased urinary nitrogen excretion is not in the amino acid fraction. This latter fraction increases only when excessively large amounts of amigen are given too rapidly as in T. A., Table VII, when up to 3 Gm. of amino acid nitrogen appeared in the urine. In the days following the administration of amigen, the urinary nitrogen excretion promptly returned to its original level, although for a day following the injection of amigen there may be some increased urinary nitrogen loss. When amigen is administered in conjunction with human plasma (Period 5, Table

TRAVENOUS ADMINISTRATION OF WHOLE BLOOD AND AMIGEN
years, carcinoma of stomach

		INTAKE					BLOOD	
MMONIA N_2 (GM.)	SUGAR (GM.)	NITROGEN INTAKE (GM.)		CALORIC INTAKE	FLUID INTAKE	WEIGHT (KG.)	H.B. (GM.)	TOTAL PROTEIN (GM.)
1.082	28.2	0		1400	4000	56	12.5	6.3
0.972	19.2	0		1000	3200	55.2		
1.08	49.1	0		1760	4450	55.4		
		I.V. WHOLE BLOOD						
		GM. N_2	VOL. (C.C.)					
0.713	29.4	12.305	500	1200	4100	54.8		
0.650	12.0	11.685	500	1200	4350	55.0		
0.37	19.0	9.820	500	1200	3800	54.9		
0.208	35.1	7.320	400	1200	3975	55.2		
	Total	41.30						
	Av. daily	10.280						
		I.V. AMIGEN						
		GM. N_2						
1.510	11.79	24.0		1750	5000	54.6	13.6	7.5
1.85	11.85	24.0		1750	4500	55.2		
1.85	10.8	18.0		1200	3700	56.6		
1.52	12.9	30.0		2000	5400	57.6		
	Total	96.0						
	Av. daily	24.0						
		I.V. BLOOD						
1.91	67.9	15.05		1000	3400	57.8		
1.37	26.5	0		1000	3400	55.2		
0.88	2.14	0		1100	3700	55.6		

VIII; Period 4, Table IX), a more marked positive nitrogen balance results. The urinary nitrogen excretion while getting amigen plus plasma was slightly higher in Table IX and slightly lower in Table VIII than when getting amigen alone. However, the results obtained in Period 5, Table VIII, may not reflect a true state of affairs, for during this period the urinary volume decreased markedly, the patient gained three kilograms and developed mild edema. Following this period the patient's condition became precarious and the study had to be discontinued. Nitrogen retention is even more marked when amigen plus whole blood is given (Table VIII, Period 4; Table IX, Period 6). Here again the urinary nitrogen loss remains about at the same level as with amigen alone, whereas the nitrogen intake is markedly increased. In Period 6, Table IX, only about 66 per cent of the injected hemoglobin from the 2,000 c.c. of blood given can be accounted for by an increase of hemoglobin level and blood volume. The cause of the anemia which developed during the study (Table IX) is not definite. It may only partially be explained on the basis of blood loss due to repeated blood specimens taken for analysis which amounted to 450 c.c. removed by Aug. 15, 1946. There were no other known sources of blood loss and examination of the stools showed no marked loss by that avenue.

TABLE VIII. NITROGEN BALANCE STUDY ATTENDING THE INTRAVENC

E. E., U. H. No. 764398, a

		URINE						
PERIOD	DATE	VOLUME (C.C.)	SPECIFIC GRAVITY	TOTAL N_2 (GM.)	UREA N_2 (GM.)	AMINO ACID N_2 (GM.)	CREATININE (GM.)	AMMON N_2 (GM.)
1	4/12/46	1680	1.022	12.56	6.8	0.47	1.02	0.59
	4/13/46	1640	1.010	7.3	3.9	0.1	0.71	0.35
	4/14/46	2140	1.012	7.5	2.5	0.0	0.77	0.47
	4/15/46	2280	1.005	6.7	2.2	0.103	0.63	0.51
			Total	34.06				
			Av. daily	8.51				
2	4/16/46	2470	1.010	14.3	6.6	0.395	0.84	0.34
	4/17/46	1880	1.017	18.1	7.3	0.27	0.85	0.40
	4/18/46	1550	1.013	15.43	5.6	0.18	0.81	0.36
	4/19/46	1880	1.018	14.86	6.0	0.29	0.77	0.40
	4/20/46	1990	1.020	17.9	7.1	0.26	0.79	1.25
	4/21/46	1430	1.020	16.12	5.7	0.20	0.72	0.97
			Total	96.71				
			Av. daily	16.12				
3	4/22/46	1350	1.020	8.6	4.5	0.2	0.614	0.58
	4/23/46	1015	1.012	4.37	2.5	0.1	0.426	0.35
4	4/24/46	2470	1.017	15.29	10.1	0.4	0.79	0.42
	4/25/46	2100	1.017	17.1	7.9	0.34	0.79	0.44
	4/26/46	1550	1.018	11.4	4.4	0.22	0.54	0.40
	4/27/46	1010	1.018	9.8	3.94	0.12	0.65	0.16
			Total	53.59				
			Av. daily	13.39				
5	4/28/46	840	1.015	9.22	3.2	0.13	0.42	0.126
	4/29/46	485	1.027	5.83	1.89	0.08	0.421	0.136
			Total	15.05				
			Av. daily	7.52				

PRESENTATION OF CLINICAL CASES: CLINICAL RESULT OF THE PREPARATION BY PARENTERAL MEANS OF POOR-RISK PATIENTS FOR SURGERY

The following case histories are presented as representative of patients requiring preoperative preparation by parenteral feedings, either as the sole source of protein and caloric intake, or as a supplement to an inadequate oral intake. A record of the pulse and blood pressure during operation, and of the postoperative clinical course, is shown with each case history.

CASE 1.—A. S., (U. H. No. 688258), a 65-year-old man, was admitted to the University of Minnesota Hospitals on Aug. 26, 1946, with a four-month history of having experienced a thirty pound weight loss amounting to 20 per cent loss of his normal body weight, anorexia, and a feeling of gaseous distress in the epigastrium. The patient had been unable to eat solid foods for one month prior to admission to the hospital. General physical examination revealed a pale appearing white man in no acute distress. Temperature

ministration of Amigen, Human Plasma, and Whole Blood
years, carcinoma of stomach

	Stool							Blood			
gar (m.)	Total N_2 (Gm.)	Caloric Intake	N_2 Intake (Gm.)		Fluid Intake (c.c.)	Weight (Kg.)	Total Protein (Gm. %)	Alb. (Gm. %)	Glob. (Gm. %)	Urea N_2 (Mg. %)	Uric Acid (Mg. %)
7.3		2002	0		3100	85.9					
4.8		1930	0		3500	86.8	4.38	2.15	2.23	12.8	4.5
7.9		1930	0		3400						
2.0		1930	0		3450		4.31	2.10	2.20	11.0	3.24
Total	1.78										
Av. daily	.44										
			I.V. 3000 c.c. 5% Amigen								
5.1		2367	18		4250						
4.2		2080	18		4000	86.8					
4.2		1460	18		3600	87.7	4.28	2.04	2.24	14	3.35
5.7		2080	18		4000	88.6					
0.5		2080	18		4000	89.5					
0.3		1488	18		4000						
Total	6.04	Total N_2	108.0								
Av. daily	1.01	Av. daily	18.0								
4.7		1296	0		2400	90.9	4.16	1.93	2.23	12.5	4.3
1.12		1296	0		2600	92.3					
Total	6.12		3000 5% Amigen I.V.	500 c.c. Blood I.V.							
Av. daily	.81										
4.62		1842	18	14.15	4000	91.1	4.22	1.95	2.27	11.0	3.5
4.3		1696	18	14.0	4000	91.6					
3.2		1746	18	13.3	3700	93 0					
2.5		1650	18	14.8	4200	93 0					
Total	2.44	Total N_2	128.25								
Av. daily	0.61	Av. daily	32.06								
				(Plasma I.V.)							
2.5		1677	18	4.63	4600	92.7					
1.82		1425	18	4.81	4250	96.1	4.43	2.62	1.81	19	
Total	2.08	Total N_2	45.44								
Av. daily	1.04	Av. daily	22.72								

was 98.6°F., pulse was 76 and blood pressure was 110/70 mm. Hg. There was a suggestive mass in the epigastrium, but no other abnormalities were noted on physical examination. Gastrointestinal x-ray studies revealed a large polypoid carcinoma of the stomach with considerable retention of barium after four hours. Hemoglobin on admission was 12.5 Gm. per cent, white blood count was 7,500 with a normal differential. Blood urea nitrogen was 15 mg. per cent, blood chlorides were 568, and total plasma proteins were 5.1 Gm. per cent. Urinalysis was negative.

The patient was prepared almost entirely by parenteral means. Whatever was taken by mouth was lost by gastric aspirations and vomitus. He received 3000 c.c. daily of 5 per cent amigen in 5 per cent glucose solution intravenously plus therapeutic doses of vitamin B, C, and K, for seven days. In addition, during this time, the patient received 500 c.c. of whole blood and 500 c.c. of human plasma.

On Sept. 3, 1946, the patient was operated upon. Exploration of the peritoneal cavity revealed a large carcinoma of the stomach with infiltration into the lesser omentum and involvement of lymph nodes along both curvatures. A gastric resection was performed removing about 80 per cent of the stomach and all palpable involved nodes. The operation

TABLE IX. NITROGEN BALANCE STUDY ATTENDING THE INTRAVEN(
C. A., U. H. No. 768842, a

				URINE						STOOL	
PERIOD	DATE (1946)	VOL. (C.C.)	SP. GR.	TOTAL N_2 (GM.)	UREA N_2 (GM.)	AMINO ACID N_2 (GM.)	CREAT-ININE (GM.)	AM-MONIA N_2 (GM.)	SUGAR (GM.)	TOTAL N_2 (GM.)	BLO DRAV (C.C
1	7/31	2450	1.015	9.70	7.60	0.290	1.52	1.47	26.46		66
	8/1	1570	1.022	4.53	4.08	0.100	0.59	0.99	58.09		
	8/2	2930	1.013	5.89	4.10	0.162	0.64	1.55	23.19		20
	8/3	3840	1.013	5.52	4.56	0.261	1.34	1.70	82.17		
	8/4	1990	1.012	5.71	4.99	0.237	0.99	1.18	33.43		
			Total	31.35						Total 0.86	
			Av. daily	6.27						Av. daily .17	
2	8/5	2450	1.010	10.05	7.35	0.382	0.71	1.41	2.11		86
	8/6	2400	1.006	13.93	11.10	0.266	1.01	1.23	1.73		
	8/7	2740	1.004	13.48	10.96	0.482	0.47	1.58	2.11		
	8/8	2860	1.007	13.38	10.81	0.295	0.83	1.15	3.09		20
			Total	50.84						Lost	
			Av. daily	12.71							
3	8/9	3450	1.005	13.58	11.30	0.173	0.90	2.00	4.35		86
	8/10	3350	1.005	7.14	4.76	0.184	0.97	1.27	1.71	0	
4	8/11	2940	1.004	8.38	6.40	0.188	0.91	1.54	1.85		66
	8/12	3470	1.005	17.14	14.99	0.413	1.01	1.70	2.78		
	8/13	3750	1.007	18.30	14.63	0.375	0.98	1.32	3.08		20
	8/14	2830	1.008	15.34	13.24	0.396	0.934	0.85	2.92		
			Total	59.16						Total 0.70	
			Av. daily	14.79						Av. daily 0.17	
5	8/15	2000	1.004	8.28	7.20	0.238	0.88	1.08	1.36		86
	8/16	3460	1.007	6.32	5.19	0.132	0.83	1.59	4.67		
			Total	14.60						Total 0.62	
			Av. daily	7.30						Av. daily 0.31	
6	8/17	2350	1.009	12.48	10.22	0.778	1.10	1.25	3.36		91
	8/18	3650	1.006	15.11	11.03	0.689	0.95	1.99	1.61		5
	8/19	3370	1.008	18.54	16.18	0.815	1.08	1.35	5.19		5
	8/20	3180	1.007	18.19	14.91	0.804	1.05	1.81	2.16		5
			Total	64.32						0	
			Av. daily	16.08							
	8/21										

lasted five and one-half hours, during which time the patient received 1000 c.c. of whole blood and 1000 c.c. of 5 per cent glucose solution. The patient's postoperative course was uneventful. His highest temperature was 101.6°F. by rectum on the first postoperative day. He was allowed out of bed on the first day after operation and left the hospital on the sixth postoperative day.

Case 2.—E. P. (U. H. No. 772109), a 49-year-old white woman, was admitted to the University of Minnesota Hospitals on November 5, 1946, and discharged Nov. 20, 1946. She gave a history that dated back one year when the onset of vomiting was first noted. At the start, this occurred chiefly at night, but as time went on it occurred after every meal. Along with the vomiting and a progressive weight loss, which amounted in all to about forty-five pounds or 30 per cent loss of her normal body weight, the patient noted epigastric distress and weakness.

MINISTRATION OF AMIGEN, HUMAN PLASMA, AND WHOLE BLOOD
years, carcinoma of esophagus

INTAKE					BLOOD								
NITROGEN INTAKE (GM.)		CAL. INTAKE (GM.)	FLUID INTAKE	WEIGHT (KG.)	HB. (GM. %)	HEMATOCRIT	TOTAL PROT. (GM. %)	ALBUMIN (GM. %)	GLOBULIN (GM. %)	UREA N_2 (MG. %)	PLASMA CL. (MG. %)	URIC ACID (MG. %)	VOL. (L.)
0		1200	3000	52.2	12.20	41.6	6.00	3.47	2.03	10.3	495	1.90	5.25
0		1600	4000	51.8									
0		1600	4000	53.0			6.25	3.55	1.97	12.8	570	2.28	
0		1600	4000	52.0									
0		1600	4000	51.2									
3000 c.c. 5% AMIGEN I.V.													
18		1600	4000	52.4	11.00	35.0	6.25	3.55	2.28	13.7	521	2.50	5.29
18		1600	4000	53.0									
18		1600	4000	53.4	9.00		6.00	3.67	2.14	15.0	602	2.90	
18		1600	4000	53.2									
al	72.0												
daily	18.0												
0		1600	4000	53.0	9.65	35.0	6.40	3.43	2.10	13.7	566	2.45	
0 5% V. GEN	500 c.c. I.V. HUMAN PLASMA												
8	6.15	1600	4500	53.0									
8	4.45	1600	4500	53.6									
8	4.60	1600	4500	54.2			5.90	2.93	2.08	13.7	586	2.00	
8	4.15	1600	4500	54.4									
al	91.35												
daily	22.84												
0		1200	3000	55.0	8.40	29.0	5.40	3.11	1.73	17.0	520	1.95	5.65
0		1600	4000	54.0									
0 5% . GEN	500 c.c. I.V. BLOOD												
8	14.95	1600	4500	54.0	8.65	30.5	5.90	3.21	2.28	15.0		2.50	6.05
8	16.05	1600	4500	54.8									
8	16.75	1600	4500	55.2									
8	14.05	1600	4500	55.2									
al	133.8												
daily	33.45												
					12.05	40.0	6.20	3.55	2.00	24.0		2.21	5.80

General physical examination revealed a cooperative white woman showing evidence of recent weight loss. Blood pressure was 130/80 mm. Hg., pulse was 80, and temperature was 98.6° F. In the midepigastrium, a hard nontender mass about 7 cm. in diameter was noted. The remainder of the physical examination was essentially negative. Gastrointestinal x-ray examination revealed a large annular mass in the distal half of the stomach, past which barium flowed with only slight difficulty. Admission laboratory study revealed a negative urinalysis; hemoglobin was 10.4 Gm. per cent; white blood count was 7,350 with a normal differential. Blood urea nitrogen was 8 mg. per cent, blood chlorides were 658 mg. per cent, and total plasma proteins were 5.8 Gm. per cent. Preoperative preparation extended over a nine-day period during which time the patient received intravenously 3000 c.c. of 5 per cent amigen in 5 per cent glucose solution plus therapeutic doses of vitamins B, C, and K, added to the fluids daily. In addition, during this time, the patient received three transfusions of whole blood, a total of 1,500 c.c. Oral intake consisted of University Hospital

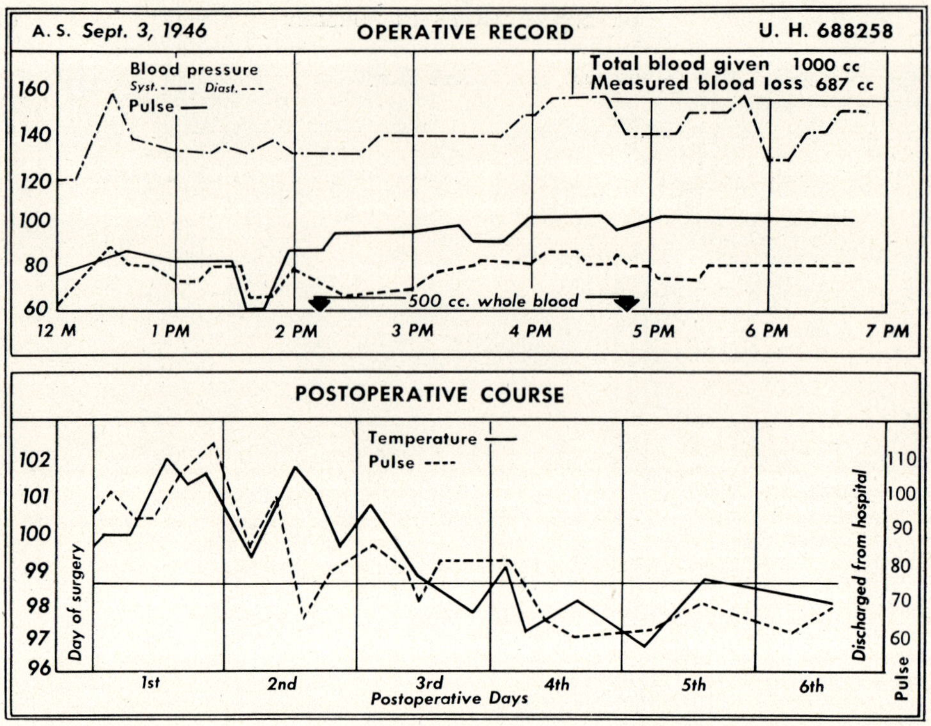

Chart 1.

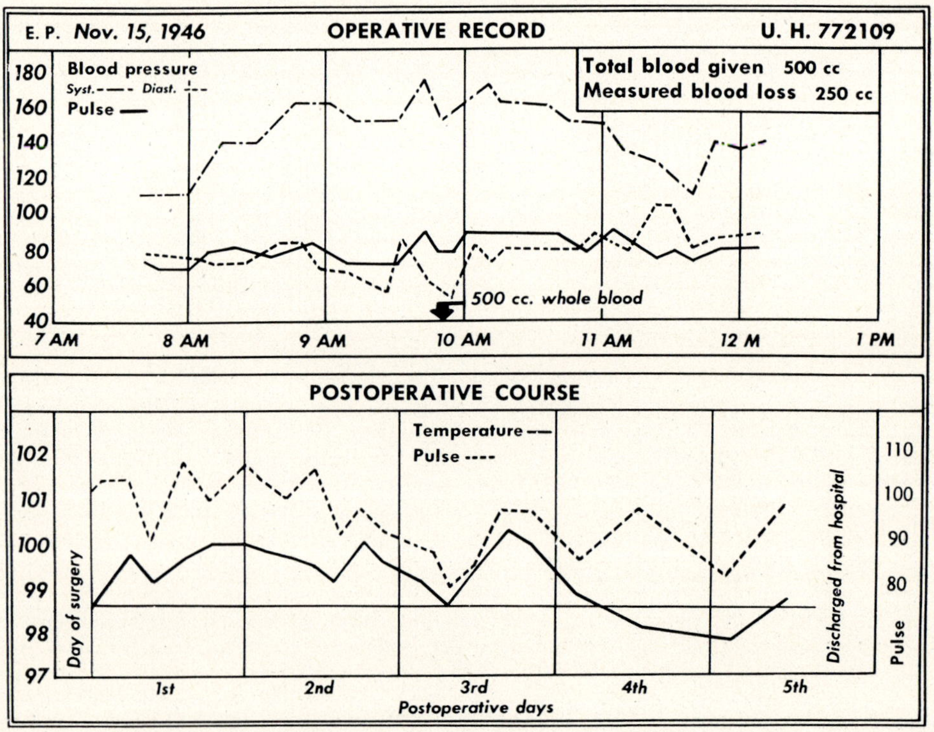

Chart 2.

Diet 2204 in amounts from 500 to 1,500 c.c. daily, plus about 500 c.c. of water and fruit juice. However, at least one-half of the daily oral intake was lost by vomiting or gastric aspirations and at times almost the entire oral intake was lost. During this period the patient's weight increased from 51 kilograms on November 6, to 54.6 kilograms on November 14, the day before surgery.

Nov. 15, 1946, the patient was operated upon. A large carcinoma involving the lower half of the stomach was found. A gastric resection removing 75 per cent of the stomach was carried out. In addition, since the gall bladder contained numerous stones, it was removed, and an appendectomy was also performed. The operation lasted four hours during which time the patient received 500 c.c. of whole blood. The measured blood loss was 250 c.c.

The postoperative course was smooth and uncomplicated. The patient was allowed out of bed on the first postoperative day and left the hospital on the fifth postoperative day.

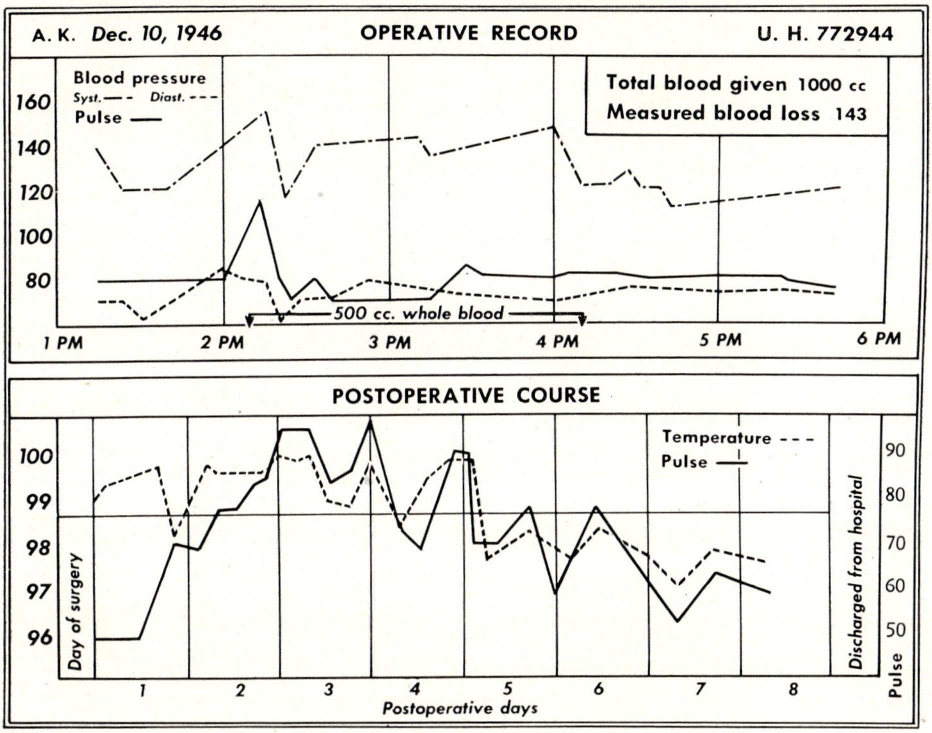

Chart 3.

Case 3.—A. K. (U. H. No. 772944), a 60-year-old woman was admitted to the University of Minnesota Hospitals on Nov. 30, 1946. The illness at time of admission dated back about seven months when the patient first became aware of vague epigastric pains and distress and of a sense of early satiety after eating. These symptoms became progressively more marked, to be followed by progressive weight loss, amounting to a total loss of fifty pounds during the illness or about 30 per cent of her normal weight, and increasingly frequent spells of vomiting. There had been no melena or hematemesis. For the month preceding admission to the hospital the patient had noted a mass in the epigastrium, which was especially prominent after eating.

General physical examination revealed a fairly comfortable, stoical, white woman. Although there was evidence of weight loss as noted by loose flabby skin, the patient did not appear markedly emaciated. Blood pressure was 130/74 mm. Hg., pulse was 72, and temperature 98.6° F. The only finding of note on physical examination was a large, firm, nontender mass in the left upper quadrant, about 8 by 16 cm. in diameter. Gastrointestinal x-ray studies on three occasions revealed an extremely dilated stomach with many retained food particles and an area of complete obstruction at the pylorus. On three examinations it was impossible to get sufficient barium past the obstructing lesion, so that a diagnosis other than high-grade obstruction could be made. Laboratory studies revealed a negative urinalysis, hemoglobin was 10.3 Gm. per cent, white blood count was 4,300 with a normal differential. Blood urea nitrogen was 17 mg. per cent and the total plasma proteins were 4.9 Gm. per cent. For nine days the patient received 3000 c.c. of 5 per cent amigen in 5 per cent glucose solution, plus therapeutic doses of vitamins B, C, and K, daily. In addition, during the nine-day preoperative preparation period, the patient received 1,500 c.c. of whole blood. The patient took about 1,000 c.c. of University Hospital Diet 2 daily by mouth, but over one-half of this was vomited or removed by aspirations.

On Dec. 10, 1946, the patient was operated upon. An obstructing carcinoma of the prepyloric area of the stomach was found with a huge dilated stomach. A 75 per cent gastric resection was performed. Because of the huge dilated stomach filled with particulate matter, it became necessary to open the stomach during the operation and suction off the retained material. This was not entirely successful because of the size of the retained food particles, and finally using a gall bladder scoop, scoopful after scoopful of this material was removed from the stomach. Aside from this irregularity, the operation proceeded uneventfully. In all it lasted four hours, during which time the patient received 1000 c.c. of whole blood and 500 c.c. of 5 per cent glucose solution. Another 500 c.c. of whole blood were given to the patient after she returned to the floor to sustain her blood pressure. The postoperative course was uneventful and uncomplicated. The highest postoperative temperature was 100.2° F. by rectum. The patient was allowed out of bed on the second postoperative day, and she left the hospital on the eighth postoperative day.

Case 4.—T. A. (U. H. No. 773208), a 53-year-old white woman, was admitted to the University of Minnesota Hospitals on Dec. 4, 1946, with a history of nausea and vomiting of one-month duration, becoming progressively more severe. For the two weeks before admission, the patient had been unable to retain anything taken by mouth. There had been a fifteen pound weight loss in the preceding month and a thirty-five pound weight loss in the preceding three months, amounting to about 25 per cent loss of her normal body weight.

On admission, physical examination revealed the patient to be somewhat dehydrated with evidence of marked recent weight loss. Her temperature was 98.8°F., pulse was 85, and blood pressure was 126/88 mm. Hg. Admission hemoglobin was 12.5 Gm. per cent, white blood count was 6,000 with a normal differential distribution. Blood urea nitrogen was 19 mg. per cent. Blood chlorides were 566 mg. per cent and total plasma proteins were 6.3 Gm. per cent.

The patient was unable to retain anything taken by mouth except small sips of water. Gastrointestinal x-ray study revealed a dilated stomach with complete obstruction in the pyloric area and the duodenum could not be visualized. The patient was placed on a nitrogen balance study (see Table VII, Fig. 7) prepared by intravenous amigen and whole blood and was operated upon Dec. 18, 1946. Exploration of the abdomen revealed an extensive carcinoma of the antrum of the stomach extending beyond the serosa. There were extensive metastases to the liver which I estimated to replace about 50 per cent of the liver tissue. In addition, there were numerous grossly involved lymph nodes extending along the greater and lesser curvatures of the stomach. However, because of the complete obstruction of the stomach, palliative gastric resection was decided upon. A 75 per cent gastric resection was carried out. The operation lasted 4.5 hours during which time 500 c.c. of whole blood and 1000 c.c. of 5 per cent glucose solution in distilled water were given. The postoperative course was routine and uneventful. The patient was allowed out of bed on the day after surgery, and each day thereafter for increasingly longer periods. The indwelling nasoduodenal tube which had been placed into the afferent loop of the gastrojejunal anastomosis at the time of surgery was removed on the third postoperative day and the patient left the hospital on the fifth postoperative day.

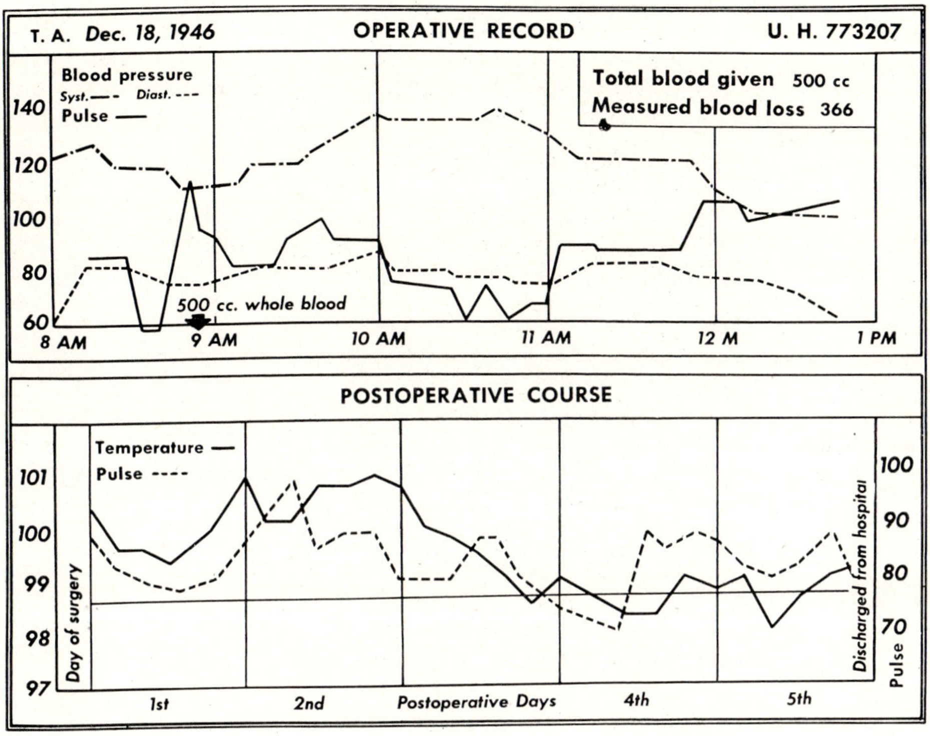

Chart 4.

Case 5.—E. B. (U. H. No. 773802), a 89-year-old white woman, was admitted to the University of Minnesota Hospitals on Jan. 7, 1947, with a history of increasing weakness, a fifty pound weight loss amounting to 33 per cent loss of her usual body weight, and constipation becoming increasingly more severe during the preceding six months. For the past six weeks, the patient had been unable to retain any solid food taken orally. A diagnosis of pernicious-like anemia had been made by one physician. Liver and iron therapy had been instituted, but in spite of this her course had been progressively downhill.

General physical examination on admission revealed an emaciated, moderately dehydrated, white woman. Blood pressure was 120/80 mm. Hg. pulse was 100, temperature was 98.6° F. There was a large, nodular mass in the right upper quadrant of the abdomen apparently separate from the liver. Barium enema x-ray study revealed a constricting carcinoma of the hepatic flexure of the colon associated with the palpable mass described. Gastrointestinal study revealed a normal stomach with some distortion of the duodenum believed to be due to extrinsic pressure. Laboratory studies revealed a negative urinalysis. Hemoglobin level was 10.6 Gm. per cent; white blood count was 17,000 with 70 per cent polymorphonuclear cells, 25 per cent lymphocytes, 2 per cent monocytes, and 3 per cent eosinophiles. Blood urea nitrogen was 24 mg. per cent; blood chlorides were 578 mg. per cent, and total plasma protein level was 5.4 Gm. per cent. After the diagnosis was established and a decision was made to operate upon the patient, an intensive course of parenteral preoperative preparation was started on Jan. 20, 1947. The patient was able to take from 500 to 800 c.c. of University Hospital Diet 2 orally daily, but vomited over one-half of the amount taken each day, and at times she retained practically none of the oral intake. Tube feedings were attempted, but this was unsuccessful because of vomiting. The patient received 1500 c.c. of 5 per cent amigen in 5 per cent glucose solution intravenously daily and a total of 2000 c.c. of whole blood during this period. On Jan. 31, 1947, the patient was operated upon.* A right hemicolectomy and end-to-end ileotransverse colostomy was performed. The operative procedure lasted 3.5 hours. At the completion of the operation, the patient's blood pressure fell to shock levels, despite a transfusion of blood. At this time it became apparent that the needle through which the blood had been given had slipped from the vein and the major portion of the transfused blood and 5 per cent glucose solution had inadvertently been administered subcutaneously. When another bottle of blood was started intravenously, the patient rallied promptly and the blood pressure returned to normal levels.

Postoperatively the patient did very nicely. Convalescence was uncomplicated. The highest postoperative temperature was 101.6° F. rectally on the first postoperative day. She was allowed out of bed this day and each day thereafter. She left the hospital on the tenth postoperative day.

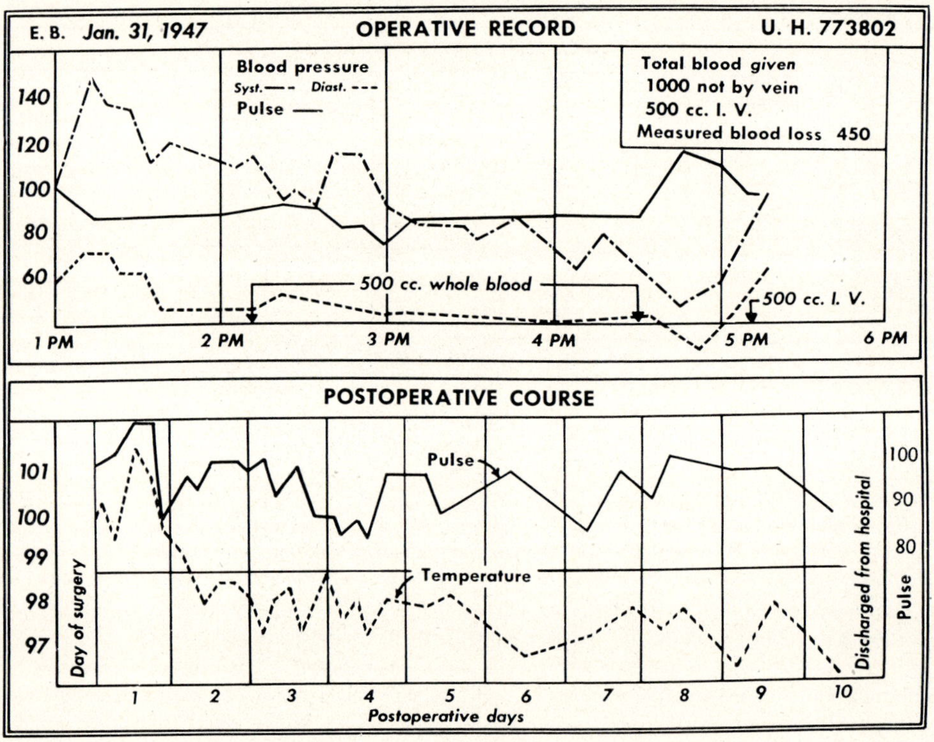

Chart 5.

Case 6.—W. J. (U. H. No. 773121) was a man admitted to the University of Minnesota Hospitals on Jan. 7, 1947, and discharged Feb. 4, 1947. He gave a history of vague epigastric pain and distress over the preceding six months associated with anorexia, weakness, and a weight loss of thirty pounds amounting to about 20 per cent of his usual body weight.

General physical examination revealed a comfortable somewhat emaciated white man. Blood pressure was 140/70 mm. Hg. pulse rate was 75 per minute, and temperature was 98.6° F. No abnormalities were noted on physical examination. Gastrointestinal x-ray study

*Operation was done by Dr. Fred Kolouch.

revealed an extensive carcinoma of the stomach. While in the hospital, the patient developed symptoms of small bowel obstruction, successfully treated by Miller-Abbott, small bowel, intubation suction. At the termination of this episode, the patient was placed on a nitrogen balance study (Table V, Fig. 5) during which time the patient's only source of protein intake consisted of whole blood transfusions. The remainder of the nutritional requirements were met by intravenous glucose and vitamins B, C, and K. The only thing allowed by mouth was sweetened strained fruit juice. At the completion of this study, Jan. 29, 1947, the patient was operated upon.

Exploration of the peritoneal cavity revealed an extensive carcinoma of the stomach involving the esophagus. There were numerous carcinomatous metastases in the mesentery of the small bowel where it joins the gut. In the lower ileum two of these metastases had become annular and obstructed the bowel. As a palliative measure, about thirty inches of lower ileum with the obstructing sites of tumor were resected, and an end-to-end anastomosis was performed. The operation lasted 2.5 hours, during which time the patient received 500 c.c. of whole blood slowly. The measured blood loss was 53 c.c.

The patient's postoperative course was uncomplicated. The highest temperature was 100° F. by rectum. He was allowed out of bed on the first postoperative day, and on the sixth postoperative day he was discharged from the hospital.

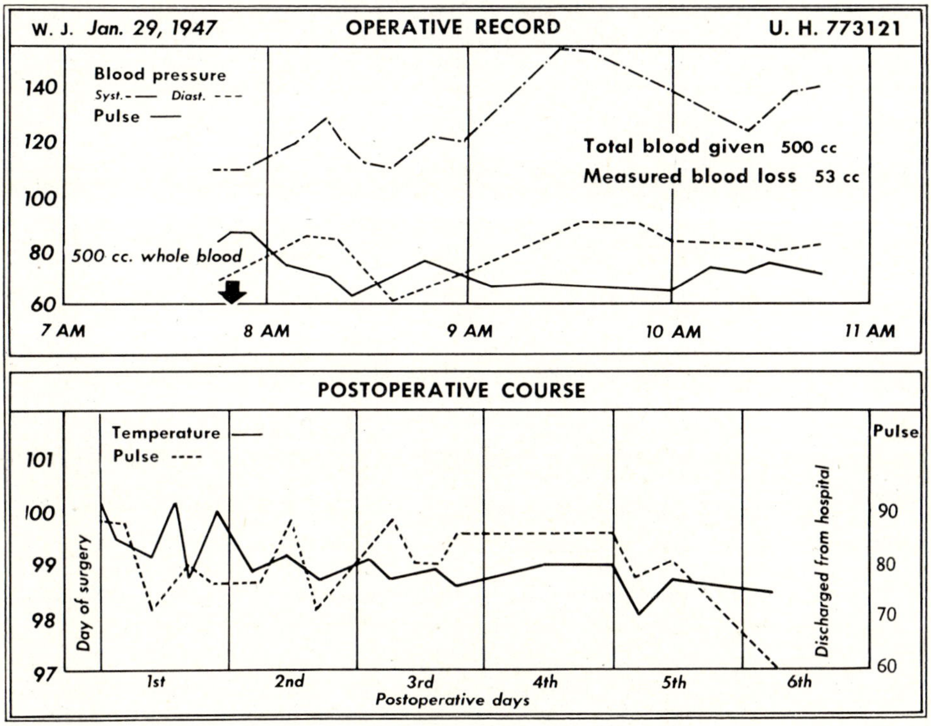

Chart 6.

Case 7.—C. N. (U. H. No. 775502), a 69-year-old woman, was admitted to the University of Minnesota Hospitals on Feb. 4, 1947. For the preceding year she had noticed a mass in the right upper quadrant of the abdomen, which had slowly progressed in size. In all, the patient had lost thirty pounds in weight, amounting to 30 per cent of her normal body weight.

General physical examination revealed an extremely emaciated, elderly, white woman. Blood pressure was 130/80 mm. Hg, pulse rate was 75, and temperature was 98.6° F. The only positive finding aside from the emaciation was a mass in the right upper abdomen about 6 cm. in diameter and apparently fixed to the liver. Laboratory studies revealed a negative urinalysis. Hemoglobin level was 5.2 Gm. per cent, red blood cell count was 3,140,000, and white blood cell count was 10,200. The blood urea nitrogen was 10 mg. per cent, blood chlorides were 634 mg. per cent, and total plasma proteins were 6.7 Gm. per cent. Barium enema x-ray study revealed a carcinoma involving the hepatic flexure of the colon. The patient was prepared for surgery by massive blood transfusions, receiving from February 5 to February 10, a total of 4500 c.c. of whole blood. Prior to starting transfusions, blood study revealed a hemoglobin level of 5.6 Gm. per cent; hematocrit reading was 23.5, plasma volume was 2.18 L., and blood volume was 2.84 L. After receiving 4500 c.c. of whole blood, repeat blood studies revealed a hemoglobin level of 16.5 Gm. per cent, a hematocrit of 58.5, a plasma volume of 2.19 L., and a blood volume of 5.29 L. In addition to the whole blood transfusions, the patient took by mouth 1000 to 1500 c.c. of University Hospital diet.

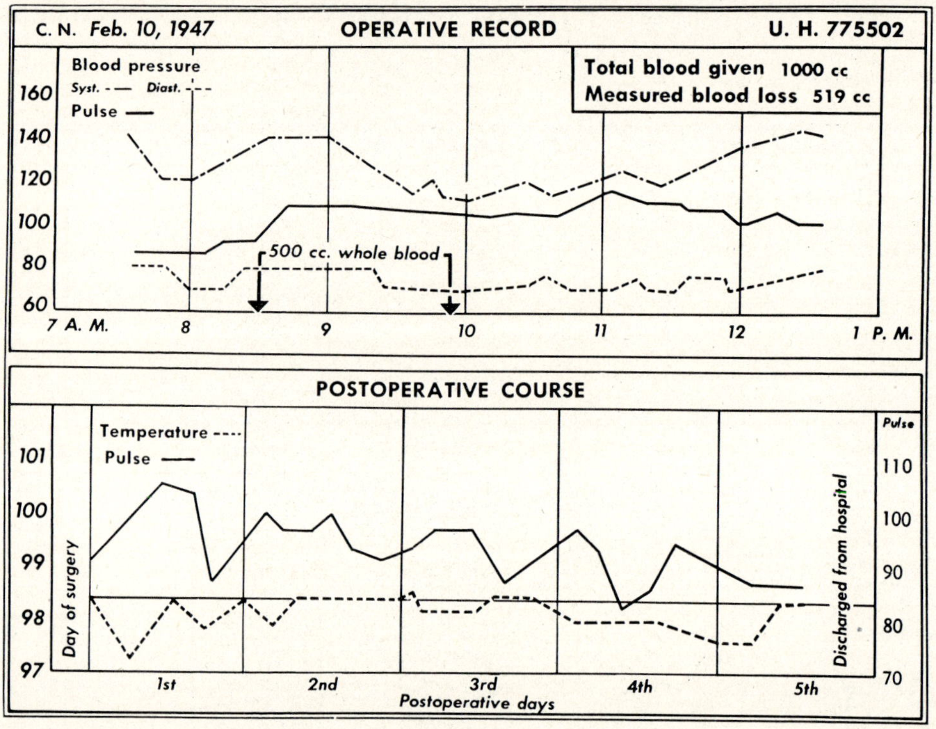

Chart 7.

On Feb. 10, 1947, the patient was operated upon.* A right hemicolectomy with excision of 20 cm. of terminal ileum and an end-to-end ileotransverse colostomy was performed. The operation lasted 4.5 hours, during which time the patient received 1000 c.c. of whole blood and 1000 c.c. of 5 per cent glucose in distilled water.

The patient's postoperative course was uneventful. The highest postoperative temperature was 98.6° F. the day after surgery, and she was discharged from the hospital on the fifth postoperative day.

Case 8.—B. T. (U. H. No. 775215), a 75-year-old white man, was admitted to the University of Minnesota Hospitals on Jan. 24, 1947. The patient apparently had been in

*Operation was done by Dr. Owen H. Wangensteen.

good health until two months prior to admission to the hospital at which time he had first noticed loss of appetite, progressively increasing weakness, and vague epigastric pain. During the period of his illness, the patient lost forty-five pounds amounting to 30 per cent of his normal body weight. General physical examination revealed a poorly nourished white man who appeared apathetic and listless, but who did not appear to be in any acute distress. Temperature was 100.4° F., pulse rate was 100, blood pressure was 110/60 mm. Hg. The remainder of the physical examination was essentially negative. Gastrointestinal x-ray studies revealed a carcinoma of the antrum of the stomach producing a fairly high-grade obstruction. Urinalysis on admission was negative, hemoglobin level was 10.9 Gm. per cent, and white blood count was 15,000. Blood urea nitrogen level was 18 mg. per cent, blood chlorides were 611 mg. per cent, total plasma proteins were 6.4 Gm. per cent. During the patient's stay on the medical service, the patient continued to have a tachycardia up to 120 per minute. Clinically the patient appeared to be a poor risk for surgery. However,

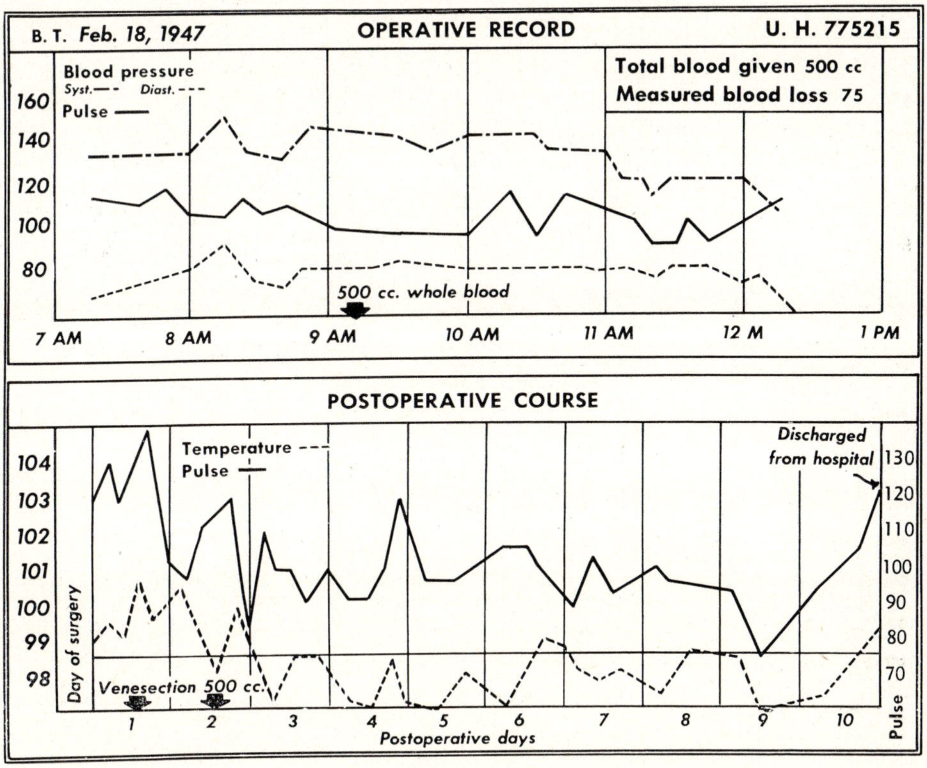

Chart 8.

because of the presence of malignant disease, surgical therapy was decided upon, and on February 6 an active period of preoperative preparation was begun. During the twelve-day period, from February 6 to 17, the patient received daily either 500 or 1000 c.c. of whole blood, a total of 6500 c.c. of whole blood being given during this period. The patient took 600 to 1000 c.c. of University Hospital Diet 2 orally, but most of it was lost by emesis or removed by gastric aspiration. During this period, the patient's weight increased from 52.2 to 57 kilograms; his hemoglobin increased to 18.8 Gm. per cent with a hematocrit of 64 on Feb. 17, 1947.

On Feb. 18, 1947, the patient was operated upon. A carcinoma of the distal one-half of the stomach was found, and a 75 per cent gastric resection was performed. The operation was uncomplicated. It lasted four hours and ten minutes, during which time the patient received 500 c.c. of whole blood. The measured blood loss was 73 c.c.

On the first postoperative day, the patient's general condition was complicated by a persistent tachycardia up to 130 and a moderate amount of dyspnea. Because of the markedly elevated hemoglobin and hematocrit, a venesection drawing off 500 c.c. of blood was performed on February 19. This produced very definite improvement in both respiration and pulse. Next day, since the hemoglobin level was still elevated at 17.9 with a hematocrit of 62.4, the venesection was repeated again removing 500 c.c. of blood. From this day onward the convalescence was uncomplicated except for a mild icterus which first appeared on February 24 and cleared in two days. This was not associated with any laboratory findings of liver damage. The patient was allowed out of bed on the second postoperative day, and left the hospital on the eleventh postoperative day.

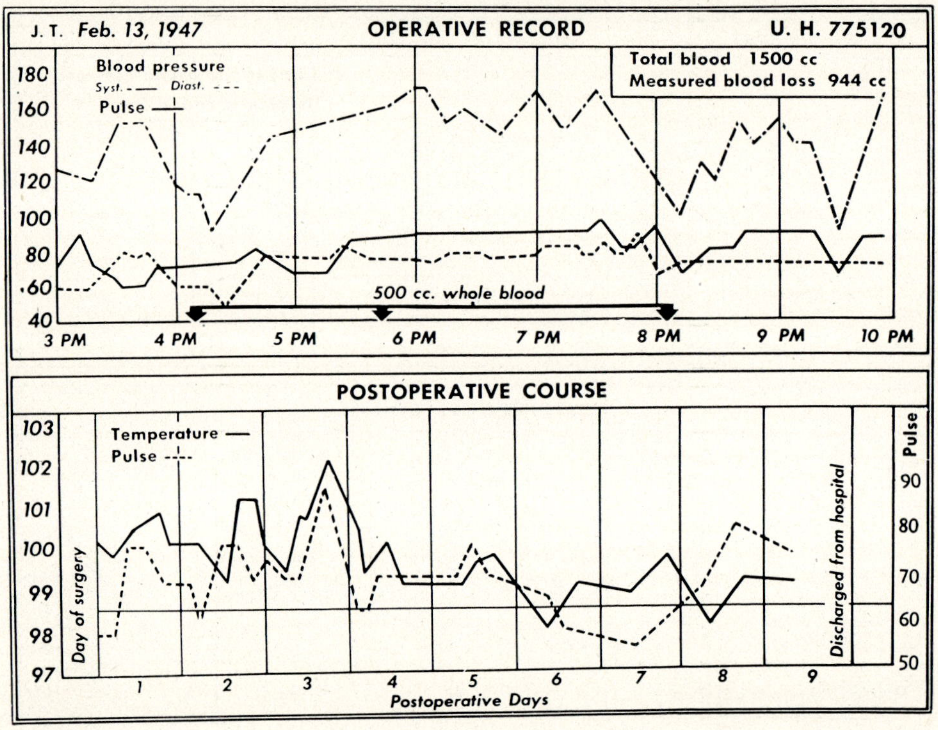

Chart 9.

Case 9.—J. T. (U. H. No. 775120), was a man who was admitted to the University of Minnesota Hospitals on Jan. 28, 1947. The illness at the time of admission had begun about six months previously with difficulty in swallowing solid foods as the first symptom. This became progressively more marked as time went on. More recently there was noted some difficulty in the swallowing of liquid foods also. In addition, the patient experienced vague, indefinite, epigastric pain becoming more severe during the illness. In all, there was noted a forty-five pound weight loss amounting to 30 per cent loss of his normal body weight.

Physical examination on admission revealed a somewhat emaciated, comfortable, and cooperative white man. Blood pressure was 140/70 mm. Hg, pulse rate was 70, temperature was 98.6° F. There were no gross abnormalities noted on examination. Gastrointestinal x-ray study revealed a definite constricting lesion of the lower esophagus associated with a filling defect of the upper portion of the stomach. Although the lesion produced considerable obstruction to the lower esophagus, barium could be seen going past the site of narrowing.

The patient was started on a nitrogen balance study on Jan. 29, 1947 (see Chart 9, Fig. 6), receiving whole blood daily as the only source of nitrogenous intake. In addition, the patient received 3000 c.c. of 10 per cent glucose intravenously, also sweetened fruit juice by mouth ad libitum. At the completion of the study on Feb. 13, 1947, the patient was operated upon.

At operation exploration of the abdomen was carried out through a transverse upper abdominal incision, at which time the diagnosis of carcinoma of the upper stomach and esophagus was confirmed. The lesion appeared to be operable and no distant metastases were noted. The incision was then extended across the eighth costal cartilage and out into the seventh left intercostal space, entering the left pleural cavity. The left diaphragm was then incised from the area of the incision down to the esophageal hiatus. Resection of the upper one-half of the stomach and lower one-third of the esophagus was carried out. The residual stomach was then mobilized and anastomosed in the chest with the proximal esophagus. In all, the operation lasted six hours and forty minutes during which time the patient received 1500 c.c. of whole blood and 1500 c.c. of 5 per cent glucose solution in distilled water. The measured blood loss was 944 c.c.

All in all the patient withstood this long difficult operation very well. The postoperative course in the hospital was smooth and apparently uncomplicated, and the patient was discharged from the hospital on the ninth postoperative day. Four days later, however, the patient was readmitted to the hospital in an acutely dehydrated state and in shock. For the preceding two days the patient had been vomiting and had been unable to retain anything taken by mouth. He responded to prompt treatment of intravenous saline solution, glucose, and plasma. X-ray studies of the abdomen revealed several dilated loops of small intestine, and a tentative diagnosis of paralytic ileus was made. During the night of admission, however, the patient passed some bloody material by rectum; on rectal examination the next day, bloody material could be noted on the examining finger whereas it had not been noted on admission. On abdominal examination, moderate distention was observed and the abdomen was somewhat more rigid than it had been on admission. The drainage from the nasogastric tube which had been passed had a definite feculent odor. In addition, during this time, the patient developed signs of vascular insufficiency to the right leg and foot with a line of demarcation appearing in the mid-calf. A clinical diagnosis of probable mesenteric thrombosis was made, and in spite of the precarious state of the patient, operation was decided upon. Exploration was carried out on Feb. 26, 1946. At abdominal exploration, gangrene of the entire small intestine beginning four inches distal to the ligament of Treitz and extending to about four inches proximal to the ileocecal orifice was noted. Resection without spillage of the entire involved small intestine and end-to-end anastomosis of the residual eight inches of small intestine were performed. The patient withstood this operation but left the operating room in a precarious state and died about twenty-four hours later.

Post-mortem examination revealed the esophagogastric anastomosis to be perfectly intact and well healed. The heart was normal, but the aorta was involved by extensive atherosclerosis. In the thoracic and upper abdominal aorta there were two large thrombi about two inches in length. These were the probable source of emboli which migrated into the superior mesenteric artery and the right femoral artery.

This group of nine poor-risk patients, all of whom had lost from 20 to 33 per cent of their normal weight, were prepared for operation principally by parenteral feedings. All survived an operation of major magnitude with two postoperative complications occurring in the group.

One complication occurred in J. T. (Case 9), who developed a thrombosis on a markedly atherosclerotic aorta which may well have occurred independently of the preoperative preparation or the operation. However, the possibility remains that the repeated blood transfusions may have augmented the known increased tendency of blood to clot postoperatively and so have produced this accident. The aortic thrombosis may have occurred early in the postoperative course with the mesenteric embolism occurring much later. Nevertheless, the patient did survive a long and difficult operation; the operative wound and anastomosis healed per primam, bearing testimony that at least functionally the protein metabolic processes were operating normally.

The other complication, that of B. T. (Case 8), was definitely related to overenthusiastic use of blood transfusions. When it was appreciated that incipient circulatory failure was resulting from the persistent plethora, and venesection was done, prompt improvement resulted. From this case, as well as C. N. (Case 6), and from balance studies V and VI, it should be appreciated that whole blood transfusions will produce increases in blood volume directly proportional to the amount of blood given, and that this increase is almost entirely in the cellular component of the blood. Almost all of the transfused red blood cells remain in the circulation at least for the first few days after transfusion. For this reason, in an instance where there are no avenues of blood loss, daily whole blood transfusions should not be kept up indefinitely. However, it should also be pointed out that patients seem to tolerate a mild plethora very well. It may even have a cushioning effect on withstanding the trauma of the operation.

DISCUSSION

From nitrogen balance studies attending the use of whole blood intravenously, as the sole source of protein intake, it was noted that uniformly no increase of urinary nitrogen excretion occurred over that noted during a preliminary basal period. In this respect whole blood behaves as does whole human plasma. In contradistinction to this response, the intravenous use of casein digests are uniformly attended with a marked pyramiding of urinary nitrogen excretion as noted in these studies and as reported by others.[12, 24, 61, 115, 129, 139, 194] From this difference in type of response, it would appear that there is a fundamental difference in the manner of utilization of these materials by the body. That this variation could be explained on the basis of time factor is entirely possible. The protein digests are apparently utilized and deaminized in a short period of time. Hence, the end results of their metabolism appear directly as an increase in urinary nitrogen excretion. On the other hand, plasma protein does not appear to be catabolized directly. It apparently leaves the circulation and becomes a part of the general body protein stores to be available on call as needed by the over-all protein economy of the body. The fact that its use is not attended by an increased urinary nitrogen excretion is further evidence that it is not broken up into its constituent amino acids as has been similarly postulated by Whipple and his coworkers.[99, 103, 128] From the work of Schoenheimer and associates[182] it appears that the half life of plasma protein is about two weeks. It may take that long for the normal course of protein metabolism to bring about the catabolism of the injected plasma protein. Elman and Davey[62] reported a delayed urinary nitrogen excretion after giving plasma intravenously to dogs, while at the time of plasma infusion no augmentation of urinary nitrogen was evident and marked positive nitrogen balance was present. However, it is also true that as the protein stores of the body are depleted, extreme conservation of available bodily nitrogen material occurs, whereas when the protein stores of the body are in a more normal state this conservation is not as marked.[23, 97, 155] In the studies herein reported, although the follow-up time was not long, no evidence of delayed nitrogen excretion after plasma infusions was noted. Certainly it would appear that plasma protein given intravenously soon leaves the circulation and becomes part of the general body protein pool and as such is utilized and slowly replaced in the continuing metabolism of the body.

With the use of whole blood for nutritional purposes, additional factors are at play. From the evidence presented, it appears that the red blood cells injected remain in the circulation and as such they probably do not directly partake of the general body protein economy. That there are no reservoirs outside of the circulation where red blood cells can be sequestered has been shown by the work of Ross and Chapin[173] and Hahn and associates[83] using red blood cells tagged with radioactive iron.

However, the red blood cells in themselves may constitute a pool of protein which on their inevitable disintegration becomes available for the body needs. With an increase of red blood cell mass, more cells will eventually disintegrate and more protein for general bodily use will be liberated. Eventually all of the injected red blood cells must disintegrate and their contained protein becomes liberated for general body needs. This is a continuing process. When the total circulating red cell mass is raised, more cells are available which have reached the end of their life span and are disintegrated. That no increased urinary nitrogen excretion is evident when the red cell mass is increased must indicate that the proteins so liberated are reutilized by the body. By supplying preformed red blood cells to the body, the protein which, as shown by Robscheit-Robbins and her co-workers,[167, 169] would by first priority have been used for building new hemoglobin is thereby spared and is available for other body uses. McDonald and associates[133] have postulated that an excess red cell mass may have an immediate sparing action on body proteins by displacing plasma volume and thereby reducing the amount of plasma protein needed to maintain circulation. Protein so spared, they stated, may be used for wound healing.

Somewhat less than the almost complete retention of red blood cells in the circulation of the recipient observed in Tables V and VI and in C. N. (Case 6), may possibly have occurred. In these studies, the total blood volume was determined by measuring the plasma volume and the hematocrit value of the peripheral blood. Snead and Ebert[191] and Hahn and associates [83, 84] have shown that red cell volumes as calculated from plasma volume and venous hematocrit give values about 25 per cent higher than when checked by viviperfusion, by radio iron distribution in tagged red blood cells, and by measurements before and after known massive bleeding.

Since the malnourished state has been shown quite uniformly to be associated with a contraction of blood volume,[2, 34, 123, 135, 155, 185, 211, 217] the use of whole blood transfusions during the preoperative preparation phase has the added beneficial effect of restoring this volume to normal levels before subjecting the patient to the trauma of operation. Lyons[123] felt that the unsteady state of patients with chronic infections and weight loss is primarily related to a reduced blood volume, a deficiency of total circulating hemoglobin, and to an excessive interstitial fluid volume. In this connection it would be of great importance to ascertain the effect on blood volume of oral dietary preparation alone, and of protein digest solutions given parenterally and orally. However, it would appear in the light of present knowledge that correction of this phase of the malnourished state can be most promptly and effectively brought about by whole blood transfusions.

That human plasma protein may not be a complete protein for the rat is suggested by the work of Hegsted and associates,[92] who found that when human plasma protein fed to rats was supplemented with isoleucine or with whole casein, better growth occurred than when equivalent amounts of protein were taken as human plasma protein alone. In contrast, Madden and Whipple,[128] Weech and Goettsch,[212] and Melnick and co-workers[138] found beef plasma protein to be the most effective of all proteins tested, in producing plasma protein regeneration in protein-depleted dogs. Similarly, hemoglobin on chemical analysis is low in isoleucine, cystine, and methionine.[18] Albanese,[6] employing the method of bio-assay in rats, which require isoleucine for growth and maintenance, found that hemoglobin failed to support weight in mature rats, unless supplemented by isoleucine. Robscheit-Robbins and associates[168] found that addition of methionine to hemoglobin solution increased its effectiveness in dogs. Miller[141] also found that dog hemoglobin given parenterally was well utilized to maintain weight and nitrogen balance in dogs. Its utilization, however, was improved by the addition of d. l. methionine, but was unaffected by the addition of isoleucine.

It would appear that in a person to be maintained by parenteral means there might be some benefit derived, from a nutritional viewpoint, of supplementing whole blood transfusions with a complete mixture of amino acids. This can be most practically done at present with a good digest of a complete protein. From studies here reported the greatest nitrogen retention occurred when whole blood plus 3000 c.c. of 5 per cent amigen in 5 per cent glucose solution was given intravenously.

At present, there are no actually objective means of deciding when a patient has had sufficient preoperative preparation. Such clinical criteria as return of appetite, loss of anorexia, and improvement of strength are helpful adjuncts and often appear when the drain of a state of negative nitrogen balance is replaced by a state of positive nitrogen balance. Certainly one should not expect marked weight gain, other than that associated with fluid replacement. The suggestion of Lyons[123] and Abbott and Mellors[2] of determining blood volume and returning a contracted blood volume to normal levels before embarking on a major operative venture is of real importance, but this does not reflect the state of the protein stores. From the results in the patients reported, all of whom had lost from 20 to 33 per cent of their body weight, it would appear that about one week of intensive, parenteral, preoperative preparation may be sufficient. During this time, such patients should receive daily whole blood transfusions supplemented by an intravenous casein digest solution in amounts up to 18 Gm. of nitrogen. Under such a regimen, and without oral supplements, positive nitrogen balance can be achieved and poor-risk patients so prepared can be operated upon with risks comparable to similar uncomplicated cases.

SUMMARY AND CONCLUSIONS

1. The importance of a clear understanding by surgeons of protein metabolism and its related problems in the care of surgical patients is stressed.

2. A consideration of hemoglobin metabolism as it relates to general protein metabolism is presented.

3. In the preoperative preparation of patients for surgery, the necessity of replenishing depleted protein stores is stressed.

4. In the malnourished poor-risk patient, who cannot maintain nutrition by oral means, parenteral preoperative preparation is necessary and effective.

5. Positive nitrogen balance in man, using human plasma given intravenously as the sole source of nitrogen intake, can be attained.

6. Positive nitrogen balance in man, using whole human blood intravenously as the sole source of nitrogen intake, appears to be attained, although the protein contained in the red blood cells is not immediately and directly available for general body protein needs.

7. After daily whole blood transfusions in man, the major part of the injected red blood cells remain in the circulation of the recipient and account for the rise of total blood volume observed. Very little change in plasma volume is observed.

8. Positive nitrogen balance in man cannot be attained when giving intravenously amounts of an acid hydrolysate of casein fortified with tryptophane containing 6 Gm. of nitrogen.

9. Positive nitrogen balance in man cannot be attained when giving intravenously amounts of an enzymatic digest of casein containing 6 Gm. of nitrogen.

10. Positive nitrogen balance in man can uniformly be attained when giving intravenously amounts of an enzymatic digest of casein containing 18 Gm. of nitrogen.

11. A difference in mode of utilization of casein digests and of whole plasma protein given intravenously is noted. A possible explanation of this difference is presented.

12. From a nutritional viewpoint, supplementation of whole blood transfusions by amino acid solutions or casein digest may have a beneficial effect on nitrogen retention.

13. Malnourished, poor-risk patients can be adequately prepared for surgery by parenteral means alone, and when so prepared will stand operations of major magnitude with risks equal to those of similar uncomplicated cases.

REFERENCES

1. Abbott, W. E., Hirshfeld, J. W., and Meyer, F. L.: Metabolic Alterations Following Thermal Burns: II. Changes in Plasma Volume and Plasma Protein in the Convalescent Phase, Surg., Gynec. & Obst. **81**: 25-30, 1945.
2. Abbott, W. E., and Mellors, R. C.: Total Circulating Plasma Protein in Surgical Patients With Dehydration and Malnutrition: Indications for Intravenous Alimentation With Amino Acids, Arch. Surg. **46**: 277-288, 1943.
3. Abderholden, E., and Rona, P.: Ueber die Ververtung die Abbauprodukte des Casein im Tierischen Organismus, Ztschr. f. physiol. Chem. **44**: 198-205, 1905.
4. Abels, J. C., Young, N. F., and Taylor, H. C.: Effects of Testosterone Propionate on Protein Formation in Man, J. Clin. Endocrinol. **4**: 198-201, 1944.
5. Addis, T., Poo, L. T., and Lew, W.: The Quantities of Protein Lost by Various Organs and Tissues of the Body During a Seven Day Fast, J. Biol. Chem. **115**: 111-116, 1936.
6. Albanese, A. A.: Studies on Human Blood Proteins: I. Isoleucine Deficiency of Hemoglobin, J. Biol. Chem. **157**: 613-620, 1945.
7. Albanese, A. A., Irby, V., and Frankston, J. F.: Effect of Carbohydrate Feeding on Urinary Output of Amino Acids and Other Metabolites, Federation Proc. **5**: 118, 1946.
8. Albright, F.: Cushing's Syndrome, Its Pathological Physiology, Its Relationship to Adrenogenital Syndrome, and Its Connection With Problem of Reaction of Body to Injurious Agent, Harvey Lect. **38**: 123-186, 1943.
9. Ashby, W.: The Determination of the Length of Life of Transfused Blood Corpuscles in Man, J. Exper. Med. **29**: 267-281, 1919.
10. Austin, J. H., and Eisenbrey, A. B.: The Utilization of Parenterally Introduced Serum, Arch. Int. Med. **10**: 305-313, 1912.
11. Barnett, C. W., Jones, R. B., and Cohn, R. B.: Maintenance of Normal Plasma Protein Concentration in Spite of Repeated Protein Loss by Bleeding, J. Exper. Med. **55**: 683-693, 1932.
12. Bassett, S. H., Woods, R. R., Shull, F. W., and Madden, S. C.: Parenterally Administered Amino Acids as a Source of Protein in Man, New England J. Med. **230**: 106-108, 1944.
13. Beams, A. J., Free, A. H., and Leonards, J. R.: Experimental Hypoproteinemia and Edema; Studies of Intestinal Absorption and Intestinal Roentgenologic Characteristics, Arch. Int. Med. **73**: 397-402, 1944.
14. Belk, W. P., and Barnes, B. C.: The Survival Time After Transfusion of Erythrocytes of Citrated Human Blood Stored at 4° to 6° Centigrade, Am. J. M. Sc. **201**: 838-841, 1941.
15. Berger, G. C. E., Sandstead, H. R., and Drummond, J.: Starvation in Western Holland, Lancet **249**: 282-283, 1945.
16. Bernard, Claude: Quoted by Foster, M., Claude Bernard, New York, 1889, Longmans, Green & Co., p. 46.
17. Best, C. H., and Taylor, N. B.: The Physiological Basis of Medical Practice, Baltimore, 1945, Williams & Wilkins Company, pp. 20-21.
18. Block, R. J., and Bolling, D.: The Amino Acid Yield From Various Animal and Plant Proteins After Hydrolysis of the Fat Free Tissue, Arch. Biochem. **3**: 217-226, 1943.
19. Blundell, J.: Principles and Practice of Obstetrics, London, 1834, E. Cox.
20. Borsook, H., and Keighley, G. L.: The Continuing Metabolism of Nitrogen in Animals, Proc. Roy. Soc., s., B. **118**: 488-521, 1935.
21. Borsook, H., and Dubonoff, J. W.: The Metabolism of Protein and Amino Acids, Ann. Rev. Biochem. **12**: 183-204, 1943.
22. Boycott, A. E., and Douglas, C. G.: Further Observations on Transfusions, J. Path. & Bact. **14**: 294-327, 1910.
23. Browne, J. S. L., Schenker, V., and Stevenson, J. A. F.: Some Metabolic Aspects of Damage and Convalescence, Proc. Am. Soc. Clin. Investigation 1944; J. Clin. Investigation **23**: 936, 1944.
24. Brunschwig, A., Clark, D. E., and Corbin, N.: Post Operative Nitrogen Loss and Studies on Parenteral Nitrogen Nutrition by Means of Casein Digest, Ann. Surg. **115**: 1091-1105, 1942.
25. Brunschwig, A., Nichols, S., Biglow, R. R., and Miles, J.: Sulfhydryl Protection of the Liver, Arch. Path. **40**: 81-84, 1945.
26. Burroughs, E. W., Burroughs, H. S., and Mitchell, H. H.: The Independence of the Endogenous and Exogenous Metabolism of Nitrogen, J. Nutrition **19**: 271-283, 1940.
27. Burroughs, E. W., Burroughs, H. S., and Mitchell, H. H.: Amino Acids Required for Complete Replacement of Endogenous Losses in Adult Rat, J. Nutrition **19**: 363-384, 1940.
28. Burr, G. O., and Burr, M. M.: A New Deficiency Disease Produced by the Rigid Exclusion of Fat From the Diet, J. Biol. Chem. **82**: 345-367, 1929.
29. Cannon, P. R.: Antibodies and the Protein Reserves, J. Immunol. **44**: 107-114, 1942.

30. Cannon, P. R.: The Importance of Proteins in Resistance to Infection, J. A. M. A. **128**: 360-362, 1945.
31. Cannon, P. R, Chase, W. E., and Wissler, R. W.: The Relationship of the Protein Reserves to Antibody Production, J. Immunol. **47**: 133-148, 1943.
32. Cannon, P. R., Wissler, R. W., Woolridge, R. L., and Benditt, E. P.: Relationship of Protein Deficiency to Surgical Infection, Ann. Surg. **120**: 514-525, 1944.
33. Cathart, E. P.: The Influence of Carbohydrate and Fats on Protein Metabolism, J. Physiol. **39**: 311-330, 1909.
34. Chang, Hsiao-Chien: Plasma Protein and Blood Volume, Proc. Soc. Exper. Biol. & Med. **29**: 829-832, 1932.
35. Chittenden, R. H.: Physiological Economy in Nutrition With Special Reference to the Minimal Proteid Requirements of the Healthy Man, New York, 1907, F. A. Stokes Company.
36. Clark, A. H.: The Effect of Diet on Healing of Wounds, Bull. Johns Hopkins Hosp. **30**: 117-120, 1919.
37. Clark, D. E., and Brunschwig, A.: Intravenous Nourishment With Protein, Carbohydrate and Fat in Man, Proc. Soc. Exper. Biol. & Med. **49**: 329-332, 1942.
38. Cope, O.: Nathanson, I. T., Rourke, G. M., and Wilson, H.: Symposium on Management of Cocoanut Grove Burns at Massachusetts General Hospital: Metabolic Observations, Ann. Surg. **17**: 937-958, 1943.
39. Cori, C. F., and Cori, G. T.: The Fate of Sugar in Animal Body: Sugar Oxidation and Glycogen Formation in Normal and Insulinized Rats During Absorption of Fructose, J. Biol. Chem. **73**: 555-566, 1927.
40. Co Tui, Wright, A. M., Mulholland, J. H., Carabba, V., Barcham, I., and Vinci, V. J.: Studies on Surgical Convalescence: I Sources of Nitrogen Loss Post-gastrectomy and Effect of High Amino Acid and High Caloric Intake on Convalescence, Ann. Surg. **120**: 99-122, 1944.
41. Croft, P. B., and Peters, R. A.: Nitrogen Loss After Thermal Burns: Effects of Adding Protein and Methionine to Diet of Rats, Lancet **1**: 266-271, 1945.
42. Cruz, W. O., Hahn, P. F., and Bale, W. F.: Hemoglobin Radioactive Iron Liberated by Erythrocyte Destruction (Acetylphenylhydrazine) Promptly Reutilized to Form New Hemoglobin, Am. J. Physiol. **135**: 595-599, 1942.
43. Cuthbertson, D. P.: The Influence of Prolonged Muscular Rest on Metabolism, Biochem. J. **23**: 1328-1335, 1929.
44. Cuthbertson, D. P.: The Disturbance of Metabolism Produced by Bony and Non-Bony Injury With Notes on Certain Abnormal Conditions of Bone, Biochem. J. **24**: 1244-1263, 1930.
45. Cuthbertson, D. P.: Observations on the Disturbance of Metabolism Produced by Injury to the Limbs, Quart. J. Med. **26**: 233-246, 1932.
46. Cuthbertson, D. P.: Further Observations on the Disturbance of Metabolism Caused by Injury, With Particular Reference to the Dietary Requirements of Fracture Cases, Brit. J. Surg. **23**: 505-520, 1936.
47. Cuthbertson, D. P.: Post Shock Metabolic Response, Lancet **1**: 433-436, 1942.
48. Cuthbertson, D. P.: Protein Metabolism, Brit. M. Bull. **2**: 207-217, 1944.
49. Cuthbertson, D. P.: McCutcheon, A., and Monro, H. N.: A Study of the Effect of Overfeeding on Protein Metabolism of Man, Biochem. J. **31**: 681-705, 1937.
50. Dacie, V. D., and Mollison, P. L.: Survival of Normal Erythrocytes After Transfusion to Patients With Familial Haemolitic Anaemia, Lancet **1**: 550-552, 1943.
51. Daft, F. S., Robscheit-Robbins, F. S., and Whipple, G. H.: New Formed Hemoglobin and Protein Catabolism, J. Biol. Chem. **103**: 495-510, 1933.
52. Daft, F. S., Robscheit-Robbins, F. S., and Whipple, G. H.: Liver Injury by Chloroform: Nitrogen Metabolism and Conservation, J. Biol. Chem. **113**: 391-404, 1936.
53. Daft, F. S., Robscheit-Robbins, F. S., and Whipple, G. H.: Plasma Protein Given by Vein and Its Influence Upon Body Metabolism, J. Biol. Chem. **123**: 87-98, 1938.
54. Davis, H. A., and Blalock, J. F.: Autologous and Homologous Transfusion of Human Ascitic Fluid, J. Clin. Investigation **18**: 219-225, 1939.
55. Davis, H. A., and Getzoff, P. L.: Hypoproteinemia in Surgical Diseases, Arch. Surg. **44**: 1071-1090, 1942.
56. Davis, N. C., and Whipple, G. H.: Influence of Fasting and Various Diets on Liver Injury Effected by Chloroform Anesthesia, Arch. Int. Med. **23**: 612-635, 1919.
57. Davis, N. C., Hall, C. C., and Whipple, G. H.: The Rapid Construction of Liver Cell Protein on a Strict Carbohydrate Diet Contrasted With Fasting: Mechanism of Protein Sparing Action of Carbohydrates, Arch. Int. Med. **23**: 689-710, 1919.
58. Editorial: Protein Requirements of Adults, Brit. M. J., pp. 19-20, Jan. 4, 1947.
59. Elman, R.: Parenteral Replacement of Protein With Amino Acids of Hydrolyzed Casein, Ann. Surg. **112**: 594-602, 1940.
60. Elman, R.: Parenteral Alimentation in Surgery With Special Reference to Proteins and Amino Acids, New York, 1947, Paul B. Hoeber, Inc.

61. Elman, R., Charnas, R., and Davey, H. W.: Ceiling of Utilization of Nitrogen, Arch. Surg. **47**: 216-220, 1943.
62. Elman, R., and Davey, H. W.: Studies on Hypoalbuminemia Produced by Protein Deficient Diets: III. The Correction of Hypoalbuminemia by Means of Large Plasma Transfusions, J. Exper. Med. **77**: 1-5, 1943.
63. Elman, R., Davey, H. W., and Kiyasu, R.: Nitrogen Balance on a Restricted Caloric Intake, J. Lab. & Clin. Med. **30**: 273-277, 1945.
64. Elman, R., and Weiner, D. O.: Intravenous Alimentation With Special Reference to Protein (Amino Acid) Metabolism, J. A. M. A. **112**: 796-802, 1939.
65. Farr, L. E., and MacFadyen, D. A.: Amino Acid Nitrogen in Urine of Children With the Nephrotic Syndrome Following Intravenous Amino Acids, Proc. Soc. Exper. Biol. & Med. **42**: 444-446, 1939.
66. Fine, J., and Seligman, A.: Traumatic Shock: Study of the Problem of Lost Plasma in Hemorrhagic Shock by the Use of Radioactive Plasma Protein, J. Clin. Investigation **22**: 285-303, 1943.
67. Fink, R. M., Enns, T., Kimball, C. P., Silberstein, H. E., Bale, W. F., Madden, S. C., and Whipple, G. H.: Plasma Protein Metabolism: Normal and Associated With Shock Observations Using Protein Labeled by Heavy Nitrogen in Lysine, J. Exper. Med. **80**: 455-475, 1944.
68. Flink, E. B., and Skubi, K. B.: Blood Transfusion Studies: II. Survival of Fresh and Stored Transfused Erythrocytes as Determined by Urobilinogen Excretion, J. Lab. and Clin. Med. **31**: 1074-1078, 1946.
69. Folin, O.: Analysis of Thirty Normal Urines, Am. J. Physiol. **13**: 45-65, 1905.
70. Folin, O.: Laws Governing the Chemical Composition of Urine, Am. J. Physiol. **13**: 66-116, 1905.
71. Folin, O.: A Theory of Protein Metabolism, Am. J. Physiol. **13**: 117-138, 1905.
72. Folin, O., and Bell, R. D.: Application of a New Reagent for the Separation of Ammonia: I. The Colorimetric Determination of Ammonia in Urine, J. Biol. Chem. **29**: 329-335, 1917.
73. Folin, O., and Wu, H.: A System of Blood Analysis, J. Biol. Chem. **38**: 81-110, 1919.
74. Frame, E. G., Russell, J. A., and Wilhelmi, A. E.: Colorimetric Estimation of Amino Nitrogen in Blood, J. Biol. Chem. **149**: 255-270, 1943.
75. Goldschmidt, S., Vars, H. M., and Ravdin, I. S.: The Influence of the Foodstuffs Upon the Susceptibility of the Liver to Injury by Chloroform and the Probable Mechanism of Their Action, J. Clin. Investigation **18**: 277-289, 1939.
76. Govaerts, P.: Du Role de la Pression Osmotique des Proteins du Sang dan la Pathogenie des Oedemes, Presse méd. **32**: 950-952, 1924.
77. Govaerts, P.: Influence Du Rapport Albumines-Globulines sur la Pression Osmotique des Proteines du Serum, Compt. rend. Soc. de biol. **93**: 441-443, 1925.
78. Greenberg, D.: The Colorimetric Determination of the Serum Protens, J. Biol. Chem. **82**: 545-550, 1929.
79. Gregerson, M. I.: Practical Method for Determination of Blood Volume With Dye 1824; Survey of Present Basis of Dye Method and Its Clinical Applications, J. Lab. & Clin. Med. **29**: 1266-1286, 1944.
80. Hahn, P. F., Bale, W. F., Lawrence, E. O., and Whipple, G. H.: Radioactive Iron and Its Metabolism in Anemia, J. Exper. Med. **69**: 739-754, 1939.
81. Hahn, P. F., Bale, W. F., Ross, J. F., Hettig, R. A., and Whipple, G. H.: Radio Iron in Plasma Does not Exchange With Iron in Red Cells, Science **92**: 131-132, 1940.
82. Hahn, P. E., Bale, W. F., and Balfour, W. M.: Radioactive Iron Used to Study Red Blood Cells Over Long Periods: The Constancy of the Total Blood Volume in the Dog, Am. J. Physiol. **135**: 600-605, 1942.
83. Hahn, P. F., Balfour, W. M., Ross, J. F., Bale, W. I., and Whipple, G. H.: Red Blood Cell Volume, Circulating and Total as Determined With Radio Iron, Science **93**: 87-88, 1941.
84. Hahn, P. F., Ross, J. F., Bale, W. F., Balfour, W. M., and Whipple, G. H.: Red Cell and Plasma Volumes (Circulating and Total) As Determined by Radio Iron and by Dye, J. Exper. Med. **75**: 221-232, 1942.
85. Hahn, P. F., and Whipple, G. H.: Hemoglobin Production in Anemia Limited by Low Protein Intake, J. Exper. Med. **69**: 315-326, 1939.
86. Harrison, H., and Long, C. N. H.: The Regeneration of Liver Protein in the Rat, J. Biol. Chem. **161**: 545-557, 1945.
87. Hartzell, J. B., Winfield, J. M., and Irvin, J. L.: Plasma Vitamin C and Serum Protein Levels in Wound Disruption, J. A. M. A. **116**: 669-674, 1941.
88. Hawk, P. B., and Bergheim, O.: Practical Physiological Chemistry, Philadelphia, 1942, P. Blakiston's Son & Co., p. 427.
89. Harvey, S. C., and Hawes, E. L.: Effect of High Protein Diet on the Velocity of Growth of Fibroblasts in the Healing Wound, Ann. Surg. **91**: 641-650, 1930.

90. Harvey, William: Exercitatio Anatomica de Motu Cordis et Sanguinus in Animalibus, 1628; translated from the Latin by Willis, R., London, 1908, J. M. Dent & Co.
91. Hawkins, W. B., and Whipple, G. H.: Life Cycle of Red Blood Cell in the Dog, Am. J. Physiol. **122**: 418-427, 1938.
92. Hegsted, D. M., McKibbin, J. M., and Stare, F. J.: The Nutritive Value of Human Plasma for the Rat, J. Clin. Investigation **23**: 705-707, 1944.
93. Heidelberger, M., Treffers, H. P., Schoenheimer, R., Ratner, S., and Rittenberg, D.: Behavior of Antibody Protein Toward Dietary Nitrogen in Active and Passive Immunity, J. Biol. Chem. **144**: 555-562, 1942.
94. Henriques, V.: Die Eiweissynthese im Tierishen Organismus, Ztschr. f. physiol. Chem. **54**: 406-422, 1908.
95. Henriques, V., and Anderson, A. C.: Ueber Parenterale Ernahrung Durch Intravenose Injektion, Ztschr. f. physiol. Chem. **88**: 357-369, 1913.
96. Himsworth, H. P., and Glynn, L. E.: Toxipathic and Trophopathic Hepatitis, Lancet **1**: 457-461, 1944.
97. Himsworth, H. P.: Protein Metabolism in Relation to Disease, Proc. Roy. Soc. Med. **40**: 27-34, 1946.
98. Hoffman, W. S., Kozoll, D. D., and Osgood, B.: Blood Chemical Changes Following Intravenous Administration of a Casein Hydrolysate to Human Subjects, Proc. Soc. Exper. Biol. & Med. **61**: 137-140, 1946.
99. Holman, R. L., Mahoney, E. B., and Whipple, G. H.: Blood Plasma Protein Given by Vein Utilized in Body Metabolism: Dynamic Equilibrium Between Plasma and Tissue Proteins, J. Exper. Med. **59**: 269-282, 1934.
100. Holt, L. E., Jr., Tidwell, H. C., and Scott, T. F. M.: Intravenous Administration of Fat: Practical Therapeutic Procedure, J. Pediat. **6**: 151-160, 1935.
101. Horwitz, A., Sachar, L. A., and Elman, R.: Effect of Parenteral Amino Acids (Hydrolyzed Casein) on Growth of Rats, Proc. Soc. Exper. Biol. & Med. **49**: 118-121, 1942.
102. Howard, J. E., Parson, W., Stein, K. E., Eisenberg, H., and Reidt, V.: Studies on Fracture Convalescence: I. Nitrogen Metabolism After Fracture, Bull. Johns Hopkins Hosp. **75**: 156-168, 1944.
103. Howland, J. W., and Harkins, W. B.: Protein Metabolism, Protein Interchange, and Utilization in Phlorhizinized Dogs, J. Biol. Chem. **123**: 99-110, 1938.
104. Hubbell, R. B., and Koehne, M.: Effects of Varying Sugar Intake on Nitrogen Retention in Children, Am. J. Dis. Child. **47**: 988-992, 1934.
105. Isaacs, R.: Formation and Destruction of Red Blood Cells, Physiol. Rev. **17**: 291-303, 1937.
106. Itami, S.: Ueber Veranderungen der Blutbildenden Organe bei Experimenteller Polycythamie, Folia haemat. **6**: 425-428, 1908.
107. Jackson, C. M.: The Effects of Inanition and Malnutrition Upon Growth and Structure, Philadelphia, 1925, P. Blakiston's Son & Co.
108. Jones, C. M., and Eaton, F. B.: Postoperative Nutritional Edema, Arch. Surg. **27**: 159-177, 1933.
109. Kenyon, A. T., Knowlton, K., Sandiford, I., Koch, F. C., and Latwin, G.: A Comparative Study of the Metabolic Effects of Testosterone Propionate in Normal Men and Women and in Eunuchoidism, Endocrinology **26**: 26-45, 1940.
110. Kenyon, A. T., Sandiford, I., Bryan, A. H., Knowlton, K., and Koch, F. C.: The Effect of Testosterone Propionate on Nitrogen, Electrolyte, Water, and Energy Metabolism in Eunuchoidism, Endocrinology **23**: 135-153, 1938.
111. Keynes, G.: The History of Blood Transfusion, Brit. J. Surg. **31**: 38-50, 1943.
112. Kochakion, C. D., and Murlin, J. R.: Effect of Male Sex Hormone on Protein and Energy Metabolism of Castrated Dogs, J. Nutrition **10**: 437-459, 1935.
113. Kremen, A. J., Hall, H., Koschnitzke, H. K., Stevens, B., and Wangensteen, O. H.: Studies on the Intravenous Administration of Whole Bovine Plasma and Serum to Man, SURGERY **11**: 333-356, 1942.
114. Landergen, E.: Untersuchungen Über die Eiweissumsetzung des Menchen, Skandinav. Arch. f. Physiol. **14**: 112-175, 1903.
115. Landesman, R., and Weinstein, V. A.: The Intravenous Use of Amino Acids for Nutritional Purposes in the Surgical Patient, Surg., Gynec. & Obst. **75**: 300-306, 1942.
116. Landsteiner, K.: Ueber Agglutinationserscheinungen Normalen Menschlichen Blutes, Wien. klin. Wchnschr. **14**: 1132-1134, 1901.
117. Larson, P. S., and Chaikoff, I. L.: Influence of Carbohydrate on Nitrogen Metabolism in Normal Nutritional State, J. Nutrition **13**: 287-304, 1937.
118. Latta, T.: Injection of Saline Solutions in Extraordinary Quantities Into the Veins in Cases of Malignant Cholera, Lancet **2**: 243-244, 1831.
119. Laycock, H. T.: Some Impressions of Slow Starvation in China, Brit. M. J. **1**: 677-678, 1944.
120. Lewisohn, R.: A New and Greatly Simplified Method of Blood Transfusion. A Preliminary Report, M. Rec. **87**: 141-142, 1915.

121. Lewisohn, R.: Blood Transfusion by the Citrate Method, Surg., Gynec. & Obst. **21**: 37-48, 1915.
122. Lucido, J.: Metabolic and Blood Chemical Changes in a Severe Burn, Ann. Surg. **111**: 640-644, 1940.
123. Lyons, C.: Penicillin Therapy in Surgical Infections in the United States Army, J. A. M. A. **123**: 1007-1018, 1943.
123a. Clark, J. H., Nelson, W., Lyons, C., and Mayerson, H. S.: Chronic Shock: The Problem of Reduced Blood Volume in the Chronically Ill Patient.
124. Madden, S. C., Carter, J. R., Kattus, A. A., Miller, L. L., and Whipple, G. H.: Ten Amino Acids Essential for Plasma Protein Production Effective Orally or Intravenously, J. Exper. Med. **77**: 277-295, 1943.
125. Madden, S. C., Finch, C. A., Swalbach, W. G., and Whipple, G. H.: Blood Plasma Protein Production and Utilization. The Influence of Amino Acids and of Sterile Abscesses, J. Exper. Med. **71**: 283-297, 1940.
126. Madden, S. C., Kattus, A. A., Carter, J. R., Miller, L. L., and Whipple, G. H.: Plasma Protein Production as Influenced by Parenteral Protein Digests, Very High Protein Feeding and Red Blood Cell Catabolism, J. Exper. Med. **82**: 181-191, 1945.
127. Madden, S. C., Noehren, W. A., Waraich, G. S., and Whipple, G. H.: Blood Plasma Protein Production as Influenced by Amino Acids, J. Exper. Med. **69**: 721-738, 1939.
128. Madden, S. C., and Whipple, G. H.: Plasma Proteins: Their Source, Production and Utilization, Physiol. Rev. **20**: 194-217, 1940.
129. Madden, S. C., Woods, R. R., Shull, F. W., and Whipple, G. H.: Amino Acid Mixtures Effective Parenterally for Long Continued Plasma Protein Production: Casein Digests Compared, J. Exper. Med. **79**: 607-625, 1944.
130. Madden, S. C., Zeldis, L. J., Hengerer, A. D., Miller, L. L., Rowe, A. P., Turner, A. P., and Whipple, G. H.: Casein Digests Parenterally Utilized to Form Blood Plasma Protein, J. Exper. Med. **73**: 727-743, 1941.
131. Magee, E. H.: Discussion of the Physiology and Treatment of Starvation, Proc. Roy. Soc. Med. **38**: 388-395, 1945.
132. McCullum, E. V.: Nature of Repair Processes in Protein Metabolism, Am. J. Physiol. **29**: 215-237, 1911.
133. McDonald, J. J., Cadman, E. F., and Scudder, J.: The Importance of Whole Blood Transfusions in the Management of Severe Burns, Ann. Surg. **124**: 332-353, 1946.
134. Mecray, F. M., Borden, R. P., and Ravdin, I. S.: Nutritional Edema: Its Effect on Gastric Emptying Time Before and After Gastric Operations, SURGERY **1**: 53-64, 1937.
135. Melnick, D., and Cowgill, G. R.: The Serum Protein Complex as a Factor in Regulating Blood Volume, Proc. Soc. Exper. Biol. & Med. **35**: 312-314, 1936.
136. Melnick, D., and Cowgill, G. R.: The Problem of Hypoproteinemia, Yale J. Biol. & Med. **10**: 49-63, 1937.
137. Melnick, D., Cowgill, G. R., and Burack, E.: The Influence of Diet Upon Regeneration of Serum Protein, J. Exper. Med. **64**: 877-920, 1936.
138. Melnick, D., Cowgill, G. R., and Burack, E.: Influence of Diet Upon Regeneration of Serum Protein, Potency Ratios of Serum Protein, Lactalbumin, and Casein and Effect of Tissue Protein Catabolism on Formation of Serum Protein, J. Exper. Med. **64**: 897-920, 1936.
139. Messinger, W. J.: Nitrogen Equilibrium and Regeneration of Serum Proteins, Arch. Int. Med. **72**: 91-103, 1943.
140. Meyers, W. K., and Keefer, C. S.: Relation of Plasma Proteins to Ascites and Edema in Cirrhosis of the Liver, Arch. Int. Med. **55**: 349-359, 1935.
141. Miller, L.: Dog Hemoglobin Parenterally Well Utilized to Maintain Weight and Nitrogen Balance: Utilization Improved With d.l. Methionine but Not With d.l. Isoleucine, Federation Proc. **5**: 73, 1946.
142. Miller, L. L., Ross, J. F., and Whipple, G. H.: Methionine and Cystine, Specific Protein Factors In Preventing Chloroform Liver Injury in Protein Depleted Dogs, Am. J. M. Sc. **200**: 739-756, 1940.
143. Miller, L. L., and Whipple, G. H.: Chloroform Liver Injury Increases as Protein Stores Decrease, Am. J. M. Sc. **199**: 204-216, 1940.
144. Mitchell, H. H.: A Method of Determining the Biological Value of Protein, J. Biol. Chem. **58**: 873-903, 1924.
145. Moore, N. S., and Van Slyke, D. D.: The Relationship Between Plasma Specific Gravity, Plasma Protein Content and Edema in Nephritis, J. Clin. Investigation **8**: 337-355, 1930.
146. Mueller, A. J., Fickas, A. D., and Cox, W. M.: Minimum Maintenance Requirements of Enzymatic Casein Hydrolysate, Bull. Johns Hopkins Hosp. **72**: 110-115, 1943.
147. Mueller, A. J., Kemmerer, K. S., Cox, W. M., and Barnes, S. T.: The Effect of Casein and a Casein Digest on Growth and Serum Protein Regeneration, J. Biol. Chem. **134**: 573-583, 1940.

148. Mulholland, J. H., Co Tui, Wright, A., and Vinci, V. J.: Nitrogen Metabolism, Caloric Intake and Weight Loss in Postoperative Convalescence, Ann. Surg. **117**: 512-534, 1943.
149. National Research Council Reprint and Circular Series No. 122, Washington, D. C., August, 1945.
150. Opie, E. L., and Alford, L. B.: The Influence of Diet on Hepatic Necrosis and Toxicity of Chloroform, J. A. M. A. **62**: 895, 1914.
151. Opie, E. L., and Alford, L. B.: The Influence of Diet Upon Necrosis Caused by Hepatic and Renal Poisons. I. Diet and the Hepatic Lesions of Chloroform, Phosphorus, and Alcohol, J. Exper. Med. **21**: 1-20, 1915.
152. Orten, A. V., and Orten, J. M.: The Role of Dietary Protein in Hemoglobin Formation, J. Nutrition **26**: 21-31, 1943.
153. Osborne, T. B., and Mendel, L. B.: Amino Acids in Nutrition and Growth, J. Biol. Chem. **17**: 325-349, 1914.
154. Osborne, T. B., and Mendel, L. B.: A Quantitative Comparison of Casein, Lactalbumin and Edestin for Growth and Maintenance, J. Biol. Chem. **26**: 1-24, 1916.
155. Peters, J. P.: Problems of Nitrogen Metabolism, Federation Proc. **3**: 197-201, 1944.
156. Peters, J. P., and Van Slyke, D. D.: Quantitative Clinical Chemistry, Vol. II, Baltimore, 1931, Williams & Wilkins Company, p. 518.
157. Ibid: P. 602.
158. Pfluger, E.: Ueber Einige Gezetze des Eiweisstoffwechsels (mit Besonderer Berucksichtigung der Lehre vom Sogenannten Circulirenden Eiweiss), Arch. f. d. ges. Physiol. **54**: 333-420, 1898.
159. Pommerenke, W. T., Slavin, H. B., Kariher, D. H., and Whipple, G. H.: Dog Plasma Protein Given by Vein Utilized in Body Metabolism of Dog: Horse Plasma and Dog Hemoglobin not Similarly Utilized, J. Exper. Med. **61**: 283-297, 1935.
160. Ravdin, I. S.: Hypoproteinemia and Its Relation to Surgical Problems, Ann. Surg. **112**: 576-583, 1940.
161. Ravdin, I. S., McNamee, H. G., Kamholz, J. H., and Rhoads, J. E.: Effect of Hypoproteinemia on Susceptibility to Shock Resulting From Hemorrhage, Arch. Surg. **48**: 491-492, 1944.
162. Ravdin, I. S., Stengel, A., and Prushankin, M.: The Control of Hypoproteinemia in Surgical Patients, J. A. M. A. **114**: 107-112, 1940.
163. Rasmussen, L. H., Abels, J. C., Pack, G. T., and Rhoads, C. D.: Metabolic Studies on Patients With Cancer of the Gastrointestinal Tract: XIV Effect of High Protein Diets on the Prevention of Postoperative Hypoproteinemia in Patients With Gastric Cancer, J. A. M. A. **124**: 358-360, 1944.
164. Reineke, E. P.: Williamson, M. D., and Turner, C. W.: Utilization of Glycoprotein of the Blood Plasma by the Lactating Mammary Gland, J. Biol. Chem. **138**: 83-90, 1941.
165. Rhoads, J. E., and Kasinskas, W.: The Influence of Hypoproteinemia on the Formation of Callus in Experimental Fractures, SURGERY **11**: 38-44, 1942.
166. Ringer, A. I.: Protein Metabolism in Experimental Diabetes, J. Biol. Chem. **12**: 431-445, 1942.
167. Robscheit-Robbins, F. S., Miller, L. L., and Whipple, G. H.: Hemoglobin and Plasma Protein: Simultaneous Production During Continued Bleeding as Influenced by Amino Acids, Plasma, Hemoglobin, and Digests of Serum, Hemoglobin, and Casein, J. Exper. Med. **77**: 375-396, 1943.
168. Robscheit-Robbins, F. S., Miller, L. L., Alling, E. L., and Whipple, G. H.: Human and Animal Globin Related to the Production of Hemoglobin and Plasma Protein, J. Exper. Med. **83**: 355-372, 1946.
169. Robscheit-Robbins, F. S., Miller, L. L., and Whipple, G. H.: Hemoglobin and Plasma Protein Production, J. Exper. Med. **83**: 463-475, 1946.
170. Robertson, O. H., and Rous, P.: Normal Fate of Erythrocytes: II. Blood Destruction in Plethoric Animals and in Animals With Simple Anemia, J. Exper. Med. **25**: 665-673, 1917.
171. Rose, W. C.: The Nutritive Significance of the Amino Acids, Physiol. Rev. **18**: 109-136, 1938.
172. Rose, W. C., Haines, W. J., and Johnson, J. E.: The Role of Amino Acids in Human Nutrition, J. Biol. Chem. **146**: 683-684, 1942.
173. Ross, J. F., and Chapin, M. A.: Absence of Red Blood Cell Reserves in Human Subjects as Indicated With Radioactive Tagged Cells, J. Clin. Investigation **21**: 640, 1942.
174. Ross, J. F., and Chapin, M. A.: Effect of Storage of Citrated Blood on the Survival of Transfused Red Blood Cells, J. A. M. A. **123**: 827-829, 1943.
175. Rous, P.: Destruction of Red Blood Corpuscles in Health and Disease, Physiol. Rev. **3**: 75-105, 1923.

176. Rous, P., and Robertson, O. H.: The Normal Fate of Erythrocytes: I. In Healthy Animals, J. Exper. Med. **25**: 651-665, 1917.
177. Sachar, L. A., Horwitz, A., and Elman, R.: Studies on Hypoalbuminemia Produced by Protein Deficient Diets: I. Hypoalbuminemia as a Quantitative Measure of Tissue Protein Depletion, J. Exper. Med. **75**: 453-459, 1942.
178. Sako, W. S.: Resistance to Infection as Affected by Variations in the Proportions of Protein, Fat and Carbohydrate in the Diet, J. Pediat. **20**: 475-483, 1942.
179. Schoenheimer, R., and Rittenberg, D.: Study of Intermediary Metabolism of Animals With the Aid of Isotopes, Physiol. Rev. **20**: 218-248, 1940.
180. Schoenheimer, R., and Rattner, S.: The Metabolism of Proteins and Amino Acids, Ann. Rev. Biochem. **10**: 197-220, 1941.
181. Schoenheimer, R., Rattner, S., and Rittenberg, D.: The Interaction of Blood Proteins of the Rat With Dietary Nitrogen, J. Biol. Chem. **144**: 541-544, 1942.
182. Schoenheimer, R., Rattner, S., Rittenberg, D., and Heidelberg, M.: The Interaction of Antibody Protein With Dietary Nitrogen in Actively Immunized Animals, J. Biol. Chem. **144**: 545-554, 1942.
183. Schmidt, C. L. A., Allen, F. W., and Tarver, H.: A Theory of Protein Metabolism: The Transformation of Proteins, Science **91**: 18-19, 1940.
184. Shaffer, P. A., and Coleman, W.: Protein Metabolism in Typhoid Fever, Arch. Int. Med. **4**: 538-600, 1909.
185. Shearburn, E. W.: The Effect of Plasma Transfusion Upon the Serum Proteins and Blood Volume of Dogs Rendered Hypoproteinemic by Diet, Surg., Gynec. & Obst. **74**: 343-347, 1942.
186. Shemin, D., and Rittenberg, D.: Some Interrelationships in General Nitrogen Metabolism, J. Biol. Chem. **153**: 401-421, 1944.
187. Shemin, D., and Rittenberg, D.: Studies on the Formation of Heme and on the Average Life Time of the Human Red Blood Cell, Federation Proc. **5**: 153, 1946.
188. Shohl, A. T., Butler, A. M., Blackfan, K. D., and MacLachlan, E.: Nitrogen Metabolism During Oral and Parenteral Administration of the Amino Acids of Hydrolyzed Casein, J. Pediat. **15**: 469-475, 1939.
189. Shohl, A. T., and Blackfan, K. D.: The Intravenous Administration of Crystalline Amino Acids to Infants, J. Nutritionu **20**: 305-316, 1940.
190. Shohl, A. T.: Nitrogen Storage Following Intravenous and Oral Administration of Casein Hydrolysate to Infants With Acute Gastrointestinal Disturbance, J. Clin. Investigation **22**: 257-263, 1943.
191. Snead, E. A., and Ebert, R. V.: Relationship of Plasma Volume and the Cell Plasma Ratio to the Total Red Cell Volume, Am. J. Physiol. **132**: 411-417, 1941.
192. Starling, E. H.: On the Absorption of Fluids From the Connective Tissue Spaces, J. Physiol. **19**: 312-326, 1895.
193. Strumia, M. M., Chornock, F. W., Blake, A. D., and Karr, W. G.: The Use of a Modified Globin From Human Red Blood Cells as a Plasma Substitute, Am. J. M. Sc. **209**: 436-443, 1945.
194. Strumia, M. M., Blake, A. D., Reider, H. C., and Chornock, F. W.: The Use of a Modified Globin From Human Red Blood Cells in Hypoproteinemias, Am. J. M. Sc. **211**: 51-62, 1946.
195. Studley, H. O.: Percentage of Weight Loss: A Basic Indicator of Surgical Risk in Patients With Chronic Peptic Ulcer, J. A. M. A. **106**: 458-460, 1936.
196. Sun, T. P.: Histophysiological Study of the Epithelial Changes in the Small Intestine of the Albino Mouse After Starvation and Refeeding, Anat. Rec. **34**: 341-350, 1927.
197. Taylor, S. G., III, and Lytle, F.: Effect of Resuspended Erythrocyte Transfusion on Serum Protein, Proc. Central Soc. Clin. Research **18**: 20-21, 1945.
198. Thompson, W. D., Ravdin, I. S., and Frank, I. L.: Effect of Hypoproteinemia on Wound Disruption, Arch. Surg. **36**: 500-508, 1938.
199. Thompson, W. D., Ravdin, I. S., Rhoads, J. E., and Frank, I. L.: Use of Lyophile Plasma in Correction of Hypoproteinemia and Prevention of Wound Disruption, Arch. Surg. **36**: 509-518, 1938.
200. Torbert, H. C.: Effect of Fasting on Serum Protein Concentration of Rat With Special Reference to Question of Existence of Immediately Utilizable Circulating Plasma Protein, J. Exper. Med. **62**: 1-10, 1935.
201. Tucker, H. F., Treadwell, C. R., and Eckstein, H.: Effect of Supplementary Cystine and Methionine on the Production of Fatty Livers in Rats on High Fat Diets Containing Casein or Edistin, J. Biol. Chem. **135**: 85-90, 1940.
202. Tsan Wen Li, and Freeman, S.: Effect of Protein Deficiency and Cholesterol Feeding on the Liver of Dogs, Am. J. Physiol. **145**: 646-659, 1946.
203. Tsan Wen Li, and Freeman, S.: Experimental Lipemia and Hypercholesterolemia by Protein Depletion and by Cholesterol Feeding in Dogs, Am. J. Physiol. **145**: 660-667, 1946.
204. Varco, R. L.: Preoperative Dietary Management for Surgical Patients With Special Reference to Lesions of the Stomach and Duodenum, SURGERY **19**: 3-78, 1946.

205. Vaughan, J.: Experience at Belsen, Lancet **248**: 724, 1945.
206. Voit, C.: L. Herman's Handbuch der Physiologie, Leipzig, 1881, quoted by Folin, O.: A Theory of Protein Metabolism, Am. J. Physiol. **13**: 117-138, 1905.
207. Wangensteen, O. H., Hall, H., Kremen, A. J., and Stevens, B.: Intravenous Administration of Bovine and Human Plasma: Proof of Utilization, Proc. Soc. Exper. Biol. & Med. **43**: 616-621, 1940.
208. Wasserman, L. R., Volterra, M., and Rosenthal, N.: Quantitative Urobilinogen Excretion Following Transfusion of Fresh and Stored Blood, Am. J. M. Sc. **204**: 356-364, 1942.
209. Watson, C. J.: Studies on Urobilinogen; An Improved Method for the Quantitative Estimation of Urobilinogen in Feces and Urine, Am. J. Clin. Path. **6**: 458-475, 1936.
210. Watson, C. J.: The Pyrol Pigments With Particular Reference to Normal and Pathologic Hemoglobin Metabolism, Downey's Handbook of Hemotology, New York, 1938, Paul B. Hoeber & Co.
211. Weech, A. A.: The Significance of the Albumin Fraction of Serum, Harvey Lect., Bull. New York Acad. Med. **15**: 63-91, 1939.
212. Weech, A. A., and Goettsch, E.: Dietary Protein and Regeneration of Serum Albumin: Comparison of Potency Values of Beef Serum, Beef Muscle and Casein, Bull. Johns Hopkins Hosp. **63**: 181-186, 1938.
213. Weech, A. A., Goettsch, E., and Reeves, E. B.: The Effect of Serum Transfusion on Plasma Protein Depletion Associated With Nutritional Edema in Dogs, J. Clin. Investigation **12**: 217-227, 1933.
214. Weech, A. A., Snelling, C. E., and Goettsch, E.: Relation Between Plasma Protein Content, Plasma Specific Gravity, and Edema in Dogs Maintained on Protein Inadequate Diet and in Dogs Rendered Edematous by Plasmaphoresis, J. Clin. Investigation **12**: 193-216, 1933.
215. Weech, A. A., Wollstein, M., and Goettsch, E.: Nutritional Edema in Dog: Development of Deficits in Erythrocytes and Hemoglobin on Diet Deficient in Protein, J. Clin. Investigation **16**: 719-728, 1937.
216. Whipple, A. O.: The Critical Latent or Lag Period in Healing of Wounds, Ann. Surg. **112**: 481-488, 1940.
217. Whipple, G. H.: Protein Production and Exchange in the Body Including Hemoglobin, Plasma Protein and Cell Protein, Am. J. M. Sc. **196**: 609-621, 1938.
218. Whipple, G. H.: Hemoglobin and Plasma Proteins: Their Production, Utilization and Interrelation, Am. J. M. Sc. **203**: 477-489, 1942.
219. Whipple, G. H., and Madden, S. C.: Hemoglobin, Plasma Proteins, and Cell Proteins: Their Interchange and Construction in Emergencies, Medicine **23**: 215-224, 1944.
220. Whitehorn, J. C.: A System of Blood Analysis: Supplement II. Simplified Method for the Determination of Chlorides in Blood or Plasma, J. Biol. Chem. **45**: 449-460, 1921.
221. Wiener, A. S.: Longevity of the Erythrocyte, J. A. M. A. **102**: 1779, 1934.
222. Wintrobe, M. M.: Clinical Hematology, Philadelphia, 1942, Lea & Febiger, p. 201.
223. Woodyatt, R. T., Sansum, W. D., and Wilder, R. M.: Prolonged and Accurately Timed Intravenous Injections of Sugar, J. A. M. A. **65**: 2067-2070, 1915.
224. Zeldis, L. J., Alling, E. L., McCoord, A. B., and Kulka, J. P.: Plasma Protein Metabolism: Chronic Depletion of Circulating Proteins During Low Protein Feeding, J. Exper. Med. **82**: 157-179, 1945.

Book Reviews

Principles in Roentgen Study of the Chest. By William Snow. Springfield, Ill., 1946, Charles C Thomas, Publisher.

This monograph is an excellent one because of its simplicity and conciseness. The author, in the beginning, describes the various types of roentgenography followed by a discussion of normal lung findings. At the end of each chapter is an excellent group of representative roentgenograms demonstrating the points which the author wants to emphasize. After the consideration of the normal anatomy and roentgenologic findings, the various disease processes are taken up separately, the first part of each chapter being given over to the subject, with reference to illustrative roentgenograms at the end of each chapter. Special chapters deal with special chest problems in children and the roentgenologic demonstration of the thoracic circulatory system and the thoracic cage itself. The monograph is profusely illustrated as demonstrated by the 508 illustrations in the 397 page monograph. Illustrations are well produced.

The only criticism that the reviewer has of the book is that bronchiectasis, which is such a frequently encountered condition, is certainly inadequately considered.

Because of the conciseness of the work, it should be of great value to every physician.

Surgical Treatment of the Nervous System. By Bancroft, F. W., and Pilcher, C., editors. Pp. 534, with 298 illustrations. Philadelphia, 1947, J. B. Lippincott Company.

This is a compilation of twenty chapters, seventeen of them written by an individual and three of them written by a senior and junior author. The associate editor wrote five chapters.

Since there are many contributors, there is considerable chapter variation in manner of presentation and quality. There are some very well written chapters, but so many are mediocre that the book as a whole is a disappointment. Perhaps the deficiencies of the book are due in part to the trying time in which it was compiled but it seems that all chapters should have a common objective, which is apparently not the case. As written, the general surgeon and general practitioner will find it a valuable reference book but with the exception of a few chapters the neurosurgeon will profit little by reading it. A similar but more comprehensive treatise written as a ready reference for the nuerosurgeon would be most valuable. Some chapters have no bibliography, others have a list of references at the end of the chapter, and a few have documented the text by specific reference to the bibliography.

Chapter 1, The General Principles of Neurosurgical Technique, is a description of standard neurosurgical technique, anesthesia in neurosurgery, technique of pneumoencephalography, angiography, etc.

Chapter 2, The Surgery of Infantile Hydrocephalus, is a discussion of the author's views concerning the diagnosis, selection of cases for operation, treatment, and prognosis. Toxoplasmosis, one of the more common causes of infantile hydrocephalus, is not even mentioned.

Chapter 3, Craniocerebral Trauma. In this chapter in addition to the usual textbook discussion of subdural hematoma, there is added a one-page discussion of subdural hematomas in children, including some information recently published in the periodic literature.

Chapter 4, Cranioplasty, is a fairly good review of modern methods of skull defect repair but would be much more easily understood if better illustrated. There is a page of colored photography which catches the eye but is very disappointing when one attempts to find the details referred to in the legend.

Chapter 5, Brain Abscess, is one of the better chapters. It is short yet contains many of the problems encountered in treating these difficult lesions. The author admits that difficult situations may be encountered and that the surgeon may make serious errors. Vincent's method of excision of abscesses is briefly discussed. Even since this book was written a more radical modification of Vincent's methods seems to be gaining favor.

Chapter 6, Osteomyelitis of the Skull, is a good discussion of sinus and mastoid infections in their relation to osteomyelitis of the skull. It seems unfortunate that a neurosurgeon sufficiently familiar with osteomyelitis of the skull could not be found to write this chapter. It is obvious that the author has had a large experience with osteomyelitis of the skull and in general the opinions expressed and the technique described conform to good neurosurgical practice, yet there are minor variations from accepted neurosurgical practice, such as chiseling on the skull which contains a traumatized brain. The important subject of bone regeneration after osteomyelitis is dismissed with a statement that in some instances bone regeneration serves to reduce or even correct the deformity.

Chapter 7, Tumors of the Skull, is a good but short chapter (seven pages). Eosinophilic granuloma, a recently described lesion of bone, is included. The use of fibrin film to repair dural defects is recommended by the author as though it were an accepted procedure.

Chapter 8, Tumors of the Meninges. After some very brief general remarks on meningiomas, the operative technique for meningiomas is discussed. In general, there is little to praise or severely criticize in this chapter, but one might disagree with some of the author's technique, that is ''Deeper dissection may be done more gently and with less trauma to the adjacent brain by a dissecting finger.'' Obviously, the author of Chapter 10 is not of this opinion, for he writes ''once the surface of the tumor is exposed, gentle dissection is less destructive and less hemorrhagic than crude finger enucleation.''

Chapter 9, Tumors of Cranial Nerves, contains many informative illustrations but like the preceding chapter gives the impression of being compiled without great effort on the part of the authors. Only one reference is given.

The upright or sitting position for operation is considered to be by far the most favorable for operation in the posterior cranial fossa; its advantages and disadvantages are discussed but the reader is not cautioned that air embolus can occur.

Total and partial removal of eighth nerve tumors is discussed but the authors do not indicate whether their own practice is to remove these tumors totally or partially. Choice of operation is dismissed with the noncommittal statement that ''surgeons differ in their views regarding the most desirable method, but sound surgical judgment demands that the method be chosen that best meets the circumstances encountered in each individual patient.''

Chapter 10, Intrinsic Tumors of the Cerebrum. The surgical pathology of most of the intrinsic tumors of the brain is briefly discussed followed by a section entitled clinical discussion, in which the results of surgery are given and a very brief discussion of the symptomatology and findings in the various types of tumor is included. Under operative methods it is obvious that only the author's individual technique is considered. A short paragraph on prevention of cortical ruptures is interesting and has merit but one wonders if the methods described are always effective in its prevention. The author is very pessimistic about the results of x-ray therapy in intrinsic tumors of the cerebrum.

Chapter 11, Tumors of the Hypophysial Region. Much of this chapter is anatomy, surgical pathology, and diagnosis of suprasellar lesions. Fig. 66 which the same author uses in Chapter 9 would have been more appropriate here. Treatment is discussed in more or less standardized fashion giving the impression that chromophylic adenoma, craniopharyngioma, and suprasellar cholesteotoma are frequently totally removed without insurmountable difficulty. Hyperthermia resulting from trauma to the hypothalamus is not mentioned.

Chapter 12, Intrinsic Tumors of the Cerebellum and Brain Stem, is an excellent chapter with absence of mediocrity found in many of the other chapters. It is documented. The author gives not only his own opinion or procedure but also that of others and discusses factors favorable and unfavorable.

Chapter 13, Vascular Anomalies of the Brain, is very much the same material contained in a paper published in 1946 by the author of this chapter. It advocates excision of these lesions if possible and three cases in which excision was performed are reported.

Chapter 14, Surgery of Disorders of the cranial Nerves, is one of the better chapters in the book. It is quite inclusive, giving not only the author's procedures but also all others, including even the most recent literature. There are a number of very informative line drawings, and a good bibliography is appended.

Chapter 15, Diseases Characterized by Involuntary Movements, is a good and well-documented discussion of these movements and their treatment. Complete detailed description of the operation is given. Much is said in evaluation of the operative treatment for these conditions and it seems to be well balanced without undue conservatism or enthusiasm for the operation.

Chapter 16, Epilepsy Due to Atrophic Cerebral Lesions, is a short but well-written chapter, most of it a description of indications for operation and technique of operation.

Chapter 17, Surgery of the Spinal Cord, is a narration for the most part of the author's opinion and practice, with no bibliography. It is well illustrated but otherwise gives the impression of having been composed without great effort.

Chapter 18, Surgical Lesions of Peripheral Nerves, is a good standard discussion with brief mention of most of the recent developments. Such problems as nerve grafts, causalgia, and phantom limb pain with cortical excision for its relief are considered and one of the admirable features is the fact that the author freely gives his opinion in many controversial matters.

Chapter 19, Surgery of the Sympathetic Nervous System, is a well-written and illustrated forty-four pages. This is one of the better chapters in the book. Much of it is description of various types of sympathectomy followed by a discussion of their application.

Chapter 20, Chemotherapy in Neurosurgery, is a very short discussion of some of the general principles of the use of sulfonamides and penicillin in neurosurgery.

It is to be hoped that this is only the first of many future editions of a comprehensive up-to-date text and reference book of neurosurgery.

Gynecological and Obstetrical Pathology. By Emil Novak, A.B., M.D., D.Sc., F.A.C.S., ed. 2, Philadelphia, 1947, W. B. Saunders Company.

This book is so well known by gynecologists, obstetricians, and pathologists that mention of its value is unnecessary. Although neither an exhaustive treatise nor a reference, the book covers the material adequately in a clear concise style. Suitable bibliographic references for additional study are supplied at the end of each chapter.

The second edition has brought the material up to date and has many new illustrations. Most of the illustrations are excellent. However, those showing the various gross vulvar lesions are unsatisfactory.

The book should appeal to pathologists as well as gynecologists and residents in training.

Radiology for Medical Students. By Hodges, F. J., Lampe, I., and Holt, J. F. Pp. 424. Chicago, 1947, The Year Book Publishers, Inc. $6.75.

This little book is the first adequate single volume presentation of the principles of present-day roentgenologic diagnosis and radiation therapy. While it is designed for the use of medical students and has been organized around the course presented at the University of Michigan it would constitute a very adequate and complete introduction to radiology for any physician who wishes to know more about the fundamentals of the radiologic approach to medical problems both diagnostic and therapeutic.

Thorough-going courses in radiology are relatively new in the medical curriculum and the authors of this book have been aware of the usual problem that arises as to whether to present merely a few fundamental considerations or to attempt to present a wealth of detail. It seems to this reviewer that the authors have made a very wise choice in steering, as far as text is concerned, a more or less middle ground. The emphasis has certainly been, particularly in the diagnostic section, on principles without too much attempt to present all of the various diagnostic possibilities and rare and unusual conditions which might be illustrated.

Very excellent and concise introductory material is presented on the history of the development of radiology and there are also excellent brief sections on the physics of diagnostic roentgenology, the physics of therapeutic radiology and, of special interest, material on the biologic and therapeutic effects of radiation. This latter material is particularly difficult of access in concise and understandable form and seems particularly valuable for inclusion in an elementary treatise of this sort.

Of special merit in the diagnostic section is the emphasis on the method of approach both in planning and in carrying out the x-ray study and in interpretation of the findings. It is this emphasis on the presentation of what might be called the underlying philosophy of radiology that principally distinguishes this book in the reviewer's mind.

The section on the tissue effects of radiation is of the greatest importance and there is an excellent presentation of the fundamental differences between radiosensitivity and radiocurability of tumors. Also very important is the emphasis on the late effects of the intensive irradiation for destruction of neoplasms of which both the physician and the patient should be aware at the time the irradiation is carried out.

No attempt has been made to be dogmatic as to the choice of therapeutic methods recommended and it is well emphasized that the radiation method is not in competition with surgery but rather that the two methods have specific indications and often are supplementary.

This volume is not intended to be in any way a handbook or atlas of radiology for the diagnosis and treatment of disease but it is a very well thought out and readable presentation of the fundamentals of the subject.

The 1946 Year Book of Neurology, Psychiatry and Neurosurgery. Edited by Neurology: Hans H. Reese, M.D., Professor of Neurology and Psychiatry, University of Wisconsin Medical School and Mabel G. Masten, M.D., Associate Professor Neuropsychiatry, University of Wisconsin Medical School; Psychiatry: Nolan D. C. Lewis, M.D., Director, New York State University; Neurosurgery: Percival Bailey, M.D., Professor Neurology and Neurological Surgery, University of Illinois. Pp. 732, with 103 illustrations. Chicago, 1946, The Year Book Publishers, Inc. $3.75.

This book is comprised of abstracts of articles which the editors consider representative of the year's literature in these fields. The editors possess wide experience and are capable of proper selection of articles and of making proper criticism of them. It is unfortunate that they do not comment more frequently and in greater detail concerning their opinions of the articles reviewed. Such an addition would give the book better continuity and the abstracts proper relative significance. The subject matter of the various fields is well covered. Both the foreign and American literature is abstracted.

The section on neurology includes articles on neuroanatomy, neurophysiology, neuropathology, convulsive disorders, diseases of the central nervous system, and neurologic diagnostic procedures. The abstracts are complete, in fact, some are too long and could be adequately reviewed with greater brevity.

The section on psychiatry includes articles on specific childhood psychiatric problems, the psychoses, the psychoneuroses, and special therapy in psychiatry. There are also many abstracts dealing with military psychiatric problems. The abstracts in this section are concise; the field of psychiatry is well reviewed.

The section on neurosurgery includes information on peripheral and sympathetic nerve surgery, purulent infections of the central nervous system, herniated discs, spinal cord and craniocerebral injuries, vascular lesions, and intracranial tumors. This is the first year that there has been a separate section of the Year Book devoted to the field of neurosurgery. The advisability of having such a section is readily apparent to the reader. It is an excellent addition and should be continued.

This year's Year Book is especially valuable since there is more comprehensive coverage of more closely allied fields of interest than in previous years. It is emphasized that all persons even with an indirect interest in neurology, psychiatry, and neurosurgery should read this book.

Diseases of the Adrenals. By Louis J. Soffer, M.D., Philadelphia, 1946, Lea & Febiger.

This book is written well and is easy and interesting to read. It contains a thorough summary of the recent advances in the study of the physiology of the adrenal cortex including the chemistry of the steroid hormones of the cortex and the function of these compounds. The physiologic concepts of adrenal cortical function are very nicely correlated with clinical conditions. The chapters dealing with Addison's disease are especially informative. The details of treatment are good, but the discussion of the treatment of crisis in Addison's disease is a bit too brief for the person who has had little experience with the disease. The discussion of the adrenogenital syndrome is rather complicated as it necessarily must be. The evaluations of diagnostic aids such as 17—ketosteroid analysis and perirenal air insufflation are conservative and fair. The indications for operation and the precautions regarding therapy immediately after removal of an adrenal cortical tumor are thoroughly discussed. In the discussion of the diagnosis of pheochromocytoma no mention is made of the histamine provocative test described by Roth. This test is simple and should be of much use in detecting this condition. The extensive bibliography covering the subject of adrenal physiology and pathology is worth a great deal. There are several errors in text references to the bibliography. This book should be very useful for physicians in general internal medicine as well as for physicians limiting their practice to metabolic diseases.

Medicine in the Changing Order. Report of the New York Academy of Medicine and the Changing Order. Pp. 240. New York, 1947, Commonwealth Fund. $2.

In 1942 the New York Academy of Medicine appointed a committee to study the problems of medical care, a committee which during the course of its deliberations was wisely designated as a Committee on Medicine and the Changing Order. This committee, made up largely of physicians, but with representation from allied professions and social groups, has had the advice and counsel of a large number of distinguished community leaders representing diversified interests and points of view. Subcommittees dealt with medical education, graduate and postgraduate medical education, internships, hospitals, administration of public health services, extension of medical services, cost of diagnostic and consultant services, industrial medicine, rural medicine, nursing, and dentistry.

The committee has already sponsored a series of distinguished monographs which represented, however, the points of view of the respective authors, not of the committee. Several of these monographs have already been reviewed in these columns. The current volume signed by the committee constitutes the report and conclusions of its deliberations. At the same time it serves as an admirable summary of the entire series.

Approaching its task from the historical perspective, the committee has analyzed the current problems and needs of medical care and in a thoroughly objective manner has attempted to appraise the various suggestions advanced for better medical service. Throughout the report, emphasis is placed upon quality as well as quantity of care, and upon the necessity of greater attention to the preventive aspects of medical service.

The report is packed with recommendations which are made boldly and without evasive qualifications. The committee supports the growing tendency toward group practice, urges more extensive voluntary health insurance aided by governmental subsidy if necessary, but rejects compulsory insurance. It advocates expansion of health services and the construction of new hospitals and health centers radiating into rural areas from metropolitan centers. Among the many other recommendations are proposals for medical and nursing education and licensing, and for hospital construction and administration.

Throughout the book runs a dominant theme of the need for greater recognition of the social obligations of medicine and attention to social and economic forces without sacrifice of the scientific aspects which have developed more rapidly in recent years. Few readers will agree with all the proposals and recommendations but all will recognize this volume as a thought-provoking and forthright analysis of medicine's obligation to adapt itself to changing social conditions.

Postgraduate Obstetrics. By William F. Mengert, M.D., Pp. 363, with 123 illustrations. New York, 1947, Paul B. Hoeber, Inc.

This book is a brief review of practical clinical obstetrics. Virtually all theoretical discussions have been eliminated. On the whole, the material is well presented and the illustrations, although limited, are good. The book considers only common complications of pregnancy.

It is a little difficult to understand how the book can be extensively used as it is too brief for medical students and too incomplete for the practitioner dealing with specific obstetric problems in practice.

The widest application of this material would probably be for the physician desiring a brief review of obstetrics before beginning practice.

Penicillin in Neurology. By A. Earl Walker, M.D., Associate Professor of Neurological Surgery, the University of Chicago, and Herbert C. Johnson, M.D., Resident Neurological Surgeon, The University of Chicago. Pp. 204 with 95 illustrations. Springfield, Ill., 1946, Charles C Thomas, Publisher. Cloth. $5.

The jacket on this volume states "this monograph presents (1) the results of studies of the dispersion and absorption of penicillin when administered by intrathecal injection and (2) the effect of the drug on nervous tissue in health and disease. On the basis of these investigations and clinical experiences, the rational use of penicillin in neurological disorders is discussed, giving the book a wide range of appeal among physicians, surgeons and research workers."

The introductory chapters are devoted to a consideration of penicillin in general and to the routes of administration of the drug with particular reference to the distribution of penicillin in the central nervous system. Then follow experimental and clinical observations detailing the toxic effects of penicillin upon the central nervous system. These and subsequent investigations indicate that toxic reactions are related to the quantity of the antibiotic introduced intrathecally and into the ventricular spaces. Therapy of suppurative meningitis is then presented with the important recommendation that penicillin must be injected intrathecally as well as administered parenterally for the most satisfactory results. There is a sound discussion of the therapy of pyogenic infections of the skull and brain, as well as the diseases of the spinal cord. A glaring weakness of this monograph is the brief and incomplete discussion of penicillin in the treatment of syphilis of the nervous system. This chapter might well have been omitted without detracting from the purpose and value of the monograph. The work concludes with a brief discussion of other antibiotics such as streptomycin, streptothricin, actinomycin, and clavacin. The volume is well indexed, profusely illustrated, and the publisher has utilized skill and good taste in producing an attractive book.

On page 150 the authors touch upon an important theme which has distressed many clinicians treating suppurative disease of the central nervous system with penicillin. They refer to discretion on the part of the physician in treating infected cases of spina bifida where there is serious derangement of the nervous system. Eradication of the infection in some cases will lead to major social and economic complications. In older children and adults suppuration of the central nerves causes irreparable damage to the central nervous system, and the use of a potent antibacterial agent like penicillin has eliminated the infection but has left patients hopelessly incompetent. However, brilliant therapeutic results frequently ensue in some of the most desperately ill patients, and the physician has no choice but to treat all of the patients with this expectation in view.

The monograph should be of interest to students in this field, and individuals in the related specialties, but the general physician can find more suitable information elsewhere.

Parenteral Alimentation in Surgery, With Special Reference to Proteins and Amino Acids. By Robert Elman, M.D., Associate Professor of Clinical Surgery, Washington University School of Medicine. Pp. 284, with 31 illustrations. New York, 1947, Paul B. Hoeber, Inc.

This monograph dealing with work for which the author was awarded the quinquennial Samuel D. Gross prize of the Philadelphia Academy of Surgery is commended to both the physician and the surgeon. The introductory chapter on the history of parenteral alimentation is interesting and informative. The early chapters of the book deal with the intriguing thesis of supplying all necessary nutritional elements by parenteral means. Chapters V through X relate to the problem of parenteral protein therapy. The material is well presented and complete, although there is a tendency to gloss over controversial material. Not enough stress seems to have been paid to blood volume changes in relation to malnourished states and in relation to the studies relating to the use of amino acid solutions.

Even though parenteral alimentation appears to be effective, and positive nitrogen balance can be achieved, the author wisely states that it should be considered as a temporary expedient for oral alimentation. It should be used as a means of clearing temporary hurdles with the ultimate aim in treatment to restore the patient as rapidly as possible to such a state that he may take all his nutritional requirements by mouth.

In spite of differences of opinion among workers in the field of protein therapy, particularly as it relates to surgical patients, this book is a very valuable contribution and marks a real advance of the science of nutrition as it can be applied clinically.

SURGERY

Vol. 23 | February, 1948 | No. 2

Original Communications

THE OPERATIVE TREATMENT OF CHRONIC GASTRIC AND DUODENAL ULCER

Christian Bruusgaard, M.D., Oslo, Norway
(From the Ullevaal Hospital, Surgical Department III)

FOLLOW-UP EXAMINATIONS OF PATIENTS TREATED WITH GASTROJEJUNOSTOMY AND PARTIAL GASTRECTOMY

I COMPILED,* in 1946, the following results and drew the conclusions listed here after clinical, roentgenologic, and in part gastroscopic follow-up examinations of a total of 600 patients treated surgically for chronic gastric and duodenal ulcer at the Oslo University Clinic Department A, and Aker Hospital. The period of observation for most of the patients was over four years.

1. Gastrojejunostomy was done in 416 patients operated upon. The mortality rate was 4.7 per cent. During the time gastrojejunostomy was used as a routine method, the mortality rate was 1.4 per cent in 139 operations.

2. Partial gastrectomy was done in 572 patients operated upon. The operative method was partial resection with gastrojejunostomy according to modifications of the Billroth II method. The mortality rate was 4 per cent in 572 resections. Partial gastrectomy with exclusion of a duodenal (pyloric) ulcer according to Finsterer's method was used in 16 per cent of the cases in this group. In one-half of the cases the resection was made through the pyloric antrum without excision of the antral mucosa, and in the other half through the pylorus or the duodenum.

Gastric Acidity.—Caffeine test meal fractionally recovered every ten minutes for two hours showed the findings listed in Table II.

Postoperative Anemia.—A hypochromic anemia not caused by gastric hemorrhage occurred in approximately 50 per cent of the women with anacid gastric contents in age groups between puberty and the menopause. In women of older age groups with anacid gastric contents and in men the percentage of hypochromic anemia was 30. This anemia responded to large doses of iron in most cases. In only 5.4 per cent did the anemia produce subjective symptoms in the patients with resection.

Received for publication, May 1, 1947.
*In Acta Chir. Scandinav. 94: Suppl. 117, 1946.

TABLE I. CHIEF POSTOPERATIVE COMPLICATIONS

COMPLICATIONS	GASTROJEJUNOSTOMY FREQUENCY (%)	GASTROJEJUNOSTOMY MORTALITY (%)	PARTIAL GASTRECTOMY FREQUENCY (%)	PARTIAL GASTRECTOMY MORTALITY (%)
Hemorrhage	2.4	0.5	2	0.2
Peritonitis	0.5	0.5	3	2.0
Severe evacuation difficulties	2.4	1.2	2	0.35

Complications Caused by the Changed Evacuation Conditions in the Stomach (Dumping Stomach).—The characteristic symptoms of "dumping stomach" are nausea, fainting, weakness, heaviness in the legs, and occasionally sweating. The symptoms cease in the course of about twenty minutes. As a rule the patient must lie down. If he eats while reclining or lies down immediately after meals, the symptoms do not appear. This trouble is closely connected with the first half hour following meals, chiefly breakfast and dinner.

TABLE II. THE FOLLOW-UP EXAMINATIONS OF THE PATIENTS

LOCATION	GASTROJEJUNOSTOMY (PER CENT ANACID)	PARTIAL GASTRECTOMY (PER CENT ANACID)
Duodenal ulcer	20	92
Ulcer of the pyloric region	40	95
Ulcer of the corpus region	57	100

There is no connection with hypoglycemia. The treatment, eating meals in a reclining position, is simple but not easy to follow under all circumstances. This complication occurred in 15 per cent of the gastrectomy patients, but in only 2 per cent was it so severe as to cause the patient to be listed as not cured after the operative treatment.

TABLE III. RESULTS OF OPERATIVE TREATMENT

TREATMENT	NUMBER OF PATIENTS FOLLOWED	PER CENT SYMPTOM-FREE
Gastrojejunostomy	234	64
Partial gastrectomy	364	84

Conclusions.—Gastrojejunostomy should not be used as the routine method for treatment of chronic gastric and duodenal ulcers. In my studies, gastrojejunostomy in the age group over 60 years gave the same results as partial gastrectomy in the treatment of duodenal ulcer. In patients over 60 years of

TABLE IV. INCIDENCE OF THE LATE COMPLICATIONS

COMPLICATIONS	GASTROJEJUNOSTOMY (%)	PARTIAL GASTRECTOMY (%)
Postoperative jejunal ulcer	8	1.8 (combined)
Recurrent ulcer in stomach and duodenum	9	
Hemorrhage	4	
Gastritis	9	4.6
Hypochromic anemia with subjective symptoms	2.5	5.4
Evacuation disturbances, intestinal disturbances, cancer in the operated stomach, intestinal obstruction	3.5	4.2

age with duodenal ulcers, whose general condition is poor or in whom technical difficulties for performing a radical gastrectomy are present, a gastrojejunostomy can be done with little risk for recurrent ulcer or stomal ulcer.

Partial gastrectomy should be the method of choice in the treatment of chronic gastric and duodenal ulcers with the limitations stipulated for the age group over 60 years. The basis for advising this operative intervention is that the mortality rate can be maintained at a reasonably low level, that is, not over 1 to 2 per cent.

FACTORS INFLUENCING THE OPERATIVE MORTALITY RATE

What can the surgeon do to lower the mortality rate? In the following paragraphs I shall give an account of the measures which we have taken at Ullevaal Hospital, Surgical Department III, in order to keep the mortality rate down. I shall report the statistics from this department for the last four years on patients with surgical ulcer. This group includes a total of 240 patients, 32 women and 208 men, operated upon between 1942 and 1945, inclusive. The sites of the ulcers as follows: 110 duodenal (54 anterior wall, 20 posterior wall, 36 kissing ulcers), 28 pyloric, 71 in the angle of the corpus, 5 in the oral half of the corpus, 13 postoperative jejunal, and 13 in both the stomach and duodenum. Fifty-five of the patients were over 50 years of age.

Preoperative Treatment.—Careful clinical, hematologic, x-ray, and functional examinations must be made before the operation is undertaken. Poor nutritional condition should be improved, if necessary, with parenteral administrations controlled by determinations of blood proteins and electrolytes. Anemia should be repaired by blood transfusions. The patient should not be operated upon during a period of intercurrent disease or of acute gastric pain while the gastritis and inflammatory process around the ulcer are most marked, but should be given a course of medical treatment, if necessary, with gastric lavage, for a few weeks before the operation.

Operative Indications.—Operation must be done in cases with perforation, grave stenosis, repeated hemorrhage, and gastric ulcers suspected of being cancer. All ulcers which give troublesome or serious symptoms in spite of expert medical treatment should be removed surgically unless there are definite contraindications. The surgical treatment should not be postponed until the ulcer becomes callous and penetrating, thus unnecessarily increasing the operative risk.

Anesthesia.—We have used spinal anesthesia with a novocain-pantocain solution of a greater specific gravity than the spinal fluid, usually 200 mg. novocain + 10 mg. pantocain. This anesthetic lasts from one and one-half to two hours. Since our operations usually last about two hours, we have used local anesthesia in the abdominal wall in order to obtain relaxation for closure. About one-half hour before we begin the closure of the abdominal wall, a solution of ½ per cent novocain and ½/1000 pantocain is injected preperitoneally and subcutaneously. This local anesthesia, which also has a general effect, has given excellent results. We have used N_2O ether anesthesia in only a few cases.

Choice of Operative Method.—Local pyloroplastic operations were used only twice during this period. The moderate mortality rate of these operations does not outweigh the more certain results obtainable by the radical operations.

Gastrojejunostomy was used in patients over 60 years of age for treatment of duodenal ulcers, when there was poor general condition or technical difficulty to add to the operative risk.

Partial (about two-thirds) gastric resection according to Billroth II has been the routine method in the treatment of gastric and duodenal ulcers. My previous investigations have shown that the different end-to-side gastrojejunostomies commonly used in the Billroth II resections all give the same satisfactory results, therefore the surgeon has free choice of method in this respect. The important point is that he chooses one method and becomes expert at it. At Ullevaal Hospital, Department III, we have used the Krönlein modification of Billroth II during this four years. After the usual resection through the upper part of the duodenum, the stomach is mobilized. The resection line is then made perpendicular to the axis of the stomach. The amount of the stomach removed in our cases has not been weighed, but the resection has been from 60 to 75 per cent of the stomach. We are of the opinion that the gastrectomy should be a 75 per cent resection to accomplish a satisfactory operation for ulcer.

The finishing gastrojejunostomy is in our cases made terminolaterally. The afferent loop is made a maximum of 20 cm. long, and placed in an antecolic position from the lesser to the greater curvature. Extensive experimental work from the University of Minnesota Hospitals by Wangensteen and his associates, has shown that a short afferent anastomotic loop is of great importance for a satisfactory result from the gastrectomy. Wangensteen in his operations uses a 2 to 5 cm. afferent loop placed in retrocolic position. I am of the opinion that our operative technique would be nearer "the satisfactory operation for ulcer" if we made our antecolic afferent loop about 10 to 12 cm. long or made a retrocolic anastomosis with an afferent loop 5 to 8 cm.

IMPORTANT TECHNICAL DETAILS IN THE PERFORMANCE OF KRÖNLEIN'S MODIFICATION OF PARTIAL GASTRIC RESECTION ACCORDING TO BILLROTH II

The freeing of the duodenum and the closure of the duodenal stump are the most important points in the accomplishment of the Billroth II resection. When there are no particular difficulties, the duodenal cuff which is to be inverted should be about 2 cm. long and should be closed with one continuous or interrupted catgut suture and two silk purse-string sutures. Callous ulcers, particularly those which penetrate into the pancreas, demand special skill and care in mobilization. In some cases it has been necessary to leave the base of the ulcer at its point of penetration into the pancreas. The mobilization of the duodenum is then continued beyond the distal edge of the ulcer, if possible, in order to obtain a cuff ½ to 1 cm. wide with which to cover the resection surface. The anterior wall of the duodenum has been used in so far as possible, and every effort has been made to avoid injury to the pancreas during the inversion of the duodenal stump. In the event that the pancreas has been injured during the procedure, or if the security of the duodenal stump closure is questionable, a drain has been placed on the duodenal stump and allowed to remain a week. In cases in which the duodenal stump closure might be insecure, an anastomosis between the afferent and efferent loops can be used to relieve the duodenum. There has been only one case of duodenal insufficiency in over 200 radical resections. In this case a duodenal fistula formed and healed spontaneously in two weeks.

Partial gastrectomy with exclusion of a duodenal (pyloric) ulcer according to Finsterer's method has been performed in only three cases, and then as a prepyloric resection. It is important to remove the mucous membrane in the excluded distal part of the stomach. The blood supply to this part of the stomach must be left intact. The closed stump of this antral pouch may be sewed to the anterior abdominal wall. The excluded central part of the stomach must not be made less than 5 cm. long.

Our material shows that a radical removal of a duodenal or pyloric ulcer can be done in almost all cases with little risk.

The Anastomotic Suture.—Before the suture is commenced it is important that the curvatures at the place of the anastomosis are made as free as possible of omental fragments.

We use three layers of sutures in the anastomosis. In the serosa we use an interrupted silk suture and a continuous catgut suture. After the seromuscular layer is divided, all the visible blood vessels are ligated with a suture ligature, a sufficient amount of the seromuscular coat being engaged to prevent the stitches from cutting through. For the third suture the mucosal layers are separated and a continuous catgut suture is made through all layers of the stomach. This suture is made carefully with comparatively small stitches. Particular care is taken with the corner stitches in order to ensure free entrance to, and exit from, the stomach. In most cases we have used clamps on the stomach and duodenum while making the anastomosis. We have not used clamps in a number of cases and have encountered no disadvantages as a result.

My earlier investigations mentioned previously showed that the immediate operative results were the same in Billroth II operations with three and with two layers of sutures in the anastomosis. Wangensteen uses one layer of interrupted silk sutures in closed gastric anastomoses. The three layer suture method has given very good immediate results in our gastric resections, and a very small amount of emptying disturbances, but experience shows that a one-layer anastomosis as done by Wangensteen can be done with the same degree of safety. Obviously, a single-row inversion provides large patulous orifices in the new stoma.

SURGICAL TECHNIQUE IN THE TREATMENT OF POSTOPERATIVE JEJUNAL ULCER

The operative treatment of postoperative jejunal ulcer should be so radical as to produce anacidity. This is attainable only by a radical gastrectomy and resection of the previously excluded pyloric antrum in cases in which Finsterer's operation has been done. The anastomosis must be a short loop anastomosis. We have tried to avoid resection of the anastomotic loop of the jejunum by using the previous anastomosis in several cases. By these procedures we have avoided the more dangerous resection of the jejunum with end-to-end suture of the resected surfaces.

Postoperative Care.—Atony of the stomach and intestines and swelling of the new anastomosis require careful regulation of the oral fluid intake and supplementary rectal and parenteral fluids, as well as blood infusions, when necessary, controlled by determinations of the patient's blood protein and electrolyte levels. The patient should have regular gastric aspirations morning and evening, or oftener, if necessary, for the first three days. We use a thin nasal tube, with no continuous suction. *The patients usually get up on the second or third postoperative day.*

THE IMMEDIATE POSTOPERATIVE RESULTS

Operative Complications.—Postoperative peritonitis occurred in one case as a Douglas abscess which healed after drainage. *Leakage from the duodenal stump occurred once after partial gastrectomy.* Serious postoperative hemorrhage occurred once, but the patient recovered after blood transfusions. Pulmonary embolism occurred once *with fatal outcome.* This patient did not get up until the seventh day, and he died the moment he arose. Thrombosis has been practically eliminated by allowing the patients to get up soon after the operation. One patient had a peculiar nutritional disturbance with muscular atrophy and paralysis after the operation.

Mortality Rate.—In the 240 stomach operations which include 2 pyloroplasties, 23 gastrojejunostomies, 3 resections for exclusion, and 212 partial gastrectomies, there has been one death (pulmonary embolism). This gives a mortality rate of 4 per thousand. The operations have been performed by nine surgeons using the same operative technique.

The operations and the operative techniques used in Department III of Ullevaal Hospital have given good immediate operative results with a low mortality rate, as is shown from my study. The operations include a relatively large number of gastrojejunostomies, 10 per cent (used for the treatment of duodenal ulcer on elderly persons), while resections for exclusion (Finsterer) have been used only exceptionally. The partial gastrectomies have been radical, about 75 per cent resections in most cases, but with a proximal anastomotic loop up to 20 cm. in length.

In spite of the satisfactory immediate results obtained there are two criticisms of the operative methods used which can be made: Gastrojejunostomy has been performed in too many cases, and the proximal anastomotic loop in the partial gastrectomies has been too long.

The end results cannot be discussed because the patients were operated upon so recently that there have been no adequate follow-up examinations.

SUMMARY

I have reported the immediate and late results in a study of gastric and duodenal ulcers treated operatively. I have discussed measures employed to achieve a lower operative mortality rate.

PRODUCTION OF ALLERGIC GASTRIC AND DUODENAL EDEMA WHICH PREDISPOSES TO THE HISTAMINE-PROVOKED ULCER IN DOGS

STANLEY R. FRIESEN, M.D.,* DAVID STATE, M.D., DONALD E. JASPER, D.V.M., MINNIE FINN, B.S., AND OWEN H. WANGENSTEEN, M.D.
MINNEAPOLIS, MINN.

(From the Department of Surgery, University of Minnesota Medical School)

GASTROINTESTINAL manifestations of allergic disease were recognized by Osler[1] in 1904, when he described visceral crises in allergic individuals to be due to infiltration of blood and serum into the wall of the gastrointestinal tract. In 1915, Crispin[2] observed by x-ray, in a patient with hematemesis, a transient lesion at the pylorus which was found at operation to be due to angioneurotic edema. Roentgenologic evidence of the disturbances which occur in allergic reactions of the gastrointestinal tract has been obtained by others,[3, 4] gastric retention being the most common finding. Hyperemia, edema, and submucosal hemorrhage in the stomach have been observed gastroscopically in experimentally reproduced gastric allergy in man.[5]

Lintz[6] observed that patients with allergy frequently show evidence of gastric or intestinal hemorrhages. Of forty-four patients with bronchial asthma examined by him, eighteen had blood in the stomach contents; ten of twenty-five, in the feces. Of 300 patients with general allergy, 95 also had gastrointestinal allergy. In thirty-two unselected patients with peptic ulcer, Kern and Stewart[7] found that 40 per cent of those patients gave a history of some type of allergic disturbance. Gay[8] was able to determine, in a small series of ulcer patients, the allergens (chiefly wheat, eggs, beef, and milk) which precipitated the ulcer symptoms in these patients, by studying the leucopenia, fall in gastric acidity, and subjective discomfort of the patients. Upon elimination of the allergens from the diet, clinical improvement in these patients was noted.

Gastrointestinal changes in experimental anaphylaxis in animals were first noted by Schittenhelm and Weichardt[9] in 1910. They observed numerous miliary hemorrhages in the mucosa and submucosa of the gastrointestinal tract in sensitized dogs reinjected with egg protein. Experimental production of gastric ulcer by local anaphylaxis utilizing the principle of the Arthus phenomenon has been described by Shapiro and Ivy.[10] These investigators injected antigen into the gastric mucosa of previously sensitized dogs and rabbits; ulcers were produced which later tended to heal.

Freeman,[11] in 1925, was the first to demonstrate that local passive sensitization of the tissue followed by intravenous injection of the sensitizing antigen

This research supported by the John and Mary R. Markle Foundation, the Augustus L. Searle Fund for Surgical Research, the Berenice Moriarity Fund. Dr. and Mrs. Harry B. Zimmermann and the Robert A. Cooper Funds for Surgical Research and The Graduate School of the University of Minnesota.

Received for publication, May 24, 1947.

*National cancer trainee.

results in edema of that tissue. He injected into the skin of a normal patient serum obtained from a patient with hay fever. After two weeks the sensitizing pollen was injected intravenously, producing edema at the local site of sensitization. This phenomenon has been demonstrated experimentally in monkeys and in man by others.[12] It has been shown that serum (obtained from an allergic patient), when injected locally into the gall bladder wall, skin, ileum, rectum, and stomach, and later followed by systemic administration of the sensitizing antigen, results in pallor, hyperemia, and transient edema.

Edema of the gastrointestinal tract is often seen in conjunction with, or as a result of, other conditions which have been found to predispose to erosion and ulceration. These include the nutritional edema of hypoproteinemia,[13] portal hypertension,[14] and systemic disease such as toxemia and septicemia.

The purpose of this study, therefore, is threefold: (1) to determine whether local antigen-antibody reactions can be utilized to produce prolonged gastric and duodenal edema, (2) to determine whether edema per se (without alteration of the general condition of the animal) favors the experimental production of the histamine-in-beeswax provoked ulcer, and (3) to determine whether local anaphylaxis produced by passive local sensitization of the gastric and/or duodenal mucosa with local antigen-antibody reaction abets the ulcer diathesis. It has been found by Hay and associates[15] that forty days are necessary to produce ulcers consistently and with regularity in dogs given histamine-in-beeswax daily. In their series, the average appearance time of the ulcers after the administration of histamine was begun was twenty-three days.

METHOD AND MATERIALS

Serum was obtained from an adult horse which had been sensitized previously to five different antigens, these being swine serum (anticholera hog serum), bovine serum (antihemorrhagic septicemia serum of bovine origin), rabbit serum, egg albumin (1:10 dilution), and skim milk. The horse was given intravenous injections of each antigen every other day for three weeks in 40 to 50 c.c. doses. Thirty-four days after the first injection, when intradermal wheals indicated marked sensitivity of the animal to all antigens, blood was drawn for serum extraction and preserved with aqueous merthiolate in 1:10,000 dilution. Antibody titers (precipitin method) of the horse serum for the different antigens were as follows:

Swine serum	1:6400
Bovine serum	1:3200
Rabbit serum	1:1600
Egg Albumin	1:6400
Skim milk*	------

Adult dogs were subjected to laparotomy under sodium pentobarbital anesthesia, and, with the exercising of sterile precautions, the horse serum was applied locally to the stomach and/or duodenum, either by direct infiltration into the submucosa (20 c.c.), or by intra-arterial (left gastric artery) injection (40 c.c.), the horse serum in the latter instance reaching the gastric wall via the blood vessels of the stomach. The area of infiltration was marked with a loose

* It was not possible to determine the antibody titer to skim milk by the precipitin method employed.

cotton stitch just into the mucosa. The size of the area sensitized was about 25 sq. cm. when direct infiltration was used, and approximately two-thirds of the stomach when intra-arterial injection was employed. After one to ten days, laparotomy was again performed and the stomach and/or duodenum opened at a site away from the previously sensitized area for observation. One of the antigens to which the dog had been sensitized was injected systemically via a tongue vein, and measurements by a caliper of the viscus wall thickness and biopsies were obtained before and after injection of the antigen up to ten hours. The abdomens of the animals were closed aseptically and the dogs were allowed to recover; some were sacrificed in twenty-four hours for measurements and biopsies of the stomach and/or duodenum. In all experiments surgical trauma was directed away from the sensitized sites (opposite gastric wall, etc.).

This method of production of the allergic phenomenon differs from that described by Shapiro and Ivy,[10] in that in this study the animal is sensitized passively and locally (stomach and duodenum) by local injection of the antibodies, followed later by systemic administration of the antigens, instead of the active sensitization of the animal followed by local injection of the antigen according to the Arthus phenomenon.

To evaluate the role of edema thus produced upon ulcer provocation, a number of dogs were sensitized in the manner described. Forty-eight hours following sensitization, daily intravenous injection of the antigen into the systemic circulation was begun; that is, a different one of the five antigens to which the horse had been sensitized was injected daily until all five foreign proteins had been administered (a total of five days). Histamine-in-beeswax mixture, prepared after the method of Code and Varco,[16] was injected intramuscularly (30 mg. base) each evening. The only restriction of food intake exercised was elimination of milk and horse meat from the diet. One series of dogs was subjected to the same procedures, using instead of the prepared horse serum with high antibody titer, normal horse serum having a negative antibody titer to the antigens employed. Animals were sacrificed after five daily injections of antigen, and sections of the stomach and duodenum were obtained for microscopic study.

EXPERIMENTS

Experimental studies were divided into two parts as follows:

I. *Production of a Prolonged Gastric and Duodenal Edema.*—Eight dogs received a local injection of 20 c.c. of horse serum with high antibody titer directly into the gastric and duodenal mucosa and submucosa. In two dogs, the duodenum was sensitized by placing 20 c.c. of horse serum within the lumen of the duodenum, an area of approximately 5 cm. being isolated by rubber-shod clamps for twenty minutes and then released. The local reaction to systemically injected antigen (20 c.c.) in these dogs was studied in fourteen experiments from one to ten days following sensitization.

Five dogs received a local injection of 20 c.c. of horse serum with negative antibody titer directly into the gastric and duodenal mucosa and submucosa, and observations were made after systemic injection of 20 c.c. antigen in one to three days following sensitization in nine experiments.

Six dogs received local intra-arterial (left gastric artery) injection of 40 c.c. of horse serum with high antibody titer. Observations, after systemic injection of antigen, were made in two to six days following sensitization in six experiments.

Two dogs received local intra-arterial (left gastric artery) injection of 40 c.c. of horse serum with negative antibody titer and were studied in forty-eight hours, after systemic injection of 20 c.c. antigen.

Two dogs underwent laparotomy in which the stomach and duodenum were opened for observations and measurements during ten hours of exposure of the mucous membrane to the air. One of these dogs received systemic injection of antigen during the time of observation.

II. *Evaluation of Role of Allergic Edema on Ulcer Production.*—Three series of experiments were carried out.

Series 1: Twelve dogs were sensitized locally with immune horse serum of high antibody titer and daily intravenous administration of antigens was begun after forty-eight hours, together with daily administration of histamine-in-beeswax mixture.

Series 2: Six dogs were used in this series. The stomach of each dog was sensitized locally with horse serum of high antibody titer, followed in forty-eight hours with daily intravenous administration of antigens. No histamine was given in this series.

Series 3: Four dogs were used in this series. Normal horse serum with negative antibody titer to the antigens employed was injected locally into the submucosa of the stomach and duodenum of each dog, followed in forty-eight hours by daily intravenous administration of the five antigens, together with daily injections of histamine-in-beeswax mixture.

RESULTS

I. *Production of a Prolonged Gastric and Duodenal Edema.*—All dogs sensitized locally by immune horse serum of high antibody titer, either by direct mucosal and submucosal infiltration or intra-arterial injection demonstrated gross and microscopic edema following systemic intravenous injection of antigens. The two dogs in which sensitization of the duodenum was accomplished by injecting immune horse serum within the duodenal lumen also developed mucosal edema after systemic injection of antigen. All five antigens were found to be effective in initiating the response, and responses were obtained from twenty-four hours to ten days following sensitization. The onset of the edema varied between fifteen minutes and one hour, and persisted for as long as twenty-four hours; the maximum effect was noted at from two to six hours. The edema represented an increase in thickness of the viscus wall from two to five times its original thickness.

The animals which received local injection (direct infiltration or intra-arterial) of horse serum with negative antibody titer and were observed after intravenous administration of antigens demonstrated no edematous reaction, and the findings were uniformly negative.

Exposure to the air of the gastric or duodenal wall for ten hours, with or without intravenous injection of antigen, in dogs not passively sensitized resulted in no more than 1 mm. increase in thickness.

Microscopic examination revealed marked "watery" edema located chiefly in the submucosa. There was no demonstrable cellular reaction and eosinophiles were not found to be increased in number.

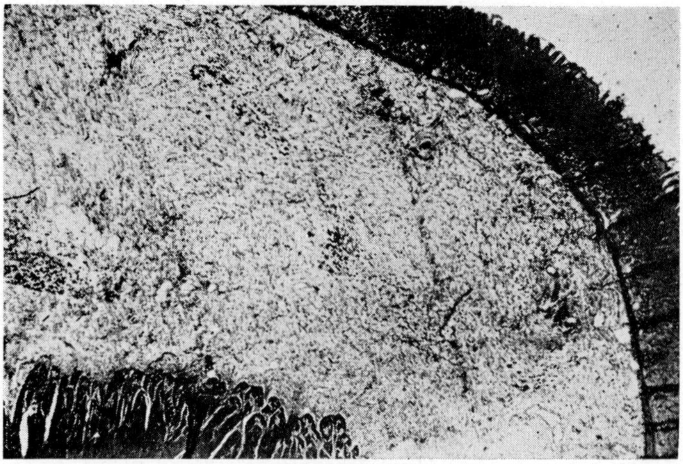

Fig. 1.—Microscopic section demonstrating submucosal gastric edema in a dog subjected to local passive sensitization and systemic injection of antigen (magnification ×7).

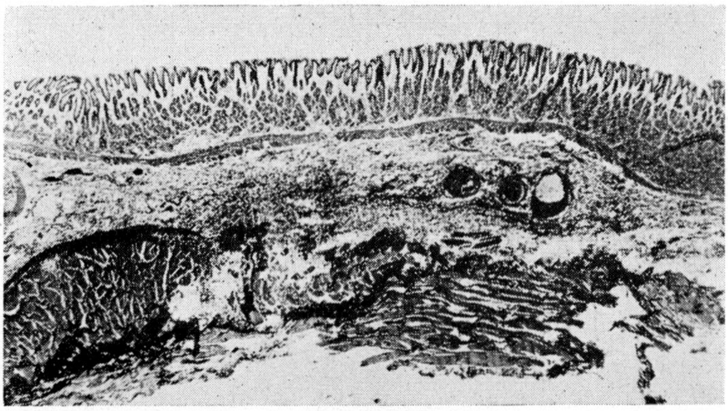

Fig. 2.—Microscopic section of normal gastric wall of a dog (magnification ×7).

II. *Evaluation of Role of Allergic Edema on Ulcer Production.*—

Series 1 (see Table I): All of the twelve dogs, subjected to the production of local anaphylaxis with concomitant administration of histamine-in-beeswax mixture, demonstrated edema with ulcer and/or erosion at the site of sensitization at the time of death or sacrifice (five days or less). Two dogs died of peritonitis after four and five days of antigen and histamine administration; one showed numerous deep duodenal ulcers in the area of edema with perforation; and the other, a perforated gastric ulcer in the area of edema.

TABLE I. DOGS SUBJECTED TO PRODUCTION OF LOCAL ANAPHYLAXIS WITH CONCOMITANT ADMINISTRATION OF HISTAMINE-IN-BEESWAX MIXTURE*

DOG	WEIGHT (POUNDS)	SENSITIZATION	NUMBER OF ANTIGENS AND INJECTIONS	NUMBER OF HISTAMINE INJECTIONS	RESULTS	REMARKS
703	29	50 c.c. left gastric artery	4	4	Gastric edema; three bleeding gastric ulcers in edematous area	Sacrificed; melena
706	35	40 c.c. submucosal infiltration: gastric and duodenal	5	5	Punctate hemorrhagic areas at edema	Sacrificed
708	26	40 c.c. left gastric artery and duodenal lumen	2	2	Three lesser curvature ulcers in edematous area	Emesis; died of aspiration pneumonia
755	32	20 c.c. submucosal infiltration: gastric and duodenal	5	5	Gastric bleeding points; duodenal ulcer; edema	Sacrificed
759	32	Same as Dog 755	5	5	Gastric erosion and ulcers in edematous area	Sacrificed
760	34	Same as Dog 755	5	5	Two small gastric ulcers in edematous area	Sacrificed
763	34	Same as Dog 755	4	4	Gastric bleeding points; perforated duodenal ulcer and other deep duodenal ulcers in edematous areas	Died, peritonitis
764	34	Same as Dog 755	5	5	Gastric ulcer in edematous area	Sacrificed
766	24	Same as Dog 755	2	2	Small gastric ulcers in edematous area	Died, pneumonia
767	29	Same as Dog 755	2	2	Gastric bleeding points and erosions in edematous areas; duodenal erosion in edematous area	Sacrificed
768	33	Same as Dog 755	5	5	Large perforated gastric ulcer in area of edema	Died, peritonitis
769	31	Same as Dog 755	5	5	Gastric ulcer in area of edema	Sacrificed

*The procedure in this series of dogs consisted of: (1) Passive local sensitization of the stomach and/or duodenum with immune horse serum of high antibody titer. (2) After forty-eight hours, daily intravenous injections of the antigens were given, accompanied by, (3) daily intramuscular injections of histamine-in-beeswax (30 mg. base).

All twelve dogs developed edema with ulcer and/or erosion in five days or less. Two dogs died of peritonitis due to perforated ulcers, one gastric and one duodenal. There was evidence of hemorrhage in five animals.

TABLE II. DOGS SUBJECTED TO PRODUCTION OF LOCAL ANAPHYLAXIS WITHOUT THE ADMINISTRATION OF HISTAMINE-IN-BEESWAX MIXTURE

DOG	WEIGHT (POUNDS)	SENSITIZATION BY SUBMUCOSAL GASTRIC INFILTRATION	NUMBER OF ANTIGENS AND INJECTIONS	NUMBER OF HISTAMINE INJECTIONS	RESULTS	REMARKS
787	29	20 c.c.	5	0	Bleeding gastric ulcer in edematous area	Sacrificed, melena
786	26	20 c.c.	5	0	Edema only	Sacrificed
796	32	20 c.c.	5	0	Edema only	Sacrificed
797	31	20 c.c.	5	0	Gastric ulcer in edematous area	Sacrificed
806	36	20 c.c.	5	0	Edema only	Sacrificed
807	30	20 c.c.	5	0	Gastric ulcer in edematous area	Sacrificed

Summary: All six dogs developed edema, three of which presented gastric ulcers, one bleeding.

TABLE III. DOGS SUBJECTED TO PRODUCTION OF LOCAL ANAPHYLAXIS WITH SENSITIZING HORSE SERUM OF NEGATIVE ANTIBODY TITER

NUMBER OF DOGS	SENSITIZATION	NUMBER OF ANTIGENS AND INJECTIONS	NUMBER OF HISTAMINE INJECTIONS	RESULTS	REMARKS
4	Stomach and duodenum	5	5	No edema, erosion, or ulcer	Sacrificed

TABLE IV. DOGS RECEIVING DAILY INJECTIONS OF HISTAMINE-IN-BEESWAX MIXTURE ALONE

NUMBER OF DOGS	SENSITIZATION	NUMBER OF ANTIGENS AND INJECTIONS	NUMBER OF HISTAMINE INJECTIONS	RESULTS	REMARKS
4	0	0	5	No erosion or ulcer	Sacrificed

Series 2 (see Table II): Three of the six dogs subjected to the production of local anaphylaxis without administration of histamine-in-beeswax mixture demonstrated definitive ulcers at the site of edema, when sacrificed after five days of antigen administration. All six showed edema at the site of sensitization. One ulcer was actively bleeding.

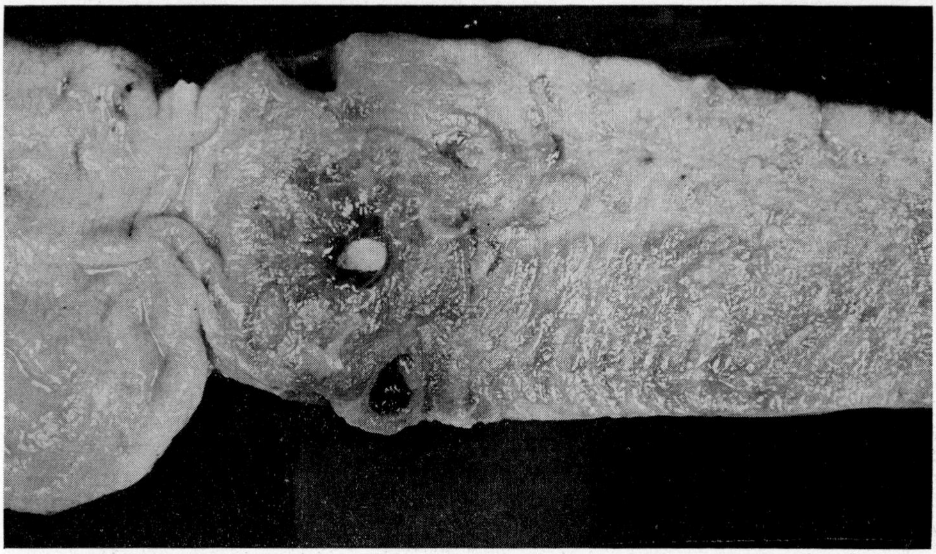

Fig. 3.—Duodenal ulcers (one perforated) in area of duodenal edema in Dog 763 (see Table I) subjected to the production of local allergic edema accompanied by four daily injections of histamine-in-beeswax mixture (magnification ×1.2).

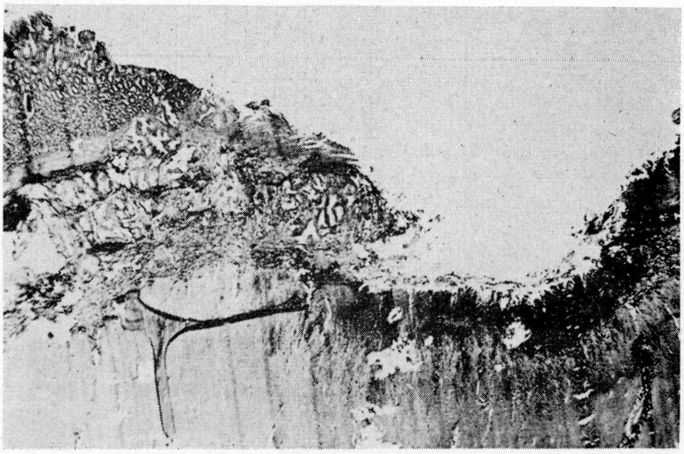

Fig. 4.—Microscopic section through edge of duodenal ulcer situated in an area of duodenal allergic edema in Dog 763 (see Fig. 3) (magnification ×7).

Series 3 (see Table III): Of the four dogs subjected to local injection of normal horse serum of negative antibody titer followed in forty-eight hours by daily systemic injection of antigen accompanied by histamine-in-beeswax administration, none showed edema, erosion, or ulcer.

Four additional control dogs (Table IV) receiving daily injections of histamine-in-beeswax mixture alone, did not present ulceration when sacrificed in five days.

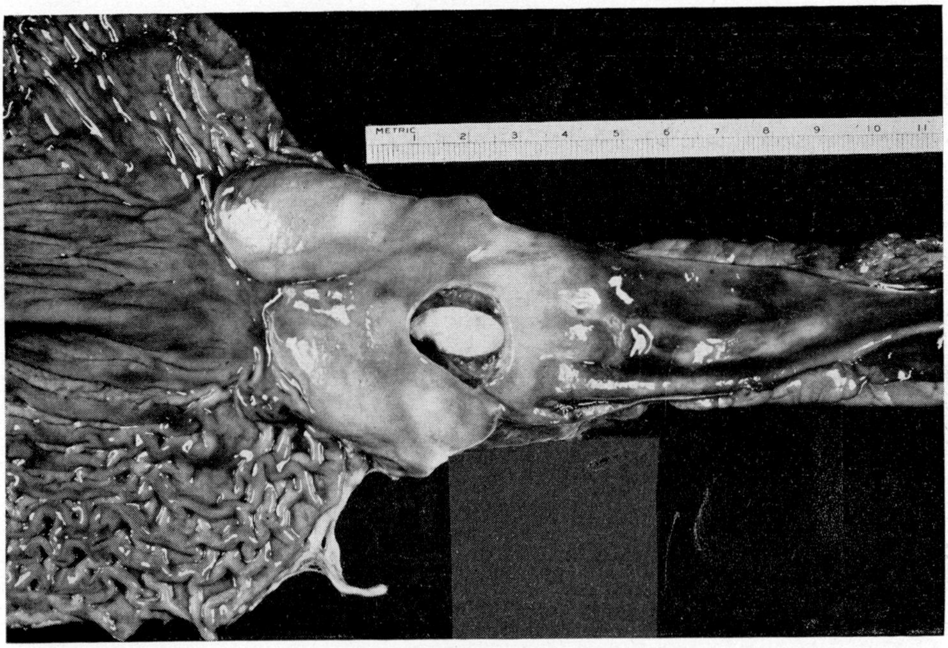

Fig. 5.—Perforated gastric ulcer in area of antral edema in Dog 768 (see Table I) subjected to the production of local allergic edema accompanied by five daily injections of histamine-in-beeswax mixture (magnification ×0.85).

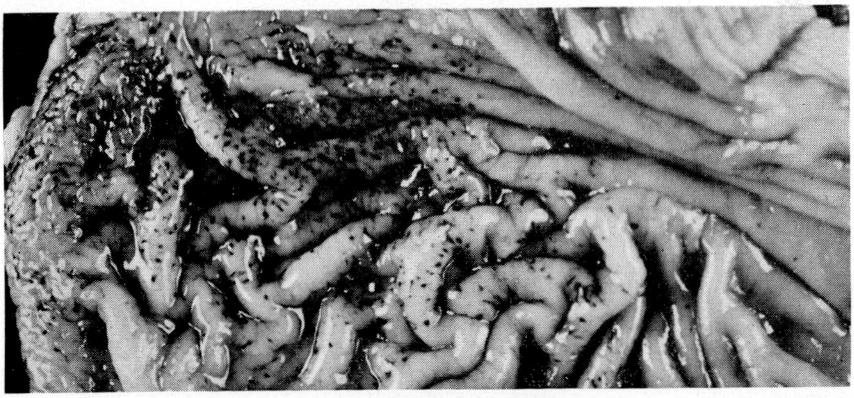

Fig. 6.—Punctate gastric bleeding points in area of gastric edema in Dog 706 (see Table I) subjected to the production of local allergic edema accompanied by five daily injections of histamine-in-beeswax mixture (magnification ×1.3).

DISCUSSION

It is seen that local antigen-antibody reaction produced by local passive sensitization and initiated by systemic administration of antigen results in marked edema of the gastric and duodenal wall. That it is a specific antigen-antibody reaction is evidenced by the circumstance that no edematous reaction takes place when the sensitizing horse serum has a negative antibody titer to the antigens in use. When the passively sensitizing serum contains antibodies to five antigens, a different antigen may be injected daily for continual provocation of the edematous response. By this method, edema on an allergic basis can be made to persist for as long as five days when five antigens are employed for its production.

By passively sensitizing an organ and then producing an allergic edema by the subsequent intravenous injection of the antigen no general manifestations of anaphylactic shock were produced. By avoiding the appearance of anaphylactic shock, the alterations caused by local edema in the stomach and duodenum could be studied without the marked alterations of the general physiology of the body accompanying anaphylactic shock.

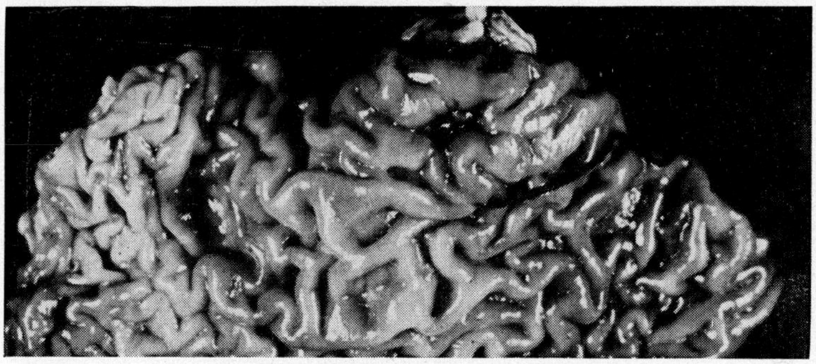

Fig. 7.—Bleeding gastric ulcer in area of gastric edema in Dog 787 (see Table II) subjected to local passive sensitization of the stomach followed by daily systemic injections of the antigens; no histamine administration; sacrificed in five days (magnification ×0.7).

It was noted in this study that swine serum antigen initiated the most marked response, and rabbit serum antigen, the least. This fact reflects the degree of sensitization of the horse used for the source of the sensitizing serum. It was observed that an antigen is unable to provoke a second response if reinjected into the same animal within a period of ten days.

It is apparent that ulcers are provoked more readily and quickly with histamine in the presence of gastric and duodenal edema resulting from experimentally produced local antigen-antibody reaction. It is noteworthy that ulcers were produced by local anaphylaxis alone and that ulcers were produced more consistently by administration of histamine in addition to the production of local anaphylaxis. No ulcers were produced by five daily injections of histamine-in-beeswax alone. From these observations it would appear that local anaphylactic edema can be an important factor in the production of ulcer.

The size of the sensitized or edematous area had no apparent relation to the incidence of ulceration; the presence or absence of an edematous area, on the other hand, had a distinct bearing upon the occurrence of ulceration. All ulcers were situated in the edematous areas.

The incidence of ulceration in the dogs subjected to local anaphylaxis without histamine administration was three of six. It is possible that this incidence would be greater if serum containing antibodies for a greater number of antigens were employed, thus increasing the number of daily injections of antigens and prolonging the duration of edema.

CONCLUSIONS

1. A method of experimentally producing a prolonged gastric and duodenal edema on an allergic basis in dogs is described. Edema resulting from local antigen-antibody reaction is produced by passive local sensitization to multiple antigens, and initiated by daily systemic administration of the different antigens.

2. Experimental gastrointestinal edema resulting from local antigen-antibody reaction favors the development of the histamine-provoked ulcer in dogs and abets the ulcer diathesis.

REFERENCES

1. Osler, William: On the Surgical Importance of the Visceral Crises in the Erythema Group of Skin Diseases, Am. J. M. Sc. **127**: 751, 1904.
2. Crispin, E. L.: Visceral Crises in Angioneurotic Edema, Collected Papers of Mayo Clinic **7**: 823, 1915.
3. Rowe, Albert H.: Roentgen Studies of Patients With Gastrointestinal Food Allergy, J. A. M. A. **100**: 394, 1933.
4. Fries, J. H., and Mogil, M.: Roentgen Observations on Children With Gastrointestinal Allergy to Foods, J. Allergy **14**: 310, 1943.
5. Pollard, H. M., and Stuart, G. J.: Experimental Reproduction of Gastric Allergy in Human Beings With Controlled Observations on Mucosa, J. Allergy **13**: 467, 1942.
6. Lintz, from Lipschutz, E. W.: Treatment of Peptic Ulcer Based on Its Etiology; Survey of Systemic Causes of Disease, M. J. & Rec. **128**: 630, 1928.
7. Kern, R. A., and Stewart, S. G.: Allergy in Duodenal Ulcer; Incidence and Significance of Food Hypersensitiveness as Observed in 32 Patients, J. Allergy **3**: 51, 1931.
8. Gay, L. P.: Gastro-intestinal Allergy; Leukopenic Index as Method of Specific Diagnosis of Allergens Causing Peptic Ulcer, J. A. M. A. **106**: 969, 1936.
9. Schittenhelm, A., and Weichardt, W.: Ueber die Rolle der Ueberempfindlichkeit bei der Infektion und Immunitat, Munchen. med. Wchnschr. **57**: 1769, 1910.
10. Shapiro, P. F., and Ivy, A. C.: Gastric Ulcer; Experimental Production of Gastric Ulcer by Local Anaphylaxis, Arch. Int. Med. **38**: 237, 1926.
11. Freeman, J.: Discussion on Paroxysmal Rhinorrhoea, Proc. Roy. Soc. Med. (Sect. Laryn.) **18**: 29, 1925.
12. Walzer, M.: Allergy of Abdominal Organs, J. Lab. & Clin. Med. **26**: 1867, 1941.
13. Weech, A. A., and Paige, B. H.: Nutritional Edema in Dog; Peptic Ulcer Produced by Same Low Protein Diet That Leads to Hypoproteinemia and Edema, Am. J. Path. **13**: 249, 1937.
14. Baronofsky, I. D., and Wangensteen, O. H.: Obstruction of Splenic Vein Increases Weight of Stomach and Predisposes to Erosion or Ulcer, Proc. Soc. Exper. Biol. & Med. **59**: 234, 1945.
15. Hay, L. J., Varco, R. L., Code, C. F., and Wangensteen, O. H.: Experimental Production of Gastric and Duodenal Ulcers in Laboratory Animals by Intramuscular Injection of Histamine-in-beeswax, Surg., Gynec. & Obst. **75**: 170, 1942.
16. Code, C. F., and Varco, R. L.: Prolonged Action of Histamine, Am. J. Physiol. **137**: 225, 1942.

ASEPTIC GASTRIC RESECTION, BILLROTH I TECHNIQUE

A. MONTEIRO, M.D., AND H. BARRETO, M.D., RIO DE JANEIRO, BRAZIL

(From the Surgical Clinic of Prof. Alfredo Monteiro, University of Brazil)

IN THE field of gastric surgery beset with doubt and slowly paced, treated with fear and sometimes with audacity, we have advanced from Torell's partial extirpation to the total resection of Graham. With conscious boldness, based increasingly more on physiopathology and clinical experience, the surgeon sought to cure malignant tumors by extirpation of the involved part of the organ. Restoration of the anatomic relations of the organ by gastroduodenostomy was the object of former surgeons who lacked the basis for further advances in gastric resection. It occurred to them as logical, when forced to resect a segment of the organ, to re-establish continuity of the lumen by preserving the same relation and form as existed before surgery was undertaken. Thus, the dominance of anatomy over physiology and pathology was clearly shown. In this manner Kocher, Pean, and Billroth proceeded in their major preoccupation of curing patients with gastric neoplasm.

Obliged to accomplish extensive resections, however, they witnessed successive failures of gastroduodenostomy because of the difficulty of uniting the cut edges, and because of the failure of union following suture of the stomach to the duodenum under tension. Billroth overcame these difficulties through gastrojejunostomy. The two techniques of Billroth are the patterns from which the other methods of gastric resection with which we are acquainted are planned.

Lately surgeons have been divided in their choice between the first and second procedures of Billroth, but it is best to accept both methods. If the first, which is an ideal procedure, is not always applicable and thus at times fails in its results, the second because it is efficient and easy of execution does not deserve such an exclusive and general indication.

In the case of ulcers and tumors the extensive resection necessary accounts for the performance of a gastrojejunostomy. We find, nevertheless, a perfect indication for gastroduodenostomy after conservative partial resections or those that offer the possibility of reconstructing the gastroduodenal lumen under favorable circumstances. The degree of hyperacidity, gastroscopic findings, etc., is useful in the determination of the extent of resection. Thus we can by semeiotic means and by exploration during the operative procedure often plan on re-establishing the continuity once the resection is performed following the Billroth I technique.

Considering the indications for this technique instead of forgetting them with those of the past we have methodized its steps under the same principles of the aseptic gastrectomy, Billroth II technique described by Monteiro in 1945.

Received for publication, June 5, 1947.

METHOD

Following the same technique as the one used for mesial section in gastric resection, Billroth II method, we free the greater curvature, placing ligatures above the gastroepiploic artery. From the site for the gastric section to the duodenum, the lesser peritoneal cavity is exposed. The assistant passes two

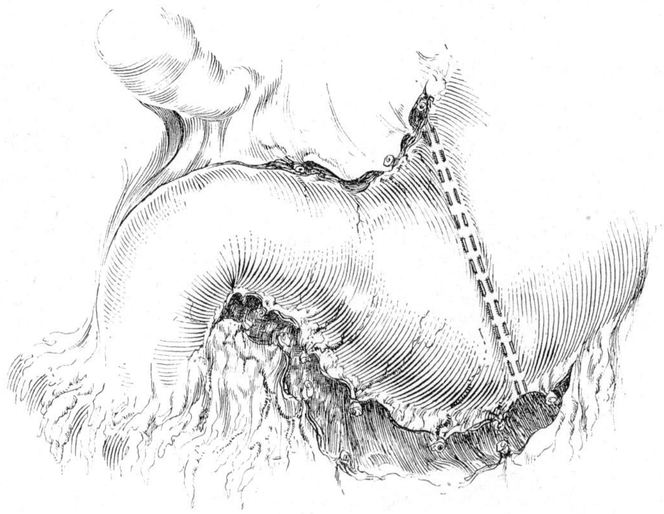

Fig. 1.—After mesial section the site for gastric section is clamped with a Von Petz instrument which leaves two rows of clips.

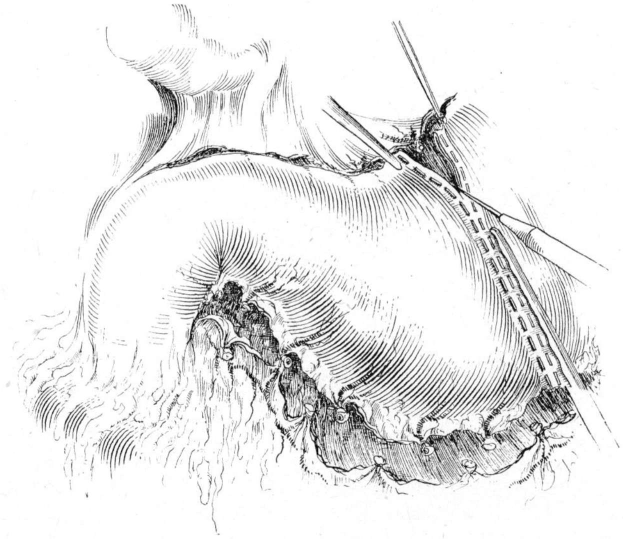

Fig. 2.—Close to the proximal margin clips is placed the anastomotic clamp. Two repair stitches are placed at the extremities and the stomach is sectioned, between clips, with the cautery.

fingers through this cavity to ascertain the pyloric vessels at the level of the lesser curvature (Finochetti). Once the vessels are tied we start freeing the portion to resect with care in hemostasis. At this moment the duodenal dissec-

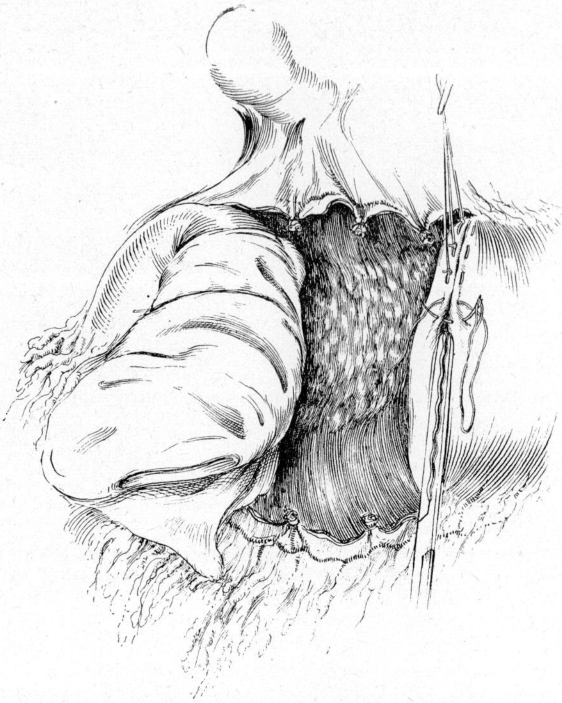

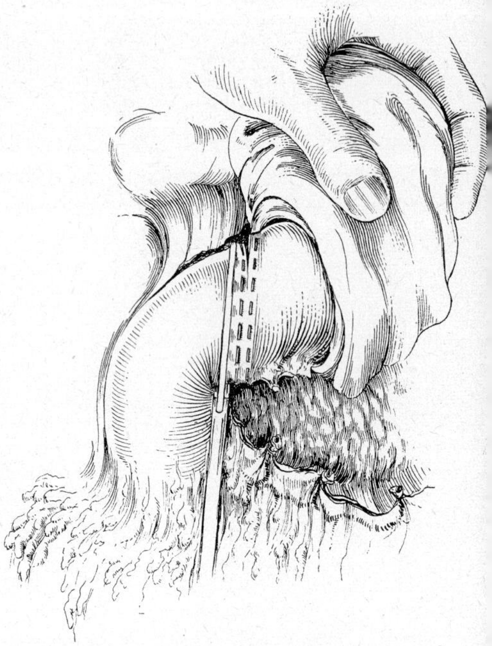

Fig. 3.—Once the distal margin is covered with gauze and riveted, the proximal margin of the stomach is inverted, which exceeds the anastomotic clamp, with Halsted stitches.

Fig. 4.—Clamping with Eugênio de Sousa's instrument, the site of the duodenum for oblique section, sectioning is carried out between clips with the cautery, after the anastomotic clamp is placed close to the distal margin.

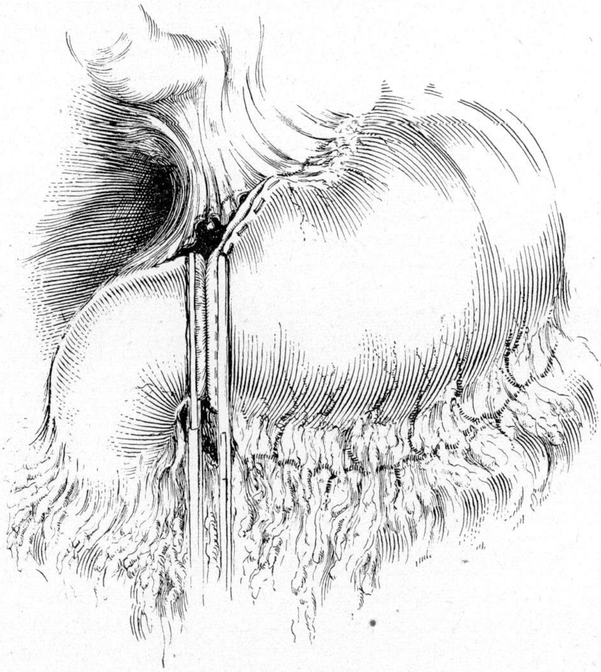

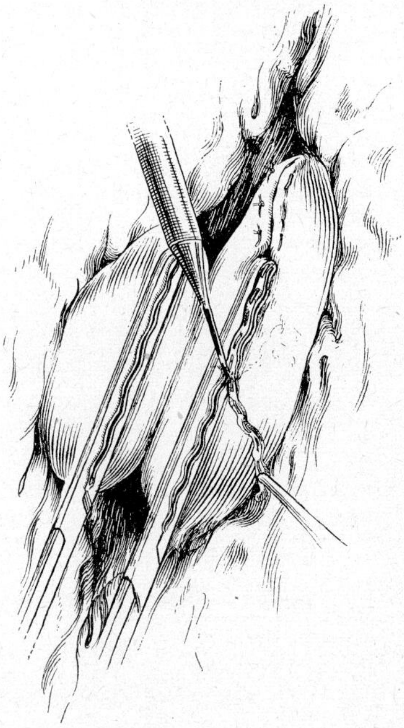

Fig. 5.—The anastomotic clamps are brought together to consider the possibility of a perfect union. Otherwise the Billroth II method can be applied.

Fig. 6.—Removal of the row of clips close to the clamp, followed by electrocoagulation of the surfaces.

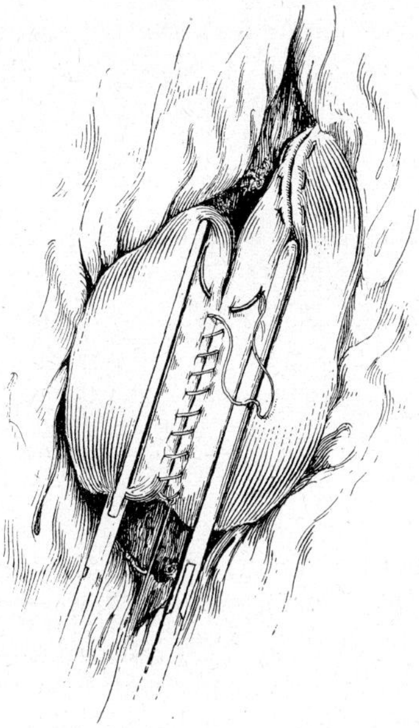

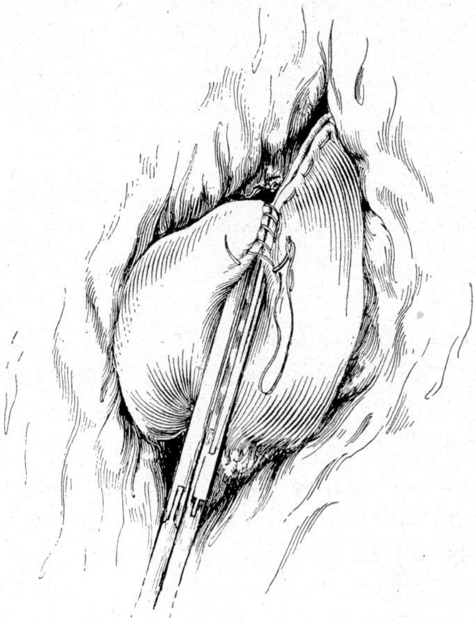

Fig. 7.—Rotation of the clamp outward, allowing the posterior seromuscular suture.

Fig. 8.—Having once outlined the superior angle, the continuous suture is followed through the anterior wall. The clamps are rotated bringing together the sectioned surfaces.

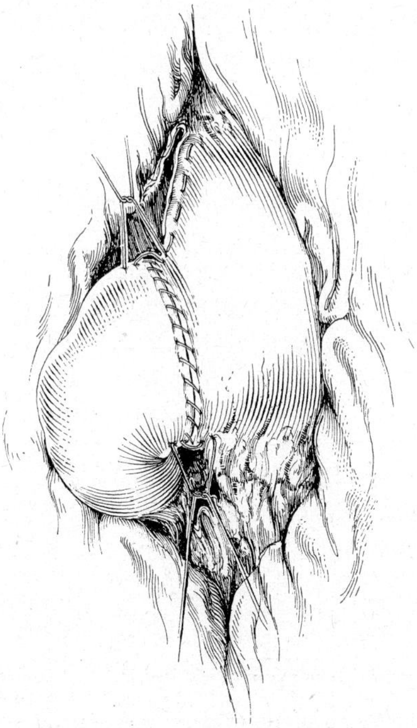

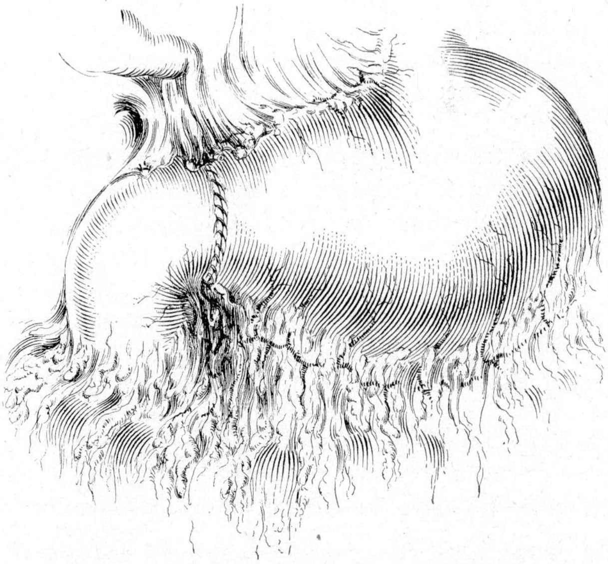

Fig. 9.—The anastomosis accomplished, reinforcement stitches are placed at the angles, especially the superior one.

Fig. 10.—View of the accomplished operation. Note the epiploplasty at the angles of anastomosis.

tion can be accomplished. When the portion of the stomach and duodenum to be resected is freed from the omentum we proceed in clamping the site for gastric section with a Von petz instrument. Repair sutures placed at the extremities of the clamped zone maintain it tense after the clamp is removed. Close to the proximal margin clips we place Monteiro's anastomotic clamp and following this we cut the stomach with the cautery. Once riveted with the distal margin covered with gauze, we invert the sectioned surface beyond the anastomotic clamp. This inversion is made with Halsted type sutures. After protecting the suture and the clamped zone we pass to the duodenal stage.

With the stomach riveted, the duodenal stage becomes easy. We use Eugênio de Sousa's clamp based on the Von Petz instrument, which facilitates the procedure. The clamping is done obliquely to afford a larger zone of anastomosis to coincide with the length of the clamp which is placed close to the distal margin clips. After sectioning between the clips with the cautery the duodenal and gastric clamps are approximated to initiate the anastomosis. The edges with the clips are removed with the cautery and the excised surfaces are electrocoagulated to effect hemostasis. By rotation the approximated clamps present the posterior walls of the stomach and duodenum for the posterior sero-, serous suture. This suture, which is done with nonabsorable thread, is started at the end of the clamp and carried through to the superior angle (lesser curvature). Without interrupting the continous suture, the clamps are rotated 180 degrees, bringing together the sectioned surfaces. We then continue the sutures through the anterior wall. We interrupt the suture after the angle and follow with another thread because of the possibility of a hemostatic failure. At the inferior angle (greater curvature) interrupted sutures are placed at the bases of the clamps. When the clamps are removed the thread is pulled taut, closing the opening. The suture line once accomplished is reinforced at the angles, especially the superior one (fatal suture angle). A segment of the omentum is tacked over the line of closure and the hepatogastric ligament is closed transversely. The lesser omentum is thus fixed to the stomach and duodenum to maintain both organs in alignment and secure better reinforcement at the superior angle. Figs. 1 to 10 show the details of the technique. The Von Petz instrument may be substituted by a temporary transfixation suture at the crushed zone held laterally by two strong clamps only at the portion of the stomach which is beyond the anastomosis. In the other technical steps the compression clamp and forceps effect a satisfactory closure of the sectioned surfaces meeting adequately the aseptic requirements.

DISCUSSION

The method proposed by us allows the surgeon a tactical decision in the operative procedure with choice of the first or second plan of Billroth's technique. Following gastric resection it is easy to perform a gastrojejunostomy when the conditon of the duodenum does not permit a gastroduodenostomy. Therefore, until the resection is accomplished one can plan one or the other procedure and especially consider the possibility of performing the Billroth I.

Hemostasis is of the utmost importance. Through experience in our clinic we have concluded that thorough hemostasis may very well account for the success obtained by the method of Monteiro. As is well known, the vessels in the stomach lie in the submucous layer. A perfect crushing will tear this layer together with the mucosa and circular fibers of the muscularis. When crushing does not accomplish hemostasis, the vessels which are withdrawn with the submucosa will continue to bleed into the cavity. Even if hemostasis is accomplished by crushing it may not be sufficient to withstand postoperative distention. This would result in secondary hemorrhages. It is logical to believe that the success of hemostasis and antisepsis in our method is based on the following fact: the Von Petz instrument performs the crushing but not a lamination that would pierce and permit the submucosa to retract. When the clips are withdrawn and the sectioned surface is electrocoagulated, hemostasis is affected by directly reaching the layers with the vessels. The surface is rendered free from bacteria by the same procedure.

We, therefore, take the liberty of recommending the avoidance of severe crushing to accomplish a successful result. Furthermore, it does not seem wise, in an effort to accomplish an aseptic procedure, to sacrifice a technique by exposing it to failure of hemostasis. All our observations account for this reasoning.

SUMMARY

Lately the surgeons are divided in their choice of one of the two techniques for gastrectomy: the Billroth I or II methods.

The best practice is to accept both procedures leaving the choice as a tactical decision.

By careful observation of the patient or during the course of the operation we can decide which technique may best be applied.

A gastroduodenostomy is often indicated and we have methodized its steps following the principles of the aseptic technique used in gastrojejunostomy.

The use of the Von Petz instrument, hemostasis with the electric cautery, and some special clamps constitute the basic points of the oblique and aseptic anastomosis.

The success of gastroduodenostomy has been, in our hands, equal to that of gastrojejunostomy, technically speaking.

REFERENCES

Babcock, W. W.: Aseptic Gastrointestinal Anastomosis, Surg., Gynec. & Obst. **75**: 485, 1942.

Balfour, D. C.: The Status of "Billroth No. I" in the Surgery of Stomach and Duodenum, Surg., Gynec. & Obst. **58**: 917, 1934.

Carey, J. B.: Gastroscopic Observations of the Post-Operative Stomach Surg., Gynec. & Obst. **65**: 447, 1937.

Desmarest, E., and Debray, G.: A propos, de 25 gastro-pylorectomies pour ul cère de l' estomac J. de chir. **32**: 1, 1928.

Donati, M.: Sobre a tecnica da resseccao gastroduodenal, j. de chir. **46**: 814, 1935.

Holman, E.: An Aseptic Resection of the Stomach for Carcinoma and Ulcer, Surg., Gynec. & Obst. **74**: 146, 1942.

Marshall, S. F., and Kiefer, E. D.: Partial Gastrectomy for Gastric or Duodenal Ulcer, J. A. M. A., **109**: 1341, 1937.

McClure, R. D., and Fallis, L. S.: Partial Gastrectomy for Peptic Ulcer, SURGERY **8**: 575, 1940.
Monteiro, A.: Asceptic Gastric Resection, Surg., Gynec. & Obst. **81**: 177, 1945.
Idem.: Gastrectomía aséptica, Rev. brasil. de cir. 1943.
Idem.: Tecnica Cirurgia, 3: 1943.
Ochsner, A., Gage, M., and Hosoi, K.: Treatment of Peptic Ulcer Based on Physiological Principles, Surg., Gynec. & Obst. **62**: 257, 1936.
Pauchet, V.: Traitement des ulcus gastriques haut situés par la résection en gouttière—"La Pratique Chirurgicale Illustree," Fasc.. VII, 131.
Richter, H. M.: Resseccao gastricą para ulcera peptica, Surg., Gynec. & Obst. **11**: 337-343, 1934.
Spivack, J. L.: Tecnica Quirurgica En Las Operaciones Ab-Dominales, ed. 3, Chicago, 1940, S. B. Debour.
Vale, C. F.: Gastric Resection for Ulcer, Am. J. Surg. **55**: 500, 1942.
Walters, W.: Factors Determining the Choice of Operation in Diseases of the Stomach and Duodenum, S. Clin. North America **18**: 1055, 1938.
Wangensteen, O. H.: Aseptic Resections in the Gastro-Intestinal Tract, Surg., Gynec. & Obst. **72**: 257, 1941.

PRIMARY NONSPECIFIC ULCERS OF THE SMALL INTESTINE*

John A. Evert, M.D.,† B. Marden Black, M.D.,‡ and
Malcolm B. Dockerty, M.D.,§ Rochester, Minn.

THE jejunum and ileum are sometimes the seat of local nonspecific inflammatory ulcers which apparently have no relation to any other disease process. Whether or not these ulcers are manifestations of a single pathologic condition, they are readily distinguishable from other ulcerative lesions of the small intestine because they are usually small and solitary and are not accompanied by pathologic changes in the remainder of the intestine. For want of a better term they have been called "primary" or "simple" ulcers. Primary ulcers produce few symptoms until they bleed, obstruct the lumen of the intestine, or perforate into the general peritoneal cavity. Usually they are recognized only at laparotomy or at necropsy performed after one of these complications has taken place.

Primary ulcers of the small intestine were first described by Matthew Baillie in 1805. Cruveilhier,[1] when writing about gastric ulcers in 1830, remarked that similar "simple" ulcers had been found in the jejunum and ileum. The first review of the subject was made by Combes,[2] who collected reports of thirty-six cases of primary ulcer of the small and large intestine in 1897. Since that time numerous reports have appeared, among which are the reviews by Morrin[3] and Ebeling.[4]

This paper presents a review of the reports of forty-five recently occurring cases of primary jejunal and ileal ulcers. It includes a review of all the reports of cases available in the literature since the appearance of Morrin's article in 1931, a series of thirty-one cases (Table I), and, in addition, a review of the records of all proved cases which have been encountered at the Mayo Clinic, a series of fourteen cases (Cases 1 to 14). Nine of the fourteen cases included in the latter series were reported by Brown and Pemberton[5] in 1936.

PATHOLOGY

A practical definition, in pathologic terms, of primary ulcer has been given by Grasmann.[6] He stated that a simple (or primary) ulcer is a defect of the substance of the mucosa and often of the deeper layers of the small intestine. It is usually localized or single, with well-defined boundaries and with little or no surrounding inflammatory reaction. The etiology of the ulcer, whether acute or chronic, is unknown and its pathogenesis is uncertain.

The ulcer has a fairly characteristic appearance pathologically. Typically the primary ulcer is rounded, with a smooth base, a so-called punched-out

Received for publication, May 19, 1947.

*Abridgment of thesis submitted by Dr. Evert to the Faculty of the Graduate School of the University of Minnesota in partial fulfillment of the requirements for the degree of M.S. in Surgery.

†Fellow in Surgery, Mayo Foundation.
‡Division of Surgery, Mayo Clinic.
§Section on Surgical Pathology, Mayo Clinic.

TABLE I. SUMMARY OF CASE REPORTS PUBLISHED SINCE MORRIN'S REVIEW IN 1931; THIRTY-ONE CASES (EXCLUSIVE OF MAYO CLINIC CASES)

AUTHOR	DATE	AGE (YR.) AND SEX	ULCER		COMPLICATION	SYMPTOMS AND THEIR DURATION	LABORATORY FINDINGS	POSSIBLE PREDISPOSING FACTORS	TREATMENT	RESULT
			LOCATION	NUMBER						
Gutierrez*	†	30, M	Jejunum	1	Perforation	Sudden onset; severe abdominal pain			Laparotomy, perforation not found	Died after 4 days
Bigger[19]	1926†	20, M	Ileum, 3 in. (7.6 cm.) proximal to valve, antimesenteric	1	Perforation	1 wk.: fatigability; sudden perforation	Wassermann negative		Excision of ulcer	Recovery
Bigger	1926†	43, M	Ileum, junction of upper and middle thirds	1	Perforation	Sudden onset; severe abdominal pain and vomiting			Excision of ulcer, enterostomy	Died after 4 days
Heinatz[20]	1928†	24, M	Jejunum, 60 cm. distal to flexure	1	Perforation	1 yr.: sour eructations and periumbilical pain 3 to 4 hr. after meals, relief by fasting; sudden perforation		Healed duodenal ulcer and active gastric ulcer	Operation	Died after 11 days
Zeno, Santorelli, and Ercole*	1931	21, F	Jejunum, 80 cm. distal to flexure, antimesenteric	1	Perforation	Abdominal pain and diarrhea; sudden perforation			Resection and end-to-side anastomosis	Died after 4 days
Lind[7]	1931	52, M	Ileum, 18 in. (45 cm.) and 28 in. (71 cm.) proximal to valve, free border	2	Perforation	8 mo.: distress after eating; 4 mo.: diarrhea; sudden perforation			Laparotomy, perforation not found	Died after 8 hr.
Babington[8]	1932	50, M	Ileum	Several	Obstruction	15 yr.: bouts of severe abdominal pain and vomiting	Wassermann negative	Giardia lamblia in intestine	Resection and lateral anastomosis	Recovery
Moiroud[21]	1932	35, M	Ileum, 60 cm. proximal to valve, free border	1	Perforation	Sudden severe abdominal pain while lifting	Typhoid agglutination negative	Effort	Closure of perforation	Died
Ebeling[14]	1933	36, M	Jejunum, 6 in. (15 cm.) distal to flexure, annular	1	Hemorrhage, obstruction	6 yr.: indigestion; 4 yr. before admission: episode of melena; 8 wk.: abdominal pain and vomiting	Wassermann negative; obstruction to barium meal		Resection and lateral anastomosis	Recovery

Adamek[22]	1934	61, F	Jejunum, distal portion	1	Perforation	Sudden severe periumbilical pain		Vascular?	Laparotomy, perforation not found	Died after 4 days
Desyacques and Doucet-Bon*	1935	45, M	Jejunum, 10 cm. distal to flexure, antimesenteric	1	Perforation, hemorrhage	Several mo.: dyspepsia; hematemesis; sudden perforation			Operation	Died after few hours
Smith[18]	1935	30, M	Jejunum, 2 feet (61 cm.) distal to flexure, antimesenteric	1	Perforation, hemorrhage	2 yr.: distress after eating; sudden perforation	Wassermann negative; occult blood test positive	Buerger's disease	Closure of perforation	Recovery
Levalle and Lubetkin[23]	1936	21, F	Ileum	1	Perforation	4 wk.: periumbilical pain in attacks; vomiting; sudden perforation			Closure of perforation	Recovery
Coletti*	1936	56, M	Jejunum, free border	1	Perforation, hemorrhage	2 yr.: vague generalized abdominal pain preceding defecation; 2 mo. before admission: severe rectal hemorrhage; sudden perforation			Excision of ulcer	Recovery
Davidovitch*	1937	23, M	Jejunum	1	Perforation	Severe abdominal pain for 3 days			Closure of perforation	Recovery
Lastra[24]	1937	47, M	Jejunum, 4 cm. distal to flexure	1	Localized perforation onto transverse colon causing adhesions, obstruction, hemorrhage	4 mo.: periumbilical pain; intermittent intestinal obstruction	Wassermann negative; occult blood test positive		Resection and end-to-end anastomosis	Recovery
Baravalle[25]	1937	37, M	Ileum, proximal portion, free border	1	Perforation	4 or 5 yr.: periodic abdominal pain 4 hr. after eating, relieved by food; sudden perforation			Closure of perforation	Recovery
Masciottra[26]	1938	56, F	Jejuno-ileal region, close to mesentery	1	Perforation	2 days: 2 episodes of severe abdominal pain, the second accompanied by symptoms of perforation		Infection of upper part of respiratory tract	Resection and end-to-end anastomosis	Recovery
Pierangeli[27]	1938	57, M	Ileum, 10 cm. proximal to valve, free border	1	Perforation	Those of sudden perforation	Wassermann negative		Closure of perforation	Recovery

*The case reports of Gutierrez, Zeno and co-workers, Zaffagnini, Desyacques and Doucet-Bon, Coletti, and Davidovitch were abstracted and quoted by Mangione.

†Reported previous to 1931 but not included in Morrin's review.

Table I.—(Cont'd)

Author	Date	Age (yr.) and sex	Ulcer: Location	Ulcer: Number	Complication	Symptoms and their duration	Laboratory findings	Possible predisposing factors	Treatment	Result
Mangione[28]	1938	46, F	Jejunum, close to flexure	1	Perforation, fistula	1 mo.: episodes of severe abdominal pain, diarrhea; mass in abdomen	Wassermann negative; occult blood test positive		Lateral anastomosis proximal to fistula	Died after 3 wk.
Tosonotti[29]	1940	15, M	Ileum, 20 cm. proximal to valve, free border	1	Perforation	Those of sudden perforation	Wassermann negative	Pleurisy with effusion	Closure of perforation	Recovery
Segelman[30]	1940	40, M	Ileum	1	Perforation	10 days; abdominal pain and fever; diagnosis: peritonitis			No operation	Died
Segelman	1940	31, M	Ileum, 25 cm. proximal to valve	1	Perforation	Those of sudden perforation	Wassermann negative; typhoid agglutination negative		Closure of perforation	Recovery
Segelman	1940	32, M	Ileum, 50 cm. proximal to valve	1	Perforation	10 days: malaise; sudden perforation			Resection and end-to-end anastomosis	Recovery
Robinson and Wise[15]	1940	52, F	Ileum, 15 in. (38 cm.) proximal to valve, antimesenteric	1	Perforation	1 mo. before admission: two episodes of periumbilical pain; sudden perforation		Heterotopic mucosa	Resection and lateral anastomosis	Died after 14 days
Robinson and Wise	1940	20, M	Ileum, middle third	1	Perforation	Those of sudden perforation			No operation	Died
Piulachs[9]	1941	46, M	Ileum, 20 and 50 cm. proximal to valve, free border	2	Perforation	Those of sudden perforation	Typhoid culture and agglutination negative		Resection and lateral anastomosis	Died after 1 day
Dowdle[10]	1942	59, M	Jejunum, 1 in. (2.5 cm.) distal to flexure, annular	2	Obstruction, hemorrhage	10 yr.: black stools; progressively severe vomiting after meals for 6 mo.	Obstruction to barium meal		Resection and lateral anastomosis	Died after 8 days
Chambers[11]	1943	34, F	Jejunum, 3 in. (7.6 cm.) distal to flexure	4	Hemorrhage	6 mo.: colicky abdominal pain; malnutrition; massive fatal intestinal hemorrhage		Tuberculosis?	No operation	Died
Marqués and Quintana[31]	1944	46, M	Jejuno-ileal region, free border	1	Perforation	Sudden perforation; lifting at time of onset of symptoms		Effort	Closure of perforation	Recovery

margin (Fig. 1), and little induration of the surrounding tissues. The serosa beneath the ulcer is whitened or reddened. The intestine is frequently narrowed by the fibrous scarring of the ulcer. When examined microscopically, the ulcer is found to have a base which does not undermine the near-by epithelium and which is covered by a thin layer of fibrin and leucocytes. The underlying inflammatory reaction involves all the layers of the intestine but does not extend far beyond the margin of the ulcer laterally. The ulcer base consists of a layer of granulation tissue which replaces the muscularis mucosae, is infiltrated by lymphocytes and plasma cells near the surface, and is underlaid by a varying amount of mature collagenous connective tissue (Figs. 2 and 3). Rarely extensive accumulations of lymphoid tissue are found in the wall of the bowel. The epithelium at the margin of the ulcer shows the changes characteristic of active proliferation, namely, small darkly stained cells with irregularly arranged nuclei and many mitotic figures. The remainder of the tissues either are normal or show minor degrees of inflammation. Enlargement of regional lymph nodes is unusual. Acute ulcers, in which little or no fibrosis has occurred, have been described but chronic ulcers are more common, even in cases in which the clinical illness has been of short duration.

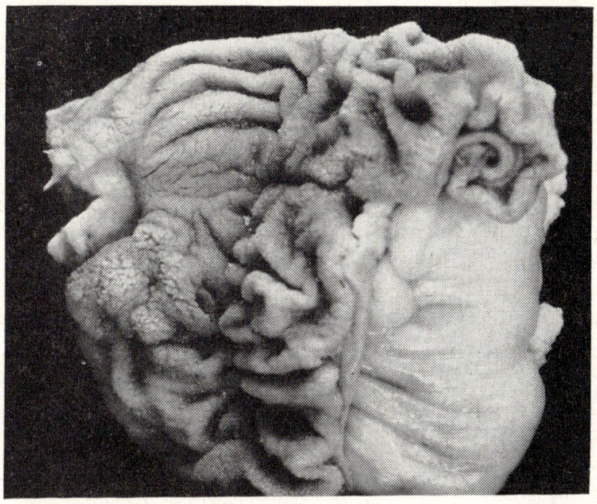

Fig. 1 (Case 13).—Portion of a primary jejunal ulcer; the punched-out margin of the ulcer is demonstrated.

Primary ulcers have been found throughout the small intestine. Of all the known cases (including those collected by Morrin), in 38 per cent the ulcer was in the jejunum and in 62 per cent in the ileum. Of the forty-five recently occurring cases, the ulcer in eleven was less than 80 cm. from the duodeno-jejunal flexure and in nineteen it was less than 60 cm. from the ileocecal valve. Brown and Pemberton commented on the frequency with which the lesion was found close to the ileocecal valve. It would also appear that the lesion is frequently found a short distance below the duodenojejunal flexure (Table II). A primary ulcer does not have any constant relation to the mesentery.

Although the primary ulcer is typically solitary as contrasted to other types of ulcers, nonspecific ulcers with a characteristic pathologic appearance have been found in localized groups. Grasmann collected reports of four cases in which multiple ulcers occurred simultaneously; Lind,[7] Babington,[8] Piulachs,[9] Dowdle,[10] and Chambers[11] have each reported cases since then, and in the Mayo Clinic series there was one such case (Case 10). When the lesions are multiple, a group of two or three is the rule.

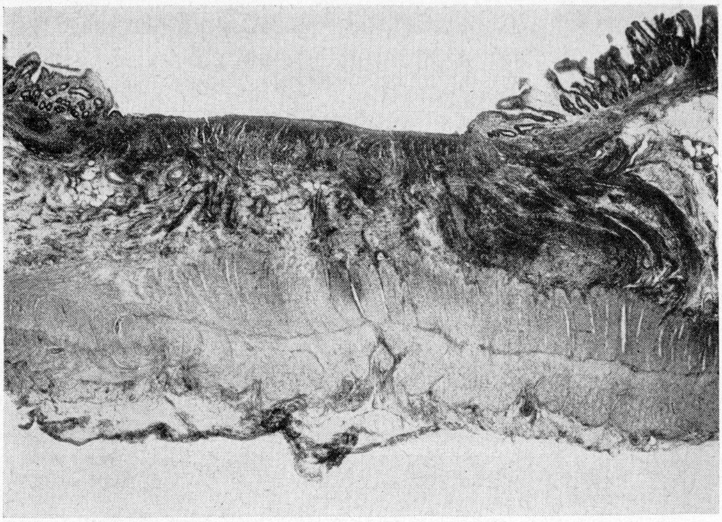

Fig. 2 (Case 5).—Primary ileal ulcer. Note well-defined margins, narrow superficial zone of necrosis, underlying zone of granulation tissue infiltrated by inflammatory cells, and deeper zone of fibrosis (hematoxylin and eosin, ×7½).

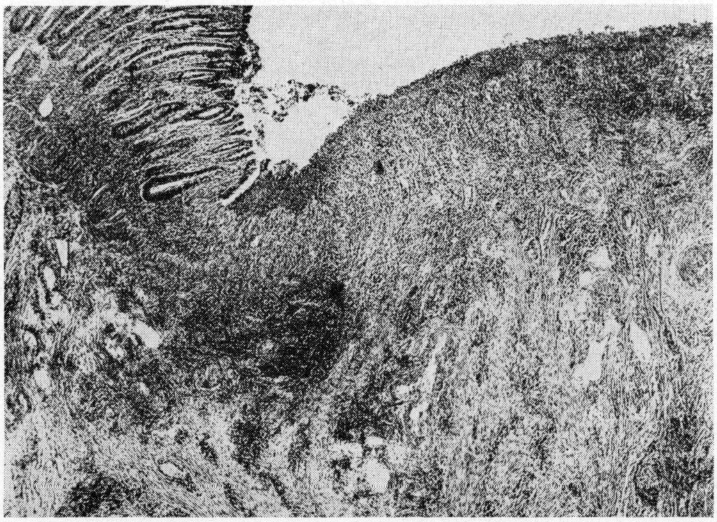

Fig. 3 (Case 13).—Primary jejunal ulcer. The granulation tissue is densely infiltrated with inflammatory cells near the surface but is blended with young connective tissue peripherally. The inflammatory cells are mostly plasma cells and lymphocytes, with a few polymorphonuclear leucocytes (hematoxylin and eosin, ×25).

TABLE II. LOCATION OF PRIMARY ULCERS IN THE JEJUNUM AND ILEUM (FORTY-FIVE CASES)

LOCATION	CASES
Jejunum	
Proximal 80 cm.	11
Unspecified	4
Middle and distal portions	2
Jejuno-ileal region	3
Ileum	
Upper and mid-portions	3
Unspecified	3
Terminal 60 cm.	19
Total	45

Primary ulcers are potentially dangerous because of the complications which may develop. In every reported case of ulcer which has caused clinical symptoms or which has been recognized at laparotomy, perforation, bleeding, or obstruction has occurred. Perforation occurred in 81 per cent of all recorded cases, bleeding in 15 per cent, and clinical obstruction in 9 per cent; from these figures it is apparent that a few patients suffered from multiple complications (Table III).

TABLE III. COMPLICATIONS IN 130 CASES

COMPLICATION	85 CASES BEFORE 1931		31 CASES 1931 TO 1944		14 CASES FROM MAYO CLINIC		TOTAL, 130 CASES	
	NUMBER	PER CENT	NUMBER	PER CENT	NUMBER	PER CENT	NUMBER	PER CENT
Perforation	75	88	27 (25 free, 2 localized)	87	3 (1 free, 2 localized)	21	105	81
Bleeding	2	2	8 (5 gross, 3 occult)	26	9 (7 gross, 2 occult)	64	19	15
Obstruction (clinical)	5	6	3	10	4	28	12	9

Perforation, which resulted most often in generalized peritonitis, was found in thirty of the forty-five recently occurring cases. In four cases, however, the perforation had been localized by inflammatory adhesions; two of these localized perforations were associated with inflammatory abdominal masses, one was associated with a jejunocolic fistula, and one was surrounded by extensive adhesions to the mesentery.

Recurrent, prolonged, and occasionally massive bleeding has been associated with primary ulcer. In seventeen of the forty-five cases just referred to, unmistakable clinical signs of loss of blood were present; in twelve of these seventeen, grossly visible blood had passed from the gastrointestinal tract. Five of the ulcers which bled were annular, two were located near the mesentery, and five were at a distance from the mesentery. In every case in which an annular ulcer was reported, there was a history of recognizable gastrointestinal bleeding.

Symptoms of intestinal obstruction were recorded in seven of the forty-five cases referred to previously. Clinical evidence of obstruction was considerably less frequent than was the pathologic finding of dilatation of the intestine proximal to a stricture at the site of the ulcer. This is well demonstrated in the series of fourteen cases studied. In nine of these cases there was pathologic evidence of dilatation of the bowel proximal to a stenotic ulcer, but in only four of the nine was there sufficient stenosis to cause clinical symptoms of obstruction.

Recurrence of primary ulcer has been reported. The patient of Gale[12] had three different episodes of perforation, each of which followed an attack of furunculosis. Fischer[13] and also Brown and Pemberton[5] (Case 5, reported herein) have reported cases in which clinical symptoms recurred after resection for ulcer.

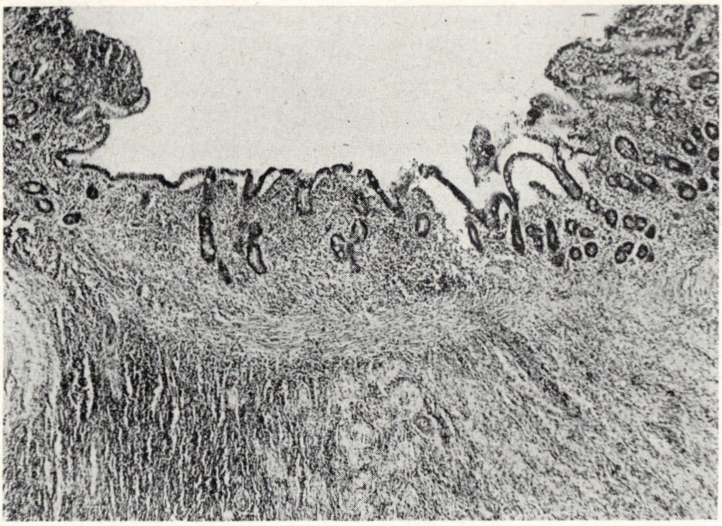

Fig. 4, (Case 11).—Primary jejunal ulcer. The surface is covered by a thin layer of mucous membrane which is not thrown into villi. The presence of well-organized granulation tissue and fibrosis beneath the ulcer indicates a process of healing (hematoxylin and eosin ×40).

From available facts, it cannot be said whether a primary ulcer of the type herein described ever occurs without producing clinical manifestations or whether an ulcer ever heals spontaneously. It would seem possible that an ulcer might occur without bringing about symptoms necessitating laparotomy and, therefore, without ever being detected. An ulcer of this description has not been reported as an incidental finding at necropsy. There is good presumptive evidence that an ulcer may heal spontaneously. For example, Oudard and Jean[14] reported the case of a patient who had a group of ulcers, one of which seemed to be in the healing stage. The appearance of the ulcer microscopically in Case 11 reported herein, in which the base of the ulcer consisted of an abnormally thin layer of mucous membrane covered by epithelium and beneath which were granulation tissue and fibrosis, suggests healing (Fig. 4). Also, it is known that many patients whose perforated ulcer is treated only by simple closure have no more symptoms.

ETIOLOGY

The cause of primary ulcer is not known. The occurrence of this type of ulcer has been attributed to infection, peptic digestion, trauma, or vascular abnormalities. No infectious agent has been found in constant association with the lesion. Syphilis and tuberculosis have been excluded as possible etiologic agents in most cases. A certain number of high jejunal ulcers have been found in association with peptic ulcers, but many more have not. The widely quoted theory that heterotopic gastric mucosa in the intestine might contribute to the formation of these ulcers, just as such tissue contributes to the formation of ulcers about Meckel's diverticulum, cannot be substantiated because microscopic amounts of gastric tissue have almost never been found[15] in association with these ulcers. At times perforation of chronic ulcer has been associated with external trauma.[16] Only rarely has an intraintestinal foreign body been found near an ulcer. Cornioley's[17] suggestion that all the ulcers are secondary to ischemia produced by localized arteriolosclerosis or embolism has not been generally accepted. In the cases studied there was no evidence of heterotopic gastric mucosa or of any vascular abnormality. Thorough discussions of etiologic theories may be found in the papers of Ebeling and of Oudard and Jean.

Oudard and Jean have concluded that these ulcers might well result from a variety of causes, for they have been associated with distinctly different diseases.

Although some of the so-called primary ulcers have probably in actual fact been caused by infections, trauma, or peptic digestion, the pathogenesis of most primary ulcers must remain obscure.

OCCURRENCE

Primary ulcer of the jejunum and ileum is rare. Morrin collected reports of eighty-five cases in the literature up to 1931, and to this number forty-five cases have since been added, making a total of 130 cases. The number of cases studied at the clinic is equivalent roughly to one per 100,000 patients registered. In ninety-seven of the known cases the patients were men, and in thirty-three they were women, a ratio of about 3:1. The youngest patient who was reported to have such a lesion was 1 year old, and the oldest, 77; the majority were adult persons. The average age of all patients was 43 years.

SYMPTOMS AND LABORATORY FINDINGS

The symptoms of primary ulcer depend chiefly on complications. For convenience of discussion, known cases may be divided into two groups according to whether free perforation did or did not occur. When free perforation occurred, the symptoms were those characteristic of any sudden perforation of a viscus into the peritoneal cavity. In contrast to gastric or duodenal perforation, jejunoileal perforation was often associated with a point of maximal tenderness to the left of the umbilicus in the reports of cases studied.[18] The perforations of primary ulcer were preceded by some sort of chronic abdominal pain in about one-half of the reported cases.

The exact diagnosis of chronic nonperforated primary ulcer has seldom been made clinically. Under certain circumstances, however, the symptoms may suggest a lesion of the small intestine. Primary ulcer has been found at laparotomy done for (1) episodes of crampy abdominal pain and vomiting suggestive of obstruction of the small intestine, (2) anemia and unexplained gastrointestinal bleeding, and (3) postprandial epigastric or periumbilical pain. In certain cases the abdominal symptoms have been so vague or so mild as to defy diagnostic classification.

In addition to clinical findings, those laboratory tests which are of specific aid in establishing a diagnosis of chronic jejunoileal ulcer depend on the fact that the ulcer may bleed or cause obstruction. Benzidine and guaiac tests for occult blood in the stool have proved to be of considerable value. In several cases a history of melena was confirmed by the results of a test for occult blood; in five of the seventeen cases, referred to previously, in which bleeding occurred, the result of the test for occult blood was the only positive evidence of bleeding. No case of primary ulcer has yet been reported in which such a test, when done, gave negative results. Brown and Pemberton, Smith and Ebeling have called attention to the value of this test as a diagnostic measure. Roentgenologic demonstration of a small intestinal ulcer is rarely possible. However, on two occasions constricting ulcers have been demonstrated by means of a barium meal.[4, 10] In the series studied herein, a constricting ulcer could not be demonstrated in any of the four patients to whom a barium meal was administered.

DIAGNOSIS

Because of the rarity of primary ulcer and the variety of clinical symptoms which it may produce, the clinical diagnosis was so obscure that it was established in only one reported case.[4] However, it is useful to think of the possibility of occurrence of these lesions in the following groups of patients: (1) patients who present a problem of gastrointestinal hemorrhage, acute or chronic, in whom there is no roentgenologic evidence of abnormality of the esophagus, stomach, duodenum, or colon; (2) patients who have symptoms and signs of peritonitis suggestive of a ruptured peptic ulcer, in whom no gastric or duodenal perforation is discovered at laparotomy, and (3) patients who present a problem of recurrent postprandial pain suggestive of peptic ulcer, in whom there is roentgenologically no evidence of gastric or duodenal ulceration.

MORTALITY RATE

The mortality rate in cases of primary ulcer is high. Morrin found reports of fifty-six fatalities among the records of eighty-five cases (66 per cent). There were twenty-one deaths among the forty-five recently occurring cases, a mortality rate of 47 per cent. In the latter series of cases, ulcers, associated with free perforation and generalized peritonitis accounted for fourteen deaths in twenty-six cases (54 per cent), and ulcers associated with local perforation or not associated with perforation accounted for seven deaths in nineteen cases (37 per cent). Among twelve patients of the recently reported series who had grossly recognizable intestinal bleeding, one had a fatal hemorrhage.

TREATMENT

The treatment in all cases in which the lesion was recognized during life was surgical (Table IV). In most cases the gravity of the complications was such that laparotomy had been done without specific preoperative diagnosis. Robinson and Wise have concluded that "the simplest procedure compatible with the condition encountered . . . should be done." In the presence of free perforation, transverse closure of the perforation would seem to be the best procedure, according to the results obtained in the twenty-six cases of the recently occurring series in which this complication was present. Nine of those twenty-six patients were treated by simple closure of the perforation, with one fatality; three were treated by excision of the ulcer and transverse closure of the bowel, with one fatality, and five were treated by resection and anastomosis, with three fatalities. The three patients whose perforated ulcers were not discovered at the time of laparotomy and the three patients who did not undergo operation all died. Three other patients died after unspecified surgical procedures.

TABLE IV. MORTALITY IN RELATION TO SURGICAL OR NONSURGICAL TREATMENT (FORTY-FIVE CASES)

COMPLICATION	TOTAL CASES	TREATED SURGICALLY		NOT TREATED SURGICALLY	
		CASES	DEATHS	CASES	DEATHS
Free perforation	26	23	11	3	3
No perforation or localized perforation	19	18	6	1	1 (died of hemorrhage)
Total	45	41	17	4	4

More extensive procedures have been used in the treatment of ulcer which has not perforated. Of eighteen such patients who underwent surgical treatment, one was treated satisfactorily by simple closure of a local perforation, three were treated, with one fatality, by lateral anastomosis without resection, and fourteen were treated by resection and anastomosis, with five fatalities. Removal of the ulcer would not appear to be strictly necessary, since those patients in whom the ulcer was not actually removed and those in whom a simple closure was done for perforation all had little further trouble. The occasional tendency to recur and the difficulty of excluding from consideration the possibility of malignancy on the basis of gross appearance, however, would suggest that resection of the diseased tissue would be the procedure of choice whenever such procedure would not materially increase the risk of operation.

REPORT OF CASES

In view of the rarity of primary ulcer the records of all the cases of primary ulcers encountered at the Mayo Clinic have been reviewed. The first nine cases in this series, which were reported in abstract by Brown and Pemberton in 1936, have been included in more detail. Five new reports of cases complete the series. These cases have been selected in accordance with the pathologic criteria stated by Grasmann. Those ulcers which seemed to be acute and which were found incidentally in cases in which death had resulted from other diseases were not included in this series. In the majority of cases reported in the literature, the complication of acute perforation was present, whereas in virtually all the cases studied at this institution, chronic complications led to the diagnosis, possibly because comparatively few emergent abdominal conditions of any type were seen here. The deaths which followed surgical treatment in this series of cases all occurred before the year 1933.

CASE 1 (Brown and Pemberton, Case 1).—An architect, 58 years old, had had recurrent attacks of severe colicky periumbilical pain for three years. The pain lasted hours at a time and recurred every few months. During the ten months before admission to the clinic, the pain had become more frequent and had been brought on by eating. The patient had lost forty-five pounds (20.4 kilograms).

The abdomen was distended and on its surface peristaltic waves could be seen. A mass was palpable in the left lower quadrant. The other findings were not significant.

At laparotomy an inflammatory ulcer was found in the distal part of the ileum. At the site of the ulcer there was an obstructing stricture and proximally there was distention of the bowel. A lateral anastomosis was performed and the site of the ulcer was not disturbed. Convalescence was uneventful. The patient was reported to be in good health six years later.

CASE 2 (Brown and Pemberton, Case 2).—A housewife, 58 years old, had had vague abdominal pains as well as numerous other complaints for many years. Three weeks before admission she began to have griping periumbilical pain accompanied by bloating of the abdomen and borborygmi.

The abdomen was somewhat tender and peristalsis could be seen on its surface. The other findings were not significant.

At laparotomy an obstructing ulcer was found 100 cm. proximal to the ileocecal valve. The mesentery beneath the ulcer was involved in an inflammatory reaction and free fluid was present in the peritoneal cavity. A lateral anastomosis was established and the site of the ulcer was not disturbed. Convalescence was uneventful but during the remaining eleven years of her life the patient continued to complain of vague abdominal pain.

CASE 3 (Brown and Pemberton, Case 3).—A janitor, 47 years old, had had dull, burning epigastric pain for three years. The pain began about one hour after eating, was relieved by so-called dyspepsia pills, and was occasionally accompanied by a sensation of bloating. During the three weeks before admission the pain had become more severe and vomiting had occurred frequently.

The patient appeared ill and was evidently in pain. Tenderness and rigidity were present in the midepigastric region.

At laparotomy two or three loops of bowel were found to be adherent about an abscess which communicated with a perforating ulcer of the ileum. The ulcer was 5 cm. proximal to the ileocecal valve. A few small edematous ecchymotic spots were seen in the near-by ileum. The perforation in the ileum was closed. Postoperatively an enterocutaneous fistula developed but the abdominal symptoms had been relieved for at least a year when the patient was last seen.

CASE 4 (Brown and Pemberton, Case 5).—A carpenter, 47 years old, had passed massive tarry stools many times during the eight years before admission. He had no gastrointestinal symptoms except occasional sensations of bloating. During the last four months before admission, he had become extremely weak.

The spleen was palpable. The hemoglobin measured 4.4 Gm. per 100 c.c. of blood. The results of guaiac tests were repeatedly positive for occult blood in the stool.

At laparotomy an ulcer which had produced a partially obstructing stricture was found halfway between the duodenum and cecum. The lesion was removed and an end-to-end anastomosis and a proximal enteric stoma were established. The ulcer was annular, measured 6 mm. in cross section, and was atypical in that the adjacent submucosa was densely infiltrated by lymphocytes. Five years afterward the patient was reported to be in good health.

CASE 5 (Brown and Pemberton, Case 6).—A grocer, 35 years old, complained of intermittent abdominal pain which had been present in increasing severity for six years. The pain was located in the upper part of the abdomen and was sometimes brought on by eating. There were sensations of abdominal bloating and anorexia. He had lost twenty-five pounds (11.3 kilograms).

The patient looked ill but no physical abnormalities were found. The value for the hemoglobin was 7.3 Gm. per 100 c.c. of blood, and the results of guaiac tests were repeatedly positive for occult blood in the stool.

At laparotomy an obstructing ileal ulcer with a punched-out appearance was found 90 cm. proximal to the ileocecal valve. The involved part of the ileum was resected, an end-to-end anastomosis was established, and a proximal enteric stoma was made. The ulcer measured 1.5 cm. in diameter and had a typical appearance pathologically as shown in Fig. 2.

One and one-half years later the patient again noticed sharp pain to the left of the umbilicus, which appeared about one-half hour after meals and was accompanied by belching. The patient was last seen two years after operation, at which time he had the same symptoms and was still anemic. Because of the similarity of the symptoms to those which occurred before operation, the patient was considered to have a recurrence of the ulcer.

CASE 6 (Brown and Pemberton, Case 8).—A laborer, 26 years old, had had increasingly severe abdominal pain for one and one-half years. The pain was located across the middle part of the abdomen, it sometimes extended to the back, and it began about one-half hour after eating. Vomiting occasionally relieved the pain. The patient had lost ten pounds (4.5 kilograms).

Physical findings were not significant. The hemoglobin was 30 per cent of normal and the results of guaiac tests were positive for occult blood in the stool.

At laparotomy a solitary ulcer was found near the mesentery of the ileum about 2 feet (61 cm.) proximal to the ileocecal valve. The mesentery beneath the ulcer was considerably thickened. The lesion was removed and a lateral anastomosis was established. The patient died four days later because of general peritonitis. The ulcer was rounded, measured 2.5 cm. in diameter, and had a typical appearance pathologically.

CASE 7 (Brown and Pemberton, Case 10).—A housewife, 24 years old, had been severely anemic most of the time for ten years. At intervals during this period she had been troubled by constipation and by severe cramps across the lower part of the abdomen. During the last three months before admission, she had passed tarry or bloody stools on several occasions and had had severe abdominal cramps accompanied by vomiting. She had lost twenty-three pounds (10.4 kilograms).

The results of physical examination were not remarkable. The content of hemoglobin was 7.4 Gm. per 100 c.c. of blood, and the results of guaiac tests were positive for occult blood in the stools.

At laparotomy a constricting ulcer of the ileum 45 cm. proximal to the ileocecal valve was found. The lesion was removed and an end-to-end anastomosis and a sidetracking lateral anastomosis were established. Three weeks later the patient died because of general peritonitis. The ulcer was annular and had a characteristic appearance microscopically.

CASE 8 (cited by Brown and Pemberton).—A farmer, 46 years old, had been pale, weak, and easily fatigued for eight months. After examination a diagnosis of pernicious anemia was established. As a phase of a method of treatment in vogue nearly thirty years ago, ileosigmoidostomy was performed. During the operation an ulcer was found in the ileum 15 cm. proximal to the ileocecal valve. The ulcer was removed. It measured 1.5 by 1 cm. and had the microscopic appearance of a simple ulcer. The patient died six days afterward because of general peritonitis.

CASE 9 (cited by Brown and Pemberton).—An insane patient, 47 years old, who was suffering from general paresis, complained of abdominal pain and became ill. Within a few hours he had a temperature of 104° F. The following day the patient died. At necropsy general peritonitis and a clean-cut perforation secondary to an acute nonspecific inflammatory ulcer of the ileum, 80 cm. proximal to the ileocecal valve, were observed.

CASE 10.—A housewife, 45 years old, had been troubled by constipation for four years and had lost twenty pounds (9.1 kilograms) because of a self-imposed diet. For eight months she had noticed increasingly severe, diffuse abdominal pain which was relieved by defecation and which sometimes awakened her at night. She had had some nausea and a sensation of abdominal fullness after eating.

The abdomen was tympanitic and tender about the umbilicus. The value for hemoglobin was 68 per cent. Other studies, including urinalysis, a flocculation test for syphilis, and roentgenography of the stomach and colon, did not give significant results.

During a period of observation the patient continued to have abdominal pain and the value for hemoglobin fell to 58 per cent.

At laparotomy two constrictions secondary to punched-out nonspecific ulcers were found 8 cm. apart about 30 cm. proximal to the ileocecal valve. One ulcer was annular and the other was oval; the diameter of each varied from 1 to 2.5 cm. The appearance microscopically was similar to that of other primary ulcers previously described. The mesenteric lymph nodes were enlarged but the remainder of the intestine appeared normal. The involved segment of bowel was resected and an end-to-end anastomosis was established. Five days later the patient died of general peritonitis.

CASE 11.—A Negro, 65 years old, who had been troubled by constipation for many years, had noticed crampy midabdominal pain for two months. The pain was intermittent, often became worse fifteen minutes after meals, and sometimes awakened the patient at night. He lost twenty pounds (9.1 kilograms).

The results of physical examination were not remarkable. The content of hemoglobin was 7.0 Gm. per 100 c.c. of blood and the result of a benzidine test was positive for small amounts of occult blood in the stool. Other studies, including urinalysis, a flocculation test for syphilis, and roentgenologic examination of the stomach, small intestine, and colon, gave essentially negative results.

At laparotomy an ulcer 1 cm. in diameter was found in the midjejunal region, away from the mesentery. The involved segment of bowel was excised and an end-to-end anastomosis was established. Convalescence was uneventful. The appearance of the ulcer microscopically suggested a process of healing, as described previously in this paper (Fig. 4).

CASE 12.—A man, 55 years old, had had four episodes of massive gastrointestinal bleeding in twelve years. On one occasion the bleeding had been manifested as hematemesis, on other occasions, as melena. He had had no abdominal symptoms save an occasional so-called gassy sensation after eating.

The findings on physical examination were not significant. The value for hemoglobin was 11.7 Gm. per 100 c.c. of blood. On roentgenoscopic examination changes suggestive of a duodenal ulcer were seen. The results of urinalysis and a flocculation test for syphilis were essentially negative.

At laparotomy no external evidence of duodenal abnormality was encountered but a chronically obstructing lesion of the jejunum about 20 cm. distal to the duodenojejunal flexure was found. The lesion was an ulcer 2 by 2.5 cm. in diameter, located adjacent to the mesentery and associated with three inflammatory lymph nodes. On microscopic examination a dense collection of lymphocytes and plasma cells beneath the ulcer, with edema of the adjacent submucosa, was seen. The involved segment of bowel was resected and an end-to-end anastomosis was established. Convalescence was uneventful.

CASE 13.—For six years a housewife, 31 years old had had epigastric pain which often began two hours after eating and which was relieved by drinking milk. The pain was present only at irregular intervals. The patient had passed bulky tarry stools and had become weak on ten different occasions. The patient's father was said to have suffered from a stomach or peptic ulcer.

Save for slight epigastric tenderness there were no significant findings on physical examination The content of hemoglobin was 9.7 Gm. per 100 c.c. of blood. Other tests, including urinalysis, a flocculation test for syphilis, tests for coagulation of blood and bleeding time, and roentgenoscopy of the stomach, small intestine, and duodenum, gave negative results.

At laparotomy an indurated constricting lesion was found in the jejunum 45 cm. distal to the duodenojejunal flexure. This lesion was removed and was found to contain an ulcer 1.5 by 2 cm. in diameter, located 1 cm. from the mesentery. Microscopically the ulcer was similar to those described previously (Fig. 3). There was no lymphadenopathy. An end-to-end anastomosis was established and the patient had an uneventful convalescence.

CASE 14.—A housewife, 60 years old, had had abdominal cramps which lasted one or two days at a time, for two years. One week before admission she became unable to move the bowels and began to have crampy abdominal pain and distention. The latter symptoms progressed and she vomited foul brown material.

The patient was a thin sick-looking woman whose abdomen was moderately distended and tympanitic. On roentgenographic examination multiple distended loops of small intestine were seen.

After nasogastric intubation the patient improved temporarily. On the sixth day in the hospital laparotomy was performed. The intestine was obstructed by adhesions about a perforating ulcer located in the terminal part of the ileum. There was no lymphadenopathy. The lesion was removed and an end-to-end anastomosis was made. The ulcer was similar to those seen in the other cases save for a more acute inflammatory process. The patient's convalescence was satisfactory.

SUMMARY

Nonspecific localized ulcerations of the jejunum and ileum are so similar pathologically as to justify their classification as a group under the name "primary" or "simple" ulcers. Although the lesions are characteristically solitary, small groups of ulcers are sometimes found. The etiology of primary ulcers is unknown. There is little direct evidence to support the theories that they are caused by infection, irritation from gastric secretions, trauma, or vascular abnormalities.

The symptoms of primary ulcer are for the most part secondary to the complications of perforation, bleeding, or obstruction. The possibility of these lesions should be considered in the presence of unexplained intestinal bleeding or of peritonitis which suggests acute visceral perforation when such perforation cannot be found in the stomach or duodenum.

The mortality rate in patients suffering from primary ulcer is high. The lesion has been recognized during life only after some complication has led to surgical intervention.

REFERENCES

1. Cruveilhier: Quoted by Grasmann.[6]
2. Combes, Charles: Des ulcerés simples de l'intestine, Thèse de dact., Faculté de Medecine et de Pharmacie de Toulouse, 1897, No. 193, pp. 185-197.
3. Morrin, F. J.: Spontaneous Perforation of Primary Jejunal Ulcers, Irish J. M. Sc. **6**: 198-213, 1931.
4. Ebeling, W. W.: Primary Jejunal Ulcer, Ann. Surg. **97**: 857-874, 1933.
5. Brown, P. W., and Pemberton, J. deJ.: Solitary Ulcer of the Ileum and Ulcer of Meckel's Diverticulum, Ann. Int. Med. **9**: 1684-1702, 1936.
6. Grasmann, Max: Zur Frage des Ulcus simplex des Dünndarmes, Arch. f. klin. Chir. **136**: 449-478, 1925.
7. Lind, S. C.: Simple Ulcer of the Intestine, Ohio State M. J. **27**: 621-627, 1931.
8. Babington, S. H.: Simple Ulcers of the Jejuno-ileum; Report of Case, California & West. Med. **37**: 191-192, 1932.
9. Piulachs, P.: Perforación de la úlcera simple de intestino delgado, Med. españ. **5**: 89-98, 1941.
10. Dowdle, Edward: Multiple, Primary Nonspecific Jejunal Ulcers, With Chronic Duodenal Dilatation, Ann. Surg. **116**: 348-354, 1942.
11. Chambers, W. T.: Case of Ulceration of Duodenum and Jejunum, M. J. Australia **2**: 316-318, 1943.

12. Gale, S. S.: Repeated Perforations of Small Intestine Due to Focal Infection, J. A. M. A. **79**: 1047-1048, 1922.
13. Fischer, Hermann: Primary Ulcer of the Jejunum, Ann. Surg. **77**: 775-776, 1923.
14. Oudard, and Jean, G.: L'ulcère simple du grêle, Arch. d. mal. de l'app. digestif. **15**: 208-228, 1925.
15. Robinson, D. R., and Wise, W. D.: Simple Non-specific Ulcer of the Jejuno-ileum, Surg., Gynec. & Obst. **70**: 1097-1099, 1940.
16. Taylor, John: Three Cases of Acute Perforating "Ulcer" of the Small Intestine, Edinburgh M. J. **32**: 255-262, 1925.
17. Cornioley, C.: L'ulcère simple de l'intestin grêle, Rev. méd. de la Suisse Rom. **50**: 91-111, 1930.
18. Smith, B. C.: Primary Perforated Jejunal Ulcer, Ann. Surg. **101**: 1225-1249, 1935.
19. Bigger, I. A.: Simple Ulcer of the Small Intestine, Virginia M. Monthly **53**: 4-6, 1926.
20. Heinatz, S. W.: Ueber das nichtoperative Ulcus pepticum jejuni, Zentralbl. f. Chir. **55**: 534-535, 1928.
21. Moiroud, P.: Perforation d'un ulcère simple de l'iléon, Bull. et mém. Soc. nat. de chir. **58**: 1157-1162, 1932.
22. Adamek: Sitzungsberichte aus chirurgischen Gesellschaften (Sitzung vom. 14, Dec. 1933), Centralbl. f. Chir. **61**: 589, 1934.
23. Levalle, R. P., and Lubetkin, C.: Ulcera solitaria del intestino delgado, Semana méd. **2**: 405-407, 1936.
24. Lastra, J. S.: Ulcera simple, estenosante del yeyuno que simula un cancer del colon transverso, Bol. Liga contra el cáncer **12**: 355-364, 1937.
25. Baravalle, C.: Un caso di ulcera rotonda del tenue perforata, Gior. med. d. Alto Adige **9**: 557-562, 1937.
26. Masciottra, R. L.: Ulcera simple perforada del yeyuno-ileon, Bol. y trab. de la Soc. de cir. de Buenos Aires **22**: 38-43, 1938.
27. Pierangeli, L. L'ulcera semplice del tenue, Arch. ital. di chir. **53**: 731-739, 1938.
28. Mangione, G.: Sull'ulcera semplice primitiva del digiuno, Arch. ital. di chir. **52**: 764-780, 1938.
29. Tosonotti, Tito: L'ulcera semplice primitiva del tenue, Policlinico (sez. chir.) **47**: 30-40, 1940.
30. Segelman, S. Y.: Simple Ulcers of Small Intestine, Novy khir. arkhiv. **48**: 45-48, 1940.
31. Marqués, V. N., and Quintana, F. I.: Ulcera simple del intestino delgado perforada, Día Méd. **16**: 1052-1055, 1944.

CARCINOMA OF THE GALL BLADDER

Report of Seventy-five Cases

Frank P. Sainburg, M.D., and John H. Garlock, M.D., New York, N. Y.

(From the Surgical Service of the Mount Sinai Hospital)

Although numerous reports concerning the subject of carcinoma of the gall bladder have emphasized the gloomy outlook in this disease, it seems justifiable to continue the analysis of large series of cases in order to arrive at some more promising active or prophylactic therapy. Reports of cure of carcinoma of the gall bladder are indeed rare. Mohardt,[1] in a comprehensive analysis of the literature, found a paucity of five-year cures, and stated that the survival rate, including all cases reported, varied from 0 to 6 per cent.

The contention by many physicians and surgeons alike that this disease is too uncommon to cause grave concern, is not borne out by the surveys made in recent years. In large series of consecutive autopsies, the percentage of occurrence of carcinoma of the gall bladder is shown to be .41,[2] .27,[3] and .33.[4] These autopsies, however, are unselected and include all age groups as well as patients who may have been operated upon previously. Thus, Graham[5] stated that carcinoma of the gall bladder constitutes 8 to 10 per cent of all carcinomas and Kirshbaum and Kozoll[2] placed the incidence at 3 per cent of carcinomas found in 13,300 autopsies.

Even more important is the frequent occurrence of carcinoma of the gall bladder in association with cholelithiasis. Graham found that in 8½ per cent of all cases of cholelithiasis, discovered at autopsy, carcinoma of the gall bladder was also present, and he quoted previous authors as finding an incidence of 5 to 14 per cent. In a more recent report,[6] figures of 4, 5, and 6 per cent were given. Warren and Balch[7] gave the incidence of carcinoma found at operation on such diseased gall bladders as 1 to 2½ per cent. As Mohardt indicated, however, the low incidence found in many recent reports on operative findings may in a large part be due to the fact that many more cholecystectomies are now performed on younger patients. It is evident, therefore, that cancer of the gall bladder is not as rare as some reports would have one believe.

REPORT OF CASES

In the fourteen years from 1933 to 1946, inclusive, seventy-five patients with carcinoma of the gall bladder were encountered on the ward services of the Mount Sinai Hospital. Sixty-five of these were subjected to operation, and the diagnosis was verified by microscopic examination. Of the remaining ten patients, five were moribund on admission and could not be dealt with surgically, and the other five died of unrelated disease. At necropsy, all ten were found to have carcinoma of the gall bladder. Follow-up was complete in all cases. One patient was alive thirteen and one-half years after operation; the remainder died

Received for publication, June 2, 1947.

within a period of thirty-five months after operation. This constitutes a five-year survival rate of 1½ per cent.

Sixty-three patients were women and twelve were men, a sex incidence of 84 and 16 per cent, respectively. This ratio of 5.2 to 1 is in accordance with that found by most observers, the average having been 4 to 1 in the collective study of Mohardt. In Table I is seen the incidence according to age. The youngest patient was 38 years old, the oldest 83 years. Over 89 per cent of the patients were between the ages of 40 and 69 years.

TABLE I. AGE INCIDENCE

AGE (YR.)	CASES	INCIDENCE (PER CENT)
30-39	1	1.3
40-49	8	10.7
50-59	29	38.7
60-69	30	40
70-79	6	8
80-89	1	1.3
Total	75	100

In an endeavor to discover some means of correlating diagnosis with the history, physical examination, and/or laboratory findings, a careful analysis of each phase of the examination was made. The past history was significant only in that thirty-two, or 42.6 per cent, had a history of one to forty years strongly suggestive of gall bladder disease, as indicated by positive cholecystograms, or because of recurrent attacks of right upper quadrant pain, fatty food intolerance, jaundice, nausea, and vomiting. The criterion of the onset of the illness in all cases, which ranged from one day to one year, was either the initial appearance of complaints or a marked transition from the longer history referable to gall bladder disease.

The predominant symptoms were as follows:

Of the total, 77.3 per cent complained of abdominal pain. This was most frequently located in the right upper quadrant, but occasionally in the epigastrium and rarely in the lower abdomen.

There was definite weight loss in 41 per cent of the patients, varying in amount from five to seventy pounds.

Jaundice was a symptom in 38.6 per cent.

Other less frequent symptoms were anorexia, nausea, vomiting, weakness, constipation, dyspepsia, diarrhea, melena, chills, and fever. Nine patients were known to have diabetes.

On physical examination the important frequent findings were a palpable mass in the right upper abdomen, 64 per cent; jaundice, 38 per cent; and a palpably enlarged liver, 28 per cent.

Laboratory diagnostic aids, such as blood counts, chemical analyses of blood and urine, and roentgen examination showed no constant aberration from the normal. The correct clinical diagnosis was made in 22.7 per cent of the patients, although its possibility was suggested in many of the others. These clinical findings compare favorably with those found by Kirshbaum and Kozoll in a series of fifty-five cases in which the correct diagnosis was also made in 22 per cent of the patients. They related the cardinal findings to be pain, jaundice, and a palpable tumor, although these were by no means always associated. Our cardinal findings are the same, in addition to weight loss.

At operation, the findings varied from the appearance of a chronic cholecystitis to a totally inoperable neoplastic mass which in different cases involved virtually every abdominal organ. In those which were entirely inoperable, a biopsy was taken and the abdomen closed (Group I). Where it was thought that the disease was beyond surgical excision, but that some palliative procedure might prolong the life of the patient, such procedures as hepaticoduodenostomy, choledochostomy, partial cholecystectomy en bloc, excision of liver and gall bladder, or simple cholecystostomy were performed (Group II). In another group of cases it was felt by the surgeon that all visible disease could be extirpated and that the patient might possibly be cured (Group III). The remainder constitute those in which the diagnosis was made by the pathologist, and in which the surgeon at the time of operation had not suspected carcinoma (Group IV). In Table II are the average postoperative survival periods for the groups mentioned. The one living patient who is included in Group IV was operated upon thirteen and one-half years ago and is now free of any evidence of disease. This patient was 53 years old at the time of operation and she had had a three-week history indicative of acute cholecystitis. This also was the postoperative diagnosis, but the microscopic sections of the gall bladder revealed an early adenocarcinoma, as well as cholelithiasis and acute cholecystitis. If this patient is excluded, the average survival in this group becomes only eleven and one-half months, rather than thirty months.

TABLE II. SURVIVAL PERIODS

GROUP I	GROUP II	GROUP III	GROUP IV*
22 cases	27 cases	8 cases	7 cases
2.3 mo.	3.4 mo.	6.7 mo.	30.5 mo.

*One patient living at present.

The microscopic diagnoses were as follows: adenocarcinoma, 82.7 per cent; squamous carcinoma, 4 per cent; carcinoma (cell type not specified), 13.3 per cent.

Cholelithiasis was found either at operation or at necropsy in fifty-five cases, or 73.3 per cent. In an additional 13 per cent where the disease was inoperable and no necropsy was performed, it is probable that stones were present. The remainder came to autopsy, but in only one case was it specifically stated that no stones were present, no reference to stones having been made in the others. In two cases, with a previous history of cholecystostomy, reformed stones were found and an associated carcinoma. This finding is similar to the experience of Finney and Johnson.[8]

DISCUSSION

With a mortality of 98.5 per cent in less than three years after operation this disease is virtually incurable. Early diagnosis is not an aid, for once the disease manifests itself by the production of symptoms it is already beyond the localized stage. This is well demonstrated in Table II where it is noted that even in eight cases fortuitously discovered by the pathologist, the average life following discovery was only thirty months, and eleven and one-half months if we exclude the only survivor. Radical and palliative procedures add only a few months to the survival period in those patients in whom the disease can be so treated. The over-all survival period following operation in all sixty-five cases is 4.4 months.

If in the light of our present knowledge we are unable to provide adequate active therapy for this disease, it seems imperative to apply preventive measures. Although the exact etiology of carcinoma of the gall bladder is as yet unknown, evidence that cholelithiasis is the most important predisposing factor is too strong to ignore. In the face of convincing statistics and experimental data, we must accept this as the most important precursor of carcinoma. Graham, in a review of statistical studies, found that the incidence of cholelithiasis in carcinoma of the gall bladder ranged from 69 to 100 per cent. Other significant series have shown 70 to 100 per cent,[7] 72.6 per cent,[2] and 80 per cent.[8] Our incidence is at least 73.3 per cent. All figures reported are many times the incidence of gallstones as reported in various necropsy statistics on patients dying from all other causes.[2, 8]

That foreign bodies in the gall bladder are capable of producing carcinoma and other less malignant forms of metaplasia has frequently been shown experimentally. Mohardt quoted the work of Kazama and Leitch, who inserted hard foreign bodies in the gall bladders of guinea pigs, resulting in carcinoma in twenty-six of ninety-eight, and eight of thirty-five animals, respectively. More recently Petrov and Krotkina[6] found five cases of carcinoma resulting from the introduction of foreign bodies into the gall bladders of fifty-one animals. They emphasized that even in these short-lived animals, it took a period of one to two years to obtain these carcinomatous changes.

That the stones are not a result of carcinoma is pointed out by Graham, who stated that in series of metastatic carcinoma of the gall bladder, the incidence of stones is only 8 per cent, well within the usual range of gallstone incidence in all patients. Papillomas of the gall bladder have been suggested as a predisposing factor; Mohardt quoted a series of 500 cases of papilloma of the gall bladder, without a single association of carcinoma in that organ.

If, then, cholelithiasis seems responsible for this malignant transformation, are we justified in performing cholecystectomies on patients with asymptomatic gall stones, as well as on patients with symptoms, because of the possibility of carcinomatous transition? The incidence of carcinoma in calculus gall bladders is variously reported as 3,[2] 5,[8] and 5 to 14[5] per cent. The mortality following cholecystectomy at various institutions compares more favorably. Mortality of 1.6 per cent following cholecystectomy for all patients, including those with jaundice, was reported by the Mayo Clinic.[9] Graham gave a figure of 1.5 per cent. In 1946, at the Mount Sinai Hospital there were 346 cholecystectomies on patients with all the various complications of stones, resulting in the death of two patients, or an over-all mortality of 0.6 per cent. It follows that cholecystectomy is indicated for calculus gall bladder on the grounds that the operative mortality is less than the mortality due to malignant transformation. This, in addition to the other frequently fatal complications of cholelithiasis, constitutes an obligation to remove all calculus gall bladders, in the absence of surgical contraindications. Although there may be such an entity as "silent" gallstones, we have no method of foretelling which will remain as such.

SUMMARY

A report is made of seventy-five patients with carcinoma of the gall bladder, sixty-five of whom were operated upon, with only one survivor (thirteen years) longer than three years. When this disease is diagnosed clinically it is virtually incurable; consequently its occurrence must be prevented. Overwhelming evidence points to gall stones as a predisposing factor in carcinoma of the gall bladder. Since the death incidence of malignant transformation in calculus gall bladders far exceeds the prevailing operative mortality of cholecystectomy, it is indicated to remove even asymptomatic calculus gall bladders on these grounds alone.

REFERENCES

1. Mohardt, J. H.: Internat. Abstr. Surg. **69**: 440-450, 1939.
2. Kirshbaum, J. D., and Kozoll, D. D.: Surg. Gynec. & Obst. **73**: 740-754, 1941.
3. Jankelson, I. R.: New England J. Med. **217**: 85, 1937.
4. Illingworth, C. F. W.: Brit. J. Surg. **23**: 4, 1935.
5. Graham, E. A.: Ann. Surg. **93**: 317-322, 1931.
6. Petrov, N. N., and Krotkina, N. A.: Ann. Surg. **125**: 241-248, 1947.
7. Warren, R., and Balch, F. G., Jr.: SURGERY **7**: 657-665, 1940.
8. Finney, J. M. T., and Johnson, M. L.: Ann. Surg. **121**: 425-435, 1945.
9. Walters, W., Gray, H. K., and Priestley, J. T.: Proc. Staff Meet., Mayo Clin. **16**: 681, 1941.

HEMORRHAGIC INFARCTION OF THE GREATER OMENTUM SIMULATING ACUTE APPENDICITIS

A Report of Two Cases

Franklin I. Harris, M.D., Theodore Diller, M.D., and Sanford A. Marcus, M.D., San Francisco, Calif.

(From the Department of Surgery, Mount Zion Hospital)

FROM time to time reports have appeared in the literature of lesions of the greater omentum, variously classified as primary acute epiploitis,[1] idiopathic segmental infarction,[2] or as infarcts due to primary torsion of a segment of the greater omentum.[3] In all of these there is a common underlying pathology characterized by vascular congestion, hemorrhagic extravasation, usually a thrombus formation, and an inflammatory response of varying degree. Evidence of torsion of the involved portion of the omentum is a relatively frequent but not invariable finding. The clinical and laboratory picture is related most closely to that found in acute appendicitis, and the diagnosis can be made only at surgery.

The etiologic factors have been well discussed by Eliason and Johnson, who reported thirteen cases and reviewed the theoretical possibilities in the causation of this unusual lesion. The opinion of these writers is that the lesion is vascular in nature, resulting either from occlusion of the blood supply due to torsion, or from primary thrombosis or embolism of the omental vessels. A third possibility, bacterial invasion of the omentum by way of the blood stream, is mentioned but is not to be confused with the type of case under discussion.

That the lesion is a primary one of the omentum is shown by the fact that only in extremely few of these cases were there evidences of other systemic or vascular lesions that might cause these changes. In one of the cases reported by Pines and Rabinovitch, for example, there was demonstrated a pre-existing Buerger's disease; Hines[4] reported a case with primary infarction due to thrombosis of the superior mesenteric and splenic veins; and in Berger's case there was cardiac decompensation with arteriosclerosis, hypertension, and syphilis. A case of Totten's[6] presented a definite although compensated aortic insufficiency incident to a pre-existing rheumatic fever.

CASE REPORT

Case 1.—L. S., a 52-year-old white man, was admitted to the hospital with a complaint of pain in the right lower quadrant of seventy-two hours' duration. The pain was described as being dull and intermittent in character, the patient being able to sleep during the remissions. There was no nausea or vomiting, and no bowel changes were noticed. Past medical history was not contributory. The patient had been trying unsuccessfully to lose weight for several weeks.

Physical examination revealed an obese man lying in bed in no great distress. There was a definite tenderness and guarding to deep palpation over the right lower quadrant, but

Received for publication, June 16, 1947.

rebound and psoas tests were negative. In addition there was a harsh blowing systolic murmur heard maximally at the cardiac apex, which was transmitted up the left sternal border to the neck vessels. Temperature on admission was 98.6° F., pulse was 108, respiration was 18, and blood pressure was 160/90. Electrocardiogram showed depression of S-T_2 and S-T_3 with flattening of T_1 and T_2, indicating suggestive evidence of myocardial damage. The urine examination was negative and the blood showed a total white cell count of 8000, with 78 per cent polymorphonuclear cells and 22 per cent lymphocytes. Kline exclusion test was negative. The persistence of the right lower quadrant pain and discomfort for seventy-two hours with moderate guarding and tenderness over McBurney's point despite a fairly normal blood count appeared to justify a diagnosis of acute appendicitis, and operation was recommended.

Through a McBurney approach and under general anesthesia the abdomen was opened. Exposure was extremely difficult because of the large amount of fat present in the body wall and in the omentum. The appendix was exposed and was disappointingly free of gross evidence of inflammation. It was removed in the routine manner and further exploration of the abdomen was undertaken.

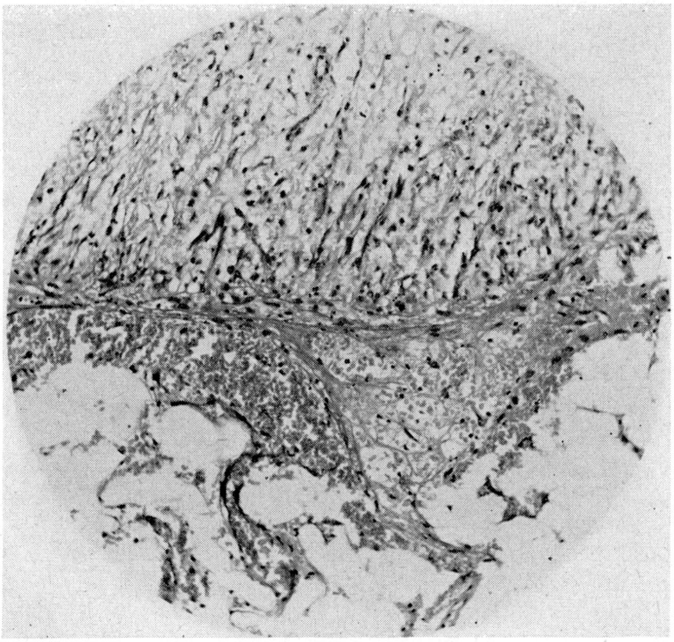

Fig. 1.—Photomicrograph of tissue taken from patient (Case 1). Note the dissolution of the fat and proliferation of fibrous tissue.

Lying immediately superior to McBurney's point and just beneath although not adherent to the parietal peritoneum was a reddish-black segment of the distal greater omentum, measuring approximately 3 by 3 cm. It resembled grossly an area of hemorrhagic necrosis but was unlike any pathologic entity previously seen by the surgeon. It was decided to remove this area of the omentum for histopathologic examination. The remainder of the abdominal exploration being negative, the abdomen was closed.

Microscopically this portion of omentum showed a diffuse acute hemorrhagic process with blood present under the peritoneal surface and extending along the septal fibrous bands. Associated with the red blood cells were groups of polymorphonuclear leucocytes, some of which were undergoing dissolution. In a few places the fat cells were considerably altered with a tendency toward granule formation in the cytoplasm. The septal fibrous bands were somewhat masked by the acute hemorrhagic process and were considerably thickened by the proliferation of connective tissue cells and by edema, in addition to the leucocytes. One sharply demarcated zone showed an avascular organization with young fibroblasts replacing fat cells. No hemosiderin or other evidence of old hemorrhage was present. Throughout the tissue the blood vessels were dilated and congested but there was no evidence of specific vascular disease (see Fig. 1).

CASE 2.—W. S., a 49-year-old white man, entered the hospital with a complaint of abdominal pain for the preceding twenty-four hours. The onset was fairly sudden and the progress of the pain was constant until, at the time of admission, he was in acute distress. The pain was diffuse at first over the entire right side of the abdomen and flank, but localized over the right lower quadrant two or three hours before entry. The pain, although constant, was characterized by spasmodic increases in intensity, at which times the patient was obliged to flex the thighs on the abdomen. There was no nausea or vomiting. Past medical history revealed a ''chronic appendicitis'' ten years previously, the recurrent attacks of which were marked by a dull pain in the right lower quadrant which soon subsided on application of an ice bag.

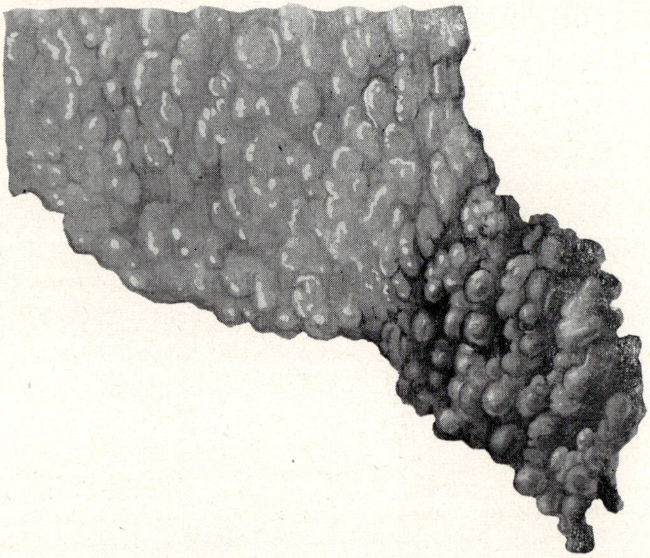

Fig. 2.—Artist's representation of specimen taken in Case 2. Note the sharp line of demarcation between normal and diseased tissue.

Physical examination revealed an obese individual and was negative except for diffuse tenderness and guarding, most marked over the right lower quadrant, with rebound tenderness and skin hyperesthesia elicited in this region. The abdomen was moderately distended and peristalsis was minimal. Temperature on admission was 100.4° F., pulse was 110, and respirations 25. The urine was negative; the blood showed a total white cell count of 5300 with 64 per cent poymorphonuclear leucocytes and 36 per cent lymphocytes. Kline exclusion test was negative. A diagnosis of acute appendicitis was made

Under spinal anesthesia the appendix was approached through a McBurney incision. Lying immediately beneath the parietal peritoneum and delivering into the operative field as this was opened was an irregularly ovoid, hemorrhagic mass measuring about 2.5 by 3 cm. (see Fig. 2). This was seen to be an appendage of the greater omentum, from the normal tissue of which it was sharply demarcated. This hemorrhagic tissue, as well as a moderately fibrotic appendix, was excised; the abdomen was closed in layers and the postoperative course was uneventful.

Microscopic examination of the tissue showed an acute diffuse interstitial hemorrhagic process with small groups of red blood cells arranged in clusters or cords between isolated fat cells. There was a superficial focal accumulation of leucocytes and fibrin among the red cells along the peritoneal aspect of the fat. All the vessels were dilated and congested, but showed no specific alteration.

Both cases simulated acute appendicitis clinically although admittedly the white blood count was low, remaining well below the average of 12,000 found in the six cases reported by Pines and Rabinovitch. In both cases tenderness and rigidity were present, nausea and vomiting were absent, fever was slight. These observations are not out of harmony with the results of the aforementioned workers or with those of Eliason and Johnson. At operation the appendix was not involved in either case, but the clinical picture is explained by the pathologic findings in the greater omentum; this also coincides with the experience of previous writers.

It can be seen from a comparison of the two cases that the pathologic process in the first instance has advanced far beyond that noted in the second, and this is borne out by the clinical history. Evidence of advanced necrosis, as described by Pines and Rabinovitch, is lacking but we believe this to be due to the recent occurrence of the hemorrhage. In neither of the cases was thrombosis a causative factor or a consequence of the production of the lesion. In neither case was there torsion of the involved omental segment, nor was there evidence that this had occurred earlier with subsequent restitution of the twisted segment.

It is interesting to observe that both patients were of a hypersthenic body habitus, and both had abdominal walls and greater omenta that were heavily laden with fat.

The absence in both cases of evidence of torsion and the inability to point out evidence of specific vascular lesions immediately raise the question of the etiologic factors involved. The presence of presumptive evidence of cardiac damage in Case 1, as shown by the electrocardiogram, could not be explained on a basis other than the mild hypertension, and the patient was well compensated. Vascular sclerosis, as indicated by eye-ground changes, was minimal; arterial emboli were unlikely on the basis of the consistently regular cardiac rhythm, by the absence of other evidence of embolic phenomena, and by the nature of the pathologic process in the infarcted area itself.

The lesion, therefore, must be regarded as a localized process. Experiments performed on animals by Pines and Rabinovitch indicate that a sudden pull along the axis of a vessel can lead to damage of the intima and production of a thrombus closely related in type to those observed in their cases. However, it is pointed out that in neither of our cases was there evidence of thrombus formation, any infarct formation being due, apparently, to the primary hemorrhage.

Totten hypothecated a state where the thin-walled omental vessels, engorged following a meal, are subjected to an unusual force incident to straining, sneezing, and so forth, which is sufficient to rupture a vessel and cause hemorrhage with the sequence of pathologic changes just enumerated. Indeed, our two cases resemble most closely (from a pathologic standpoint) the second of the two cases reported by him. Neither of our patients, however, offered any history of previous violence or straining, such as was recorded in the case of Totten.

It is believed by us that an extremely fatty omentum, as was seen in both our cases by increasing the gravitational pull acting on the omental vessels may act in conjunction with the factors mentioned to cause rupture of a vessel.

CONCLUSIONS AND SUMMARY

1. Two cases of primary hemorrhagic infarction of a segment of the greater omentum are presented, together with a discussion of the pathologic changes found in each case.

2. Possible factors in the causation of this lesion are reviewed.

3. The inability to differentiate this condition from the clinical manifestations of acute appendicitis or other intra-abdominal conditions is emphasized.

4. It is believed by us that the correct diagnosis may be suspected if consideration is given to the fact that the syndrome occurs more commonly in hypersthenic, obese individuals.

REFERENCES

1. Eliason, E. L., and Johnson, J.: Primary Acute Epiploitis, SURGERY **6**: 68-73, 1939.
2. Pines, B., and Rabinovitch, J.: Idiopathic Segmental Infarction of the Greater Omentum, Surg., Gynec. & Obst. **71**: 80-85, 1940.
3. Barsky, E. K., and Schwartz, A. M.: Primary Omental Torsion. Review of the Literature and Report of Two Cases, Am. J. Surg. **38**: 356-363, 1937.
4. Hines, L. E.: Hemorrhagic Infarction of the Greater Omentum, Illinois M. J. **66**: 166-167, 1934.
5. Berger, A. R.: Hemorrhagic Infarction of the Greater Omentum, Arch. Surg. **36**: 497-499, 1938.
6. Totten, H. P.: Primary Idiopathic Segmental Infarction of the Greater Omentum, Am. J. Surg. **56**: 676-679, 1942.

A COMPARATIVE STUDY OF THE ACTION OF DEMEROL AND OPIUM ALKALOIDS IN RELATION TO BILIARY SPASM

EDWARD A. GAENSLER, M.D., JOHN M. McGOWAN, M.D., M.S. (SURGERY), AND FRANCIS F. HENDERSON, M.D., BOSTON, MASS.

(From Dr. Henderson's Laboratory, Fourth Surgical Service, Boston City Hospital, and Tufts Medical School)

THE chemical structure of demerol* was originally designed to resemble that of atropine and papaverine combined.[1] This was done in order to combine the neurotropic action of the atropine and the musculotropic action of papaverine in the hope that a double acting smooth muscle relaxing drug would result. Animal experimentation soon demonstrated its unexpected analgesic properties as well. Further investigation revealed that the opium alkaloids were shown to be related chemically to demerol.[2] The central analgesic action of demerol has since been well established, and it is because of this property that it finds its greatest use today. It has found a place in the clinician's armamentarium where analgesia approaching that of morphine is desired without the undesirable side effects of the latter, such as respiratory depression, constipating action, urinary retention, and depression of cough reflexes. This is most notably true in obstetrics, in pre- and postoperative care, particularly in the face of pulmonary pathology, and in poor-risk or elderly patients. The original findings of its nonaddicting properties have not been substantiated. Tolerance, physical dependence, and habituation have been shown to develop with its prolonged use.[3-10]

It is our purpose in this paper to attempt an evaluation of the spasmolytic properties of demerol with particular reference to the biliary tract and to the second portion of the duodenum.

REVIEW OF THE LITERATURE

The spasmolytic action of this drug was first demonstrated in animals by Eisleb and Schaumann.[1, 2] Strips of large intestine of the guinea pig which had been made spastic by such substances as acetylcholine, barium chloride, or histamine were promptly relaxed by demerol. It was noted, however, that the effect was variable in different sections of the intestine. Furthermore, the drug's action on quiescent segments was not tested, or at least not reported. Gruber, Hart, and Gruber[11] after extensive investigation on the pharmacologic action of demerol in this country confirmed the antagonism to spasm from histamine, barium chloride, or acetylcholine. They demonstrated, however, that in the intact intestine in dogs, as well as in isolated duodenal and ileal strips of cats and rabbits, the drug regularly increased tonus and peristalsis and decreased the organ's volume at the same time. The latter action they attributed also to smooth muscle spasm. Furthermore, they showed that demerol has no relaxing

Received for publication, May 19, 1947.

*1-Methyl 4-phenyl piperidine 4-carboxylic acid ethyl ester hydrochloride, also known in various countries and at various times as Eucolat, Dolantol, Dolantin, Pethidine, and meperidine hydrochloride.

effect on bowel made spastic with morphine. The former finding was amply confirmed by Yonkman and his co-workers,[12] but they claimed that demerol relaxed the spasm produced by morphine in the intestine. This was also confirmed by Dryer.[13] Barlow[14] found antagonism to histamine, barium chloride, and, in addition, to pilocarpine and physostigmine. He, however, found a spasmolytic effect on quiescent ileal strips of rabbits. Observations made in Great Britain by Duguid and Heathcote[15] showed the drug to be one-half as effective as papaverine in reducing amplitude of contraction of an isolated gut segment. On the acetylcholine activated intestine, they found atropine to have 500 times as much relaxing quality as demerol. As the drug was also found to slow respirations, depress the blood pressure, and decrease the amplitude of heart beat, they concluded that demerol is a depressant to all forms of muscular tissue. Batterman and Himmelsbach[8] summarized these results of animal investigation and pointed to the variable and conflicting results of the effect of demerol not only on smooth muscle of the intestinal tract, but on that of other organs as well, such as the uterus.

In man there have been but few studies to substantiate the expected relaxing effect on the intestinal and urinary tracts, which is the basis of its use in biliary, intestinal, and renal colic. Decrease in tonus and decrease in amplitude of contraction with use of demerol on the human ureter has been demonstrated in one study.[16] Investigations of the gastrointestinal tract have been confined to balloon recordings either by intubation or through incidental fistulas. Batterman[17] reported an antispasmodic effect in 84 per cent of twenty-seven human subjects studied. His records, however, showed a decrease in motility rather than in tone. This is in contrast to his clinical experience in which he found the drug nonconstipating. The decrease in motility was most marked in the stomach and pylorus and slight in the ileum and colon. There was no report of studies on the duodenum in his paper. His results have been confirmed by other investigators.[13, 14] Yonkman[18] found that the drug did not decrease tone but decreased large intestinal contractions. He could not, with demerol, prevent the tonic action of morphine. No studies on the biliary tract have been reported.

Clinically, the use of demerol in pain due to spasm of smooth muscle of intestinal, biliary, and renal colic has been advocated on the basis of the experimental results described, or with an eye to its chemical structure and intended effects. Frequent final recourse to morphine for this type of pain is admitted by some authors.[19] Others recommend demerol as the drug of choice for this type of pain and mention excellent and even dramatic results with its use, but no detailed statistics are given.[8, 17, 20, 21] Noth and his co-workers[7] reported relief in only three of five cases of biliary colic.

We have undertaken a study of demerol and its pharmacodynamic action on the biliary tract and second portion of the duodenum for several reasons: (1) We have not been able to confirm the clinical results of others of dramatic relief with demerol in biliary colic; (2) it has been our impression for some time that demerol has no beneficial spasmolytic action on the biliary tract and that the relief, if any, is due to its central analgesic action; and (3) previous experimental work has appeared inconclusive to us. Further, the spasmolytic action of demerol is attributed to its atropine-like and papaverine-like structure. Both these drugs have been shown by Butsch, Walters, and one of us (J. M. M.)[22] to be ineffective in biliary spasm.

METHOD

In a previous publication Butsch, Walters, and one of us (J. M. M.)[23] has described a method of measuring pressure in the common bile duct of man. Measurement of pressure changes was found to be an excellent method of studying changes in the tone of the musculature of the second portion of the duodenum.[24] It was found that spasm of the muscle of the second portion of the duodenum occluded the lower end of the common bile duct with a sphincter-like action. It was concluded that while the sphincter of Oddi may exist as a separate entity its function is physiologically synchronous with that of musculature of the second portion of the duodenal wall. For this reason the term, duodenal spasm, refers to spasm of the sphincter mechanism of the biliary tract (sphincter of Oddi). It was found that spasm of the second portion of the duodenum was produced by codeine, dilaudid, pantopon, and morphine. This spasm produced enough back pressure in the biliary tract, in some cases, to produce an attack of biliary colic. The nitrite drugs, aminophylline and epinephrine, were found to relax this spasm, while papaverine and atropine were without effect. This same method of pressure studies has been found useful in determining the optimum time for removal of the T tube.[25-27]

Pressure studies made include (1) resting intrabiliary pressure, (2) perfusion pain level, and (3) pressure changes resulting from the action of various drugs. Ten postoperative patients with T-tube biliary drainage were studied. Pressure studies were made under various conditions in order to compare the action of demerol with opium alkaloids on the sphincter mechanism at the lower end of the common bile duct. These patients had been subjected to an exploration of the common bile duct for such varied pathology as cholelithiasis with "gravel," dilation of the common duct, common duct stone, history of jaundice, pancreatic fibrosis, and chronic pancreatitis. It is to be noted that in five of these ten patients common duct stones were found at operation.

The pressure apparatus used was similar to the one previously described.[23] Briefly it consisted of a water manometer with a thinly blown glass bulb as float. An aluminum extension and writing arm was attached to this float and arranged to record the pressure in millimeters of water on a slowly revolving smoked drum. The manometer was connected to the T tube emerging from the abdominal wall and to a bottle of sterile physiologic saline solution used to fill the system. A marker was used on all kymographic recordings. The base line was adjusted to correspond to the level of the xiphoid process of the patient, which was considered the zero level. The patient's resting intrabiliary pressure was recorded on the drum for about one-half hour before any drug was given. Three deep inhalations of amyl nitrite were then given to determine the presence or absence of initial spasm.[25] Following this the various drugs under investigation were administered. This procedure was carried out on the patient for the first time two weeks postoperatively and repeated until the biliary dynamics returned to normal.[26, 27] Weekly cholangiograms (using diodrast) were made in order to detect any missing stone and to follow the progress of any obstructing lesion such as ampulla edema, spasm, or pancreatitis, and to study the effect of the various drugs.

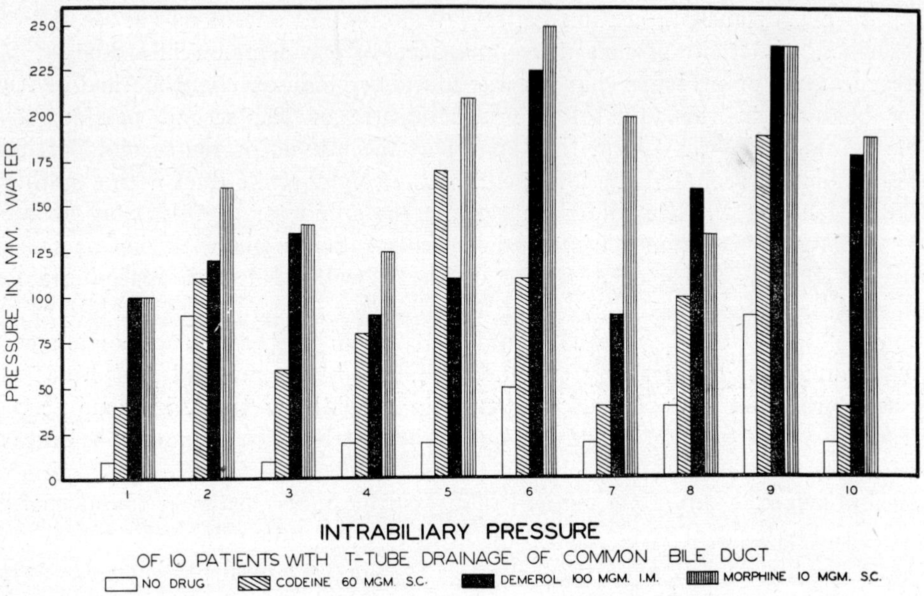

Fig. 1.—Comparison of the spasmogenic action of codeine, demerol, and morphine on the sphincter mechanism of the common bile duct as measured by changes in the intrabiliary pressure in man.

RESULTS

Demerol was found to produce spasm of the sphincter mechanism of the common bile duct (duodenal wall). The resultant spasm, as evidenced by a rise in intrabiliary pressure, was found to begin within five minutes after administration of 100 mg. of the drug intramuscularly. Pressure then rose

TABLE I

PATIENT	RESTING INTRA-BILIARY PRESSURE	PEAK READING WITH CODEINE (60 MG. S.C.)	PEAK READING WITH DEMEROL (100 MG. I.M.)	PEAK READING WITH MORPHINE (10 MG. S.C.)
1	10*	40*	100*	100*
2	90	110	120	160
3	10	60	135	140
4	20	80	90	125
5	20	170	110	210
6	50	110	225	250
7	20	40	90	200
8	40	100	160	135
9	90	190	240	240
10	20	40	170	190
Mean value		94	144	175

Note: These figures represent peak values in millimeters of water taken from kymographic tracings. They were taken from numerous records selected for comparison.

quickly to a peak usually reached at the end of twenty minutes. Some spastic effect was found to last for as long as 1½ to 2 hours (Figs. 2 and 3). The intensity of the spasm was intermediate between that of codeine and that produced

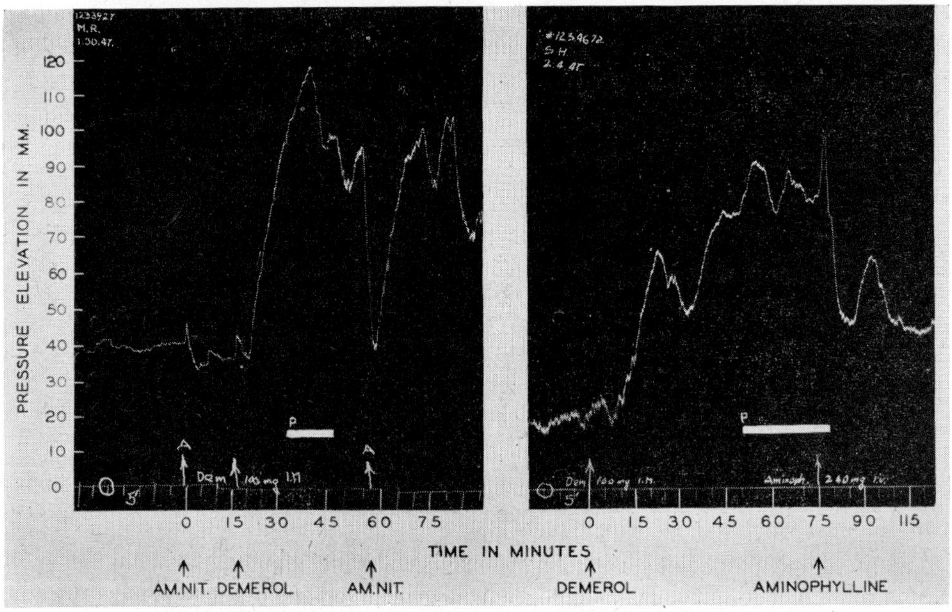

Fig. 2.—Kymograph tracings showing pressure changes associated with two instances of biliary colic produced in different patients by the administration of 100 mg. of demerol intramuscularly. Relief in the first case was obtained with inhalations of amyl nitrite and in the second with 240 mg. of theophylline with ethylenediamine (aminophylline) given intravenously. *P*, pain. The base line or zero level in this and succeeding illustrations is at the level of the xiphoid with the patient in the prone position.

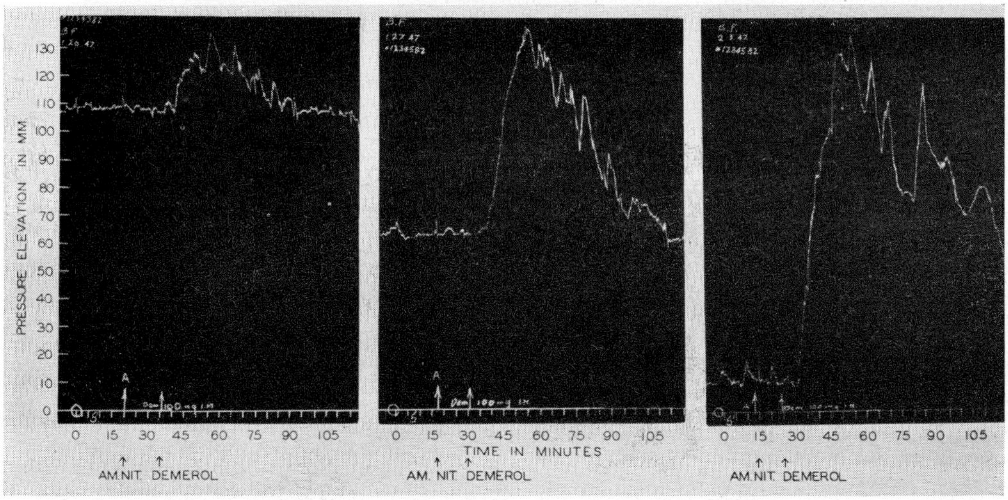

Fig. 3.—Three tracings taken two, three, and four weeks postoperatively in the same patient. No pressure reduction to amyl nitrite initially indicates edema rather than spasm as the cause of the elevated resting pressure. Here edema decreased gradually postoperatively as noted in each succeeding graph. Demerol produced the same peak elevation from a variable resting level.

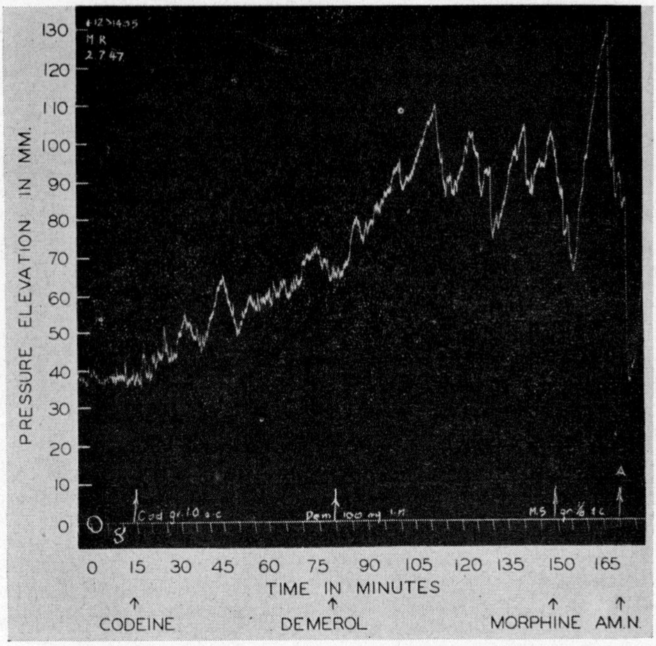

Fig. 4.—Codeine, demerol, and morphine administered consecutively in the same patient, illustrating the spasmogenic properties of these drugs in the order named. Relief of spasm by amyl nitrite occurred at the end.

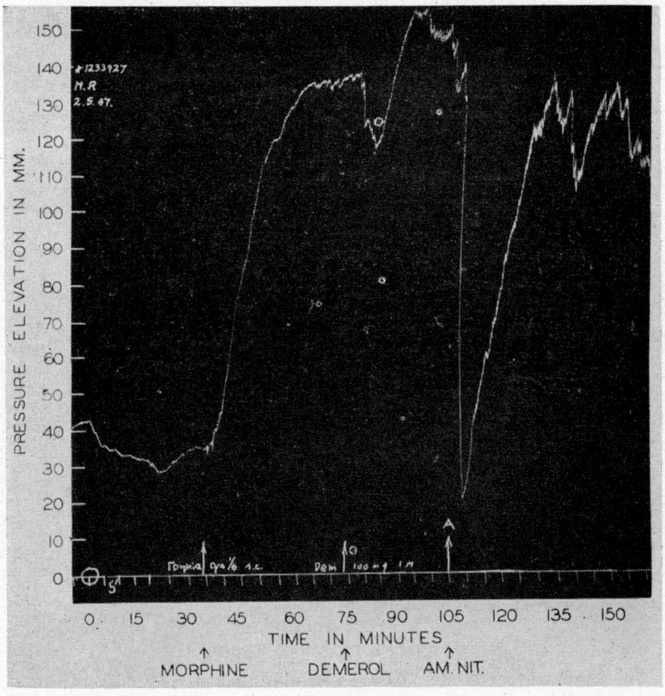

Fig. 5.—Demonstration of the inability of demerol to relieve morphine-induced spasm. In this particular patient demerol produced more spasm than did morphine. Relief was obtained with amyl nitrite.

by morphine (Figs. 1 and 4).[22] Generally the intensity of spasm approached that of morphine. Table I illustrates this point. The average intrabiliary pressure elevations, above normal, recorded in millimeters of water for the three drugs studied, are as follows: codeine, 94; demerol, 144; morphine, 175. In one instance demerol was even more spasmogenic than morphine (Figs. 1 and 5).

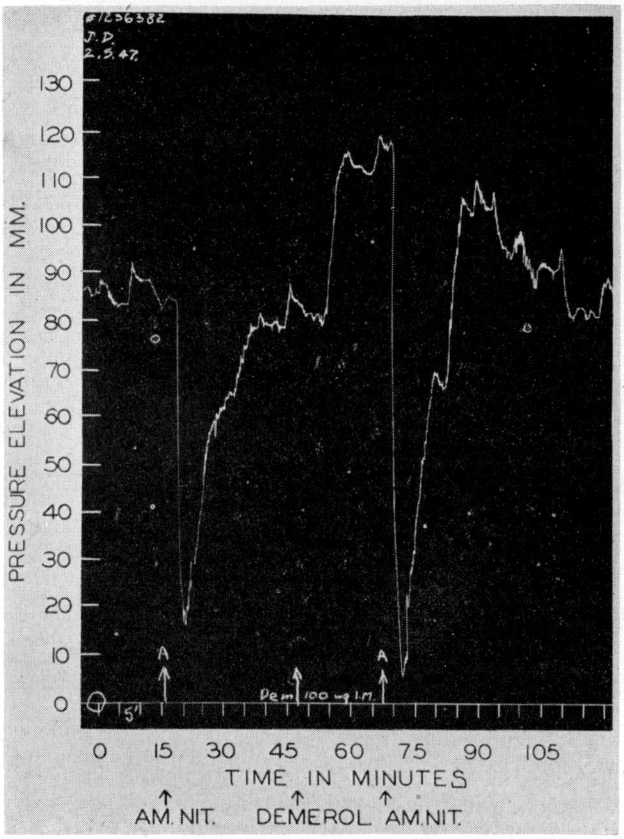

Fig. 6.—Example of natural duodenal spasm (not drug) relieved by amyl nitrite and increased rather than relieved by demerol.

When the drugs were given consecutively to the same patient, the spasmogenic effect of the second drug was found to be superimposed on that of the first (Figs. 4 and 5). In some cases pressure elevation was present from edema of the ampulla of Vater. Such a pressure elevation naturally does not decrease with amyl nitrite (Fig. 3). The ampulla edema gradually decreased with continued T-tube biliary drainage. Fig. 3 shows that the degree of edema does not effect the pressure elevation due to demerol. As the edema and resting pressure level decreased with T-tube drainage, the height of pressure elevation from demerol remained the same. This means that a patient with biliary colic from back pressure as a result of obstruction due to a stone or edema is not, so far as biliary dynamics are concerned, made worse by demerol. In other words, if a patient with biliary colic is given amyl nitrite and no relief is obtained, one may then assume that the back pressure is due to some cause other than spasm and may administer demerol or an opiate derivative for relief of pain and know that the biliary dynamics will not be further disturbed.

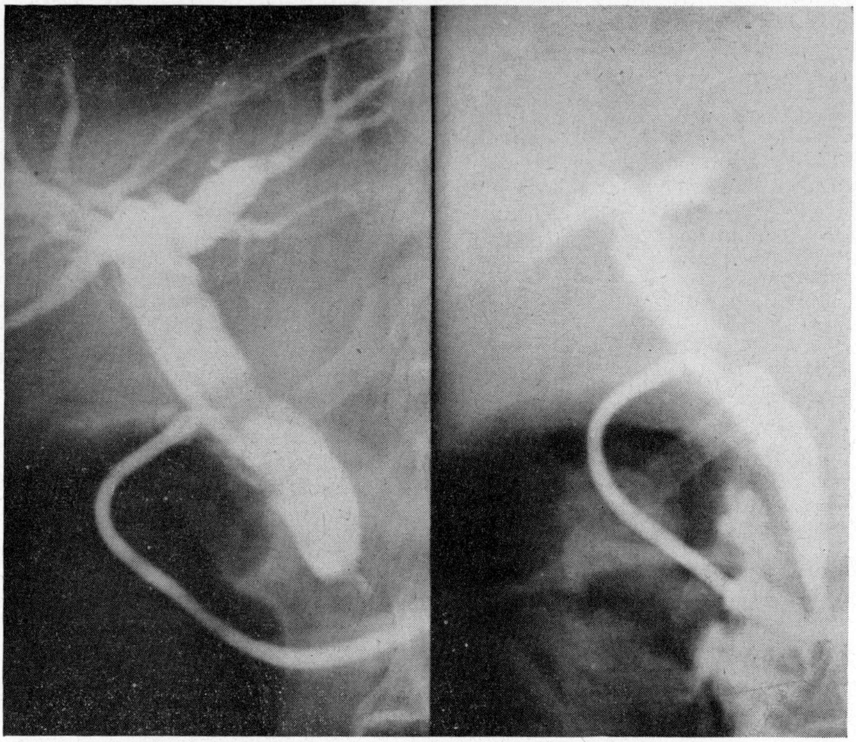

Fig. 7.—*A*, Cholangiograms of the same patient as illustrated in Fig. 6. There is marked spasm at the lower end of the common bile duct with dilatation above (hydrohepatosis). No diodrast reached the duodenum. *B*, The second plate was taken one minute following inhalation of amyl nitrite. The sphincter has relaxed and contrast media is flowing freely in to the duodenum.

Demerol, hence, was found regularly to increase the spasm already produced by a previous dose of codeine (Fig. 4). Demerol given after morphine was found not to relieve the spasm (Fig. 5). The spasm produced by demerol was regularly but only briefly relieved by either inhalations of amyl nitrite or intravenous injection of theophylline with ethylenediamine (aminophylline) (Figs. 2, 4, 5, 6).

Two patients experienced a typical attack of biliary colic with nausea and cramping right upper quadrant pain following administration of demerol about two weeks postoperatively. These attacks were relieved by amyl nitrite inhalation in one case and by aminophylline intravenously in the other (Fig. 2).

In addition to its failure to relax morphine spasm, demerol was found to be ineffective against natural spasm. On the contrary, it further increases this spasm (Fig. 6). Cholangiograms taken five to thirty minutes after intramuscular administration of 100 mg. of demerol repeatedly demonstrated these spasmogenic qualities of the drug. Relief with amyl nitrite was well visualized (Fig. 5). The pain threshold as determined by perfusion pain levels was regularly raised by demerol, its action in this respect being intermediate between that of morphine and that of codeine. In other words, it does not produce as much spasm as morphine but it does not relieve pain quite as well, either. The only side effects noted with administration of demerol intramuscularly were perspiration and slight dizziness. These were found in 100 per cent of the subjects studied.

CONCLUSION

Demerol is not the answer to the quest for an ideal spasmolytic analgesic agent for use in biliary colic and postoperative biliary pain. If biliary colic is due to spasm, nitroglycerin, gr. 1/250,[25] in doses of one to two granules under the tongue will relieve the attack. This should be tried first in such instances. If the pain is due to biliary obstruction other than spasm, no relief will be afforded by the nitrites and there will not be harmful aggravation of the local pathology by the administration of spasmogenic analgesic. In such an instance, morphine or demerol may be given for the relief of this severe type of pain. For postoperative use demerol is not contraindicated if relief of pain cannot be obtained by the nitrite drugs. It does not elevate the pressure above the secretion pressure of the liver (300 ml. as had been shown in the case of morphine[23] and, therefore, will not tend to produce jaundice. If following cholecystectomy, biliary fistula is feared or is present, demerol should be used with as much caution as any drug which raises intrabiliary pressure.

SUMMARY

1. Contrary to common belief, demerol has been shown to be a spasmogenic rather than a spasmolytic agent on the sphincter mechanism at the lower end of the common bile duct (Oddi) in ten unselected patients with T-tube drainage of the common duct.

2. The spasm produced was intermediate in intensity between that produced by codein and that of morphine; it was sufficiently severe in two cases to produce a typical attack of biliary colic.

3. Demerol was shown to increase rather than relieve natural spasm as well as spasm produced by codeine.

4. The effect produced by demerol was regularly but briefly relieved by amyl nitrite or theophylline with ethylenediamine (aminophylline).

5. Demerol should be used with as much caution as the opiates in postcholecystectomy pain.

REFERENCES

1. Eisleb, O., and Schaumann, O.: Dolantin, ein Neuartiges Spasmolytikum und Analgetikum, Deutsche med. Wchnschr. **65**: 967-968, 1939.
2. Schaumann, O.: Ueber eine neue Klasse von Verbindungen mit Spasmolytischer und Zentral Analgetischer Wirksamkeit unter Besonderer Beruecksichtigung des 1-Methyl-4-Phenyl-Piperidine-4-Carbonsaeure-Ethylaesters (Donlantin), Arch. f. exper. Path. u. Pharmakol. **196**: 109-136, 1940.
3. Andrews, H. L.: The Development of Tolerance to Dermerol, J. Pharmacol. & Exper. Therap. **75**: 338-341, 1942.

4. Kucher, I.: Zwei Faelle von Dolantinsucht, Klin. Wchnschr. **19**: 688-689, 1942.
5. Von Bruecke, S.: Ueber Dolantinabusus und einen Fall von Dolantindelir, Wien. klin. Wchnschr. **53**: 854, 1940.
6. Himmelsbach, C. K.: Studies on the Addiction Liability of "Demerol" (D-140), J. Pharmacol. & Exper. Therap. **75**: 64-68, 1942; Further Studies on the Addiction Liability of Demerol, ibid. **79**: 5-9, 1943.
7. Noth, P. H., Hecht, H. H., and Yonkman, F. F.: Demerol: A New Synthetic Analgesic, Spasmolytic and Sedative Agent; II Clinical Observations, Ann. Int. Med. **21**: 17-34, 1944.
8. Batterman, R. C., and Himmelsbach, C. K.: Demerol—New Synthetic Analgesic; Review of Its Present Status and Comparison With Morphine, J. A. M. A. **122**: 222-226, 1943.
9. Anslinger, H. J.: Demerol, Correspondence, J. A. M. A. **132**: 43-44, 1946.
10. Wieder, H.: Addiction to Meperidine Hydrochloride (Demerol Hydrochloride), J. A. M. A. **132**: 1066-1068, 1946.
11. Gruber, C. M., Hart, E. R., and Gruber, C. M., Jr.: The Pharmacology and Toxicology of the Ethyl Ester of 1-Methyl-4-Phenyl-Piperidine-4-Carboxylic Acid (Demerol), J. Pharmacol. & Exper. Therap. **73**: 319-333, 1941.
12. Yonkman, F. F., Noth, P. H., and Hecht, H. H.: Demerol: New Synthetic Analgetic, Spasmolytic and Sedative Agent; Pharmacologic Studies, Ann. Int. Med. **21**: 7-16, 1944.
13. Dryer: Personal Communication as quoted by Batterman and Himmelsbach.[8]
14. Barlow, O. W.: Studies on the Pharmacology of 1-Methyl-4-Phenylpiperidin-4 Carbonic Acid Ethylester (D-140, Demerol): II. Pharmacology, Toxicology and Addiction Liability (to be published). As quoted by Batterman and Himmelsbach.[8]
15. Duguid, A. M. E., and Heathcote, R. St. A.: Pharmacological Action of Ethylmethylphenylpiperidine Carboxylate, Quart. J. Pharm. & Pharmacol. **13**: 318-331, 1940.
16. Climenko, D. R., and Berg, H.: The Influence of Demerol on the Contractions of the Ureters, J. Urol. **49**: 255-258, 1943.
17. Batterman, R. C.: Clinical Effectiveness and Safety of a New Synthetic Analgesic Drug, Demerol, Arch. Int. Med. **71**: 345-356, 1943.
18. Yonkman, F. F.: The Actions of Demerol and Morphine on the Gastro-Intestinal Musculature, Anesth. & Analg. **23**: 207-210, 1944.
19. Hoffman, R.: Demerol, A New Departure in Analgesia: An Evaluation of Present Therapeutic Claims, Anesth. & Analg. **22**: 336-340, 1943.
20. Batterman, F. C.: Demerol: A New Synthetic Analgesic: Its Indications as a Substitute for Morphine, Connecticut M. J. **8**: 13-17, 1944.
21. Curry, J. J.: Clinical Appraisal of Demerol, Benadryl and Pyribenzamine, M. Clin. North America **30**: 1138-1146, 1946.
22. Butsch, W. L., McGowan, J. M., and Walters, W.: Clinical Study of Certain Drugs in Relation to Biliary Pain and to Variation in Intrabiliary Pressure, Surg., Gynec. & Obst. **63**: 451-456, 1936.
23. McGowan, John M., Butsch, Winfield, and Walters, Waltman: Pressure in the Common Bile Duct of Man: Its Relation to Pain Following Cholecystectomy, J. A. M. A. **106**: 2227-2230, 1936.
24. McGowan, John M., Knepper, Paul, Walters, Waltman, and Snell, Albert: Relation of Spasm of the Second Portion of the Duodenum to Biliary Colic, Surg., Gynec. & Obst. **66**: 979-987, 1938.
25. McGowan, John M., and Henderson, Francis: Prevention and Management of Pain Following Cholecystectomy, New England J. Med. **222**: 948-953, 1940.
26. McGowan, John M.: Dynamics of Biliary Drainage: Its Relation to Cholangitis and Pancreatitis From Stricture of the Ampulla of Vater, SURGERY **18**: 470-478, 1945.
27. McGowan, John M., Keeley, J. K., and Henderson, Francis F.: Pathological Physiology of Biliary Drainage: The Description of the Use of a New Type of T-tube and the Criteria for Its Removal, Surg., Gynec. & Obst. **84**: 174-180, 1947.

SURGICAL MANAGEMENT OF ACQUIRED STRICTURE OF THE ESOPHAGUS WITH ESOPHAGOBRONCHIAL FISTULA AND BRONCHIECTASIS OF ENTIRE RIGHT LUNG

REPORT OF CASE

O. THERON CLAGETT, M.D.,* AND HERBERT W. SCHMIDT, M.D.†
ROCHESTER, MINN.

BRONCHIECTASIS involving an entire lung does not occur frequently although it is not a rare condition. Strictures of the esophagus occurring as a result of ingestion of lye are, unfortunately, rather common. Acquired fistulas between the esophagus and the major bronchi or trachea are unusual. The occurrence of all three of these conditions in the same patient is certainly remarkable and presents formidable problems in regard to management. A report of such a case in which surgical management was successful appears warranted.

REPORT OF CASE

A white man, 25 years of age, registered at the Mayo Clinic on Aug. 24, 1946. At 2 years of age he had accidentally swallowed lye, and a stricture of the esophagus had developed. This had been treated with repeated esophageal dilatations and the patient had been able to take a fairly normal diet. At the age of 12 years he had pneumonia. The periodic esophageal dilatations were not performed during this illness and the esophagus became completely closed. Gastrostomy had been performed and all food and liquid had been given by this route for the thirteen years previous to admission to the clinic. Since the age of 2 years, when the patient had swallowed lye, he had been troubled with a mild, chronic cough productive of some mucopurulent material. After the patient had pneumonia at the age of 12 years, the cough became much worse. Three to four ounces (90 to 120 c.c.) of thick, purulent, blood-streaked sputum were raised daily. The patient had never been able to work. Clubbing of the fingers had developed after the pneumonia. Recently there had been rather severe hemoptysis. The patient had noted that if the feedings given through the gastric stoma were too thin or if they were too large he would cough up some of the food that had been administered. A diagnosis of bronchiectasis of the right lung and of a fistula between the right bronchus and esophagus had been made elsewhere.

On physical examination the patient was observed to be a tall, very thin, white man, weighing only 110 pounds (49.9 kilograms). There was no expansion of the right side of the chest, and the interspaces were narrowed. The right side of the chest was dull to percussion. Numerous coarse râles were heard on auscultation. There was marked clubbing of the fingers and toes. A gastric stoma, with tube in place, was noted in the left upper part of the abdomen. Physical examination was not remarkable otherwise.

The concentration of the hemoglobin was 14.2 Gm. per 100 c.c. of blood. The leucocyte count was 14,600 per cubic millimeter of blood with a normal distribution. The sedimentation rate was 32 mm. in one hour (Westergren method). Examinations of sputum for acid-fast bacilli gave negative results. Roentgenograms of the chest revealed an extensive suppurative process involving the entire right lung (Fig. 1). Bronchographic studies demonstrated diffuse saccular bronchiectasis of the right lung. There was a small area of cylindric bronchiectasis in the left base. An attempt was made to examine the upper part of the esophagus with

Received for publication, May 26, 1947.
*Division of Surgery, Mayo Clinic.
†Division of Medicine, Mayo Clinic.

radiopaque oil, but it was impossible for the patient to swallow enough oil to permit demonstration of anything. Apparently the upper part of the esophagus was completely closed. Barium was injected into the stomach through the gastric stoma, and the lower part of the esophagus was visualized satisfactorily. A fistula from the esophagus to the right bronchus was demonstrated.

Esophagoscopy was attempted. There was scarring at the level of the cricoid cartilage. About 3 cm. below the cricopharyngeus muscle the esophagus narrowed to a tiny slit and it was impossible to pass the esophagoscope beyond that point. Bronchoscopy was then performed. A large amount of pus was seen coming from the right lung. There was considerable inflammatory reaction in the right main bronchus. The fistulous communication with the esophagus could not be visualized. Subsequently esophagoscopy was again performed and attempts were made to pass filiform bougies through the strictured esophagus, but without success. A cystoscope was inserted into the stomach through the gastric stoma and attempts were made to pass ureteral catheters up the esophagus. Complete obstruction was met about 8 to 10 cm. above the cardia.

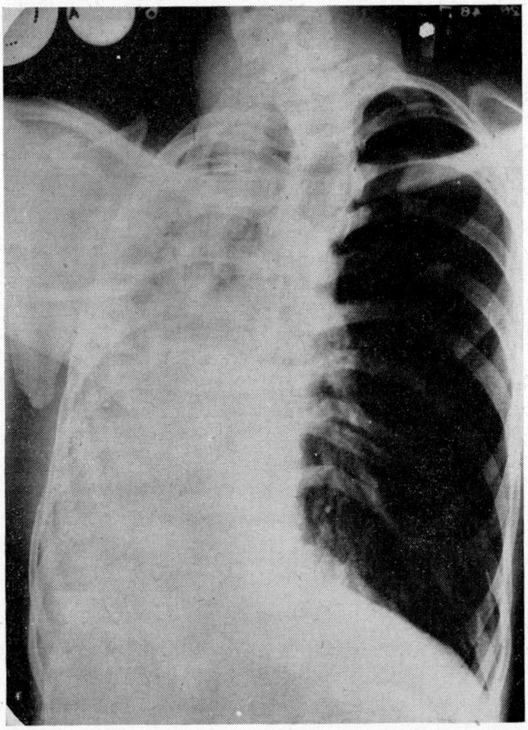

Fig. 1.—Extensive suppurative process throughout the entire right lung before operation.

All attempts to open the esophagus having failed, it was decided that the patient should undergo surgical exploration. After thorough preparation, including administration of penicillin, operation was performed on Oct. 10, 1946. A long, curved incision was made around the tip of the scapula on the right. The fifth rib was resected and the pleura opened. The lung was densely adherent to the parietal pleura over its entire surface and was mobilized with some difficulty. In some places it was necessary to carry out the dissection along an extrapleural line of cleavage. The hilar dissection was difficult, but each vessel was dissected out individually, doubly ligated, and sectioned. The posterior surface of the right main bronchus was densely adherent to the esophagus. The esophagus was so scarred that it was impossible to establish definitely the location of the fistula. The bronchus was severed, the lung removed, and the stump of bronchus closed with a single row of interrupted silk sutures.

Below the level of the bronchus the esophagus appeared normal externally, but when its lumen was opened several short strictured portions were observed; a ureteral catheter could be passed into the stomach, however. A cystoscope was inserted through the gastric stoma, and the end of the ureteral catheter was picked up and brought out of the stomach through the gastric stoma. The esophagus above the bronchus was so scarred and fibrotic that it could hardly be recognized. A lumen was found finally and a ureteral catheter passed up toward the mouth. An esophagoscope was inserted, and this catheter was picked up and brought out through the mouth. A strong silk fishline suture was attached to the ureteral catheter and one end was drawn out through the mouth, the other out through the gastric stoma. Attempt was then made to repair the esophagus as well as possible, with pleura being used to cover the defects. The bronchial stump was also covered with pleura. The operation required about four and one-half hours. The patient was given 2,500 c.c. of blood during the operation.

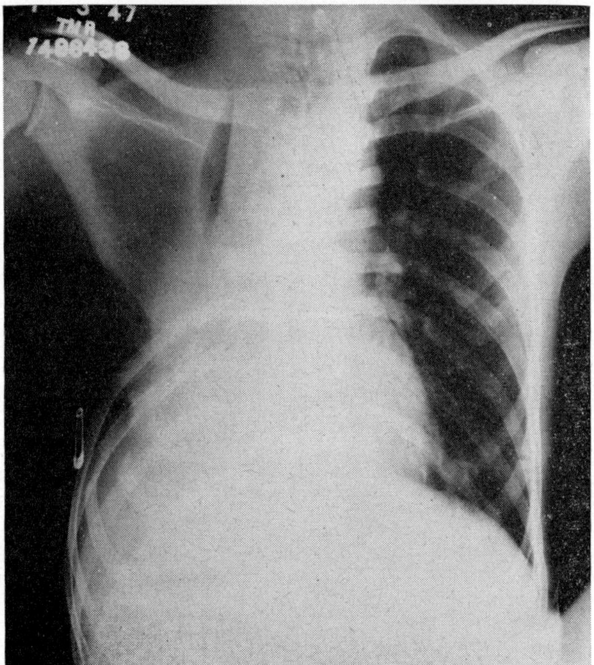

Fig. 2.—Appearance after pneumonectomy and thoracoplasty on the right.

Bronchoscopy was performed at the conclusion of the operation. A large amount of thick, mucopurulent material was aspirated from the trachea and the left bronchus. The patient was taken from the operating room in good condition. The immediate postoperative course was satisfactory, and the highest temperature was 102° F. On the seventh postoperative day evidence of considerable pneumothorax on the right developed. It was thought likely that the esophagus was leaking. There was no evidence of any leakage from the bronchial stump. It had been anticipated that such a leak might occur and cause empyema. On Oct. 19, 1946, with the patient under local anesthesia, the anterior end of the incision was opened and the pleural space evacuated of all its contents. The wound was left open to permit free drainage. One month later thoracoplasty was performed, the first seven ribs being removed (Fig. 2). Since permanent interruption of the phrenic nerve had been performed at the time of pneumonectomy, thoracoplasty obliterated the remaining pleural space. On Nov. 26, 1946, progressive dilatation of the esophagus was instituted by passing dilators over the silk thread that had been left in place in the esophagus. The first dilatation was performed with a 22 French sound and subsequently larger sounds were used. The cavity caused by empyema became obliterated rapidly and was completely healed on Jan. 18, 1947. On dismissal of the patient the esophagus had been dilated up to the size of a 33 French sound and the patient was able to swallow all liquids and soft foods without difficulty (Fig. 3). He had no cough. He had gained weight and the general condition was excellent. Esophageal dilatations were continued by local physicians. The patient is now able to work for the first time in his life and is employed full time in a grocery store.

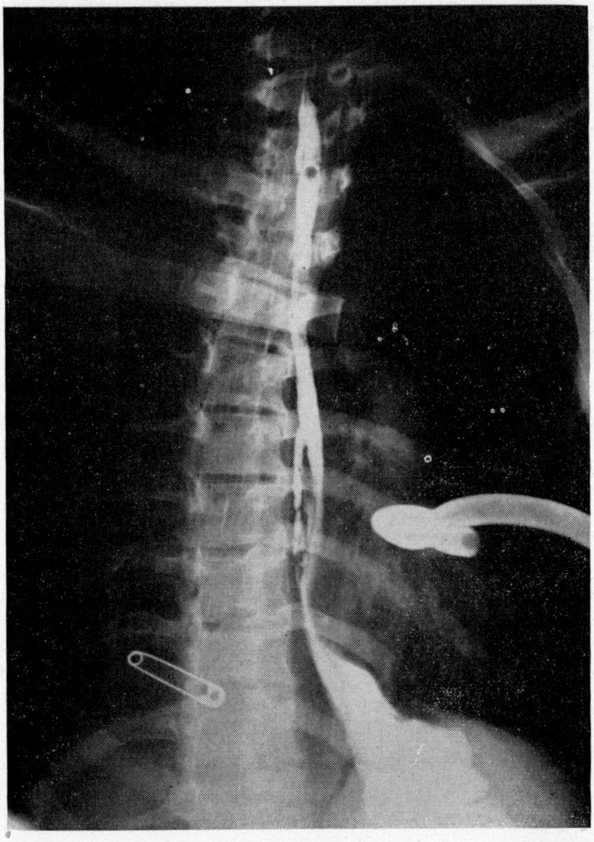

Fig. 3.—Appearance of the esophagus after closure of the fistula and progressive esophageal dilatations.

COMMENT

From the history in this case it seems likely that the bronchiectasis may have originated at the time the lye was accidentally swallowed. Possibly some of the lye was aspirated into the right bronchus, setting up an inflammatory process there, or some gastric contents may have gotten into the tracheobronchial tree during the vomiting that undoubtedly followed the swallowing of the lye. In a child 2 years old such an etiologic factor seems reasonable. There was no history of cough before the time lye was swallowed. We cannot be sure just when the fistula between the esophagus and right main bronchus developed; it had not been noticed before the attack of pneumonia which occurred when the patient was 12 years of age, but it was apparent soon afterward. We believe that the development of the fistula may have caused the severe pneumonia that occurred in the bronchiectatic lung. The symptoms of bronchiectasis had been progressive since the development of the fistula and may have been due, in some part at least, to aspiration of food into the right lung when the feedings through the gastric stoma were too large or too liquid in character.

We had hoped that we might be able to get a string through the esophagus before attempting pneumonectomy, but this was impossible; if it had been possible the operation would have been somewhat easier than it was. The extent of the esophageal stricture and the involvement of the upper part of the esophagus almost to the cricoid cartilage precluded any attempt to excise the stricture and re-establish esophagogastric continuity by bringing the stomach high in the chest and anastomosing it to the upper part of the esophagus according to the method reported by Kay[1] and by Sweet.[2] This would not have been feasible in any event because the right lung was completely destroyed in so far as respiratory function was concerned, and an operation through the left side of the chest could not be considered. After careful consideration of the whole problem, we felt that our only chance of helping this patient lay in performing pneumonectomy on the right side and in attempting, at the same time, to repair the esophageal fistula and to reopen the strictured esophagus, if possible. The magnitude of such an operation is obvious. As we anticipated, it was a difficult procedure throughout. We were gratified that we were able to reopen the strictured esophagus and get a silk thread through from the mouth to the gastric stoma so that dilatation of the esophagus could be performed subsequently.

A strictured esophagus that can be re-utilized as a tube to convey food from the mouth to the stomach will function far better than an artificially made esophagus or an esophagogastric stoma made after esophageal resection. Uncomplicated cicatricial strictures of the esophagus can almost always be managed by dilating the stricture over a previously swallowed twisted silk thread. If anything will pass the strictured region, thread can be swallowed. If 15 feet (4.5 meters) of thread are swallowed at the rate of 1 foot (30 cm.) an hour the distal end will become anchored in the loops of the jejunum. Graduated Plummer dilating sounds can then be used to dilate the stricture, the thread serving as a guide. If there has been complete closure of the esophagus, a gastric stoma will be necessary. At the time of operation a thread can usually be passed into the stomach by attaching it to a flexible bougie and carefully introducing this instrument past the strictured region into the stomach, where the surgeon can disengage the thread and carry it out through the gastric stoma. At other times it is possible to thread a small ureteral catheter into the cardia in a retrograde fashion as has been described herein. Once a thread has passed through the lumen of the esophagus and has become engaged, repeated dilations are usually easy. The risk of these procedures is small and the results are excellent. One concern of ours in this particular case was whether or not a repaired esophagus would withstand the trauma of esophageal dilation. This concern proved to be unnecessary since the patient stood the dilations very well.

We were not surprised that empyema developed. It would have been remarkable if it had not occurred. We had planned, in any event, to perform thoracoplasty, since we felt this would result in considerable support for the esophagus so that rupture of the esophagus during dilatations might be prevented.

The postoperative result has been excellent. The patient is able to swallow most foods. The gastric stoma has not been closed, but all feedings are taken in a normal manner. The patient is completely relieved of cough. For the first time in his life he is able to work.

Fortunately, problems of this kind do not occur frequently. It is gratifying that advances in thoracic surgery have made it possible to handle problems of this magnitude.

REFERENCES

1. Kay, E. B.: Surgical Lesions of the Esophagus Seen in an Army Thoracic Center, SURGERY 21: 143, 1947.
2. Sweet, R. H.: Subtotal Esophagectomy With High Intrathoracic Esophagogastric Anastomosis in the Treatment of Extensive Cicatricial Obliteration of the Esophagus, Surg., Gynec. & Obst. 83: 417-427, 1946

RESTORATION OF THE THUMB

By Transplantation, Plastic Repair, and Prosthesis

Arthur J. Barsky, M.D., New York, N. Y.

IN DESCRIBING losses of the thumb, certain terms are used, perhaps arbitrarily, and it might be well, therefore, to define these terms at the outset. A *partial loss* is one that involves no more than the distal phalanx. A *subtotal loss* involves approximately both phalanges of the thumb. A *total loss* means that not only are both phalanges missing, but that all or most of the metacarpal of the thumb is also absent.

PARTIAL LOSSES OF THE THUMB

Occasionally the amount of thumb loss is so slight that operative restoration is not practical. Much more frequent are cases in which there has been a loss of the distal phalanx which has healed with the formation of an adherent scar over the stump. In repairing such a condition, the surgeon is usually forced to choose between length of finger and preservation of highly specialized sensation. It is possible to lengthen the finger by utilizing a flap of skin, but if this flap is taken from a distant region (that is, not the skin of finger or palm), although in time it will develop primary sensation (heat, cold, pressure, pain), it will never develop stereognosis (see Figs. 1 to 3). Stereognosis, the highly refined perception which enables one, by touch alone, to distinguish and understand the form and nature of objects, might well be called the ''eyes'' of the fingers. It is dependent upon specialized touch corpuscles present in the digits and the palm. The pulps of the thumb and fingers, especially the first two fingers, are richly supplied with these corpuscles, but they are lacking in most skin areas of the body. Thus, if the tip of a thumb or finger is replaced by a skin graft or flap from a distant area, this fine perception can never develop.

A partial loss of the thumb which has healed with scarring on the distal and palmar aspects of the amputation stump therefore constitutes a troublesome problem. In such instances I believe it is ill-advised to attempt to replace the tip with a free graft or a distant flap. Occasionally flaps from the palm of the hand itself may be used successfully to replace a missing finger tip, but when a thumb is involved this is usually not feasible because of the difficulty of obtaining skin from the hypothenar eminence or base of the palm. It is my belief that, with rare exceptions, it is advisable in such a case to shorten the thumb and to use the normal palmar skin to replace the scar and cover the distal end of the thumb stump. This may even necessitate shortening the thumbnail.

Occasionally one encounters an individual who has sustained a partial or subtotal loss of the thumb, and whose index finger, although possessing normal sensation, is functionless because of bone, joint, and tendon damage. In such a case the end of the index finger may be transplanted to repair the thumb

Received for publication, June 4, 1947.

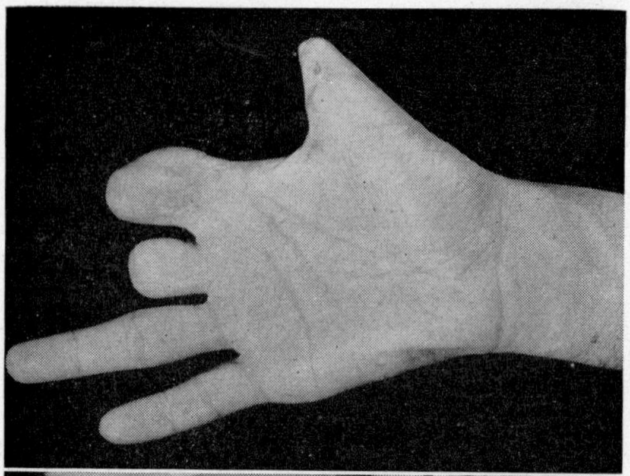

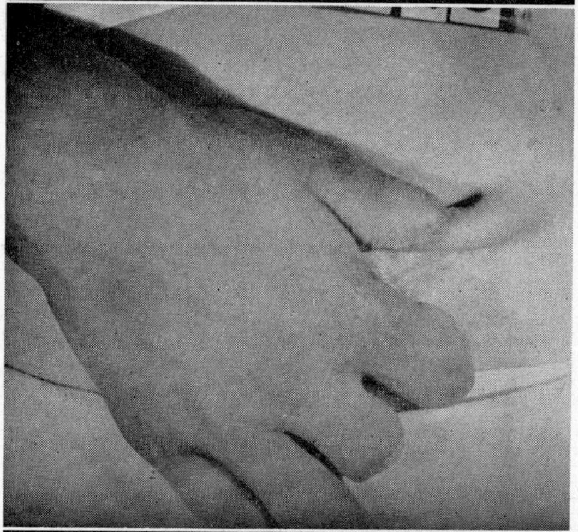

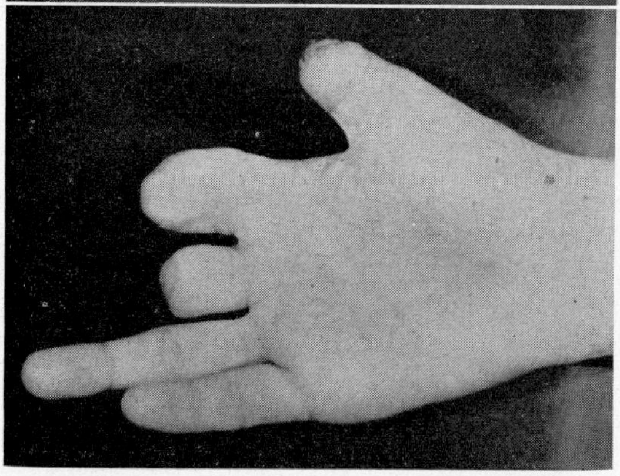

Fig. 1.—Partial loss of the thumb.

Fig. 2.—Abdominal flap migrated to the thumb in one stage. The pedicle of the flap is tubed and the donor area on the abdomen is closed. (Closed flaps of this nature, when properly planned and executed, are practically certain to take. They should be used in preference to open flaps.)

Fig. 3.—Final stage. The pedicle should be left attached to the finger for about three weeks. If there is any doubt as to the circulation, it may be tested by injecting sodium fluorescein intravenously and using ultraviolet light to observe the fluorescence. Clamping off the flap for a few minutes daily a few days before severing the flap is often useful.

(see Figs. 4 to 10). I had the opportunity of carrying out such a transplantation in the case of a young officer who had sustained a gunshot wound of the left hand.* The projectile had shattered the distal portion of the thumb and had

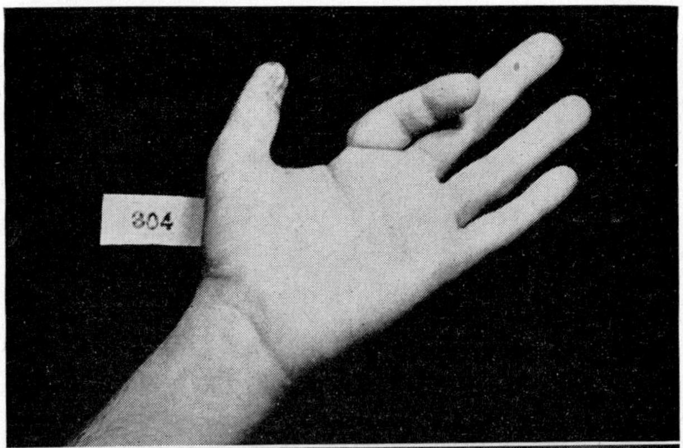

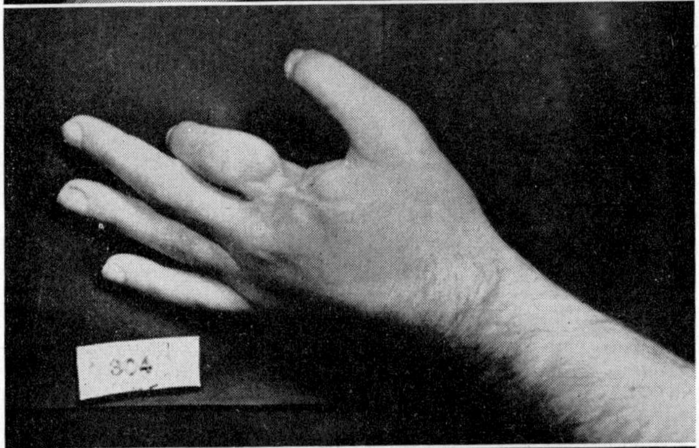

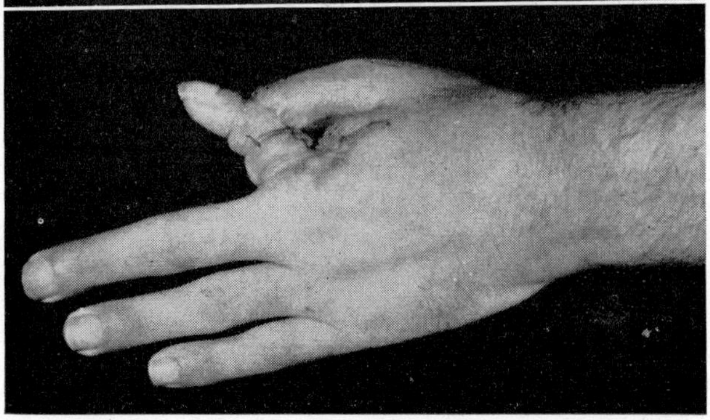

Figs. 4 and 5.—Palmar and dorsal views of a shrapnel wound of the hand. The distal phalanx of the thumb has been badly shattered and is covered with an unstable scar. There has been a compound fracture through the proximal finger joint of the index finger, with involvement of both flexor and extensor tendons. However, the index finger has normal sensation.

Fig. 6.—View illustrating the condition after healing of the first operation. The proximal two phalanges of the index finger have been fileted through a mid-dorsal incision and the index finger tip has migrated to the thumb after removing the useless tissue at the end of the thumb.

*This case was reported at the second annual meeting of the American Society for Surgery of the Hand, Chicago, Ill., January, 1947.

then passed through the proximal joint of the index finger, destroying the joint, the flexor and extensor tendons, and the skin covering. The circulation of the index finger was not affected and its digital nerves were also intact.

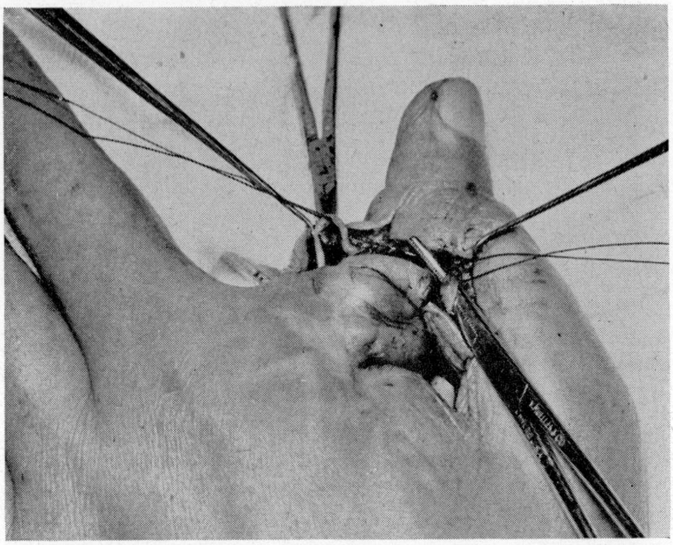

Fig. 7.—Photograph taken at the second operation, that of nerve suture. The digital nerve of the ulnar side of the thumb is elevated by the lower hemostat, while the upper hemostat shows the digital nerve on the ulnar side of the index finger. The nerves on both sides were united.

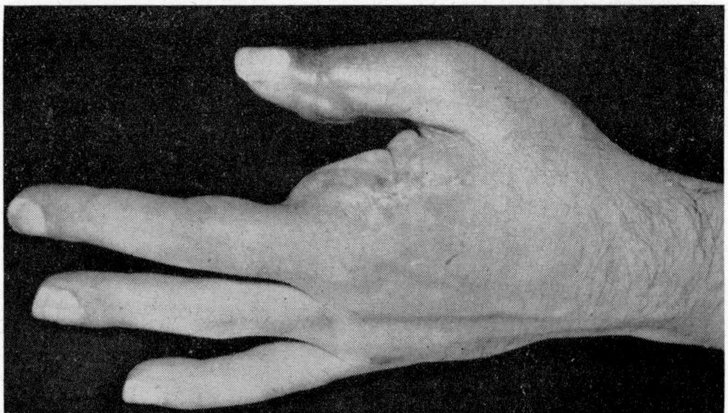

Fig. 8.—The thumb after the pedicle of the index finger was severed.

Since this index finger was practically useless, it was decided to transplant a portion of it to the thumb, to increase the usefulness of the thumb. All operative procedures were carried out under local anesthesia, procaine 2 per cent. At the first operation a middorsal incision was made on the index finger from the proximal to the distal finger joints. As this incision was made, the extensor tendon was reflected to one side, and the digital nerves and vessels were preserved. The bones of the proximal two phalanges were fileted, thus leaving a tube of skin, its distal end consisting of the index finger tip with its phalangeal bone, digital vessels, and nerve. At this first operation the distal end of the thumb stump was freshened by doing a guillotine amputation through the distal joint. The distal end of the bone of the proximal phalanx itself was not disturbed. The long extensor tendon of the thumb was identified. The finger tip was then migrated to the thumb stump, and after uniting the extensor tendon of the index finger with that of the thumb, the remainder of the suturing was carried out as shown in Fig. 6.

I should like to emphasize at this point that the tendon suture was not carried out with the idea of restoring motion to this transplanted finger tip, but for the purpose of stabilizing the joint.

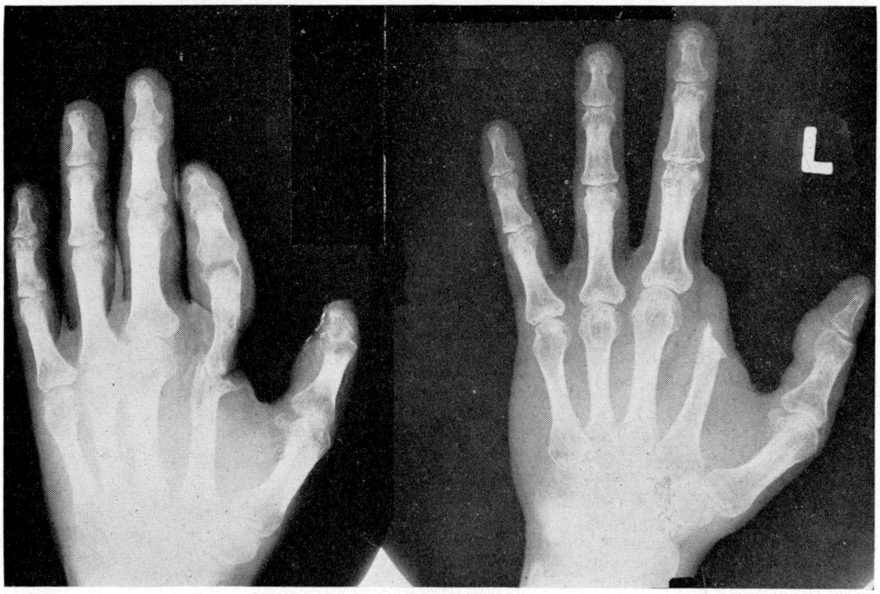

Fig. 9.—X-ray view taken before operation.
Fig. 10.—X-ray view taken after the transplantation had been completed. After this view was taken, the distal two-thirds of the second metacarpal was removed.

The migrated finger tip healed in place uneventfully. Approximately six weeks after the first operation, nerve suture was performed (see Fig. 7). Mid-lateral incisions were made on the pedicle of the index finger and the digital nerves exposed well proximal to the distal joint. In a similar manner, through mid-lateral incisions on the proximal phalanx of the thumb, the digital nerves of the thumb were exposed and dissected out distally to their ends. Fig. 7 shows the digital nerve of the thumb on one side and the digital nerve of the index finger on the other. Using 000000 black silk on atraumatic needles, nerve suture was carried out, uniting the proximal end of the digital nerve of the thumb to the distal end of the nerve of the index finger. The same procedure was, of course, carried out on both sets of digital nerves. The nerve suture was so located that it could be embedded in a healthy fat pad, and was located as far distally as possible so that the new growth of axons would be as short as possible. At this same operation the digital arteries in the pedicle of the index finger were tied off in order to compel the finger tip to derive its entire circulation from the vessels of the thumb. It is no doubt possible to sever the pedicle at this stage, but I preferred not to do so in this instance. In approximately five weeks the patient developed a good return of sensation in the migrated tip. This sensation was, of course, associated as coming from the thumb tip.

The third operation was performed about six weeks after the second. At this stage the pedicle of the index finger was severed, and the flexor profundus tendon of the index finger sutured to the long flexor tendon of the thumb. Here again, it is emphasized that this was done for the purpose of stabilizing the joint, and not with the idea of giving motion to the finger tip. Fig. 8 shows the result obtained after the transplantation. Figs. 9 and 10 show x-ray views of the finger before and after the transplantation. The second metacarpal bone was trimmed down after this later x-ray picture was taken.

When last seen, in June, 1946, this patient had a stable, useful thumb, with good sensation.

I believe that a slight variation of this method could be used to obtain a movable joint. In order to do this, the joint of the index finger, with the distal part of the middle phalanx, would have to be transplanted after ablating the proximal half of the middle phalanx and the entire proximal phalanx of the index finger. Thumb amputation would then be carried out through the middle of the proximal phalanx. After migration and bony union had taken place, tendon transplantation could be carried out.

This method could also be used to transplant a finger from one hand to the other. Naturally one would hesitate to sacrifice a normal finger in order to reconstruct a thumb, but in the case here reported the index finger was useless.

Transplantation of the toe as substitute for a finger, following the method of Nicoladoni, is also a procedure which under certain special conditions might be attempted. Kuslik reported a successful case using Nicoladoni's procedure. The operation is best performed under local anesthesia. A transverse incision is made across the stump of the finger and its extensor tendon isolated. The distal end of the phalanx is exposed and the periosteum removed. An incision is made at the base of the second toe (the one generally used), and a skin flap formed after dividing both dorsal interosseous arteries. The extensor tendon of the toe is incised proximally as far as possible. A cuff of periosteum is turned back distally for about 1 cm. from the point at which the bone of the toe is divided. The distal end of the bone of the toe phalanx is dislocated into the wound and approximated to the freshened end of the bony stump of the finger. The periosteum of the toe is sutured to that of the finger, thus helping to maintain the bones in contact. The extensor tendons are then sutured in such a fashion that the suture line is proximal to that of the periosteum. The skin flap of the toe is then sutured to the skin of the finger and the wound closed on the palmar surface of the finger and the dorsal surface of the toe. A plaster bandage is then applied.

In Kuslik's case, immobilization was maintained for about one month. However, ten days postoperatively, pressure was applied to compress the plantar circulation and force dependence on the finger circulation. One month after the first stage, the second stage was carried out. The remainder of the toe was divided, the flexor tendons united, and the skin incisions closed.

Six technical details recommended by Kuslik are:

1. A plantar toe pedicle is advised because the plantar arteries are better developed than the dorsal. The patient will also be more comfortable if the finger is placed over the toe rather than under it. Both plantar arteries should be preserved.
2. The levels of the periosteal, tendon, and skin sutures should not coincide.
3. The periosteal cuff formed on the phalanx of the toe will facilitate better contact and immobilization of the bones.
4. The plaster bandage should be applied from the shoulder blade downward, covering the upper and lower extremities on the side of the operation.
5. The pedicle must not be severed too early.
6. The recipient must be kept warm.

I have had the opportunity of transplanting the toe only once, and in this particular case the result was not successful, because of three factors. First, the apposition between the finger and the toe was not close enough to fulfill the requirement of primary tissue contact. Second, the early stages of immobilization caused the patient such discomfort and she was so restless that there was a slight disturbance of the contact. Third, because of this discomfort the pedicle of the toe was severed, perhaps too early, on the sixteenth day.

SUBTOTAL LOSSES OF THE THUMB

In subtotal losses of the thumb where there remains a mobile metacarpal covered with a good scar, and where the patient is able to grasp, surgery may not be necessary. However, as a general rule, the prehensile function of the hand is much improved if the web is deepened. This may be accomplished quite simply by the Z-plastic operation, with transposition of flaps.

If conditions permit, subtotal losses of the thumb may be repaired by migration of another finger, as described previously. It is essential that such a restored finger have sensation, for without it the finger cannot function efficiently. The skin will become atrophic and may even ulcerate. A restoration of this type should therefore always include nerve transplantation and suture.

Phalangization of the thumb metacarpal is often very helpful in aiding the prehensile function of the thumb. This may be brought about by using either a flap or a free graft. My own preference is for a flap, because a flap will permit the use of heavier skin, which will be more durable than a free graft. Figs. 11, 12, and 13 show a case of this type. While it is desirable to obtain as deep a web as possible, muscular attachments should not be sacrificed. If they have already been damaged, a tendon transplant to bring about opposition, as described by Bunnell, is advocated.

TOTAL LOSSES OF THE THUMB

Total loss of the thumb, including loss of the metacarpal, reduces the efficiency of the hand by approximately 40 per cent. Such a hand lacks opposition and therefore cannot perform those functions which require prehensile movements. On the other hand, it is sometimes astonishing how much dexterity a patient who has lost the entire thumb may develop. Some patients, thus, do not wish to have any surgery done, nor do they desire a prosthesis.

The simplest form of prosthesis is basically somewhat similar to the "sailor's palm." Although the sailor's palm was not designed for prehensile movements, it can easily be seen that if the palmar portion is elongated, the fingers

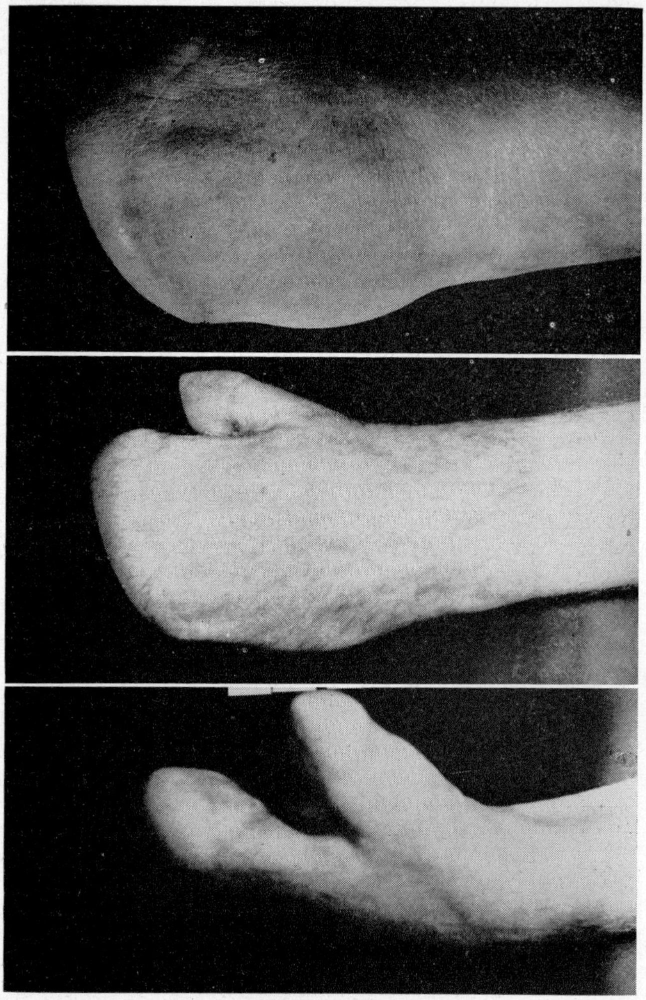

Fig. 11.—A loss of all five fingers. The metacarpals are all intact.

Fig. 12.—The result obtained by phalangization of the first metacarpal.

Fig. 13.—The amount of abduction present. This type of thumb reconstruction restores some of the prehensile functions of the hand, whereas previously the main member could be used only as a paw.

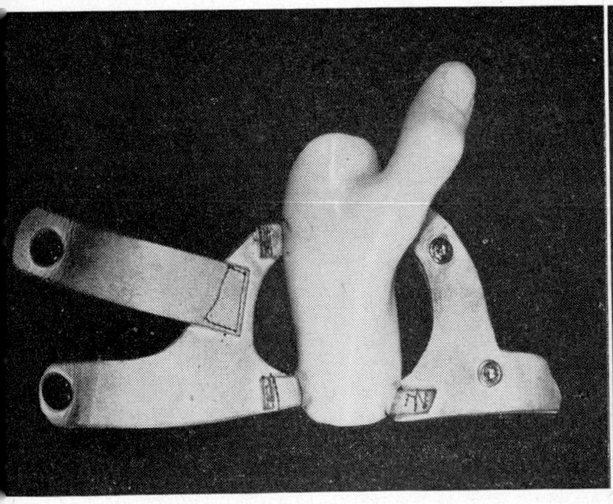

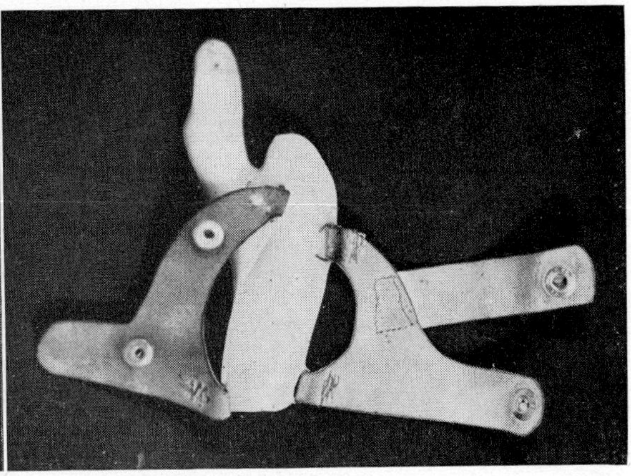

Fig. 14.—A working prosthesis. This thumb prosthesis is not to be confused with one which serves only to restore appearance.

Fig. 15.—Inside view of the prosthesis. Note that the palmar tip of the thumb is slightly roughened to prevent slipping.

Fig. 16.

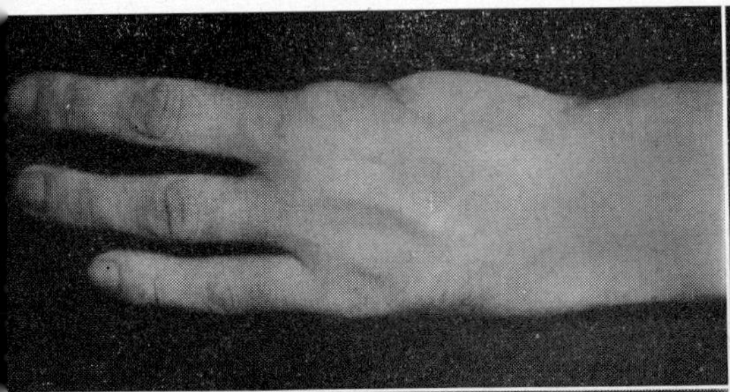

Fig. 17.

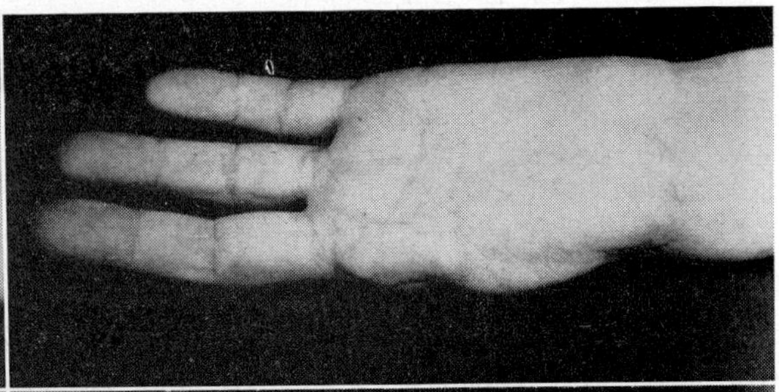

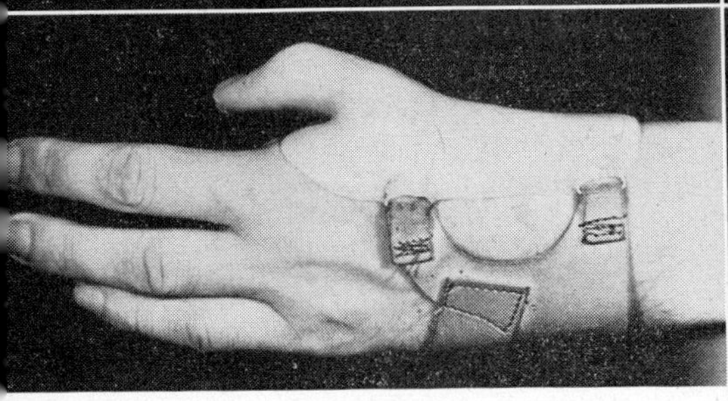

Fig. 18.

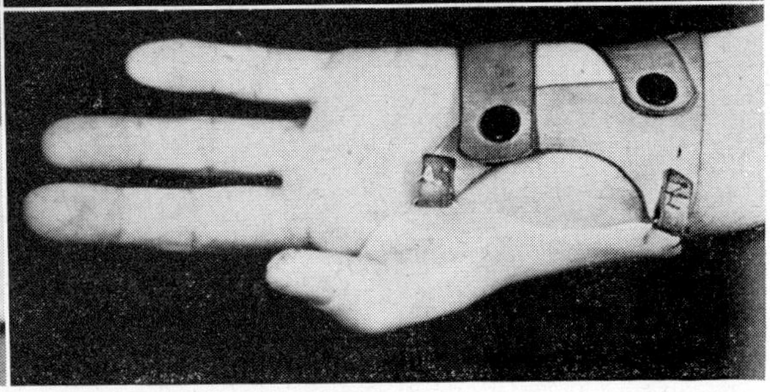

Fig. 19.

Fig. 16.—Loss of the thumb and index finger. Before a prosthesis can be used, the base upon which it is placed must be a stable skin covering with normal subcutaneous tissue. No sharp, bony spurs or irregularities should be permitted to remain, for they will only cause pain and discomfort, will interfere with the use of the prosthesis, and will discourage the patient.

Fig. 17.—A palmar view of the same hand.

Fig. 18.—The work prosthesis strapped in place.

Fig. 19.—A palmar view of the prosthesis in place. Note that snap fasteners have been used on the straps in preference to buckles.

may flex upon the post for grasping. The simplest type of prosthesis which we have used consists of a restoration made of acrylic resin, with its distal end slightly roughened to prevent slipping, and made with a sort of bracelet arrangement to attach the prosthesis to the hand. This thumb prosthesis is shown in Figs. 14 and 15. It is, of course, a work prosthesis, not a "dress" prosthesis. Its effectiveness is directly related to the patient's desire to use it. Those patients who have had the desire and the persistence to learn to use a prosthesis have found it very helpful (see Figs. 16 to 19). In this connection, it is well to

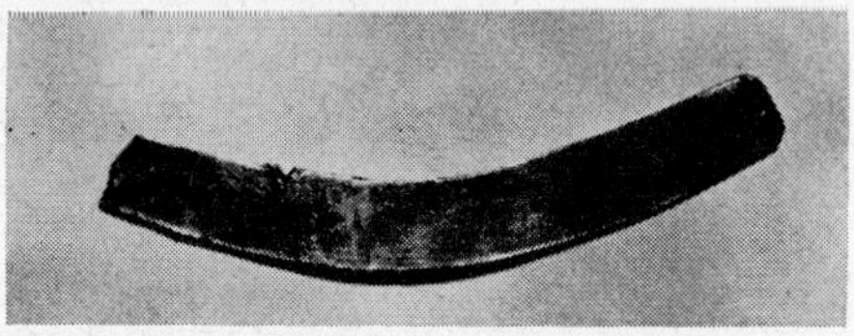

Fig. 20.—A curved lead pattern. This is sterilized and the graft fabricated according to it. The lead pattern is prepared beforehand and varies not only according to the size of the hand but also in length, depending upon the presence or absence of an index finger and upon the location of the recipient site.

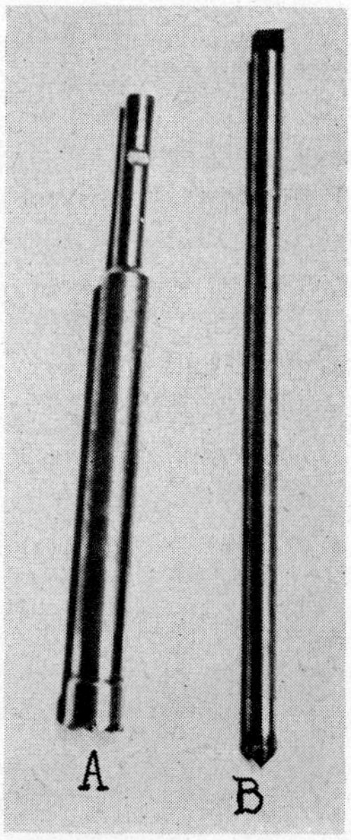

Fig. 21.—*A*, The peg-former; *B*, the drill used to prepare the donor site. The drill is marked off in centimeters. It cuts only at the end and therefore cannot become entangled with the soft tissue.

note that it is not wise to urge a patient to have a prosthesis made. On the contrary, it is best to explain carefully and honestly the advantages and disadvantages of the mechanical device, and at the same time to point out the possibilities and limitations of surgical restoration of the thumb. The patient who is permitted to make his own choice is much more satisfied with the result, and much more interested in developing skills, than the patient who reluctantly consents to corrective steps urged by the surgeon.

Surgical restoration for total loss of the thumb may be accomplished in a number of ways. The presence of even a small proximal portion of the metacarpal which has mobility greatly increases the usefulness of the surgical restoration. It may sometimes be possible, in restorations where the entire

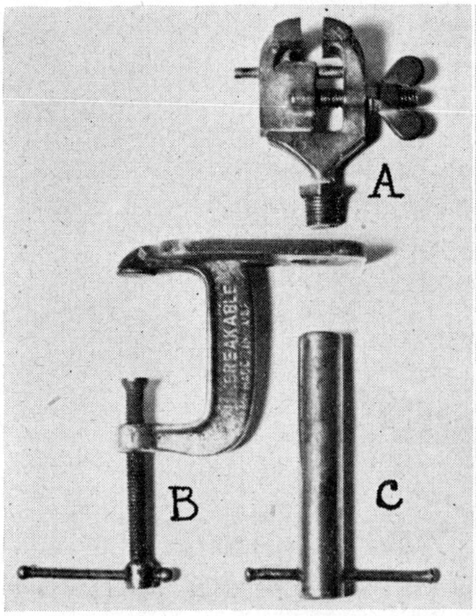

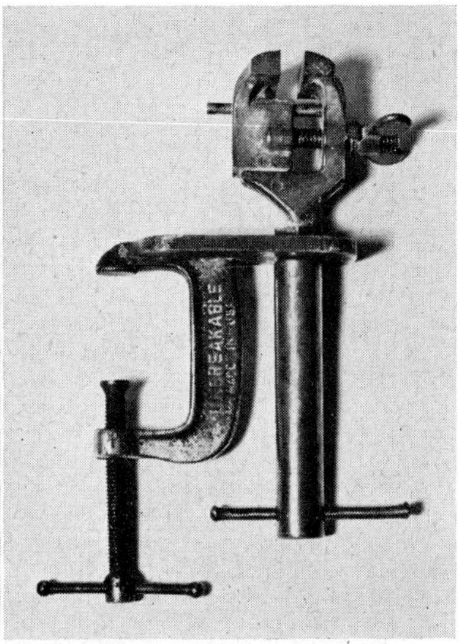

Fig. 22.—The component parts of the bone vise. When the vise head (*A*) is attached to the handle (*B*), the vise may be held in the hand.

Fig. 23.—The vise assembled so that it may be clamped to a table. By loosening the handle, the vise may be adjusted at any horizontal position.

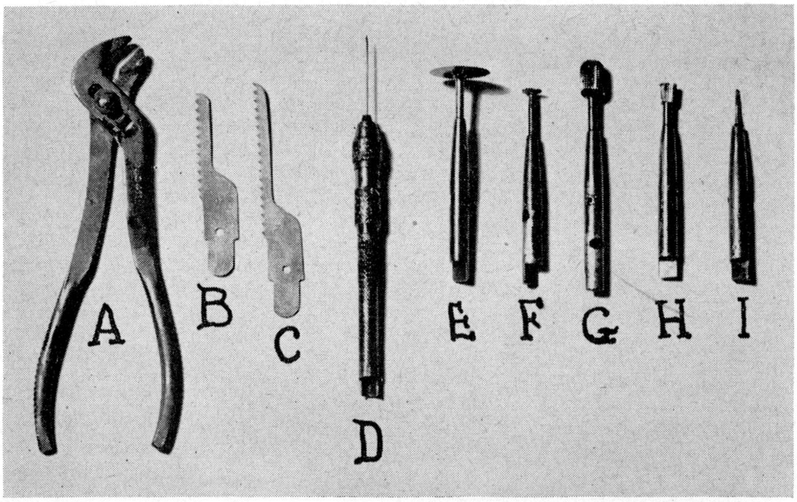

Fig. 24.—The shaping of the bone graft is expedited by the use of power instruments. *A*, A small bone-grasping forceps. These are mechanics' small ignition pliers. *B* and *C*, Small blades used in the reciprocating saw hand piece. *D*, The small chuck which fits into the rotary hand piece. This is used for driving in the Kirschner wires under power. *E* and *F*, Small circular saws used to cut and shape the graft. *G* and *H*, Rotary files. *I*, A fissure burr used to make the end cuts when taking a tibial graft. Note that these instruments fit directly into the rotary saw hand piece and avoid the used of a heavy, cumbersome chuck.

metacarpal is gone, to provide motion by making a false joint and carrying out tendon transfer.

If the index finger is present and if, after due consideration, it is thought advisable to use this finger to replace a lost thumb, the first step is to phalangize the metacarpal of the index finger. The index metacarpal is separated from the third metacarpal, but the structures of the index finger, that is, the flexor and extensor tendons, the vessels, and the nerves, are kept intact. It is neces-

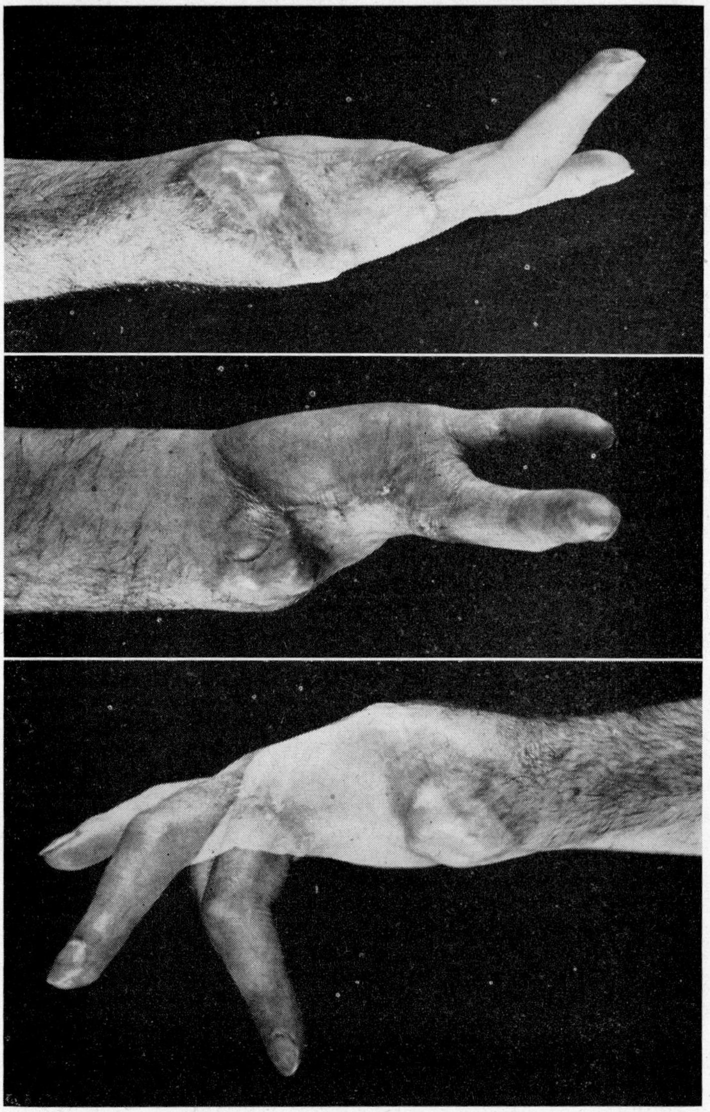

Fig. 25.—Loss of the thumb and index and middle fingers following a hand-grenade explosion.

Fig. 26.—Palmar view. Note the thin, tight scar over the rough bony prominences.

Fig. 27.—Double exposure, showing the range of motion.

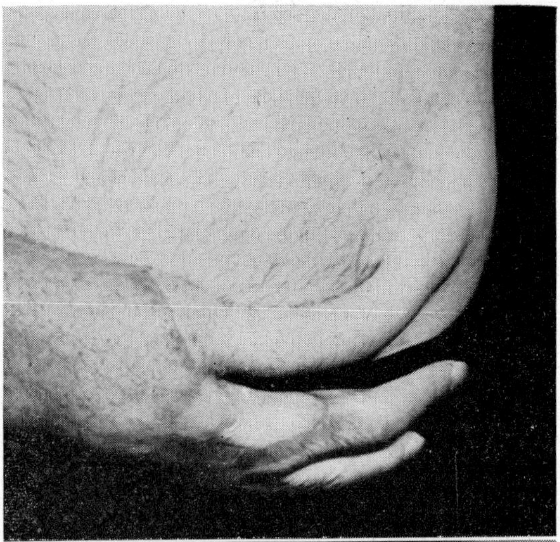

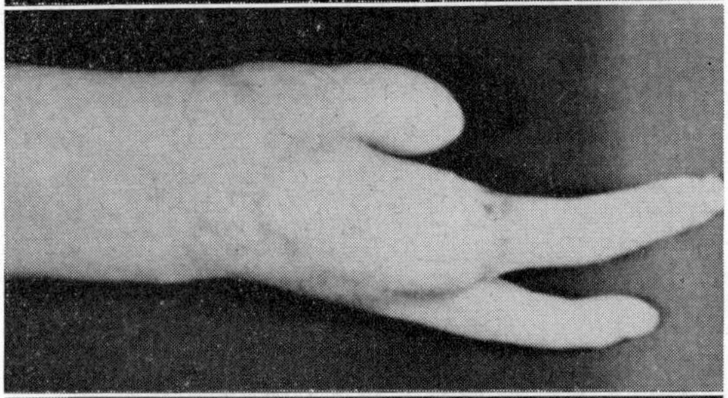

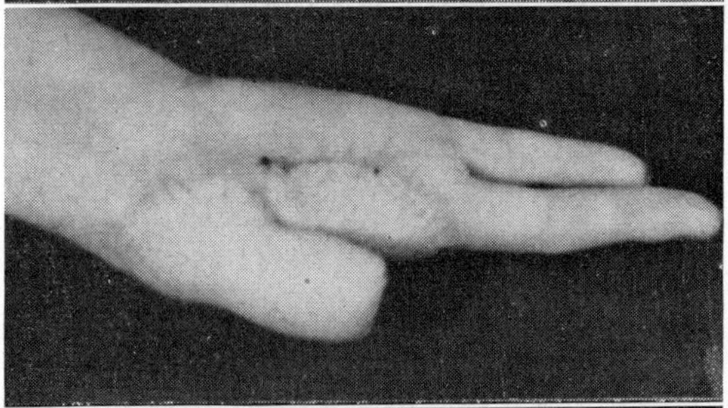

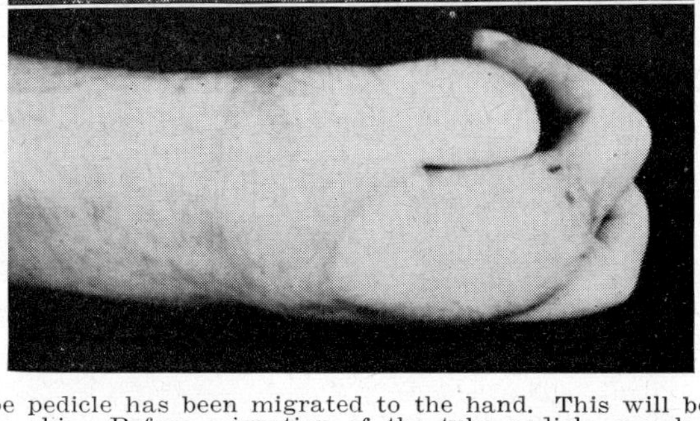

Fig. 28.—A tube pedicle has been migrated to the hand. This will be large enough to replace all the unstable skin. Before migration of the tube pedicle, rough bony spurs were removed.

Fig. 29.—Dorsal view after insertion of the bone graft.

Fig. 30.—Palmar view. Note that the flap has replaced all the unstable scar with heavy skin and good subcutaneous padding.

Fig. 31.—The range of motion after healing. It was necessary to release the flexor tendons of the ring finger to bring about this degree of flexion.

sary to split the digital nerve of the index finger from the common digital nerve which supplies the ulnar side of the index finger and the radial side of the middle finger. The raw area between the second and third metacarpals

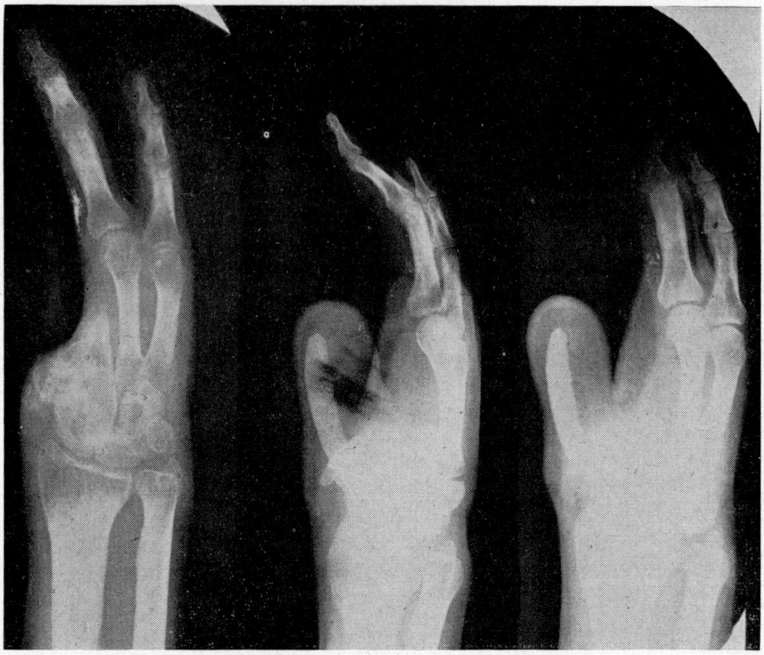

Fig. 32.—X-ray view taken before operation.

Fig. 33.—X-ray view taken after insertion of the bone graft. Curved iliac bone was used and fastened in place with two Kirschner wires.

Fig. 34.—Another postoperative x-ray view.

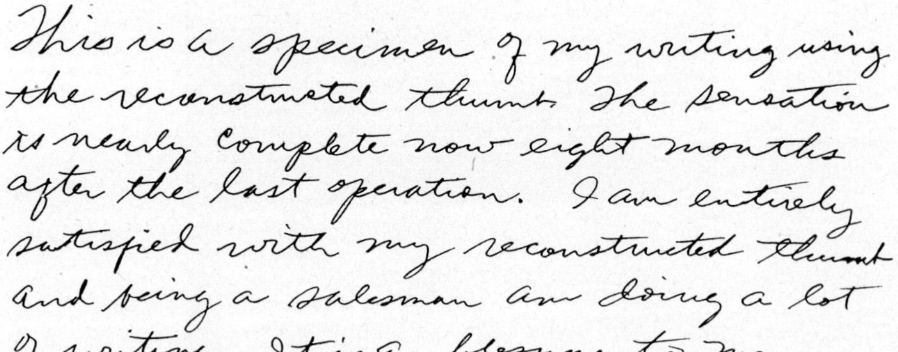

Fig. 35.—Specimen of the patient's handwriting made eight months after the final operation.

should be covered with a flap of skin. This flap should be of generous size to permit the migration of the metacarpal of the index finger to the position of the thumb. At a subsequent operation the index metacarpal is migrated to the position of the thumb and so rotated that the index finger is placed in the position of opposition. At the same time the metacarpal should be shortened.

In those cases where it was considered desirable to provide a thumb, that is, simply an immovable post in the position of opposition, we have used a procedure which is well standardized. An abdominal tube pedicle is prepared at the first operation.* At a second operation, one end of the tube is migrated

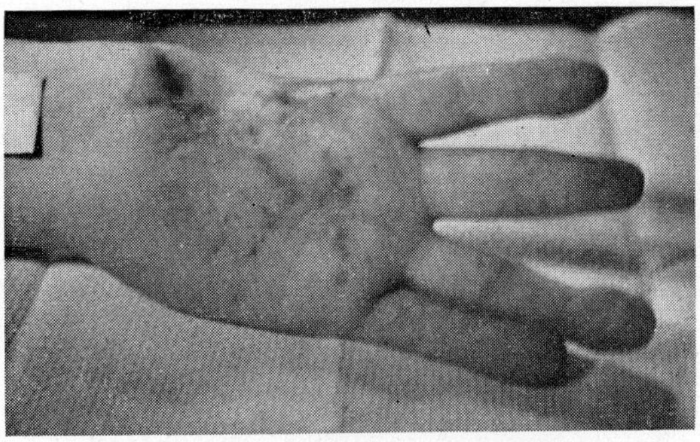

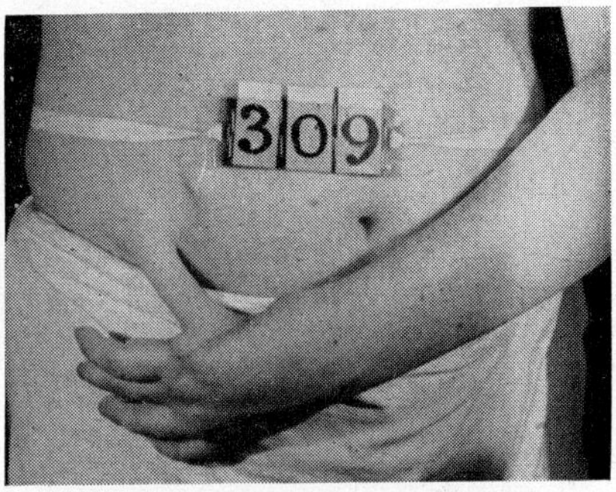

Fig. 36.—Total loss of the thumb.
Fig. 37.—Tube pedicle attached to the thenar eminence.

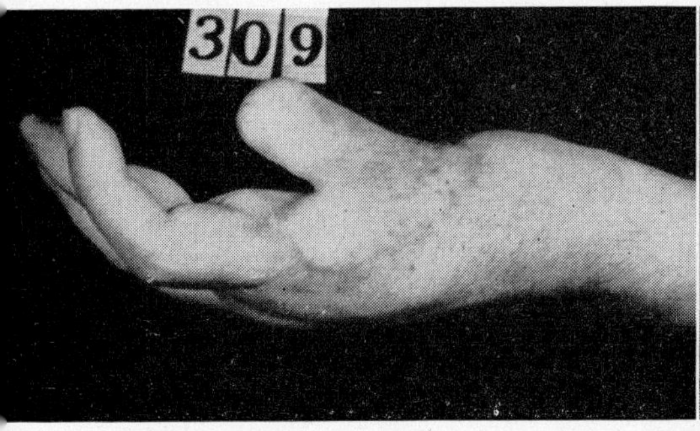

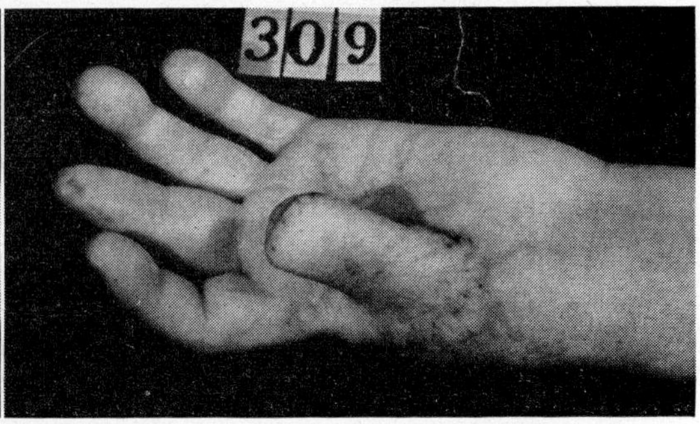

Fig. 38.—Postoperative view from the radial side after the implantation of a straight tibial bone graft. The cleft is in line with the long axis of the forearm.

Fig. 39.—A palmar view. An attempt is made to locate the thumb in a position of opposition, the tip being opposite the cleft between the index and middle fingers.

to the thenar eminence. It is desirable to locate the scar in a neutral position, that is, away from areas of friction and use. At a third stage, the abdominal end of the pedicle is divided. Since the distal end of the tube is a terminal structure, it may be well to clamp off the pedicle prior to severing it. A rubber-covered clamp should be applied distal to the site at which the pedicle is to be divided. At the first trial, the clamp is applied only for a few minutes. If the portion of the pedicle attached to the hand does not become cyanotic, the pedicle may be clamped on succeeding days for longer periods of time. If there remains any doubt about the vigor of the circulation, it is best to sever the pedicle partially and to wait about one week before detaching it completely.

*It is possible to migrate the flap in one stage, tubing the pedicle, but I believe that if this is done in two stages, the flap has a much better circulation at its distal end.

A bone graft may be inserted in the pedicle at the third stage operation, but I have found it more desirable to implant the bone at a later stage. The reason for this is that the distal end of the tube may heal slowly, and if a bone graft has been inserted, there is a possibility that the skin will break down and

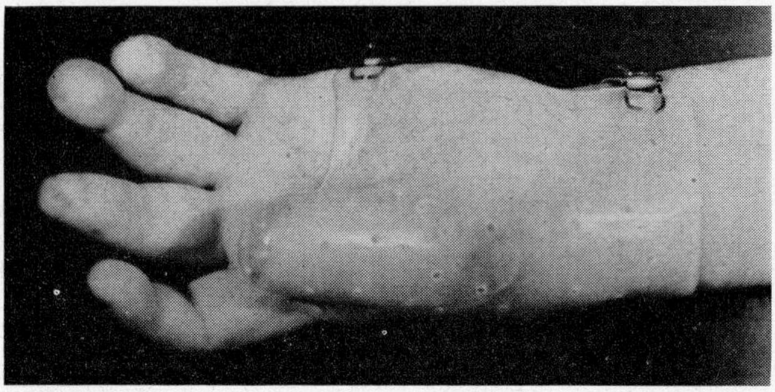

Fig. 40.—The same patient wearing the combined splint and protector. This simple device is made of a transparent synthetic resin.

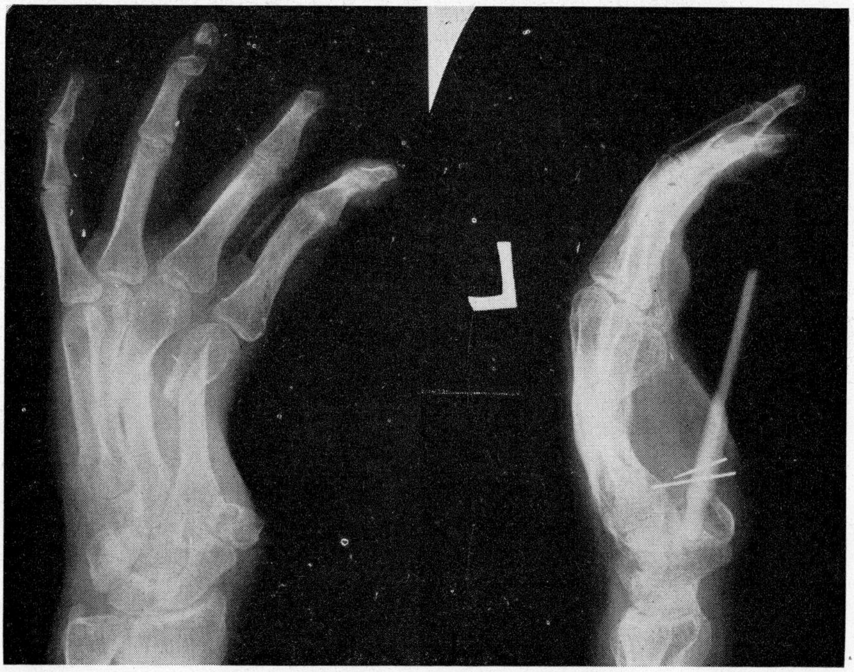

Fig. 41.—Preoperative x-ray view.

Fig. 42.—Postoperative x-ray view showing the straight tibial bone graft immobilized by two Kirschner wires. If the wires cause no trouble and do not loosen, they may be left in situ, otherwise they are easily removed.

endanger the result. I have tried various sources for bone grafts: tibial bone, both straight and angulated; the curved portion of the ilium; and finally, a rib graft. I believe that the angulated or curved graft is most desirable, and that the iliac graft is preferable to the tibial, since the former heals more readily. The rib graft has no particular advantage.

The angulation or curve of the graft should be designed prior to the operation. Fig. 20 shows a simple lead pattern that is used to shape the graft. Fig. 21 shows a peg-former (*A*) and end-cutting drill (*B*).

Straight grafts from the tibia are cut with the twin-bladed rotary saw from the upper part of the anteromedial surface. The anatomic margins are avoided. A heavy rotary burr is used to cut the ends of the graft. When an angulated graft is taken from the tibia, the reciprocating saw is used. A curved graft taken from the crest of the ilium is removed by means of a wide, sharp chisel. When rib is used (preferably the eleventh or twelfth), it is removed in the usual manner, using Doyen rib elevators and rib shears.

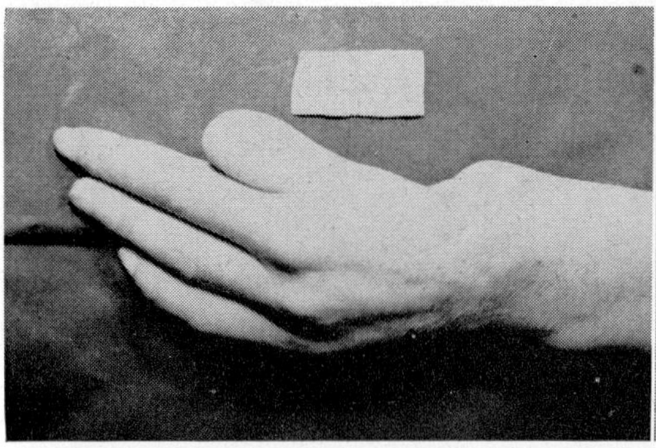

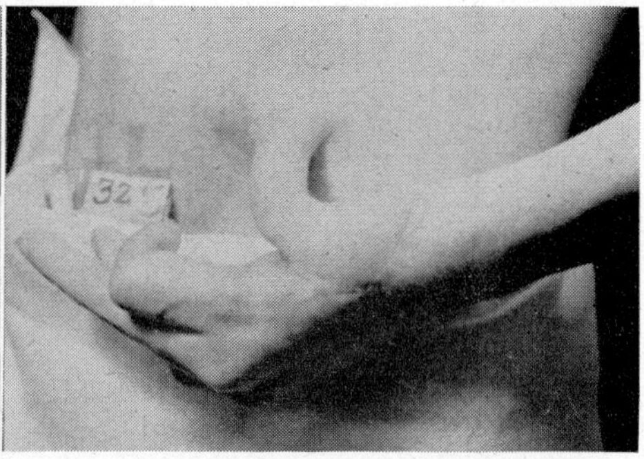

Fig. 43.—Another case showing total loss of the thumb. The bone graft in this case was on angulated tibial graft.

Fig. 44.—Tube pedicle migrated to the hand.

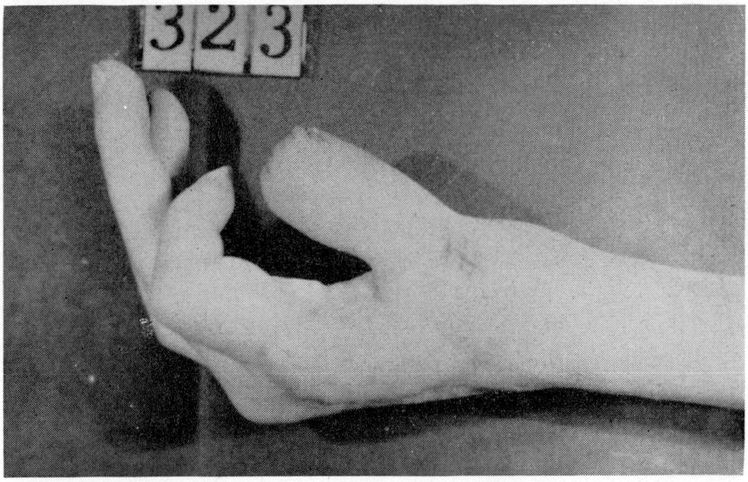

Fig. 45.—Postoperative result.

The placement of the bone graft requires great care, for unless the thumb post is in the proper position, its efficiency is markedly decreased. It should be so placed that the cleft between the post and the index finger, when viewed from the radial side of the hand, is aligned with the long axis of the forearm, and when viewed from the palmar aspect of the hand, the post should be in a position of opposition to the cleft between the index and middle fingers (or to the radial and adjacent fingers if the index is missing). The post must not be too long, for in this case it will tend to interfere with the closing of the fingers. When the post is of the proper length, the patient may pinch against it with the index and middle fingers by *fixing* the two distal joints of each finger and moving the metacarpal phalangeal joints. When the post is to be cleared by the fingers, the two distal joints are flexed first, following which the metacarpal phalangeal joints are flexed.

When the proper site for insertion of the bone graft has been located, the drill is inserted into the carpal bones or into a remnant of the metacarpal if it is present. The drill is driven down to a predetermined depth; this is easily ascertained from the markings on the drill, as shown in Fig. 21, *B*.

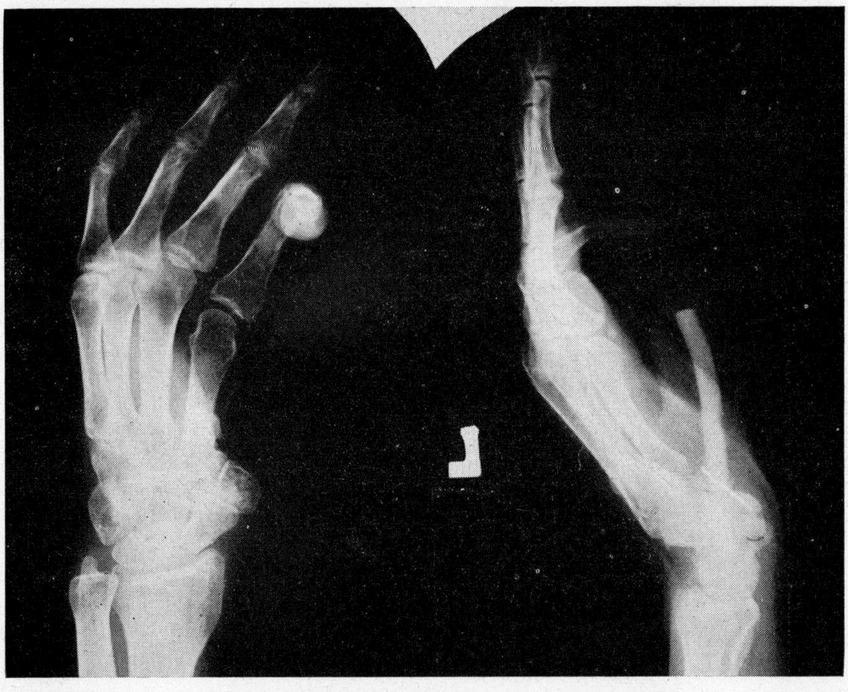

Fig. 46.—Preoperative x-ray view.
Fig. 47.—Postoperative x-ray view showing the angulated tibial graft.

The shaping of the bone graft is expedited by the use of a simple bone vise and power-driven instruments (see Figs. 23 and 24). The general shaping of the bone graft is done with a rotary file. All sharp edges are smoothed and the distal end is carefully rounded. The graft is then placed in the bone vise, proximal end upward, and the peg-former (see Fig. 21, *A*) in the rotary saw handle is driven down on the graft to form a peg of the same diameter and length as the drill hole. The graft is then placed in the hole which has been prepared for it, and if it fits satisfactorily, it may be fastened in situ. All our grafts have been fastened with stainless steel Kirschner wire, using a simple,

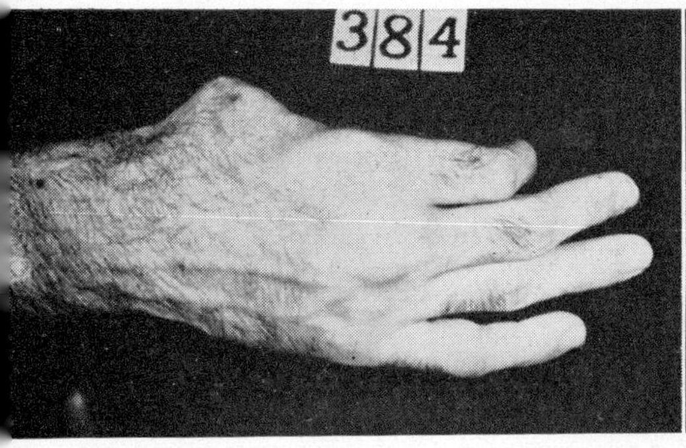

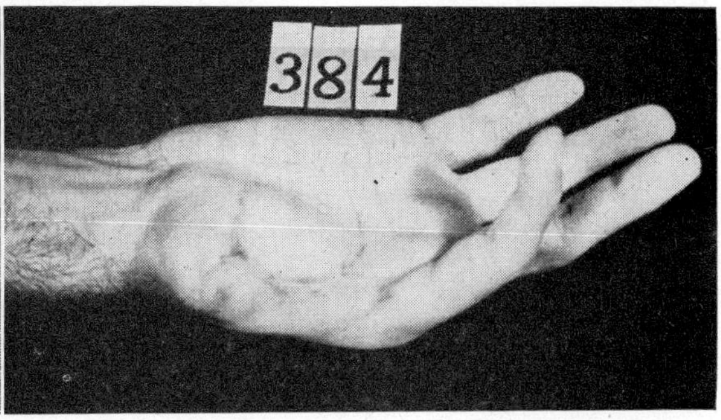

Fig. 48.—Dorsal view of a hand in which the restoration was carried out by using a rib graft.

Fig. 49.—Palmar view of the same hand.

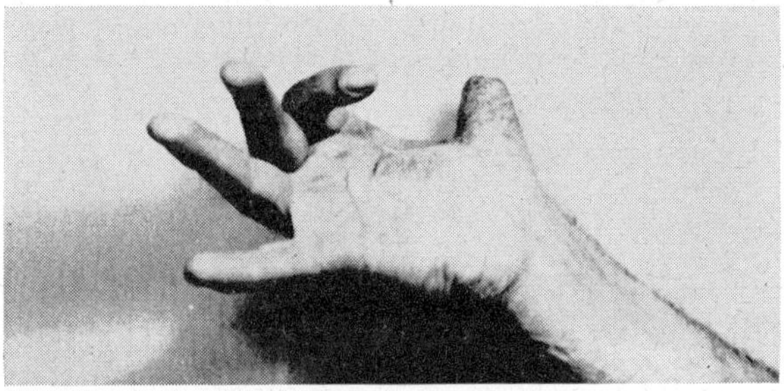

Fig. 50.—The reconstructed thumb. The thumb should never be made too long, lest it interfere with function.

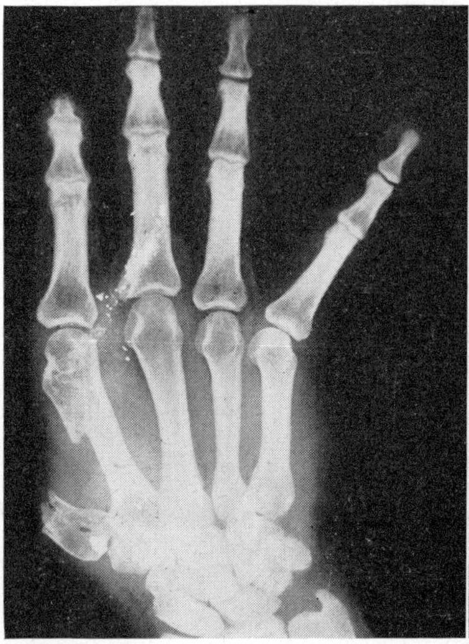

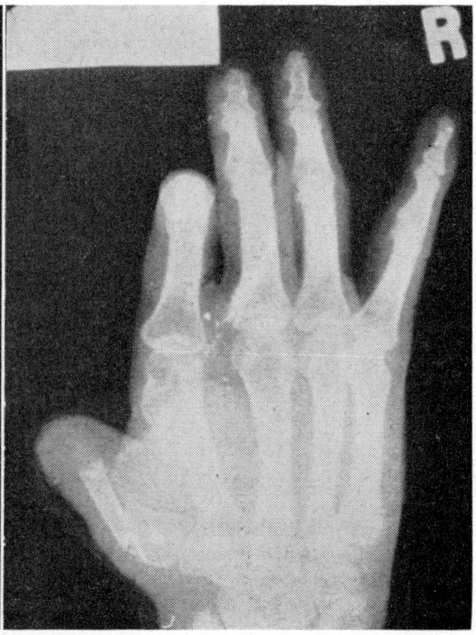

Fig. 51.—Preoperative x-ray view.

Fig. 52.—Postoperative x-ray view showing the rib graft.

efficient device to drive the wire in under power (see Fig. 24, *D*). Anyone who has attempted to use the conventional egg-beater type of hand drill to insert Kirschner wire in a small bone realizes how inefficient and laborious such a procedure can be. With a power-driven device, the placement of the wires can be carried out with ease and precision. Two wires are usually sufficient to hold the graft securely. The wires are left in indefinitely. However, if they should loosen, or if x-ray examination should show absorption around them, they should be removed.

The skin covering should be sutured carefully over the bone graft and a simple plaster splint applied to immobilize the thumb and wrist. This cast is removed after about three weeks and replaced by a protector, as illustrated in Fig. 40. This protector serves to immobilize the graft and to prevent injury to the skin of the restoration. It must be stressed that the development of sensation in the skin of the restoration may take as long as a year. During this time, the restoration may be damaged. Protection during the interval while sensation is developing is therefore important, and the patient should be cautioned in the care of the restored thumb.

Figs. 25 to 52 show a number of thumb restorations, using different types of bone grafts.

Complications.—In nine cases in which the thumb was restored, only one complication developed: ulceration of the distal end of the thumb before the implantation of the bone graft. This was attributed to early severance of the tube, without progressive clamping off of the circulation.

SUMMARY AND CONCLUSIONS

A successful new technique for restoring the thumb by means of a finger transplantation and nerve suture is presented. This technique is applicable to certain special cases which are discussed.

Other methods of restoration of the thumb in cases of partial, subtotal, and total loss are described and illustrated. The use of different types of bone grafts is discussed. A practical work prosthesis is shown.

Loss of the thumb is so crippling a disability that every effort toward restoration should be made. In properly selected cases, a carefully thought-out and well-executed restoration will result in a marked improvement in the functioning of the hand.

REFERENCES

Apetrosyan, K. A.: Plastic Reconstruction of Fingers by Means of Transplantation of Toes, Ortop. i travmatol. **13**: 74-78, 1939.

Barsky, A. J.: Plastic Surgery, Philadelphia, 1938, W. B. Saunders Company.

Blair, V. P., and Byars, L. T.: Toe to Finger Transplant, Ann. Surg. **112**: 287-290, 1940.

Bolté, R.: Use of First Metacarpus in Plastic Restoration of Thumb; Case, J. de l'Hôtel-Dieu de Montréal **7**: 359-365, 1938.

Bunnell, Sterling: Physiological Reconstruction of a Thumb After Total Loss, Surg., Gynec. & Obst. **52**: 245-248, 1931.

Bunnell, Sterling: Surgery of the Hand, Philadelphia, 1944, J. B. Lippincott Co.

Cannon, B., and Graham, W. C.: Plastic and Reconstructive Surgery, Mil. Surgeon **97**: 137-139, 1945.

Dial, D. E.: Reconstruction of Thumb After Traumatic Amputation, J. Bone & Joint Surg. **21**: 98-100, 1939.

Dzbanovskiy, V. P.: Transplantation of Toe to Replace Thumb, Nicoladoni Method, Vestnik khir. **55**: 626-629, 1938.
Esser, J. F. S., and Ranschburg, P.: Reconstruction of a Hand and Four Fingers by Transplantation of the Middle part of the Foot and Four Toes, Ann. Surg. **111**: 655-659, 1940.
Gillies, Harold: Autograft of Amputated Digit; A Suggested Operation, Lancet **1**: 1002-1003, 1940.
Gioia, T.: Phalangization of First Metacarpus to Substitute for Thumb, With Report of Case, Semana méd. **1**: 490-497, 1943.
Gordon, Stuart: Autograft of Amputated Thumb, Lancet **2**: 823, 1944.
Jones, R. M.: Successful Suture of Finger Flexor Tendon, Lancet **2**: 111, 1944.
Köster, K. H.: Plastic Operations in Loss of Thumb, Acta orthop. Scandinav. **9**: 115-131, 1938.
Kuslik, M. I.: Transplantation of a Toe According to the Method of Nicoladoni, Arch. Surg. **32**: 123-130, 1936
Labok, D. M.: Simultaneous Osteocutaneous Graft in Reconstruction of the Thumb, Khirurgiya **2**: 73-75, 1944.
Meyer-Wildisen, R.: Plastic Surgery to Restore Function After Loss of Thumb, Helvet. med. acta **6**: 872-873, 1940.
Neuhof, H.: Transplantation of Toe for Missing Finger; End-Result, Ann. Surg. **112**: 291-293, 1940.
Novitskiy, S. T.: Total Transplantation of Large Toe to Replace Thumb, Vestnik khir. **57**: 352-361, 1939.
Palmstierna, K.: Plastic Surgery of the Thumb, Nord. med. (Hygiea) **1**: 243-244, 1939.
Parin, B. V.: Restoration of Lost Fingers, Trudy Molotovsk. gos. med. Inst. **21**: 125-142, 1942.
Petersen, N.: Plastic Reconstruction of the Thumb, South African M. J. **17**: 137-138, 1943.
Shirokov, B. A.: Phalangization of First Metacarpal Bone in Plastic Restoration of Thumb; Anatomic Basis of Author's Method, Khirurgiya **7**: 115-122, 1939.
Soraluce, J. A.: Transplantation of Large Toe to Replace Thumb; Case, Semana méd. españ. **3**: 81-84, 1940.
Wittek, A.: Successful Substitution of Second Metacarpal Bone for Missing Thumb; Case. Chirurg **13**: 577-581, 1941.

TYPHOID OSTEOMYELITIS OF THE RIBS TREATED WITH STREPTOMYCIN AND SURGICAL EXCISION

A Case Report

HENRY P. ROYSTER, M.D., CHARLES K. KIRBY, M.D., AND ROBERT G. WILBUR, M.D., PHILADELPHIA, PA.

(From the Surgical Clinic of the Hospital of the University of Pennsylvania and the Harrison Department of Surgical Research, Schools of Medicine, University of Pennsylvania)

STREPTOMYCIN has been shown to be of great value in the treatment of certain infections, while in others its effectiveness is still in doubt.[1, 2] The sensitivity of many gram-negative bacilli to this new antibiotic has led to the hope that it will be useful in controlling typhoid infections. In vitro, *Eberthella typhi* is sensitive to concentrations of streptomycin readily obtained in the blood stream of patients receiving divided doses of 2,000,000 to 3,000,000 units daily.[3, 4] In some studies there has appeared to be definite improvement in patients with acute typhoid fever while in others the evidence of benefit is not clear cut.[1, 5] Streptomycin has had only a transient effect in reducing the number of organisms in typhoid carriers,[6, 7] and its use in other typhoid sequelae has not been reported.

Typhoid osteomyelitis is now rarely seen although Murphy,[7] in 1919, found that it occurred in nearly 0.82 per cent of 18,840 cases of typhoid fever. It has long been recognized[8] that typhoid bacilli may remain in the bones for many years before clinical evidence of osteomyelitis is present. In the typhoid era surgeons found that only radical operations were effective in controlling this lesion.

CASE REPORT

W. K., a white man, 73 years of age, was admitted to the Hospital of the University of Pennsylvania on Oct. 24, 1946. Chief complaint was a draining sinus in the right anterior part of the chest wall. The onset of the illness was in September, 1944, when the patient became ill with what was proved to be typhoid fever. His wife, who was discovered to be a carrier, was presumably the source of infection. The acute illness, with high fever, anorexia, and weight loss, lasted for two months, and he recovered sufficiently so that he considered himself to be in normal health. In late November, 1944, he noticed that there was a tender swelling over the anterior surface of the lower right part of the chest which gradually increased in size and became fluctuant. His physician aspirated this and obtained pus, which on culture was positive for *E. typhi.* A roentgenogram of the affected area showed no evidence of bone or lung involvement.

Since this lesion did not regress under conservative measures, the patient was then operated upon in another hospital. An incision was made over the right lower part of the chest and pus was drained. The distal ends of ribs eight, nine, and ten were exposed, and several necrotic fragments of bone were removed. The wound was packed and partially closed.

Subsequent to this operation the wound did not heal, and he was admitted to the same hospital one year later, in April, 1946. Through an incision in the same area more bone

Received for publication, April 28, 1947.

was resected, and a portion of the adjacent sternum, which had apparently been infected, was curetted. During this operation the chest cavity was accidentally entered. The wound was packed open as before. The patient was very ill following this operation, but he was soon convalescent. However, the wound did not heal, and it was still draining on admission to this hospital. There had been no cough, hemoptysis, or other evidence of pulmonary disease.

Physical examination disclosed a well-nourished man of about 73 years whose only significant findings were confined to the right lower anterior part of the chest. At the level of the anterior portion of the seventh rib there was a transversely placed sinus 6 cm. in length discharging yellowish-white pus. Immediately superior and medial was another small sinus. There were signs of underlying thickened pleura. A probe could be passed through the larger sinus medially and posteriorly for 4 cm.

Laboratory examinations were as follows: Hemoglobin, 72 per cent; white blood cells, 10,000. Urinalysis was negative. Culture of the wound yielded hemolytic *Staphylococcus aureus* and *E. typhi.* The nature of the *E. typhi* strain was further confirmed by the agglutination reaction. The Widal test was positive for *typhoid H* in a dilution of 1:640. Roentgen examination revealed that there were bands of adhesions and thickened pleura in the right costophrenic sinus. Lipiodol injection of the sinus showed no communication with the lung. Stool and urine cultures were negative for *E. typhi,* and on this organism streptomycin sensitivity tests showed that inhibition took place at concentrations of from 0.5 to 5.0 units per cubic centimeter. A culture taken from tissue at the time of operation after five days of streptomycin therapy was positive for *E. typhi.*

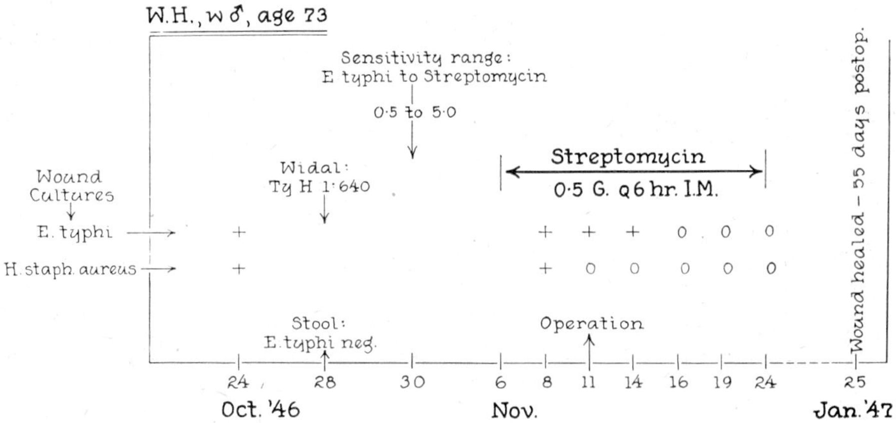

Fig. 1.—Protocol of patient with typhoid osteomyelitis of the chest wall.

Course.—Streptomycin administration was begun on Nov. 6, 1946, five days before operation and continued until Nov. 23, 1946, thirteen days after operation. One-half gram of the drug was given every six hours intramuscularly, and the total amount was 36.0 Gm., or 36,000,000 units, injected over a period of eighteen days. On Nov. 11, 1946, eighteen days after admission, extensive resection of the diseased area in the right lower chest wall was performed. The draining sinuses and associated scar were completely excised through a long transverse incision and a shorter vertical one in the form of a "T" placed parallel with and adjacent to the sternum. The costal cartilages and anterior bony ends of ribs five to ten, inclusive, were excised. The right lateral margin of the sternum was also resected, along with the upper portion of the rectus sheath. An en bloc dissection was carried out, and normal tissue surfaces remained in the wound everywhere except at the center where thickened pleura attached to the lung was only partially removed. The entire cavity was packed with iodoform gauze and the skin edges approximated except for two openings where the ends of the packing protruded. Considerable bleeding took place, estimated at over 500 c.c., and this was replaced by blood transfusion during the procedure.

The postoperative course was satisfactory. The wound drained a large amount of serosanguineous material, and the packing was completely changed on the fifth day after operation. On Nov. 20, 1946, nine days postoperatively, enough granulations had appeared to make packing unnecessary. At this time the wound was free of pus and necrotic tissue. Cultures of the wound showed that *E. typhi* had disappeared by the fifth postoperative day and had not returned up to the day of discharge, November 24, thirteen days after operation.

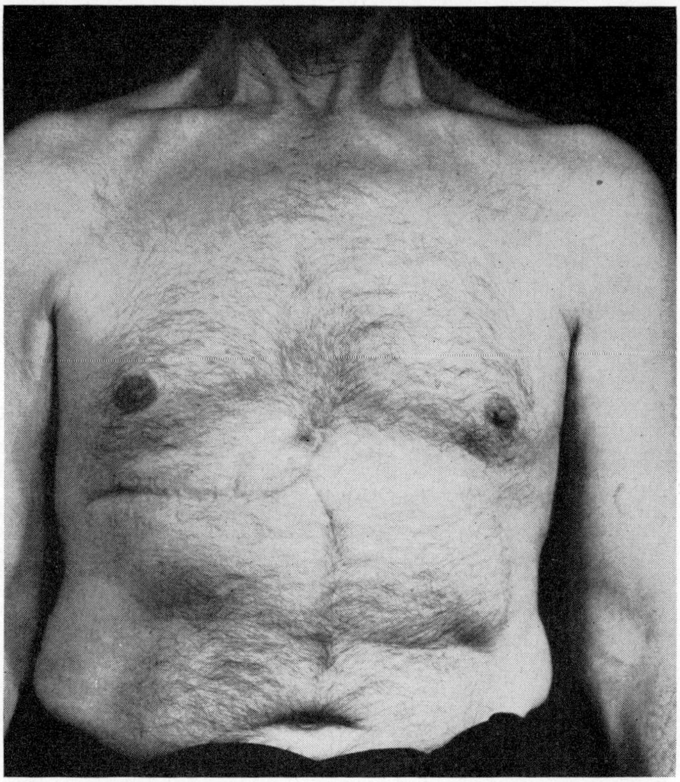

Fig. 2.—Patient W. H., with typhoid osteomyelitis of right anterior part of chest wall. End result five months after radical operation and streptomycin therapy.

The patient was followed in the outpatient clinic at intervals for redressing, and it was noted that the wound had healed over completely by Jan. 5, 1947, fifty-five days after operation. By April, the wound had remained closed for three months, and the patient was entirely asymptomatic.

COMMENT

Keen,[9] in reviewing his extensive experience with typhoid fever and its sequelae, concluded that "the tendency to chronicity, to persistent sinuses and especially to recurrences, are among the most marked characteristics of bone disorders following typhoid."

The sensitivity to streptomycin of the typhoid bacillus isolated from this patient suggested that the likelihood of cure following operation might be enhanced by the use of streptomycin, as in the use of penicillin for staphylococcal osteomyelitis.[10] Because of the chronicity of this lesion and the presence of sequestra and fibrosis, cure or marked improvement was not expected with streptomycin alone. During the five-day interval of streptomycin therapy before operation there was no change in the quantity or quality of the purulent wound drainage, and typhoid bacilli were cultured from the chest wall.

SUMMARY

1. Streptomycin may be a valuable adjunct to the surgical treatment of typhoid osteomyelitis.

2. The use of streptomycin in one patient with typhoid osteomyelitis suggests that it will not replace adequate excision, just as penicillin does not replace surgery in the treatment of staphylococcal osteomyelitis.

REFERENCES

1. Keefer, C. S., Blake, F. G., Lockwood, J. S., Long, P. H., Marshall, E. K., Jr., and Wood, W. B., Jr.: Streptomycin in the Treatment of Infections, J. A. M. A. **132**: 4, 1946.
2. Nichols, D. R., and Herrell, W. E.: Streptomycin, Its Clinical Uses and Limitations, J. A. M. A. **132**: 200, 1946.
3. Robinson, H. J., Smith, D. G., and Graessle, O. E.: Chemotherapeutic Properties of Streptomycin, Proc. Soc. Exper. Biol. & Med. **57**: 226, 1944.
4. Zintel, H. A., Flippin, H. F., Nichols, A. C., Wiley, M. M., and Rhoads, J. E.: Studies on Streptomycin in Man. I. Absorption, Distribution, Excretion and Toxicity, Am. J. M. Sc. **210**: 421, 1945.
5. Reiman, H. A., Elias, W. F., and Price, A. H.: Streptomycin for Typhoid: A Pharmacologic Study, J. A. M. A. **128**: 175, 1945.
6. Rutstein, D. D., Stebbins, R. B., Cathcart, R. T., and Harvey, R. M.: The Absorption and Excretion of Streptomycin in Human Typhoid Carriers, J. Clin. Investigation **24**: 898, 1945.
7. Murphy, J. B.: Bone and Joint Disease in Relation to Typhoid Fever, Surg., Gynec. & Obst. **23**: 119, 1916.
8. Winslow, N.: Typhoidal Osteomyelitis, Ann. Surg. **77**: 319, 1923.
9. Keen, W. W.: Surgical Complications and Sequels of Typhoid Fever, Philadelphia, 1888, W. B. Saunders Company.
10. Lockwood, J. S., White, W. L., and Murphy, F. D.: The Use of Penicillin in Surgical Infections, Ann. Surg. **120**: 311, 1944.

EXPERIMENTAL OBSERVATIONS IN THE TREATMENT OF CRANIOSYNOSTOSIS

FRANC D. INGRAHAM, M.D., DONALD D. MATSON, M.D., AND EBEN ALEXANDER, JR., M.D., BOSTON, MASS.

(From the Department of Surgery, Harvard Medical School, and the Neurosurgical Service, The Children's Hospital)

INTRODUCTION

ANY abnormality, whether congenital or acquired, which interferes with unrestricted growth of the human brain during the first years of life, results in corresponding interference with the neurologic functions which are elaborated during the same period. A large group of clinical entities has been described, exhibiting varying degrees of cranial deformity, amblyopia, and mental deficiency, whose common underlying pathology is restriction of normal brain growth due to premature fusion of the cranial sutures. These bony lesions may be grouped together under the term "craniosynostosis." Although the etiology of this condition is poorly understood,[1-3] the actual pathologic physiology, as a primary mechanical disturbance of cranial growth with secondary compression or distortion of the central nervous system, is generally recognized.

In the normal human skull, the separate bones of the calvarium begin to fuse with one another in the third and fourth decades of life and are usually not completely fused until the seventh or eighth decades. Normally, only the suture between the two frontal bones (metopic) fuses before birth or during the first few years of life. Occasionally this suture persists for a longer period, but as such is of no clinical significance.

In craniosynostosis, one or more of the sutures becomes prematurely obliterated, due presumably to some inherent mesenchymal defect rather than to any known pre- or postnatal disease process. The coronal and sagittal sutures are the most frequently involved and are of greatest clinical significance.

This abnormal fusion may occur before birth or during the first months of life. During the first six months the brain normally increases about 85 per cent in weight, and during the first year about 135 per cent.[4, 5] In the first six months more than 40 per cent, and during the first year more than one-half, of all postnatal increase in the circumference of the skull normally occurs.[5] It is during this first year of life, therefore, that unrestricted growth is particularly important.

TREATMENT

Craniosynostosis, because of its mechanical nature and apparent lack of primary pathology in the nervous system, suggests itself as a favorable and challenging lesion for surgical therapy. A number of different surgical procedures have been attempted to relieve the constriction caused by premature synostosis. Linear craniectomy,[6, 7] subtemporal decompression on one or both

Received for publication, May 15, 1947.

sides,[8, 9, 10] elevation of large bone flaps on one or both sides,[11] removal of plaques of bone,[12] creation of artificial sutures,[13] and "morcellation" of the entire calvarium above the cerebellar region[14, 15, 16] have all been employed. These operations have met with a certain amount of success in the relief of intracranial pressure and probable preservation of function in older children. However, during the first months of life these procedures would appear to be unsatisfactory because of the extremely rapid regrowth of bone which fuses artificially created defects at this age.

If unrestricted growth of the brain for an adequate length of time is to be insured in infants with craniosynostosis, repeated decompression or repeated creation of artificial sutures must be carried out. It has seemed desirable, therefore, to devise a method of producing artificial channels similar in distribution to the normal sutures which have prematurely fused, in which fusion could safely be delayed or indefinitely prevented. Such a means would then sustain during continued growth the immediate decompression obtained at the time of operation.

Theoretically, at least, one should attempt to reproduce as nearly as possible the normal pattern of growth. The possibility, therefore, of creating artificial sagittal and coronal sutures and preventing their subsequent closure for prolonged periods and perhaps indefinitely has commanded our attention. Since new bone arises from the outer layers of the dura as well as from the periosteum and eventually fills in any defect in the calvarium of young infants, it would appear necessary to introduce some substance between the margins of an artificially created suture, which would either delay this regeneration or prevent solid union of the new and old bone.

Any form of living tissue introduced into the gap could lead to formation of scar tissue, with resultant solid fibrous union, in which new bone formation could follow the invasion of osteoblasts from the bone margins. It seemed more profitable to investigate the possibility of introducing an inert foreign substance which would mechanically prevent the closure of such an artificial suture. Such a foreign substance should be well tolerated by bone as well as by dura and scalp; it should be light, suitable for sterilization, easily shaped, and resistant to undesirable physical or chemical changes when buried in the body.

EXPERIMENTAL INVESTIGATIONS

The problem first approached in the laboratory was to study the reaction of inert foreign substances placed between the margins of artificially created channels in the cranium. The following substances were investigated:

1. Fibrin film (obtained from the fractionation of human blood plasma)
2. Oxidized cellulose gauze (Oxycel)
3. Tantalum
4. Methyl methacrylate (Lucite)
5. Polyethylene (Polythene)

Observations on eleven dogs and sixteen monkeys are included in this study. Most of these animals were used for other experimental procedures as well, but in no instance did the other experiments involve the cranium or its contents. Employing aseptic technique, midline incisions under intravenous nembutal were made, and the scalp was reflected to expose the vertex. Burr holes were made in the frontal region and in the postparietal region, approximately 1.5 cm. to either side of the midline. The frontal and postparietal burr holes on each side were connected by an ordinary saw cut, made with a standard Gigli saw. The saw cuts averaged 2.5 to 3.0 cm. in length. The edges of the saw cut were trimmed to right angles, by removing any roughened edges of bone with a sharp scalpel. This resulted in a gap averaging 2 mm. in width. Bone wax was used sparingly to control bleeding. Drill holes were made with a 1 mm. dental drill about 3 mm. from the lateral edge of the saw cut for the

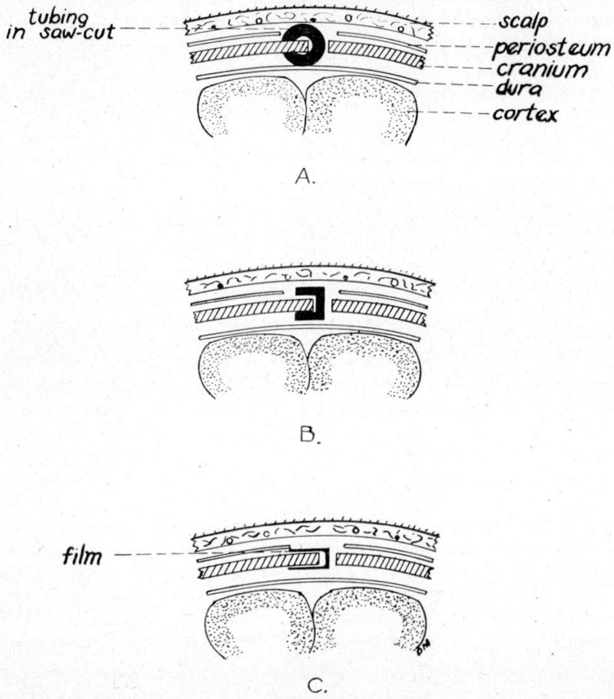

Fig. 1.—Schematic cross-section representation of the methods used to implant inert foreign substances into artificial sutures in the cranium of experimental animals. *A*, Tubing (polyethylene, fibrin film) inserted over bony margin of the saw cut; *B*, "U"-shaped insert (tantalum, Lucite); *C*, thin plastic film (polyethylene).

passage of 4-0 silk sutures. Two sutures were used in each case to hold whatever substance was introduced in the saw cut in position. On the right side of each animal, one of the substances just listed was introduced into the gap. On the left side, a saw cut of similar length and width was made in a similar location as a control (Figs. 1 and 2). The dura was not opened in any instance.

The monkeys were all small adults *(Macacus rhesus)* in good health with the exception of two animals who died early, presumably of tuberculosis. Among the monkeys there was no postoperative infection. Among the dogs there were two instances of superficial wound infection. Both adult and very young dogs were used. Specimens were studied at intervals varying from 32 up to 315 days. Observations of the gross appearance of the foreign substance, the bone, overlying scalp, and underlying dura were made at the time of death or sacrifice in each case. Histologic studies were made of cross sections through the saw cuts containing each type of substance and through selected controls.

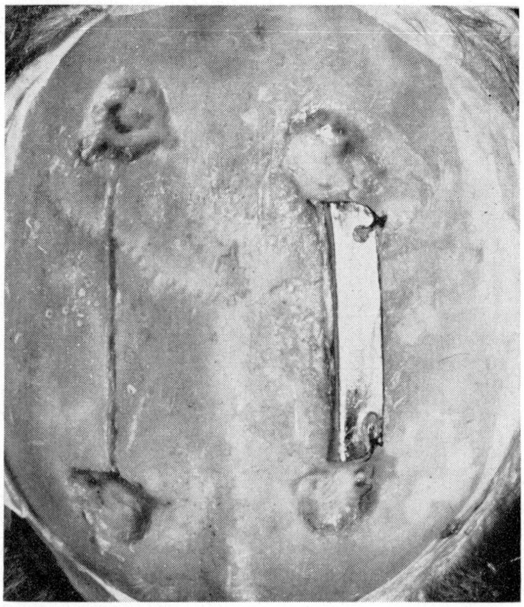

Fig. 2 (Monkey 57).—Appearance of the cranium thirty-nine days after insertion of a piece of tantalum over one margin of a saw cut. There is no evidence of new-bone growth or foreign body reaction. This figure illustrates the manner in which various inert substances were implanted in artificial cranial channels. Control saw cut is shown on the left.

RESULTS

Controls.—In the monkeys, the control saw cuts showed bony fusion in all those examined after 100 days. Of those examined before 100 days, one at thirty-nine days showed no bony fusion; one at seventy-five days showed complete closure, and another at ninety-one days showed only partial bony union. The remaining thirteen control specimens, ranging from 114 to 315 days, showed solid bony healing. Microscopic examination of the control saw cuts was made in several instances. Illustration of the healing in 114 days is shown in Fig. 3.

In the dogs, control specimens were examined at periods varying from 32 to 118 days. In every instance there was bony healing across the control saw cut. In young puppies the healing was particularly rapid. In most instances, in both the dogs and the monkeys, the burr holes also were partially or completely bridged by thin layers of new bone in specimens examined after 100 days.

Fibrin Film.—Fibrin film, made from pure fibrin derived from the fractionation of human blood plasma, has been shown by Ingraham, Bailey, and Cobb[17] to be well tolerated in experimental animals and in human patients.

They also demonstrated that this film was eventually completely absorbed. The possibility of delaying the closure of artificial sutures by interposing several thicknesses of fibrin film was therefore examined. Tubes were made by wrapping the fibrin film around glass rods of various sizes under sterile conditions. The wall of the tubing varied in thickness according to the number of layers of wrapping, usually 1 to 2 mm. At operation the tube was slit longitudinally and slipped over one margin of the saw cut, as shown in Fig. 1, *A*. It was held in position by two silk sutures, as previously noted. Fibrin film was implanted in this manner in three monkeys, and the specimens examined after 207, 209, and 257 days.

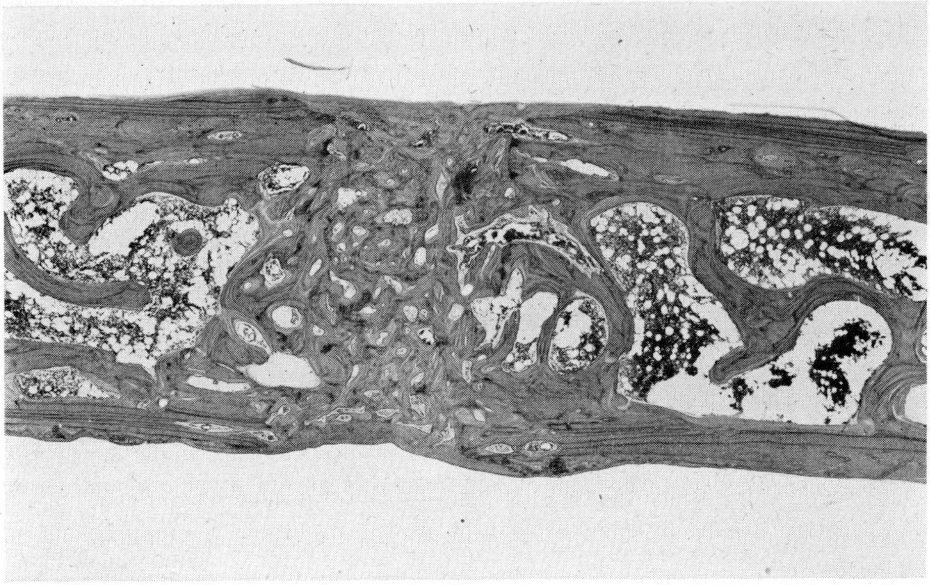

Fig. 3 (Monkey 53).—Low-power photomicrograph (×20) of cross section through control saw cut at 114 days. Solid fusion by dense new-bone formation across the gap has taken place.

In each instance there was no evidence of fluid and no gross evidence of foreign body reaction at the time of sacrifice. No trace of the fibrin film could be made out. In one of the specimens—that examined in 209 days—the saw cut was bridged by bone which was very thin compared to the new bone bridging the control saw cut. In the other two specimens, solid bony union of the saw cuts was present, no difference between this side and the control saw cut being discernible grossly.

Microscopic sections revealed no trace of the fibrin film. No evidence of foreign body giant cells or round-cell infiltration could be made out. The gap between the cut edges of the bone was filled with dense fibrous tissue in which osteoid tissue and new bone had formed (Fig. 4).

Conclusion.—Although several layers of fibrin film introduced into a saw cut possibly produced slight delay in bony union as compared with the control saw cut, there was essentially no difference at the end of six to seven months. There was no unusual tissue reaction to the fibrin film.

Oxidized Cellulose Gauze.—Frantz and Lattes[18, 19] found that Oxycel—oxidized cellulose gauze—introduced experimentally into fracture sites in long bones prevented or markedly delayed callus formation; this occurred only when the gauze was soaked with blood when it was inserted, not when it was dry. Because of this finding, it was thought desirable to test this substance in artificial saw cuts in the cranium. Consequently, blood-soaked Oxycel was introduced into the gap of saw cuts made in the cranium of four puppies. These specimens were examined in forty-two to forty-four days. At this time no gross evidence of residual Oxycel could be demonstrated. There was no gross inflammatory or unusual foreign body reaction demonstrable. There appeared to be solid fibrous union, which was grossly as strong as the early bony fusion on the control side.

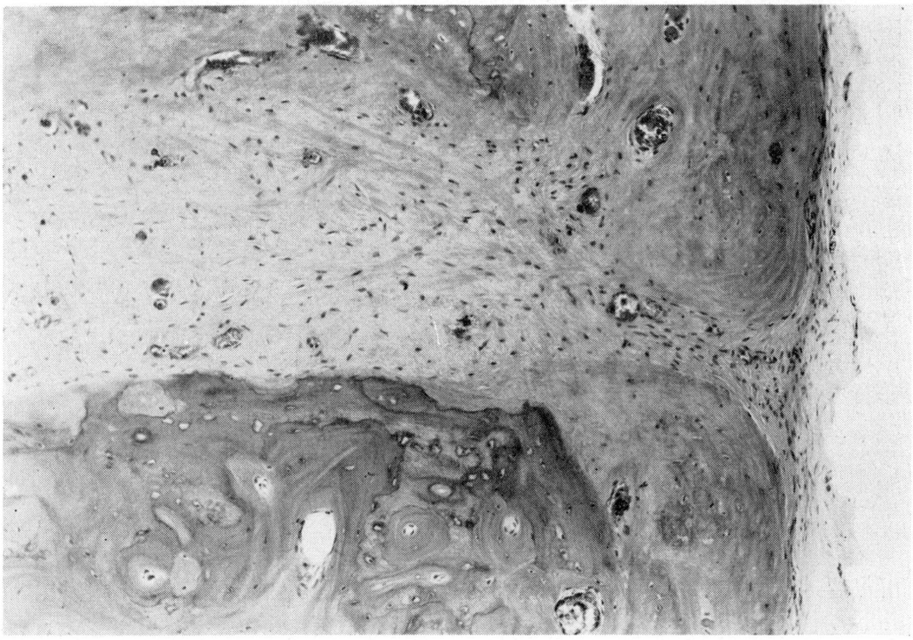

Fig. 4 (Monkey 58).—Photomicrograph of the periosteal margin of a cranial saw cut 207 days after insertion of several layers of fibrin film showing osteoid tissue invading the dense fibrous tissue in the gap. No trace of the fibrin film remains.

Microscopic sections showed the gap between the margins of the bone filled with dense fibrous tissue. Occasional small spaces which had been occupied by Oxycel were still present, and adjacent to them foreign body giant cells, young fibroblasts, and new capillaries could be found (Fig. 5).

Conclusion.—Because of the early dense fibrous healing across the saw cut, almost as rapid as that seen in the controls of the same length of time, it was felt that further experimentation with this substance as a material for delaying closure of artificial sutures was not indicated.

Tantalum.—The element tantalum has received an ever-increasing use in surgery during the past decade. During World War II, its application in the closure of cranial defects was developed into a standard, widely employed procedure. Its inertness in the body, and particularly its tolerance by bone, has been well established.[20, 21, 22] Tantalum can be formed in thin sheets which are malleable, but difficult to shape easily at the operating table. Tantalum is a heavy substance, opaque to x-ray, and expensive.

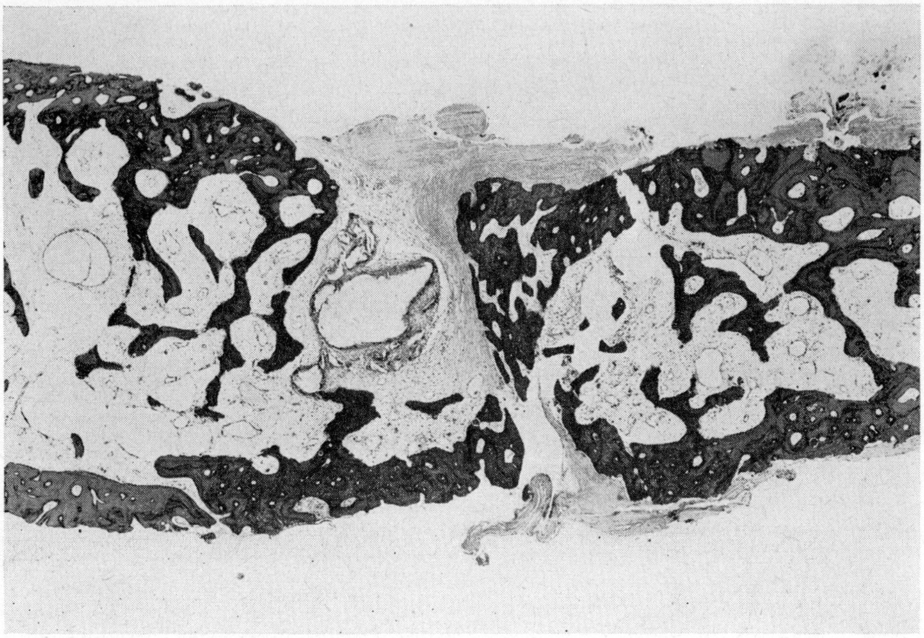

Fig. 5 (Dog 141).—Low-power photomicrograph (×20) of cross section through saw cut forty-two days after implantation of blood-soaked oxidized cellulose gauze. In the middle of the gap between the bony margins a space is visible in which the remains of the oxidized gauze were located. Dense fibrous tissue has invaded the gap. Grossly, this fibrous union was as solid as the control on the opposite side of the cranium.

In five monkeys, tantalum was inserted into the gap between the margins of a cranial saw cut. A piece of tantalum plate .015 in. in thickness was used, fashioned in the shape of a "U," the arms of which were approximately 4 mm. in width, the base a little more than the thickness of the cranium, that is, approximately 3 mm. This U-shaped piece of tantalum was inserted over the lateral margin of the saw cut, in the manner shown in Figs. 1, *B* and 2. It was held in place with two silk sutures. Specimens were examined after 39, 75, 91, 248, and 289 days.

Gross examination of these specimens in every case revealed no evidence of infection or foreign body reaction. There was a thin, filmy, fibrous tissue envelope around the tantalum, which did not contain any fluid. The inner surface of this envelope was smooth and glistening. It extended between the tantalum and the bone, between the tantalum and the dura, and between the tantalum and the scalp. There was no evidence of new bone formation in this fibrous envelope.

Microscopic examination of cross sections through the saw cut after removal of the tantalum showed the thin, densely packed fibrous tissue membrane which completely surrounded the tantalum with a smooth, serosa-like inner surface adjacent to the metal (Fig. 6). Blood vessels were found in the deeper layers of the membrane. At the angles of the saw cut new bone formation had taken place, with many osteoblasts in evidence, but no evidence of any bone growing across the gap around the tantalum, either on the periosteal or dural surface (Fig. 7). It was noted that the membrane on the outer surface of the tantalum was thinner than that between the tantalum and the bone.

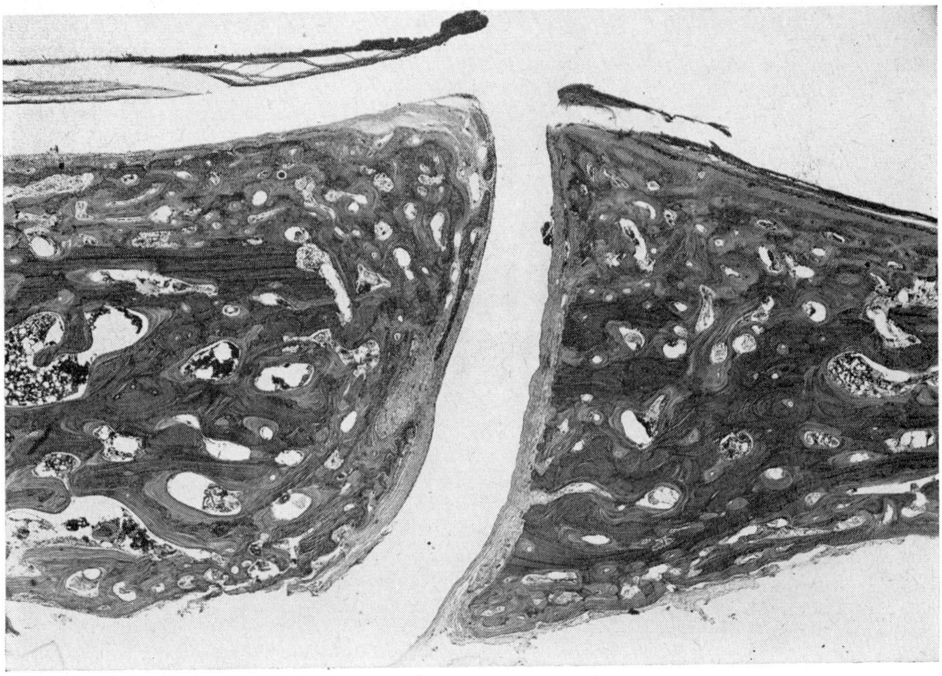

Fig. 6 (Monkey 59).—Low-power photomicrograph (×20) of cross section through saw cut in which a U-shaped piece of tantalum had been inserted over one margin 248 days previously. The fibrous tissue membrane between the bone ends and the site of the tantalum is easily visible. New bone formation at the margins of the saw cut has taken place but there is no invasion of the membrane over the tantalum.

Conclusion.—The tolerance of tantalum by bone and other tissues in the body has been confirmed. A nonadherent fibrous tissue envelope surrounded the metal. There was no attempt at new bone formation across the foreign body to bridge the saw cut. This substance would, therefore, seem suitable for permanent implantation. It is possible that the use of annealed tantalum foil might obviate some of the undesirable technical properties of tantalum plate. However, its weight and opacity to x-rays probably make tantalum a less desirable substance than others investigated.

Methyl Methacrylate (Acrylic Resin, Lucite, Plexiglas).—Methyl methacrylate, a synthetic plastic, has been shown, like tantalum, to be well tolerated in the tissues of human patients and experimental animals.[22-29] It has been used largely in the making of dental prostheses, and more recently in cranioplasty and other conditions where a rigid substance was required for burial within the body. Methyl methacrylate is a transparent, hard substance, which can be cast into desired forms. It can subsequently be molded to a slight degree by heating to temperatures just below that of boiling water. However, it is difficult to manipulate to any considerable degree once it has been cast in a given shape. It is light, nonopaque to x-rays, and relatively inexpensive. Its lack of undesirable reactions in contact with bone has been demonstrated repeatedly, as pointed out by Woolf and Walker.[22]

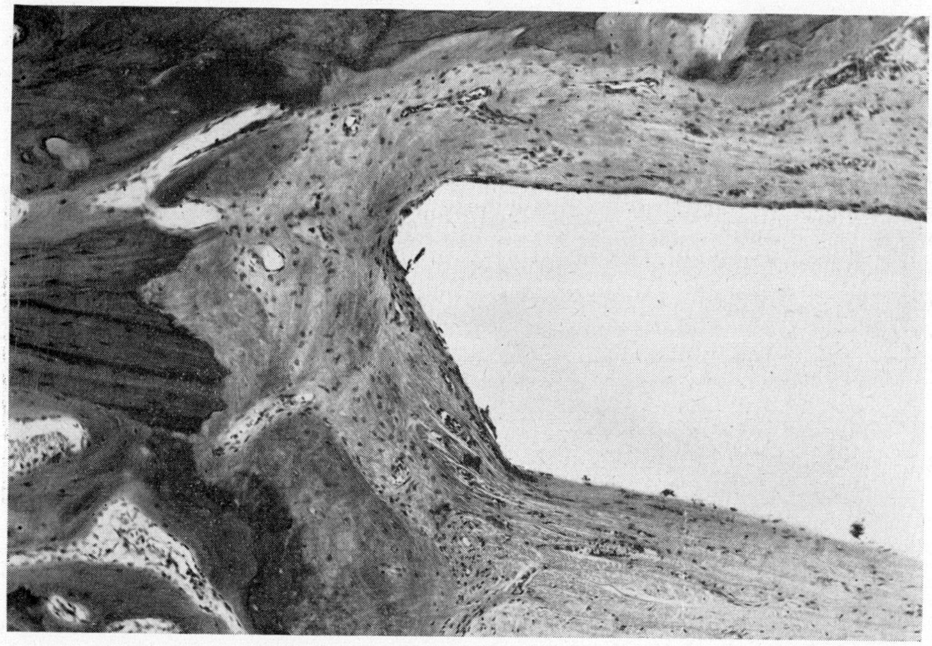

Fig. 7 (Monkey 59).—High-power photomicrograph at the edge of a tantalum implant after 248 days. Note the presence of osteoid tissue adjacent to the old bone. This has been laid down in the outer layers of the dense fibrous tissue membrane surrounding the tantalum.

U-shaped pieces of Lucite were fashioned, with the arms of the "U" 4 to 5 mm. in width and the base a little more than the thickness of the cranium in the monkey, that is, 3 to 4 mm. The Lucite itself was about 1.5 mm. in thickness. These U-shaped pieces of Lucite were dipped in water just below the boiling point at the operating table and bent slightly to conform to the contour of the skull. They were then inserted over the lateral margin of the saw cut, as illustrated in Fig. 1, *B*. The plastic was held in place with two silk sutures. Lucite was inserted in this manner in two monkeys, and the specimens were examined in 172 and 188 days.

There was no gross evidence of inflammatory or foreign body reaction adjacent to this plastic. It was enclosed in a fibrous tissue envelope of about the same thickness as that surrounding tantalum. There was no fluid in the envelope. The surface of the membrane adjacent to the plastic was nonadherent, smooth, and glistening. There was no invasion of the fibrous tissue membrane around the plastic by new bone, either on the periosteal or dural surface. Therefore, no bridging of the artificial gap had resulted.

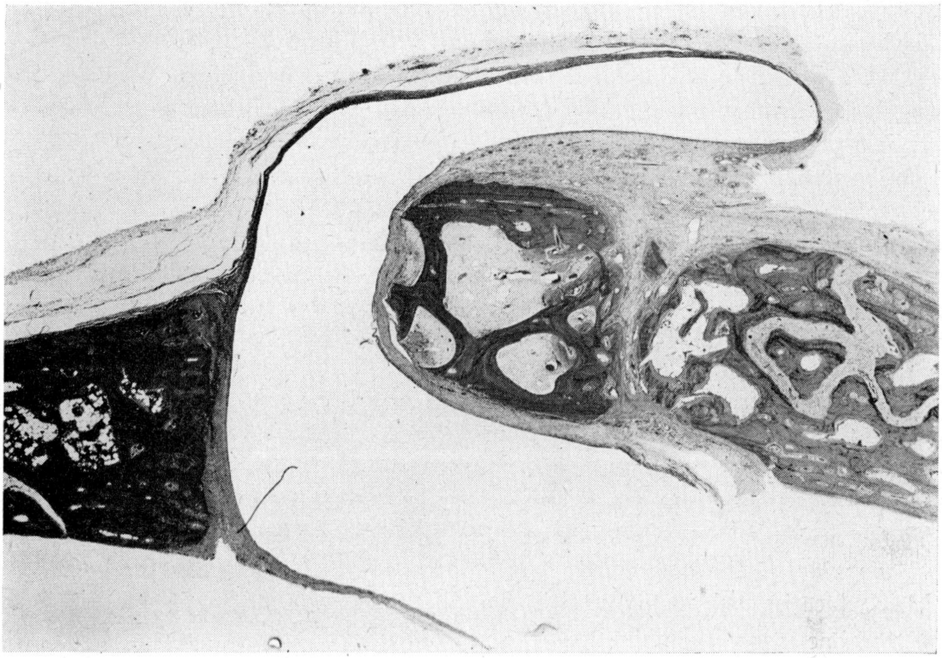

Fig. 8 (Monkey 67).—Low-power photomicrograph (×20) of cross section through cranial saw cut in which a U-shaped piece of methyl methacrylate (Lucite) had been inserted 171 days previously. The fibrous tissue envelope surrounding the plastic is clearly visible. Dense fibrous tissue has invaded a drill hole through the bone on the right. A silk suture had been passed through this drill hole to hold the plastic in place.

Histologic examination of cross sections through the saw cut after removal of the Lucite revealed a well-defined dense fibrous tissue membrane completely enveloping the plastic in the saw cut. The border adjacent to the plastic had a smooth, even surface. There were small blood vessels in the deeper layers of the membrane. There was no evidence of round-cell infiltration and there were no foreign body giant cells adjacent to the plastic. The membrane was about twice as thick between the plastic and the bone as it was over the outer surface of the plastic. Small islands of new bone formation were seen underneath the membrane at the margins of the saw cut, but no attempt had been made to bridge the gap over the surface of the plastic, either on the dural or periosteal aspect (Fig. 8).

Conclusion.—The tolerance of methyl methacrylate by bone and other tissues of the body has been confirmed. No evidence of bony fusion across the plastic inserted in a saw cut occurred in six months' time. Lucite proved a difficult substance to mold into shapes suitable for this procedure, and it made a palpable swelling beneath the scalp. Because of its rigidity and brittleness, its applicability to placement over the margins of artificial sutures in very young, rapidly growing infants seems doubtful.

Polyethylene (Polythene).—Polyethylene is a pure synthetic plastic substance, a simple polymer of ethylene. It is a tough, thermoplastic resin, slightly cloudy in appearance, which is flexible, resistant to water, and chemically inert. It is light, resistant to temperature changes found within the body, and can be produced easily and inexpensively in flexible tubes and films of any desired size. Its tolerance by the body when buried in the central nervous system or over its surface has been reported by Ingraham, Alexander, and Matson.[26, 30] It can be sterilized by boiling, in which case it retains the shape assumed during the process of boiling, or by immersion in 1:1000 solution of Zephiran for periods of eighteen hours or longer. It cannot be autoclaved. Preliminary experiments with this material seemed to indicate that it would be a particularly suitable substance to introduce into artificial sutures to delay bony healing indefinitely; therefore, it was implanted in cranial saw cuts in seven dogs and six monkeys.

Tubes of pure polyethylene with a wall thickness of 1 mm. were slit longitudinally and inserted over the lateral edge of a saw cut in six monkeys and four dogs, as shown in Fig. 1, *A*. The plastic was held in position with two silk sutures. Polyethylene film, 0.020 in. in thickness, was used over one margin of a saw cut in two puppies (Figs. 1, *C* and 9) and it was placed over both margins of the saw cut in one puppy. The polyethylene film was also held in place in each instance with two silk sutures.

Specimens were examined after the following number of days: 32, 42, 45, 68, 70, 113, 114, 115, 118, 199, 268, 292, and 315. With the exception of one puppy, who suffered a superficial postoperative wound infection, there was no gross evidence of inflammatory or unusual foreign body reaction around the plastic material. The plastic in every case was enveloped by a thin fibrous tissue membrane which was somewhat thicker in specimens older than 100 days than in those examined earlier. In every case the membrane was nonadherent to the plastic, and its surface was smooth and glistening. There were no fluid collections in these fibrous envelopes around the plastic material. The bone edge adjacent to the plastic appeared eburnated and smooth, as shown in Fig. 10. The bone edges adjacent to the plastic were movable to a slight degree, as if a false joint had been formed. In one of the puppies, new bone formation had occurred across the periosteal surface of the film at one end of the saw cut. This was nonadherent to the plastic and had not united with bone on the opposite side, so that there was no actual bony fusion across the artificially created suture. Presumably, this bone grew from periosteum back of the edge of the plastic. There was no new bone formation underneath the plastic where the periosteum had been removed. There was no new bone formation in this case or in any other, on the dural surface.

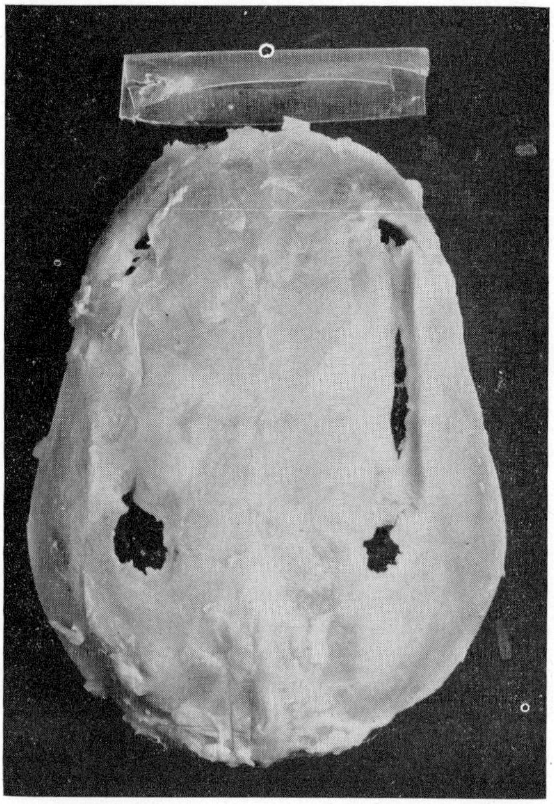

Fig. 9 (Dog 144).—Appearance of calvarium thirty-two days after insertion of polyethylene film in saw cut of a young puppy. On the left the control saw cut has already healed solidly. The piece of film has been removed from the saw cut on the right. There was no attempt at new-bone formation bridging the plastic.

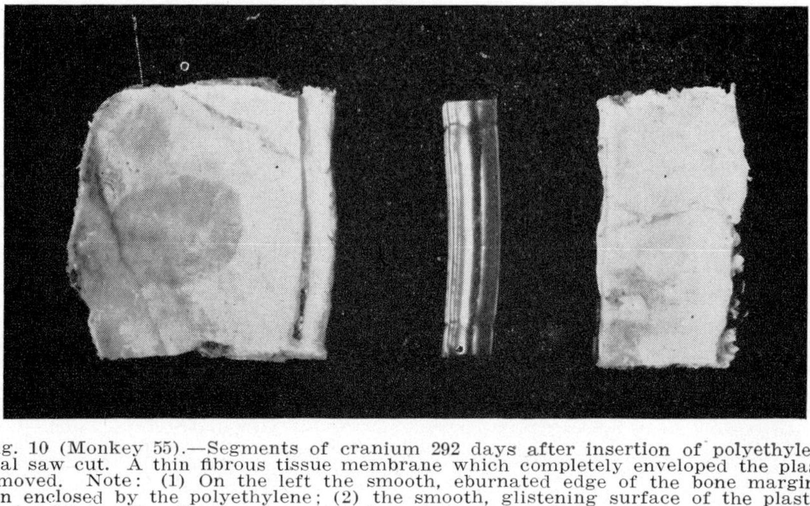

Fig. 10 (Monkey 55).—Segments of cranium 292 days after insertion of polyethylene tube in cranial saw cut. A thin fibrous tissue membrane which completely enveloped the plastic has been removed. Note: (1) On the left the smooth, eburnated edge of the bone margin which had been enclosed by the polyethylene; (2) the smooth, glistening surface of the plastic after being buried 9½ months. There was no new-bone formation in the membrane around the plastic, either adjacent to the edges of the bone or on the pericranial or dural surface.

In one very young puppy, when the cranium was examined after 115 days, marked asymmetry in the growth of the skull was noted. The side where the polyethylene had been inserted in the saw cut was more than 1.5 cm. wider than the opposite half of the cranium at a corresponding point. Specimens of polyethylene removed after periods up to 315 days showed that the plastic had become slightly more translucent and slightly more rigid. However, the material appeared as tough as before, maintained its smooth glistening surface, and was still flexible (Fig. 10).

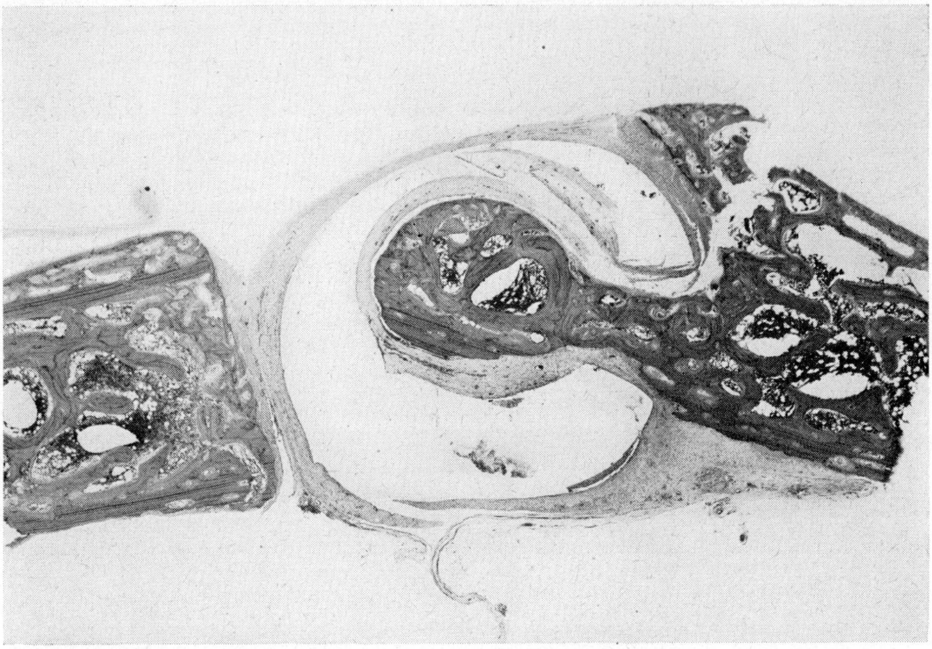

Fig. 11 (Monkey 53).—Low-power photomicrograph (×20) of cross section through the site of implantation of a section of polyethylene tubing over one margin of a saw cut in the parietal bone.

Note: (1) The fibrous tissue envelope completely surrounding the plastic; (2) the smooth, eburnated surface of the bone adjacent to the plastic, resulting in the formation of a false joint.

Histologic examinations of cross sections through the area of the saw cut after removal of the polyethylene were made. These showed that a fibrous tissue membrane enveloped the plastic tubing or film in every case, isolating it from the cut ends of the bone as well as from the dura beneath and the scalp above (Figs. 11 and 13). This fibrous tissue envelope did not contain fluid. It consisted of densely packed, longitudinally arranged fibroblasts. The surface adjacent to the plastic consisted of elongated, flattened cells, having the appearance of serosa. The deeper layers of the membrane contained small blood vessels. The membrane was considerably thicker between the plastic and the bone than on the outer surface of the plastic. The membrane surrounding the fairly thick-walled polyethylene tubing was considerably thicker than that surrounding the thin film. There was no invasion of this membrane ad-

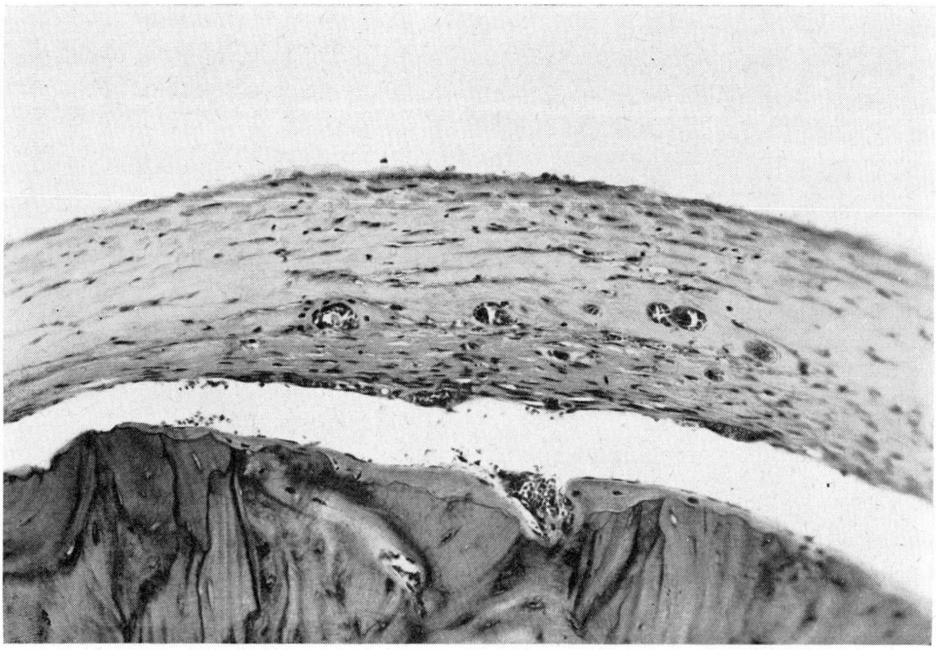

Fig. 12 (Monkey 53).—High-power photomicrograph of the membrane between the cut surface of bone and polyethylene tubing which was removed from the space at the upper margin of the picture. The compact arrangement of the fibrous tissue is evident. The complete lack of inflammatory or foreign body giant cells in the membrane adjacent to the plastic should be noted.

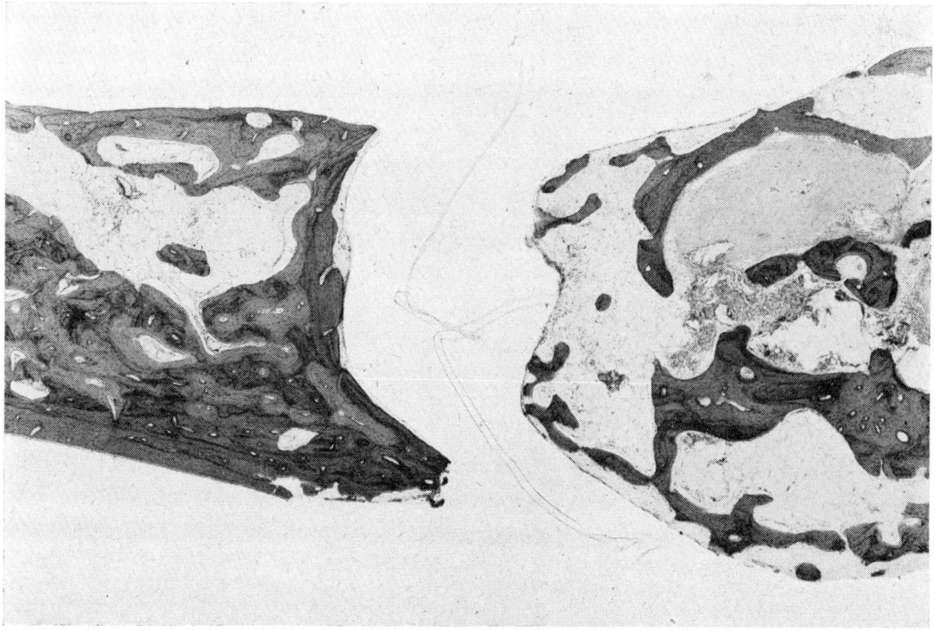

Fig. 13 (Dog 138).—Low-power photomicrograph (×20) of cross section through cranial saw cut in which may be seen a piece of polyethylene film which had been inserted 115 days previously. The thin filmy membrane which has formed over the cut surface of the bone is also visible. The dense fibrous tissue in the marrow at the right is adjacent to remnants of the silk suture passed through the bone at this point.

jacent to the plastic by inflammatory cells or foreign body giant cells (Figs. 12 and 14). The bone edges adjacent to the plastic, particularly the edge enclosed by the plastic tube, assumed a smooth, eburnated appearance; that is, dense bone similar to that of the inner and outer tables formed across the cut edge, in a smooth rounded pattern conforming to the inner surface of the plastic tubing (Figs. 11 and 12).

It is interesting to note that there was considerably more fibrous tissue reaction and cellular infiltration around the silk sutures used to hold the plastic in place than there was around the plastic itself. New bone did not grow into the fibrous envelope which surrounded the plastic, in any instance.

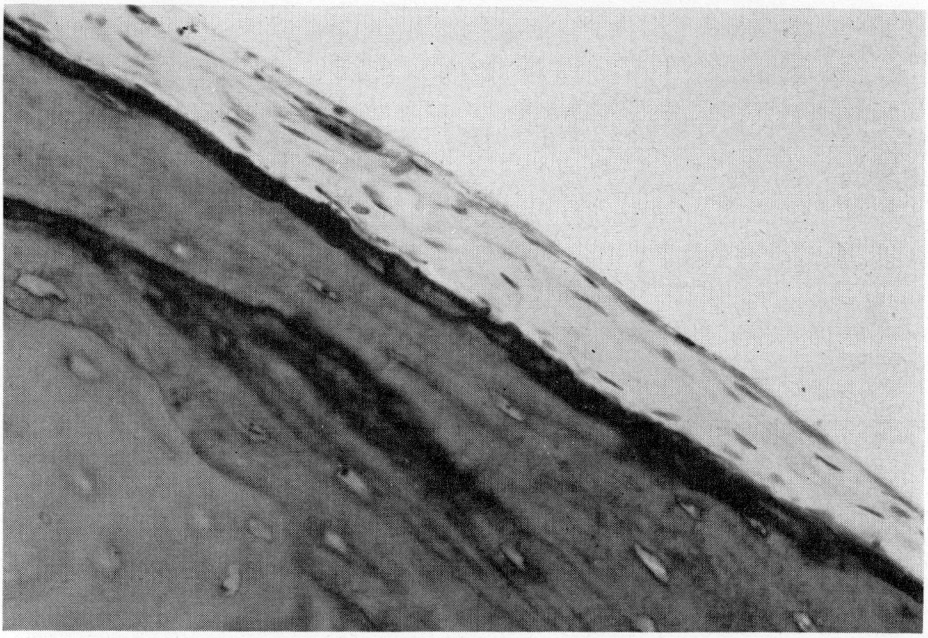

Fig. 14 (Dog 138).—High-power photomicrograph showing the character of the membrane which has formed between the cut surface of bone and a piece of .020 in. thick polyethylene film implanted 115 days previously.

Conclusion.—Polyethylene has proved a foreign substance which, because of its flexibility, transparency, and availability in various sizes of tubing and film, seems particularly adaptable technically to introduction into the gap of artificially made sutures in the cranium in order to inhibit bony healing. Its tolerance by the tissues is equal to that of tantalum and methyl methacrylate; its physical properties make it more suitable than either of these substances.

SUMMARY

1. Craniosynostosis is an obscure inherent mesenchymal defect in which premature closure of cranial sutures produces a variety of deformities of the head and results in mechanical restriction of normal brain growth during infancy.

2. It is particularly important during the first twelve months of life that expansion of the brain be allowed to proceed uninhibited if cerebral deficiency and blindness are to be avoided.

3. Because of the rapid regeneration of bone in this age group it seems desirable to devise a means of creating artificial sutures analogous to those which have fused prematurely and whose closure can be delayed indefinitely or permanently prevented.

4. The interposition of various foreign substances to accomplish this delayed closure of artificial cranial sutures has been investigated in dogs and monkeys. Fibrin film, oxidized cellulose gauze, tantalum, methyl methacrylate, and polyethylene were studied.

5. Of this group, the synthetic plastic, polyethylene, possesses the most desirable physical properties. It can be obtained and used as flexible hollow tubing or as a thin film. The latter form is more suitable for the application considered in this report. Polyethylene is well tolerated by bone and other body tissues. In periods up to nine and one-half months it remained physically inert in the body.

6. Preliminary observations of clinical trials of this method in six infants with craniosynostosis have been favorable. These will be reported in detail at a later date.

REFERENCES

1. Greig, D. M.: Oxycephaly, Edinburgh, M. J. **33**: 189, 280, 357, 1926.
2. Greene, H. S. N.: Oxycephaly and Allied Conditions in Man and in Rabbit, J. Exper. Med. **57**: 967, 1933.
3. Park, E. A., and Powers, G. F.: Acrocephaly and Scaphocephaly With Symmetrically Distributed Malformations of the Extremities, Am. J. Dis. Child. **20**: 235, 1920.
4. Coppoletta, J. M., and Wolbach, S. B.: Body Length and Organ Weights of Infants and Children. A Study of the Body Length and Normal Weights of the More Important Vital Organs of the Body Between Birth and Twelve Years of Age, Am. J. Path. **9**: 55, 1933.
5. Faber, H. K., and Towne, E. S.: Early Craniectomy as Preventive Measure in Oxycephaly and Allied Conditions With Special Reference to the Prevention of Blindness, Am. J. M. Sc. **173**: 701, 1927.
6. Bauer, K. H.: Die zirkuläre Kranitomie als Entlastungstrepanation bei drohender Turmschädelerblindung und bei nightokalisierbaren Hirngeschwülsten, Deutsche Ztschr. f. Chir. **237**: 402, 1932.
7. Lane, L. C.: Pioneer Craniectomy for Relief of Mental Imbecility Due to Premature Sutural Closure and Microcephalus, J. A. M. A. **18**: 49, 1892.
8. Bedell, A. J.: Oxycephalus: Report of Three Cases With Operation in One, J. A. M. A. **68**: 1979, 1917.
9. Bennett, A. E., Keegan, J. J., and Hunt, H. B.: Oxycephalus: Premature Synostosis of Cranial Sutures; Prevention of Blindness by Craniectomy and Decompression; Two Case Reports, J. Nerv. & Ment. Dis. **84**: 274, 1936.
10. Sharpe, W.: Oxycephaly, Cranial Deformity of, Operative Treatment. Case Reports, Am. J. M. Sc. **151**: 840, 1916.
11. Dandy, W. E.: Operation for Scaphocephaly, Arch. Surg. **47**: 247, 1943.
12. Patterson, H.: Oxycephaly. Unpublished observations.
13. Faber, H. K., and Towne, E. B.: Early Operation in Premature Cranial Synostosis for the Prevention of Blindness and Other Sequelae; Five Case Reports With Follow-up, J. Pediat. **22**: 286, 1943.
14. King, J. E. J.: Oxycephaly: A New Operation and its Results (A Preliminary Report), Arch. Neurol. & Psychiat. **40**: 1205, 1938.
15. King, J. E. J.: Oxycephaly (Surgical Therapy in Four Cases), Ann. Surg. **115**: 488, 1942.
16. Woodhall, B.: Oxycephaly: Results of Treatment by the King "Morcellation" Method, J. Pediat. **20**: 585, 1942.
17. Ingraham, F. D., Bailey, O. T., and Cobb, C. A., Jr.: The Use of Fibrin Film as a Dural Substitute, J. A. M. A. **128**: 1088, 1945.

18. Frantz, V. K., and Lattes, R.: Oxidized Cellulose-absorbable Gauze (Cellulosic Acid), J. A. M. A. **129**: 798, 1945.
19. Lattes, R., and Frantz, V. K.: Absorbable Gauze in Bone Surgery. Experimental Studies Suggesting Clinical Application in Reconstruction of Joints, Ann. Surg. **124**: 26, 1946.
20. Delarue, N. C., Linell, E. A., and McKenzie, K. G.: Experimental Study on the Use of Tantalum in the Subdural Space, J. Neurosurg. **1**: 239, 1944.
21. Woodhall, B., and Spurling, R. G.: Tantalum Cranioplasty for War Wounds of the Skull, Ann. Surg. **121**: 649, 1945.
22. Woolf, J. I., and Walker, A. E.: Cranioplasty; Collective Review, Internat. Abstr. Surg. **81**: 1, 1945.
23. Beck, D. J., Russell, D. S., Small, J. M., and Graham, M. P.: Implantation of Acrylic-resin Discs in Rabbits' Skulls, Brit. J. Surg. **33**: 83, 1945.
24. Elkins, C. W., and Cameron, J. E.: Cranioplasty With Acrylic Plates, J. Neurosurg. **3**: 199, 1946.
25. Harmon, P. H.: Methacrylate Resins in Surgery, Modern Plastics **20**: 56, 1942.
26. Ingraham, F. D., Alexander, E. Jr., and Matson, D. D.: Synthetic Plastic Materials in Surgery, New England J. Med. **236**: 362, 402, 1947.
27. Mackenzie, C. M., Sharpless, D. H., and Millard, P.: Tissue Reactions to Vitallium and Acrylic Implants, Northwest Med. **44**: 277, 1945.
28. Shelden, C. H., Pudenz, R. H., Restarski, J. S., and Craig, W. McK.: The Lucite Calvarium—a Method for Direct Observation of the Brain; the Surgical and Lucite Processing Technique, J. Neurosurg. **1**: 67, 1944.
29. Shoreston, J.: Primary Skull Closure With Acrylic Plates, Proc. Congress C. M. F. Army Surgeons, Rome, 1945, pp. 123-124.
30. Ingraham, F. D., Alexander, E. Jr., and Matson, D. D.: Polyethylene, a New Synthetic Plastic for Use in Surgery. Experimental Applications in Neurosurgery, J. A. M. A. **113**: 82, 1947.

CYST FORMATION AT THE OPERATIVE SITE FOLLOWING CEREBELLAR OPERATIONS (PSEUDOMENINGOCELE)

WILLIAM T. PEYTON, M.D., AND DONALD R. SIMMONS, M.D.
MINNEAPOLIS, MINN.

(From the Division of Neurosurgery, Department of Surgery, University of Minnesota Hospitals)

AN OCCASIONAL troublesome complication following operations for lesions in the posterior cranial fossa is the collection of a large amount of fluid under the occipital muscles at the operative site. In the last ten years, this complication has been present in fourteen patients who have had operations in the posterior fossa at the University of Minnesota Hospitals. The seriousness of this complication is illustrated by the fact that it caused a considerable increase in the period of hospitalization in most of these cases, and in three of them a second operation was performed because of the protrusion at the operative site. One patient died as a result of this complication. The results obtained by the use of a simple pressure dressing over the protruding area indicate that these protrusions may be treated quite successfully by this method.

A review of the literature from 1916 to 1946 reveals very few references to cyst formation at the operative site following intracranial surgery, but the fact that this complication has been occasionally mentioned indicates that it has been seen and recognized by others. Schloffer[1] in 1923 reported a case of meningioma of the right parietal area which was completely removed in two stages. Following removal of the tumor, there was a marked increase in the cerebrospinal fluid pressure which was relieved by periodic lumbar punctures with drainage of from 20 to 125 c.c. of cerebrospinal fluid during each puncture. There was marked protrusion of the scalp over the operative site which was reduced with each lumbar puncture. This protrusion persisted for a period of eight months following operation, but gradually disappeared. One year following the removal of the tumor this patient was perfectly well. The protrusion in this case did not follow a cerebellar exploration, as was true in our cases, but otherwise it was similar. Cushing apparently has made no direct mention of this problem, but that he was aware that such cyst formation followed cerebellar operations is evidenced by comments in at least two of his papers dealing with cerebellar tumors.[2, 3] In discussing the postoperative course of individual cases in these papers he mentioned several times that there was no protrusion at the operative site. Bucy[5] has reported that Cushing applied the term "pseudomeningocele" to this condition. Since the protrusion is apparently due to a collection of cerebrospinal fluid in a cystic cavity under the suboccipital muscles, this term seems appropriate for the condition and we have continued its use.

Pseudomeningoceles were present in fourteen of our patients who had cerebellar operations within the last ten years. In the group there were six cases

Received for publication, May 28, 1947.

of cystic astrocytoma of the cerebellum, one hemangioma of the cerebellum, one pinealoma, and two cases of obstruction of the aqueduct of undetermined etiology. In seven of these cases a curved incision extending from one mastoid process to the other was used; in four cases a straight midline incision was used; in two the incision was of the hockey stick type for unilateral cerebellar exploration; and in one case the type of incision was unknown. The dura was closed in six cases; in two cases it was left open. It appears then, that pseudomeningoceles may occur with any type of incision, and that closure of the dura will not prevent their occurrence.

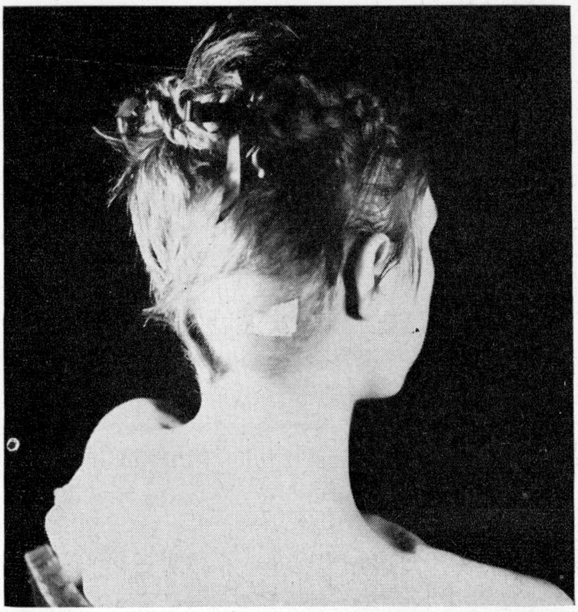

Fig. 1.—A typical pseudomeningocele which occurred following a right suboccipital craniotomy for removal of a meningioma from the posterior fossa.

Eight patients in this group were operated upon before 1944 when pressure dressings were first used to treat pseudomeningoceles. Five of these eight patients were treated either by repeated aspirations of the cystic cavity or by lumbar puncture with drainage of cerebrospinal fluid to decompress the pseudomeningocele. In three of the cases no aspirations were performed. In one case a cerebrospinal fluid fistula developed as a result of the pseudomeningocele and the patient died of meningitis secondary to this fistula. Three of these eight patients were reoperated upon because the nature of the pseudomeningocele was not recognized, and it was thought that they had increased intracranial pressure due to recurrence of the tumor. In each of these three cases a cystic cavity filled with clear colorless fluid was found under the occipital muscles, and there was no recurrence of the tumor. The cysts were lined by thick, glistening, white membranes. Biopsy of the cyst walls revealed that they were composed of collagenous connective tissue. No communication was found at operation between the cyst cavity and the subarachnoid space, but that such a communication does exist in these cases is shown by the fact that the cyst can be completely collapsed by aspiration of cerebrospinal fluid by the lumbar route. In addition, the fluid in the pseudomeningocele is chemically identical with the cerebrospinal fluid removed at the same time from the lumbar subarachnoid space.

Six patients with pseudomeningocele have been seen since 1944. All of these have been treated by the application of a pressure dressing over the pseudomeningocele. In five of these patients, the pseudomeningocele quickly disappeared following the application of the pressure dressing. In one case the pressure dressing failed to cure the condition, but this failure was probably due to the fact

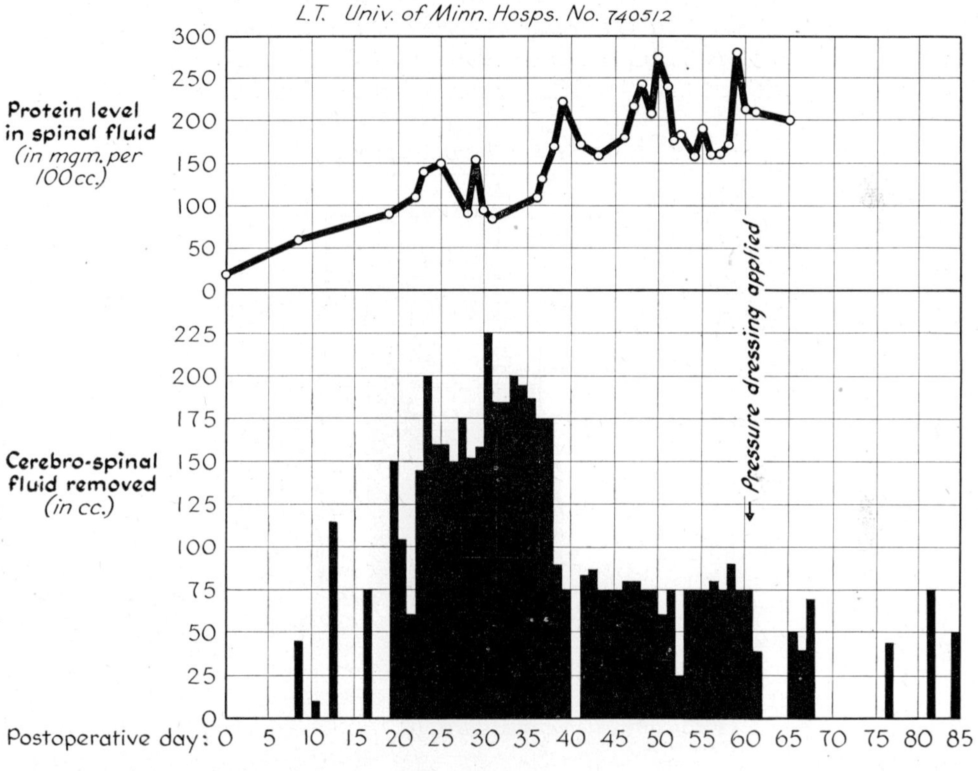

Fig. 2.—Graph showing amounts of fluid removed to decompress the pseudomeningocele before and after the application of pressure dressings.

that the tumor could not be completely resected. The patient continued to have increased intracranial pressure following the operation. The first two patients of this group who were treated by the application of a pressure dressing were first treated by repeated aspirations of cerebrospinal fluid. Figs. 2 and 3 are graphs summarizing the treatment of these two patients by aspiration of cerebrospinal fluid. These graphs also illustrate how effectively the pseudomeningoceles were treated by the use of a pressure dressing. In the first of these two cases (Fig. 2) there was so little accumulation of fluid following the application of a pressure dressing that subsequent aspirations were done only seven times.

We realize now, although we did not at the time this patient was being treated, that even these aspirations were unnecessary. In the second case (Fig. 3) there was accumulation of fluid in the cystic cavity only twice after the pressure dressing was applied, and these two recurrences of the pseudomeningocele occurred when the child pulled off the pressure dressing.

Pseudomeningoceles must be due either to an increased secretion or to diminished absorption of cerebrospinal fluid, or possibly to both of these factors. Flexner[5] has shown that the formation of cerebrospinal fluid is a linear function of the difference between the effective hydrostatic pressures in the capillaries of the choroid plexus and in the ventricles. Weed[6, 7] has demonstrated that an increase in the hydrostatic pressure of the cerebrospinal fluid increased the absorption of the fluid. In cerebellar operations, large skull defects are produced so that it is possible for a large amount of fluid to accumulate at the site of the operation without bringing back to normal the hydrostatic pressure in the

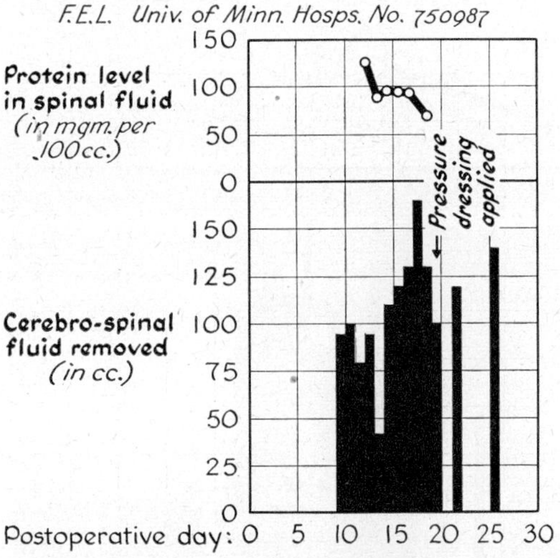

Fig. 3.—Graph showing amounts of fluid removed from pseudomeningocele.

craniospinal cavity. Thus, fluid accumulates to form a cyst, or pseudomeningocele, until the area of the wound becomes tense and the hydrostatic pressure of the cerebrospinal fluid is raised to a level at which normal relationships between absorption and secretion are resumed, but because the cyst causes stretching of the soft tissues the pseudomeningocele may become progressively larger. Application of a pressure dressing over the pseudomeningocele arrests the process because its support of the soft tissues over the skull defect causes an increase in hydrostatic pressure of the cerebrospinal fluid without protrusion of the operative site.

The most satisfactory method for applying moderate pressure to the suboccipital area is by the use of an elastic bandage as illustrated in Fig. 4. Some patients complain of mild headache for the first twenty-four to forty-eight hours after the bandage is applied, but there is no other discomfort. The length of time that the dressing is needed varies from patient to patient. The procedure which we have used and found to be satisfactory is to apply the dressing for five days and then to discontinue its use unless there is recurrence of the pseudomeningocele. If there is recurrence, the dressing is used for an additional two or three days. Again its use is discontinued to discover whether the tendency to cyst formation has been eliminated. This procedure is repeated until the tendency to develop a pseudomeningocele has completely disappeared. Frequently it is found that the pseudomeningocele recurs only at certain times during the day, so that a compression dressing is necessary only at these times. It has been found unnecessary for the patient to remain in the hospital if tendency to form pseudomeningocele is prolonged, for a member of the patient's family can be easily taught to apply the pressure dressing. Only a moderate amount of pressure is needed to control the protrusion so that the bandage should be applied snugly, but not so tightly that there is danger of pressure necrosis to the underlying skin. However, if there is any doubt about the condition of the skin, the dressing may be removed daily and immediately replaced.

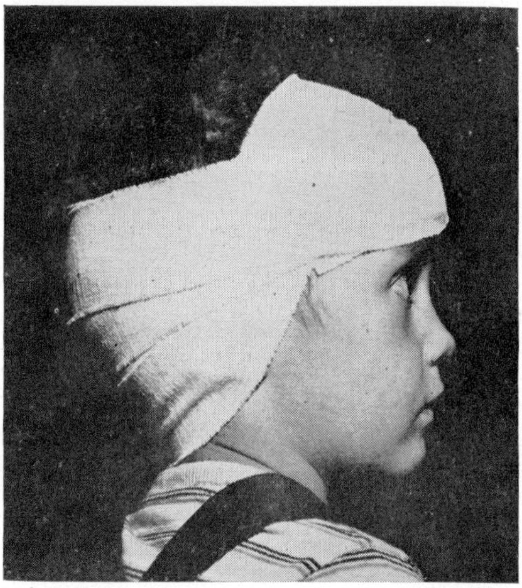

Fig. 4.—A patient with a pseudomeningocele with pressure dressing in place.

Following is the case report of a patient with a pseudomeningocele. This case illustrates the ease with which this complication may be treated with pressure dressings.

B. R., a 33-year-old white woman, was operated upon Aug. 6, 1945. A straight midline cerebellar incision was used and a large meningioma was found, having its origin from the inferior surface of the tentorium on the right side of the posterior fossa. The tumor was completely removed and the dura, subcutaneous tissues, and skin were closed in layers. The patient's immediate postoperative course was uneventful, and she was discharged from the hospital on the fourth postoperative day.

On the eighth postoperative day, the patient noticed some protrusion at the operative site. This increased until the eighteenth postoperative day when she returned to the outpatient clinic because she had become alarmed about this swelling. The area was tense and protruded about 3 cm. An elastic bandage was applied over the protruding area and was left in place for twenty-four hours. At the end of this twenty-four hour period the operative area was soft and flat. The pressure dressing was then removed, but within three hours the swelling had recurred. The bandage was again applied and left in place for three more days. At the end of this time, the dressing was again removed, but the pseudomeningocele recurred within a few hours. The dressing was then reapplied and left in place for another three days. It was then removed. This period of compression apparently was sufficient, for there was no further protrusion at the operative site. The patient was followed in the outpatient service for one year after operation and remained completely free of symptoms.

SUMMARY

Pseudomeningocele or cyst formation at the operative site following cerebellar operations has received little mention in the literature, but apparently is frequently encountered by neurosurgeons.

We have encountered this complication fourteen times during a ten-year period.

A simple but efficient method for the elimination of meningoceles has been found in the application of a pressure dressing.

REFERENCES

1. Schloffer, H.: Zur Frage des Hirndruckes und der Liquorsekretion nach Radikaloperation, Med. Klin. **19**: 4, 1923.
2. Cushing, H.: Experiences With Cerebellar Medullablastomas—a Critical Review, Acta path. et microbiol. Scandinav. **7**: 1, 1930.
3. Cushing, H.: Experiences With Cerebellar Astrocytomas—a Critical Review of 76 Cases, Surg., Gynec. & Obst. **5**: 129, 1931.
4. Bancroft, F., and Pilcher, C.: Surgical Treatment of the Nervous System, Philadelphia, 1946, J. B. Lippincott Company, p. 226.
5. Flexner, Louis B.: The Water of the Cerebrospinal Fluid—Variations in Its Rate of Flow With Variations of Ventricular Pressure, Am. J. Physiol. **106**: 170, 1933.
6. Weed, Louis H.: Forces Concerned in the Absorption of the Cerebrospinal Fluid, Am. J. Physiol. **114**: 40, 1935.
7. Weed, Louis H.: Meninges and Cerebrospinal Fluid, J. Anat. **72**: 181, 1937.

FOREIGN BODY LOCALIZATION IN THE SOFT PARTS

A Simple Method Requiring no Especial Training or Equipment

Clarence E. Gardner, Jr., M.D., Durham, N. C.

(From the Department of Surgery, Duke University School of Medicine)

THE search for and removal of foreign bodies in the soft parts can be one of the most difficult and exasperating of surgical problems. Methods described to assist in the procedure have become numerous and complex and often require elaborate equipment and specialized training which is not available in the ordinary hospital. A procedure is here described which is simple and satisfactory and requires no especial equipment or training.

Reed and Black,[1] in a review of the literature in 1938, classified the methods of foreign body localization under ten different principles of which 110 methods were reported. Since then the literature has contained many references to refinements in these methods, and the introduction of at least one new principle.[2]

The method here described is to us the simplest and most satisfactory and is the one least mentioned in the literature. It consists in the insertion under fluoroscopic control of two long slender needles at right angles into the tissues at a distance from the proposed incision so that they cross in the approximate location of the foreign body. An anteroposterior and lateral x-ray film is then exposed and with the needles still in place the field is draped and the area explored at operation. The foreign body can usually be quickly found because of the ease in localizing it in relation to the fixed point of the two crossed needles. If difficulty is still experienced, the needles are withdrawn and two more inserted in the same manner so that they cross again at the approximate location of the foreign body. The wound is then covered, anteroposterior and lateral x-ray views again taken and, with the needles acting as fixed points for localization, we have never failed to find even the tiniest of foreign bodies.

Most of the methods used in foreign body localization rely upon skin markings made with the aid of x-ray examination. The difficulty with this method is that the foreign body may shift in relation to the skin mark if the patient is not in exactly the same position on the operating table as under the x-ray screen. Furthermore, during the course of operation both foreign body and the skin marks shift as tissues are retracted.

The method described eliminates this error, for the two crossed needles anchor the tissues, and their relation to the foreign body does not change. It is only when the needles become loosened in the tissues during the dissection and no longer act as fixed points that they may need to be withdrawn and reinserted for a second x-ray exposure.

Although the method has been previously described,[3, 4] we developed the technique independently in military service and have subsequently used it in civilian practice. The following case report in which a thoracentesis needle

Received for publication, May 5, 1947.

broke off flush with the inner margin of a rib is an example of an extremely difficult foreign body to find, in which the method was used with excellent results.

CASE REPORT

T. P. (No. B 91370), a 15-year-old Negro girl, was hospitalized elsewhere when a lumbar puncture needle inserted into the right thorax for thoracentesis broke off at its hub. Immediate exploration through a 3 cm. incision was unsuccessful and the patient was brought to us. Fluoroscopy showed an 8 cm. needle entirely within the right thorax except for its distal end, which was in the chest wall between the eighth and ninth ribs at the posterior axillary line (Fig. 1). Its most superficial end appeared to be on a level with the mid-portion of the rib (Fig. 1, *c*). Two long 22 gauge needles were thrust through the soft tissues of the chest wall starting them about 3 cm. from the skin incision so that the needles crossed in approximately the location of the needle (Fig. 1, *A*, *B*, and *C*). This was done under the fluoroscope. Using the point where the needles crossed as the fixed

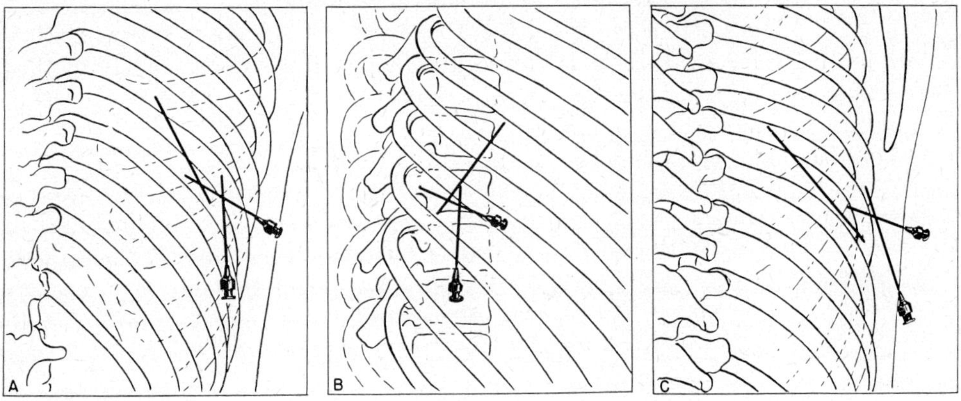

Fig. 1.—Drawings made from tracings of anteroposterior, lateral, and oblique x-ray films after two slender needles had been inserted through the soft tissues of the chest wall so that they crossed in approximately the same position as the end of the broken needle. *A*, anteroposterior; *B*, lateral; *C*, oblique.

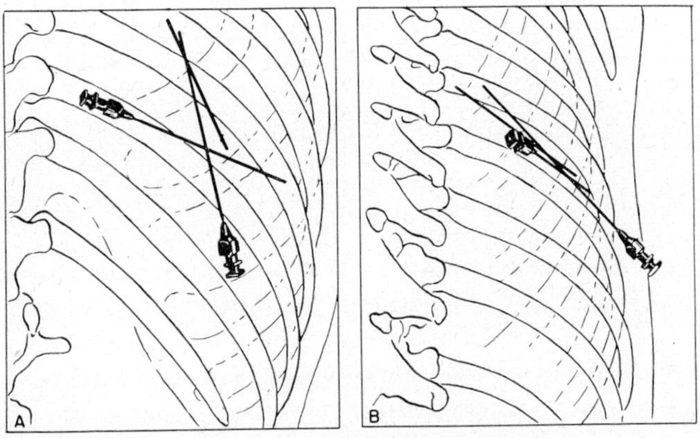

Fig. 2.—Drawings of the anteroposterior and oblique x-ray views made on the operating table after the first set of localizing needles had been loosened and a second set had been inserted through the intercostal space so that they crossed at the approximate location of the broken needle. The end of the broken needle was immediately located by searching along the horizontal of the two localizing needles 1 cm. lateral and 2 mm. above the fixed point found by the crossing of the two needles.

point it was seen that the end of the foreign body was located about 1 cm. caudad, 1 cm. posterior, and ½ cm. deeper than the fixed point. Exploration in this area failed to locate the foreign body quickly and the needles became slightly loosened during the procedure. These needles were withdrawn and two lumbar puncture needles were inserted starting at a distance of some 4 cm. from the wound and inserting the needles into the thoracic cavity crossing them through the interspace at the point where the foreign body was thought to be. Study of anteroposterior and oblique x-ray films (Fig. 2, *A* and *B*) showed that these needles crossed at exactly the same level as the end of the foreign body and that the end of the foreign body was located along the horizontal of the two needles 1 cm. lateral to the crossing and about 2 mm. cephalad. Exploration at this point immediately revealed the broken end of the needle with only about 2 mm. of its length superficial to the pleura. When the needle was withdrawn a little air sucked into the pleural cavity. This was quickly stopped by suturing the muscles over the opening. The previous wound in the skin and subcutaneous tissues was then excised and closed and the patient allowed to return to the original hospital.

SUMMARY

A simple and satisfactory method of localizing foreign bodies in the soft parts, without the need of elaborate equipment or an especially trained staff, is presented.

REFERENCES

1. Reed, E. K., and Black, L. F.: Foreign Body Localization in Military Roentgenology, Radiology **31**: 567, 1938.
2. Moorhead, J. J.: A Foreign Body Finder: The Locator, J. A. M. A. **121**: 123, 1943.
3. McNealy, R. W., and Willims, J. D.: Small Foreign Bodies in Extremities; Improved Method for Their Removal, Am. J. Surg. **18**: 268, 1932.
4. Hotchkiss, W. S.: A Practical Method for Localizing and Removal of Foreign Bodies, Virginia M. Monthly **71**: 37, 1944.

SUBCUTANEOUS EMPHYSEMA FOLLOWING CHEST TRAUMA

Analysis of Twenty Cases

William Sheinfeld, M.D.,* Brooklyn, N. Y.

(From the Surgical Service of the Coney Island Hospital)

SUBCUTANEOUS emphysema following thoracic trauma is not infrequent and is often seen after blunt chest injuries as well as after penetrating wounds. In the majority of instances active therapy directed toward controlling the spread of emphysema is unnecessary as the process is a self-limited one and subsides spontaneously. There are cases, however, where the emphysema is progressive, respiration becomes much embarrassed, and the circulation is interfered with. Such cases, unchecked, may result in death. An understanding of the pathologic physiology involved is necessary to treat this condition adequately. The tempo of events may be very rapid or last over a period of days. One must realize that other important lesions may be present in various combinations and that the emphysema may be but one phase of a complicated clinical picture.

There are two pathways by which air will reach the subcutaneous tissues from the lungs. Each involves a different mechanism and depends on a different type of pulmonic injury. Nevertheless, one, or the other, or both mechanisms may operate in any one or several cases.

Mechanism 1.—With rib fractures, the parietal pleura, visceral pleura, and underlying lung may be lacerated. Air will pass from the injured lung into subcutaneously lacerated soft tissues via the pleural space with or without an x-ray-apparent pneumothorax in the early phases of the condition. Later x-ray examination may reveal a small pneumothorax or pleural or pulmonary changes not manifested early. In some instances a minimal or partial pneumothorax will be seen early. In expiration, air escapes into the pleural space; with inspiration, it is forced into the soft tissues by the expanding lung, thereby causing and extending the subcutaneous emphysema. This may continue until an obvious pneumothorax forms which will compress the lung and interrupt the further escape of air from it, or until the laceration in the lung becomes sealed over. With a penetrating injury, air may also be sucked into the thoracic parieties from the exterior. This explanation was presented by Stenbuck[1] in 1937.

That air can get from the lung to the subcutaneous tissues without connecting adhesions or x-ray-determined pneumothorax after injury is suggested by the following:

In five of our penetrating thoracic injuries there was x-ray-demonstrable pneumothorax in none, extensive subcutaneous emphysema in three, moderate emphysema in one, and slight emphysema in one.

It is unlikely that the lung was uninvolved in all five cases or that the exterior was the sole source of emphysema by the very nature of the injuries,

Received for publication, May 9, 1947.

*Associate Surgeon, Coney Island Hospital.

that is, three stab wounds, one transfixion on a spike, and a nail penetration. Furthermore, in one case, pulmonary infiltration and pleural thickening were demonstrable by x-ray examination, indicating that the lung had been injured.

In six cases of unilateral rib fractures, in nonpenetrating injuries, four left and two right, the emphysema was present essentially on the side of the fractures. In four cases, pneumothorax was noted on the same side; in three cases there was homolateral pleuritis or pleural fluid; and in two cases, pulmonary infiltration. In one case of multiple right and one left rib fracture there was extensive right subcutaneous emphysema, right pneumothorax, pleuritis, and diminished aeration of the right lower lung. Such correlation of phenomena strongly suggests the local mechanism just elucidated.

Mechanism 2.—This explanation has been given a number of times in the several articles on the subject by Macklin,[2] and Macklin and Macklin.[3, 4] The demonstrations and data presented were very convincing and reference is made to their publications for details. In essence, as a result of a variety of factors, that is, external trauma with or without rib fracture, overinflation of the lungs as a result of inhalation anesthesia, resuscitative measures, atelectasis for one cause or another with compensatory emphysema, straining, and a congenital predisposition on the part of the subject, rupture of overdistended alveoli take place. These are usually multiple and may be demonstrable by microscopic and special techniques elaborated by Macklin and Macklin, occasionally by ordinary observation. Air escapes from the alveoli into the perivascular sheaths of capillaries and larger blood vessels. As a result of inspiration and expiration further expulsion of air takes place.

Air bubbles coalesce and are pushed along throughout the lung substance down toward the lung root into the mediastinum. They may infiltrate across the other side into the opposite lung root. The mediastinal pressure builds up. Occasionally the air remains trapped and causes marked cyanosis and dyspnea because of the avascularity of the lung involved, and the pressure on the great mediastinal veins impeding the return flow of blood to the heart. Death may result. There are three main routes of egress from the mediastinum; the subcutaneous tissues of the neck, the pleural cavities, and the retroperitoneal space. Air may escape into any one or more of these, and will cause subcutaneous emphysema, pneumothorax, or retroperitoneal emphysema. Subcutaneous emphysema may become generalized. Even when air enters one of the escape routes, pressure symptoms may still occur and constitute a threat to life.

In eight of our cases collected, this mechanism alone, or possibly in conjunction with the first described, may have operated. The symptomatology and course of events are best explained on the basis of this concept. The following two cases are presented in some detail as they appear to illustrate the second mechanism described.

CASE REPORTS

CASE 1 (No. 117493).—W. G. was admitted Oct. 22, 1946 and discharged Nov. 12, 1946. This patient was a 62-year-old white man who fell off a steam-heat radiator and struck the right side of the chest against it. He then complained of pain in the right side of

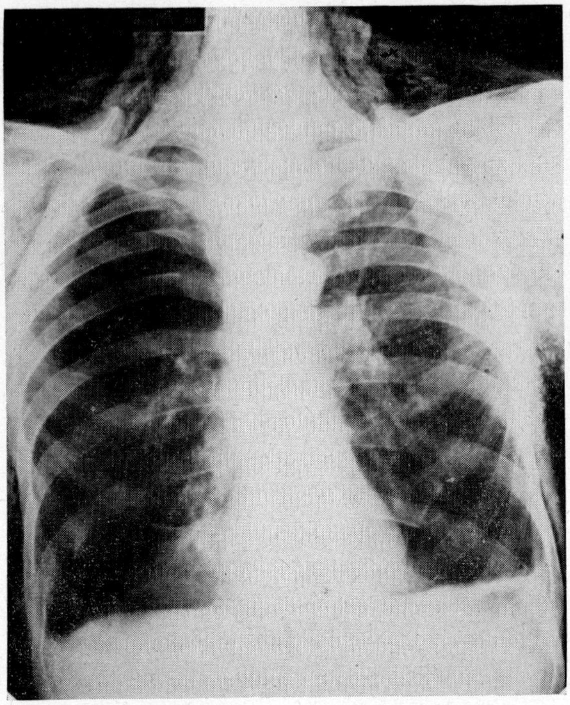

Fig. 1 (Case 1).—X-ray view taken Oct. 22, 1946, showing marked subcutaneous emphysema of thoracic wall and cervical areas.

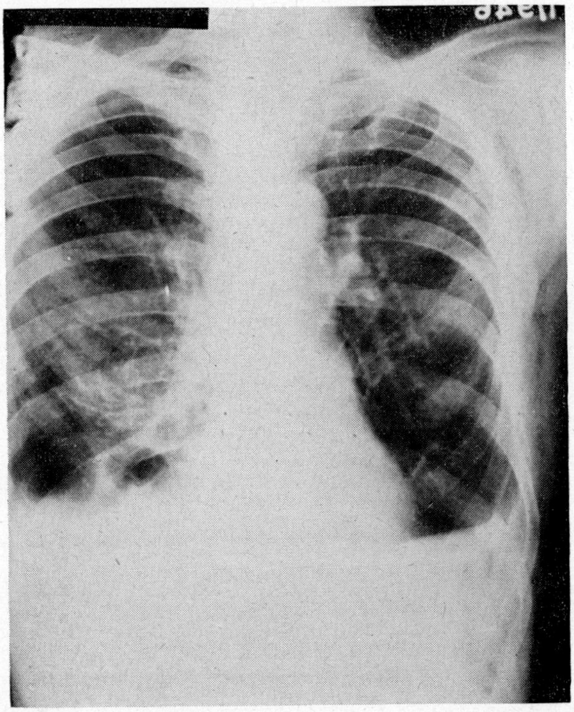

Fig. 2 (Case 1).—X-ray view taken Oct. 29, 1946, showing diminished subcutaneous emphysema, partial pneumothorax of the right lower lung, and pleural thickening of both bases.

the chest and some difficulty in breathing. His physician noticed increasing crepitation of the chest wall over a two-day period and referred him for hospitalization.

Physical examination on admission Oct. 22, 1946, revealed moderate respiratory distress. Subcutaneous emphysema was present over the entire chest, subcostal margins, and flanks. There was no skin laceration. The remainder of the examination was essentially irrelevant. Laboratory data: Hemoglobin was 13 Gm.; white blood cells, 9000; blood Wassermann, negative; x-ray examination on Oct. 23, 1946, showed a marked degree of subcutaneous emphysema in the thoracic wall and in the cervical regions of both sides, particularly on the *left*. There were complete fractures of the right seventh, eighth, ninth, and tenth ribs in the axillary region (Fig. 1).

Course in the Hospital.—The chest was strapped over the area of the rib fractures but the strapping was poorly tolerated and had to be discontinued. For the next few days the emphysema continued to extend until on Oct. 27, 1946, it became universal, involving the entire body from the scalp to the ankles. The eyelids were puffed up and closed. Cyanosis, dyspnea, and orthopnea developed. At this time there was no demonstrable pneumothorax on either side, no mediastinal shift, and no significant pulmonary changes. It was apparent that active treatment was necessary and further expectant therapy dangerous to the patient's life. Accordingly, under novocain infiltration, a small horizontal one-inch, suprasternal incision was made. The incision was carried down through all the layers of fascia and subcutaneous tissue to the trachea. The finger was then bluntly introduced into the superior mediastinum behind the sternum. Air bubbled out through the incision continuously during the operation. A Penrose drain was introduced into the space which had been opened. Within ten minutes the dyspnea and orthopnea were relieved. Recovery thereafter was continuous and within one week there was almost complete disappearance of the subcutaneous emphysema. For the first ten days a low-grade febrile course persisted and penicillin was administered throughout this time. Chest x-ray view on Oct. 29, 1946, showed a considerable degree of subcutaneous emphysema of the entire thorax and cervical region (less than on the previous film), a partial pneumothorax at the right lower lung, and pleural thickening of both bases (Fig. 2).

CASE 2 (No. 118268).—J. S. was admitted Dec. 17, 1946, and discharged Jan. 10, 1947. This patient was a 57-year-old man who was attacked by two bandits, and sustained ten fractured ribs about equally distributed on either side.

Examination on admission disclosed subcutaneous emphysema of the entire chest wall, front and back, extending up to the face and down to the iliac crests. It was most marked posteriorly. Pain was present on inspiration but dyspnea and cyanosis were absent.

X-ray examination on admission showed marked subcutaneous emphysema of the chest wall, cervical area, and the *mediastinum* (Figs. 3 and 4). There were multiple bilateral rib fractures with slight displacement of some fragments. There was partial atelectasis or hemorrhage in the right lower lung.

Course in the Hospital.—The chest was strapped and the patient treated expectantly. For two days there was extension of the emphysema and then it began to subside. Recovery was uneventful. X-ray examination of the chest on Jan. 2, 1947, revealed minimal degree of pulmonary infiltration at the right base. The right diaphragm was elevated. X-ray examination on Jan. 8, 1947, was essentially negative.

Table I is a summary of the pertinent data in twenty cases of subcutaneous emphysema following chest injury encountered at the Coney Island Hospital in the past nine years.

Five were penetrating chest wounds. X-ray-demonstrable pneumothorax was not present in any. There was a small pleural effusion in one case, and slight pulmonary infiltration in the right upper lobe with pleural thickening in another.

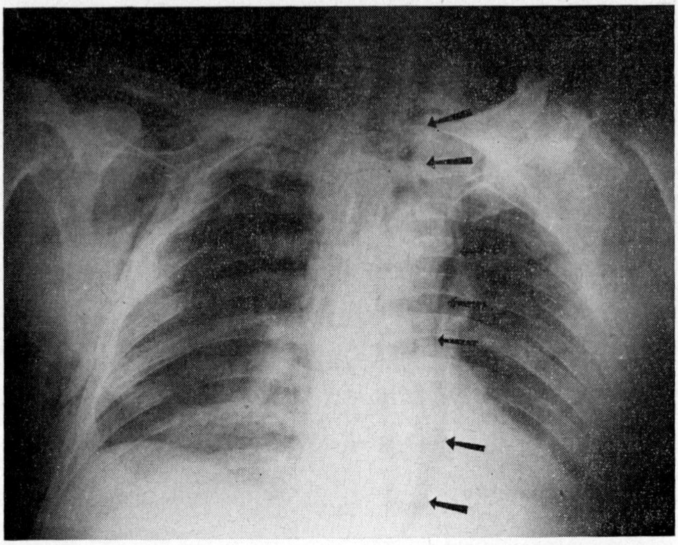

Fig. 3 (Case 2).—X-ray view showing subcutaneous emphysema of chest wall, cervical area, and mediastinum.

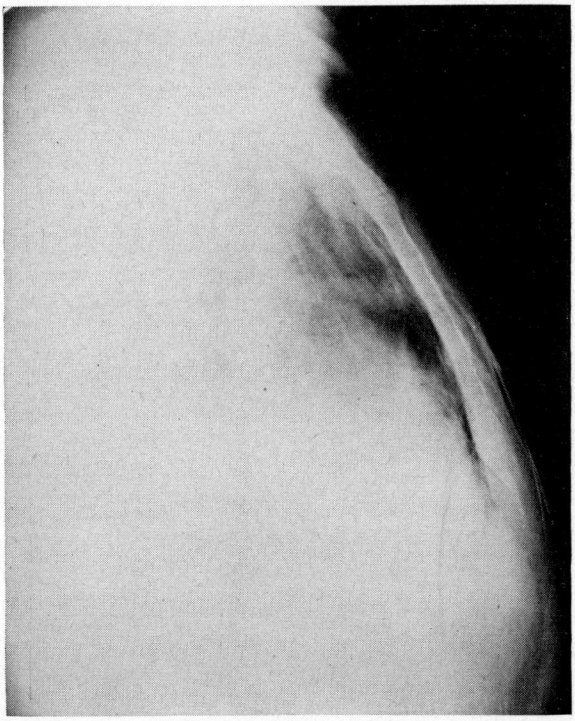

Fig. 4 (Case 2).—Lateral X-ray view showing subcutaneous and mediastinal emphysema.

TABLE I. SUMMARY OF DATA IN TWENTY CASES OF SUBCUTANEOUS EMPHYSEMA FOLLOWING CHEST TRAUMA

CASE NO., AGE, SEX	INJURY	EMPHYSEMA (SITE, EXTENT, COURSE)	PNEUMOTHORAX (EARLY, LATE)	PLEURAL FLUID, PLEURITIS	PULMONARY CHANGES (EARLY, LATE)	RESPIRATORY EMBARRASSMENT	COMMENT
1. C. P. (82221), 26, ♂	Stab wound of 4th right interspace posteriorly	Marked over right posterior chest; uneventful recovery in 5 days	0	Small amount of fluid	0	0	
2. F. W. (88332) 28, ♂	Stab wound of 2nd left interspace parasternally	Marked on left anterior chest from clavicle down; spread to face and subsided spontaneously	0	0	0	0	
3. C. W. (81435), 29, ♀	Stab wound of 4th left interspace of anterior axillary line	Moderate over anterior left chest, supraclavicular area and left posterior chest wall; uneventful recovery in several days	0	0	0	0	
4. N. A. (65278), 17, ♂	Nail laceration of left axillary area, 3rd interspace	Relatively slight, in left axillary area; uneventful recovery	0	0	0	0	
5. F. G. (64857), 13, ♂	Fell on spike; laceration of right anterior and posterior chest	About laceration sites, front and back of chest; no spread, uneventful recovery in 9 days	0	Slight right pleural thickening	Alveolar hemorrhage of right upper lung, early; slight pulmonary infiltration of right upper lung, late	0	These first 5 cases were all penetrating chest injuries
6. S. C. (78590), 67, ♂	Struck by train; multiple left rib fractures, fractured skull	Over left lateral aspect of chest	Left (small) early	Small amount (early blood?)	0	+	Patient died several hours after admission in coma; dyspnea of cerebral origin, death due to head injury
7. D. J. (102859), 76, ♂	Hit by an auto; fracture of left clavicle and right scapula, laceration of scalp, shock, B.P. 85/50, no rib fracture	Extensive over both sides of neck and in right axillary region; spread to abdomen and gluteal area	Right (early)	0	0	++	Death in 24 hr. with marked respiratory embarrassment; while death may have been due to shock and head trauma, the pulmonary complication may have played a large part, decompression of the mediastinum might have relieved the respiratory distress

TABLE I—CONT'D

CASE NO., AGE, SEX	INJURY	EMPHYSEMA (SITE, EXTENT, COURSE)	PNEUMOTHORAX (EARLY, LATE)	PLEURAL FLUID, PLEURITIS	PULMONARY CHANGES (EARLY, LATE)	RESPIRATORY EMBARRASSMENT	COMMENT
8. B. R. (101878), 45, ♂	Struck by car; unconscious, shock, head trauma, multiple bilateral rib fractures	Moderate of left side of chest	0	+ Moderate amount	Some pulmonary infiltration (hemorrhage?)	Developed on day after admission +	Death 24 hr. after admission; respiratory difficulty became marked on day after admission and pulse markedly irregular; while death was probably due to shock and head trauma, the possibility of increased mediastinal pressure is present
9. C. H. (64507), 33, ♂	Struck by car; unconscious, head trauma, right rib fracture	Extensive over anterior and posterior chest, neck, down to below mid-trunk; progressive for 24 hr. down to inguinal areas, then subsidence and rapid convalescence	Possible right (minimal and early)	0	Bilateral emphysema	0	Emphysema spread through mediastinal route (most probable); spontaneous recovery
10. A. S. (61537), 49, ♂	Struck by auto; multiple left rib fractures, laceration of left chest, contusion of left kidney	Entire left chest wall and neck involved; subsided after several days	+ Late left	Pleural thickening and fluid, left lower lung, late	Clouding lower ½ left lung (hemorrhage?) early	0	
11. A. G. (114085), 48, ♂	Struck by auto; fracture 5th & 6th left ribs, linear skull fracture	Anterior chest wall up to clavicle, subsided spontaneously	++1 Left early	+ Left (late)	Collapse of left lung (early)	0	Spontaneous subsidence; early moderate pneumothorax and lung collapse may have caused early stopping of emphysema
12. P. M. (64464), 38, ♂	Struck by auto; unconscious, multiple right rib fractures	Moderate right thoracic wall and right cervical region; subsided spontaneously after several days	+ Right early (minimal)	0	Bronchitic change; right lower lung early	+ on admission, subsided spontaneously	Hemoptysis on admission; signs of peritoneal irritation, exploratory laparotomy revealed some free blood
13. W. W. (64718), 65. ♂	Multiple bilateral rib fractures, patient in shock	Extensive right chest wall; progression for 2 days then subsidence and recovery	+ Right (slight) early	Moderate right fluid late	Diminished aeration of right lower lung, early; persistence of lung clouding (late); hemor-	0	Spontaneous recovery with expectant treatment

14. I. A., (68828), 51, ♂	Fell from a chair, striking chest; multiple left rib fractures	Moderate of left posterior chest, spontaneous subsidence in 8 to 9 days	0	0	Atelectasis of left base (early), also infiltration of lung	0	
15. P. K. (62883), 58, ♂	Hit by auto; multiple right rib fractures	Moderate in axillary area of right chest; spontaneous recovery	0	0	0	0	Associated fracture of transverse process of spine
16. T. C. (64190), 58, ♂	Auto accident; bilateral multiple fracture of ribs, fracture of pubis, sacrum, and contusion of kidney	Moderate amount in left chest; early subsidence	Right early (slight), left early *considerable*	Left pleural thickening, late	Diminished aeration of right lower lobe *early;* diminished aeration of left lower lung *late*	0	Case of bilateral rib fractures and bilateral pneumothorax
17. S. G. (113975), 46, ♂	Auto accident; multiple bilateral upper rib fractures, fracture of right scapula and clavicle, head injury	Both sides of neck and right upper chest	Right + (partial) early	Fluid right, late	Atelectasis right upper lung (early)	0	
18. R. W. (117123), 25, ♂	Severe beating; multiple right rib fractures	Extensive over chest, anterior and posterior from jaw down to iliac crests; spontaneous subsidence in about a week	0	0	Minimal infiltration, right lung field (late)	0	–
19. W. G. (117493), 62, ♂	Fell off radiator and struck right chest; multiple right rib fractures	Extensive over chest, spread and involved entire body, universal, after 5 days, then respiratory distress became marked; relieved by mediastinal decompression, incision into superior mediastinum through suprasternal approach; gradual subsidence in following week	Partial pneumothorax right base (late)	Diaphragmatic pleural thickening, bilateral (late)	–	Cyanosis dyspnea, orthopnea +	Case reported in greater detail in text
20. J. S. (118268), 57, ♂	Severe beating; multiple bilateral rib fractures	Entire chest front and back, face, lower abdomen, and back; spontaneous recovery after 4 to 5 days	0	0	Partial atelectasis or hemorrhage of right lower lung (early); pulmonary infiltration of right base (late)	0	Pneumomediastinum demonstrated on x-ray films; case reported in greater detail in text

Fifteen were blunt chest injuries. In fourteen of these there were fractured ribs, multiple in thirteen cases, and bilateral in five. One patient had no rib fracture, but had a fractured right scapula, left clavicle, and a right pneumothorax.

X-ray-demonstrable pneumothorax was present in ten cases. It was noted early in eight, one of which was bilateral, and late in two cases. In six cases it was on the same side as unilateral rib fractures; it was bilateral in a case of bilateral rib fracture; it appeared twice on the right side in cases of bilateral rib fractures, and in both of these cases the emphysema was most marked on the right side of the chest. Once it was noted without any rib fracture.

In six of the cases of unilateral pneumothorax the subcutaneous emphysema was mostly on the same side. In the other four cases the emphysema was generalized. In the nonpenetrating wounds, pleural fluid or pleural thickening was found eight times. In six instances this was a late occurrence and was absent on the early x-ray views. It was on the same side as the unilateral rib fractures three times, was bilateral in the case of universal emphysema, appeared in the case without rib fracture, and was seen three times in the cases of bilateral rib fracture.

Pulmonary infiltration suggestive of pulmonary interstitial hemorrhage, diminished aeration, or patchy atelectasis was seen in nine cases. It was seen late in four lungs (early x-ray pictures failed to show it). Early lung changes occurred in eight lungs. Partial collapse of the lung occurred twice. Respiratory embarrassment was present in five cases. It was marked in one fatal case and developed in the second fatal case, possibly playing a part in the mortality. In the other three cases it was marked only in the case of universal emphysema.

The emphysema was extensive in twelve cases, moderate in six, and slight in two. Active treatment toward relieving the emphysema was necessary once and might have been of value in two of the fatal cases (death was probably due to the associated injuries).

DISCUSSION

Numerous instances of interstitial pulmonary, mediastinal, and subcutaneous emphysema following a variety of causes have been reported in the literature. For the most part, with the exception of cases of direct chest trauma, these cases have been explained or proved to be caused in the manner described under Mechanism 2.

Cowart[5] described two cases of mediastinal emphysema following chest contusions with spontaneous recovery in each. Lilienthal[6] quoted a case from Dr. Fred Zimmer, where generalized subcutaneous emphysema after multiple rib fractures with marked dyspnea was successfully treated by open thoracotomy. Friedman and King[7] reported a case of mediastinal and extensive subcutaneous emphysema following an automobile accident. Dyspnea was marked at first. Oxygen was given and spontaneous recovery ensued.

Cases have occurred after general anesthesias. Thornton, Jr., Adams, and Livingstone[8] reported a fatal case. At autopsy, marked mediastinal and pulmonary interstitial emphysema were demonstrated. Another fatal case was cited by Barret and Thomas.[9] A convulsion complicated an endotracheal general anesthetic. General subcutaneous emphysema rapidly developed, and death ensued before effective therapeutic measures could be instituted. These authors also reported another case of emphysema successfully treated by needle aspiration and general measures.

Bronchoscopy has, on a number of occasions, been followed by a rapidly developing generalized subcutaneous emphysema, dyspnea, and cyanosis. Jones[10] reported two patients, desperately ill, but each recovering after needling and general supportive measures. Hammond[11] incised the neck, opening the perivascular spaces and the superior mediastinum with a successful outcome in a severe case. Fisher and Macklin[12] reported a fatal case following a peanut inhalation, with resultant atelectasis and subsequent bronchoscopies. At autopsy, mediastinal and interstitial pulmonary emphysema with rupture of multiple alveoli were demonstrated.

Cases complicating influenza pneumonia,[13] bronchopneumonia,[14] and asthma[15] have been collected and published.

The literature is a vast one, and only a few illustrative reports are quoted. However, the underlying principles of disturbed physiology appear to be similar in the numerous instances of this clinical syndrome.

TREATMENT

The method of approach in curing subcutaneous emphysema will depend upon the type of injury and its extent.

1. In true mediastinal emphysema, mediastinal decompression should be employed. This can best be done by incision over the jugulum and adequate drainage of the air from the mediastinum. Occasionally needle aspiration, suprasternally or parasternally, may suffice.

2. A needle or trocar may be introduced into the pleural space, and underwater drainage established. This will interrupt the further extension of air across the pleural space into the subcutaneous tissues.

3. Pneumothorax with moderate positive pressure may be used to compress the lung, and thus prevent further air leakage from it.

4. Thoracotomy with suture of the parietal pleura alone may be enough.

5. Suture of lung laceration may be done. This will be necessary rarely.

6. Combination of these methods, in cases of extensive and rapidly forming emphysema, may be utilized.

7. Expectant treatment may be enough when careful observation shows there is little or no progression.

The course of events may be relatively slow, and adequate treatment may be decided upon after ample deliberation. On the other hand, progress may be very rapid, and one's resources may be severely taxed to apply an effective combination of methods. Adequate oxygen concentration and a free airway must be assured.

REFERENCES

1. Stenbuck, J. B.: Traumatic Subcutaneous Emphysema of Thoracic Origin, New York State J. Med. 37: 395-399, 1937.
2. Macklin, C. C.: Transport of Air Along Sheaths of Pulmonic Blood Vessels From Alveoli to Mediastinum, Arch. Int. Med. 64: 913, 1939.

3. Macklin, M. T., and Macklin, C. C.: Malignant Interstitial Emphysema of Lungs and Mediastinum as Important Occult Complication in Many Respiratory Diseases and Other Conditions, Medicine **23**: 281-358, 1944.
4. Macklin, C. C., and Macklin, M. T.: Air Block in Lung Blast? Lancet **1**: 602, 1942.
5. Cowart, J. T.: Mediastinal Emphysema; Report of Two Cases Due to Chest Trauma, U. S. Nav. M. Bull. **43**: 119-121, 1944.
6. Lilienthal, H. K.: Thoracic Surgery, Philadelphia, 1925, W. B. Saunders Company, p. 250.
7. Friedman, B., and King, S. D.: Recovery Following Conservative Therapy, California & West. Med. **58**: 66-69, 1943.
8. Thornton, T. F., Jr., Adams, W. E., and Livingtone, H. M.: Mediastinal and Subcutaneous Emphysema Following Intratracheal Insufflation Anesthesia, Anesth. & Analg. **23**: 177-188, 1944.
9. Barret, N. R., and Thomas, D.: Massive Surgical Emphysema During Course of General Anaesthesia, Brit. M. J. **2**: 692-693, 1944.
10. Jones, R.: Massive Surgical Emphysema, Pneumothorax and Pneumoperitoneum, Brit. M. J. **2**: 530-531, 1945.
11. Hammond, A. E.: Emergency Cervical Mediastinotomy in Case of Massive Mediastinal and Subcutaneous Emphysema Secondary to Removal of Foreign Body From Bronchus, Ann. Otol., Rhin. & Laryng. **53**: 829-836, 1944.
12. Fisher, J. H., and Macklin, C. C.: Pulmonic Interstitial and Mediastinal Emphysema, Am. J. Dis. Child. **60**: 102, 1940.
13. Torrey, R. G., and Grosch, L. C.: Acute Pulmonary Emphysema Observed During the Epidemic of Influenzae Pneumonia at Camp Hancock, Ga., Am. J. M. Sc. **157**: 170, 1919.
14. Chanduri, K. C.: Following Bronchopneumonia, Indian J. Pediat. **10**: 176-179, 1943.
15. Schwartz, E.: Spontaneous Mediastinal and Subcutaneous Emphysema Complicating Bronchial Asthma, J. Allergy **16**: 279, 1945.
16. Hamman, L.: Mediastinal Emphysema; Frank Billings Lecture, J. A. M. A. **128**: 1-6, 1945.
17. Donaldson, J. K.: Surgical Disorders of the Chest, Philadelphia, 1944, Lea & Febiger.

CARCINOSARCOMA OF THE MAMMARY GLAND

BÉLA HALPERT, M.D., AND MILLINGTON O. YOUNG, M.D.,* OKLAHOMA CITY, OKLA.
(From the Department of Pathology, The School of Medicine of the University of Oklahoma)

IN A comprehensive review, Saphir and Vass[1] assembled the available reported cases of carcinosarcomas, and tabulated 153 according to the sites of occurrence. They concluded that perhaps only three or four of them might be designated as true carcinosarcomas. Among the thirty-two cases recorded as primary in the mammary gland, Saphir and Vass apparently believed none to be true carcinosarcomas; they considered twenty-one as "duct carcinomas." Since then Harrington and Miller,[2] Smithy,[3] Govan,[4] Mosto,[5] and Adair and Herrmann,[6] have reported cases of carcinosarcoma of the mammary gland. In this paper an additional case is presented, and because of the rarity of the neoplasm and the theoretical implications, the data are recorded in some detail.

REPORT OF CASE

A 43-year-old Negro woman was admitted to the University of Oklahoma Hospitals, April 8, 1944, complaining of a mass in the left mammary gland, first noticed four months previously, and twenty pounds loss in weight during the previous year. The patient stated that two months before admission, she slipped and fell on ice, striking the left breast. Following the fall the mass became painful and increased in size. On March 18, 1944, a physician incised the mass and "some pus and a large amount of blood" were obtained. The mass remained tender and the wound failed to heal, draining a brown purulent material.

At the time of admission the patient was obese and did not appear ill. The temperature was 100.6° F. In the upper inner quadrant of the left mammary gland there was a firm, warm, tender mass 8 cm. in diameter attached to the overlying skin. From an elevated, ulcerated area of the skin 2 by 2 cm. over the mass, a foul sanguinopurulent liquid exuded. The lymph nodes in the axilla were not palpable. The remainder of the physical examination yielded no pertinent information.

Urinalysis gave essentially negative results. The red blood cell count was 4,580,000; the hemoglobin content was 15.2 Gm.; the white blood cell count was 8,100, with polymorphonuclears 55, lymphocytes 40, monocytes 4, and eosinophiles 1 per cent. The Mazzini test of the blood was negative. A roentgenogram of the chest disclosed no evidence of pulmonary metastasis. A biopsy from the ulcerated area revealed a rapidly growing malignant neoplasm.

On April 14, 1944, a radical mastectomy was performed. The postoperative course was uneventful, except for some separation of the incision which necessitated a skin graft on May 8. The patient was discharged on May 19. Subsequently, she was given roentgen radiation over a period of twenty-seven days (May 31 to June 26) to four fields, two over the left upper thorax, one over the left axilla, and one over the left supraclavicular region (total dose 1,600 r. to the two anterior fields and 2,200 r. to the two fields over the axilla and supraclavicular regions; distance 50 cm.; 170 kv. over the two anterior fields and 200 kv. over the left axilla and supraclavicular regions; 18 ma.; Thoraeus filter).

When seen on Jan. 3, 1945, the patient had gained fifteen pounds in weight. There was some edema of the left arm and no evidence of any local recurrence. A roentgenogram of the chest disclosed numerous round areas of increased density scattered throughout both lung fields interpreted as pulmonary metastases. The patient died in another hospital on March 11, 1945. No necropsy was performed.

Received for publication, June 10, 1947.
*Now at the Department of Surgery, Yale University School of Medicine, New Haven, Conn.

The biopsy specimen consisted of two mottled brown and yellow-gray fragments of tissue together 2.5 by 1.5 by 0.8 centimeters. Microscopic preparations stained with hematoxylin and eosin disclosed sheets of large neoplastic cells with marked variation in size and shape of the nuclei and many in a state of division. In places, clusters of apparently epithelial cells were seen surrounded by cells in a streamlike arrangement within a fibrillar ground substance into which faded the cytoplasm of the cells. Occasional cells had giant proportions with several nuclei. Areas of necrosis and hemorrhage were frequent, and a broad zone of fibrinopurulent exudate covered part of one surface.

The specimen obtained at operation consisted of the left mammary gland with the underlying pectoral muscles and axillary contents. The nipple was inverted, freely movable, and centrally located in an elliptical portion of dark brown skin 20 by 15 centimeters. In the upper inner quadrant in the skin overlying a fluctuant mass 8 cm. in diameter, there was an ulcerated area 2 by 2 cm. with everted, heaped-up margins. On the cut surfaces this led into a craterlike cavity 6 cm. in diameter filled with green, yellow and brown tissue debris surrounded by a soft, pale yellow-gray margin of neoplastic tissue 1 cm. wide (Fig. 1). Continuous with the necrotic area, there was a gray-pink neoplastic field 4 by 3 centimeters. Detectable lymph nodes in the axillary content were in great part replaced by adipose tissue, and there seemed to be no neoplastic involvement.

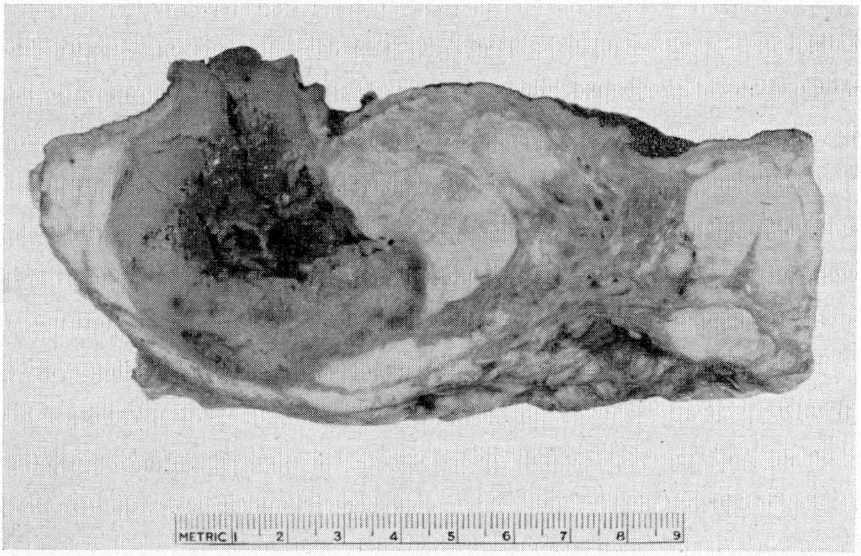

Fig. 1.—Appearance of the growth on the cut surfaces. An ulcerated area in the everted, heaped-up margins leads to a craterlike cavity 6 cm. in diameter filled with tissue debris and lined by neoplastic tissue.

In microscopic preparations stained with hematoxylin and eosin, representing many parts of the growth, there were sheets, columns, or nests of neoplastic epithelial cells in a stroma composed of neoplastic cells with large vesicular, round, oval, or irregularly shaped nuclei in a streamlike or interlacing arrangement. The cell nuclei varied markedly in size, and a number were seen in a state of division. The cytoplasm of these cells faded into a fibrillar ground substance similarly arranged in streams or whorls. The epithelial elements in the obviously nonepithelial stroma were composed of cells with large, vesicular, deeply stained nuclei with pink or lavender stained cytoplasm having clearly discernible borders or within a halo of cytoplasm. Some of the cells had huge nuclei or multiple nuclei with some in multicentric cell division. Although the epithelial and nonepithelial elements blended imperceptibly in places (Fig. 2), elsewhere the stroma was obviously provided by the nonepithelial growth (Fig. 3). Areas of necrosis and hemorrhage were frequent and extensive. The

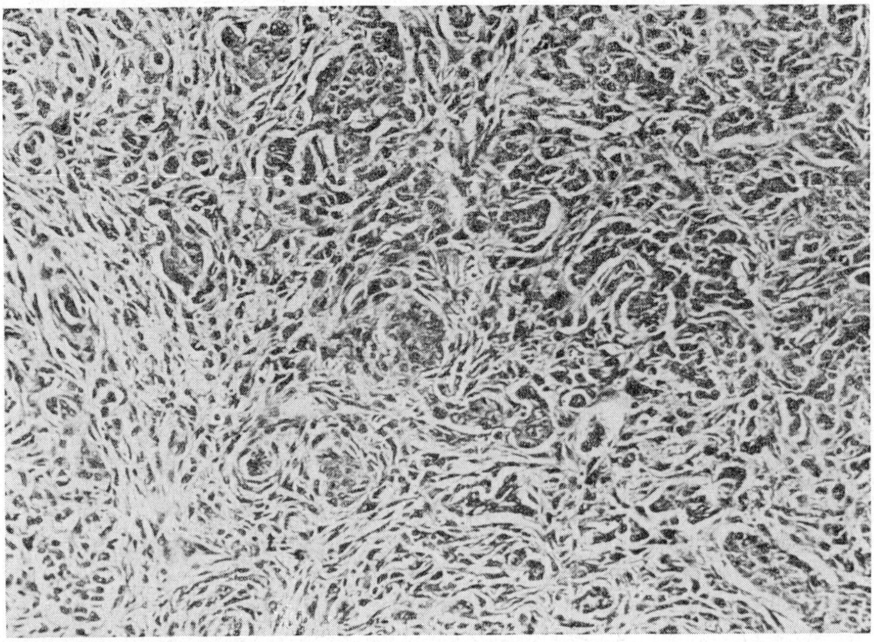

Fig. 2.—The cancerous growth is composed of epithelial elements, carcinoma, in a sarcomatous stroma. The two tissue elements in places blend imperceptibly (×150).

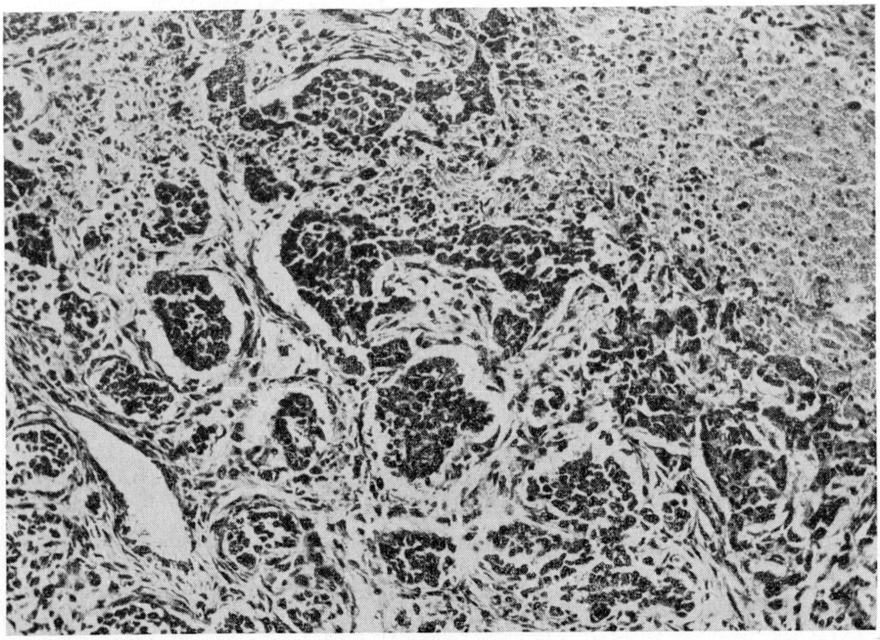

Fig. 3.—The epithelial elements of the cancerous growth are clearly discernible from the sarcomatous stroma (×150).

distribution of the obviously epithelial and nonepithelial elements varied in different portions of the growth. In the periphery of the growth in places there appeared to be a condensation of the fibrous connective tissue. Occasional groups of intact acini and ducts of the mammary gland were seen surrounded by a loose connective tissue fading into the neoplastic tissue. Preparations from the axillary lymph nodes disclosed marked adipose tissue replacement of the lymphatic pattern and no neoplastic involvement.

COMMENT

There is ample evidence that cancerous growths composed of both carcinomatous and sarcomatous elements occur. In the mammary gland, they have been seen in mice,[7] rats,[8] and men. Neoplastic proliferation of the epithelium in the mammary gland seems to furnish an incentive for neoplastic growth of the stroma as in fibroadenomas. A pure fibroma of the mammary gland is exceedingly rare.[9] Therefore, the interpretation as to the origin of carcinosarcomas needs not necessarily be complicated, although the possibilities enumerated by Harrington and Miller[2] must be kept in mind. Perhaps the simplest concept is to assume that the epithelial element, the carcinoma, is dominant and that the connective tissue element, the sarcoma, is subservient and forms the stroma. Carcinoma always stimulates the surrounding connective tissue to provide a stroma for it. In this instance the stimulation was such that a sarcomatous stroma was produced. The sarcoma, on the other hand, provides its own stroma, and, therefore, is unlikely to initiate the growth of a carcinoma. According to this concept, the carcinomatous metastases might induce the proliferation of a sarcomatous stroma while sarcomatous metastases would be free of carcinoma. Unfortunately, in our case there was no opportunity to study the structure of the metastatic growths.

SUMMARY

A carcinosarcoma of the mammary gland is reported in a 43-year-old Negro woman. The morphologic appearance of the rare cancerous growth suggested that the epithelial element, the carcinoma, was dominant and that the connective tissue element, the sarcoma, formed the stroma.

REFERENCES

1. Saphir, O., and Vass, A.: Carcinosarcoma, Am. J. Cancer **33**: 331-361, 1938.
2. Harrington, S. W., and Miller, J. M.: A Mixed Tumor (Carcinosarcoma) of the Breast, SURGERY **7**: 122-128, 1940.
3. Smithy, H. G.: Mixed Malignancy of the Breast, SURGERY **16**: 854-864, 1944.
4. Govan, A. D. T.: Two Cases of Mixed Malignant Tumour of the Breast, J. Path. & Bact. **57**: 397-404, 1945.
5. Mosto, D.: Carcinosarcoma de la Glandula Mamaria, Rev. Asoc. méd. argent. **59**: 1410-1411, 1945.
6. Adair, F. E., and Herrmann, J. B.: Sarcoma of the Breast, SURGERY **19**: 55-73, 1946.
7. Williams, A. C., Silcox, L. E., and Halpert, B.: Carcinoma of the Mammary Gland in an Inbred Stock of Albino Mice, Am. J. Cancer **24**: 823-830, 1935.
8. Dunning, W. F., Curtis, M. R., and Maun, M. E.: Spontaneous Malignant Mixed Tumors of the Rat, and the Successful Transplantation and Separation of Both Components From a Mammary Tumor, Cancer Research **5**: 644-651, 1945.
9. Halpert, B., and Dial, D. L.: Fibroma of the Breast, Am. J. Path. **9**: 905-908, 1933.

A NEW MATERIAL AND TUBE DESIGN IN GASTROINTESTINAL INTUBATION

ARTHUR L. KASLOW, M.D., HOLLYWOOD, CALIF.

(From the Section of Internal Medicine, Wm. E. Branch Clinic, the Hollywood Presbyterian Hospital, and the Cedars of Lebanon Hospital)

PROLONGED use of the rubber stomach or intestinal tube passed intranasally is frequently the cause of bitter complaint on the part of the patient due to obvious irritation in the nasopharynx and esophagus. The natural quality of rubber material is a high degree of stickiness, a property which makes it useful in tires to prevent slipping, but truly uncomfortable and irritating in the nose and throat.

Holinger and Loeb[1] recently reported four cases of severe infection of the cricoid cartilage following ulceration of the postcricoid mucosa in the anterior wall of the esophagus caused by the irritation of intranasal tubes made of rubber. A survey of the literature reveals twenty-four cases of serious pharyngeal infections following the usual rubber intubation procedure through the nose.

Repeated trial and observation have shown that intestinal intubation at times is a lifesaving procedure. Eliason and Welty,[2] in a ten-year survey of intestinal obstruction, concluded that where suction drainage by means of the Jutte, Levine, or Miller-Abbott tube was carried out in 124 of 292 cases (as an adjunct in treatment of obstruction from all causes) it was of value in 80 to 90 per cent of cases. In fact, in 25 per cent of the cases in which suction drainage was carried out, no subsequent operative procedure was required. They felt that it was particularly valuable in obstructive cases developing postoperatively where fresh adhesions are the basis for the obstruction. In most of these cases intubation eliminates the necessity for a subsequent operation. The statistics they presented are convincing proof of the lifesaving possibilities of intraintestinal intubation. When the Miller-Abbott tube was used for intraintestinal suction in 1937 for the first time, the 31 per cent mortality that existed with the use of the intragastric tube from 1934 to 1937 was reduced by 50 per cent. In sixty-five cases where intraintestinal intubation was used after 1937 the mortality was only 15 per cent. Intubation can prevent surgical intervention in a partial intestinal obstruction apparently by reducing intraintestinal tension.

It is because such important uses have been firmly established for intestinal intubation that a new material was sought that would justify more frequent and early use of the intranasal tube. This is important since there is a great deal of reticence among doctors to use an intranasal tube except in serious circumstances. This is understandable since there is a marked discomfort inflicted on the patient by the use of the rubber tube. The present report deals

Tubing provided by Don Baxter Company, Glendale, Calif., and Clinical Plastic Products, Los Angeles, Calif.

Received for publication, April 22, 1947.

with a tube made of plastic material which reduces to a negligible degree the nasal and pharyngeal discomfort. This material has so little irritative effect that its early use in gastric or intestinal difficulties due to irritation or stasis is urgently recommended since it will cause little or no irritable complaint from the patient.

Of all plastic materials tested, the one that proved to be most useful and least irritating was a smooth transparent plastic of the Koroseal type. From this material, modifications of the stomach and intestinal tubes now made of rubber were developed and are discussed herein.

All plastic tubes to be described are of a smaller caliber than rubber tubes (14 to 16 Fr. diameter) and can readily be passed through the nose. The tubes are of a clear colorless transparency, have a moderate amount of pliability with a satisfactory amount of elasticity, and above all possess a smooth glasslike slickness.

ADVANTAGES OF PLASTIC OVER RUBBER

The advantages of this plastic material over rubber are fivefold:

1. Plastic tubes have a smoother surface than rubber, thereby reducing friction in the nose and throat while passing the tube, as well as minimizing the irritation on the pharynx while swallowing after the tube is in place.

2. The smoother plastic material cannot kink or twist on itself tightly enough to obstruct the flow in either direction. As many as three tight knots were experimentally tied in a length of tubing, yet suction could be maintained to carry on the withdrawal of intestinal contents. This is due to the negligible amount of stickiness of plastic material whereas rubber has a marked amount.

3. The colorless transparency gives continuous visualization of the stomach or intestinal contents as siphoned out. The nature of the material can in this way be continuously observed and alteration in treatment made frequently. With opaque rubber tubes, definite periods of collection of intestinal contents in bottles are necessary to see the type of drainage taking place.

4. The absence of deterioration of plastic when in contact with oil or ointments permits the use of ointments having greater lubricating properties in passing the tube. More tenacious ointments can also be applied after the tube is in place. This adds considerably to the comfort of the patient since it minimizes the irritation of the tube on the nasopharyngeal tissues. The only types of lubricant that can be used on rubber tubes are water-soluble types and these tend to disappear rapidly.

5. The inexpensive cost permits expendability. The cost of this tubing is much less than for an equal length of rubber tubing. In time it will be economically feasible to discard the plastic tube after one use. The discard of gastric and intestinal tubes will save much time and labor which is at present expended needlessly in the cleaning of the tubes by supply room personnel after each use. The use of a fresh noncontaminated tube on each new patient will also mark a step forward in medicine. At times re-used rubber tubes have such disagreeable odors that it is not very convincing to the patient when he is told that the ill-smelling tube about to be used on him has been sufficiently

cleansed in order to be used safely again. There is no odor to the plastic tube such as rubber tubes possess.

GASTROINTESTINAL TUBE

This design of a plastic gastrointestinal tube differs somewhat from the present types made of rubber. It is a single-lumen plastic tube ten feet long with a weighted balloon attached to its end. The balloon is weighted by being partly filled with 5 c.c. of liquid metallic mercury. The balloon is a separate chamber and has no connection to the lumen of the tube, nor does it require any inflation or deflation after passage through the nose. The end of the tube is weighted in this manner so that gravity and peristalsis will move the tube through the intestinal tract in the same manner that a bolus of food is swept along. X-ray studies clearly show the location of the mercury-filled balloon at all times.

Proximal to the attachment of the balloon are perforations directly into the lumen of the tube into which the intestinal contents are sucked.

The distal tip of the tube is made of a loop of small caliber plastic tubing which is soft and flexible. This tip is unlike a metal ball and has no traumatic effect either in passing through the nasopharynx or on the gastrointestinal mucosa. Perforations in the tip permit suction of gastric or intestinal contents from the distal end of the tube as well as from the area behind the balloon.

The simplicity of this tube eliminates a good deal of nurse and doctor care, since once it is passed there is no necessity of constantly watching the tube for the proper time to inflate the balloon in order to move it through the intestinal tract. To pass the tube the patient is placed in a semisitting position with the head tilted back. The balloon and tubular tip is then passed through the nasal orifice. The mercury in the balloon runs into the dependent part of the chamber when it reaches the back nasopharynx and aids in directing the tube down the esophagus. After the passage of the tube into the stomach, or to the 1½ foot mark, the patient is placed on his right side. In a short period of time, gravity or peristalsis pulls the weighted balloon into the pylorus (see Fig. 1). Having passed through the pyloric sphincter it readily moves into the duodenum. In repeated trials the tube has been inserted up to ten feet into the intestinal tract in a much shorter period of time than the presently used rubber tubes require.

In over 110 cases of intestinal intubation with this plastic tube it has been shown that there are many advantages in simplicity of handling and there is a remarkable absence of discomfort to the patient after as long as fifteen days of constant use.

STOMACH IRRIGATION TUBE

This design of a stomach irrigation tube consists of a double-lumen tube in which a narrow tube is inserted through and beyond a larger diameter tube. Both tubes are of plastic material. The smaller tube extending beyond the large tube has perforations only at its distal end so that cleansing fluids instilled through it will run directly into the stomach. The larger tube has per-

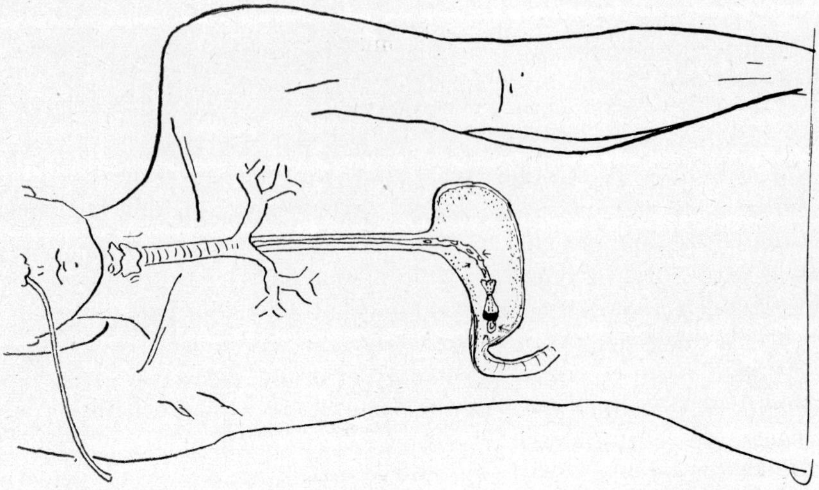

Fig. 1.—Weighted tip of tube showing structure; gravity tends to direct tip toward pylorus.

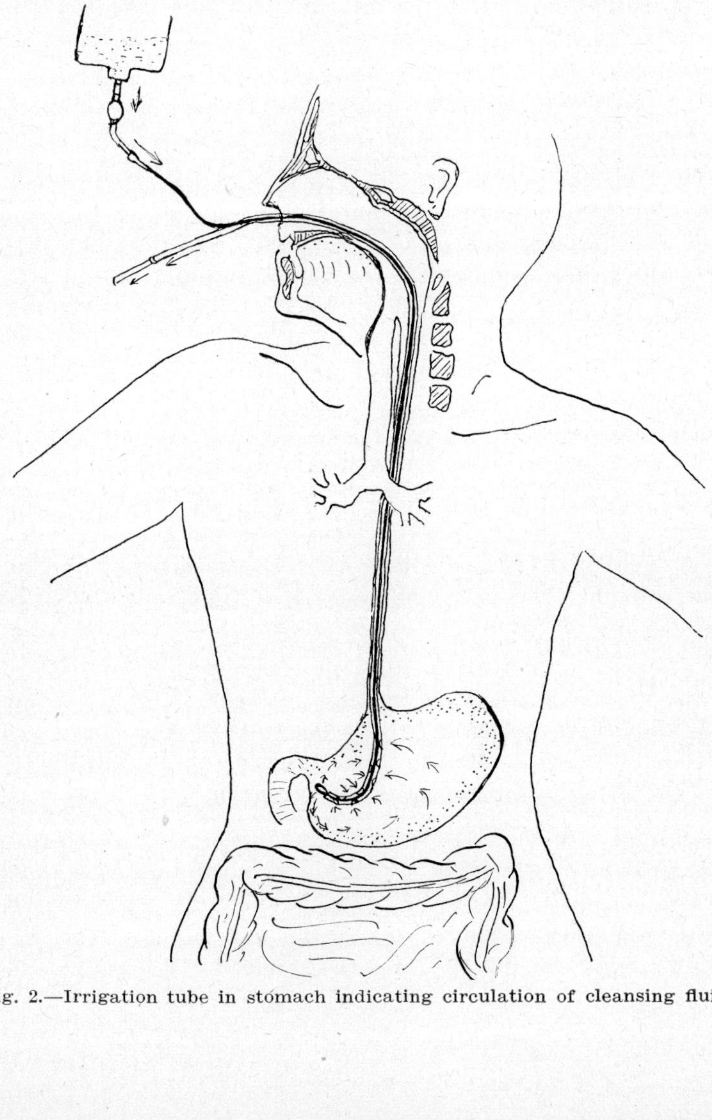

Fig. 2.—Irrigation tube in stomach indicating circulation of cleansing fluid.

forations proximal to its end so that suction applied to it sucks back the washings of the cleansing fluids ejected from the smaller tube (see Fig. 2).

This tube is especially useful in those cases requiring repeated *lavage* over a period of time, where it is necessary to spare the patient as much discomfort as possible due to debility or shock. It has been used with good cleansing results in postoperative nausea and vomiting, partial intestinal obstruction, barbiturate poisoning, gall bladder distress with nausea and vomiting, and as a cleansing procedure following food poisoning. Recently it has been used with success as a continuous irrigation of the stomach for four days in a case of severe nephritis in which anuria was imminent. The patient survived the acute phase of the disease.

By this tube arrangement cleansing fluids, such as bicarbonate of soda or saline solution, are continuously instilled into the stomach while a Wangensteen suction drains the washings back. This is a true irrigation device. Furthermore, it can be set up and left functioning without constant nursing attention. Irrigation with the present single-lumen tube requires the pushing back and forth of the column of material already in the tube with each use of the syringe.

One liter or more of cleansing solution is attached to the small lumen tube and allowed to run in by gravity, while an alternate suction or Wangensteen suction is attached to the larger suction tube. Irrigation and lavage in this manner is very gentle and is carried out without the discomfort to an already irritable stomach of spasmodic gushes of fluid into it. It also offers the advantage of continuous operation day and night, without disturbing the patient, simply by adding fluids to the irrigation bottle. Due to its negligible discomfort to the patient, the device described here has uses other than that of an irrigation apparatus where prolonged use of a nasal tube is required. It has been used in gall bladder drainage by allowing a solution of magnesium sulfate to drip through the small tube into the duodenum, while the bile is drained back through the larger tube.

It has been used for intragastric as well as intraintestinal feeding for periods lasting up to ten days. Feeding can be more easily accomplished by gravity feeding through one lumen while medication is administered through the other tube. This eliminates the need to disconnect the tube to give medication.

SUMMARY

Stomach and intestinal tubes made of plastic material have been extensively used and found to be comparatively free of discomfort compared to rubber tubes.

A simplified tube used for intestinal intubation is presented to indicate its greater ease in handling.

A two-way stomach tube that permits continuous irrigation and *lavage* is discussed. Other uses for such a tube are mentioned.

REFERENCES

1. Holinger, Paul H., and Loeb, William J.: Feeding Tube Stenosis of the Larynx, Surg., Gynec. & Obst. **83:** 253-259, 1946.
2. Eliason, E. L., and Welty, R. F.: A Ten-Year Survey of Intestinal Obstruction, Ann. Surg. **125:** 57-63, 1947.

ELECTRIC LIFT

An Aid in the Treatment of Decubitus Ulcers

Joseph G. Kostrubala, M.D., and Albert G. Wagner, M.D., Hines, Ill.

REPORTS of surgical treatment by excision and plastic closure of decubitus ulcers in paraplegic patients indicate an increasing number of successful results. Most of the reports to date come from military hospitals where these patients were first received and treated. Eventually all veterans with spinal cord injuries will of necessity be admitted for treatment to the several paraplegic centers in the Veterans Administration Hospitals. It is in such centers that surgical treatment of bed sores poses a formidable problem as far as the local treatment is concerned.

Suitable and frequent changes of dressings are a necessity and are extremely difficult to accomplish because the patients are paralyzed and the lesions are most frequently found about the pelvic girdle. Extensive bed sores can be compared with deep burned lesions and require properly applied pressure dressings. Uninvolved bony prominences must be given special attention while a dressing is applied, and should be well padded to prevent additional ulcerations. After plastic closure has been accomplished, voluminous pressure dressings must also serve as a splinting device to produce at least partial immobilization. At least two assistants are needed during application of a dressing and even then, the process is tedious and the dressing not entirely satisfactory.

A well-organized and properly equipped dressing room is indispensable on a large service where many pre- and postoperative dressings are done each day. The main feature of this dressing room is the electric hoist which enables one doctor or one nurse to change an extensive dressing properly without exertion. The results where these hoists have been used were so uniformly gratifying and the acceptance by the patients of this method so enthusiastic, that it was thought advisable to present it graphically in detail. The accompanying illustration is self-explanatory.

The procedure usually carried out is as follows: The litter with the patient is wheeled into the dressing room to a position directly under the hoist. With the patient in prone position, a 9 inch belt is placed under the chest, a 6 inch belt under each thigh, the snaps secured, and the separator placed between the two cables that support the thighs. The lever is pulled that raises the patient to the desired height and the old dressings are removed. Aseptic technique is easy to carry out while the patient is suspended. When the patient is redressed, he is lowered to the litter by pulling the proper lever of the hoist.

Among the variations from this usual procedure, the following may be noted: At times, a patient in bed or on a Stryker frame may be brought in directly without placing him on a litter. It is obvious that the door to the dressing room must be wide enough to admit a hospital bed. Although the prone

Published with the permission of the Chief Medical Director, Department of Medicine and Surgery, Veterans Administration, who assumes no responsibility for the opinions expressed or the conclusions drawn by the authors.

Received for publication, May 21, 1947.

position is most satisfactory, should a spastic condition of the patient require that he be raised with the hips flexed, he may be placed into the apparatus lying on his side, a pillow between the knees, one belt around both thighs, and the upper belt around the chest. If spasms are too frequent to allow the patient to remain suspended during the entire change of dressing, he is raised long

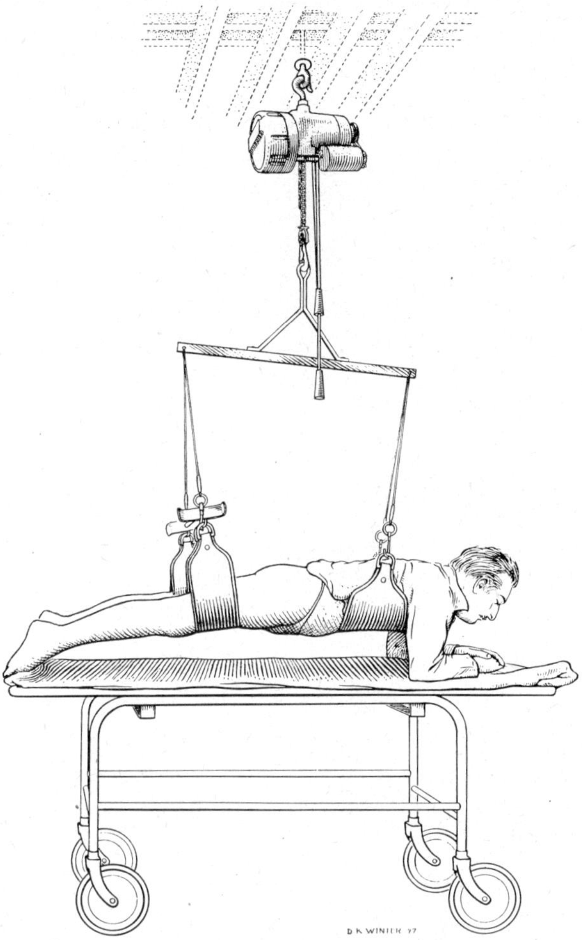

Fig. 1.—The paraplegic patient is elevated to a sufficient height from the cart allowing direct access to all parts of the pelvis. Local treatment of the decubitus ulcers and proper application of dressings are markedly facilitated. The electric lift shown is ⅛ ton "Budgit" hoist manufactured by Manning, Maxwell & Moore, Inc., Muskegon, Mich.

enough to remove the outer bandage material and lowered for the necessary observation and treatment and raised again to permit reapplication of the dressing.

SUMMARY AND CONCLUSIONS

1. The importance of proper dressings should be recognized as a very important part of the surgical treatment of decubitus ulcers. Because of the paralytic condition present and the location of the ulcers, proper application of dressings is extremely difficult to attain.

2. A dressing room featuring the use of an electric hoist is presented which markedly reduces the difficulties of handling the patient and allows easy application of dressings.

3. With slight variations, this type of hoist may also be used in the operating room for immediate postoperative dressings. It may be anticipated that this method may well serve other uses, such as the treatment of burns about the pelvic girdle and in certain orthopedic conditions requiring unobstructed access to the pelvic region.

Case Reports

ASSOCIATED PANCREATIC NECROSIS AND BILIARY DISEASE

A Case Report

Joel W. Baker, M.D., and Milton W. Durham, M.D., Seattle, Wash.

THE case we are presenting for review is of interest in that: first, the problem of acute pancreatitis associated with cholelithiasis is presented; second, the nonsurgical removal of persistent postoperative stones in the common duct is accomplished.

CASE REPORT

M. B. (Clinic No. 124482), a 38-year-old Jewish housewife, was first referred to the Mason Clinic, April 9, 1946, with the chief complaint of intermittent, severe, right upper quadrant pain associated with nausea and vomiting of four days' duration.

The family history was noncontributory. She had suffered no previous injuries or serious illnesses in the past; she had had no previous surgical operations. She had been perfectly well until five years prior to admission. At that time she first noticed loose stools, especially in the morning. The stool was not watery, but was soft and bulky. The increase in bowel movements gradually continued until two years prior to admission she was having seven to ten soft loose stools daily, and at the same time noticed onset of right upper quadrant pain with nausea and vomiting which spontaneously subsided after a few bouts. There was an increase in the frequency and severity of the attacks until for the four days prior to hospital admission she had suffered continuous attacks.

Systemic review revealed no significant facts except that the patient had always been obese, for many years having weighed over 200 pounds.

Physical examination revealed a moderately ill, obese woman, 5 feet 5 inches tall and weighing 211 pounds. Temperature on admission was 98° F., pulse 70, respirations 16, and blood pressure 150/90. There was an icteric tinge to the sclera, and a very slight icterus of the skin. Chest examination was negative. The abdomen was obese. There was tenderness in the right upper quadrant and in the epigastrium, but because of the thickness of the abdominal wall, neither muscular rigidity nor masses could be demonstrated. The remainder of the general physical examination revealed no significant findings. The significant laboratory tests were an icterus of 55, bile in the urine, demonstrated multiple stones in the gall bladder, and a normal leucocyte count.

Three days after completion of the laboratory results, and a total of six days after the first visit, she was admitted to the hospital in an emergency with severe exacerbation of the right upper quadrant pain. The last attack had been of nine hours' duration, associated with continuous nausea and the vomiting of greenish bile-stained material. The attack was the same as those previously described, except with increasing severity and radiation to the back. Stools during this period had been persistently white with dark urine. A repeated complete physical examination showed no change from the previous examination except that the temperature on admission was 95.4° F. (checked), pulse 60, respiration 16. There was more marked tenderness in the right upper quadrant and epigastrium and some tenderness in the left upper quadrant. Repeated blood and urine examination revealed no

Presented in a Dry Clinic at the annual meeting of the Pacific Coast Surgical Association, Seattle, Wash., Feb. 18, 1947.

Received for publication, June 10, 1947.

essential change from the previous reports except an increase in the leucocyte count to 13,000 with 84 per cent neutrophiles; the icterus index had increased to 75 units.

The clinical impression was that the patient suffered from (1) an acute exacerbation of chronic cholecystitis with demonstrated stones, and (2) common bile duct obstruction due to lithiasis, and with extreme obesity to complicate the surgical management of the condition. On admission she was given glucose infusions plus demerol hypodermically for pain. The following day the temperature ranged between 97 and 98.6° F., the pulse from 70 to 80, and the patient showed clinical improvement.

Choledochostomy and cholecystectomy were advised. On April 18, 1946, nine days after the first examination, the patient was operated upon under inhalation anesthesia. When the peritoneum was opened there were immediately apparent multiple miliary areas of fat necrosis (Fig. 1), averaging 5 to 10 mm. in diameter, and one of these areas was removed for biopsy and photograph. These covered the greater omentum, the gastrocolic omentum, and the fat around the duodenum and the duodenohepatic ligament. The head of the pancreas was the size of a baseball, was diffusely firm, and was intimately adherent by fresh adhesions to the overlying colon and other structures. The gall bladder was moderately distended with a slightly thickened wall, but without exudate. It was packed with multiple,

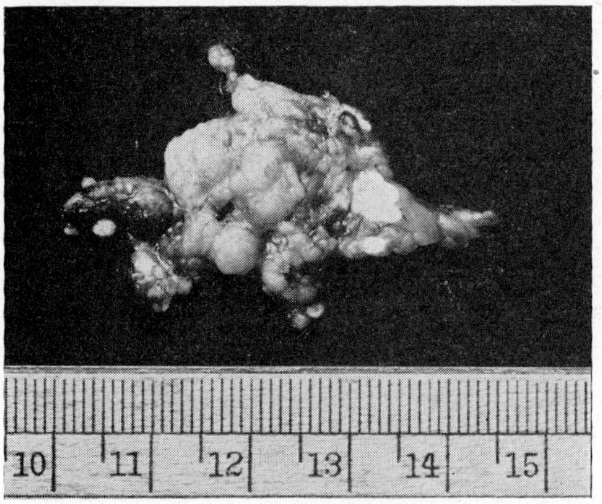

Fig. 1.—Biopsy of omentum showing fat necrosis. Microscopic study was reported as caseous necrosis of omentum.

small faceted stones with several of these impacted in the cystic duct, which was long and small. The common duct was not visualized nor was it openly explored, because of the edema of the duodenohepatic ligament, the encroachment upon it by the enlarged pancreas, and the critical state of the patient. During the induction stage of the anesthetic the patient vomited bile and gastric secretion; she had a dusky color from this point throughout the remainder of the operation. It was felt that she may have aspirated some of the gastric content. This, plus the proved high mortality rate in acute pancreatic necrosis and the individual technical problem here involved, influenced us to resort to simple cholecystostomy. By removing the stones from the cystic duct, indirect drainage of the common bile duct was provided. To insure that this was accomplished a continuous flow of common duct bile into the gall bladder via the cystic duct was demonstrated. The gall bladder was then drained with a No. 12 Pezzer catheter and brought out through a stab wound in the right flank. The patient's condition upon completion of the operation was satisfactory, with a stable blood pressure and pulse, and with a fair amplitude of respiration.

A serum amylase determination, neglected preoperatively, was made immediately after the operation, and was found elevated to 432 units. Although considered as critically ill postoperatively, the patient made an uneventful convalescence. During this period the

Pezzer catheter continued to drain from 100 to 300 c.c. of moderately clear bile daily, although cramps ensued if the tube was clamped. There was a rapid diminution in the icterus so that by the ninth postoperative day the icterus index was reported as 19 and the serum amylase as 122. The stool examination showed an excess of neutral fat present. Microscopic report of the biopsy of omentum was "caseous necrosis of the omentum."

The cholangiogram at this time (Fig. 2) showed multiple nonopaque areas in the distal third of the common duct which had the appearance of stones; the oil entered the duodenum readily and the maximum diameter of common duct was 13 mm. Observation films at five and ten minutes and one hour showed residual fluid in the common duct. This was due in part to the fact that some emptied from the gall bladder. It was noted that injection of the oil caused severe, upper right quadrant pain.

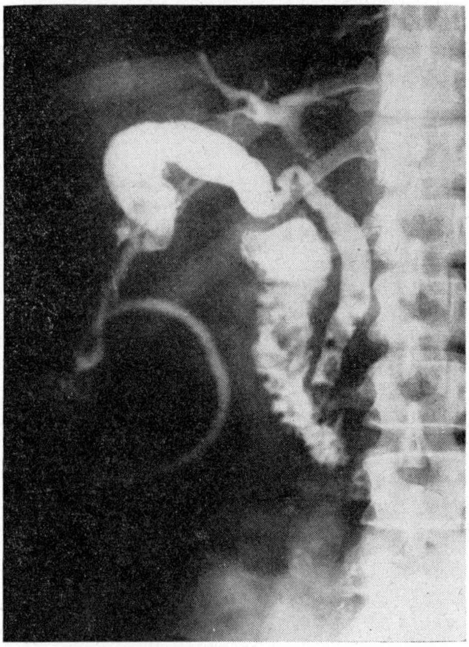

Fig. 2.—Cholangiogram on twelfth postoperative day showing multiple nonopaque areas in distal third of common duct.

The patient was discharged from the hospital on the fifteenth postoperative day with a final diagnosis of chronic cholecystitis and cholelithiasis, residual choledocholithiasis, and acute pancreatic necrosis. The Pezzer catheter was connected to an infant hot-water bottle to collect conveniently the biliary drainage, and the patient was instructed to irrigate the tube daily with normal saline solution to insure against encrustation. At home the patient continued to regain strength and was much improved except that if the catheter was clamped off or became plugged at any time, she immediately suffered exacerbation of the right upper quadrant pain which was relieved by opening the tube. A second stage choledochostomy to remove the residual stones was planned after sufficient time should have elapsed for the pancreatitis to subside.

It was at this time that Harris and Moncus[1] suggested the injection of 1:500 solution of nupercaine in normal saline solution for relief of spasm of the sphincter of Oddi, and reported one instance in which this method had allowed passage of a residual common duct stone.

On May 15, twenty-nine days after operation, the catheter in the gall bladder was injected with 30 c.c. of 1:500 nupercaine solution in normal saline solution, and irrigated with normal saline solution afterward without pain. Thirteen days later the patient reported to the hospital at 9 P.M. with a severe episode of right upper quadrant pain similar to that she had had preoperatively. Nupercaine solution, 30 c.c. injected into the Pezzer catheter promptly relieved the pain and a third injection of nupercaine solution carried out thirteen days later produced no pain.

At this time a repeat cholangiogram (Fig. 3) was obtained, and showed the maximum diameter of the common duct to be 12 mm., with a small nonopaque area in the distal common duct. In fifteen minutes, 20 per cent of the oil had escaped into the duodenum, and in thirty minutes, 50 per cent. The multiple, nonopaque shadows previously noted had disappeared except for one remaining. Irrigation with nupercaine was carried out at ten-day intervals and thirty days after the second cholangiogram a third x-ray series demonstrated the diameter of the common duct to be reduced to 10 mm., and the previously noted

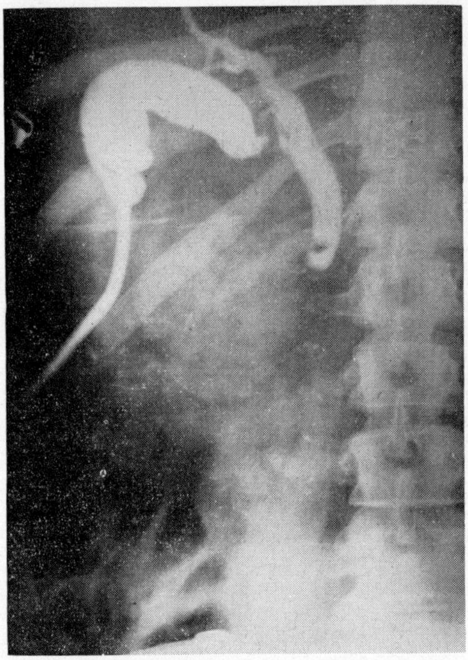

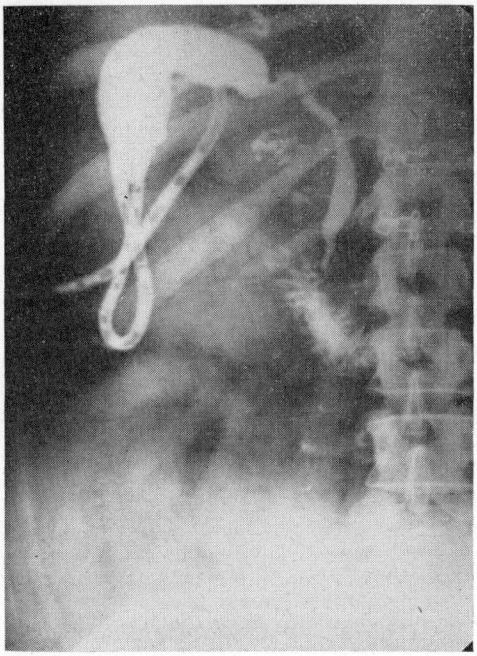

Fig. 3.—Cholangiogram taken after three irrigations of cholecystostomy tube with 1:500 nupercaine in saline solution carried out over a twenty-six day period, showing one remaining nonopaque area in distal common duct.

Fig. 4.—Final cholangiogram taken thirty days after that shown in Fig. 3, during which period the Pezzer catheter had been irrigated with nupercaine solution three more times. The filling defects shown previously are no longer present and the diameter of the common duct is reduced to 10 mm.

filling defect no longer present. Oil entered the duodenum immediately, with 60 per cent emptying in ten minutes. The tube was clamped off during the day and biliary drainage at home which had been averaging 300 c.c. daily, promptly diminished to only 10 or 15 c.c. during the night. The patient was without distress. The Pezzer catheter was removed on Aug. 1, 1946, three and one-half months postoperatively. The patient continued well for the ten months following that time.

Comment.—The association of inflammatory disease of the pancreas and infection of the biliary tract is recognized, but the teleological relationship is not satisfactorily understood. Investigators have reported biliary tract disease in from 16[2] to 81 per cent[3] of cases of pancreatitis, with an average incidence in large series of 55 per cent.[4, 5] The exact evaluation of the relative involvement of the biliary tract and of the pancreas has assumed greater importance in the last ten years since it has been demonstrated that under conservative treatment the mortality of acute pancreatitis is less than with emergency surgical intervention. The development of a reliable and rapid determination of the serum amylase has afforded us a valuable guide to severity in early cases. On our service we feel that acute cholecystitis should be handled as a surgical emergency and operation deferred only for necessary preparation or for nonsurgical complications. Since associated acute pancreatitis is one of the latter, we have the additional rule that a serum amylase determination be made before emergency laparotomy for the acute crisis of the upper abdomen. Like many rules that are made to be broken, we slipped in this instance—a mistake that fortunately turned out satisfactorily.

The second point of interest concerns the stones necessarily left in the common duct at the time of emergency cholecystostomy. Previous attempts to remove overlooked or secondary stones in the duct, usually following primary choledochostomy, by chemical means have in most instances been fraught with failure until Harris and Moncus,[1] applying a new principle, suggested relaxation of the sphincter of Oddi, rather than chemical dissolution of the stones. The practical application of this principle is successfully demonstrated in the case herein presented. Whether success following pressure irrigation with nupercaine solution should be attributed to the relaxation of the sphincter by the anesthetic agent or whether the anesthetizing of the ductal tree permits greater pressure to be used remains unproved. Preliminary studies on a small series indicate a lower perfusion pressure following nupercaine injection, but no lessening of the pain threshold, thus indicating that relaxation of the sphincter of Oddi is the mode of action. Further studies on this are continuing.

REFERENCES

1. Harris, Franklin I., and Moncus, Sanford I.: Common Duct Stone Relieved by Injection of Nupercaine Solution Into T-Tube, J. A. M. A. **131**: 29-30, 1945.
2. Weiner, H. A., and Tennant, Robert A.: Statistical Study of Acute Hemorrhagic Pancreatitis, Am. J. M. Sc. **196**: 167-176, 1938.
3. DeTakats, Geza, and MacKenzie, Wallace D.: Acute Pancreatic Necrosis and Its Sequelae, Ann. Surg. **96**: 418-439, 1932.
4. Puestow, Charles B., Louby, William E., and Risley, Thomas S.: Acute Pancreatitis, Am. J. Surg. **72**: 818-825, 1945.
5. Lamson, R. Starr: Acute Pancreatitis, Ann. Surg. **116**: 367-372, 1942.

Recent Advances in Surgery

CONDUCTED BY ALFRED BLALOCK, M.D.

MESENTERIC CYSTS

A REVIEW OF THE LITERATURE AND REPORT OF A CALCIFIED CYST OF THE MESENTERY

ARKELL M. VAUGHN, M.D., WILLIAM M. LEES, M.D., AND JAMES W. HENRY, M.D., CHICAGO, ILL.

(From the Departments of Surgery and Pathology, Loyola University School of Medicine and Mercy Hospital)

CYSTS of the mesentery have been described as the rarest of all abdominal tumors,[20] notwithstanding a score or more yearly case reports in recent years. The preoperative diagnosis of this condition is a difficult problem and requires ingenuity and experience. Because of the rarity of correctly diagnosed cases preoperatively, we should like to present this case and bring the literature up to date in so far as it is possible, with poor scientific communications between countries isolated by World War II.

HISTORY AND INCIDENCE

The first observation of this entity was made by the Florentine anatomist, Benevieni in 1507 who called these cysts found at autopsy, "anatomic curiosities."[10] In 1842, Rokitansky[38] gave the first recorded description of a chylous cyst. Tables I and II record chronologically contributions of various authors on the subject and their estimates as to the incidence of mesenteric cysts. Further incidence is illustrated by the following:

1. Judd and Crisp[36] stated that in 820,000 admissions to the Mayo Clinic, only twenty-five mesenteric tumors were found and of these only eight were cysts, an incidence of less than one in 100,000 admissions.

2. Roller[40] quoted the following reports: The Massachusetts General Hospital has a record of only six cases from 1900 to 1926. The University of California Hospital has a record of one cyst and one tumor of the mesentery in 93,511 admissions since 1906. The Children's Hospital of Los Angeles has three cases, occurring in the years 1932 to 1935, in a total of 12,425 admissions during the same period. Los Angeles General Hospital has a record of one case in 188,921 admissions in the five-year period, 1930 to 1935.

3. Olesen[41] reported no cases found at Los Angeles Hospital from 1912 to 1929.

4. Costello[17] reported one case in 28,312 admissions to Women's and Children's Hospital of Toledo, Ohio.

TABLE I

DATE	SURGEON	CONTRIBUTION
1507	Benevieni	First observed a mesenteric cyst at autopsy
1803	Portal[22]	Classified these cysts
1842	Rokitansky[38]	First described chylous cysts from autopsy
1880	Tillaux	First successfully operated on a cystic mesentery tumor[1]
1883	Pean	First marsupialized such a tumor successfully and later Bramann, Kilian, Millard, and Marklen also treated patients surgically[1]
1886	Augagneur[23]	Found 18 out of 90 cases of mesenteric tumors to be cystic
1887	Hahn[24]	Classified cysts as blood, chylous, serous, and echinococcus
1891	Arekion[25]	Referred to 81 case reports
	Bianchi[35]	Found 95 cases to this date
1892	Braquehaye[26]	Added 23 cases and said the total to date was 104
1897	Moynihan[27]	Added 9 cases and reviewed the literature
1900	Dowd[9]	In a classical review added 32 published cases making the total 145
1906	Porter	Estimated the total number of reported cases at 200[1]
1910	Timball[11]	Added 30 cases
1912	Friend	Collected 52 cases of chylous cysts[1]
1913	Benedict	Added 44 cases
1921	Carter[19]	Stated that not over 300 cases had been reported
1924	Higgins and Lloyd[14]	Reported that 250 cases had been recorded
1930	Flynn[20]	Judged that there were 200 to 300 cases published
1932	Warfield[1]	Found 129 cases reported since 1920 and estimated total to be about 500
1941	Loeb[3]	Estimated 550 to 600 cases reported

5. Porter[42] stated that no mesenteric cysts were found in 15,000 autopsies at the University of Minnesota and only two cases were observed in 200,000 clinical case reports at St. Mary's and St. Luke's Hospitals in Duluth, Minn.

6. Roller[40] found three cases in 900 surgical admissions to the University of Pennsylvania in two and one-half years (1931 to 1933).

7. As far as we can determine, our case is the third one of a mesenteric cyst in about 750,000 admissions to Mercy Hospital, Chicago, in the past ninety-eight years. Hueper[43] reported a case of mesenteric cyst (mesenteric enterocystoma) from this hospital in 1927. The patient was a boy, aged 5 years, who had a cyst the size of a hen's egg, located between the leaves of the mesentery 2½ inches from the ileocolic juncture, but not connected to the ileum. A third case was reported by Sawyer[44] in a personal communication. This case, however, was never reported in the literature.

TABLE II. FOUR HISTORICAL PERIODS OF MESENTERIC CYSTS ACCORDING TO BRAQUEHAYE[26] AND OTHERS

PERIOD	DATE	CHARACTERISTICS OF PERIODS
1	1507-1850	The lesion was found only at autopsy
2	1850-1880	Occasional operations were performed but usually on an incorrect preoperative diagnosis and none of the patients is reported to have survived
3	1880-1900	Operations for this lesion were followed by a few recoveries
4	1900-Date[34]	The condition was admirably described by Dowd, and surgeons took cognizance of such an entity and diagnosed several cases preoperatively

Therefore, it is reasonable to say that mesenteric cysts are sufficiently uncommon to arouse considerable interest. Warfield[1] emphasized that many surgeons of wide experience have neither observed nor operated upon a patient. The consensus of opinion in the literature is that the condition occurs twice as frequently in women and is rarely found in the colored races. Of all mesenteric tumors the cystic variety is four times more common than the solid. Most textbooks on surgery refer to the subject only briefly, if at all. Surgeons compose the majority of authors who write on this subject and most of them report a single case. Several have reported two cases; Roller[40] had three and DePenna[21] reported four. Hinkel[16] and others stated that the diagnosis is rarely made before surgery but this is not entirely so since diagnosed cases are reported by Haworth,[28] Bertolini,[29] Naumann,[32] Aloi,[30] Finucci,[31] Levison and Wolfsohn,[33] Kross,[15] and others.

ETIOLOGY AND CLASSIFICATION

Various classifications of mesenteric cysts have been offered as aids to a better understanding of the subject. Portal[22] was the first to make such a proposal in 1803. In 1842, Rokitansky[38] said that the tumors arose from degenerated lymph nodes. Braquehaye[26] listed the cysts according to their contents as sanguineous, lymphatic, parasitic, etc. In 1897, Moynihan[27] elaborated somewhat on this same classification and suggested several causes for the formation of these cysts. Dowd[9] in 1900, first attempted to name the various types of cysts according to their origin. It was his opinion that many of the cysts were of embryonic origin and he presented much evidence in proof of this opinion. He further stated that we can include all mesenteric cysts in three categories: (1) embryonic cysts, (a) hydatid cysts, (3) cystic malignant disease. Dowd also urged all investigators to obtain microscopic and chemical analyses of these cysts so that we can better understand the problem.

Many authors since have amplified Dowd's classification and the literature contains many theories as to the genesis of mesenteric cysts but the subject is still rather confusing. For a more detailed version of this phase of the problem we refer the reader to an original article by Warfield,[1] who presented an excellent discussion of the entire subject. More recent ones are Swartley,[10] Loeb,[3] Lahey and Eckerson,[2] Berger and Rothenberg,[13] and Roller,[40] who feel that mesenteric, omental, and retroperitoneal cysts should be classed together. Hill (quoted by Dunne[7] and Larkin[12]), in 1930, presented a classification which is widely accepted at present. This is also a modification of Dowd's classification. Hill said that all mesenteric cysts are of two types:

A. Simple
1. Serous
2. Chylous
3. Irregular types

B. Neoplastic
1. From ectoderm (dermoid)
2. From mesoderm (lymphangioma)
3. From entoderm (enterocystoma)
4. From fetal inclusions (teratoma)

Newer work on these cysts reveals that some are due to diverticula from the intestine in the embryo. It was suggested by Guthrie and Wakefield[4] that these diverticula may extend into the mesentery and become pinched off. Some are absorbed and others remain to form cysts. Intestinal epithelium was found in the majority of twenty-two human cysts and according to these authors substantiates the theory of embryonic origin of mesenteric cysts.

SIGNS AND SYMPTOMS

Mesenteric cysts may occur anywhere from the duodenum to the rectum. Over one-half of the cysts occur in the small bowel and one-fourth of them in the mesentery of the ileum.[1] The contents of the cysts may be clear, milky, sebaceous, bloody, yellow, or brown. These cysts are usually benign but malignant degeneration can occur and may be either carcinoma or sarcoma. Recently, there have been several reports describing such changes.[6, 37]

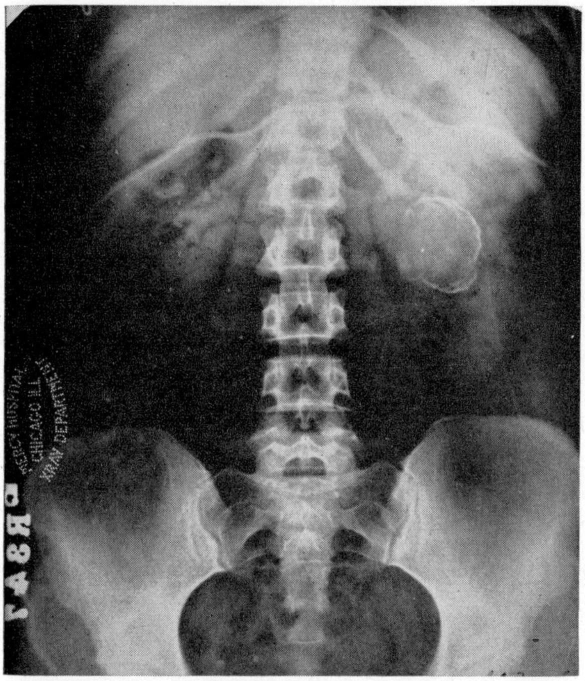

Fig. 1.—Scout roentgenogram of abdomen showing calcified mesenteric cyst in left upper quadrant.

Other than pain the symptoms are those due to complications, principally obstruction. Roller[40] stated that acute, chronic, or intermittent intestinal obstruction is responsible for 40 per cent of all complications. Pain is present more frequently in this type of cyst than in any other type of cystic abdominal tumor. Increase or decrease of the patient's weight is not of any great significance. An abdomen in acute surgical condition may present itself if rupture of a mesenteric cyst occurs. A careful history will reveal the probable cause of such an episode.

DIAGNOSIS

The principal point in the diagnosis of mesenteric cysts is to bear in mind the possibility of such a condition causing the symptoms present in a patient

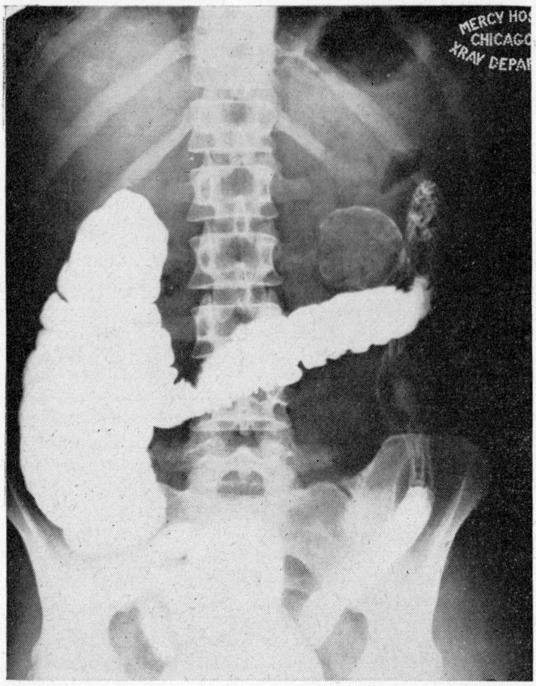

Fig. 2.—Roentgenogram of barium enema showing mass outside gastrointestinal tract.

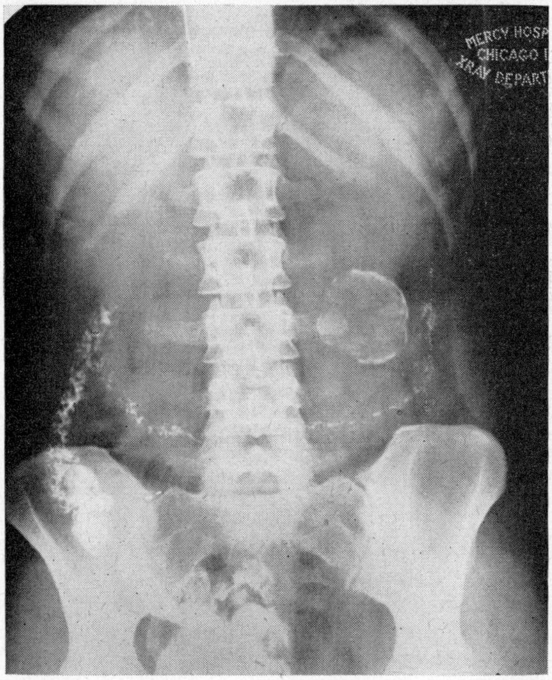

Fig. 3.—Roentgenogram following evacuation of enema.

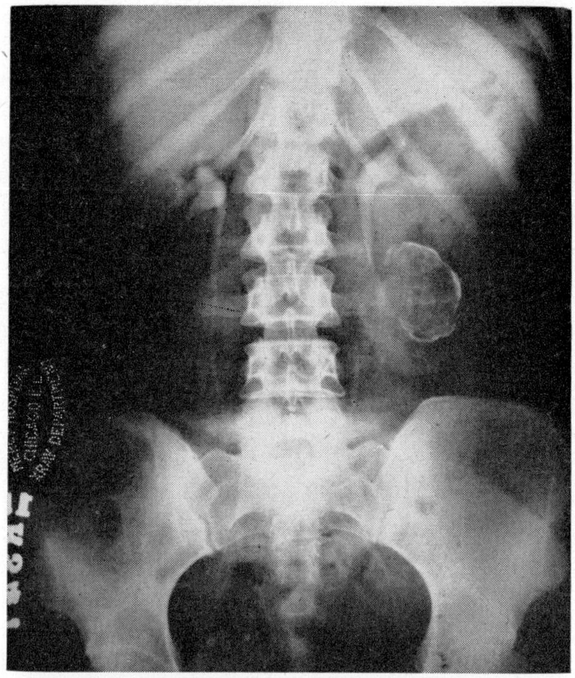

Fig. 4.—Intravenous pyelogram showing mass outside the kidney—ureter—bladder tract.

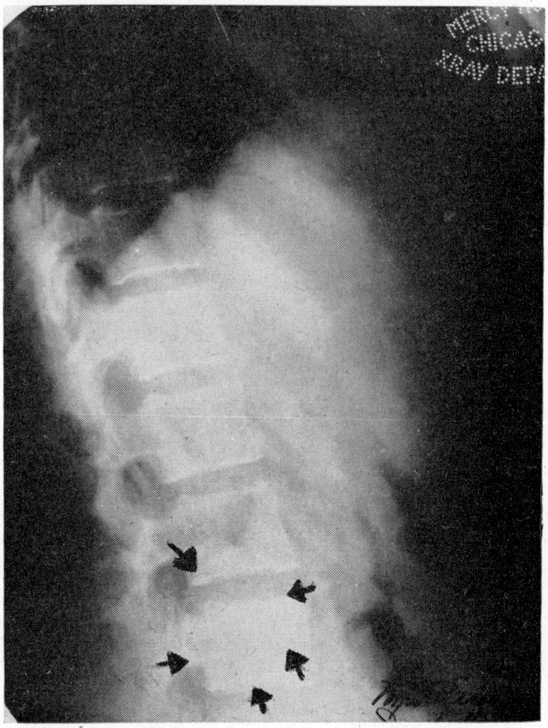

Fig. 5.—Lateral roentgenogram further localizing the calcified mass.

with an abdominal mass. Many grow to a fairly large size with the patient complaining only of an increase in girth of the abdomen. A rounded abdominal mass, which may be soft or firm, tender or not should at least suggest the possibility of a mesenteric cyst. A single scout film of the abdomen is seldom of great assistance in the diagnosis since many of these cysts are not radiopaque and cast no shadow. Very occasionally, as in our case, the cyst wall contains sufficient calcium to be outlined on the x-ray plate (Fig. 1). One of the cysts in Hinkel's report[16] also contained calcium. It is important to rule out a connection with the bowel lumen, which can be done with a barium meal or enema (Figs. 2 and 3). A pyelogram will aid in ruling out any connection with the kidney (Fig. 4). Both anteroposterior and lateral films aid in locating the cyst (Fig. 5). Hinkel also suggested pneumoperitoneum as a possible diagnostic aid. These results plus a careful history and physical examination should lead to a correct diagnosis in most instances.

TREATMENT AND MORTALITY

Treatment appears to be the one phase of the subject that most authors agree upon. In the order of desirability the treatment is as follows:

1. Total removal or enucleation is the operation of choice.

2. Enucleation with subsequent intestinal resection made mandatory by involvement of the blood supply to a portion of the bowel.

3. Marsupialization is the least desirable method and is resorted to only when point 1 or 2 is not possible due to too extensive involvement of the bowel. A draining sinus often accompanies this procedure but usually heals in one to three months.

4. Aspiration is mentioned only to be condemned as a method of treatment. It may be used for diagnostic purposes after the tumor has been isolated at operation, or to facilitate removal by reducing the size of the cyst.

Atchley[39] reported the mortality as a whole to be about 35 per cent. Roller[40] stated that the mortality following removal of the cyst without intestinal resection is about 9 per cent; with resection 25 to 30 per cent; and with marsupialization about 16 per cent.

CASE REPORT

E. M., aged 32 years, a white woman, para i, gravida i, entered Mercy Hospital, Jan. 20, 1946. The patient was well up to four to five years prior to hospital admission. At that time she complained of headaches associated with vomiting. Medical work-up resulted in the conclusion that no migraine was present. This cleared up gradually and three years before admission she began to have pain in the region of the sixth thoracic vertebra which radiated superiorly to the occiput. This pain was not related to the previously mentioned headache. A physician consulted at this time suspected some focus of infection but the patient refused another work-up and became well in six to eight weeks without medication. Seven years before admission the patient was in an automobile accident and sustained contusions and abrasions to the left leg, thigh, hip, and shoulder and left side of the chest and a fractured nose. Six months before she noticed a "shooting pain" which began in the left sacroiliac region and left lower quadrant of the abdomen and radiated down the anterior aspect of the thigh to the knee.

The past history was negative except as described. The family history was noncontributory.

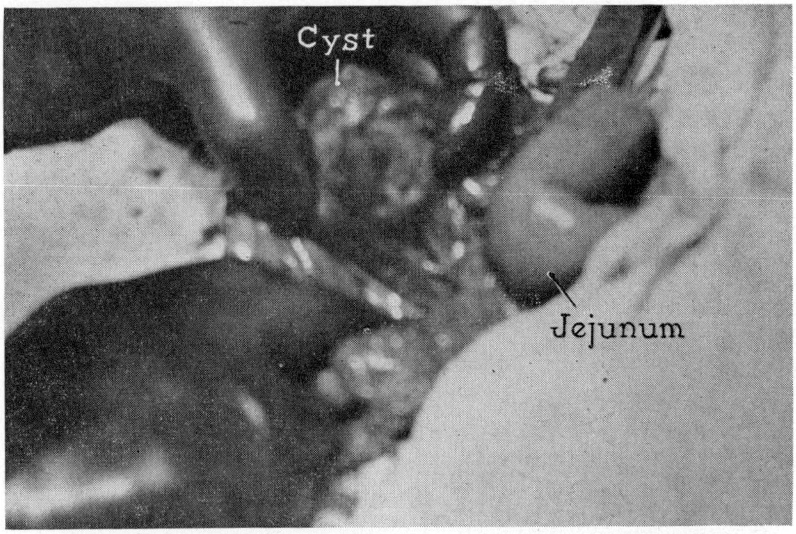

Fig. 6.—Photograph at operation showing calcified mesenteric cyst being dissected from its bed near the duodenojejunal ligament (Treitz).

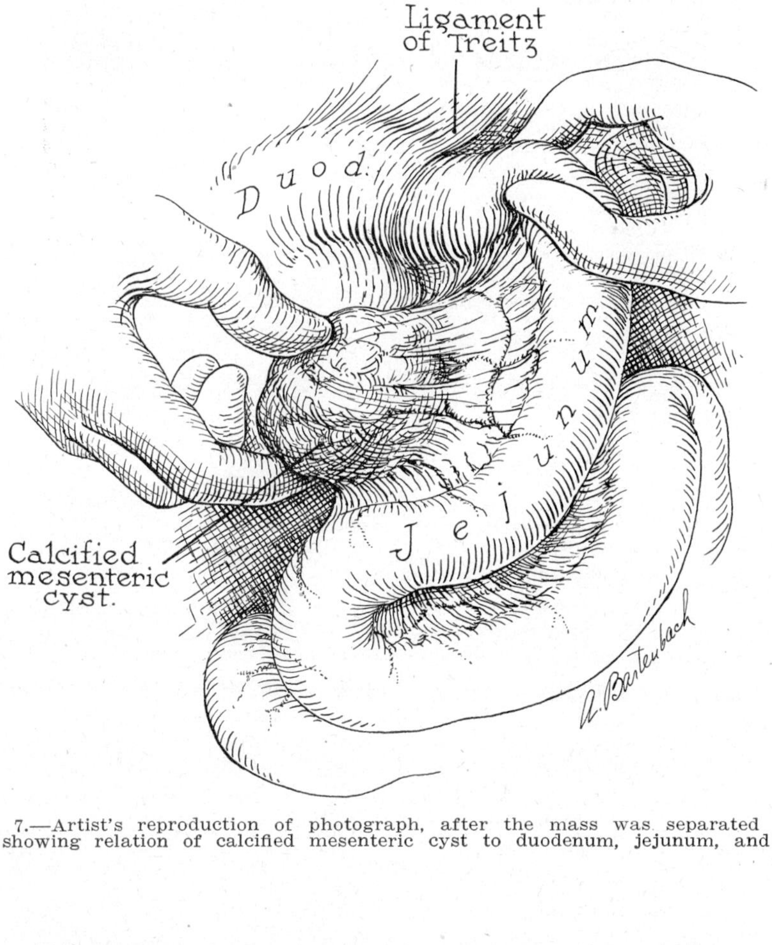

Fig. 7.—Artist's reproduction of photograph, after the mass was separated from the jejunum, showing relation of calcified mesenteric cyst to duodenum, jejunum, and ligament of Treitz.

The essential findings on physical examination were in the abdomen, which was soft, with tenderness elicited in the left upper quadrant. There was no rigidity except voluntary when the left upper quadrant was palpated. There was a firm, smooth, freely movable mass about the size of an orange just to the left and above the umbilicus. All tenderness was centered about this mass. The mass was more easily palpable when the patient lay on the stomach, whereupon the mass moved forward and lay against the anterior abdominal wall. The liver, kidneys, and spleen were not palpable.

Because of the firmness it was thought that the mass was calcified and the impression was listed as calcified cyst or hematoma of mesentery. A pedunculated pancreatic cyst, hypernephroma of left kidney, calcified accessory spleen, and retroperitoneal sarcoma were to be ruled out.

Urologic Consultation.—Pyelogram revealed a calcified cyst not attached to the kidney. The impression was calcified mesenteric cyst.

Laboratory Reports.—There were red blood cells, 4,380,000; white blood cells, 6,000; hemoglobin, 13 Gm. (84.4 per cent). Urine (voided specimen) was negative except for six to ten white blood cells per high-power field and rare red blood cells. Blood chemistry was essentially normal with nonprotein nitrogen 28.5, urea nitrogen 14, creatinine 1.6, chlorides 480, sugar 73, calcium 10, serum protein 6. Basal metabolic rate was minus 21 per cent.

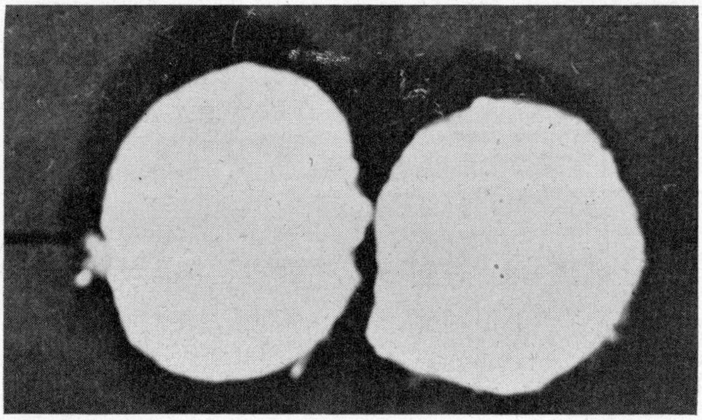

Fig. 8.—Photograph of calcified mesenteric cyst.

On Jan. 25, 1946, exploration of the abdomen was carried out. A left paramedian incision was made and the tumor was found in the left upper quadrant, surrounded by omentum and adhesions. Careful dissection revealed the mass to arise from the base of the jejunal mesentery close to the ligament of Treitz. Although the jejunum was adherent to the superior aspect of the mass, further dissection revealed it to be an inflammatory attachment and not a true outpouching of the jejunal wall (Figs. 6 and 7). Removal of the cyst was carried out uneventfully and no opening into the bowel could be demonstrated. The serosa of the jejunum was closed with interrupted silk sutures and hemostasis was secured without involving any of the major vessels to the bowel. The appendix was quickly removed and the abdomen closed in layers without drainage.

The patient had an uneventful convalescence except for a mild cystitis due to a postoperative catheterization which quickly cleared up. She was ambulatory on the eighth postoperative day and left the hospital on the twelfth postoperative day. Follow-up twelve months postoperatively revealed the patient working every day, although still complaining of occasional headaches associated with nausea.

Pathology.—The cyst was semisolid in consistency and roughly ovoid in contour, measuring 5.2 by 4.4 by 3.8 cm. (Fig. 8). The outer aspect of the cyst was smooth in areas and elsewhere shaggy reddish-gray. On sectioning, a fairly thick wall measuring up to 0.3

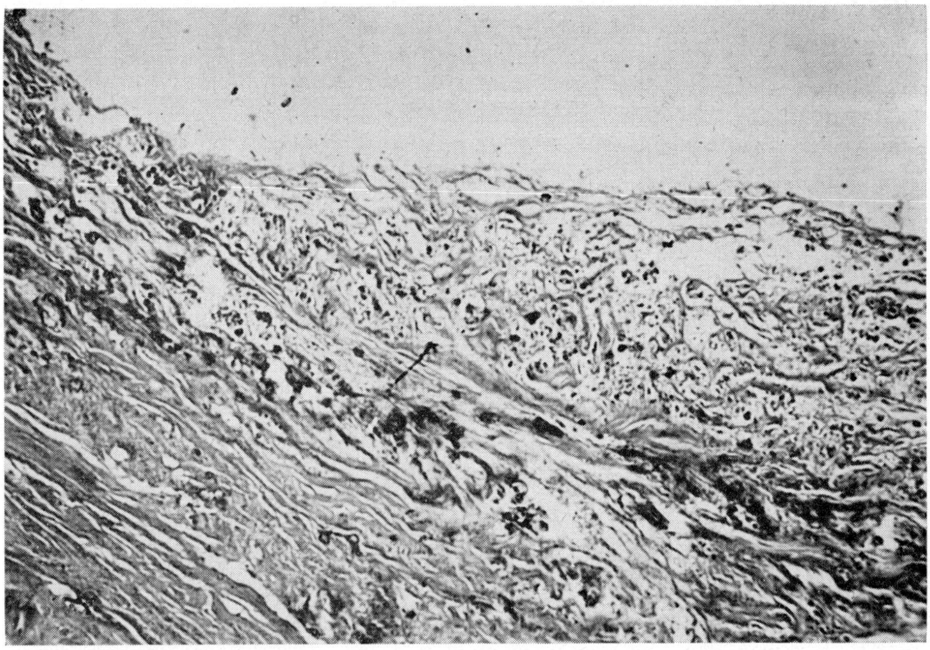

Fig. 9.—Section through inner half of cyst wall (×260): Prominent calcium deposition; dense collagenous fibrous tissue wall, and "frayed" inner aspect with chronic inflammatory and fat-laden macrophages within interstices of connective tissue.

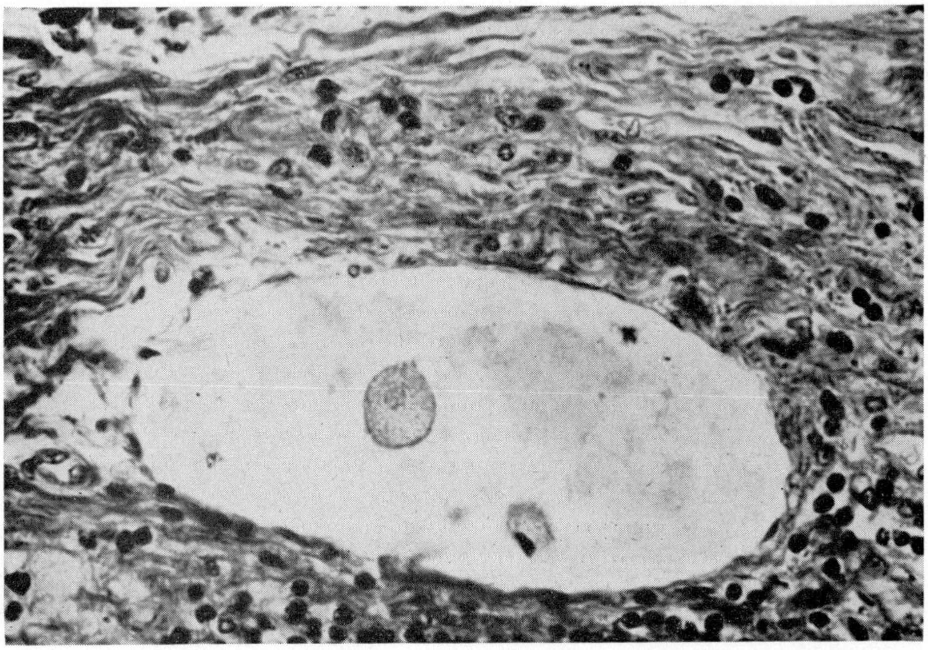

Fig. 10.—Section through endothelial lined lymphatic channel (×675) with two fat-laden "foamy" macrophages; chronic inflammatory cells in dense collagenous tissue of cyst wall is shown.

cm. was revealed. In many areas the wall was quite rigid and sectioned with a distinct grating sensation due to gritty calcific deposits; elsewhere the wall was densely fibrous in nature and pliable. The interior of the cyst was filled with soft, yellowish-gray material of the consistency of cottage cheese and slightly greasy. Removal of the contents disclosed a fairly smooth, grayish-white to pale tan inner lining with occasional roughened areas.

Multiple microscopic preparations of the cyst wall revealed it to be composed of fairly dense collagenous connective tissue with scattered foci of chronic inflammatory cells, predominantly lymphocytes, with occasional plasma cells, monocytes, and neutrophiles (Fig. 9). Calcific deposition occurred irregularly throughout the inner half of the wall. Fat laden, ''foamy'' macrophages were prominent in many areas along the innermost aspect of the wall and within a few endothelial lined channels (Fig. 10). The latter were situated at the outer confines of the wall. Formidable lymphoid tissue aggregates were nowhere apparent and the inner expanse of the wall was devoid of identifiable endothelial or epithelial lining elements. In the smoother portions of the interior aspect, condensations of collagenous fibrous tissue were apparent but no particular affinity for silver stains was demonstrable. Smears and cultures of the cyst content in addition to Gram-Weigert and modified Ziehl-Neelsen preparations of various aspects of the wall disclosed no organisms.

COMMENT

It is our impression that this cyst was of the lymphogenous type because of the inspissated chyliform content and prominent lymph channels in the wall of the cyst, some with ''foamy'' fat-ingested macrophages.

Due to the appearance of the contents of the cyst an underlying tuberculous factor was considered; however, the lack of caseative features to the contents, the failure to demonstrate tubercle bacilli, and the lack of tuberculous granulation tissue in the wall tend to rule out tuberculosis.

If this cyst were of the enterogenous type we would expect to find epithelial inclusion from the intestine plus a more mucoid type of content.

Because of the history of trauma several years previously the possibility of traumatic fat necrosis of the mesenteric fat and pseudo-encystment or localized hematoma were considered. The lack of altered blood pigments and foreign body giant-cell reaction in the cyst wall mitigate against these possibilities.

SUMMARY AND CONCLUSIONS

1. A case of mesenteric cyst is reported as the first calcified mesenteric cyst in ninety-eight years at Mercy Hospital, Chicago, in over 750,000 admissions.

2. Mesenteric cysts are rare and calcified mesenteric cysts are extremely rare.

3. The history of these cysts dates to 1507, when they were first found at autopsy and considered ''anatomic curiosities.''

4. Their history is divided into four periods, beginning with 1507 to the present.

5. The etiology, pathology, and classification remains obscure.

6. Cysts in the region of the jejunum and upper ileum are chiefly mesenteric in distribution, while in the ileocecal region they lie in the submucous or muscular layers of the intestinal wall.

7. Complications are serious. An acute abdomen may be the existing condition when first seen by the surgeons.

8. Mesenteric cysts must be included in differential diagnosis of obscure abdominal pathology.

9. It is possible to diagnose these cases if a careful history, physical examination, and laboratory checkup are done.

REFERENCES

1. Warfield, J. O: Ann. Surg. **96**: 329, 1932.
2. Lahey, F. H., and Eckerson, E. B.: Ann. Surg. **100**: 231, 1934.
3. Loeb, M. J.: New York State J. Med. **41**: 1564, 1941.
4. Guthrie, R. F., and Wakefield, E. G.: Proc. Staff Meet., Mayo Clin. **18**: 52, 1943.
5. Schunke, G. B., and Waugh, J. M.: Proc. Staff Meet., Mayo Clin. **16**: 676, 1941.
6. Peterson, E. W.: Ann. Surg. **112**: 80, 1940.
7. Dunne, R. E.: J. Connecticut M. Soc. **3**: 54, 1939.
8. Snyder, J. W.: South. Surgeon **8**: 240, 1939.
9. Dowd, Charles: Ann. Surg. **32**: 515, 1900.
10. Swartley, W. R.: Ann. Surg. **85**: 886, 1927.
11. Timbal, R.: Rev. de chir. **41**: 45, 1910.
12. Larkin, F. L.: Pennsylvania M. J. **43**: 1446, 1940.
13. Berger, L., and Rothenberg, R. E.: SURGERY **5**: 522, 1939.
14. Higgins, T. T., and Lloyd, E. I.: Brit. J. Surg. **2**: 95, 1924.
15. Kross, I.: Rev. Gastroenterol. **9**: 281, 1942.
16. Hinkel, L.: Am. J. Roentgenol. **48**: 167, 1942.
17. Costello, R. C.: Ohio State M. J. **38**: 543, 1942.
18. Frazier, C. H.: J. A. M. A. **61**: 97, 1913.
19. Carter, R. M.: Surg. Gynec. & Obst. **33**: 544, 1921.
20. Flynn, Charles W.: Ann. Surg. **91**: 505, 1930; Tr. South. S. A. **42**: 241, 1930.
21. DePena, P.: Arch. latino am. de pediat. **18**: 144, 1924.
22. Portal, A.: Cours d'antomie medicale ou elemens de l'anatomie de l'homme, t.v., Paris, 1803, Baudonin.
23. Augagneur, V.: Tumeurs du mesentere, Thése d'Agregation, Paris, 1886.
24. Hahn, E.: Berlin klin. Wchnschr. **24**: 408, 1887.
25. Arekion, H. F.: Étude sur les kyster du mesertere, Thése Paris, 1891.
26. Braquehaye, Jules: Arch. gén. de méd. **2**: 291-313, 572-592, 1892.
27. Moynihan, B. G.: Ann. Surg. **26**: 1, 1897.
28. Haworth, J. K.: Lancet **1**: 1269, 1920.
29. Bertolini, A.: Osp. maggiore **9**: 278, 1921.
30. Aloi, V.: Riforma med. **43**: 1011, 1927.
31. Finucci, V.: Policlinico (sez. chir.) **37**: 506, 1930.
32. Naumann, H.: Arch. f. klin. Chir., Berlin **117**: 819, 1921.
33. Levison, C. G., and Wolfsohn, M.: California & West. Med. **24**: 480, 1926.
34. Ney, G. C., and Wilkinson, A. L.: Ann. Surg. **54**: 115, 1911.
35. Bianchi, G.: Riforma med., Napoli **7**: 457, 1891.
36. Judd, E. S., and Crisp, N. W.: Proc. Staff Meet., Mayo Clin. **7**: 555, 1932.
37. Masson, J. C., and Rienets, J. H.: S. Clin. North America **2**: 743-751, 1931.
38. Rokitansky, Lehrbuch I.: Pathologie und Anatomie, Vienna, 1842.
39. Atchley, R. I.: J. Oklahoma M. A. **22**: 125, 1929.
40. Roller, Charles S.: Surg., Gynec. & Obst. **60**: 1128, 1935.
41. Olesen, L. A.: California & West. Med. **30**: 261, 1929.
42. Porter, M. F.: Tr. West. Surg. & Gynec. Ass., p. 242, 1905.
43. Hueper, W. C.: J. Lab. & Clin. Med. **12**: 427-430, 1927.
44. Sawyer, C. F.: Personal communication.

Book Reviews

Handbook of Fractures. By Duncan Eve, Jr., M.D. Pp. 263, with illustrations. St. Louis, 1947, The C. V. Mosby Company.

This handbook was prepared by the author for students, practitioners, and surgeons in general, omitting lengthy discussions of the manner of injury together with the signs and symptoms of fractures, and placing emphasis on the details of treatment. The text is adequately illustrated with photographs, roentgenograms, and drawings.

The author devotes three chapters at the beginning to immobilization methods, open reduction and internal fixation, and compound fractures; the remainder of the handbook is then broken up into chapters dealing with fractures in the various regions of the body. In general, the author outlines the one or two procedures which he himself generally uses in connection with a given fracture, and therefore has found from experience to be satisfactory. In those instances in which open reduction seems indicated, he outlines briefly the technique and procedure for the operation.

The book is interestingly written and well illustrated; the methods and procedures described are basically sound and conservative. As one reads and reviews it, he senses that the author is writing from a wealth of experience and that his judgment is mature and sound. It will prove a useful guide to anyone undertaking to deal with the average run of fracture problems in the hospital or in civil practice.

Outline of the Spinal Nerves. By John Favill, Clinical Professor of Neurology, University of Illinois. Pp. 190, with 12 illustrations. Springfield, Ill., 1946, Charles C Thomas, Publisher.

This book is composed for the most part of lists of nerves and muscles with certain information about each.

Part I consists of a list of the spinal nerves with the muscles innervated by the dorsal and the ventral division of each.

Part II is composed of lists of all nerves with the muscles supplied by each nerve, the segments contributing to the innervation of each muscle and other information about lesions of each nerve.

Part III lists all muscles with the nerves which innervate them, also the segmental innervation of each muscle, also its origin, insertion, action, function, test for loss of function, and the effect if it is paralyzed.

Part V is thirty-three pages of what the author calls supplementary data.

It is obvious that this is a reference book. Most of the material in it is anatomic detail learned by the freshman medical student in Gross Anatomy but soon forgotten, reviewed by the neurologist in training, but again only partially retained. It should be a great convenience to the neurologist or neurosurgeon to have these data collected and condensed in this form for easy reference.

Five Million Patients. By Allen W. Freeman, M.D. Pp. 299, no illustrations. New York, 1946, Charles Scribner's Sons. $3.

This is the autobiography of the author beginning with his entrance into medical school in 1901 and ending presumably with his retirement from Professor of Public Health Administration at Johns Hopkins in 1945.

After graduation in 1905, and one year of internship, he engaged in private practice until June, 1907, when he was appointed City Medical Inspector of Richmond, Va. He remained in public health work, becoming Assistant Commissioner of Health for the state of Virginia in 1908, Epidermiologist in the United States Public Health Department in 1915, Commissioner of Health of Ohio in 1917; he was a major in the Reserve Corps of the Army from July, 1918, to December, 1918, and then resumed his duties as Commissioner of Health of Ohio until he was appointed Resident Lecturer in Public Health Administration at Johns Hopkins in 1921. After one year as lecturer he became Professor at Johns Hopkins, where he remained until retirement in 1945.

The book consists of 111 chapters, each relating some episode in the author's life which he considered important or at least interesting. Physicians will find it more entertaining than enlightening, but it does give an account, easy to read, of many phases of public health in an earlier period.

Those untrained in medicine and also public health nurses, social workers, etc., will find this book interesting and profitable reading.

COMMUNICATION

THE NEW YORK HOSPITAL
JANUARY 8, 1948.

ALTON OCHSNER, EDITOR
OCHSNER CLINIC,
NEW ORLEANS, LA.

DEAR DR. OCHSNER:

In Volume 22, August, 1947, page 341, of SURGERY my article entitled "One-stage Push-back Operation for Congenital Insufficiency of the Palate" was published. In this article the technique of lengthening the palate by freeing of the palatine artery from its bony canal was described. Since publication it has come to my attention that this same operative technique was reported by Dr. Hector Marino of Buenos Aires, Argentina, in the *Revista de Cirugia*, Volume 23, November-December, 1944, page 363, and I wish to give prior credit for the establishment of this technique to Dr. Marino.

Very truly yours,
HERBERT CONWAY, M.D.
New York, N. Y.

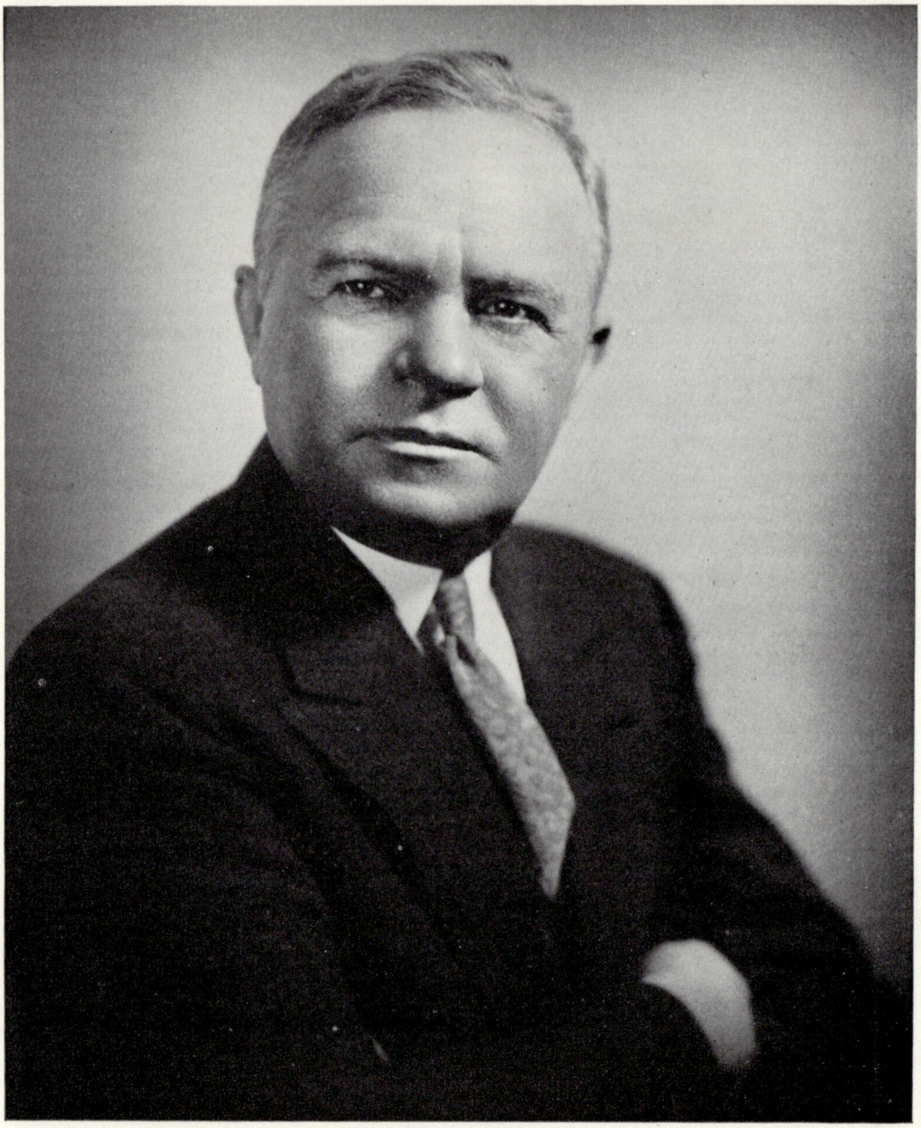

George J. Heuer

SURGERY

Vol. 23 | March, 1948 | No. 3

George J. Heuer Birthday Volume

GEORGE J. HEUER'S CONTRIBUTIONS AND HIS PLACE IN AMERICAN SURGERY

William DeWitt Andrus, M.D., New York, N. Y.

HAVING been closely associated with George J. Heuer for twenty-five years, I feel well qualified to speak of his personality, his detailed clinical and operative skills, and his teaching methods, and have therefore sought the aid of a number of his contemporaries who occupy high academic and professional posts throughout the country in estimating his place in American surgery. All have responded most willingly and the collected opinions in themselves constitute a glowing tribute.

Undoubtedly Dr. Heuer has made some of his greatest contributions as a teacher—both in the undergraduate and graduate fields—for unlike his preceptor, William Halsted, he is equally effective with residents and medical students. He brought to his rounds and clinics not only profound knowledge and concise formulation of subject matter, but often a certain light touch, accompanied by a twinkling eye, which served both to put a student at his ease who was making a creditable effort and to bring confusion to a bluffer or the overconfident. He always held as a major tenet of his teaching philosophy that the student should be given the greatest possible degree of independence in the way in which he learned, but as a corollary he expected diligence and a certain amount of insight. Neither the student nor the members of the resident staff could expect help unless they had already exerted themselves. No one could listen to his discussion of a case without realizing the breadth of experience which seemed immediately available in his clinical judgment. His diagnoses seemed almost occult at times, but were obviously the result of his enormous clinical contacts which had accumulated and been digested over a period of years. On occasion he could be somewhat disdainful of a diagnosis made by a lucky guess, expecting such to be arrived at by an orderly reasoned process and weighing of possibilities.

In his teaching he sought a balance between the new and the proved, and while not slow to adopt sound innovation, always insisted on the most careful evaluation based on actual experience. Though always tolerant, he frequently pointed out the fact that patients were cured sometimes before the advent of sulfonamides, for example, and urged careful consideration of the dangers as well as the potential benefits of a drug or procedure before its adoption.

While all those under him worked hard, the department as a whole has been administered much more by leadership than by domination. Many matters were decided in group conferences, and all came to feel both that they knew what was going on in the department and that they had a share in its progress. He had himself experienced the Prussian rigidity of organization in Kuttner's clinic in Breslau where he had served as exchange resident in 1914, and the contrast to the atmosphere of Dr. Halsted's department made a lasting impression and was one reason for his preference for administration through the respect of the staff rather than by rigid discipline. How well he succeeded in this was frequently illustrated in his rounds where anyone—staff member, resident, intern, or student—felt free to present a differing opinion, which however he was then called upon to support. A foreign visitor commenting on the atmosphere of the rounds and of the department as a whole once said to me that it helped him to understand what liberty meant and to show him that it could be combined with discipline. The leadership which he provided was always one that brought his subordinates into the picture with as much responsibility as they could assume. Thus, he rarely gave a direct order but rather prefaced what he had to say by, "Don't you think that it might be well to do so and so . . . ," or "Do you like to do thus and so . . ." in a given case. This sometimes provoked discussion but certainly gave the recipient an idea of what was wanted and at the same time a feeling of a shared responsibility. Dr. Heuer believed firmly in the value of responsibility in promoting the progress made by members of the resident staff and commented on the way in which individuals burgeoned when advanced in status.

When he began his professorship in Cincinnati, the resident system, while well established at Johns Hopkins and a few other university clinics, was looked upon as impractical, if not perhaps undesirable, for other hospitals. It was felt that such a system was adaptable only to a rather narrow academic atmosphere and unsuited to the problems of the ordinary city hospital, for example. This constituted a challenge which he accepted with enthusiasm, and to many his greatest contribution has been the demonstration that the resident system was not only practical under quite diverse circumstances, but that it produced results in care of patients and in operative mortality which surpassed those of other types of organization. The details of the development of the resident system in Cincinnati are treated elsewhere by his first resident, B. Noland Carter, and the adoption of the resident system throughout the country is due in no small measure to this demonstration of its efficacy.

In 1935, participating in a symposium on the teaching of surgery before the American Surgical Association, Dr. Heuer presented a paper entitled "Graduate Teaching of Surgery in University Clinics" in which he traced the spread of such teaching throughout the country and analyzed its status at that time. In the conclusions which he drew from this study he stated, "The study shows that . . . there are still lacking sufficient opportunities to meet demands of men seeking a higher degree in surgery and to meet the needs of the country in respect to trained surgeons." This symposium gave impetus to the founding of The American Board of Surgery, and Evarts Graham credits the stimulation of Dr. Heuer's address on this occasion with a large share in bringing this about. The widespread adoption of the resident system and particularly the high standards set by this Board eventually requiring what amounts to a thorough residency or its equivalent has been the source of intense satisfaction.

Except for a maintained interest and stimulation and an occasional appearance to demonstrate an operative method, Dr. Heuer has not been very active in the experimental laboratory during the last years of his tenure. His earlier work on pneumonectomy in dogs with particular reference to the healing of the bronchial stump was fundamental, however, and so exhaustive that little save minor alterations of the technique has been added since it appeared. He stimulated others to study the effects of removal of the lung on the remaining pulmonary tissue from both the anatomic and functional standpoint.

He later attacked several clinical problems in patients, including some of the earlier attempts to modify high blood pressure by means of operations on the nervous system, in one group of cases denervating the renal pedicle, in another performing extensive anterior root section. All of these patients were carefully observed, and while the procedures are no longer employed for this condition the observations were fundamental. With Harold Stewart and the writer he became interested in pericardiectomy for chronic constrictive pericarditis, and over a period of several years more than twenty such procedures have been carried out in consecutive cases without a death during the operation or in the hospital after operation. This work has been typical of his interests in bettering the operative results in various fields and the improvement obtained has been due not only to his own operative skill but also to a keen analysis of and attention to the critical features of the procedure, those responsible both for its good effects and for its mortality.

To his pupils and to many others, however, Dr. Heuer's ability as an operator has been his most outstanding achievement. Completely unruffled and at ease in the most trying situations, never seeming to hurry yet constantly moving forward, undertaking the most diverse and major procedures, yet always at home in each one, he has inspired everyone who watched. His own contemporaries and many others bear witness to this quality. One of them, the head of a university clinic, writes, "I can repeat what I have said many times, that Dr. George Heuer is the most skillful surgeon I have ever seen do an operation. Other surgeons have perhaps equalled his skill in some of the particular fields of surgery, but I know no other surgeon who has shown such superior ability to operate in any part of the body. I have seen Dr. Heuer do all sorts of surgery with the exception of ophthalmological surgery and much of it was done in its early stage of development. I can remember no instance in which he was in trouble and did not have complete control of the situation." A similar opinion is expressed by many others, and one says, "I think that George Heuer is probably the best living exponent of the meticulous surgical technique first introduced into American surgery by his teacher, Dr. Halsted, and certainly he has improved on Dr. Halsted's technique. Dr. Heuer is noted for his sound surgical judgment, his ability to not go to the extreme, so frequently found with surgeons, and for his fearlessly espousing the thing he thought was right. He has certainly placed his love of surgery and of the teaching of surgery before all personal considerations. There is lots more I could say about him but there are so many other people who can say better than I." A third states, "I regard George Heuer as one of the ablest general surgeons of his generation in the United States and without a superior in the training of surgeons in the surgical clinics of this country. I first saw him work in the Evacuation Hospital No. 1 during World War I and his surgical judgment and technique were superb. To me his most productive period was at the University of Cincinnati where he revolutionized the surgery of the Cincinnati General Hospital and did an outstanding job in building up the teaching, research and training facilities of the surgical department. Later he established similar standards at the New York Hospital, and his accomplishments in these two institutions served to stamp him as one of America's ablest leaders in the field of surgical education."

When one attempts to define the secret of his great success as a surgeon one thinks at once of his knowledge of the operation itself gained from great experience, but added to this was the fact that he constantly learned, as he went along, always adapting the procedure to the existing situation. This he was able to do as he operated in a deliberate but by no means slow fashion, without any apparent tension. The atmosphere of quiet assurance was transmitted to his assistants and while alert, no one felt on edge; each was therefore able to contribute his best effort to the matter in hand.

One of the surgeons and professors of surgery in the country whom Dr. Heuer himself most admires writes of him as follows: "The feature which I think impressed everybody the most about him has been his great interest in the training and development of young surgeons. I am familiar with the difficulties which he encountered in introducing the resident system at Cincinnati. It was a new idea to everybody there that surgical patients could be entrusted to the care of residents without any increased danger. The great success of the program did much to help the cause of adequate surgical training throughout the country from which the public is now profiting greatly. Everybody also realized that he stood among the top surgeons of the world in technical ability and even brilliant operating skill. I always think that the fact that he was so excellent an operating surgeon and yet could champion the program of having the residents do much of the surgery helped greatly to have the program of resident training instituted more generally in other places in the country. One could safely assume that a surgeon of his skill would not be willing to advocate turning over the care of surgical patients to residents unless they were fully qualified to do the work in a thoroughly satisfactory way. I also have always placed a very high value on his original contributions and experimental work. His early experiments on pulmonary resections in dogs did much to encourage the more radical resections of pulmonary tissue in human beings."

Dr. Heuer's papers have been examples not only of scholarly writing but also of exhaustive treatment of his subject. The practice which he acquired in preparing manuscripts for Dr. Halsted's approval contributed to this skill, and he has frequently told of his experience with the first papers that he submitted, which were returned liberally pencilled—to be followed in rapid succession by the receipt of a *Webster's Unabridged Dictionary* and a copy of Quiller Couch's book on the art of written English. He was very critical of the writing of members of his staff, and the excellence of his papers has set a goal toward which his men have always aspired.

Dr. Heuer retired from his post at Cornell Medical College, July, 1947, after twenty-five years of full professorship there and at the University of Cincinnati. During this time more than one hundred surgeons have either gone through his residency or have obtained the major part of their training under him. Were his contribution limited to this, his high place in American surgery would be assured. His pupils join in honoring him on this occasion as teacher, investigator, and truly great surgeon.

TWENTY-FIVE YEARS OF A GRADUATE SCHOOL OF SURGERY FOUNDED BY GEORGE J. HEUER

B. Noland Carter, M.D., Cincinnati, Ohio

(From the Department of Surgery, College of Medicine, University of Cincinnati and the Cincinnati General Hospital)

IN VIEW of great contemporary interest in thorough surgical training, and also because well-organized graduate schools of surgery which have had continuous existence for so long as a quarter of a century are comparatively few in number, an account of the founding of such a school at the Cincinnati General Hospital appears appropriate at this time. The Graduate School of Surgery of the University of Cincinnati was founded by George J. Heuer in 1922, and has enjoyed an unbroken tradition of surgical principles and teaching throughout twenty-five years. The school stands as a monument to Dr. Heuer's recognition of the need for proper facilities for thorough surgical training, to his untiring efforts toward supplying that need, and to the results which have ensued from application of the fundamental principles which he established. His stature as an educator and a preceptor is fully as great as his reputation as a practicing surgeon.

Having been trained in the resident system under William Halsted at the Johns Hopkins Hospital, and having served there in the capacity of resident surgeon from 1911 to 1914, Dr. Heuer brought this method of training to Cincinnati upon his appointment to the chair of surgery in 1922. Modifications of the original system to meet expanding needs for surgical training were made under Dr. Heuer and his successors, but its fundamental concepts have remained unchanged to the present time. In 1932 Dr. Heuer was called to the chair of surgery at Cornell, where he introduced and expanded the methods of training surgeons which he had established at Cincinnati. Mont Reid, another of Dr. Halsted's residents, and one of Dr. Heuer's associates, succeeded him as head of the school, augmenting the system of training while adhering to its original ideals. Dr. Reid was responsible for the continuing and advancing high standards of the school from the time of Dr. Heuer's departure until his own death in 1943. Since Dr. Reid's death the two other directors of the school have been individuals who received their training under Dr. Heuer, thereby maintaining the continuity of tradition and principles of the original training program.

THE HALSTED SYSTEM

Since the resident system of training which Dr. Heuer inaugurated at the Cincinnati General Hospital was patterned after that introduced into this country by Dr. Halsted around 1890, a description of the Halsted system seems warranted. At that time there existed in the United States no organized postgraduate training programs designed for young doctors who wished to become proficient in surgery. With the introduction and spread of the principles of asepsis and the expansion of surgical knowledge, increasing numbers of men turned their attention to this phase of medicine.

Dr. Halsted had been greatly impressed with the training given in the European clinics, and had noted the greater surgical proficiency of men trained in such clinics, particularly those of Germany and Switzerland, as compared with that of surgeons in this country. He believed that this difference was largely due to the more efficient and prolonged training offered abroad, and accordingly set about founding a system of training at the Johns Hopkins Hospital which should be comparable in scope to that offered in the best European clinics. His ideal was to establish a training which ". . . will produce not only surgeons, but surgeons of the highest type, men who will stimulate the first youths of our country to study surgery and to devote their energies and their lives to raising the standards of surgical science."[1]

In bare outline, the system adopted was pyramidal in structure, with a "resident" or house surgeon at the apex, and an indeterminate number of assistant residents under him. There was no regular progression of assistant residents to the top position, no specifically assigned services through which they rotated, nor any prescribed limits to their training. Since the house surgeon might retain his position for an indefinite period of time, opportunities for advancement were sharply limited, and many assistant residents left the institution before attaining to positions of real responsibility. The resident surgeon was in charge of, and responsible to the attending staff of the hospital for, all patients admitted on the surgical service. His position thus involved administrative duties as well as operative experience, and he was further expected to teach and direct the assistant residents under him.

This type of experience afforded exceptionally fine training for the man who reached the position of resident surgeon, and the prerogative of indefinite tenure of office enabled him to perfect his judgment as well as his technique before venturing to accept a position elsewhere. The chief defect in the program lay in its static quality, which prevented more than a very few men from obtaining the desired level of training. The assistant residents were given little authority or experience, frequently remained at one level of proficiency for long periods of time, and occasionally left the clinic before adequate training had been obtained.

To those who actually reached the position of resident, the advantages of this type of training were manifest, as may be seen by their subsequent interest and efforts in spreading its ideals. Of the seventeen men who held the residency under Dr. Halsted, five founded resident training programs, and an additional six held professorial positions in first class medical schools. The first graduate school to be founded by a Halsted resident, similar in scope and aims to that of "the Professor," was that introduced at the Peter Bent Brigham Hospital by Harvey Cushing in 1912. The second such training program to be established in the United States was that founded by Dr. Heuer at the University of Cincinnati in the Cincinnati General Hospital in 1922. In the ten-year interval between the founding of these two schools less than half a dozen schools for graduate surgical training were begun, and none of these were comparable in scope to that of Dr. Halsted. Several reasons for this apparent lack include the facts that at the time the long period of training was not deemed necessary or advisable, the necessary facilities of university controlled hospitals were not available, and in the stage at which surgery then existed, the need for such training was not recognized.

THE GRADUATE SCHOOL OF SURGERY, UNIVERSITY OF CINCINNATI

At the time that Dr. Heuer brought the Halsted method to Cincinnati, only the system of postgraduate instruction offered at Peter Bent Brigham Hospital was comparable in caliber and scope to the original. Dr. Heuer followed the Halsted program very closely at first, having brought with him from Baltimore several men who had begun their training at Johns Hopkins. Only four men comprised the original group, a resident and three assistant residents.

The informal type of training which Dr. Heuer had originally advocated, with the assistant residents fulfilling whatever duties the resident deemed most necessary, was soon found inadequate for the rapidly increasing number of men seeking training. By 1924 nine men were in training, and by 1927 the resident staff numbered twelve. Under such conditions the necessity for more specific duties became apparent, and rotation through the various surgical services was begun. At first the assistant residents served on several of these, each man going through as many as seemed indicated. Later a more closely organized schedule of training was established, with each man spending a definite period of time on each service. Only minor changes have been made since Dr. Heuer's departure for Cornell; the services which are now offered appear in Table I.

TABLE I. SCHEDULE OF SERVICES

SERVICE	TIME (MO.)	NUMBER OF MEN
Surgical pathology	6	1
Experimental lab.	6	1
Dunham Hospital	6	1
General Surgery	6	2
Urology	6	1
Fractures	6	1
Holmes Hospital	6	2
Emergencies	6	1
Neurosurgery	6	1
Children's Hospital	6	1
Gynecology	6	1
First Ass't Res.	6	1
Residents	12	2
Total	7 years	16 men

Ideally, seven years are involved in the completion of all the prescribed services. Actually, however, all men do not participate in all services, nor is the period of time devoted to each always as long as is indicated in the table. The services do not necessarily follow one another in the order given. A brief description of each may show more clearly the experience which is afforded the assistant resident assigned to it.

Surgical pathology is combined with the tumor service, and the assistant resident on this service is responsible for the gross and microscopic description and diagnosis of all tissues removed in the operating rooms and outpatient clinics. He is in daily association with a trained pathologist, with whom, in addition, he and the other surgical assistant residents hold biweekly conferences. He attends the Tumor Clinic twice weekly, and is responsible for the supervision of a special ward for the care of certain of the cancer patients.

In the experimental laboratory the assistant resident becomes familiar with the techniques and procedures of laboratory investigation. He acts as assistant to members of the senior staff of the department of surgery in the pursuit of their experimental studies, and is stimulated to develop a problem of his own during the period spent in the laboratory. He is enabled and encouraged to develop his technique in the performance of various surgical procedures on animals.

The Dunham Hospital is located several miles from the Cincinnati General Hospital, and is the County Hospital for tuberculosis. Men assigned here assist in thoracic surgery as related to tuberculosis, and perform some thoracic operations under supervision. Additional experience in thoracic surgery is obtained elsewhere in the training program.

General surgery is divided between two assistant residents. One takes the adult male wards; the other, the adult female and children's wards. At the end of three months they alternate. These men act as first assistants to the operators of their own patients. As they advance in training, they are permitted to operate under guidance. They are responsible to the resident for the management of all cases on their wards; assist in the teaching of senior medical students assigned as clinical clerks on surgical wards; and directly supervise the work of the interns.

Although urology is a division of general surgery, its attending staff comprises urologists, and it does not have a separate resident system. The assistant resident in surgery serves as urology resident for six months. He learns to do all of the urological studies, and is permitted to do part of the major surgery under supervision. He also manages the urologic dispensary and handles the bulk of consultation work.

The fracture service is also a branch of general surgery, and is without a separate resident staff. All patients with fractures, except those involving the skull, are seen in the admitting ward by the assistant resident assigned to fractures, who is responsible for their subsequent treatment and care. All patients needing skeletal traction are treated by him, as are all compound fractures. The attending staff operate upon those needing open reduction until the assistant resident is capable of operating independently.

The Holmes Hospital is a private institution where two assistant residents are posted. These men are assistants in all types of surgery except eye, ear, nose, and throat. The experience obtained here is extremely valuable and highly prized, and serves to give the assistant resident an opportunity to come in contact with private patients.

The assistant resident assigned to emergencies answers all calls from receiving ward physicians who seek surgical consultation. Patients with emergency cases of traumatic or inflammatory nature are first seen by this individual, who gives them complete study and prepares them for emergency therapy. He acts as first assistant to the resident in the surgical treatment of all these cases night and day. In the discretion of the resident, he is permitted to perform operations independently. He is also in charge of the surgical dispensary in the mornings, where he sees elective surgical patients.

Operative work in neurosurgery is shared between the attending staff and the resident. Most of the work assigned to the resident is concerned with acute head injuries and peripheral nerve injuries. All house cases require complete neurologic study by the assistant resident assigned to this service.

The surgical service of the Children's Hospital is managed by an assistant resident rotating through that service from the Cincinnati General Hospital. He has all the privileges of a resident, taking care of emergency and elective surgery under the necessary supervision. The assignment usually comes late in his training as it is a post of great responsibility.

Gynecology, like urology, is a division of general surgery, but attended by a separate staff. Their resident is one of the surgical assistant residents. He works in the dispensary, performs physical examinations on admitted patients, and is permitted to perform major surgery for the usual pelvic and perineal disorders. The opportunity for such extensive experience in gynecologic surgery is a valuable adjunct to the training of a general surgeon, and is rather unusual in graduate schools of surgery. In view of the fact that a considerable number of trainees enter private practice in moderate-sized communities, this gynecologic training is of great importance.

The *first* assistant resident is next in line for the residency, and acts as an assistant to the resident. He relieves the resident of a number of the night emergencies, and of routine operative work when the latter is required for more difficult or important work. He arranges clinical material for student classes, makes complete rounds on mornings when the resident is occupied in the operating room, and takes charge when the resident is off duty.

The resident operates every day except Sunday from 8:00 A.M. until the work is finished. He sees all emergency patients and assigns the operator or operates himself. He answers all consultation requests by other services and arranges for the proper staff man to see the patients in question if it is necessary. He may choose to be first assistant in any case in which the operation is done by a staff member. He conducts members of the staff to the wards for advice or when they may wish to inspect the wards. He must check the work of all assistant residents under him. Although his responsibility is great, he knows that there is a staff man available should advice or technical assistance be necessary. The resident conducts a meeting of the entire house staff five evenings each week, at which time daily progress of every patient on the service is checked. During these meetings plans for further investigation are made, operations scheduled, and dismissals and follow-up dates for Sunday morning clinics made.

Appointments to the resident staff are made on a yearly basis, renewal of appointment being dependent on demonstration of ability. Should a man have been assigned to all services, he would have spent seven years by the conclusion of his residency. Since some of the services overlap and are not necessarily repeated, nor is always the full six months spent on each service, it is exceptional for a resident to spend more than six years in training. A typical program is represented in Table II, which does not contain all the services listed in Table I. Several of the services now offered were included in the general service at the time this man was in training; the Dunham Hospital had not yet been established, and neurosurgery was then part of general surgery. In Table III the actual clinical experience of yet another resident is represented. In Table III under "patients admitted or treated," patients examined or treated in the various dispensaries were not included, and in "operations done," only hospitalized patients were counted.

TABLE II. EXAMPLE OF A RESIDENT'S TRAINING IN THE GRADUATE SCHOOL

SERVICE BEGINNING:	SERVICE	TIME (MO.)
Sept. 1	Surgical pathology	6
March 1	General surgery	6
Sept. 1 (2nd year)	Urology	6
March 1	Emergencies	6
Sept. 1 (3rd year)	Holmes Hospital	6
March 1	Children's Hospital	6
Sept. 1 (4th year)	Fractures	6
March 1	Gynecology	6
Sept. 1 (5th year)	Resident	12
	Total	5 years

As is apparent, with the introduction of a specific course of instruction a more definite time limit for the completion of training was necessarily set. Because of the regular progression through most of the special services, and also because of the increased number of men completing the training each year, it became necessary to limit the term of the resident to one year, instead of leaving it to the option of the incumbent.

Dr. Heuer's goal was to fulfill the ideals which Dr. Halsted had established in the founding of the resident system at Hopkins, and although he modified the actual program in order to give more thorough training to a greater number of men, he never lost sight of the aims and principles on which the original system was founded. As the demand for training became more widespread, the curriculum was altered, expanded, and made more specific. In place of the informal

TABLE III. CLINICAL EXPERIENCE OF A TRAINEE IN THE GRADUATE SCHOOL

SERVICE	TIME (MO.)	PATIENTS ADMITTED OR TREATED	OPERATIONS ASSISTED	OPERATIONS DONE	TOTAL OPERATIONS
General surgery	6	624	355	108	463
Orthopedics	6	196	142	22	164
Holmes Hosp.	6	132	112	0	112
Fractures	4	410	14	1	15
Asst. Res.	2	452	24	129	153
Gynecology	6	700	165	98	263
1st Asst. Res.	9	2,430	No record	359	359
Emergencies	6	164	103	26	129
Resident	12	2,890	22 (staff)	685	707
Total	4 yr. 9 mo.	7,998	937	1,428	2,365

type of instruction offered by the earlier plan, Dr. Heuer inaugurated several regularly held formal meetings. These include ward rounds conducted by a member of the attending staff three afternoons weekly, and the biweekly clinical-pathologic conferences held under the joint direction of members of the attending staffs in surgery and pathology. There is also a weekly seminar at which the members of the resident staff discuss with members of the senior staff the current work of the department and relate to it recent or pertinent literature.

Recently, by cooperation with the department of anatomy, a specialized course in dissection under joint supervision of members of the departments of surgery and of anatomy has been offered to a limited number of assistant residents. Dissection under supervision for three hours once weekly is supplemented by additional independent work. Upon completion of the course, assistant residents aid in teaching the course in regional surgical anatomy given junior medical students.

A more direct outgrowth of the informal discussion method of teaching appears in the conduct of surgical grand rounds. At these weekly meetings of the entire resident and attending staff, emphasis is placed on informal discussion of cases following their formal presentation by a member of the house staff. Notes on cases to be presented are compiled in a concise yet complete manner and distributed at the meeting, and exchange of opinion predominates in the ensuing discussions. The director of the surgical pathology laboratory attends these meetings, emphasizing the correlation of his specialty with surgical principles and procedures. The hospital roentgenologist is also present to discuss roentgenologic diagnosis. Frequently several members of the medical service attend and present other aspects of the total clinical picture in any given case.

With all the modifications which Dr. Heuer introduced in order to facilitate the expansion of the scope and quality of the training, the lofty ideals remained essentially those of Dr. Halsted. Among the most emphasized of these ideals was that of the desirability of the assumption of great responsibility by the resident surgeon. In 1927 Dr. Heuer wrote, "The assumption of this heavy responsibility which develops on the senior graduate student or resident surgeon is, in our opinion, one of the greatest features of this course."[4] The chief resident is responsible, as has already been indicated, for the care of all patients admitted on the surgical service; and having assisted at operations and operated under supervision during the first four of five years of his training, he performs major surgical procedures on his own responsibility and makes decisions as to the pre- and postoperative care of the patients in the hospital. Not only are his clinical duties stressed, but also his responsibilities with regard to the direction of the assistant residents under him. He is expected to guide and advise the younger men, both through example and informal discussion.

Despite the increase in the number of men accepted for training, no compromise with the quality of their education has been made. The period of time required for the completion of the work remains from five to seven years, during which time experience in the various surgical specialties as well as general surgery is acquired. The comprehensive nature of the program was designed not only for the acquisition of skill, but particularly for the development of judgment. Dr. Heuer believed that, "Perhaps most striking in the longer courses is the emphasis placed upon individual responsibility as a means of developing character, surgical diagnosis, technic, and judgment."[5] He insisted upon the necessity for repetition of experiences in order that the individual might learn to exercise care and accuracy in diagnosis and treatment.

Although the Graduate School of Surgery at the Cincinnati General Hospital is an outgrowth of the Halsted system in that it comprises Dr. Halsted's ideals, the ever-increasing demand for surgical training has necessitated revision and expansion, which have been effected without any compromise of quality. In 1933 Dr. Heuer stated his ideals as follows:

> I have my own idea what, from an educational viewpoint, these men should be. They are men who have had a rather broad fundamental training in the sciences related to medicine, and a specialized training after their graduation in medicine in surgical pathology, surgical diagnosis, preoperative and postoperative treatment, and in operative surgery. Their training in general surgery has included the specialties in urology, orthopedic surgery, and gynecology. Their operative experience has been large, and acquired by assisting their seniors, by the performance of surgical operations under their direction, and by the independent performance of major surgical operations. In addition to this clinical training, they have acquired experience in and become imbued with the desire to pursue research, and they have acquired experience in teaching and in departmental organization. More and more I am realizing that all this is not enough; that the men I would seek to develop shall have acquired a spiritual experience as rich as their surgical experience, which enables them to follow only the highest ideals of medicine.[6]

With but minor variations the system and ideals are today as Dr. Heuer envisoned and established them.

Although it is difficult to evaluate anything as intangible as the influence which a set of ideals may exert, the growth and spread of the resident system since its inception at Johns Hopkins, and particularly the acceleration of this spread since the founding of the Graduate School of Surgery at the University of Cincinnati by Dr. Heuer, lead us to believe that this school has played a not inconsiderable part in the expansion. The impetus for the increased awareness of the need for, and subsequent development of, such systems stems in large part from Dr. Heuer's vital interest in the training of surgeons. Twenty-two years elapsed from the initiation of the resident system at Hopkins until the founding of the Brigham Hospital. Using the list of schools approved by the Society of University Surgeons, it appears that in the ten years which separate the founding of the latter school and that at Cincinnati, four schools were established, but beginning two years after the founding of this clinic, and continuing down to 1936, fifteen fully accredited schools came into being. Men who have been graduated from this clinic and from others similar in purpose have set out to raise the standards of surgical education all over the country. In place of half a dozen schools affording postgraduate training of any sort whatever, as was the condition in 1922 when Dr. Heuer came to Cincinnati, there are now twenty-two clinics offering the intensive and specialized training required for accrediting by the Society of University Surgeons, and nearly 300 which meet the requirements of the American College of Surgeons. Although sufficient opportunity for first-class surgical training is not yet available for all who desire it, significant strides have been made since Dr. Halsted's first efforts in that direction over fifty years ago, and since Dr. Heuer's continuing emulation of his ideas and ideals during the past twenty-five years. Perhaps no single individual has done more than Dr. Heuer in laying before the eyes of his colleagues the need for such training programs.

RESULTS OF THE RESIDENT SYSTEM OF TRAINING

It is impossible to trace the ever-widening sphere of influence of Dr. Halsted's teaching, for in addition to the men who actually trained under him in the capacity of resident or assistant resident, there is the "second generation" of men trained by the first group. Without taking account of the intangible influences which may have been exerted, it may be stated that over half of the twenty-five most outstanding graduate schools in the United States were founded by either first or second generation Halsted pupils.

Dr. Halsted's purpose in founding the resident system of graduate surgical training was to produce "surgeons of the highest type" who would by precept or example raise surgical standards throughout the country. His goal was realized in that two-thirds of his seventeen residents became full or associate professors of surgery and one-third entered private practice. Six graduate schools of surgery were founded by five Halsted residents, Dr. Heuer having played a major role in the establishment of two such training programs; and a sixth resident, Mont Reid, continued in the tradition by following Dr. Heuer as head of the Cincinnati school.

The parallel between the results obtained by Dr. Heuer in his graduate schools of surgery at Cincinnati and by Dr. Halsted is striking, for of the thirty-three men who have held the position of resident at the Cincinnati General Hospital, including the six "war residents" who did not serve the full period of time, as well as the two present incumbents, two-thirds are engaged in teaching, and one-third are exclusively in private practice. Of those who are teaching, eight are full or associate professors, seven are assistant professors, and the others, largely the group of more recent graduates, hold lesser teaching positions. Of the sixty-four assistant residents, seventeen are still in training here, having returned from military service to complete their postgraduate work, and thirteen are still in service. Nineteen of the remaining thirty-four hold teaching positions, and fifteen are in private practice. Of the latter group, ten were here for only three years or less; hence they cannot be regarded as "graduates" of the school. Of further interest is the fact that forty, or 60 per cent, of the entire group of sixty-five residents and assistant residents who are not either in training or in service are actively engaged in postgraduate surgical training programs approved by the American College of Surgeons.

A further indication of the value of the training may be seen by a tabulation of the recognition accorded the sixty-five men not still in training or in service through membership in national surgical societies. Thirty-two, or half, are diplomates of the American Board, either of surgery or of the surgical specialties, in spite of the fact that many of the more recent graduates are not yet eligible for examination by the Board. Twenty-six men are Fellows of the American College of Surgeons, fourteen are members of the Society of University Surgeons, seven of the Central Surgical Society, five of the American Surgical Society, four of the Western Surgical Society, four of the Southern Surgical Society, three of the Society of Clinical Surgeons, two are full members and five associate members of the American Association of Thoracic Surgeons, and one is a member of the American Association for the Surgery of Trauma.

Although the majority of men trained at the Graduate School of Surgery of the University of Cincinnati have remained in the state of Ohio, the geographic distribution by states, exclusive of the men still in training or in service, shows dissemination throughout twenty-three states (Fig. 1).

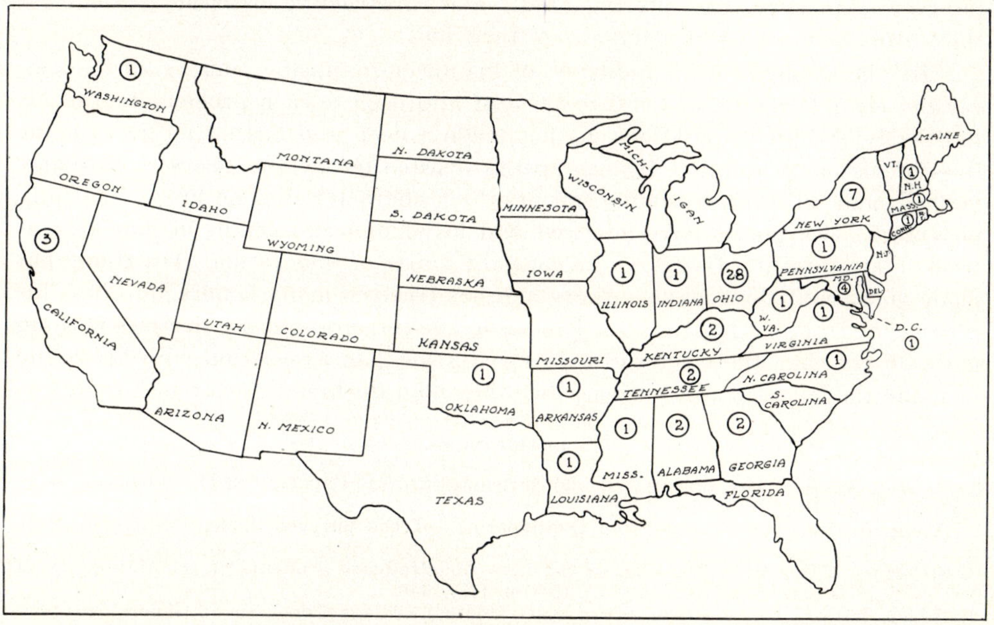

Fig. 1.—Geographic distribution of men trained in the Graduate School of Surgery, Cincinnati General Hospital.

Of the 100 living men who had received training under the resident system at Cincinnati, 70 per cent entered some branch of military service. Three lost their lives during the war and thirteen are still in service. Of the remaining fifty-four, one was director of the surgical consultant division of the Surgeon General's Office, two were surgical consultants to Service Commands, twelve became chiefs of surgical service in general hospitals, four were chiefs of service in the various surgical specialties, and five were assistant chiefs of surgical service. Three men were division surgeons, two were chiefs of surgical sections, and one was engaged in research programs both in this country and in the European Theater of Operations. Over half of those who entered the service (55.5 per cent) rose to positions of considerable responsibility. Such statistics serve as only a rough indication of the value of the type of training offered in the graduate school.

An account of the activities of a school of surgery founded and nurtured by Dr. Heuer would not be complete without some mention of his personal relations with the men who have been privileged to work under his direction. The splendid record of his pupils, so many of whom are included among the present and future leaders of surgery, and the magnitude of his accomplishments in furthering the application of basic surgical principles speak for themselves, but even more important are the personality and character of the man who has so unselfishly spent his life pursuing his ideal of giving young men an opportunity to obtain a superb training in surgery. It can be truthfully said that of the many interests in Dr. Heuer's surgical life the foremost has been his surgical schools. He has always intensely concerned himself with each of "his men," spending much time and thought in planning their careers, stimulating them to improve themselves, and offering kindly and constructive criticism, not only of their professional activities, but also of their ideals.

By the example of his industry, of his uncompromising honesty, of his logical and clear thinking, of his directness of approach to each problem, and of his faultlessly executed operations, he has made a deep and lasting imprint on the lives of his many pupils. He has always insisted on meticulousness, on orderly method, and on clear reasoning, all of which characteristics he himself so fully possesses. His pupils have admired and loved him and found in him a great teacher, an unfailing friend, and a constant source of inspiration. Dr. Heuer has made many contributions to surgery and has received many honors, but upon his retirement from his position as "Professor" I feel sure that he cherishes nothing more dearly than the memories of the years spent in association with his young men and the love and admiration which they hold for him.

REFERENCES

1. Halsted, W. S.: The Training of the Surgeon, Surgical Papers, vol. II, Baltimore, 1924, Johns Hopkins Press, p. 527.
2. Heuer, G. J.: The Training and Qualifications of the Surgeon, South. M. J. **23**: 22-29, 1930.
3. Stevenson, Jean M.: The Plan of Services for Graduate Students at the University of Cincinnati, J. A. Am. M. Coll. **15**: 169-173, 1940.
4. Heuer, G. J.: University of Cincinnati Medical College Teaching of General Surgery, in Methods and Problems of Medical Education, 8th ser., New York, 1927, Rockefeller Foundation.
5. Heuer, G. J.: Graduate Teaching of Surgery in University Clinics, Ann. Surg. **102**: 507-515, 1935.
6. Heuer, G. J.: Teaching of Graduate Surgery, J. A. Am. M. Coll. **8**: 205-213, 1933.

SOME EXPERIENCES WITH ANASTOMOSIS OF THE COMMON BILE DUCT TO THE DUODENUM, AND REPAIR OF STRICTURES OF THE COMMON BILE DUCT

M. M. Zinninger, M.D., Cincinnati, Ohio

(From the Department of Surgery, College of Medicine of the University of Cincinnati, and the Cincinnati General Hospital)

STRICTURE of the common bile duct frequently leads to partial or prolonged invalidism of the patient, and its repair may tax the resourcefulness and ability of the surgeon. The latter must also be aware that a well-planned and executed operation followed immediately by a good result may not eventually be really successful. All too often, after months or even after years, the stricture may recur and jaundice develop. This seems to be due to the fact that bile has a tendency to produce adhesions and fibrosis unless it is contained within an epithelial lining. For this reason, in making anastomoses of epithelial-lined structures for purposes of conduction of bile, it is desirable that mucosa-to-mucosa approximation be obtained, and that healing occur promptly without suppuration or formation of excessive granulation tissue. The more rapidly healing occurs so that the suture line is covered with epithelium, the less likely is contracture to occur. The use of indwelling catheters, tubes, etc., has the same purpose in mind, that is, to maintain patency of the tube until epithelization of the line of anastomosis is complete, thus reducing the likelihood of contracture.

That stricture of the bile ducts is difficult to manage is shown by the large number of operative procedures that have been recommended and used in an effort to obtain uniformly better results. None of them seems wholly satisfactory, and no one is applicable in all cases. I shall not attempt to review all the methods that have been used or described, but shall confine my remarks and comments to only a few. It is generally agreed that end-to-end anastomosis of the duct usually with a permanent or temporary indwelling tube or catheter is the method of choice when it can be accomplished. The maneuver recomded by Cattell[1] to achieve this result, namely mobilization and freeing of the descending duodenum to expose the retroduodenal portion of the common bile duct, can aid greatly in obtaining a greater length of duct than would otherwise be available. By the use of this procedure he has been able to accomplish end-to-end suture much more frequently than any other surgeon who has written on this subject. The methods of Allen[2] and Cole and associates[3] for reconstruction of the duct when only a stump of hepatic duct remains have also proved highly successful in their hands. These methods are more or less similar in that they make use of a loop of jejunum, defunctionalized by the Roux Y procedure, to replace part of the missing bile duct system and conduct bile from the hepatic ducts to the intestine. They differ in certain important details, Allen using a removable rubber tube, and Cole and his co-workers a permanently placed vitallium tube. Both of these authors pointed out the danger of possible ascending infection from the intestine into the biliary tract as a result of direct anastomosis of the bile duct system to duodenum or jejunum without the use of a defunctioned loop of bowel, and their operations have been devised to obviate this danger.

While it is my opinion that ascending infection is a real hazard, I have nevertheless performed direct anastomosis of the common or hepatic ducts to the duodenum a sufficient number of times without evidence of subsequent development of infection in the liver to make me believe that the danger is not so great as to warrant discarding completely this operative procedure. Many of the patients I have seen have been subjected to a number of previous operations, so that the entire upper abdomen was a mass of adhesions. Under such circumstances, the direct anastomosis of the hepatic duct to the duodenum is a procedure of considerably less magnitude than is the freeing and partial transplantation of the jejunum; moreover, the operative field can often be limited to a comparatively small area in the epigastrium usually no entrance into the free peritoneal cavity being made. If the results obtained are satisfactory, this smaller operative procedure may be of some importance to a patient whose general physical condition may not be and often is not particularly good. As a result of what has transpired in some of these cases, it is my belief that a direct anastomosis of this sort may be well tolerated by the patient as long as the opening remains sufficiently large so that any intestinal content that enters the biliary tree can easily return to the intestine. On the other hand, if stricture recurs so that the contents of the biliary tract are partially blocked, signs and symptoms of ascending infection develop, but are always associated with signs of bile duct obstruction. These signs are very similar to those seen when a stone in the common duct acts in a ball valve fashion, that is, there is pain, nausea, vomiting, chills and fever, followed by jaundice.

As evidence that direct anastomosis of this sort is not necessarily followed by ascending infection I should like to cite the following four cases.

CASE 1.—C. S., a white woman, 30 years of age, was admitted to the hospital Nov. 1, 1940. She had been in an automobile accident Feb. 21, 1940, at which time abdominal injuries were sustained. On February 26, an exploratory operation for so-called ''intestinal obstruction'' revealed several areas of rupture of the liver. In June, 1940, for reasons not entirely clear, a therapeutic abortion was performed. Following this procedure a transient, painless jaundice developed. In August, 1940, jaundice recurred and remained continuously present until the time of admission. There was no pain, nausea, or vomiting. There had been several shaking chills followed by fever. The icteric index varied from 110 to 150 units. There was a trace of bile in the duodenal contents. All studies suggested an obstructive jaundice. She was operated upon Nov. 16, 1940. The liver appeared normal, the gall bladder moderately distended and hard. There seemed to be a small area of fibrosis just where the common duct disappeared behind the duodenum, with some yellowish discoloration suggestive of an old hematoma or fat necrosis. The common duct was opened transversely just above the duodenum. There were no stones. At the site of the fibrotic area, the common duct was completely stenosed. The duodenum was opened, and a choledochoduodenostomy was performed using a continuous circular suture of catgut, reinforced by anterior Lembert sutures of silk. Several cigarette drains were placed down to the site of anastomosis.

There was a little bile drainage from the wound November 18, which quickly ceased. The patient was discharged from the hospital Dec. 7, 1940. On that day the icteric index was 16 units. The patient has remained quite well ever since. There were no chills and no jaundice up till June, 1946, when she was last heard from.

CASE 2.—C. D., a white man, 32 years of age, was first admitted to the Cincinnati General Hospital, January, 1936, with probable acute cholecystitis, and discharged the following day against advice. He was readmitted Sept. 21, 1936, with jaundice, pain, nausea, and vomiting and operated upon Sept. 28, 1936, by a staff surgeon. The gall bladder was thin, contained no stones, and was removed. The common duct was opened, two faceted stones and much gravel were removed, and the duct was washed until clean. The ampulla was dilated to 6 mm. diameter and the common duct was closed and drained with a catheter inserted into it through the stump of the cystic duct. The patient had a stormy postoperative course. The tube drained poorly, there were acholic stools, and considerable abdominal pain and nausea for some time. He was discharged apparently well on Oct. 28, 1936, but returned five days later with an abscess of the abdominal wall. This was opened, bile and pus being drained. The patient improved and was discharged on the seventh day, Nov. 9, 1936.

He remained fairly well but with a number of attacks of pain, chills, fever, nausea, and jaundice. He was readmitted Sept. 26, 1938, with an icteric index of 68. He was reoperated upon Oct. 5, 1938. The common duct was found to be dilated and filled apparently solidly with small stones and puttylike material. It was again cleansed as thoroughly as possible, the ampulla dilated, and the common duct drained with a catheter. The postoperative course was uneventful.

He was readmitted on the Medical Service, July 10, 1939, with a history of recurrent pain and inconstant jaundice. At this admission the icteric index was 75 units. He was treated by repeated duodenal drainages and left the hospital improved, on the tenth day, against advice.

He was admitted to the Holmes Hospital as my patient May 29, 1941, again complaining of jaundice, epigastric pain, and loss of weight. Operation was performed June 3, 1941. The common bile duct was the size of a thumb and felt like a solid structure. It was opened transversely. Claylike material completely filled it from the ampulla to the right and left hepatic ducts. This was scooped out and the ducts carefully washed with salt solution. The ampulla was dilated to 6 mm. diameter, but since the widest diameter of the common duct was 14 to 15 mm. it was thought that this funnel-shaped area might predispose to stasis. Therefore a loop of jejunum was brought up and anastomosed to the opening in the duct with a continuous circular suture of catgut, reinforced with interrupted sutures of silk.

He developed a hematoma in the wound, but no dangerous bleeding. The hematoma became mildly infected and continued to drain for some time, but finally healed leaving a small ventral hernia. The jaundice quickly subsided and the patient has remained well since. He was last seen in June, 1947.

CASE 3.—G. W., a white woman, 68 years of age, was admitted to the Cincinnati General Hospital, Jan. 8, 1942, with jaundice of six weeks' duration. The icteric index on admission was 80 units. The jaundice had been relatively painless and progressive. There was considerable difference of opinion regarding the cause of jaundice, but when the roentgenogram showed a dozen or more stones, some in the gall bladder and others in a rather linear arrangement, the majority opinion was common duct stone. This patient was quite obese, had had several hospital admissions for cardiac decompensation, and was a poor operative risk; it was decided to carry out the simplest operative procedure possible. Operation was performed Jan. 24, 1942. The gall bladder was enlarged and contained numerous stones. The common duct was dilated and there was a hard mass in the region of the ampulla. The gall bladder was opened. It contained bile-stained fluid and a number of stones. No free bile was obtained although it was thought that all stones had been removed. The common bile duct was therefore opened. It contained thick, dark bile, but no stones could be found. The ampulla admitted a tiny probe with difficulty. The apparent diagnosis was carcinoma of the ampulla or head of the pancreas. Since radical operation did not seem feasible, the common duct was anastomosed to the duodenum and the gall bladder was drained. Subsequent events proved it would have been better to have removed the gall bladder, for the patient continued to have an external mucous fistula with multiple infections of the anterior abdominal wall; roentgenograms showed that one stone had been left behind. The jaundice cleared, however, and digestion remained good. There were no chills. She died at home in the spring of 1943, apparently in cardiac decompensation. There was no autopsy.

CASE 4.—J. A. McD., a white man, 68 years of age, was first operated upon Oct. 11, 1943, with diagnosis of subacute cholecystitis and cholelithiasis. The gall bladder was removed and a T tube inserted into the common duct. Apparently no stones were found in the common duct. The patient was discharged in December, 1943, with bile draining from the wound. When the wound closed he developed chills, fever, and jaundice. He was readmitted in May, 1944. The sinus tract was followed to the common duct and according to the operative note a T tube was inserted into the common duct and through what was thought to be an inflammatory stricture into the duodenum. All bile continued to drain through the T tube. A roentgenogram with lipiodol injection, May 29, 1944, showed an obstruction of the common duct near the ampulla. This same observation was made in August, 1944, at which time I was asked to see him. During this time he had lost markedly in weight and strength. The appetite was poor, the stools acholic. All bile still drained through the T tube. There was marked edema of the ankles. After a number of blood and plasma transfusions, and refeeding of his own bile, plus vitamin K therapy, he was operated upon Aug. 10, 1944. The common duct was opened and explored. No stones could be found. No tumor mass could be felt, but a probe could not be forced through the lower end of the common duct into the duodenum. The diagnosis was not clear. The common duct was anastomosed to the duodenum, however, the T tube being left in place. It was removed three weeks later and the wound healed promptly. The jaundice cleared, the stools became acholic, and the patient did remarkably well. There were no chills or fever. He remained well until late February, 1945, when, following an automobile accident, he developed pains in the lower abdomen. He was admitted to the hospital March 5, 1945. A radiologic study of the upper gastroenteric tract showed that some barium entered the biliary tract, but left it completely within six hours. There was, however, a filling defect in the second portion of the duodenum suggestive of infiltration from a carcinoma of the pancreas. He soon started to vomit and was reoperated upon to relieve the duodenal obstruction. A large retroperitoneal mass was found with the duodenum stretched over it. A simple gastroenterostomy was performed. There was little relief obtained from this procedure. He continued to vomit irregularly, although there was no jaundice. He developed a severe right parotiditis, March 10, 1945. By March 21 he seemed better though he continued to have irregular fever and was mentally confused. He finally died April 19, 1945, apparently of pneumonia. Autopsy was not obtained.

In all four of these cases a direct anastomosis of the common bile duct to the intestine was made for the relief of jaundice or external biliary fistula. None of these patients showed signs of ascending biliary tract infection, although two of them were operated on and have remained well for approximately six years each. The other two lived only about one year each, dying of other causes. In each instance the common duct was opened by a transverse incision for exploration because it was believed that an anastomosis of the common duct to the intestine would be required, and it is easier and simpler to make such an anastomosis when the incision in the common duct is transverse to its long axis than when it is parallel to it. In each instance the anastomosis was made with continuous suture of catgut to give an accurate mucosa-to-mucosa approximation, reinforced by an anterior row of interrupted silk sutures. Chills and fever did not occur in any of these patients though two of them have had choledocho-intestinal anastomosis for more than five years. The remaining two patients each lived less than one year after the anastomosis, both of them with carcinoma, and both dying of causes not directly related to the anastomosis. In these, it might be argued that a radical operation for cancer of the pancreas or ampulla should have been undertaken but it is my opinion that neither patient would have been a suitable risk for such an operation. In Case 3, the diagnosis of cancer was made and it was decided that radical operation should not be attempted. In Case 4, the malignant nature of the obstruction of the bile ducts was not recognized at the time the anastomosis of the bile duct to the intestine was made, but even if the carcinoma had been recognized no further procedure would have been done at that time because the patient was in such poor physiologic balance as the result of the prolonged loss of bile.

During the eight-year period 1938 through 1945, I operated upon nine patients with stricture of the bile duct following operative injury to the duct. None of these patients died, and all of them are well or in reasonable state of well-being at the present time. The last operation in this group was performed in February, 1945, so that the period of postoperative observation is more than two years in all cases. Various methods have been used in the repair of the duct, but in the most difficult cases direct anastomosis of the duct to the duodenum has been performed. A brief résumé of each case follows, the cases being listed chronologically.

CASE 1.—P. F., a white woman, aged 41 years, was admitted to the hospital Feb. 19, 1938, because of jaundice, anorexia, nausea and vomiting, and abdominal pain. According to her story she had been operated upon eight months previously for uterine bleeding. A hysterectomy was done, after which the surgeon palpated the gall bladder and felt stones in it. He therefore made an upper right rectus incision and removed the gall bladder. There was considerable drainage of bile for a while, but this ceased and the patient felt quite well for several months. Then she developed anorexia and nausea, and jaundice appeared and deepened progressively. At the time of admission she was intensely jaundiced, dehydrated, and emaciated. After suitable preparation she was operated upon Feb. 25, 1938. The upper end of the common duct was a dilated bulbous structure containing colorless, mucoid bile. The distal end of the duct was found imbedded in scar tissue with a defect of approximately 1 cm. between the two ends. An end-to-end anastomosis with interrupted silk sutures was done over a catheter, 4 inches of which was allowed to extend through the ampulla into the duodenum. There was considerable drainage of bile for nearly three weeks postoperatively, but it eventually ceased and she was discharged April 2, 1938.

She returned July 22, 1938, with recurrence of jaundice. The catheter was still in place. She was operated upon again July 27. Apparently the catheter, which had not been anchored, had slipped down until its upper end was below the anastomosis and a stricture had reformed. A reanastomosis was done in the same manner and the patient left the hospital in good condition Aug. 13, 1938. The catheter was passed a few days before she left the hospital.

She was readmitted one year later, July 4, 1939, with jaundice, pruritus, and vomiting which disappeared after medical management. She remained well until January, 1942, when she was again admitted with jaundice, itching, and anorexia. The wound was reopened Jan. 31, 1942, at which time the lower end of the common duct could not be found. Only a bulbous stump at the hilum of the liver representing the proximal stump could be located. This was opened, a vitallium tube was inserted and held with a purse-string suture, and the lower end of the tube was placed in the duodenum, the latter sutured to the scar tissue on the undersurface of the liver. There was no leakage of bile postoperatively and she was discharged Feb. 15, 1942.

She remained well for about one year, returning in April, 1943, with jaundice and pruritus. Roentgenograms showed that the vitallium tube had been passed. She improved and was discharged seven days later. In December, 1943, however, the jaundice became quite deep and I operated on her for the fourth time. When the lower surface of the liver was freed from the duodenum only a tiny opening was found. This was dilated and a vitallium tube re-inserted and anchored in place with several heavy silk sutures.

This tube also passed within a few months, however, and she returned to the hospital in July, 1944, with itching and mild jaundice. This time a T tube was inserted into the hepatic ducts, the lower end extending into the duodenum.

This tube was allowed to remain in place for thirty months, during which time she remained well. The tube was removed Jan. 29, 1947, and the patient has remained well up till July, 1947.

Comment.—This case, I believe, was not well managed. The most favorable opportunity was present at my first operation, and the method chosen at that time was not the most suitable. It might have succeeded had the catheter been anchored so that it could not slip below the anastomosis before healing had occurred. Better still would probably have been the use of a T tube with the side arm emerging from the duct above or below the line of anastomosis as recommended by Lahey.[4] With each succeeding operation, there has been more scar tissue until now there is a huge mass of scar and adhesions between the liver and duodenum. If still another operation is necessary, I believe the method of using a defunctioned loop of jejunum as described by Allen offers the best hope of a lasting cure.*

CASE 2.—J. S., a white man, aged 50 years, was admitted to the Cincinnati General Hospital, Jan. 10, 1939, with history that he had had attacks suggestive of cholecystic disease beginning in 1925, with one acute attack in 1930. Early in 1937 a cholecystectomy was performed for cholecystitis and cholelithiasis at another hospital. The operation was said to have gone smoothly. There was considerable drainage of bile from the wound after operation, but eventually it ceased, the wound healed, and the patient was discharged. The wound opened and closed several times thereafter. In November, 1937, about eight months postoperatively, jaundice appeared, and in January, 1938, the wound was reopened. The common duct, described as being very tiny in diameter, was probed (and drained?). Since the second operation the jaundice was intermittent, but more or less continuously present. The patient had lost about forty-five pounds in weight, from 160 to 115 pounds. There was no fever and no chills. The icteric index varied from 40 to 50 units. Cholesterol was 266 mg. per cent, and Van den Bergh positive direct and indirect. The patient left the General Hospital because he wished to be operated upon elsewhere. I operated upon him March 4, 1939. The common duct seemed to be completely obliterated in its mid-portion, though the proximal end was not distended. Fortunately the lower end was intact and it was opened and dilated. The scarred area was excised and the two ends approximated over a T tube. Lipiodol injected through the T tube in September, 1939, went directly into the duodenum and the ducts were not visualized. The tube was removed Sept. 25, 1939, and the patient has been without jaundice, chills or fever since. In November, 1944, a roentgenologic examination of the gastrointestinal tract made because of symptoms of peptic ulcer revealed some distortion of the second part of the duodenum. In April, 1947, he was admitted to the hospital for hematuria. At that time there were no symptoms or signs of disease of the biliary tract.

Comment.—Although there had been two previous operations it was fortunately possible to find the lower end of the common duct easily, and a successful result was obtained after simple reanastomosis over a T tube.

---

*In September, 1947, the patient developed signs of ascending cholangiitis without much jaundice. Allen's operation using a defunctioned loop of jejunum was performed and she was well up to Jan. 15, 1948.

CASE 3.—H. G., a white woman, 33 years of age, was admitted to the hospital Nov. 29, 1940, deeply jaundiced. She was operated upon for the first time April 11, 1939, a cholecystectomy being performed for a small contracted gall bladder containing stones. The common duct was palpated but not opened. The operation was said to have progressed smoothly. There was prolonged bile drainage and bile was still draining when she was discharged May 2, 1939. She was readmitted Aug. 7, 1939, because of intermittent drainage of bile and a history of becoming jaundiced when the fistula closed. She was reoperated upon Aug. 11, 1939, and according to the operative note the common duct was found to be small and contracted. It was opened and dilated with considerable difficulty because of scar tissue. A T tube was inserted. Postoperatively there was considerable drainage of bile through and around the tube. The patient was discharged Sept. 9, 1939, with the T tube in place, but clamped off. There is no record of when the T tube was removed, but about the middle of 1940 she developed chills, fever, diarrhea, and jaundice. I saw her for the first time in November, 1940, at which time she was deeply jaundiced, dehydrated, and emaciated. I operated upon her Dec. 3, 1940, and could find nothing but scar tissue where the common duct should have been. A bulbous structure containing colorless, mucoid bile was finally located in the hilum of the liver, which undoubtedly represented the proximal end of the common duct. A direct anastomosis was made to the duodenum without any tube. The operation was technically quite difficult because of the short proximal stump. She had a stormy postoperative course with drainage of considerable bile and duodenal contents, but eventually the wound healed and she was discharged Jan. 4, 1941.

She remained well for almost three years but was readmitted to the hospital Dec. 27, 1943, complaining of indigestion and intermittent jaundice of several months' duration. She was not jaundiced at this time, the icteric index being 10 units. She was reoperated upon Dec. 29, 1943, and a stricture found at the site of the previous anastomosis. This was dilated, and a vitallium tube inserted, one end into the hepatic duct, the other end into the duodenum. The operation was technically very simple. She had a smooth postoperative course with no bile drainage and has remained well since. She was last examined in June, 1947, at which time she was apparently entirely well 3½ years after the last operation.

Comment.—This patient was quite difficult to manage from a technical point of view at the time of the first operation in December, 1940. All of the common duct was gone except a tiny bulbous nubbin at the hilum of the liver so that anastomosis to the intestine was exceedingly difficult. In addition she was in a deplorable physical and physiologic state. The end result has been quite gratifying and there is reason to believe that she will remain well with a direct anastomosis of the duct to the duodenum over a vitallium tube.

CASE 4.—H. K. W., a white woman, aged 43 years, was admitted to the Cincinnati General Hospital, Dec. 8, 1941, complaining of chills and fever and intermittent jaundice. According to her story she developed symptoms of cholecystic disease in 1939, and was operated upon in 1940, at which time she had jaundice and acholic stools. At this time a cholecystectomy and common duct exploration were done. Following this operation she continued to have intermittent fever and jaundice; early in 1941 she was reoperated upon and an attempt made to anastomose the common duct to the duodenum. This was evidently unsuccessful because she entered the General Hospital in December, 1941, deeply jaundiced. I operated on her Dec. 12, 1941. No common duct could be found, and when the end of the hepatic duct was found in the hilum of the liver, it was discovered that the bulbous end was at the junction of the right and left hepatic ducts. A funnel-shaped vitallium tube was introduced so that the funnel-shaped end collected bile from both right and left ducts, and was held in place by a purse-string suture (this procedure is represented diagrammatically by Pearse[5]). The distal end of the tube was inserted into the duodenum and the latter structure was sutured to the scar tissue in the hilum of the liver. The postoperative course was smooth with practically no leakage of bile and the patient was discharged on the seventeenth day, Dec. 29, 1941. She has remained entirely well since. She has moved to California and the last report I had was June 13, 1947. Her only complaint at that time was obesity and high blood pressure. A recent roentgenogram had showed that the tube was still in place.

Comment.—This patient has remained well for $5\frac{1}{2}$ years after direct anastomosis of the hepatic duct to the duodenum over a vitallium tube, and is presumably cured.

CASE 5.—V. U., a white woman, aged 34 years, was admitted to the Cincinnati General Hospital March 13, 1941, with a diagnosis of chronic cholecystitis and cholelithiasis. She was operated upon by the resident surgeon March 28, 1941. At the time of division of the cystic duct for removal of the gall bladder it was recognized that the common duct had also been divided. This was immediately anastomosed over a T tube, the side arm of which was allowed to come out through the stump of the cystic duct. The tube was removed May 3, 1941. The patient remained well for about six or eight months and then developed intermittent chills, fever, and jaundice.

She was readmitted April 27, 1942, moderately jaundiced. I operated on her May 15, 1942, at which time the two ends of the common duct were found and anastomosed over a vitallium tube. The postoperative course was smooth and she remained well until early in 1946, when she developed signs and symptoms of biliary cirrhosis. She has had several admissions to the hospital on the Medical Service. The liver function tests have shown moderate impairment of liver function and a diagnosis of biliary cirrhosis has been made. She was last seen in May, 1947, at which time she was feeling quite well, five years after operation.

Comment.—This case represents a good result obtained by end-to-end suture of the duct over a vitallium tube. One would have expected a good result from the first anatomosis over a T tube. It shows that one cannot predict with assurance what may be expected to happen after any given procedure.

CASE 6.—K. D., a white woman, aged 32 years, was admitted Oct. 14, 1942, because of intense jaundice and itching. About ten weeks earlier the patient had had a cholecystectomy performed at another hospital. At the time of operation the surgeon was apparently somewhat confused about the relationship of the ducts but finally convinced himself that everything was all right. Jaundice developed rapidly after operation, however, and soon became quite marked. On October 15 the icteric index was 176 units. At operation, Oct. 17, 1943, no common duct could be found except a small bulbous area at the hilum of the liver, at the junction of the right and left hepatic ducts. This was opened and a funnel-shaped vitallium tube inserted as in Case 4, the lower end being inserted into the duodenum, and this structure then sutured to the scar tissue at the hilum of the liver. The postoperative course was uneventful, the jaundice decreased rapidly, and the patient was discharged on Nov. 4, 1942. About ten days after discharge she had a chill and fever, which rapidly subsided.

She was readmitted about one year later, Jan. 5, 1944, with pain, nausea, jaundice, and itching which had been gradually increasing for several months. Roentgenograms showed the tube in place. She was reoperated upon Jan. 8, 1944. From the outside the anastomosis looked all right, but it was taken down and the tube removed. The latter was found to be filled solidly with puttylike biliary concretion. It was carefully cleansed, resterilized, and reinserted. This was accomplished with some difficulty as the funnel-shaped end did not seem to go freely into the hepatic end of the duct, and subsequent events make me wonder whether a small amount of duct were invaginated with the tube. The lower end of the tube was replaced in the duodenum. The operation was simple from a technical point of view. The postoperative convalescence was smooth and the patient was discharged Jan. 22, 1944, the fourteenth day.

She remained well only a short while and was readmitted May 27, 1944, again with jaundice and itching. She was operated upon May 30, 1944. There were many adhesions and a great deal of scarring. On removing the vitallium tube, a great deal of granulation tissue was found filling the lower end of the common duct proximal to the tube. This was curetted, the duct washed and dilated, and a T tube inserted into it, the other end placed in the duodenum and a tight closure made around the side arm of the tube which was brought out through the wound. The postoperative convalescence was uneventful and the patient was discharged Jan. 17, 1944. It was planned to leave the T tube in place for a period of months, possibly one year or longer.

In the spring of 1945 at a routine follow-up examination the patient announced that she was several months pregnant. After some consultation a therapeutic abortion was recommended, but the patient refused to have the procedure done. The pregnancy was without incident and the baby was born Dec. 30, 1945. During this period the T tube was kept clamped off continuously except for a period once a month when it was opened temporarily. On several occasions there was irritation of the skin around the tube. This was treated with zinc peroxide ointment, which had to be discontinued because it caused deterioration of the rubber. At one time it was doubtful whether the tube would last throughout the pregnancy. It was amazing how far down the tract became epithelized by growth from the abdominal skin. It was my hope that the duct was also becoming completely epithelized. About three weeks after termination of the pregnancy, on Jan. 21, 1946, the tube was removed. The tract continued to drain bile-stained duodenal contents except when sealed off with a gauze or cotton pack held in place by adhesive, and the patient had to change this dressing every three or four days. She has had two bouts of chills, fever, and jaundice, one requiring hospital care in April, 1947. This subsided promptly following chemotherapy, was probably due to cholangiitis, and suggests to me that the stricture may be recurring. According to more recent reports, however, she has been well for the past few months up until late August, 1947.

Comment.—It is unfortunate that in this instance the vitallium tube used in the first operation became plugged with bile pigments, for if it had not I believe a good result would have been attained. Many others who have used vitallium tubes have had the experience of having them become plugged in this fashion. The reason for the occurrence of this deposition of pigment is obscure, but is probably related to the chemical constitution of the bile. At the present time there is no known method of preventing it with certainty, and for this reason many surgeons are abandoning the use of vitallium tubes in repairing the bile ducts, and relying on the older method of some sort of removable tube.

This patient's trouble after the second operation in which the vitallium tube was removed, cleansed, and replaced was probably due to improper replacement of the tube in the proximal end of the duct, due to my unwillingness to cut the duct sufficiently widely to allow the insertion of the funnel-shaped end of the tube. I still do not feel satisfied that this patient will remain well and as in Case 1, if further operative intervention is necessary, I believe that the procedure described by Allen should be employed.

Case 7.—P. D., a white woman, aged 47 years, was admitted Nov. 9, 1943, because of a complete external biliary fistula. June 19, 1943, she had had a cholecystectomy for acute cholecystitis. Apparently she had a very stormy postoperative course, and was reoperated upon July 10, although it is not clear just what was done. Eventually she recovered, but with a complete biliary fistula.

Lipiodol injection through the fistula showed a tortuous tract up to the hilum of the liver and then outlined a dilated biliary tree. At operation Nov. 13, 1944, a catheter was inserted into the fistula as a guide and an attempt made to follow it to the common duct. The catheter slipped out, however, and the tract became smaller and smaller till it finally was lost. In spite of what was thought to have been adequate preparation with vitamin K and blood transfusions, there was continuous oozing from the wound, which was very troublesome. It seemed impossible to find the upper end of the common or hepatic ducts. Since there had been little or no obstruction, the ducts proximally were not greatly dilated nor was there much bile dammed in them. Occasionally there was a small spurt or ooze of bile, but every time the area was searched for the duct, only excessive bleeding occurred. Finally without clear visualization a vitallium tube was inserted into what was thought to be the proximal end of the duct. The other end was placed in the duodenum since the lower end of the duct could not be found. The result was unsatisfactory, and the patient was discharged Nov. 29, 1943, with some bile still draining from the wound but some reaching the intestine. The fistula closed in a few weeks but the patient then developed chills, fever, pain, and jaundice.

She returned to the hospital March 23, 1944. At this time she was moderately jaundiced, the icteric index being 25 units. She was reoperated upon March 30, 1944, and again the proximal end of the duct could not be clearly visualized. After a long time had been spent searching for the duct and when the patient's condition was becoming serious from loss of blood, a T tube was placed in what was thought to be the proximal end of the duct, the lower end of the tube being inserted into the duodenum. Bile drained around, but not through, the tube so the latter was removed and the patient discharged April 16, 1944, with a complete external biliary fistula. This fistula also closed, but soon thereafter chills, fever, malaise, and jaundice recurred.

She returned again Oct. 17, 1944, and was operated upon October 20. This time by carefully peeling the scar from the undersurface of the liver by sharp dissection, it was possible to isolate the proximal hepatic duct. A T tube was inserted into the duct, the lower end being inserted into the duodenum. It looked as though this were going to succeed and the patient seemed to be progressing satisfactorily though slowly. There was some drainage around the tube, but this gradually decreased. However, our troubles were not over. Just before the patient was discharged from the hospital, a lipiodol injection through the tube was done. To our surprise this showed that the lipiodol entered the colon as well as the duodenum and bile ducts. Barium by mouth was given and showed a large duodenocolic fistula. Just how this fistula developed remains unclear. It may have been due to an injury to the colon in freeing it which remained unrecognized at the time of operation. It is possible that I mistook colon for duodenum and inserted the lower arm of the T tube into it, though this seems unlikely for in freeing the duodenum from the liver the remains of the anastomosis of the bile ducts to it still remained in the form of a tiny hole. The fact that practically everything the patient ate went directly from the duodenum to the colon was explained to her, but she nevertheless insisted on leaving the hospital without further operation because she felt well.

She returned Dec. 29, 1944, however, because of diarrhea, vomiting, and loss of weight. There had been no chills or fever and only slight jaundice. On Dec. 30, 1944, she was reoperated upon, the colon freed from the duodenum, and the opening in the colon closed. The bile ducts were anastomosed to the duodenum over a T tube. In a few days it was obvious that this suture had not held, the T tube fell out, and there was profuse drainage of bile and duodenal contents. Fortunately the closure of the colon held, and since the operation had been performed practically extraperitoneally there was no peritoneal reaction and the abdominal wound held. On Jan. 6, 1945, a jejunostomy was done for feeding. The abdominal wound was kept as dry as possible with continuous suction. In a few days the wound began to heal, and she was finally discharged Feb. 7, 1947, eating normally, with all wounds healed and in reasonably good condition.

Since then her progress has been only fair. She has had some attacks of pain in the upper abdomen, and bouts of fever, chills and jaundice, so that I think certainly she will have further trouble. At last report in the spring of 1947 she was getting along fairly well.

Comment.—In this case the poor result was, I believe, largely due to poor operative technique. It was the only instance I have met in which it was impossible clearly to identify the duct proximally. In spite of the fact that the duct had been opened, there was no continuous flow of bile to identify it, and every attempt to locate it led to bleeding so brisk as to obscure the field. At the third attempt, the scar tissue was stripped off the undersurface of the liver up into the hilum in a broad sheet by sharp dissection until the duct was located. The duodenocolic fistula was probably also a technical error, although injury or opening into the colon was unrecognized at the time.

CASE 8.—A. L., a white woman, aged 22 years, was admitted Feb. 18, 1944. This patient had had a cholecystectomy performed elsewhere in October, 1942. The operation was said to have progressed smoothly. Postoperatively, however, there was considerable difficulty. The patient developed a large mass in the right upper quadrant, which was drained after some days and proved to be a large intra-abdominal collection of bile. Following this procedure an external biliary fistula developed, which drained only a moderate amount of bile. Lipiodol injection in January, 1943, showed that this fistula communicated with the hepatic flexure of the colon. At that time I recommended operation, but the patient was feeling well and refused to have anything done. The fistula closed and she got along fairly well for some time, but then over a period of six to nine months she developed attacks of fever, pain in the right upper abdomen, and moderate jaundice. Finally she began to lose weight and strength and agreed to operation.

She was operated on February 21, 1944. There were numerous adhesions, and a small fistulous tract only one millimeter or so in diameter extended from the common bile duct over the duodenum to the colon. This was excised and the distal end inverted into the colon. The proximal end of the duct was thick, but not much dilated. The distal collapsed end was found, with a defect of 1 to 2 cm. between the two ends. By mobilization, the two ends could be brought together and an end-to-end suture of interrupted fine silk was done over a vitallium tube. The postoperative course was smooth and uneventful and the patient was discharged March 4, 1944. She has remained entirely well since. She went through a pregnancy the following year, the baby being born by cesarean section Sept. 8, 1945. She was last heard from in June, 1947, 3½ years after operation, at which time she said her health was splendid and the only complaint was the gain in weight.

Comment.—This is the type of good result that can be expected when the most desirable method can be used, namely, direct anastomosis of the ducts over a tube.

CASE 9.—A. T., a colored woman, aged 45 years, was admitted to the Cincinnati General Hospital Feb. 9, 1945, because of an external biliary fistula and jaundice. She had had a cholecystectomy elsewhere for cholecystitis and cholelithiasis on Dec. 16, 1944. She developed jaundice a week or ten days after operation, which became progressively worse. Jan. 29, 1945, she was reoperated upon, at which time a dilated common duct was found apparently after some difficulty. The surgeon inserted a catheter into the duct, because he believed the patient's condition precluded further surgery at the time. On February 9 she was transferred to the General Hospital and I operated upon her ten days later, Feb. 19, 1945. The operation was difficult from the very beginning. The fresh adhesions and scar tissue were extremely vascular so that it was impossible to keep a dry field. By following down the undersurface of the liver into the hilum the proximal end of the common duct was found, but the distal end could not be located. A T tube was inserted into the proximal duct, the other arm put into the duodenum through a stab wound, and the duodenum sutured to the common duct. Biopsy of the liver showed focal necrosis. The postoperative course was uneventful and the patient was discharged March 12, 1945, with the tube in place but clamped off.

Lipiodol injection shortly before discharge showed that the material entered the duodenum and practically none entered the ducts. The T tube was allowed to remain in place for about eighteen months and was removed in September, 1946. The external wound healed in about six weeks after removal of the tube and when last seen in June, 1947, the patient was apparently entirely well.

DISCUSSION

Four of these nine patients had direct anastomosis of the two ends of the duct and this method proved fairly successful. In Case 1 stricture recurred after two attempts by this method, and anastomosis of bile ducts to the duodenum was then used, also with only a fair result. In Cases 2 and 8 the result was satisfactory after one attempt, while in Case 5 it was successful after a second trial. In five cases, Cases 3, 4, 6, 7, and 9, the lower end of the common duct was not found, and in Case 1 after the first two operations it was not found, so that ultimately in these six cases anastomosis of the common duct to the duodenum was used. This procedure was apparently entirely successful in three patients, and at least fairly successful in the remaining three, for all of them are alive and reasonably well from 2½ to 5½ years after the last operation. I have learned, however, that even after two to three years one cannot call a satisfactory result a cure.

Patients with stricture or absence of the common duct require a great deal of painstaking attention in the preoperative preparation, in the operative technique, and in postoperative care. Usually they are in poor physiologic balance, and blood and plasma should be used freely in preparing them for operation. Vitamin K parenterally in large doses should be given. If the patient can tolerate it, the diet should be rich in carbohydrate and protein. If the patient is unable to eat well, these substances should be given parenterally. If the patient has an external biliary fistula, collection of the bile and refeeding either by mouth or with the use of a stomach tube is of great help, otherwise a commercial form of bile salts should be given by mouth. A Levine tube for continuous gastric suction after operation should be in place in the stomach before the operation is started. It is also probably wise to prepare the patient with chemotherapy for one or two days before operation, and to continue this treatment through the first few postoperative days, although this method was not used in most of my patients.

One or two hints about the operative technique should be emphasized. The most important thing is to find the proximal end of the common duct. In order to do this it is helpful, after preliminary exposure has been made, to locate the undersurface of the right lobe of the liver, and follow down along it with sharp dissection, always staying as close as possible to the liver without actually incising it, approaching the region of the hepatic ducts in the hilum from the front and a little to the right side. If there is more or less complete obstruction, the bulbous end of the common duct will appear through the scar tissue as a bluish-tinged cystlike structure, and this should be exposed, also by sharp dissection, to its most distal or dependent part before it is opened. To find the lower end of the duct may be even more difficult. Cattell stated that it can almost always be found by mobilizing the duodenum and reflecting it to the left to pick up the retroduodenal position of the duct, which is usually below the level of scar formation. I have not had occasion to use this method, but recently watched one of my associates do so. After he had spent considerable time in thus isolating the lower end, he found that it was impossible to free it sufficiently to allow it to reach up to the very short proximal stump which was high up in the hilum of the liver. I have usually contented myself in making a reasonably careful search for the lower end of the common duct, but if it has not been found crainiad to the upper curve of the duodenum, I have abandoned the search and anastomosed the proximal end to the duodenum. In view of the excellent results reported by Cattell, I now wonder if I have been sufficiently diligent in searching for the distal end. As a result of the trouble experienced with vitallium tubes, namely, difficulty in keeping them in place for a sufficient period of time, and possible danger of their becoming plugged with concretions of biliary origin, I believe that in the future I shall use removable tubes of one sort or another, probably either a T tube or fenestrated catheter. Unless technical difficulties prevent, I am sure that every effort should be made to produce a mucosa-to-mucosa suture between bile duct and intestinal epithelium. It is better, I believe, to have a little mucosal eversion and some bile leakage, than to have a tight serosal approximation, so that there is no leakage of bile in the immediate postoperative period, but possibly an anastomosis which is partly lined by serosa and which will later contract if epithelization does not occur promptly. Finally, if it is impossible to anastomose duct-to-duct, and duct-to-intestine anastomosis becomes necessary, while I agree that it is theoretically better to use a defunctioned loop than a direct anastomosis, I still believe that the simpler technical procedure of direct anastomosis may be accepted for use in greatly debilitated or poor-risk patients because of the lessened operative hazard. In this group of patients it has been fairly satisfactory and has not been followed by evidence of ascending infection into the liver except in those cases in which stricture has recurred.

SUMMARY AND CONCLUSIONS

Thirteen cases of anastomosis of the common duct to the intestine or repair of a stricture of the common duct are reported, all of them my own personal cases. In the first four, a relatively normal duct was used in making the anastomosis. In the remaining nine cases a duct injured at a previous operation was present.

There were no operative deaths in the thirteen cases though two patients, both of whom had cancer, died subsequently of causes not directly related to the operative procedure on the common duct.

In ten of the thirteen cases, the last operation performed was some type of anastomosis of the hepatic or common duct to the duodenum without the use of a defunctionated loop, and in seven of these the result has been entirely satisfactory. Two of these seven patients died within one year of operation, but the others are well 2½ to 6 years after operation. Three patients in this group of ten have been reasonably well $2\frac{1}{3}$ to $3\frac{1}{2}$ years after operation, but all of them have had one or more attacks of chills, fever, and jaundice and may require further operation.

In three of the thirteen cases a satisfactory result was obtained by end-to-end suture of the duct, $3\frac{1}{2}$, 5, and 8 years after operation.

Two patients have gone through normal pregnancies after operation.

Certain technical details such as the importance of mucosa-to-mucosa suture, and the methods of finding the proximal end of the duct, have been discussed. While vitallium tubes have functioned successfully in a number of instances, in others they have not remained in situ, and in one case the tube became plugged with concretions, necessitating its removal.

As a result of this experience, it is my opinion that:

1. End-to-end suture of the duct is the most desirable method, but frequently it is technically impossible to achieve.

2. Mucosa-to-mucosa approximation should be a most important consideration, and should be attained if possible regardless of the method of anastomosis used.

3. While ascending infection is a hazard in anastomosis of the duct to the duodenum; it nevertheless is followed by a successful result in a sufficiently large proportion of cases, so that it should not be wholly abandoned as a method. At least it may be used as the first method attempted in patients who have a great deal of scarring and adhesions, and who are debilitated as a result of prolonged obstruction of the ducts. It is relatively simple, and in this small group of cases was attended by no operative mortality.

4. Removable tubes probably are more suitable than vitallium tubes in preserving patency of the anastomosis till epithelization has occurred.

5. No standard method is applicable to all cases but each should be treated as seems indicated in that particular case.

REFERENCES

1. Cattell, R. B.: Strictures of the Biliary Ducts, J. A. M. A. **134**: 235-240, 1947.
2. Allen, A. W.: A Method of Re-establishing Continuity Between the Bile Ducts and the Gastro-intestinal Tract, Ann. Surg. **121**: 412-424, 1945.
3. Cole, W. H., Ireneus, Carl, Jr., and Reynolds, J. R.: The Use of Vitallium Tubes in Strictures and Absence of the Common Bile Duct, Ann. Surg. **122**: 490-521, 1945.
4. Lahey, F. H.: Strictures of the Common and Hepatic Ducts, Ann. Surg. **105**: 765-786, 1937.
5. Pearse, Herman E.: Vitallium Tubes in Biliary Surgery, Tr. Am. S. A. **40**: 1031, 1942.

THE PROBLEM OF GASTRIC CANCER IN A UNIVERSITY HOSPITAL

H. GLENN BELL, M.D., SAN FRANCISCO, CALIF.

(From the Department of Surgery, University of California Medical School)

IT WAS my privilege to be the first University of Cincinnati graduate to train for six years under George J. Heuer after he came to Cincinnati as professor of surgery. That training enabled me to come to the University of California in July, 1930, to start a similar type of resident training program. It is most fitting that Dr. Heuer's residents should commemorate his retirement with a volume such as this.

The fact that cancer of the stomach is curable should be more widely emphasized. Physicians as well as laymen display an unenlightened attitude toward this dread disease. The only known cure at the present time is radical removal of the malignant process. It is granted that cures are few, but every patient should be given the chance, small though it is, for a cure. Unless distant metastases are unequivocally proved, every patient with a diagnosis of cancer of the stomach should have an exploratory operation to determine whether the lesion is resectable.

During the past seventeen years 540 patients with carcinoma of the stomach have been seen at the University of California Hospital. Out of this whole group 69.2 per cent were subjected to surgery, and gastric resection was accomplished in 34.4 per cent of cases (Table I). One must realize that most of these cases occur in the older age group in which the natural hazards of surgery and anesthesia are increased. In a well-recognized hospital where the personnel are interested and adequately trained to accomplish such drastic surgery, the mortality rate can be kept within a reasonable limit. A tremendous improvement in anesthesia during the past few years has made it possible for many of these patients to be carried through successful surgery. Many of the elderly patients are operated upon under local anesthesia. It will be noted in Table I that during the past five years the operative mortality has decreased from 22.2 to 11.9 per cent.

The only hope for increasing the number of cures is by earlier recognition of the disease and early operation. Of those patients operated upon, 49.7 per cent had a resectable lesion (Table II). The resectability rate calculated on all patients in the series was 34.4 per cent. It is in this 34 per cent that we may expect our five-year survivals or cures. Entirely too many cases come to attention at the clinic in such an advanced stage that they are already beyond help. Out of this whole group, 30.7 per cent of patients had an inoperable lesion and received only supportive medical treatment. In 65.5 per cent of all cases the lesion was not resectable.

TABLE I. FIVE HUNDRED FORTY CASES GASTRIC CARCINOMA, 1930 TO 1947—OPERATIVE MORTALITY

	NUMBER OF CASES		MORTALITY 1930 TO 1941 (PER CENT)	MORTALITY 1942 TO 1947 (PER CENT)
	NUMBER	PER CENT		
Gastric resection	186	34.4	20.6	11.7
Palliative surgery	79	14.6	23.7	10.0
Exploratory laparotomy	109	20.1	23.2	13.2
Total surgery	374	69.2	22.2	11.9
No treatment	166	30.7		
Total	540	100	22.2	11.9

It is quite apparent from Table III that the most favorable location of a gastric lesion is the pyloric end of the stomach. Perhaps this is due to the fact that symptoms of obstruction occur earlier and are called to the attention of both the patient and the doctor. Of patients with carcinoma at the pyloric end of the stomach who were operated upon over five years ago, 18.9 per cent lived five years or longer. Thirty patients in this group who were operated upon less than five years ago are still alive and well.

TABLE II. FIVE HUNDRED FORTY CASES GASTRIC CARCINOMA, 1930 TO 1947—RESECTABILITY

	PER CENT
Resectability rate (calculated on all patients)	34.4
Resectability rate (calculated on patients operated upon)	49.7
Not resectable	65.5
Inoperable (only medical treatment)	30.7

During this same seventeen-year period, gastric resection was done in seven cases of sarcoma of the stomach. Two of these patients lived well over five years, one dying at six years of intercurrent disease and one being still alive nine years after the resection.

TABLE III. FIVE HUNDRED FORTY CASES GASTRIC CARCINOMA, 1930 TO 1947—SURVIVAL FOLLOWING GASTRIC RESECTION

LOCATION OF TUMOR	TOTAL CASES	NUMBER RESECTED		OPERATIVE MORTALITY (PER CENT)	LIVED 5 YR. OR LONGER		LIVING LESS THAN 5 YR.	DIED LESS THAN 5 YR.
		NO.	PER CENT		NO.	PER CENT		
Cardia	113	24	21.2	33.3	0		2	22
Body	63	17	27.0	11.7	0		4	13
Pyloric end	259	137	52.9	13.8	14	18.9	30	93
Diffuse	105	8	7.6	12.5	0		2	6
Total	540	186	34.4	16.1	14	7.5	38	134

There is still too much delay between the time of suspicion of a gastric lesion and the time of exploratory laparotomy. Much of this delay is caused by the physicians themselves, and some is due to procrastination on the part of the patient.

To illustrate the delay as we see it in a teaching hospital to which patients are referred from all parts of the state, I should like to describe briefly the history of a woman who was seen here in April, 1946.

CASE REPORT

Except for an occasional spell of high blood pressure, this 74-year-old widow had been well until June, 1945, when she noticed increasing weakness with some accompanying loss of appetite. Her local physician told her it was her ''nerves,'' and made no examination. In December, 1945, the patient felt extremely weak, and at about this time she began to notice distress in the upper mid-epigastrium. She described this as a ''hurting'' sensation which was very deep; it was not sharp nor a real pain. Another local physician made a hemoglobin determination and told her she had anemia. She was taken to a hospital for two weeks and was given five liver shots, but no special diet. No x-ray studies nor further laboratory tests were done. In January, 1946, the patient had an attack of severe nausea and vomiting. The vomitus was whitish and contained no blood nor coffee-ground material. She was kept in the hospital again for several days on a fluid, food-free regimen. No x-ray studies were done.

In March, 1946, the patient came to California still feeling extremely weak and bothered by epigastric distress, which might come on at any time but was most marked after she had eaten any spicy foods. In April, 1946, the first x-ray examination was made and a diagnosis of carcinoma of the stomach was made. The doctor who ordered the roentgenograms told the family that their mother had a carcinoma of the stomach which was inoperable, and that nothing could be done about it but to take her home and let her die. The son, however, asked to have his mother sent to the University of California Hospital, where she was admitted on April 20, 1946. The positive findings were a blood pressure of 160/80, a hemoglobin of 46 per cent, a red blood cell count of 2,870,000, and a white blood cell count of 4,100. Gastric analysis showed no free hydrochloric acid. X-ray examination showed a filling defect in the pyloric end of the stomach.

This patient was operated upon on April 27, 1946, under local anesthesia. A carcinoma of the pyloric end of the stomach was found, and a subtotal gastric resection was done without difficulty. There was no evidence of local spread of the carcinoma, and the lymph nodes on the greater and lesser curvature were not involved. The liver was free from metastases. When last seen in July, 1947, this patient had no complaints referable to the stomach. She had regained her strength, the blood count was normal, and she was eating without difficulty.

Delays such as are illustrated by this case history are deplorable, and it seems to me that there must be something wrong with the teaching in our medical schools throughout the country for physicians at large to have such a fatalistic attitude toward carcinoma of the stomach. To be certain, it has been only one year since this patient was operated upon, but is not that one year of comfort worth something? It is my feeling that this woman, who is now 75 years of age, has a good chance of attaining her life expectancy and of dying from the cardiac disease, rather than from a recurrent malignancy.

Granting that the percentage of five-year survivals is extremely small, since there is no other known treatment for carcinoma of the stomach no patient should be denied this small chance for a cure. With the improvement in recent years in operative technique and in anesthesia, and the decrease in the operative mortality rate, I feel we are justified in doing everything we can to bring these patients to surgery earlier while there is still a possibility that the lesion may be a resectable one.

LYMPHOSARCOMA OF THE GASTROINTESTINAL TRACT

David Henry Poer, M.D., Atlanta, Ga.

LYMPHOSARCOMA involving the alimentary tract is admittedly a rare disease, and only a few such sarcomas may be seen during the entire clinical experience of one surgeon. Nevertheless, its role as a masquerading lesion and its different prognosis and management bids us re-evaluate our present data regarding diagnosis and treatment. This paper reports a case of lymphosarcoma of the duodenum presenting as perforated peptic ulcer. A brief review of the general problem of gastrointestinal lymphosarcoma is given, with a consideration of incidence, location of involvement, similarity to other conditions, diagnosis, and surgical management.

INCIDENCE

The incidence of lymphosarcoma of the gastrointestinal tract is extremely low. Taking the stomach alone as an indication, this lesion comprises approximately one-half of all sarcomas of this organ, which form only 1 to 2 per cent of all gastric neoplasms.[1, 2] While its occurrence rate in the small gut may be somewhat higher, the over-all low percentage of neoplastic involvement of this region will make it even more rare in this location. While carcinoma is found more frequently in the large intestine, sarcoma may occur in the small and large intestine and rectum.

PATHOLOGY

Sarcoma of the gastrointestinal tract may occur in three forms: spindle-cell type, generally arising from muscle, slow of growth and metastasizing late; round- or mixed-cell sarcomas, an ill-defined group; and lymphosarcoma, which is the most important of the three. This last group may be further divided into malignant lymphocytoma, giant follicular lymphoblastoma, and the more common reticulum-cell lymphosarcoma.[3]

In lymphocytoma, the normal architecture is replaced by mature lymphocytes, and the picture resembles that seen in lymphatic leucemia, the differentiation being made by examination of the blood. This condition may terminate as lymphatic leucemia. Follicular lymphoblastoma or giant follicle lymphoma is an intermediate type in which the follicles are very large and present an increase in both lymphoblasts and reticulum cells. It has a tendency to revert to either true lymphocytoma or reticulum-cell sarcoma. It is of low malignancy and is extremely radiosensitive. The third type with the reticulum cell as its unit is included with the lymphosarcomas, even though the tumor arises from reticulum cells in the node or follicle. Microscopically, it is characteristic, revealing an abundance of reticulum formation, in contrast to the widely separated, sparse original reticulum demonstrated in the other two types. It is a highly malignant disease, with an average duration of less than two years.

Grossly, the pathologic findings depend largely upon the original site of tumor growth and the manner in which it spreads. In the intestine, the growth may be polypoid or more commonly intramural. In the former instance, the projection inward of the mass may give rise to partial obstruction or serve as the leading point of an intussusception or volvulus.[4] Polypoid growths may be multiple, whereas the annular type is usually single, and may be localized or extensive enough to involve a considerable segment of bowel. It is the annular, intramural growth that affords the most variables. As the tumor spreads through the bowel layers, the muscular and submucosal layers are replaced, and the growth comes to lie beneath the serosa, which is rarely penetrated. Three processes may then take place: the submucosal portion of the tumor may break through, ulcerate, and undergo partial destruction and ulceration; there may be a gradual dilatation of the gut as the nervous and muscular layers are replaced by the growth, giving the bowel the appearance of a thick-walled hose pipe,'' an appearance which is said to be diagnostic (excluding tuberculosis); and last, there may be an actual stenosis of the gut with the narrowed lumen causing partial intestinal obstruction.[2]

SITES OF INVOLVEMENT

The relative incidence of involvement of different portions of the gastro-intestinal tract has been reported by a number of writers.[2, 5-9] In their review of their own and other statistics, Ullman and Abeshouse concluded that lymphosarcoma is more frequent in the small than in the large intestine, not excluding the rectum. The small intestine was the site of the lesion in seventy-seven cases, the large intestine (including the cecum) in thirty-two cases, and the ileocecal region in eight cases. The most common location for the tumor was the ileum, and next in order the jejunum, then the cecum. However, when the entire alimentary canal is considered, the stomach is the most frequent site. Some authors (Libman in particular[10]) found the duodenum involved as frequently as the ileum. It may be concluded, therefore, that lymphosarcoma may occur anywhere along the gastrointestinal tract, and that next to the stomach, the ileum is the most frequently involved.

DIAGNOSIS

The diagnosis of lymphosarcoma revolves about the presenting symptoms and altered physiology. The provisional diagnosis is almost always the most common one for the particular group of signs and symptoms. The differential diagnosis, however, is usually very difficult and may indeed be impossible without laparotomy. The possibility of lymphosarcoma may be suggested by several factors: The age of the patient is significant, lymphosarcoma being suspected in the young, carcinoma in the group past 40 years of age. Carcinoma is essentially an obstructive lesion, of relatively slow growth, whereas lymphosarcoma progresses rapidly, and rarely gives rise to a complete obstruction. A more rapid downhill course is to be expected with lymphosarcoma, cachexia and marked toxemia being quite common. Melena is occasionally seen when the lesion is gastric, but in the intestines is more commonly indicative of carcinoma. With gastric and duodenal lymphosarcoma, dypepsia and ulcerlike symptoms may predominate. Last, the marked radiosensitivity of lymphosarcoma will also serve to differentiate it from carcinoma. It is upon this fact that Cheever, in 1932, stated the rationale for laparotomy in all cases of an abdominal mass suspected of being neoplastic, in the hope of finding a certain percentage of lymphosarcomas which might be given radiation therapy and offer the patient a considerably longer period of survival.

SYMPTOMATOLOGY

Lymphosarcoma may present first by almost any symptom referable to the gastrointestinal tract. A review of case reports of this lesion will exemplify the diverse symptomatology and chief complaints of patients with this disease. The onset may be insidious, with weight loss, anorexia, fatigue, and other general constitutional symptoms, or may be ushered in by an acute abdominal catastrophe, such as perforation or massive hemorrhage.[19, 20]

Archer and Cooper stated that in lymphosarcoma of the stomach, the symptoms are usually those of nonobstructive peptic ulcer.[11] Hematemesis and melena are rare but may occur. Involvement of the duodenum may give rise to the same symptoms as these or may be obstructive, depending upon the character of the growth, whether intraluminal, intramural, or infiltrative.[21]

In the small intestines, the symptomatology again depends primarily upon the characteristics of the growth. Polypoid tumors may serve as the starting point for intussusceptions and present acute obstruction, as reported by Cutler and associates.[4] They may also give rise to low grade obstruction from chronic intussusceptions. Even if obstruction is not the primary factor, most patients with this lesion in the small bowel will have nausea, vomiting, and bouts of abdominal pain.[12] Gross blood and even tarry stools may occasionally be seen. Speese[13] pointed out that the symptoms might be slight at the onset, but would later develop into pain, associated nausea, anorexia, vomiting, constipation, distention, and perhaps a palpable abdominal tumor. He classified lymphosarcomas of the bowel in seven groups, depending upon the presenting signs and symptoms: latent tumor, found at necropsy; tumors discovered first by general abdominal distention and palpable tumor (these being rather rare); the acute tumors which begin with intussusception, rapid obstruction, or perforation; those which present the picture of tuberculous peritonitis; tumors in which jaundice is the first symptom; tumors which simulate ovarian cysts; and last, those which mimic appendicitis. Involvement of the cecum is manifest in the majority of cases by cramplike abdominal pain, palpable tumor, and loss of weight.[12] Diarrhea and melena are infrequent. Tumors of the colon distal to the cecum are relatively more rare and present much the same picture as cecal lymphosarcoma. Location in the rectum is revealed by blood in the stool in the majority of instances, and in almost every case the tumor can be reached by the examining finger.

The involvement of superficial lymph nodes is occasionally seen and, in the presence of a palpable abdominal tumor or one demonstrable roentgenographically, strongly suggests the diagnosis of lymphosarcoma.[2] Palpable inguinal nodes are present in about one-half the cases of lymphosarcoma of the rectum.

The hematologic picture is not diagnostic in this condition.[7] In certain cases, in which the tumor is a malignant lymphocytoma, the blood may show the typical findings of lymphatic leucemia. This may occur with other forms of lymphosarcoma, but not nearly as frequently.

ROENTGENOLOGIC FINDINGS

Roentgenologic examination may aid considerably in the diagnosis of lymphosarcoma. In the stomach, tumefaction and ulceration may be evident, riving rise to large ulcer craters similar to carcinoma.[11] Large rugae may be visualized along with separation of the individual folds. Duodenal involvement may present the deformity characteristically seen with ulcer, with evident spasm or ulceration or both.[14] Some lymphosarcomas of the stomach may present nothing diagnostic in the roentgenographic appearance of the stomach and peristalsis may not be interfered with as much as in the presence of carcinoma.[15]

Intestinal lymphosarcoma will give varied roentgenographic findings. Obstruction may predominate and distention of intestinal loops be seen. Intussusceptions may be demonstrated by contrast media, provided they occur low enough to be reached by barium enema, that is, colocolic and ileocolic. Polypoid tumors may be seen as filling defects or show chronic obstruction with motility series. Commonly seen is a partial stenosis of intestine, with proximal dilatation.[22] Less frequently one sees a dilatation of bowel in the region of tumor, said by many authors to occur more often than stenosis and to be diagnostic for lymphosarcoma. Rowe and Neely[16] and Greenfield[17] have stated that the typical roentgenographic picture of lymphosarcoma of the small bowel may be obtained by "stasis ray" of the small intestine, and they feel that the more frequent use of this method will lead to earlier diagnoses and demonstration of the lesion.

CASE REPORT

R. W. S., a 40-year-old man, was admitted to the hospital on Sept. 9, 1939, in acute distress and complaining of severe abdominal pain, of seven hours' duration. This began suddenly as epigastric distress, and rapidly became generalized, steady and excruciating. There had been no nausea, vomiting, or other gastrointestinal symptoms. No history of previous similar symptoms referable to the abdomen was elicited; appetite had been good, with only occasional indigestion, relieved by self-medication. Remainder of past history was negative.

Examination showed temperature, 97.0° F.; pulse, 84; respirations, 20; blood pressure, 150/85. The patient was a well-developed and nourished adult man in acute distress and complaining bitterly of abdominal pain. The heart and lungs were normal. The relevant portion of the examination was limited to the abdomen, which presented boardlike rigidity, rebound tenderness, and generalized tenderness. There was a loss of liver dullness on percussion over the right upper quadrant and thorax. Peristalsis was not heard, and there was tenderness bilaterally on rectal examination.

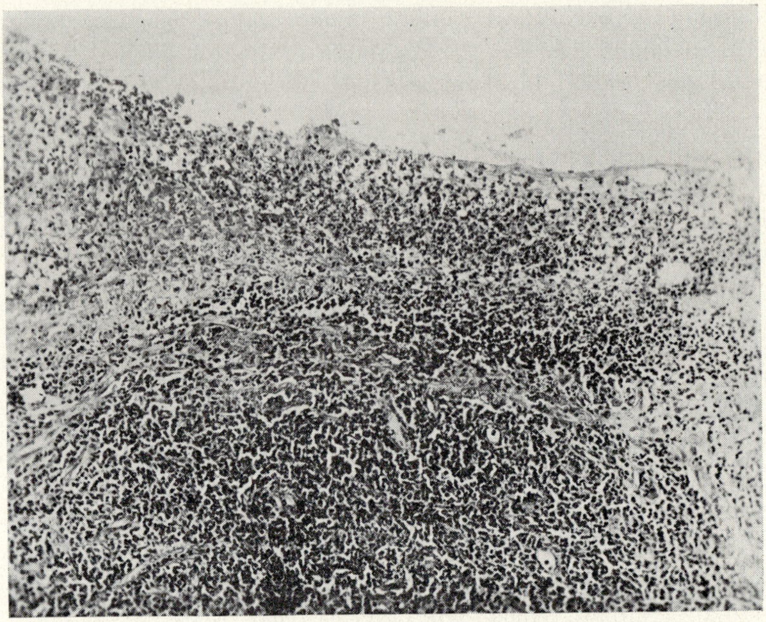

Fig. 1.—Section of floor of necrotic wall of duodenal ulcer removed at operation, showing infiltrating tumor underneath.

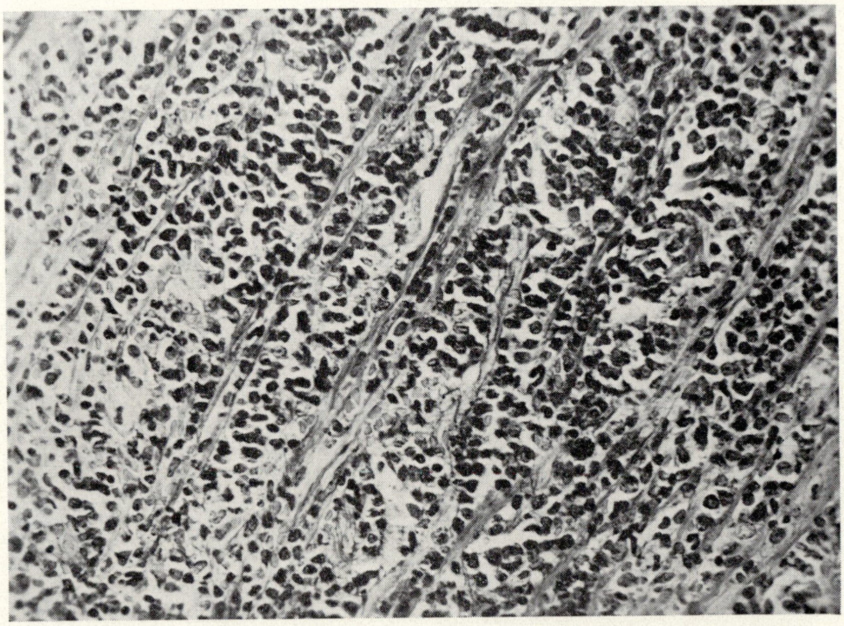

Fig. 2.—Diffuse infiltrating lymphosarcoma in duodenal wall.

Clinical impression was that this patient presented a typical picture of perforation of a viscus, more likely a peptic ulcer of stomach or duodenum. He was prepared and immediate operation performed under general anesthesia.

A high right rectus incision was made, and when the peritoneum was opened, gas escaped and gastric contents were seen. These were removed by suction and sponging, and after adequate retraction the area of perforation was visualized. In the first portion of the

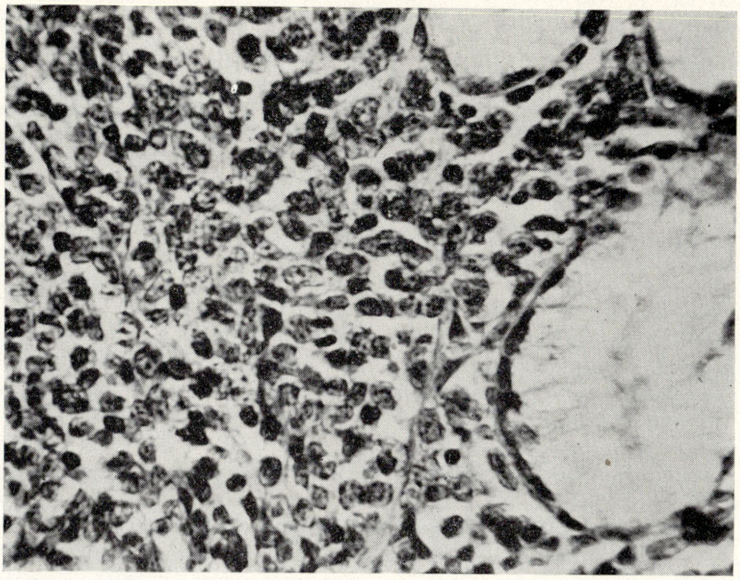

Fig. 3.—High magnification of lymphosarcoma in duodenal wall, showing numerous mitotic figures.

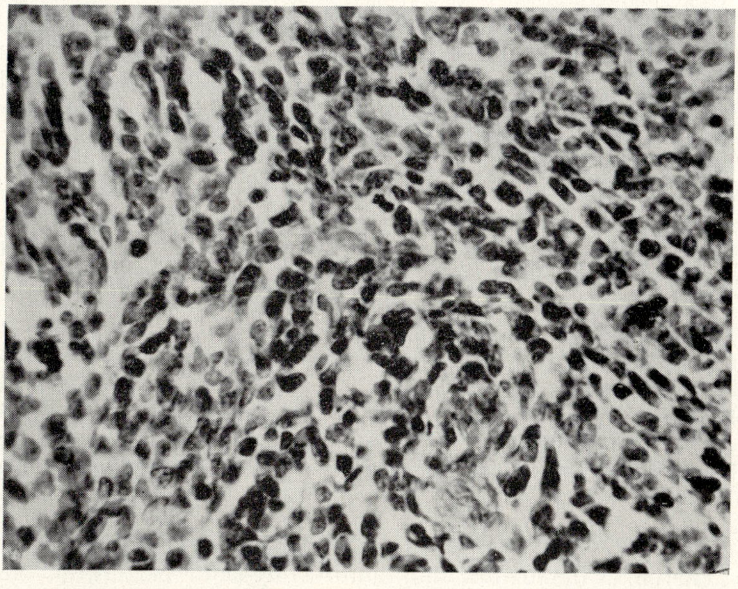

Fig. 4.—High magnification of section from nodule removed from abdominal wall seven months after original operation, showing diffuse lymphosarcoma.

duodenum an indurated area approximately 3 cm. in diameter was found, in the center of which there was a perforation. The area was isolated by packs and excision of the ulcer performed, removing a diamond-shaped portion of duodenal wall. The edges were then approximated by transverse closure, using three layers of interrupted silk sutures. The abdomen was closed in the routine manner without drainage.

Postoperative course was uneventful. Temperature did not exceed 102° F. and by the third hospital day the patient was taking fluids by mouth and a soft diet. He was discharged home on the eighth hospital day with a well-healed wound and free of symptoms.

Laboratory findings during the hospital stay were within normal limits. Pathologic report revealed fibrosis incorporating deep-staining masses of cells which were chiefly inflammatory in nature, consisting of fibroblasts, plasma cells, red cells, and an occasional eosinophile; no evidence of malignant change in margins of this ulcer. Diagnosis was that of duodenal ulcer with thickening and inflammatory hyperplasia of borders.

Course.—For several months after dismissal from the hospital, the patient felt well and had few complaints. Weight was maintained and general health was apparently good. About the fourth month after operation he began noticeably to lose weight, and complained of vague epigastric discomfort, which soon became a painful cramp, relieved by food. Gastric analysis five months after admission revealed free acid of 56 and total acid of 59. Roentgenographic study revealed evidence of a small filling defect and deformity of duodenum in the first portion. The patient was given symptomatic treatment. During the next month, downward progression was noted, with weight loss, poor appetite, development of progressively intense icterus, and liver enlargement. At six months, there was noted a mass in the field of previous operation, extending down about three fingerbreadths from costal margin. Bilateral inguinal adenopathy was present. At seven months, a nodule was seen in the skin of the anterior abdominal wall, at the site of a retention suture used in closure at operation. This was removed under local anesthesia and submitted for pathologic diagnosis. There was found very pronounced active lymphoid structure not typical of a lymph node. Most of the cells were rounded or oval but some were elongated in the manner of fibrous tissue. There were numerous mitoses noted and the picture as a whole was one of monotony found in lymphosarcoma. Upon re-examination of the original section removed from the duodenum seven months previously, essentially the same structure was seen in this section.

At this time it was obvious that the patient presented the picture of generalized lymphosarcomatosis, with intraabdominal spread, and involvement of inguinal nodes and abdominal wall. Deep roentgen therapy was given over a period of nine weeks, with a total of 3,100 r being received in three areas, the greater portion over the upper anterior abdomen. During this time the patient gained twenty-two pounds, felt better generally, and the icterus lessened.

Death occurred July 11, 1940, ten months after the original hospital admission, from bronchopneumonia superimposed upon general sarcomatosis. Autopsy revealed extensive involvement of all structures adjacent to the duodenum, biliary obstruction, and spread downward in the abdomen to periaortic nodes and bladder.

Microscopic sections were identical with that seen in nodule removed from the abdominal wall, and revealed the markedly invasive quality of the growth. Roentgen therapy had brought about partial remission in some areas, with fewer mitotic figures seen.

Detailed examination of the duodenum, pylorus, and stomach showed no extension into the stomach proper, but an extension of the tumor proximally to the pylorus and posteriorly into the pancreas and structures of the hepatic ligament. The entire first portion of the duodenum had its wall almost completely replaced by malignancy with thickening and fixation, involving the biliary and pancreatic ducts.

Summary.—A case is presented of a 40-year-old man with lymphosarcoma of the first portion of duodenum, first manifest by acute perforation, and steadily progressing over a ten-month course with generalized spread and only fair response to roentgen therapy. Diagnosis was first established seven months after the onset of symptoms by biopsy of nodule in the abdominal wall at the site of the previous operative wound.

DISCUSSION

From the case report just given, it is obvious that no preoperative diagnosis was possible, since the disease was first brought to the attention of the attending surgeon because of an acute abdominal catastrophe. Furthermore, the patient had had no premonitory symptoms, such as one might expect with ulcer.

At operation, since the lesion presented the identical picture of the many times more common duodenal ulcer, nothing unusual was suspected. It is a well-established surgical dictum that perforating lesions of the stomach should always be subjected to biopsy. Here, however, perforation occurred in a region seldom involved by malignancy. Nevertheless, as had been the practice of the surgeon in similar cases, excision of the ulcer was performed.

Unfortunately, a mistaken pathologic diagnosis of the tissue removed led to a diagnosis of benign ulcer and a policy of temporization. Not until four months had passed did the symptomatology of the true lesion begin to manifest itself. Roentgen examination at this time revealed the duodenal deformity, and the weight loss, digestive upset, and lymphadenopathy pointed clearly toward malignancy. By this time the lesion was inoperable. Response to radiation therapy was not typical of the remission seen in most radiosensitive lymphosarcomas.

From this case, and from a review of literature dealing with this subject, certain generalizations can be drawn regarding this class of tumors, and the possibility of making the correct diagnosis and instituting definitive treatment:

The presence of a tumor of the gastrointestinal tract in a relatively young individual, particularly with associated weight loss, anorexia, pain, bleeding, or lymphadenopathy, should suggest lymphosarcoma as one possibility.

Wherever feasible, biopsy should be taken of perforating lesions, in the event that an infrequent case of lymphosarcoma might be discovered and indicate decidedly different treatment, both surgical and radiologic.[18]

All palpable abdominal tumors should be explored, and a diagnosis should be established by an excisional biopsy and examination by a skilled pathologist.

Lymphosarcoma of the gastrointestinal tract carries a quite different prognosis from other tumors and demands different treatment. The marked radiosensitivity may bring about a remarkable regression of far-advanced lesions.

The ileum, stomach, and cecum are the most frequently involved sites, although the disease may occur at any level of the gastrointestinal tract. It occurs more frequently in the small than the large intestine.

Whereas local spread and metastasis occur rather late in carcinoma, the reverse is the rule with lymphosarcoma, in which local spread is rapid, and metastases to distant organs are not unusual.

Although most cases of this disease will have some premonitory symptoms, the occasional case that first presents by an acute abdominal condition should make one mindful of the possibility of its occurrence and occasion an adequate biopsy. In reducing small intestine intussusception, one should palpate carefully for possible submucosal tumors.

SUMMARY

A brief résumé of the problem of lymphosarcoma of the gastrointestinal tract has been presented, with consideration of the pathologic features, incidence, differential diagnosis, and roentgenographic findings. A case of lymphosarcoma of the duodenum, masquerading as perforated peptic ulcer, is presented.

REFERENCES

1. Taylor, E. S.: Primary Lymphosarcoma of the Stomach, Ann. Surg. **110**: 200-221, 1939.
2. Ullman, A., and Abeshouse, B. S.: Lymphosarcoma of the Small and Large Intestines, Ann. Surg. **95**: 878-915, 1932.
3. Boyd, William: A Textbook of Pathology, Ed. 6, Philadelphia, 1947, W. B. Saunders Company.
4. Cutler, G. D., Stark, R. B., and Scott, H. W., Jr.: Lymphosarcoma of the Bowel in Childhood, New England J. Med. **232**: 665-670, 1945.
5. Cheever, D.: Clinical Aspects and Treatment of Primary Lymphosarcoma of the Stomach and Intestines, Ann. Surg. **96**: 911-923, 1932.
6. McSwain, B., and Beal, John M.: Lymphosarcoma of the Gastro-intestinal Tract, Ann. Surg. **119**: 108-123, 1944.
7. Sugarbaker, E. D., and Craver, L. F.: Lymphosarcoma: A Study of 196 Cases With Biopsy, J. A. M. A. **115**: 17-23, 112-117, 1940.
8. Stout, A. P.: Is Lymphosarcoma Curable? J. A. M. A. **118**: 968-970, 1942.
9. Gall, E. A., and Mallory, T. B.: Malignant Lymphoma: Clinicopathological Survey of 618 Cases, Am. J. Path. **18**: 381-429, 1942.
10. Libman, E.: Sarcoma of the Small Intestines, Am. J. M. Sc. **120**: 309, 1900.
11. Archer, V. M., and Cooper, G., Jr.: Lymphosarcoma of Stomach: Diagnosis and Treatment, Am. J. Roentgenol. **42**: 332, 1939.
12. Usher, F. C., and Dixon, C. F.: Lymphosarcoma of the Intestines, Gastroenterology **1**: 160-178, 1943.
13. Speese, J.: Sarcoma of the Small Intestine, Ann. Surg. **59**: 727-738, 1914.
14. Giere, C. N.: Lymphosarcoma Diagnosed Gastroscopically, J. A. M. A. **117**: 173-175, 1941.
15. Holmes, G. W., Dresser, R., and Camp, J.: Lymphoblastoma, Radiology **7**: 44-50, 1926.
16. Rowe, E. W., and Neely, J. M.: Primary Malignancy of the Small Intestine, Radiology **28**: 325-338, 1937.
17. Greenfield, H.: Early Roentgen Diagnosis of Jejunal Lymphosarcoma: Report of Case, Am. J. Roentgenol. **36**: 674-677, 1936.
18. McNealy, R. W., and Hedin, R. F.: Perforation of Gastric Carcinoma, Surg., Gynec. & Obst. **67**: 818, 1938.
19. Koucky, J. D., Beck, W. C., and Atlas, J.: Acute Perforation of Lymphosarcomatous Ulcer of the Stomach, Ann. Surg. **114**: 1112-1116, 1941.
20. Davis, E.: Lymphosarcoma With Perforation of Gastric and Intestinal New Growth, Brit. M. J. **2**: 64, 1937.
21. Svien, H. J., and Rivers, A. B.: Lymphosarcoma Causing Obstruction at the Duodenojejunal Angle: Report of Case, Am. J. Digest. Dis. **1**: 45-47, 1942.
22. Shulman, S.: Primary Lymphosarcoma of the Jejunum, Am. J. Surg. **46**: 182-184, 1941.

AMNIOTIC HERNIA

Henry G. Hollenberg, M.D., Little Rock, Ark.

THE congenital disorder referred to here as amniotic hernia goes by a large variety of names. It may be well to refer to Fig. 1 to see exactly what is meant. Cullen[1] in his monumental work on the umbilicus called it an amniotic hernia or an amniotic umbilicus. Ladd and Gross[2] referred to it as an omphalocele. Other terms used are congenital umbilical hernia, umbilical eventration, funicular hernia of the umbilicus, exomphalos, and hernia into the umbilicus. The term amniotic hernia most clearly defines it, I believe.

Under any name it is to be differentiated from the common variety of umbilical hernia of infants and adults as well. The incidence of occurrence is estimated at 1 in about 6,000 births, while the common umbilical hernia is perhaps 1 in 50 at birth. The pertinent difference is that in the usual hernia the bowel is covered with peritoneum and skin and may be treated without operation or may be operated upon at any time, unless, of course, there is strangulation. In this disorder the abdominal contents are visible through only a thin, transparent, and avascular membrane. It is an emergency condition demanding prompt operative repair because otherwise it is inevitable that there will be rupture with evisceration or else a drying of the membrane with cracking and development of peritonitis. Indeed, in one of the cases which I shall describe the rupture had occurred before birth.

There are various degrees of severity. The least severe is that where a loop of bowel protrudes into the cord through a relatively small (1 to 2 cm.) hiatus in the fascia. This condition is quite properly called a herniation into the cord. In this paper I propose to deal largely with the most severe form where there has been a failure of development of the abdominal wall, resulting in a hiatus some 10 cm. in diameter and with a great part of the abdominal organs in this protruding amniotic sac. It is not uncommon for other congenital defects to be present.

Inasmuch as this is a developmental disorder, some reference to the embryology involved is in order. The amnion is first seen in the human embryo of less than 1 mm. in length as a separate cavity on the dorsum of the embryo. As development proceeds the amnion encircles the embryo, attaching to the body stalk. As the body stalk becomes the umbilical cord, the amnion forms the outer layer of the cord and attaches to the skin around the umbilicus. In the 10 mm. embryo the small bowel has begun to elongate and to be present in the cord. In the 18 mm. embryo the small bowel, cecum, and some colon are all in the exocoelomic cavity which is in the cord outside the embryo. The liver, however, is not normally in the cord at any time. In the 45 mm. embryo, which is at about 9 or 10 weeks, the bowel has normally receded into the abdomen and remains there.[2, 3] The presence of bowel in the cord at birth is, therefore, a

Read at the annual session of the Southern Surgeons' Club, May 20, 1947, Atlanta, Ga.

severe aberration. And the presence of liver, spleen, or stomach is not accountable because of the persistence of any developmental situation, but is the result of true herniation into the sac during the latter months of gestation.

The membrane which covers these herniations is variously described as amnion and peritoneum. Grossly it is a single layer.

I have had the occasion to treat several infants with the herniation into the cord of a loop or two of small bowel or small and large bowel. If the hiatus in the fascia is small, it is an exceedingly simple operation and the results are uniformly successful. The only question in this type is whether or not the smaller ones should be operated upon. If the skin edges will come together as the cord dries and if the bowel can be held in the abdomen during this ten-day period, there will be normal healing of the skin. A subcutaneous hernia may result. I recommend, however, that all of the patients be operated upon immediately if there is any doubt because the bowel cannot be held back with

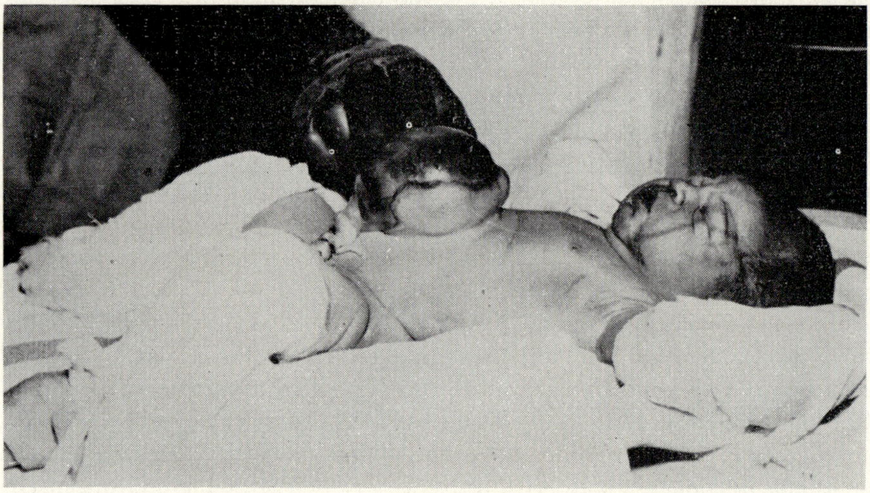

Fig. 1.—Amniotic hernia in an infant being prepared for operation within an hour after birth. There was no skin extending on the sac on the other side.

certainty in a crying infant. There may be a rupture of the sac by such crying or by the trauma of the external dressing. This is the type of hernia where bowel may be included in the cord tie and with disastrous results. Most obstetricians are alert to this danger. I had a case of this kind at our St. Vincent Infirmary in 1946. The infant was admitted five days after birth, moribund from intestinal obstruction since birth. The cord was dry and intact but a bit infected. When it was manipulated a little, feces escaped and deflation promptly occurred. This infant died in a few hours, however. Another infant was admitted twelve hours after birth with a proper tie of the cord and obvious herniation into the stump. When the dressings were first removed to examine him, this sac ruptured and bowel protruded. The bowel was not grossly contaminated and operation was accomplished within the hour. He left the hospital the next day to be returned to his mother for feeding and made an uneventful recovery.

Of the type shown in Fig. 1 and containing liver, I have had four cases in the past eight years—one at our St. Vincent Infirmary, two at the Arkansas State Children's Hospital, and one, strangely enough, in the Army at the Bushnell General Hospital. The illustrations, herewith, are all of the last case.

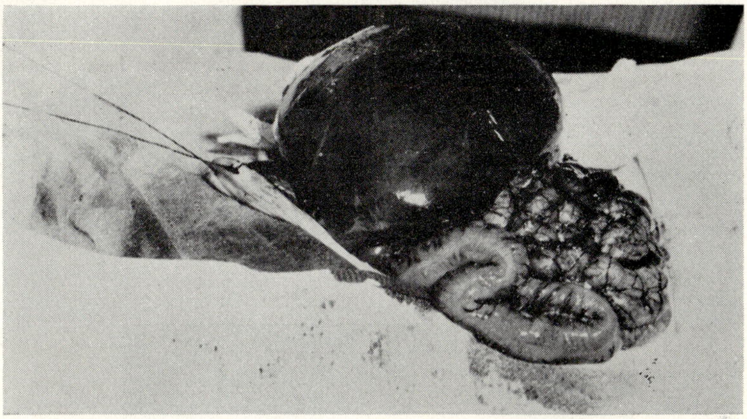

Fig. 2.—Complete evisceration during operation. This undesirable situation can hardly be prevented once the sac has been opened. The enormous size of the liver is apparent. There is no place for it within the abdomen.

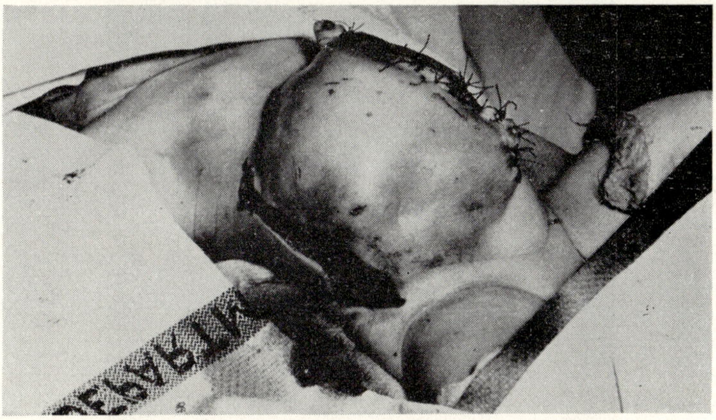

Fig. 3.—Closure at end of operation. The relaxing incision was used only on one side and only in this one case. It helps very little in our experience and may complicate later procedures.

One of these infants was born with a rupture of the sac and an evisceration of liver, and all bowel. The presence of well-organized fibrin indicated that rupture occurred well before the day of delivery. He was in excellent condition and was operated upon immediately. Another infant was seen five days after birth. The membrane had become dry and opaque but had been kept fairly clean and had not cracked through. All of these patients made uneventful recoveries following operation and remained well for one or two years. It is interesting that none had any other congenital disorder which was ever recognized.

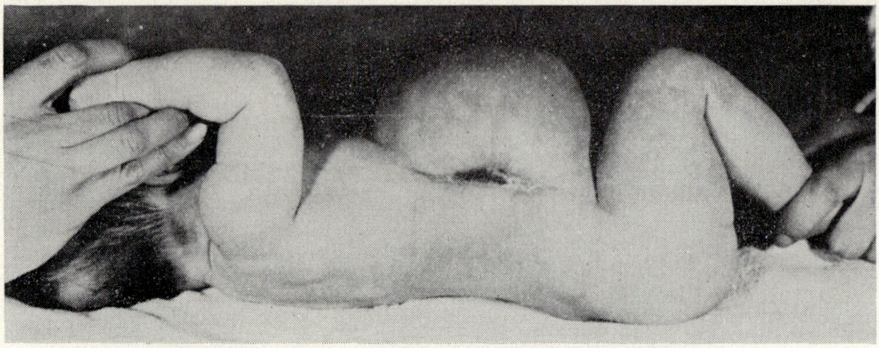

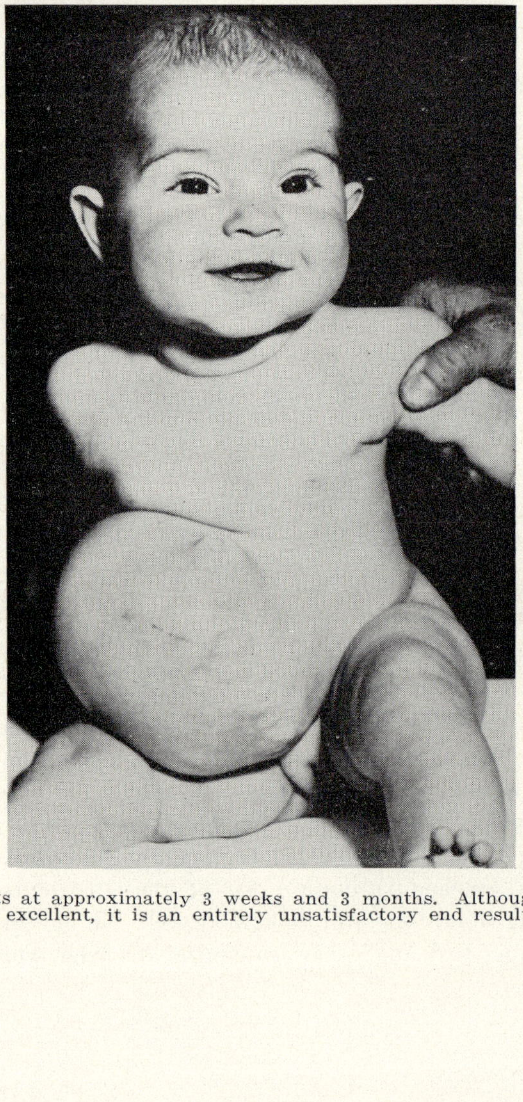

Figs. 4 and 5.—Results at approximately 3 weeks and 3 months. Although the general health is excellent, it is an entirely unsatisfactory end result.

There are several important technical points. Operation should be done as promptly as possible following delivery. Babies at birth are prepared for an ordeal and stand the procedure well. I have done them all under local anesthesia and very little of that. There is no such thing in my experience as opening one end and closing bit by bit without evisceration. All of the contents eventually escape during the procedure, as shown in Fig. 2. The umbilical vessels and urachus must be carefully tied but cause no special concern. Every millimeter of skin at the edge must be saved. It is the most difficult abdominal closure that I have ever encountered. Relaxing incisions on the sides are always described but help very little. I have used it only on one side in one case. At the area shown in Fig. 3, there was no recognizable muscle and poor fascia. In order to get any relaxation it is necessary to incise through skin and peritoneum and one then has the problem of evisceration through two incisions. This might be avoided by making the incision further back. The greatest difficulty is in closing the skin over the liver rather than over the bowel. Some operators have excised part of the liver. This is too radical. All the patients have died after such a resection. The liver is proportionately larger in infancy than later. These livers seem to be larger than in the normal infant. The wound must be closed from the upper end down and one has to be content with a covering of skin and subcutaneous fat only and a single layer of stitches in the skin. The liver must be covered over first and the bowel replaced last. The so-called "umbrella trick" is invaluable. This maneuver consists in placing a single layer of gauze over all the eviscerated organs and tucking the edges under the sides of the incision. The organs can then be better replaced and the skin covered over. The gauze is the umbrella. Getting the gauze out is the trick. It is very traumatizing to bowel but accomplishes the purpose.

In these four cases there were no immediate postoperative complications, although these infants are prone to have such complications of the chest or abdomen. However, the result as seen in Figs. 4 and 5 is most deforming and unsatisfactory. The contour of the baby's abdomen is somewhat like that of a woman at term but with the protuberance even greater and higher. It is difficult to apply any sort of an abdominal support which does not cause improper pressure.

The important part of any treatment is the end result. The end results in these cases which started so favorably are bad. Of the four patients, three have died in their second year. I do not have a follow-up on the fourth. One died of intestinal obstruction. This is not surprising with only skin covering all the bowel. The other two died of pneumonia. This too is significant when one considers that the liver has never had its normal position, the diaphragms are not properly developed, and there is no firm abdominal wall to support a cough.

These late fatal complications can be overcome only by some procedure which will construct an abdominal wall and perhaps by some form of mechanical support which will gradually force the liver back into the abdominal cavity.

Dr. Ladd has corresponded with me on this matter. He states that he knows of only one or two cases of this type in which the infant has survived any appreciable period of time. He and others suggest that on about the tenth postoperative day a series of operations be begun to bring the fascia together. Only a little can be done at one end at each sitting. When one recalls how far laterally the edge of the fascia is situated and how difficult it is to bring only skin together, it is difficult to visualize a successful accomplishment of this plan. However, I intend to try it at my next opportunity. Other ideas such as a free transplant of fascia or a dermal graft do not appeal to me but may have merit.

The problem of the construction of abdominal wall in these cases is a real challenge and I shall look forward keenly to the ideas that others may put forward.

ADDENDUM

Since this article was received for publication, Dr. Robert E. Gross, of Boston, Mass., has presented a new method for the operative treatment of these large hernias containing liver. He has utilized the method with complete success in three cases.

The sac and abdominal wall are thoroughly cleansed with soap and water and half-strength iodine. The skin is completely divided along the circumference of the sac leaving a tiny rim of skin fastened to the sac and taking great care not to enter into the abdominal cavity at any point. The skin is then mobilized over a large area in all directions sufficient to allow it to be brought up and cover the entire amnion and stump of the cord. The effect at the completion of this operation is similar to that following the operation depicted in this article. Adhesions, however, do not develop between the liver, bowel, and the skin covering because of the presence of the amnion, and a second operative procedure at the end of some six or nine months can much better be done with a layer closure.

This method obviously avoids many defects in other plans of treatment. While there are certain risks in regard to infection, to the formation of subcutaneous cysts, and to the possibility of sloughing of skin, the advantages greatly outweigh the disadvantages. The method would hardly be applicable in such a hernia which is ruptured or in one which has been neglected and is grossly infected.

REFERENCES

1. Cullen, T. S.: The Umbilicus and Its Diseases, Philadelphia, 1916, W. B. Saunders Company.
2. Ladd, W. E., and Gross, R. E.: Abdominal Surgery of Infancy and Childhood, Philadelphia, 1947, W. B. Saunders Company.
3. Gray, Henry: The Anatomy of the Human Body, Philadelphia, 1924, Lea & Febiger.

THE IMPORTANCE OF ACCURATE PATHOLOGIC CLASSIFICATION IN THE PROGNOSIS OF RENAL TUMORS

N. Chandler Foot, M.D., and Gustavus A. Humphreys, M.D., New York, N. Y.

(From the Department of Surgery, Cornell University Medical College and The New York Hospital)

INTRODUCTION

During the period of fourteen years from 1932 to 1946, 75 patients with renal tumors were admitted to the Cornell Urological Service of the New York Hospital and in 58 of these the diagnosis was confirmed by nephrectomy and pathologic examination; on pyelographic examination, the remaining 17 showed very suggestive pictures, but as most of them also exhibited evidence of advanced metastasis, palliative rather than radical treatment was indicated. A review of the 58 well-documented cases has been undertaken and the correlation of clinical and pathologic findings with the end results attempted.

Although a few tumors were discovered relatively early in the course of investigation for some other complaint and before hematuria was apparent, operation was omitted in none unless proved metastasis was present. There was one exception to this rule: a patient in whom a craniotomy revealed a probable single metastasis from a renal-celled carcinoma and craniotomy was followed by nephrectomy. The operation of choice was nephrectomy, which was performed in all but two instances through a flank incision; the exceptions were carried out transperitoneally. It is not the purpose of this article to detail the surgical signs, symptoms, or operative technique; we intend to confine ourselves solely to the correlative analysis just indicated.

The series has been grouped according to the pathologic diagnosis in each instance: it comprises 39 renal-celled, 2 tubular, 5 transitional-celled, and 3 epidermoid carcinomas; 4 embryonal tumors (two of them muscular), two nonmalignant transitional-celled papillomas, and one Wilms' tumor. Classification of renal tumors into these categories appears to be significant and helpful in judging the prognosis—more so than when older and purely descriptive classification is used. (Hypernephroma, clear-celled carcinoma, granular-celled papillary carcinoma, etc.)

There is justification on histogenetic, pathologic, and clinical grounds for classifying renal tumors under two main heads: those of mesodermal origin and those obviously arising in entodermal conduction apparatus (calyces, pelves, ureters). As will be discussed later, it is found that tumors of the former category offer a much better prognosis than do those of the latter, which appear to be hopeless if they are metaplastic.

A brief classification might be couched as follows:

A. Tumors Derived From Mesodermal Renal Cap
- Simple adenoma
- Renal-celled carcinoma, including some tubular forms

B. Tumors Derived From Entodermal Outgrowth From Cloaca
   Transitional-celled papilloma
   Transitional-celled carcinoma, epidermoid carcinoma, and some tubular carcinomas (of collecting tubules)

C. Tumors Derived From Embryonal Tissue Such as Mesonephros
   Embryonal carcinoma (juvenile and adult forms), mixed embryonal tumors, including that of Wilms

D. Tumors Derived From Perirenal Capsule
   Fatty, connective tissue, muscular and nervous growths.

Our investigation at once brings out the fact that renal-celled carcinoma is by far the commonest tumor of our service; its nearest competitor is the transitional-celled carcinoma, which takes first place among neoplasms of the urinary bladder.

Renal-celled carcinoma was first known as "hypernephroma," so named by von Grawitz[1] in 1884, who believed it to be the product of displaced suprarenal primordium. Later, Ewing[2] distinguished a microscopically different, but grossly similar tumor as "clear-celled carcinoma," basing his nomenclature upon the prevalence of clear cells grouped into tubules and papillae. Without going into details as to the dispute concerning the origin of this growth (which followed Stoerk's[3] claim that it was derived from renal parenchyma) it may be said that authorities are beginning to call it "renal-celled carcinoma." Although there is a similarity to suprarenal cortex in its histology, it is readily distinguished from true cortical suprarenal tumors. Unlike them it causes no hormonal symptoms such as virilization or devirilization. It is therefore presumed that it originates from cells of the mesodermal portion of the renal parenchyma.

In discussing this subject Stoerk said in a footnote: "It is quite incomprehensible to me that the similarity between the cells of this tumor and those of the adrenal is constantly being stressed. . . . . I cannot observe the slightest similarity. That of the cellular architecture of many Grawitz tumors to that of the outer zones of the adrenal is, of course, admitted without comment."

His conclusions were: "I have endeavored to make it evident that there is no convincing similarity between tumors derived from suprarenal or renal tissue; secondly, that the most variable forms of Grawitz tumor prove to be histological variants of the same archtype and, thirdly, that Grawitz tumors of the kidney are of nephrogenic origin. The last conclusion might be formulated to the effect that almost all epithelial tumors of the kidney might in the end produce the picture of the Grawitz tumor."

Renal-celled carcinomas are characterized microscopically by the presence of large, vacuolated or clear cells arranged in cords, tubules, or more rarely, papillary formation. The cells may occasionally possess considerable granular cytoplasm and when this is conspicuous they resemble tubular carcinoma or the growth which Ewing called "granular-celled papillary carcinoma." The similarities may be confined to occasional fields only, but the inference that all of these formerly separate groups may be essentially one large family, as Stoerk claimed it to be, is clear. Two of our specimens exhibited vacuolization of cells, or even of areas in carcinomas that were otherwise predominantly tubular structures composed of granular elements.

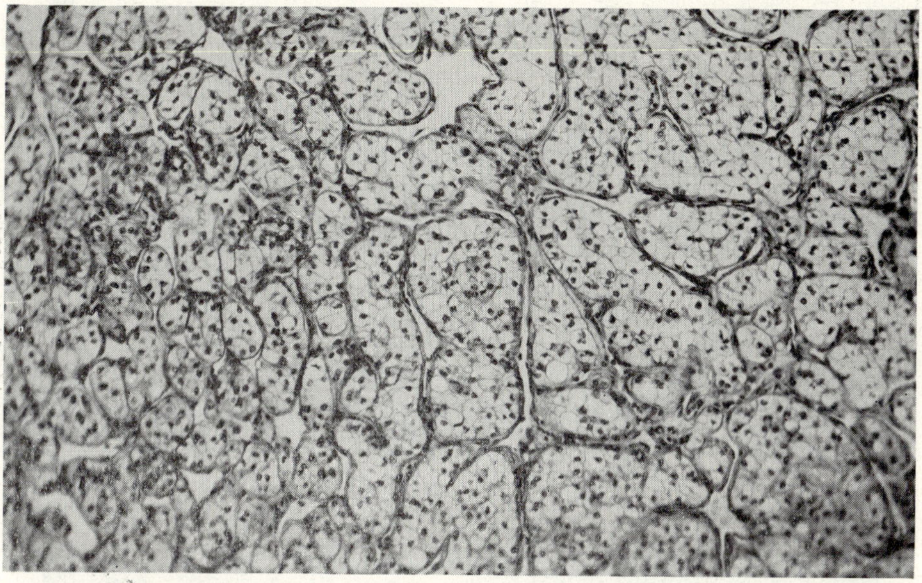

Fig. 1.—Microscopic field from a renal-celled carcinoma in a patient with a history of five-year survival after operation. Note its appearance and compare with Fig. 2. (All photomicrographs taken at ×150, by Department of Medical Photography, Cornell University Medical College.)

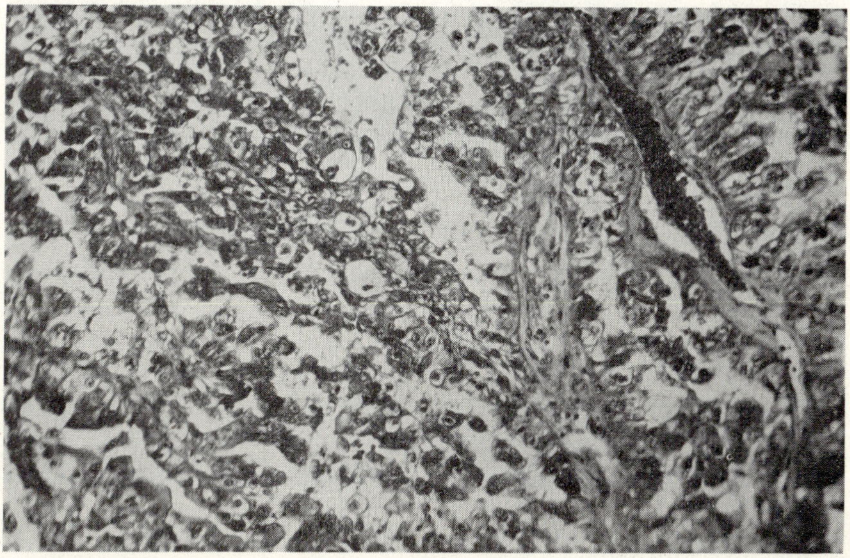

Fig. 2.—Field from a highly malignant and rapidly fatal renal-celled carcinoma. Note tubules, papillae, and generally disorderly architecture.

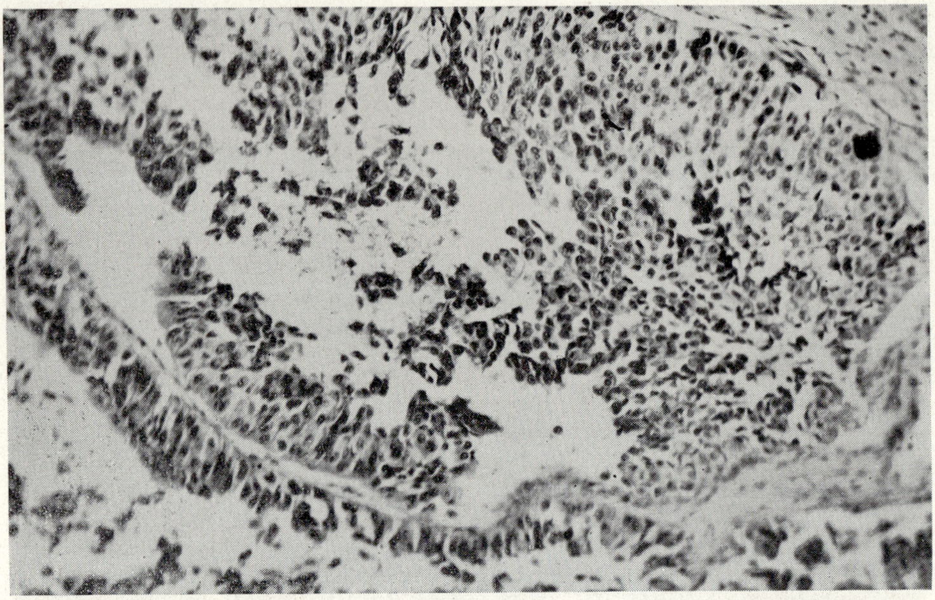

Fig. 3—Nonmalignant papilloma of renal calyx; note the excellent differentiation.

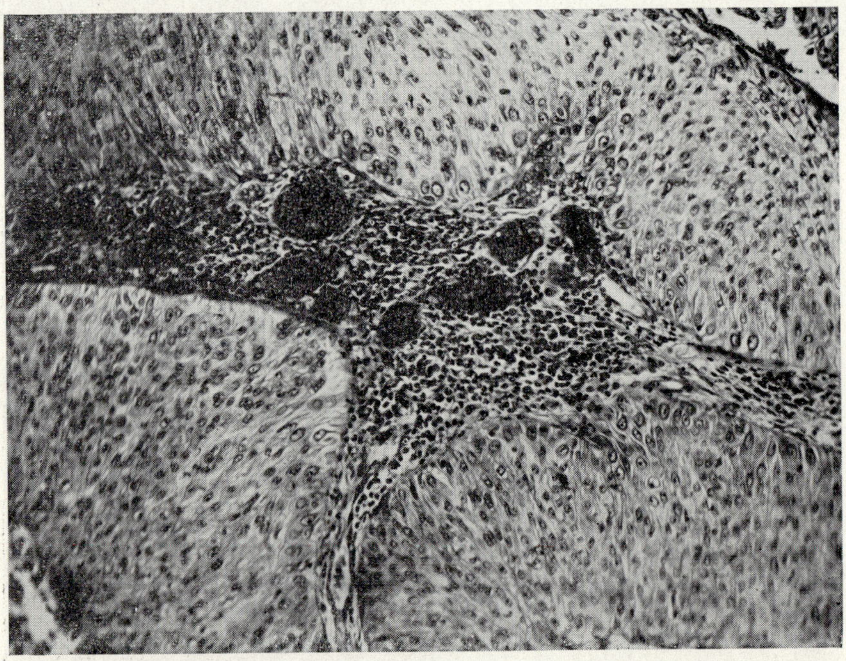

Fig. 4.—The malignant variety of the preceding type. Compare its lack of differentiation, its piling-up of cells, and numerous mitotic figures. This transitional-celled carcinoma was also situated in a large renal calyx.

Our transitional-celled tumors were either nonmalignant papillomas or carcinomas arising from the transitional epithelium of the urinary tract derived from entodermal hind-gut. The epidermoid carcinoma, as its name implies, is composed of epidermal epithelium derived from the transitional cells through a process of metaplasia that is exceedingly common in this tract and which does not necessarily lead to the production of malignant growths. (See Foot.[4])

CLINICAL FINDINGS

In evaluating our census of renal growths it will be seen that the renal-celled type outnumbers all others by a ratio of two to one; it has also offered a better life expectancy than have the other types. In order to test the survival rate of all groups of patients operated upon prior to 1943, known survival was listed after communicating with the patients or their families on the fifth anniversary after operation, either through personal interview or letters of inquiry. Deaths were listed after information was obtained from the family, or through examination of burial permits from the Mortuary Division of the New York Department of Health. All other cases were set down as "unproved," including those patients known to be alive shortly before the anniversary, as well as those lost to "follow-up" during the disruptions attributable to the war. Although much more accurate data might be obtained through the review of a longer series of cases, we believe that the trend established in ours is of considerable significance (Table I).

TABLE I

	TOTAL STUDIED	TOTAL OPERATED UPON PRIOR TO 1943	TOTAL PROVED 5 YR. SURVIVALS	TOTAL PROVED DEAD	TOTAL UNPROVED 5 YR. SURVIVALS	PER CENT OF 5 YR. PROVED SURVIVALS TO PROVED DEAD
Mixed embryonal	3	3	1	2	0	33
Embryonal carcinoma	4	4	0	2	2	0
Epidermoid carcinoma	3	3	0	3	0	0
Transitional carcinoma	4	4	0	3	1	0
Transitional papilloma	2	2	2	0	0	100
Tubular carcinoma	2	2	1	0	1	100
Renal-cell carcinoma	39	24	9	11	4	45

Reviewing these findings, pertinent facts may be adduced to assist in interpretation. The embryonal group showed but one five-year survivor, whose tumor was a leiomyosarcoma of pure composition, discovered incidentally during nephrectomy for tuberculous kidney. With that exception there were no known five-year survivals in that group, or among the epidermoid or transitional carcinomas of the kidney. The average expectancy here averages slightly over one year. By contrast, transitional-celled papilloma presents an excellent prognosis; although this is based upon only two examples, it is believed that it parallels that of similar tumors in the urinary bladder. Were these to be grouped with renal carcinoma (as they are in some classifications) the expectancy for the entire group might be improved. This would, however, be based upon a fallacy. Transitional papillomas of the bladder usually have been found to respond to treatment, while the carcinomas of that type have a poor prognosis despite operation.

The renal-celled group, on the contrary, offer a fair expectancy of a five-year survival (45 per cent). On the basis of prognosis tubular carcinomas, probably closely related to these, appear to be equally favorable. Again the number comprised in our series is too small to be at all decisive. The figure of 45 per cent five-year survivals among the renal-celled tumors is probably on the conservative side, as one of these listed as "known dead" had a cerebral metastasis removed prior to nephrectomy and died four years after the latter from a local recurrence of the cerebral metastasis. There were also two patients who died of cardiovascular disease which was present at the time of operation and in each of these no evidence of recurrent tumor was forthcoming. Two of the "unproved" patients were known to be living shortly before their fifth anniversary and may still be alive, although we cannot prove it. Further accumulation of data on the entire series, after more time has elapsed, might raise the survival rate to 50 per cent. That the "cures" are not all permanent is demonstrated by one patient who died seven years after operation from pulmonary metastasis. No inference is drawn as to whether or not operation influenced the prognosis favorably in any of these cases, as we have no comparable group available in which the tumor was permitted to run its course without operative treatment. However, our belief that radical surgical intervention should be offered all patients is substantiated by the literature.[5] From the clinical standpoint the classification employed proves to have an important bearing upon the prognosis; from the standpoint of pathology it was found that certain features of the renal-celled group might be relied upon to indicate a prognosis within the category.

PATHOLOGIC STUDY

The entire series of tumors was reviewed microscopically and the diagnoses confirmed or corrected; it was found that cases prior to 1940 had been classified according to Ewing's ideas as either hypernephroma or clear-celled carcinoma; later the term "renal-celled carcinoma" was adopted. All this group was consolidated under the renal-celled category and some examples which had mistakenly been assigned to other diagnostic groups were replaced where they belonged.

Next, all examples of renal-celled carcinoma were assembled in a table recording the name of the patient, the type and date of operation, the presence or absence of metastases (as proved by x-ray examination or necropsy), and the date and given cause of death. In columns parallel to these were recorded various histologic features of the tumors: the size of the type cell, the nature of its cytoplasm (clear or granular), the size and regularity of outline of the nuclei, the architecture of the growth (cords, tubules, papillae, etc.), the character of the stroma and septa and, finally, the presence or absence of inflammation and hemorrhage. After filling out this chart for the twenty-four tumors examined (from patients with documented histories) it was found that little of a definite nature could be adduced from the minutiae of the statistics.

It was, however, ascertained that a prognosis might be forecast with considerable accuracy, by examining the sections from the standpoint of regularity of architecture, absence of tubules and papillary growth, and the stoutness of the connective tissue septa. Tumors showing very variable cells or nuclei (anisocytosis and metaplasia) and readily discoverable mitotic figures were invariably found to have resulted fatally within a short time. In order to test the validity of these points, a series of sections from twelve cases was selected by one of us (G.A.H.) and submitted to the other for evaluation, with the understanding that they would represent an equal number of five-year survivals and proved deaths. Ten of the twelve were accurately assigned to the two categories, "good" and "bad"; one of the mistakes represented sections from a patient who had lived nine years, only to die of metastasis from a tumor that was unequivocally malignant in appearance. This naturally threw the remaining case into the wrong tray, as six had already been assigned to the "bad" category. Working from the opposite angle, the clinician was able to predict with astonishing accuracy, the probable structure, degree of differentiation, and microscopic appearance of the cells that would probably be found in sections from a given tumor. This further reinforces the idea that there is a definite correlation between the histologic picture and the clinical prognosis in the case of renal-celled carcinoma of the kidney.

In order to assist the reader in making a microscopic evaluation as to the prognosis in renal-celled carcinoma, it might be well to list favorable and unfavorable features. The relatively nonmalignant tumor shows: solid cords of large, clear cells with nuclei that are usually small and regular in size and shape; the growth is generally traversed by heavy septa of connective tissue; there is little microscopic evidence of hemorrhage and inflammation and the tumor is well delimited from the surrounding tissue, which it fails to infiltrate. The picture of tumors with an unfavorable prognosis reveals: cells of variable size often arranged in tubular or papillary formation; the nuclei are anisometric and mitotic divisions are readily noted, rather than being very difficult to find, as they are in the less malignant varieties. The septa are not stout, but poorly formed and usually infiltrated by lymphocytes or even polymorphonuclear leucocytes. Hemorrhage and necrosis are often noted. In short, well-differentiated tumors offer the best prognosis, while those with metaplasia and rapid growth (many mitoses) are to be feared. As a corollary of this, these tumors may be graded on the basis of differentiation, presence or absence of mitoses, and the nature of the stroma; Broders' method is, therefore, applicable in this case although it might work less satisfactorily in the case of other types of renal tumor.

CONCLUSIONS

1. In a series of 66 renal tumors, the renal-celled type of carcinoma (hypernephroma, clear-celled carcinoma) outnumbers the other forms 2:1.

2. Practically all other types of malignant renal tumor have at best a life expectancy of less than one year.

3. In the case of renal-celled carcinoma a prognosis may be based upon the microscopic appearance of the tumor with a reasonable degree of accuracy. The well-differentiated examples have a good chance of living five years or more.

4. A classification fundamentally based upon the embryologic origin of the tumor (entoderm or mesoderm) is the most reliable regarding correlation between pathologic findings and clinical outcome.

5. Entodermal tumors and those developing in more or less mixed mesonephric rests bear an almost hopeless prognosis; with mesodermal tumors the outlook appears to be better, particularly in the case of well-differentiated examples.

REFERENCES

1. von Grawitz, P.: Die Enstehung von Nierentumoren aus Nebennierengewebe, Arch. f. klin. Chir. 30: 824, 1884.
2. Ewing, J.: Neoplastic Diseases, all editions, Philadelphia, W. B. Saunders Company.
3. Stoerk, O.: Zur Histogenese der Grawitz'schen Nierengeschwülste, Beitr. z. path. Anat. u. z. allg. Path. 43: 393, 1908.
4. Foot, N. C.: Glandular Metaplasia of the Epithelium of the Urinary Tract (reference to literature and to epidermoid metaplasia included), South. M. J. 37: 137, 1944.
5. Welch C. E., and Nathanson, I. T.: Life Expectancy and Incidence of Malignant Disease; IV. Carcinoma of the Genito-urinary Tract, Am. J. Cancer 31: 586, 1937.

OBSERVATIONS OF SURGICAL TRAINING

RALPH F. BOWERS, M.D., MEMPHIS, TENN.

(From the Veterans Administration Medical Teaching Group, Kennedy Hospital)

HALSTED introduced a method of training surgeons shortly before the turn of the century which, collecting few advocates at its inception, gained momentum in the 1920's and finally achieved widespread recognition in the middle 1930's. Historically, this so-called resident system can be traced to a somewhat similar system in vogue in Germany and Austria at a time when German and Austrian surgery was at its height and set a high standard for the surgery of the period 1880 to 1914. Whether or not Halsted copied this continental system is a controversial subject, but certainly one can safely conclude that his annual sojourns to European clinics were a source of stimulation to him and influenced the teacher Halsted materially. It is also believed that his original aim was to produce teachers of surgery, primarily, and that these teachers in their dissemination throughout the country would spread the gospel for development of good surgery and surgical research. Dr. Heuer is of course one of these stalwarts who introduced the system in two of our large cities. His everlasting belief in the method has resulted in the training of a large number of surgeons. In time, students of Halsted satellites began to spread and to function as teachers.

In the 1930's, however, the need for a great number of teachers diminished simply because each new "mother university clinic" was feeding teachers into the communities and a saturation point was beginning to be reached. In 1935 to 1937, with the great impetus of the American Surgical Association and other surgical societies, the American Board of Surgery was founded, setting up the formal training requirements of the surgeon and empowered to check on his ability by critical examination which if successfully passed certifies him as a qualified surgeon. This first real attempt to show the lay community surgeons who could be trusted in the matter of diagnosis, pre- and postoperative care, and safe operating skill is already a significant landmark in the progress of surgery. The first generation of Halsted disciples must have all experienced a sense of satisfaction with this tribute to their method of teaching surgery which had now received acclaim by the surgical professional public. Now that the saturation point of surgical teachers is at hand, the natural flow of this talent will be into the community hospitals and clinics where teaching is not of major importance compared to the routine care of patients. This new migration of surgeons must necessarily raise the standards of surgery more generally throughout the country.

The following observations are collected from firsthand experience of working side by side with surgeons representing almost all types of teaching institutions. Statistically, the observations are not significant; I know of no method by which this can be statistically studied. Lacking that, however, general observations by an unbiased observer in the United States Army

Published with the permission of the Chief Medical Director, Department of Medicine and Surgery, Veterans Administration, who assumes no responsibility for the opinions expressed or conclusions drawn by the author.

Surgical Service and the Veterans' Administration Hospitals may be of value. It was my privilege to function as surgical chief in three general hospitals. The 9th General Hospital experience was not of great value in this respect because the capabilities of the surgeons during my chiefship were known and the men were similar in their training and ability to function. The tenure as Chief of Surgery at Lovell General and Walter Reed General Hospitals was at the height of these hospitals' activities, which included all conditions of surgery even those of women and children and in great numbers. Here, naturally, were sent general surgeons, orthopedists, urologists, neurosurgeons, thoracic surgeons, and gynecologists. To obtain the best surgical care with the surgeons sent to these hospitals, the foremost problem of the chief was to decide the surgical dependability of his staff and allot chores accordingly and regardless of rank.

At no time did the office of the Surgeon General interfere with this progress. On the contrary, his surgical and surgical specialty consultants were of great value in accomplishing these good results. The consultants, in my opinion, did a splendid job in allocating surgeons finally, oftentimes amid great confusion. The nature of their work, however, allowed them only a superficial estimation of an individual surgeon's true worth, compared to that of a chief who was working with these men daily and nightly. Some of the consultants were uncanny in their correct selection with so little actual knowledge of the man. Also, evidence is now being accumulated from work done in a large nondomiciliary Veterans Administration hospital in which surgeons from many different schools and clinics are functioning. The postwar confusion and overcrowding in our civilian hospitals have made it possible to work with the cream of the crop of prewar medical graduates, who have had various periods of time in training in the best of our university clinics and other clinics. Carefully selected, none of them is an exception to the usual product of his respective school or clinic. All are in training at this hospital with the same competitive atmosphere which exists in our university clinics.

It should be pointed out that allowance must be made for the personalities of the men, and it is realized that a few very good men have been observed who did not have the advantages of proper training and, conversely, a few very poor men came from institutions of the best opportunity for good training. There are not many of these. The virtues or failures in these few men were attributable to the men rather than the surgical school.

UNIVERSITY CLINICS

By and large, the best surgeons come from the University clinics. But the degree of surgical efficiency in men from the different clinics varies greatly, although this group represents those schools claiming the method of the Halsted resident system. If surgeons sent out from these schools are a reflection of the worth of the teaching method used, then there is great variation of local factors existing in the different schools. The study of these different surgeons is extremely interesting and no one knows what the perfect graduate resident surgeon should be like. We all expect him to be, first, a fundamentally sound clinical surgeon, capable of handling all surgical problems with logic and skill; second, that he might be desirous of teaching good surgery; third, that he might be capable of either doing surgical research work or stimulating others to do it; and, last, from the nature of his residency that he be able to organize teamwork with other surgeons, nurses, and orderlies which will result in better care of surgical patients. Because surgery is a dangerous form of therapy, it is mandatory that he meet the first category or he fails.

This mirror reflects fairly accurately the desires and capabilities of the surgical departments. These surgical schools demonstrate characteristics which alter the type of surgeon finishing his residency. They may be conveniently classified as follows:

1. The resident is a first-class clinical surgeon.
2. The resident's qualification is that of a surgical researcher.
3. The resident is a prolific writer, but not a top-grade clinical surgeon or researcher.
4. The resident is a good organizer of surgical work.
5. The resident represents a type exuding medical political influence.
6. The resident is a good clinician and excellent teacher.

Undoubtedly, many combinations exist in some instances, but rarely are all six characteristics present.

1. *First-Class Clinical Surgeon.*—Students from the group of first-class clinical surgeons are surgically dependable, can be turned loose with a lot of patients under their care, and very good results follow. Some from this school are unable to organize the work of others successfully and their scope for handling large sections of the hospital is distinctly handicapped. They are the people who give good personal care. They are resourceful, rarely get into serious difficulty, and know the practical points of obtaining good results. They are usually equipped with different surgical methods and can use the different methods to advantage.

2. *Surgical Researcher.*—The pupils from the surgical research type of school are stimulating and interesting. They are likely to be of the prima donna type and are not as dependable as those of the first group. Unquestionably they can discuss the theoretical aspects of selected subjects with great thoroughness and persuasiveness, and at the same time minimize the importance of and demonstrate little knowledge of the routine surgical problem. Among them are a few who believe that they have received a halo from their teacher which will permit discussions and opinions that oftentimes approach the ridiculous. Close scrutiny of their past experience reveals that they not only did not handle such a case, but never saw one. There are a few from this school who are surgically meek; large surgical services can find little use for these. One or two students have unhesitatingly requested to work on a laboratory problem instead of clinical work, if facilities were available. Although it is not an observation collected from working side by side with this group, one realizes that in their number perhaps may lurk the small group of

surgical savants, discoverers, and real contributors of the surgical future. These students are usually not good teachers.

3. *Prolific Writer.*—The students of the type who are prolific writers include some good average surgeons. They tend not to care so much for the personal side of the work but rather to keep their eye cocked continuously for the unusual, the rare—something about which they can write a paper. In this search for literary achievement, they experience episodes in surgery that ultimately better their technique and, often with chagrin, their surgical judgment. They are all inveterate readers. A few will become impressed from reading the literature and become diverted to the detriment of their surgical judgment. These few are in the group who will deny in 1950 that they vigorously supported an incorrect procedure in 1940. Most of them are good speakers, they are good at planning meetings, and are good teachers, if the one in charge of the student will insist that he teach correct facts.

4. *Organizer of Surgical Work.*—The good organizer type is usually well founded in fundamental principles. This surgical department will often collect good teaching clinicians and excellent researchers. The pupil demonstrates a mixture of the two influences. The surgeon is likely to have a too limited experience because of the organizer's flair for dividing his surgical department into specialties and subspecialties, and the student has more useful knowledge in some case groups than he does in others. He is distinctly mindful of statistics, often altering judgment which could be moulded by knowledge and common sense to such an extent that a poor procedure and unsound choice of action is pursued. He fails to allow the exigencies of the individual case to aid him in the choice. Conversely, and sometimes with what appears to be bitter defensive stubbornness, he selects a plan because the statistics will reflect that plan's efficiency in a large group of cases, yet in a particular case a keen clinical observer could solve the problem because he applied his course to the individual patient's needs rather than to what ought to happen by statistical prognostication. On this case a well-balanced, less highly trained individual will often offer the better solution because he merely uses his knowledge, common sense, and desire to get the patient well. This surgeon thinks in terms of large groups rather than an individual patient. He can carry out orders well and is dependable. All correspondence and paper work are of the first order. Records are meticulously compounded and filed. Imagination and originality are not among his assets, and he therefore seldom offers the bold courage and resourcefulness necessary for the development of distinctly new ideas. He is master of any procedure which he learned in his training period, conversing about it in almost textbook diction. For some undetermined reason, he is more often in the class of "hard luck" surgeons than his confreres.

5. *Medical Political Influence.*—Fortunately, only a small group of men with political influence is observed. They are not good, dependable surgeons. Their main fault lies in their attempts to woo their supervisor by nonprofessional extracurricular activities. They are masters at work delegation, but always in a manner in which the creditable work accomplished is the concern

of the delegator rather than the delegatee. They establish contacts easily, but drop them just as promptly if considered unworthy. If given the responsibility of a ward or section, they are continuously in trouble with important clinical matters, but have convinced their associates and nurses that the poor results are inevitable, occurring in all other sections handling similar conditions. Their occasional pursuit of the literature is in the form of a search to find someone who at some time or place has put down on paper the unsuccessful plan used in this incident. The finding of this literary antique is the cause of real joy and full rationalization of a mistake. Consequently, this man neither improves nor can be expected to improve. He contacts all surgeons with "big names," quotes them voluminously but with great inaccuracy. He is undoubtedly the poorest of the group of university trained men. He is also dangerous. This surgeon, when exposed in his unhappy surgical career, seeks transfer and escape from scrutinization, but always convincingly points out what the original place loses in his ultimate departure. In this gesture he usually attracts a small group of confederates who are often either totally ignorant or are of the same type. His only forte is in his ability to delegate responsibility to others, and ride to what he considers fame by their efforts.

6. *Good Clinician and Good Teacher.*—The pupils of the type of good clinicians and good teachers are the best in the group. They have been trained by a broad-minded man who allows them to increase their surgical responsibility as time advances. Hard work and long hours accompany their triumphant advancement. Fundamentals are well rooted, and the pupil is not allowed to advance without them. His appointment for senior resident is made upon strict, ruthless honesty. If the school contains good clinicians as well as teachers, then the ultimate in surgical training is reached. He is capable, dependable, strictly adheres to an almost idealistic standard and will spend hour upon hour accomplishing these ideals. Nothing is too much trouble for him, if that is necessary to have things right. He is meticulous, uses splendid judgment, is a good technician, appraises the need of pre- and postoperative treatment logically, keeps excellent records, and is a great stimulation to those under him. He definitely exhibits surgical poise, has lost the confusion and erratic bewilderment of the novice, is a great teamworker, and is often a great teacher.

He is an inveterate searcher for surgical knowledge and approaches all cases, even the simplest, with a desire and attitude that he not only can but will learn something from them. He is the type of surgeon who lives for surgery even without great financial gain. He has fun in his work, and it is fun to work with him. Mistakes are honestly bared, studied, and ways and means for nonrepetition of them are planned. A great many in the group are interested in clinical research, are always considering certain newer phases as an *Arbeit,* can collect data with critical analysis, and are honest enough intellectually to abandon the project unless it proves to be a worthy one. Their observations are the best. Few are extremely interested in animal experimentation, more or less as a hobby or a correlated aid to their clinical progress. They do not attempt new difficult procedures without learning principles in the laboratory first if possible. As a group they are good handlers of men and know how to get the job done. They are always searching for that little added maneuver to help the situation. Their only fault lies in their respect for idealism. When the facilities are not really adequate, their artistic pride is sometimes injured to the point where they are unable to function. In this they appear to lack resourcefulness. Actually, they are resourceful but their large previous experience with good facilities has tended to spoil them, and it is the compromise of their ideals that frightens them. Fortunately, there was not much of this, because the Army surgical facilities in spite of great hazards were most often adequate and good.

CLINICS WITHOUT UNIVERSITY TYPE TEACHING

The second best group of surgeons are fed to the public by the clinics without university-type teaching. In these the Halsted residency does not exist because the material is mainly private patients. It is replaced by a fellowship, or quite often the term "residency" is incorrectly applied. The period of training is shorter, and the mass of material often larger than in the university clinic. The trainees are allowed very little ward or operating room responsibility of their own. The patients are distinctly not the trainee's. Surgeon-patient relations and advancement in responsibility of care can reach only to a degree, rather than to completion of these very essential requirements for the thorough training of the surgeon. The candidate has ample opportunities to observe, study, and do the simpler forms of the work on these patients, and under excellent supervision. He is allowed to open and close wounds, do dressings, run the ward, and observe great numbers of cases. Surgical pathology is well presented to him. But he does not have the sole responsibility of care as the resident under the Halsted resident system does.

This surgeon is different in type, therefore, because of the difference in the mode of teaching. The caliber of the candidate is not the same, as recourse to these clinics for training is often precipitated in the candidate's failure to secure an appointment of the Halsted type. Naturally, the university clinics will accept what they believe to be the very top man. But they cannot accommodate all. Therefore, this clinic receives good men, some of the top class, but not the uniformly high caliber as of the university clinic.

He is usually not a good technician unless he has had a chance to perfect his technique by practice outside of the clinic. His judgment wavers, is apt to be poor because of hasty decisions. He is the most dogmatic of the group of younger surgeons observed. He valiantly wishes to carry the flag of his parent clinic, by insisting that only certain methods can be employed, even at a time when the parent clinic has abandoned the method for a newer, more efficacious one. He seems to call upon his memory for what to do rather than the spontaneity of thought and action of the man trained by advancing responsibility. He is aping good surgeons rather than subconsciously following his own individual surgical thoughts. Bewilderment is sometimes seen, but more often an overbalanced, superior attitude drives the man to prevent self-acknowledgment of his failure to function as a matter of ingrained surgical security. This aspect can be most detrimental to his progress because it teaches the man to bluff his way along until his experience will allow this sense of surgical confidence. Also, it is detrimental to good surgical results. If the chief has not been able to realize this attitude quickly many troubles ensue. On the other hand, this man improves more than any and once past his defensive, superior, bluffing attitude, quickly becomes one of the best surgeons of the group if allowed responsibility under a chief with a sympathetic understanding. He then perceives the fun of surgery and becomes very useful. He never becomes quite as dependable as the university type, but approaches it closely, depending upon the integrities of the individual. These men are interested mainly in statistical clinical research, seldom in animal experimentation. Their imagination and originality are lacking.

They are opportunists in that once a new surgical fad appears they are the first to sense it and take it up with great enthusiasm. Although boasting and impression stamping are common among university trained men with a bit of temerity, they are boldly broadcast by the clinic man in an attempt to seal his surgical presence as one of approval. Diagnostically, he is not good unless one of the conditions studied as pets in his parent clinic is at hand. During the war, at first his emergency experience was rather hectic and presumably new to him, but he learned this aspect quickly and in a short time did it well. He was the most difficult surgeon to teach the sane approach to the problem of débridement. He understood the later reconstructive phases better. He tends to minimize the importance of meticulous surgical technique and frequently is very conscious of the time consumed in an operation. He often decries the fact that it would take a good surgeon one hour to do a procedure that he was accustomed to observe being done in one-half hour and believes, therefore, that the slower operator was not a good one. He is definitely rougher in handling tissues than the university man, and as a young surgeon is sometimes not willing or able to adjust himself to the more gentle way. He is a great medical society meeting man, a good builder of contacts, and has instinct to spread gospel, the contents of which are not clear in his own mind. Beneath the crust these are good surgeons and from observations of their progress in these various institutions one can easily become convinced that if it were possible to add the last two years of any good Halsted residency training to the clinic training presently in vogue, the good men of this group would be top notch in quality. Also, it can be safely stated that a good many of these men left the Army much better surgeons than upon their induction.

GENERAL PRACTICE SURGEONS

Little need be said of the group of general practice surgeons because as a rule the members have had no formal training or, if so, there was no uniformity to the training and it was obtained in a short period with rotating internship, preceptorship, or apprenticeship. They are not good surgeons but an occasional well-balanced man is observed. Very few of course were sent to general hospitals for work in surgery. Some of them are fair "appendix-hernia" types of surgeons, most of whom employ antiquated, rough methods. They demonstrate great respect for the attending danger of surgery and are not anxious to assume responsibility beyond their experience. A fair number are in the older age group and are either fixed in their surgical ways or resignedly accept their role as surgeons for only minor conditions for which they have a repertoire of stereotyped procedures that they use automatically but in which experience has taught them to have implicit faith. They observe the more difficult surgical work in the institution very much as they would a museum specimen, and obviously do not plan to attempt it on their return to their communities. They know little about surgical diagnosis, anesthesia, or surgical technique. A few ideas of pre- and postoperative care are usefully obtained from them. It is not so difficult to teach these men the problem of débridement, possibly because they realize its use in their practice. One or two men have sought training in institutions following the war. These are the poorest surgeons of the group and cannot be depended upon for surgical responsibility in any other than minor conditions. Actually, a great number of these are general practitioners who do a little surgery on the side. If the few observed are any indication of the surgical value of these men, one must conclude that the methods of training in producing them are decidedly inferior and if possible should be abandoned.

SPECIALTIES

Since Halsted's time, overspecialization has entered the picture of surgical teaching and its influence is now being reflected in the pupils. Formerly, the well-known surgical specialties, namely, genitourinary, ear, nose and throat, eye, orthopedics, and gynecology existed with liberal allocation of some of their simpler cases throughout the specialty designated as general surgery. Today the pigeonholing has increased at the expense of general surgery until there is a virtual dilemma in attempting to organize the pedagogic course of the well-balanced general surgeon. Extinction of the general surgeon must follow if this trend increases, yet obviously the community need of the general surgeon will remain for many decades at least. Depending upon the medical school, neurosurgery, chest surgery, vascular, rectal, abdominal, head and neck, malignancy, sympathetic nervous system surgery, and probably others have appeared to confound the aims of the surgical teacher. In the former group of specialties it is a matter of rotation of the men through the specialty as assistant residents to gain at least a fundamental knowledge of their diagnostic and operative features. This appears to be sound and allows the general surgeon entering communities not staffed by these specialists to function at least safely and judiciously in the most common conditions seen. They, of course, are not as well qualified as the specialty resident, but it is the most feasible solution to the problem. Not all Halsted residencies permit this desirable rotation and the pupils have a very narrow range of operability. Indeed, some of the observations border on the ridiculous. If the present specialization program gains momentum the ridiculous state will certainly be reached, and the fruits of our teaching efforts must be lacking in satisfactorily supplying good general surgeons throughout the country.

Instances depicting this state are being daily observed. The well-trained man capable of doing major abdominal procedures doesn't know what a sprained ankle, knee, back, or wrist means. He understands total gastric resection problems but is poorly informed about fissure and fistula in ano, hemorrhoids, or pilonidal sinus. He does not know Colles' fracture except by name. A compound fracture cannot be treated by anyone except an orthopedist, yet the Army depended largely upon general surgeons for the great bulk of its orthopedic work. The work was very well done in the Army. The specialist does not know the fundamental physical diagnostic maneuvers of the shoulder, ankle, elbow, wrist, knee, hip, or back, yet the patient must consult him frequently for advice about these regions. Flatfeet is a foreign subject. Good abdominal surgeons are observed who do not understand how to do a decent pelvic examination, and must call the gynecologist to remove an ovarian cyst instead of an appendix producing the symptoms in the right lower quadrant. The gynecologist must call a surgeon if he inadvertently injures a bowel because he is not capable of its repair. The general surgeon must not follow a brain injury for the signs of increased intracranial pressure because the neurosurgeon instead of teaching the pupil to use the not-too-difficult methods of observation with sense has frightened the surgeon to the point of feeling inadequate, and the patient suffers because there is often no neurosurgeon available. The indications and technique of diagnostic and therapeutic burr holes are simple enough to be commonly used by any well-trained general surgeon. Tension pneumothorax treatment should be under control in every general surgeon's mind. Thoracotomy and closed aspiration drainage must be used by the general surgeon because of the paucity and poor allocation of thoracic talent. Amputation of an extremity is a source of amusing controversy. The general surgeon may amputate it for severe infection or traumatic mangling, but the orthopedist otherwise believes it to be in his domain. Consequently, amputation is not well understood by either surgeon or orthopedist. The orthopedist in many instances in military life delegated the problems of amputation to general surgeons, then returned to civilian life to denounce the general surgeon's interest in the subject. The oncologist desires all tumors in his section and offers to rotate surgeons through his subject, but there are so many special sections that the period of time must be relatively short if men are to rotate through all specialties. Some of these so-called "cancer surgeons" observed know the problem of melanoma well, but state that a radical operation for cancer of the breast can be done without bothering the pectoralis minor muscle, and their idea of radical surgery is really a minor procedure compared to the radical cancer surgery of the well-trained general surgeon. The cancer specialist cuts triumphantly across neoplasm; the good general surgeon thinks he has failed miserably if he does so. The cancer specialist works under the impression that he will remove all he can with ease and destroy the remaining neoplastic disease with radiation, although the particular type of neoplasm might not be amenable to radiation according to the best standards of radiotherapists.

There are other examples but nothing is gained by compilation. This discourse does not deal with the present controversy of overspecialization, but the previously mentioned facts observed by working with these men are examples of the dangers existing in the modern teaching program for general surgeons. The section training, although excellent it may be in the short time available, produces several detrimental aspects to the teaching of surgery.

1. The resident is aware of the fact that none of the specialists' problems will be admitted to his wards. Therefore, the student resident is robbed of the opportunity to develop himself diagnostically as well as if some of all general surgical problems are allowed his observation and study.

2. When he returns to the general surgical section for the final months he sees no traumatic head or extremity conditions, no chest conditions, no perivascular conditions, no tumors, etc., and, accordingly, ceases to study and think about these conditions. In a short period his unfamiliarity with some of these subjects results in lassitude, inertia, and eventual abolishment from his mind many conditions in which he should be well drilled. In other words, we teach him intensively in the sections so that he may return to general surgery and forget them.

3. Some of the specialty teachers have so impressed the young resident with the magnitude of his subject that the student leaves the section with an attitude of awe, respect, admiration for his teacher, and regret that he the student cannot really learn something worth while about the specialty. This attitude is without question responsible for the subsequent fright and "hands off" policy of the resident surgeon.

These comments are not to be construed as derogatory for the development of specialties in surgery. If teaching is not a part of the institution's program, it little matters. But if teaching is attempted and professed, it may well appear that a rejuggling of our specialty schedule to some extent at least is necessary if it is hoped to graduate well-trained surgeons. The problem is a serious one demanding current consideration.

"I WANT MY BOARDS"

The recognition of the Board certificate is certainly sound, desirable, and if continued free of political manipulation will undoubtedly better the surgical population throughout the land. Its effects will be of inestimable value. But it has added one serious blow to the philosophical attitude of many men who are seeking training in surgery. The historical episodes of men performing feats of self-denial and sacrifice, who in the pre-Board era would undergo hardships to train themselves properly in this dangerous form of therapy, are numerous. They realized that there was no rosy path to satisfactory development of surgical diagnostic and technical skill. Surgeons are not born today; they are made by hard work, study, and repetition of technical and all other phases of surgery until the young student blossoms as a man of surgical poise, with the knowledge, experience, and skill to substantiate this desired state.

The difference between the early trainee and a great number of them today is great. In the Army hospitals huge numbers of men sought aid under the guise of training when actually it was later found that they were accumulating time and perhaps some knowledge "toward my Board." The university clinics and Board-recognized Veterans Administration hospitals are besieged with stacks of applications from candidates for residencies. Many frankly discussed matters of further training in Army military hospitals. After interviewing several hundred of them, the distasteful truth reveals the fact that the man who really desires training is a rarity. Those interviewed are not necessarily the low men in the class, but are in the top third of the class from the best medical schools in our country. The frequent response to the query of purpose of application is, "I want my Boards," "I need two more years for my Boards," "The Board tells me I have to have two years and six months," etc.—and one gains the impression that the majority mean just that. Probably the influence of the Board is extremely good because without it these men could adopt the age-old adage that "I have a medical diploma and license which give me the right to operate, too." The sad implication exists in the fact that these men do not seek a position to train themselves well and do not realize that if good training is obtained their Board certificates will surely follow. They apply for the Board and not for the training. Their actions justify these comments. Other observers may state that this attitude is forced upon the men in the postwar confusion. This is not true, because the younger Army Specialized Training Program applicant demonstrates the attitude in the same manner as his war-torn, surgically frustrated predecessors. These examples tend to demonstrate these points:

1. The man is unwilling to observe, study, and work on cases day and night if that is necessary. He does not want to be bothered with what he can learn at night, and feels quite satisfied with diurnal opportunity only. He is approaching mentally the forty-hour week for learning. He says he has finished work at 5:00 P.M.—instead, he is definitely "through" at 5:00 P.M., and thinks little about surgery and its problems until the next day unless driven to it.

2. He feels no inadequacy or chagrin about missing a diagnosis, an operative indication, an important operation, or follow-up study because of his inertia or apparent disinterest.

3. He believes it is unnecessary for him to observe a sick patient continuously, or to perform laboratory tests except those required, or properly to examine physically a condition for which he depends upon the laboratory, x-ray examination, or other device to clarify the diagnosis and tell him the proper procedure. He demonstrates no alarm when he fails to solve logically a problem, because that problem required the utilization of his knowledge, skill, experience, and common sense rather than a test tube method. He adopts the attitude that if he missed the point in the case that inevitably all others would miss the point, and does not recognize the worthiness and skill required by the one who solves it for him. The correct solution in the hands of the second surgeon becomes a matter of luck. He does not recognize the fact that the power of observation has clarified many problems and does not attempt to labor to better his power of observation.

4. He is thoroughly convinced that he should learn the subject in a much shorter period of time, and would not linger longer in training if the board did not demand it.

5. A smaller group feel that to learn operative technique is all that is necessary for a surgical education.

6. He is not developing as keen a sense of responsibility in the care of his patients as his predecessors.

7. He is eager to be spoon-fed, shown movies, and given lectures, and does not admit in his mental attack that these are only guides to the opportunity awaiting him for self-advancement in the outpatient clinic, the ward, and the operating room.

8. Last, he wishes to carry the mantle of senior surgical resident without developing himself in a way to justify the undertaking of that responsibility.

9. He is training himself to pass a Board rather than the most successful satisfaction of training himself to be the best surgeon he can make out of himself.

These attitudes are, of course, not applicable to all residents, fortunately, but they are observations that are real, too numerous, and are contagious. A great many men of this caliber pass the Boards because, recognizing their deficiencies, they study arduously and assemble a great mass of facts which are useful in passing an examination; but this knowledge is short-lived because it is not a part of the man but rather a lever for Board-passing. It is also a matter of frequent observation to notice that the well-trained surgeon will often not cram for a Board examination because he knows he deserves the certificate, and occasionally fails, where, conversely, the poorly trained man will pass without as much proportional failure.

CONCLUSION

An analysis of these observations cannot definitely point to a correction of what may be lacking in our surgical teaching. It suggests:

1. That in certain institutions our teaching prowess gained in momentum during the pioneer days of the Halsted resident system.

2. That this efficient system of teaching gained widespread adoption and produced a great number of well-trained surgeons.

3. That great variation of the method exists in the teaching policies of the institutions professing its use.

4. That pupils from these schools in the great experiment of work observed in our Army and Veterans Hospitals demonstrate varying degrees of surgical proficiency which closely parallel the teaching merits of the parent school.

5. That training in our large nonuniversity clinics is excellent to a certain period of development of the surgeon, but lacks the advancing responsibility to mould the finished surgeon.

6. That preceptorship and apprenticeship are not producing good surgeons.

7. That overspecialization has detrimentally altered the training of a well-balanced general surgeon.

8. That the Board certificate, although definitely improving the standard of surgical practitioners, is unknowingly and detrimentally influencing the attitude of men undergoing surgical training.

9. That serious consideration and action on the part of surgical teaching institutions be employed to offset the ultimate decline in caliber of our finished surgical resident.

EVOLUTION OF TREATMENT OF CAPILLARY HEMANGIOMAS OF THE FACE WITH FURTHER OBSERVATION ON THE VALUE OF CAMOUFLAGE BY PERMANENT PIGMENT INJECTION (TATTOOING)

HERBERT CONWAY, M.D., NEW YORK, N. Y.

(From the Department of Surgery of The New York Hospital and Cornell University Medical College)

THE successful obliteration of capillary hemangiomas of the face long has presented a challenge to the medical profession. The variable popularity of the myriad treatments of the conservative type is mute evidence that none of these have been rewarded regularly by success. The fact that capillary hemangiomas do not undergo malignant change seems to increase the therapeutic challenge presented by the unfortunate wearer of the birthmark. Conservative methods of treatment have been directed at the destruction of the lesion, its obliteration by fibrosis of the abundant capillaries resident in the derma or in the subdermal tissues. Among such methods of treatment are the following: electrodesiccation, cauterization, distance application of ultraviolet light, carbon dioxide snow, liquid air, ignipuncture, electrolysis, Kromayer therapy, x-ray therapy, and radium therapy. Since such treatments must be applied to the lesion through the overlying skin, it is easy to understand why scarring, the result of injury to or destruction of the skin, follows so often. This objection also is relevant to the surgical attack upon the lesion for it is not possible to excise these capillary hemangiomas without sacrifice of the overlying skin.

My experience in the management of patients with port-wine stains covers a period of twelve years during which these patients have been observed in the plastic surgery clinic of The New York Hospital. The large number of patients who gave history of a series of treatments of the conservative type as listed in the preceding paragraph and whose lesions either had not been effaced or had been replaced (therapeutically) by a scar more seriously disfiguring than the original lesion, led me at first to the surgical excision of capillary hemangiomas. Advances in the technique of tissue shifting and grafting seemed to offer promise. However, the replacement of a large vascular lesion of the derma with a free graft of skin failed to provide the patient with the ideal result for, often, the graft appeared as a facial blemish no less noticeable than the port-wine stain. In recent years there has been a trend away from the use of large free grafts, the advancement of facial and cervical skin in several successive operations being employed in its stead. For smaller lesions the advancement of regional flaps is ideal. In the excision of the larger lesions usually it is necessary to employ small free grafts to surface residual defects about the eyelids or mouth. However, small grafts of suitable matching color may be obtained readily from postauricular areas, the eyelids, or the supraclavicular areas. There has been recent reactivation of interest in another conservative method of management, namely, tattooing, or the injection of permanent, insoluble pigments into the derma overlying the capillary hemangioma. The use of this permanent camouflage for port-wine stains, the only objectionable feature of which is their color, was suggested first in 1835 by Pauli.[1] In 1946, Brown, Cannon, and McDowell[2] reactivated interest in the use of this treatment for capillary hemangiomas and in 1947 Docktor and I[3] reported seven cases in which the treatment had successfully disguised the color of these lesions. The management of twenty-eight cases up to the present time has not dampened enthusiasm for the tattoo treatment. However, experience has been gained which indicates that not all port-wine stains respond equally as well to their camouflage by tattoo. The reason for this lies in the basic difference in the pathology of the lesions. Andrews[4] classified capillary hemangiomas as (a) subepidermal, those in which the abnormal capillaries lie under the epidermis in the subpapillary zone of the skin; (b) dermal, those in which the abnormal capillaries are chiefly in the midcutis, and (c) subdermal, those in which the abnormal capillaries are in the subcutaneous tissue, subadjacent to the derma. Since the inert pigments used in tattooing must be deposited in the derma if they are to remain permanently, it is apparent that this can be accomplished with ease in the subdermal variety of port-wine stain, effectively though less easily in the dermal variety, and not at all effectively in the subepidermal type. It is this variation in location of the abnormal capillaries which accounts for the differences in response of port-wine stains to camouflage by tattoo.

Since experience in the management of port-wine stains in the plastic surgery clinic of The New York Hospital has evolved according to a pattern which parallels the evolution of treatment of these lesions, four illustrative cases have been selected for report herein. These are examples of (a) excision of the port-wine stain and replacement by free whole-thickness graft of skin, (b) gradual partial excision with advancement of skin of the face and neck and with use of free whole-thickness skin graft to replace residual lesion, (c) partial excision and advancement of skin of the face or neck with tattooing of residual hemangioma, and (d) the camouflage of the entire lesion by tattooing.

CASE REPORTS

Excision of Port-Wine Stain and Replacement by Free Whole-thickness Graft of Skin

CASE 1 (N. Y. Hosp. No. 227002).—R. S., a 20-year-old girl, presented herself for treatment in February, 1939. The lesion was the dermal type of capillary hemangioma and it extended irregularly over an area of the left cheek and left upper lip, measuring 3 by 7 cm. (Fig. 1, *A*). Six radium treatments had been given at another institution six years earlier. There had been no improvement in the appearance of the lesion following this treatment. At operation on Feb. 22, 1939, the lesion was excised and a patterned whole-thickness graft of skin, cut from the lateral abdominal region, was applied. The graft was a success but its failure to match the color of the skin of the face left the patient with a deformity no more desirable than the original port-wine stain (Fig. 1, *B*). The patient found it necessary to continue the wearing of heavy cosmetics in order to hide the appearance of the graft.

In 1947, following the development of the coloring of skin grafts by permanent pigment injection, this patient was recalled to the clinic. In two treatments, flesh-colored tints were tattooed into the derma of the graft so that it matched the color of the skin of the face very well. Still, the ''patched'' appearance of the face left the result somewhat short of ideal (Fig. 1, *C*).

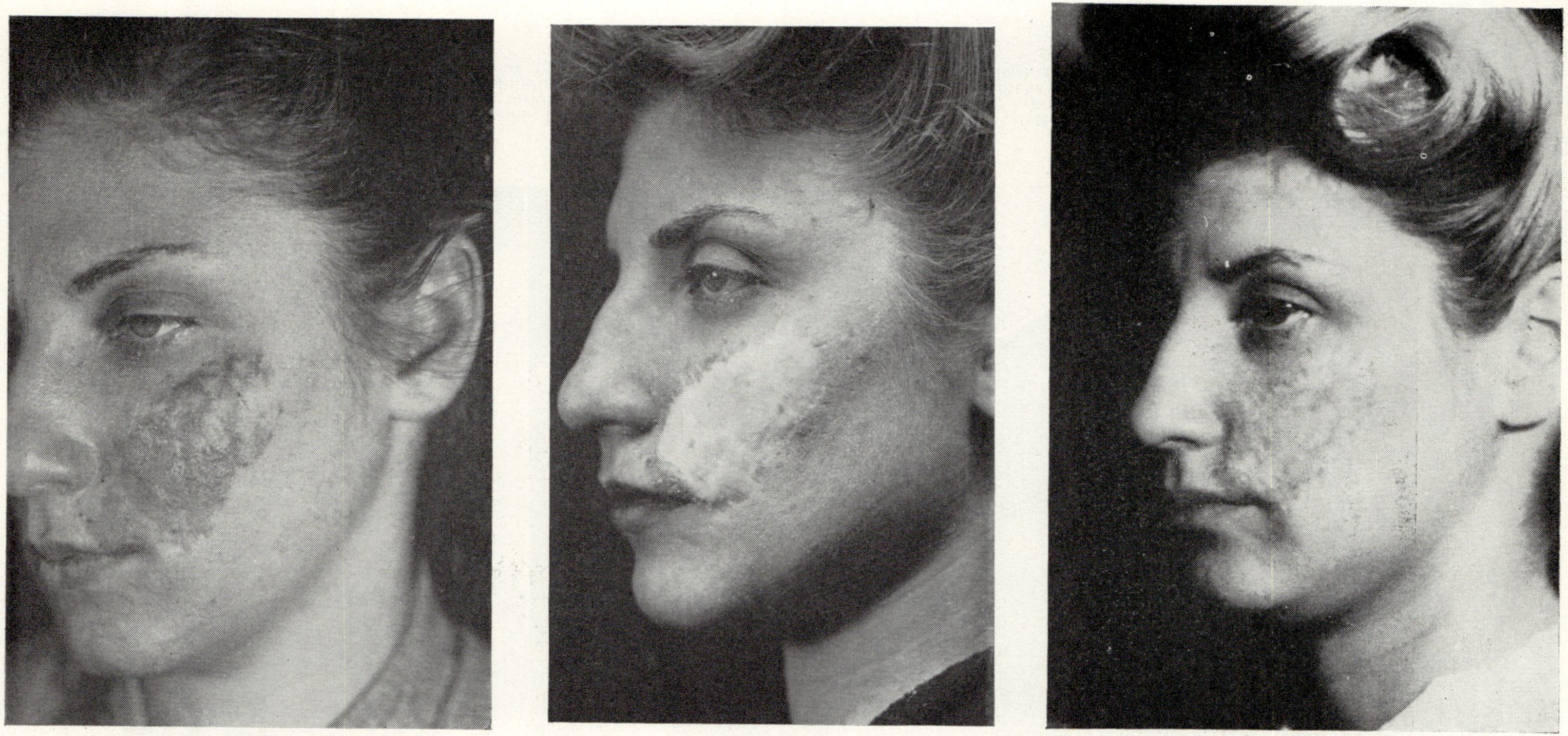

A. B. C.

Fig. 1 (Case 1).—*A*, Dermal type of capillary hemangioma of the cheek. *B*, Appearance after excision of the capillary hemangioma and replacement by a free whole-thickness graft taken from a protected area of the surface of the body. Note that the failure in color match represents a facial blemish no more desirable than the original port-wine stain. *C*, Appearance after tattoo treatment of the skin graft by injection of permanent pigments (flesh color) into its derma.

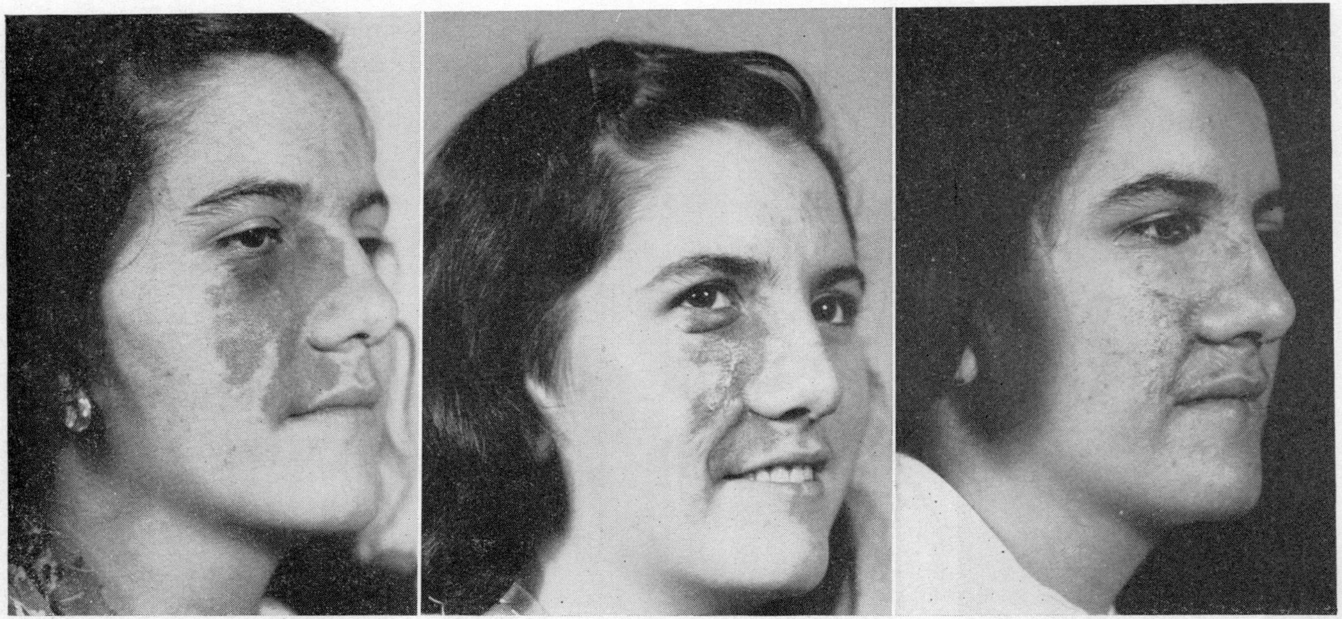

A. B. C.

Fig. 2 (Case 2).—*A*, Capillary hemangioma of the subepidermal type over the right cheek, lower eyelid, side of nose, and upper lip. *B*, Appearance after first stage of gradual partial excision with medial advancement of skin of the cheek. *C*, Appearance after excision of the residual capillary hemangioma of the lower eyelid and nose and of the upper lip. The defects after excision were surfaced with whole-thickness grafts cut from behind the ears. The color match was ideal.

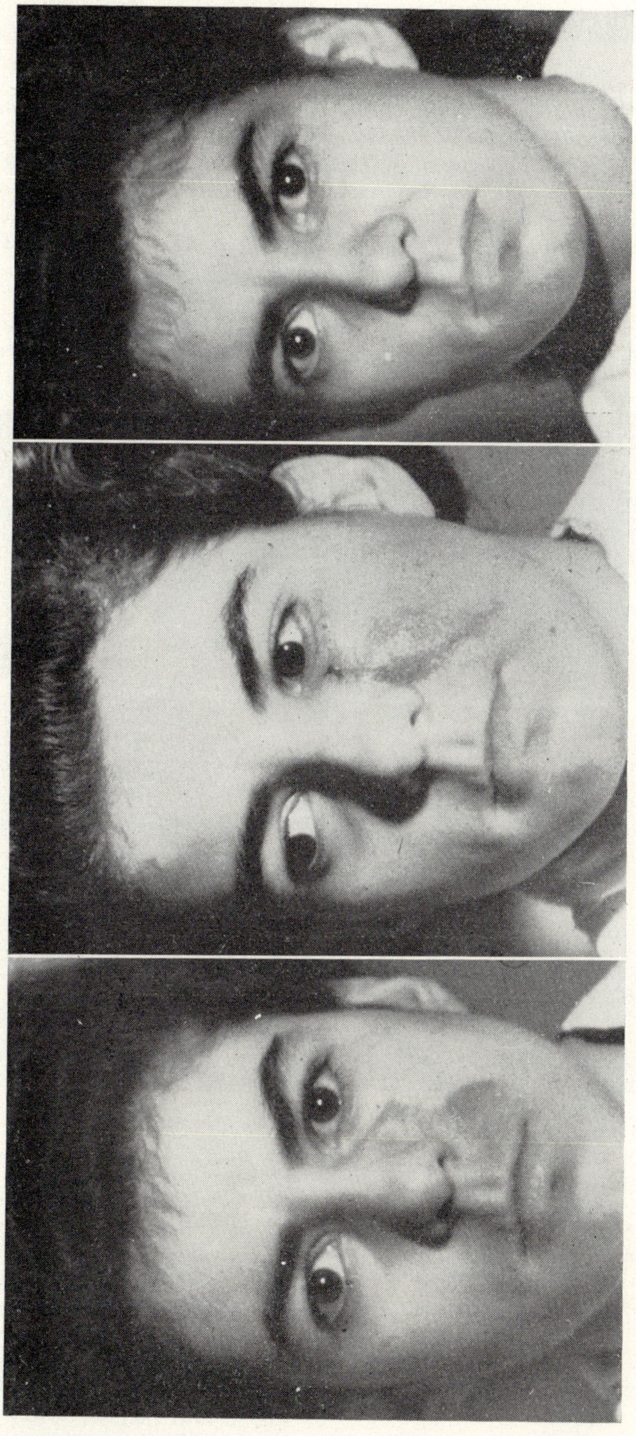

A. *B.* *C.*

Fig. 3 (Case 3).—*A*, Dermal type of capillary hemangioma of the cheek. *B*, Appearance after excision of the major portion of the lesion. By undercutting and advancement of the malar skin the line of suture was brought directly into the nasolabial fold. Since further excision with primary suture might result in distortion of the lip, the residual angioma medial to the nasolabial line was treated by tattoo. *C*, Appearance after permanent camouflage by tattoo of residual capillary hemangioma of the upper lip, medial to the nasolabial fold.

Gradual Partial Excision of Large Port-wine Stain With Advancement of Skin of the Face and the Use of Small Free Whole-thickness Skin Grafts to Replace Residual Lesion

CASE 2 (N. Y. Hosp. No 451337).—M. P., a 20-year-old girl, presented the appearance shown in Fig. 2, *A*. The lesion was a large capillary hemangioma of the subepidermal type over the right cheek, lower eyelid, side of the nose, and the upper lip. On July 31, 1946, first stage gradual partial excision was done. Approximately 2.5 cm. of transverse measurement of the lesion was excised. Skin of the cheek was widely undercut and advanced medially. The extent of the excision is shown in Fig. 2, *B*. This photograph was taken after this first operation. On Sept. 25, 1946, second stage gradual partial excision was done. The central third of the lesion was excised and, after wide undercutting of facial and cervical skin, the lateral cutaneous margin was approximated to the skin of the side of the nose. On Dec. 4, 1946, the residual hemangioma of the right lower eyelid and the lateral aspect of the nose were excised. They were replaced by a whole-thickness graft measuring 4 cm.

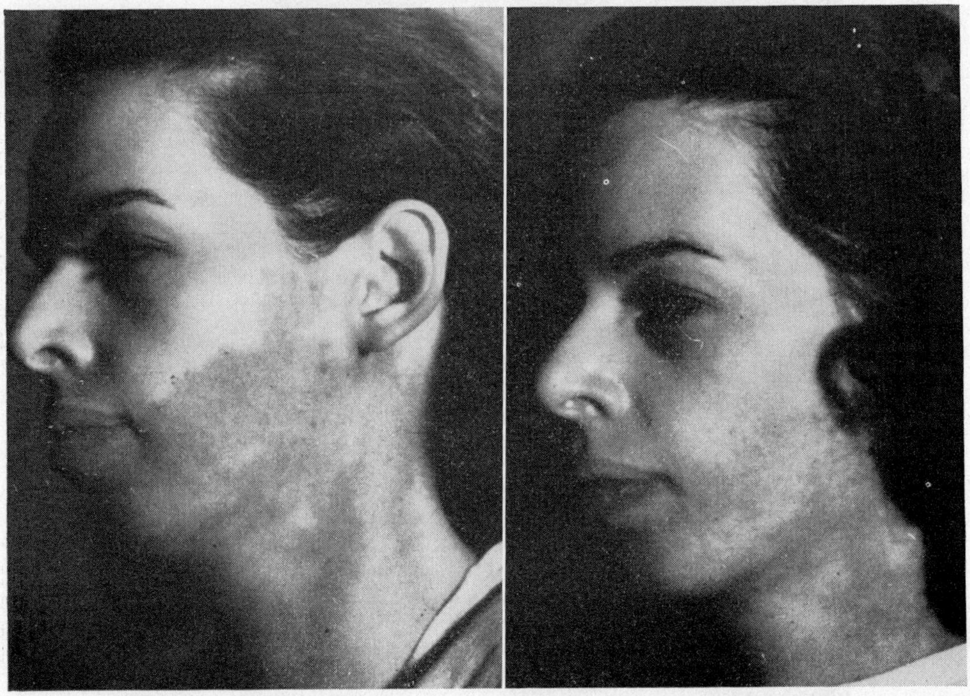

A. *B.*

Fig. 4 (Case 4).—*A*, Extensive subdermal capillary hemangioma of the neck and cheek. *B*, Appearance after permanent camouflage by nine tattoo treatments.

in its greatest vertical dimension and 5 cm. in its greatest transverse dimension. This graft was taken from the posterior aspect of the right ear and from the cephaloauricular angle. Its pattern was such that it was not possible to suture the margins of the donor wound without distortion of the external ear. Because of this, a thick-split graft was cut from the upper thigh and applied to the donor wound. Interpalpebral synechiae were established. On Jan. 8, 1947, the residual hemangioma of the upper lip was excised. The defect was covered with a second whole-thickness graft taken from behind the left ear. This graft measured only 2.5 by 1.5 cm. and its donor wound was closed by suture. On Feb. 3, 1947, the synechiae holding the eyelids closed were divided. The appearance of the patient in March, 1947, is shown in Fig. 2, *C*. The result was quite satisfactory since small grafts obtained from behind the ears matched the color of the skin of the face.

Partial Excision of Dermal Capillary Hemangioma of the Cheek With Advancement of the Skin of the Face and Camouflage of Residual Hemangioma by Tattooing

CASE 3 (N. Y. Hosp. No. 460250).—C. F., a 16-year-old girl, presented a capillary hemangioma of the left cheek of the dermal type (Fig. 3, *A*). At operation in December, 1946, all of the lesion with the exception of a small area on the upper lip, medial to the nasolabial line, was excised. The skin of the cheek was undercut widely and advanced to a line of suture which was placed exactly in the nasolabial line (Fig. 3, *B*). Further excision with primary suture might have endangered full function of the lips. The residual hemangioma was camouflaged by tattooing (Fig. 3, *C*). The inert pigments blended well with the adjacent skin and the result was ideal.

Permanent Camouflage of Large Subdermal Capillary Hemangioma of the Cheek, Lips, and Neck by Tattoo

CASE 4 (N. Y. Hosp. No. 481788).—R. M., a woman 27 years of age, presented an extensive port-wine stain of the subdermal type over the left cheek, chin, and neck (Fig. 4, *A*). It was treated by the injection of inert pigments (tattooing) into the derma overlying the lesion. This lesion, the surface area of which was seventeen square inches, was satisfactorily camouflaged in nine treatments given at two- to three-week intervals (Fig. 4, *B*). The treatments were given without anesthesia. Pigments injected were white mixed with very small amounts of green and brown. The tattoo treatment was especially adaptable to this subdermal type of port-wine stain.

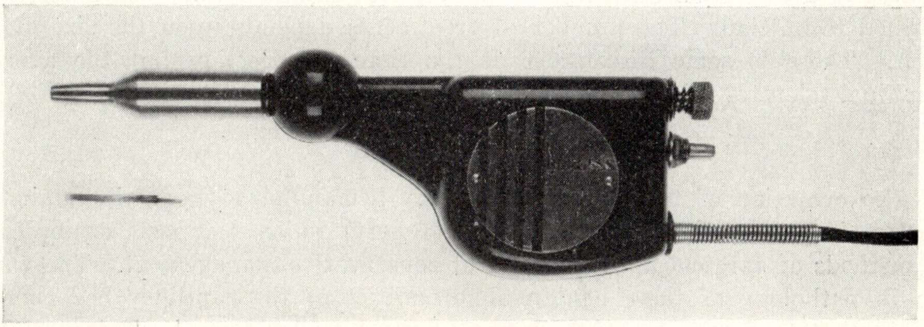

Fig. 5.—Electromagnetic device with five small needles which is used in the permanent pigment injection (tattooing) of capillary hemangiomas. (From Conway and Docktor, Surg., Gynec. & Obst., 1947.)

TECHNIQUE

The technique of intradermal injection of insoluble pigments (tattooing) for permanent camouflage of port-wine stains follows. The area to be injected is washed with soap and water, painted with aqueous solution of merthiolate, and draped with sterile towels. Instruments and pigments are sterilized. The technician wears sterile rubber gloves. The area should be free from infection. It has been found expedient to use the standard electromagnetic device to which six needles are attached. This is shown in Fig. 5. With sterile water the pigments are mixed into a thick paste which is picked up in the cup of the needle holder when the needles are withdrawn into its shaft. The current which causes rapid oscillation of the needles is operated by a foot control. The needles are inserted into the skin at an angle of approximately 60 degrees so that the pigment will be injected obliquely at varying depths in the derma. The basic pigments which are in use at present include the following: white, titanium (or zinc oxide U.S.P.); yellow, oxide of iron; red, mercury sulfide (or cinnabar); blue, cobalt blue; black, black oxide of iron; green, hydrated chrome oxide.

Combinations of these pigments usually will produce the desired tints. In addition ocher, sienna, and other earthy metallic oxides may be used. All of these pigments are inert and insoluble. They may be sterilized in 70 per cent alcohol or may be autoclaved. The mixture of colors must be suited to the individual case. For the covering of capillary hemangiomas, white is the basic pigment, occasionally mixed with a very small amount of red, green, or brown. At the first treatment, a small area is injected and a record is kept of the color combination. Three to four weeks are allowed to elapse before judgment is passed on the effect of treatment. Usually there is some absorption and some desquamation of pigment. A second or a third treatment over the same area may be necessary before the desired result is obtained. Following the treatment a sterile dressing is applied. The patient is seen in twenty-four hours, at which time a crust is present over the area which has been injected. As this peels away during the next six to ten days the effect of the injection may be observed. Once the proper mixture of pigments is decided upon, treatments may be given at two-week intervals until the skin over the entire lesion has been injected. An area of 2 to 3 square inches may be injected in about forty-five minutes by a skilled technician. The number of treatments depends upon the size of the lesion. There is some discomfort at the time of injection but the average individual tolerates this without anesthesia.

SUMMARY

The evolution of treatment of capillary hemangioma (port-wine stain) of the face is presented through four case reports which represent examples of the methods of surgical approach and of conservative management. The variation in pathology of these benign abnormalities of the capillary bed consists only in that they may be subepidermal, dermal, or subdermal. This variation must be taken into consideration in the plan of treatment. The tattoo treatment results in effective permanent camouflage of port-wine stains of the dermal or subcutaneous variety. The subepidermal variety is effectively eradicated only by excision of the port-wine stain and reconstruction of the face by advancement of regional skin supplemented on occasion by free, whole-thickness graft of skin.

REFERENCES

1. Pauli: Application de tatouage a la cure des naevi materni, Siebold's Journal **15:** 1, 1835.
2. Brown, J. B., Cannon, B., and McDowell, A.: Plastic and Reconstructive Surgery **1:** 106, 1946.
3. Conway, Herbert, and Docktor, John P.: Neutralization of Color in Capillary Hemangiomas of the Face by Intradermal Injection (Tattooing) of Permanent Pigments, Surg., Gynec. & Obst. **84:** 866-869, 1947.
4. Andrews, G. C.: Diseases of the Skin, Philadelphia, 1932, W. B. Saunders Company, p. 833.

THE SURGICAL TREATMENT OF ACUTE CHOLECYSTITIS

Frank Glenn, M.D., New York, N. Y.

(From the Department of Surgery of The New York Hospital and Cornell University Medical College)

THE early surgical treatment of acute cholecystitis, although still controversial in some medical circles, is generally accepted today as contributing to the best interests of the patient. One of the early advocates of this therapy was George J. Heuer, in whose honor this volume is dedicated. His early training under William S. Halsted provided him with his first opportunity for seeing the uneventful postoperative course of a patient operated upon for acute cholecystitis. This was followed in turn by his own successful experience of operating upon such patients in a relatively limited number before he went to Cincinnati. As professor of surgery at the University of Cincinnati and surgeon-in-chief to the University Hospital, an opportunity was afforded him again to put into practice what he believed to be a sound policy in the treatment of these patients in the early acute phase of the disease, and over a period of eleven years he demonstrated that both morbidity and mortality rates were extremely low for those patients with acute cholecystitis who were operated upon when well prepared. At the same time, he observed that the gall bladder in acute cholecystitis might proceed in its pathologic course to gangrene and perforation in the presence of subsiding and minimal signs and symptoms.

In 1932, when Dr. Heuer became surgeon-in-chief of the New York Hospital, he inaugurated in this hospital a policy of early operation for these patients. Up until this time there had been a general aversion to operating upon patients with acute cholecystitis and only an occasional incidental operation for it had been done. Dr. Heuer's policy was considered a radical change.

The experience accumulated on the surgical service of the New York Hospital from 1932 to 1947, a period of fifteen years, serves as a basis for this discussion. It is an admirable record. The accomplishment is by and large the result of the policy established by Dr. Heuer and constituted a departure from the custom of the community of New York City.

This policy has resulted in an experience of 586 patients with acute cholecystitis being treated surgically over a fifteen-year period. From an over-all standpoint the results have been gratifying, but there is room for improvement, since seventeen of these patients died following operation. Some of them might have survived had operation been performed earlier—either years earlier when the biliary tract disease was in its early phase, or days earlier before the acute attack had progressed to a stage where complications such as gangrene and perforation had taken place. The mortality rate of 2.8 per cent should therefore be reduced in the future. Acute cholecystitis is a phase of gall bladder disease that may occur in the early decades of life. In women, in particular, it may first appear during or following the first pregnancy and recur at varying intervals thereafter. It may be said that onset takes place in an older age group in men, but no age is exempt. Over 95 per cent of the patients operated upon have had gallstones, which would indicate them as the most important single factor in the precipitation of acute episodes. The diagnosis is not difficult.

Surgical treatment of acute cholecystitis at the New York Hospital provides for operation when the patient is adequately prepared, unless some coexisting condition not immediately reparable contraindicates operation. The operation of choice is cholecystectomy, and this was accomplished in 513 patients, or an incidence of 87.5 per cent. Cholecystostomy is a compromise procedure, but when indicated, may be a lifesaving one, and has been resorted to in seventy-three cases, or 12.4 per cent. If there is evidence suggesting common duct obstruction due to stones, then the procedure of choledochotomy is added. Fortunately, this increase in operative burden has been employed in only forty-five patients, or 7.6 per cent. The procedure to be employed is decided upon during the operation. The patient's immediate welfare is always the first consideration, to secure the greatest possible benefit with the least hazard. At the same time, the indicated procedure is done even though it may add some risk, as for example exploration of the common duct when obstructive jaundice believed caused by calculi is present.

TABLE I. ACUTE CHOLECYSTITIS, NEW YORK HOSPITAL (SEPT. 1, 1932 TO SEPT. 1, 1947)

Total cases	586
Deaths	17
Mortality rate	2.8%
Operative Procedures	
Cholecystectomy	513
Cholecystostomy	73*
Common duct exploration	45

*This number constitutes 12.4 per cent of total operations.

Cholecystostomy is clearly indicated under certain circumstances, such as when the patient is too ill to withstand a cholecystectomy, or when cholecystectomy presents too great difficulties. In the older age group, where extreme debilitation is encountered most frequently, and among those whose illness is the result of too long delayed operation, the simpler procedure of cholecystostomy should always be employed. It can be done under local anesthesia, disturbing the patient very little. Not only may it be lifesaving, but decompression of the biliary tract may avert progressive liver damage if complete biliary obstruction is present. In seventy-three patients, cholecystostomy was performed, with a mortality of eight, or 12.8 per cent. This high mortality rate is indicative of the serious condition of the patients when operation was undertaken.

The gross appearance of the presenting pathologic changes contributes to the type of operation to be done. For example, if gangrene and perforation accompany generalized peritonitis, the operative procedure should be limited to cholecystostomy and drainage of the operative area. If there are gangrene and perforation which have resulted in localized peritonitis or abscess in the region of the extrahepatic portion of the gall bladder, then cholecystectomy or cholecystostomy may be done according to the ease with which the procedure can be carried out. If there is extensive abscess formation, or if the omentum is adherent and obscures the structures in the region of the biliary fossa, it is probably the better part of wisdom to leave these undisturbed and to limit the procedure to cholecystostomy. Also if the patient is unusually ill and if postoperative complications appear in the offing, cholecystectomy should not be attempted. On the other hand, a small abscess, the result of perforation of the gall bladder, is no contraindication to cholecystectomy. It is not an infrequent experience to encounter abscesses located between the liver and the gall bladder wall. The patient with simple acute cholecystitis and/or hydrops of the gall bladder is generally best treated by cholecystectomy, which is readily accomplished.

Common duct exploration in acute cholecystitis has been limited in our clinic to those patients with unequivocal indication of common duct obstruction, and a distinction should be made between a mild degree of jaundice associated with inflammatory reaction throughout the bilary tract which is frequently associated with acute cholecystitis and true common duct obstruction. The incidence of postoperative complications in patients requiring common duct exploration appears higher than when such is not necessary. At the same time, it may be said that these patients are usually in the group that is more seriously ill. For the jaundiced patient that is extremely ill, decompression, that is, cholecystostomy, may be utilized as a compromise immediate procedure, having in mind of course, following the subsidence of the jaundice, the exploration of the common duct with the patient in a greatly improved condition. The presence of jaundice requires the determination of the blood prothrombin and the evaluation of any bleeding tendency, and in the presence of acute disease time may not be afforded for this. Therefore, for such patients the use of whole blood transfusions and parenteral administration of vitamin K may prevent serious postoperative hemorrhage. This same group of patients often have liver damage and special consideration must be accorded them as indicated.

The common duct was explored in forty-five of these patients, an incidence of 7.6 per cent. Stones were found in thirty of these, or an incidence of 66.6 per cent of those explored. The exploration of the common duct in the patient without stones does not apparently add materially to the postoperative complications. This should be kept in mind when deciding whether or not to explore the common duct, because failure to remove a common duct stone may lead to catastrophe. It has been our policy in such a situation to explore the duct when in doubt.

Cholecystectomy is the operation of choice in acute cholecystitis. The removal of the gall bladder interrupts the pathologic process and averts the danger of gangrene and perforation. This procedure is sometimes contraindicated, as:

1. In the presence of peritonitis due to perforation of the gall bladder. These patients are gravely ill and the simplest procedure to tide them over the immediate situation is indicated.

2. Conditions which make it difficult to identify the important structures of the biliary fossa. The acutely inflamed gall bladder, with many adhesions between it and the adjacent viscera, may so distort the anatomic relationships that they become obscure, and as a result injury to the hepatic vessels or the common duct may result.

3. The presence of a severe jaundice caused by obstruction in the common duct is a contraindication to an extensive operative procedure. It is usually better to drain the gall bladder and thereby relieve the jaundice than to subject the patient to a long procedure that may be required in searching for a stone.

4. In those patients whose general condition is so grave that a general anesthesia and a prolonged operation are not justified. This is seen most frequently in the aged and debilitated, when the acute cholecystitis is superimposed upon such systemic disorders as cardiovascular and renal disease. Under such circumstances a compromise must be sought in the form of surgical treatment that adds as little a burden as possible to the individual and yet tides him over the immediate crisis.

TABLE II. ACUTE CHOLECYSTITIS, NEW YORK HOSPITAL (SEPT. 1, 1932 TO SEPT. 1, 1947), IN PATIENTS 50 YEARS OF AGE OR OVER

Total cases	205
Deaths	13
Mortality rate	6.1%
Operative Procedures	
Cholecystectomy	165
Cholecystostomy	40*
Common duct exploration	24

*This number constitutes 19.5 per cent of total operations.

Over the fifteen-year period, 586 patients with acute cholecystitis have been treated surgically. During this same period a total of over 2,600 patients were treated surgically for biliary tract disease. Of the 586 patients, 205 were 50 years of age or over. In this group of 205 there were 13 deaths, or a mortality rate of 6.1 per cent; 165 were subjected to cholecystectomy, 40, or 19.5 per cent, to cholecystostomy. Twenty-four had, in addition, exploration of the common duct. The mortality rate of 6.1 per cent in this group of patients indicates the decidedly greater risk associated with them than with those under 50 years, who had a mortality rate of 1.04 per cent.

In patients over 50 years of age, acute cholecystitis is a more serious disease than in the younger group. The mortality rate is over five times greater. It has been our experience that changes in the vascular system, namely, arteriosclerosis, hypertension, and diabetes, are greater in those who have biliary tract disease than in a corresponding number without it. The trend of our population toward the older age group indicates that we may anticipate an increasing number of these geriatrical problems unless they can be reduced by preventive surgery. For biliary tract disease, it means operating in the earlier decades when acute cholecystitis represents an early phase of the disease. If our contention is correct, a deleterious effect upon the vascular system may be interrupted.

TABLE III. SUMMARY OF DEATHS AFTER OPERATION

	SEX	AGE (YR.)	BILIARY DISEASE HISTORY (IN YR.)	DURATION OF ATTACK	JAUNDICE	FINDINGS	OPERATION	CAUSE OF DEATH
1	F	66	8+	3 days	+	Acute cholecystitis with perforation, peritonitis	Cholecystectomy with drainage	Peritonitis
2	F	67	4+	7 days	0	Acute cholecystitis with gangrene	Cholecystostomy	Peritonitis, bacteremia
3	F	50	20+	10 days	+	Acute cholecystits, cholelithiasis, common duct obstruction	Cholecystostomy	Bacteremia, stone in common duct, thrombosis hepatic artery
4	M	72	7+	8 days	+	Acute cholecystitis, cholelithiasis	Cholecystostomy	Hepatic failure, biliary cirrhosis
5	F	57	Inadequate history	4 days	0	Acute cholecystitis, cholelithiasis	Cholecystectomy, drainage abscess	Subhepatic abscess*
6	F	70	12+	8 hr.	0	Acute cholecystitis, cholelithiasis	Cholecystectomy	Coronary occlusion, cardiac failure
7	F	64	2+	2 days	+	Acute cholecystitis	Cholecystectomy with drainage	Adrenal insufficiency
8	F	54	4+	3 days	+	Acute cholecystitis, common duct obstruction	Cholecystectomy, common duct exploration	Leakage from cystic duct, subphrenic abscess, pancreatic necrosis
9	F	72	?	3 days	0	Acute cholecystitis, carcinoma of cecum	Cholecystectomy, ileocolostomy	Intestinal obstruction, hypertensive cardiac disease
10	M	69	8	2 days	+	Acute cholecystitis	Cholecystostomy, peritoneal drainage	Bile peritonitis
11	F	61	10	5 days	0	Acute cholecystitis	Cholecystectomy	Anoxia, brain damage, anesthesia
12	M	71	Inadequate history	4 days	+	Acute cholecystitis, cholelithiasis, perforation of gall bladder	Cholecystostomy	Peritonitis, uremia*

*No autopsy.

There are those who question the advisability of operating upon the patient with acute cholecystitis. These figures, however, seem to justify the policy to which we have adhered for several years. And what is more important, we believe we have saved patients from the catastrophe of perforation following gangrene. This is in direct contrast to the so-called conservative policy that considers such patients to be medical problems and leaves them in their homes where complications may develop and be unrecognized. We consider these patients as surgical and admit them to the hospital where they are under constant observation, and where laboratory data, temperature records, and personal observation by more than one individual are of greater value in determining the course of events in the pathologic process that is going on. When such a patient is in satisfactory condition for operation, it is then deliberately done.

It should be stressed that very few patients with acute cholecystitis fail to give a long history of symptoms relative to the biliary tract. For those over 50 years of age there is often a history of disease of over twenty years. For those under 50 years, it is much less. However, the young woman recently pregnant who enters the hospital with acute cholecystitis—and I look upon her as an example of the early phase of chronic biliary tract disease—usually gives a history of indigestion, abdominal discomfort, and sometimes nausea and vomiting dating back to the early weeks of her first pregnancy. Many of these patients on x-ray examination are found to possess a nonfunctioning gall bladder or a poorly functioning one containing stones. Their symptoms previously had not been acute and they tolerated them. When they have acute attacks, they consult a physician. In the years past, they were commonly advised that they would recover, and most of them did, but only to have one attack after another.

A summary of deaths after operation follows. These twelve of the total seventeen deaths in the series were in patients 50 years of age and over, and one may consider that earlier operation might have reduced this number—years earlier, as far as biliary tract disease itself is concerned, and days earlier in the case of the acute attack.

The remaining 381 of the 586 patients were under 50 years of age. There were 4 deaths, a mortality rate of 1.04 per cent; 347, or 91.1 per cent, were subjected to cholecystectomy, and 33, or 8.6 per cent, were treated by cholecystostomy. Twenty-six, or 6.8 per cent, had in addition to one of the pro-

TABLE IV. ACUTE CHOLECYSTITIS, NEW YORK HOSPITAL (SEPT. 1, 1932 TO SEPT. 1, 1947), IN PATIENTS UNDER 50 YEARS OF AGE

Total cases	381
Deaths	4
Mortality rate	1.04%
Operative Procedures	
Cholecystectomy	347
Cholecystostomy	33*
Common duct exploration	26

*This number constitutes 8.6 per cent of total operations.

TABLE V. SUMMARY OF DEATHS AFTER OPERATION IN PATIENTS UNDER 50 YEARS OF AGE

	SEX	AGE (YR.)	BILIARY DISEASE HISTORY (IN YR.)	DURATION OF ATTACK (IN DAYS)	JAUNDICE	FINDINGS	OPERATION	CAUSE OF DEATH
1	M	41	5	1	+	Acute cholecystitis	Cholecystectomy	Cardiac and renal failure, liver death
2	F	49	15	3	+	Acute cholecystitis	Cholecystectomy	Subdiaphragmatic abscess, peritonitis
3	F	49	12	2	0	Acute cholecystitis, stones in common duct, acute pancreatitis	Cholecystectomy, choledochotomy	Pulmonary emboli 27th P. O. day*
4	M	44	4	10	0	Acute cholecystitis	Cholecystectomy	Hypertension, cardiorenal failure
5	F	49	3	3	0	Acute cholecystitis, cholelithiasis	Cholecystostomy	Coronary occlusion*

*No autopsy.

cedures just listed, exploration of the common duct. This is a far more favorable outcome than our experience with the group of patients over 50 years of age.

In the community of our practice at the New York Hospital, it has become well known among our patients that if they have an attack of acute cholecystitis they will be advised to have the gall bladder removed, unless there is a contraindication. This is a step forward because it interrupts the disease early if acute attacks occur in the late twenties and early thirties. These patients have done remarkably well following operation. Since 1932, we have not lost a single patient under 40 years of age following operation for acute cholecystitis, except one child with acute typhoid cholecystitis. The patients who die following operation are in the upper age group for the most part, and death is the result of complications (often involving the circulatory system) including embolism, the result of a phlebitis. Those patients with chronic biliary tract disease, who have as a complication acute cholecystitis, may have a complication of acute cholecystitis, namely, gangrene perforation, with a resulting local or general peritonitis. There are, we feel, patients who die as a result of complications when treated by the conservative policy in their homes or even in hospitals. The five deaths in the group under 50 years of age, listed in Table V, indicate that the biliary tract disease had been of long standing.

The evolution and development of the surgical treatment of biliary tract disease is not yet complete. Cholecystostomy for the removal of stones had been a common practice prior to Langenbach's report of cholecystectomy for chronic cholecystitis and cholelithiasis in 1884. Not long thereafter, Kümmell (1890) reported an exploration of the common duct with removal of stones. Over the past seventy-five years an increasing experience coupled with improved medical facilities has made diagnosis in biliary tract disease less difficult. As a result, a greater proportion of patients is seen by the surgeon earlier than in years past. Operative procedures are now well standardized, and when carried out in carefully selected and well-prepared patients are associated with minimal risk.

The policy inaugurated by Dr. Heuer and followed by his staff at the New York Hospital over a period of fifteen years has been presented. The results of operating on patients in the younger group in the acute phase of the disease support the contention that this is the optimum time for surgical intervention. Furthermore, operation in the acute phase for those over 50 years will reduce the morbidity and mortality rates of biliary tract disease.

REFERENCES

1. Heuer, George J.: Introductory Remarks to The Surgical Treatment of Acute Cholecystitis (by Frank Glenn), Surg., Gynec. & Obst. **83**: 50-54, 1946.
2. Heuer, George J.: The Factors Leading to Death in Operations Upon the Gallbladder and Bile-Ducts, Ann. Surg. **99**: 6, 1934.
3. Heuer, George J.: The Surgical Aspects of Acute Cholecystitis, Ann. Surg. **105**: 5, 1937.
4. Langenbach, Carl: Ein Fall von Exstirpation der Gallenblase wegen chronischer Cholethiasis. Heilung, Berl. klin. Wchnschr. **19**: 725, 1882.
5. Kümmell, H.: Zur Chirurgie der Gallenblase, Deutsche. med. Wchnschr. **16**: 237, 1890.

FURTHER OBSERVATIONS ON THE TREATMENT OF BLEEDING PEPTIC ULCER

Cranston W. Holman, M.D., New York, N. Y.

(From the Department of Surgery of The New York Hospital and Cornell University Medical College)

"THE principle established in wounds of war and accidents of civil life—that active hemorrhage must be controlled before progress can be made in saving life—is equally applicable in the type of hemorrhage under discussion." In these words, Dr. Heuer summarized his opinion concerning the treatment of a patient who was then rapidly being exsanguinated by a bleeding peptic ulcer. This patient had been admitted to the surgical ward four days previously, several hours after having vomited a pint or more of blood. The day following admission, his condition seemed improved, the blood pressure had stabilized, and he was content with the somewhat restricted diet. Unfortunately, on the following morning when the nurse delivered the breakfast tray, the patient was found pale, anxious, and in a cold sweat. At the sight of food he promptly vomited a basinful of blood. A transfusion restored the blood pressure, but only for a short time, and, in spite of continuous blood administration, the patient gradually failed, lapsed into coma, and died twenty-four hours later—five days after the onset of bleeding. Quite obviously, he had lost blood more rapidly than was possible to replace it. As in the past, it was expected and found at autopsy that the patient had bled from a sizable vessel, the pancreaticoduodenal, which lay in the base of a calloused ulcer on the posterior duodenal wall.

The sequence of events in this patient is typical of several that we witnessed each year under a conservative therapeutic regime for massive hemorrhage. Following the sadly similar results in two other patients admitted to the hospital in successive weeks, Dr. Heuer suggested a survey be made of our results in the treatment of bleeding ulcer, in the hope that from such a study, an improved program of therapy might be formulated for the use of the resident staffs. This first survey[1, 2] not only served to focus attention on bleeding ulcer and emphasize its gravity, but also led us to abandon conservative treatment in favor of immediate operation for certain groups of patients.

The primary purpose of this paper is to compare the results under this more radical therapy (adopted in 1940) with the results under the earlier conservative therapy (1932 to 1939, inclusive). Although such a report is valuable chiefly to those directly concerned with its source material, this one may claim a wider interest since it is free from the variables that distort a comparison of results from different clinics: (1) differences in professional skill, (2) variations in the class of patient, and (3) inconsistencies in the interpretation of what constitutes a severe hemorrhage or a satisfactory

This study was supported in part by the United Hospital Fund of New York.

therapeutic result. In the cases in this report, only the therapy was changed. The patients all were ward patients, all had such severe bleeding that they had to be hospitalized, and their care was directed by supervised resident surgeons, all trained by the same standards.

During the earlier period, from 1932 to 1939, inclusive, all patients admitted because of severe hemorrhage from ulcer (161 in number) were treated in a more or less standard, conservative way. This consisted of complete bed rest, nothing by mouth, adequate sedation, and supportive parenteral fluids until it was evident that the bleeding had stopped. Those who continued to bleed under this treatment or who were near exsanguination on admission also received repeated small blood transfusions. A few patients who continued to bleed after prolonged therapy, five in number, were operated upon as a last resort. During this period, twenty-one patients died—a mortality of 13 per cent—a fair average of other reported results (Table I).

TABLE I. MORTALITY

AUTHOR*	NUMBER OF CASES	DEATH	MORTALITY PER CENT
Aitken	255	27	11.0
Allen and Benedict[3]	138	20	14.5
Babey and Hurst	82	4	5.0
Burger and Hartfall	137	31	22.5
Chiesman	191	48	25.0
Conybeare†	600	22	3.7
Christiansen	289	23	7.9
Davies and Nevin	391		21.0
Fowler and Hurevitz	72	17	23.0
Hellier	202	30	14.8
Meulengracht	273	3	1.0
Thorstad	208	21	10.0
Umber	433	41	9.5
New York Hospital	161	21	13.0

*References in this table accompanied by superior figures will be found in the regular Reference list; the remainder are listed in *References to Table I.*

†Conybeare stated that the mortality from hemorrhage in chronic ulcers is between 5 and 10 per cent.

It was quite obvious that, although most patients recovered satisfactorily under this treatment, a not insignificant number, 13 per cent, would die unless more active measures were taken to control the bleeding.

The first problem was one of recognizing those patients who would not benefit from conservative treatment. Critical analysis of our patients revealed a definitely poor prognosis for two groups: those who failed to improve within twenty-four to forty-eight hours after they had been placed on a strict medical regime (in this series 48 per cent of these patients died if conservative treatment were continued), and those who suffered the first hemorrhage while they were under a strict medical regime for a heretofore uncomplicated ulcer. (In the first period, there were six of these patients, five of whom died under conservative therapy and one of whom recovered following immediate gastric resection for control of hemorrhage.) Since there has been little comment in the literature about the latter type of patient, the following case history may serve as an example.

CASE REPORT

A man, 49 years old, had had recurrent bouts of epigastric postprandial pain for five years. Three days before admission to the hospital, he developed severe, persistent, epigastric pain associated with nausea, but no vomiting, hematemesis, or melena. Physical examination was not remarkable except for tenderness and some muscle spasm in the epigastrium. Hemoglobin was 110 per cent; red blood cells 6 million; stool showed no blood.

A diagnosis of penetrating ulcer was made, and the patient was given a restricted diet with complete relief of symptoms in twenty-four hours.

Seven days after admission, the patient suddenly felt weak and several hours later passed several tarry stools. Twenty-four hours later he felt greatly improved, and the blood studies showed hemoglobin of 60 per cent and red blood cells of 3 million. The condition remained unchanged for four days, when suddenly, on the twelfth day after admission, he vomited about one pint of blood and went into shock. During the next forty-eight hours the patient continued to bleed, and, in spite of numerous blood transfusions, he developed signs of bronchopneumonia and died.

Autopsy revealed a huge ulcer situated on the posterior wall of the duodenum, adherent to the pancreas. The ulcer crater measured 3 cm. in diameter, and in its base was a large eroded vessel, which on dissection proved to be the pancreaticoduodenal artery.

In addition, it was found that the age of the patient might have a significant bearing on the prognosis. In general, the older the patient the higher the mortality,[3-5] in patients under 30 years of age the mortality was 6 per cent, in contrast to 20 per cent in those 50 years and older.

In view of these findings, it was decided that, in the future, any patient who fell into either of the two groups described, particularly if he were over 40 years of age, would be operated upon immediately if the condition in any way warranted the risk. It might be said that an analysis of the clinical course of the patients who had died revealed that, with few exceptions, there was a period when operation might have been done with a reasonable hope of success.

A survey of the period from 1940 to 1946, inclusive, when the newly instituted treatment was followed, showed a most gratifying fall in the mortality from the previous 13+ per cent to 5+ per cent. During this time, 206 patients were hospitalized because of bleeding, 11 of whom died. Of these, 19 were operated upon during active bleeding, with 4 deaths, a mortality of 20 per cent. (Two of these fatalaties were patients operated upon late in the course of the bleeding, after nine and twenty-seven days, respectively.) Of the total, 84 patients were operated upon after recovery from bleeding, with a 3.6 per cent mortality; 96 were discharged from the hospital without operation.

The success of this treatment depends upon (1) an early recognition of those patients who will not respond to conservative therapy, and (2) operation on these patients as soon as possible after the onset of bleeding, preferably within forty-eight hours. It should be emphasized that, once it has been decided to operate for control of active bleeding, any delay with the hope that the patient will spontaneously stop bleeding only increases the risk of surgery.

Finsterer[6] maintained that the optimum time for surgery on the actively bleeding ulcer is within forty-eight hours after onset of hemorrhage. Following that rule, he reported an operative mortality of 5 per cent in contrast to a

30 per cent mortality if operation is delayed. Others, as Gordon-Taylor[7] and Oliani,[8] had similar experience. Our experience is even more striking: 10 per cent mortality for those operated upon early; 70 per cent for those operated upon late.[9] It would almost seem that, if for some reason operation is delayed and is then later contemplated as a means of last resort to save the patient's life, it might be better to hope instead that the patient is one of the 50 per cent who recover on conservative therapy.

As to the type of surgical procedure to choose: even though these patients are critically ill and appear none too robust for extensive operative procedures, gastric resection is tolerated surprisingly well if a large amount of blood is given before, during, and after operation. Certainly, resection is the ideal procedure to insure both immediate control of bleeding and a satisfactory permanent result. Indirect methods, such as gastroenterostomy and plastic procedures on the duodenum, have been found of little value.[10]

In the postoperative period, special effort should be made to restore the hemoglobin to a normal level as quickly as possible. Since the diet is necessarily restricted, and since, in addition, many patients have been on a limited diet for long periods before the onset of bleeding, parenteral vitamins should also be given. Penicillin should be administered both before and after operation.

It is possible at this time also to make a preliminary report on a five-year follow-up study on all patients hospitalized for bleeding. As is well known, a true evaluation of the therapeutic results in peptic ulcer can scarcely be made until after five years of observation, and a longer period is preferable. All the patients reported on in this follow-up study were admitted to the hospital five years or more before because of bleeding; no patient is included in this report merely on the basis of a previous history of bleeding.

Table II summarizes the patients studied. Three groups are of particular interest: (1) of the 134 patients who were discharged from the hospital after recovery from the bleeding without operation, 5 (3.7 per cent) died from

TABLE II. BLEEDING PEPTIC ULCER, FIVE-YEAR FOLLOW-UP

TREATMENT	NUMBER	RESULT	NUMBER
No operation	134	Asymptomatic	32
		Bleeding	66
		Pain	31
		Death from bleeding	5
Gastroenterostomy	14	Asymptomatic	5
		Bleeding	7
		Pain	1
		Death	1
Pyloroplasty	1	Asymptomatic	0
		Bleeding	1
		Pain	0
		Death	0
Gastric resection	53	Asymptomatic	46
		Bleeding	2
		Pain	5
		Death	0

recurrent hemorrhage; 66 (50 per cent) had recurrence of the bleeding; 31 (23 per cent) had sufficient pain to require continued medical therapy; and only 32 (24 per cent) are free from pain and bleeding. (2) In contrast, of the 53 patients on whom a gastric resection was performed, none died; only 2 (3.8 per cent) had recurrence of bleeding; 5 (9.4 per cent) had pain; and 46 (87 per cent) are asymptomatic. (3) Of the 15 patients who had indirect operative procedures performed, such as gastroenterostomy or pyloroplasty, 1 (6.6 per cent) died from recurrent bleeding; 7 (46 per cent) had recurrence of bleeding; 1 (6.6 per cent) had pain; and 5 (33 per cent) are asymptomatic. In a somewhat similar group of 29, who were hospitalized because of bleeding but in whom either a gastroenterostomy or pyloroplasty had been done in the past, it was found that 24 had recurrence of bleeding, 2 had pain, and 3 are asymptomatic.

These findings, and the findings of others,[3, 11, 12] may help to formulate a policy for the management of those patients who have recovered from the hemorrhage that brought them to the hospital. That over 50 per cent of these patients will bleed again, a few fatally, and that 75 per cent will have symptoms that require medical attention, are potent arguments for surgical therapy. However, other factors, such as the duration and location of the ulcer and its previous response to medical therapy, must also be considered. Although each individual case must be judged on its own merits, it would seem reasonable to advise operation on those patients who have been known to have a symptomatic ulcer, particularly if they are men over 40 years of age.

Gastric resection, with an expected satisfactory result in 85 per cent of the cases, certainly offers the best protection against future hemorrhage. Lesser procedures, excluding vagotomy about which we have no information as yet, are patently not advisable. The respective percentages speak for themselves: recurrent bleeding in less than 5 per cent after gastric resection, in contrast to 45 per cent after the lesser procedures.

REFERENCES

1. Holman, C. W.: Severe Hemorrhage in Gastric and in Duodenal Ulcer: Study of Ninety Cases, Arch. Surg. **40**: 150-160, 1940.
2. Holman, C. W.: Treatment of Bleeding Peptic Ulcer, Internat. Clin. **3**: 164-170, 1940.
3. Allen, A. W., and Benedict, E. B.: Acute Massive Hemorrhage From Duodenal Ulcer, Ann. Surg. **98**: 756, 1933.
4. Bulmer, E.: The Mortality From Hematemesis: Analysis of Five Hundred and Twenty-Six Cases, Lancet **2**: 168, 1927; Mortality From Hematemesis: Supplementary Analysis, ibid. **2**: 720, 1932.
5. Hinton, J. W.: Massive Hemorrhage in Peptic Ulcer, Ann. Surg. **101**: 856, 1935.
6. Finsterer, H.: Operative Treatment of Severe Gastric Hemorrhage of Ulcer Origin, Lancet **2**: 303, 1936.
7. Gordon-Taylor, C.: Problem of Bleeding Peptic Ulcer, M. Press **202**: 313-319, 1939.
8. Oliani, E.: Ulteriori 200 casi di intervento per ulcera gastrica duodenale, Policlinico **38**: 288-291, 1931.
9. Heuer, G. J.: The Surgical Aspects of Hemorrhage From Peptic Ulcer, New England J. Med. **235**: 777-783, 1946.
10. Nielsen, N. A.: About the Choice Between Medical and Surgical Treatment of Ulcus Ventriculi and Duodeni, Acta chir. Scandinav. **55**: 57, 1923.
11. Westermann, J. J.: Surgical Aspects of Bleeding Gastric and Duodenal Ulcers, Ann. Surg. **101**: 1377, 1935.
12. Jordan, S. M., and Kiefer, E. D.: Complications of Peptic Ulcer: Their Prognostic Significance, J. A. M. A. **103**: 2004, 1934.

References to Table I

Aitken, R. S.: The Treatment of Profuse Bleeding From the Stomach and Duodenum, Lancet 1: 839, 1934.

Babey, A. M., and Hurst, A. F.: The Incidence, Mortality and Treatment of Hemorrhage in Gastric, Duodenal and Anastomotic Ulcer, Guy's Hosp. Rep. **86**: 129, 1936.

Burger, G., and Hartfall, S. G.: Hematemesis in Peptic Ulcer, Guy's Hosp. Rep. **84**: 197, 1934.

Chiesman, W. E.: Mortality of Severe Hemorrhage From Peptic Ulcers, Lancet 2: 722, 1932.

Conybeare, J. J.: Prognosis of Gastric and Duodenal Ulcer, Lancet 2: 1017, 1935.

Christiansen, T.: On Massive Hemorrhage in Peptic Ulcer, Acta med. Scandinav. **84**: 374, 1935; Uremia as Cause of Death in Massive Hemorrhage From Peptic Ulcer, ibid. **85**: 333, 1935.

Davies, T. A. L., and Nevin, R. W.: Prognosis of Hematemesis: Statistical Review, Brit. M. J. 2: 858, 1934.

Fowler, W. M., and Hurevitz, H. M.: Bleeding Peptic Ulcer, J. Iowa M. Soc. **25**: 115, 1935.

Hellier, F. F.: Etiology and Mortality of Hematemesis, Lancet 2: 1271, 1934.

Meulengracht, E.: Behandlung von Hamatemesis und Melana mit uneingeschranker Kost, Wien. klin. Wchnschr. **49**: 1481, 1936.

Thorstad, M. Jordan: The Problem of the Bleeding Peptic Ulcer, SURGERY **12**: 964, 1942.

Umber, F.: Zur Prognose und Behandlung grosser Ulkusblutungen, Deutsche med. Wchnschr. 2: 1265, 1935.

ROLE OF THE GLOSSOPHARYNGEAL NERVE IN THE CAROTID SINUS REFLEX IN MAN; RELIEF OF CAROTID SINUS SYNDROME BY INTRACRANIAL SECTION OF THE GLOSSOPHARYNGEAL NERVE

BRONSON S. RAY, M.D., AND HAROLD J. STEWART, M.D., NEW YORK, N. Y.

(From the Departments of Surgery and Medicine of The New York Hospital and Cornell University Medical College)

THE complexity of the anatomic arrangement and the physiologic reactions of the carotid sinus reflex in man have raised many questions, one of which is the role of the glossopharyngeal nerve. In an earlier report[1] it was shown that although certain transitory effects in blood pressure and cardiac rate followed intracranial division of the nerve for relief of pain, subsequent procainization of the homolateral carotid sinus showed the same qualitative effects as occur normally when the sinus is procainized. In 1944 the results of intracranial division of the glossopharyngeal nerve in two patients with hypersensitive carotid sinus reflexes were reported[2] and the present communication is an amplification of that earlier account. These experiences throw additional light on the mechanism of the reflex and indicate a method of treatment which has certain advantages over local denervation of the carotid sinus. With one exception[20] there appears to have been no other experience with division of the glossopharyngeal nerve for correction of the hypersensitive carotid sinus reflex.

While a detailed review of the many contributions to the knowledge of the carotid sinus reflex in experimental animals and in man is unnecessary for this discussion a brief account of certain aspects bears repetition.

The carotid sinus comprises the first portion of the internal carotid artery and perhaps short contiguous portions of the common and external carotid arteries. Specialized nerve endings in the walls of these vessels are sensitive only to stretch or pressure while others respond only to chemical stimulation. Impulses arising from chemical stimulation may be dependent upon the adjacent carotid body[3] whereas impulses resulting from stretch or pressure traverse direct afferent pathways. The afferent nerves of the reflex arc pass centrally to connect with many autonomic efferent pathways. While there are undoubtedly many other afferent mechanisms contributing to autonomic effects, most observers feel that the carotid sinuses and the aortic arch with their associated carotid and aortic bodies exert a major regulatory influence on the central cardiovascular and respiratory control. Stimulation of the sinus by chemical means, by increased pressure from within or by direct pressure from without, causes the heart rate to slow, the blood pressure to fall, and respirations to increase at least until compensated for by other mechanisms.

Normally, constant stimuli from the carotid sinuses exert a tonic inhibitory effect on autonomic centers.[4] When abnormal sensitivity of a sinus reflex exists in man the evidence indicates that the increased afferent impulses result in a variety of symptoms of autonomic overactivity depending on which of the efferent pathways are implicated. In persons more severely afflicted, one of the prominent symptoms is syncope. Through the contributions of Weiss and his associates[5] the syndrome of carotid sinus syncope is well established. The diagnosis is made from the history and from reproduction of the attack by pressure over the abnormal carotid sinus. On the basis of changes in cardiac rate and blood pressure and on the effects of certain drugs on these manifestations during stimulation of the carotid sinus, three types of the syndrome have been described[5]: (1) the "vagal type" in which syncope results from cerebral anoxia due to reflex cardiac asystole, (2) the "depressor type" in which syncope results from cerebral anoxia due to fall in systemic blood pressure alone, and (3) the "cerebral type" in which syncope ensues without significant change in cardiac rate or in blood pressure. The first type is by far the commonest.

Surgical removal of the nerve plexus from the walls of the carotid sinus and from the Y of the common carotid bifurcation has been commonly practiced for relief of hypersensitive carotid sinus. This operation is designed to sever all afferent nerve connections and has a fair degree of success but has sometimes failed apparently because of incomplete removal of all nerves or because of local nerve regeneration.

There are four nerves which contribute to the innervation of the carotid sinus and adjacent carotid body, namely, the glossopharyngeal, vagus, cervical sympathetic, and hypoglossal. The branch to the hypoglossal is inconstant and the part played by this nerve is probably not important. The other three nerves show considerable variation in their gross anatomic arrangements but great constancy in their connections to the carotid sinus and the intercarotid plexus. Embryologically the mesoderm of the third branchial arch artery and the ectoderm of the glossopharyngeal nerve possess an early juxtaposition in the region which is the anlage of the carotid body and carotid sinus; elements from the sympathetic and the vagus enter only at a comparatively late stage of development.[6] From anatomic dissection[7] it has been shown that a distinct and constant branch of the glossopharyngeal nerve connects with the sinus and intercarotid plexus. The importance of this nerve is supported by its striking constancy in all species of animal.[8]

On the basis of animal experimentation Hering[9] believed that the reflex from the carotid sinus was transmitted by a branch of the glossopharyngeal nerve which he named the "sinus nerve" (also known as the nerve of Hering). De Castro[10] on the other hand concluded, as a result of his investigations, that impulses from the carotid sinus reach medullary centers partly through the glossopharyngeal nerve but more particularly by way of the vagus. Kahn[11] believed from his studies on dogs that the main afferent pathway from the carotid sinus is through the glossopharyngeal nerve but on some occasions the vagus takes part. Others[12, 13] have postulated a three-fold afferent supply through the glossopharyngeal, vagus, and sympathetic nerves. Wright[14] believed connections also existed with the hypoglossal nerve. Code and Dingle's investigations[15] designed to settle the discrepancies of previous workers led them to conclude that in dogs the glossopharyngeal connections of the carotid sinus nerve transmit the bulk of the cardiovascular components of the sinus reflex.

Bucy[16] in 1936 raised the question of the possibility that in man interruption of the carotid sinus nerve by intracranial section of the glossopharyngeal nerve could be expected to alter the systemic blood pressure. He cited his experiences with four cases in which the glossopharyngeal nerve was divided intracranially for relief of glossopharyngeal neuralgia and reported a subsequent rise in blood pressure of a few days' duration in each. The conclusions which these observations implied are that in man the major afferent impulses of the sinus reflex are transmitted through the glossopharyngeal nerve.

In a report[1] we made in 1942 it was shown that temporary rises in blood pressure and cardiac rate followed intracranial division of the glossopharyngeal nerve for pain in three cases but no changes occurred in a fourth case. In fifteen additional cases since that time transient rise in blood pressure and cardiac rate have been similarly observed in all but three after intracranial division of the glossopharyngeal nerve. In most of these cases the return of blood pressure and cardiac rate to the preoperative level occurred in one to three days. This is in slight contrast to Bucy's report which showed a return of the blood pressure to normal over a longer period. The resumption of normal blood pressure and cardiac rate is obviously the result of compensation by other regulatory mechanisms, only a part of which is the contralateral carotid sinus reflex.

From additional observations[1] it was shown that postoperatively pressure over the carotid sinus on the side of the nerve section caused no alteration in blood pressure or cardiac rate. However, procainization of the carotid sinus on the side of the nerve section caused a rise in blood pressure similar to that which occurs characteristically with the intact carotid sinus reflex, although the response was quantitatively less than is usually seen. In the cases reported, the procainization tests were made one and five years, respectively, after operation but similar tests have since been made on two other patients two and three weeks, respectively, after intracranial division of the glossopharyngeal nerve and the same effects noted. Therefore, the question of regeneration is eliminated. Also, procaine in an amount equal to that used in blocking the carotid sinus was injected into the trapezius muscle in the latter two patients and no change occurred in the blood pressures or cardiac rates, thus excluding the possible factor of systemic action of the procaine.

These observations indicated, therefore, that in man the afferent impulses of the carotid sinus reflex are not transmitted solely through the glossopharyngeal nerve though the study does not differentiate between other possible pathways for impulses arising from pressure and chemical stimuli. A single observation in another case suggested the vagus nerve as an additional pathway for these impulses. In one patient (Case 13, previously reported)[1] traumatic paralysis of the vagus nerve at the jugular foramen had occurred at the time of intracranial division of the glossopharyngeal nerve. Postoperative procainization of the homolateral carotid sinus did not result in elevation of blood pressure and cardiac rate as had been seen when the test was employed in the presence of an intact vagus nerve after glossopharyngeal nerve section.

An unusual clinical syndrome linking the glossopharyngeal nerve to the carotid sinus reflex has come to attention in the combined glossopharyngeal tic douloureux and cardiac arrest. The first two cases of this kind were reported briefly in 1942 by Riley and associates[17]; another case (unpublished) of Browder's[18] was observed by one of us (B.S.R.) in 1942, and a fourth case has been reported by us.[19] In this syndrome paroxysms of pain occur in the pharynx and base of the tongue in the region supplied by the glossopharyngeal nerve and simultaneously there is cardiac slowing or arrest, fall in blood pressure, and sometimes syncope. Atropinization of the patient will abolish the cardiac effects, and division of the glossopharyngeal nerve intracranially abolishes the entire syndrome.

With so much evidence pointing to the important role of the glossopharyngeal nerve in the carotid sinus reflex in man, but with insufficient evidence to conclude that this nerve alone comprised the principal afferent pathway in the case of the hypersensitive carotid sinus syndrome, the crucial experiment called for intracranial division of the nerve in a patient with the syndrome. In 1942 Herbert and associates[20] briefly reported their experiences with division of the glossopharyngeal nerve in a 64-year-old man with a hypersensitive carotid sinus. Their observations up to fifteen days postoperative showed the carotid sinus reflex previously induced by pressure over the sinus was abolished on the side of the nerve section.

The following are accounts of three cases in which the glossopharyngeal nerve was divided intracranially on one side for relief of the carotid sinus syndrome.*

CASE REPORTS

CASE 1.—W. R. (Hist. No. 144171), a 71-year-old man, admitted to the New York Hospital in October, 1942, had suffered occasional attacks of syncope for ten years and during the several weeks prior to admission the attacks had increased in frequency from one to four per day. The attacks were characterized by sudden feeling of dizziness, weakness, and confusion. All attacks came while he was walking and although he never fell he often felt that he might were he unable to sit down or hold on to a support. After a few minutes the faintness would pass leaving him with palpitation and a throbbing pain in the top of the head. The whole episode lasted ten to fifteen minutes.

The physical examination disclosed little of significance besides generalized arteriosclerosis. The carotid arteries were sclerotic and moderately enlarged, particularly on the right side in the region of the sinus. The heart was slightly enlarged to the left but otherwise normal. The blood pressure was 124/80 and the form of the electrocardiogram was essentially normal.

Special preoperative tests made with the patient in sitting position were:

1. Pressure over the left carotid sinus caused slowing of the auriculoventricular discharge with blocking of the P wave for four beats then ventricular escape, followed by prompt return to normal sinus rhythm on release of pressure (Fig. 1, *A*). There was a fall in blood pressure, feeling of dizziness, and near syncope.

2. Pressure over the right carotid caused asystole for six seconds followed by ventricular escape, then prompt return to normal rhythm on release of pressure (Fig. 1, *B*). There was a fall in blood pressure and complete syncope.

3. The administration of atropine (0.0006 Gm.) intravenously produced incomplete vagal release. Because of his age the dose was not increased. At the height of the atropine effect, pressure on the left carotid sinus (Fig. 1, *C*) induced very slight slowing of the sinus rate with slight fall in blood pressure. Pressure on the right carotid sinus (Fig. 1, *D*) induced sinus bradycardia with slight fall in blood pressure. Syncope did not occur.

*Two of these cases were reported by Ray and Stewart in 1943.[2]

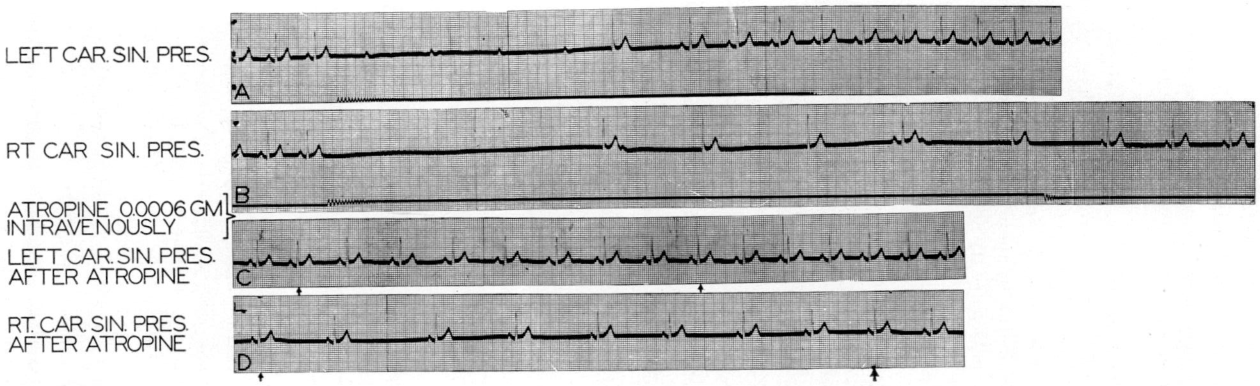

Fig. 1.—In this figure are shown electrocardiograms relating to Case 1 (W.R.). In this figure as well as in those following, the standardization was such that one millivolt produced 1 cm. deflection of the string. Divisions of the ordinates equal 10^{-4} volts. Divisions of the abscissas equal 0.04 second. Lead II is recorded in all instances. In this and the following figures the signal at the bottom of the record indicates when pressure was applied and when released. *A* shows the electrocardiogram taken during pressure over the left carotid sinus. *B* shows Lead II taken during right carotid sinus pressure. *C* shows the effect of left carotid sinus pressure and *D* the effect of right carotid sinus pressure after 0.0006 Gm. atropine intravenously. In *C* and *D* arrows indicate the onset and offset of pressure.

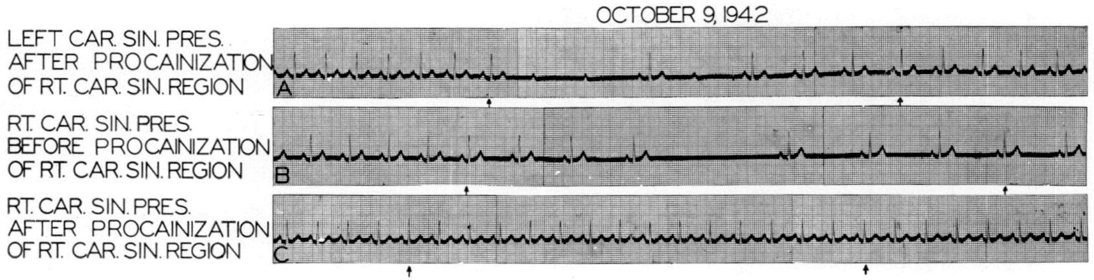

Fig. 2.—In this figure are shown data relating to Case 1. *A* shows the effect of pressure on the left carotid sinus (unanesthetized) after procainization of the right carotid sinus region. *B* shows the electrocardiogram taken during pressure on the right carotid sinus before procainization of this region, and in *C* the electrocardiogram was taken during pressure on the right carotid sinus after its procainization. In this figure arrows indicate the beginning and end of pressure.

4. After procainization of the right carotid sinus region there was slight rise in blood pressure and cardiac rate. Response to pressure on the left (unanesthetized) carotid sinus (Fig. 2, *A*) was the same as on previous occasions. Pressure on the right (anesthetized) sinus did not cause change of any kind (Fig. 2, *C*), whereas pressure applied to this sinus before its procainization showed it to be hypersensitive (Fig. 2, *B*).

At operation (October, 1942) the right glossopharyngeal nerve was divided intracranially. There was only slight transitory rise in blood pressure and increase in cardiac rate following division of the nerve. Recovery from operation was prompt and uncomplicated.

Immediately following operation and during the four and one-half years since operation, pressure over the right carotid sinus (on the side of the nerve section) has failed to cause any alteration in cardiac rate (Fig. 3, *A*), blood pressure, respirations, or state of consciousness. Sensitivity of the left carotid sinus has remained unaltered from its preoperative state (Fig. 3, *B*). In the five years since operation there have been a few mild attacks of faintness which are believed due to the hypersensitivity of the left sinus but the attacks have not been of sufficient degree to require section of the other glossopharyngeal nerve.

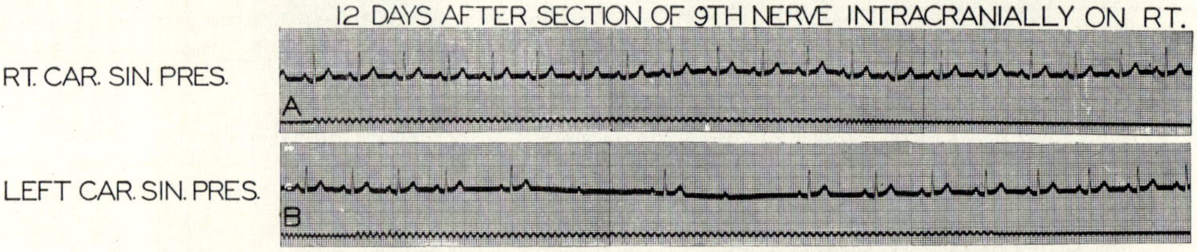

Fig. 3.—In this figure are shown data relating to Case 1. *A* shows the effect of pressure over the right carotid sinus after section of the right ninth nerve intracranially, and *B* the effect of pressure over the left carotid sinus at this time.

Postoperative procainization of the right carotid sinus (on the side of the nerve section) caused a rise in blood pressure of twenty points systolic and five points diastolic without change in cardiac rate. At another time, injection of the deltoid muscle with an equal amount of procaine did not cause any change in blood pressure or cardiac rate, thus eliminating the possibility of any systemic effect of the procaine in producing the changes noted with the former injection.

Case 2.—G. S. (Hist. No. 347441), a 78-year-old man, admitted to the New York Hospital in February, 1944, had for five years experienced syncope whenever a moderate swelling just beneath the angle of the right jaw was deliberately or inadvertently pressed upon. The attacks were characterized by a momentary feeling of swooning followed by loss of consciousness and falling unless he was supported.

The physical examination revealed only generalized arteriosclerosis in a man otherwise well preserved and in good physical condition. The carotid arteries were sclerotic and on the right side the carotid sinus was about twice normal size. The latter enlargement corresponded to the swelling of which the patient was aware. The heart was slightly enlarged to the left but otherwise normal. The blood pressure was 160/90. The form of the electrocardiogram, except for left axis deviation, was within normal limits.

Special preoperative tests made with the patient in sitting position were:

1. Pressure over the left carotid sinus caused ventricular asystole for eight seconds during which there were two or three auricular contractions (Fig. 4, *A*). The blood pressure fell and there was a feeling of dizziness but no syncope.

2. Pressure on the right carotid sinus caused marked sinus bradycardia followed by asystole for four and six-tenths seconds followed by ventricular escape after which, on release of pressure, there were two nodal beats before return to normal (Fig. 4, *B*). The blood pressure fell and complete syncope with a few convulsive twitchings occurred followed by prompt recovery on release of pressure.

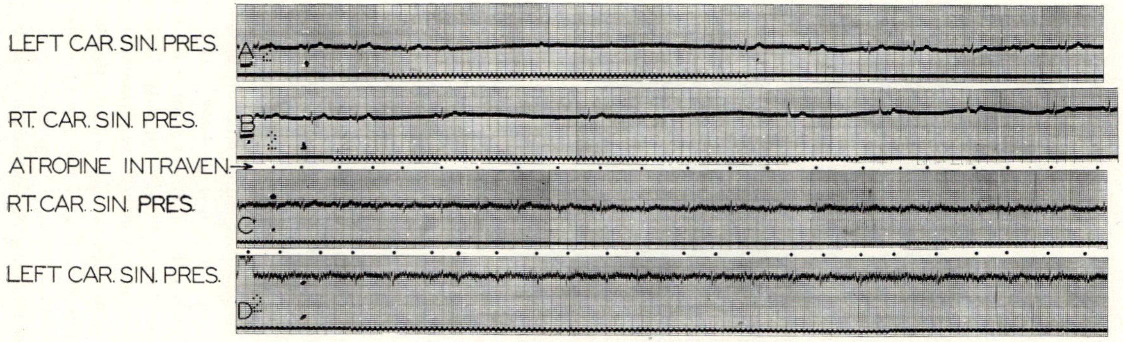

Fig. 4.—In this figure are shown data relating to Case 2 (G.S.). *A* shows the effect of pressure over the left carotid sinus, and *B* of pressure over the right carotid sinus. *C* and *D* show the effect of pressure over the right and left carotid sinuses, respectively, after the administration of 0.0009 Gm. atropine intravenously. In *C* and *D* dots identify the QRS complexes as there were muscle tremors wi.h the patient sitting up in bed.

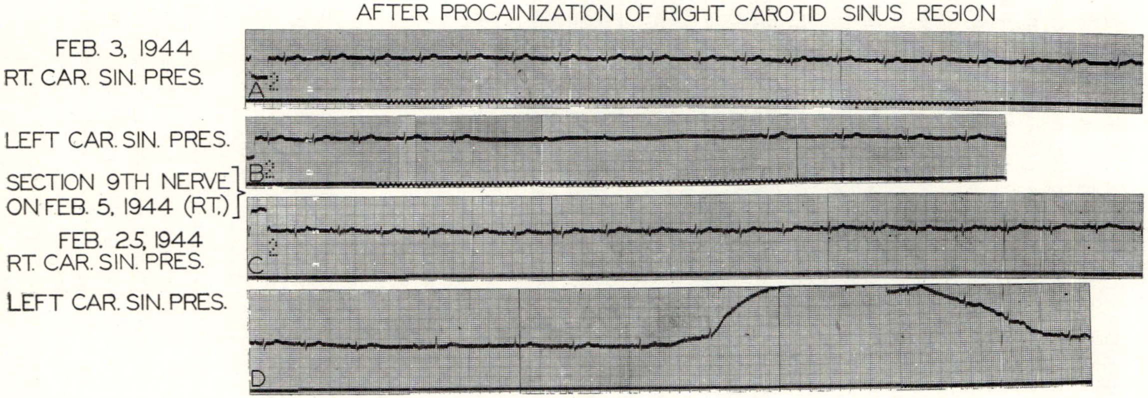

Fig. 5.—In this figure are recorded other data relating to Case 2. In *A* and *B* are shown the effects of pressure over the right and over the left carotid sinus, respectively, after procainization of the right carotid sinus region. In *C* and *D* are recorded the effects of pressure on the right and on the left carotid sinuses, respectively, twenty days after section of the right glossopharyngeal nerve intracranially.

3. The administration of atropine (0.0009 Gm.) intravenously abolished all effects of pressure over the right (Fig. 4, *C*) and the left (Fig. 4, *D*) carotid sinuses.

4. After procainization of the right carotid sinus region there was a rise of fifteen points in systolic pressure and slight increase in cardiac rate. Response to pressure on the right anesthetized sinus caused no change of any kind (Fig. 5, *A*), while pressure on the left unanesthetized carotid sinus was the same as on previous occasions (Fig. 5, *B*).

At operation (February, 1944) the right glossopharyngeal nerve was divided intracranially. There followed a prompt rise in blood pressure from 160/90 to 220/120 and a gradual return to normal over the next twelve hours. There was no change in cardiac rate. Recovery from operation was prompt and uncomplicated.

During the three and one-half years since operation the patient has had none of the former attacks of syncope and no longer protects himself against pressure over the enlarged right carotid sinus. Massage and pressure over the right carotid sinus on the side of the nerve section cause no alteration in cardiac rate (Fig. 5, *C*), blood pressure, respirations, or state of consciousness as long as the pressure does not occlude the internal carotid. The responses to pressure over the left carotid sinus, as compared to the preoperative responses, were the same or of less degree when tested on numerous occasions (Fig. 5, *D*).

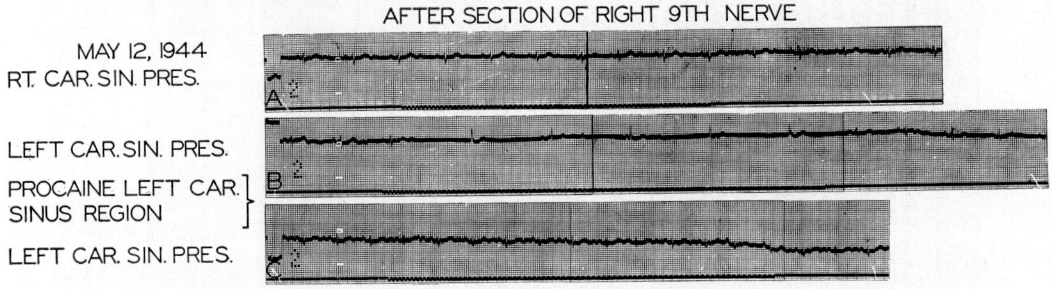

Fig. 6.—In this figure also are shown data relating to Case 2. In *A* is shown the effect of pressure over the right carotid sinus region, and in *B* the effect of pressure over the left carotid sinus region eleven weeks after section of the right glossopharyngeal nerve intracranially. *C* records the effect of pressure over the left carotid sinus after procainization of the left carotid sinus region.

However, in the early postoperative period it was found that with the patient in sitting position heavy pressure over the right carotid sinus, on the side of the nerve section, of sufficient degree to occlude the internal carotid for six to ten seconds sometimes caused a fall in systolic pressure of forty to fifty points without altering cardiac rate or state of consciousness.

Three months postoperatively pressure over the right carotid sinus had no effect on heart rate (Fig. 6, *A*) or on blood pressure. The left carotid sinus possessed the same degree of sensitivity as before operation (Fig. 6, *B*). After a control record was taken (Fig. 6, *B*) anesthetization of the left carotid sinus region (on the side opposite the nerve section) with 24 c.c. of 1 per cent procaine produced a complete Horner's syndrome, marked deviation to the left of the protruded tongue, pronounced hoarseness, and difficulty in swallowing indicating paralysis of the sympathetics, hypoglossal, vagus, and presumably the glossopharyngeal nerves. With the beginning of these effects, blood pressure rose from 170/100 to 236/120 then shortly dropped to 75/50 followed by pallor, sweating, and mental confusion. The electrocardiogram during this period showed no significant change in cardiac rate or rhythm. The head was lowered and after twenty minutes the symptoms of shock passed and the blood pressure rose abruptly to 240/120. The neurologic signs of complete anesthetization of the carotid sinus region were still present and now with the patient in sitting position, massage and pressure insufficient to occlude the artery were applied over the procainized carotid sinus; this did not produce any change in cardiac rate (Fig. 6, *C*), blood pressure, or state of consciousness. However, when heavy pressure was made sufficient to occlude the internal carotid artery for eight seconds, the systolic pressure fell from 230 to 180, although cardiac rate and state of consciousness remained unaltered. This latter response was comparable to the fall in systolic pressure observed on occlusion of the right internal carotid artery following division of the glossopharyngeal nerve on that side.

Comment.—The postoperative tests demonstrate two things. In some patients following either denervation of the carotid sinus by glossopharyngeal nerve section or procainization of all local nerve connections, compression of the sinus may cause fall in blood pressure, apparently the result wholly of carotid occlusion and unrelated to the carotid sinus reflex. This observation may have a bearing on the "depressor type" of sinus reflex, which may not in all cases be due to the sinus reflex but to anoxia of the brain from carotid occlusion. It would likewise invalidate pressure over the carotid artery as a test of the completeness of carotid sinus denervation in some cases.

The test also demonstrates the inability of bilateral carotid sinus denervation (glossopharyngeal nerve section on one side and procainization of the sinus region on the other) to prevent shock from procaine reaction.

CASE 3.—E. C. (Hist. No. 463127), a 74-year-old man, admitted to the New York hospital in December, 1946, had had about twenty-five attacks of syncope in the previous two and one-half years. The attacks came without warning, usually when standing but occasionally when sitting. After a fleeting sensation of faintness he would fall but always recovered in a matter of seconds and seem none the worse for the experience. During one attack he had hurt his head in a fall and this led to his consulting a physician who made the diagnosis of carotid sinus syndrome by compressing the left carotid sinus and reproducing an attack.

The physical examination revealed only arteriosclerosis compatible with his age. The carotid arteries were not remarkable on palpation. The heart was only slightly enlarged to the left. The blood pressure was 162/92. The electrocardiogram showed only moderate changes in the T waves and RT segments compatible with coronary artery disease. The electroencephalogram was normal.

Special preoperative tests made with the patient in sitting position were:

1. Pressure over the left carotid sinus caused complete auriculoventricular block for eighteen seconds with only one auricular contraction in that time (Fig. 7, *A*). The systolic blood pressure fell from 140 to 86 and the patient became semi-conscious.

2. Pressure over the right carotid sinus caused moderate slowing of the cardiac rate from 79 to 40 per minute (Fig. 7, *B*). The blood pressure fell from 140 to 115 and there was no syncope.

3. The administration of atropine (0.0009 Gm.) intravenously abolished the alteration in cardiac rate following pressure over the right (Fig. 7, *C*) and the left (Fig. 7, *D*) carotid sinus almost entirely but not the fall in blood pressure. Syncope did not occur. A repetition of the tests on the following day showed that the left carotid sinus (Fig. 7, *F*) remained more sensitive than the right (Fig. 7, *E*).

4. On Dec. 10, 1946, pressure over the right (Fig. 8, *A*) and left (Fig. 8, *B*) carotid sinus showed that the left remained more sensitive than the right. After procainization of the left carotid sinus region there was a rise in systolic blood pressure from 115 to 150 and in cardiac rate from 79 to 84. Pressure over the anesthetized left sinus (Fig. 8, *C*) was unaccompanied by any changes, while pressure over the right sinus caused the same changes as noted on previous occasions (Fig. 8, *D*).

At operation (January, 1946) the left glossopharyngeal nerve was cut intracranially. There was a prompt rise of twenty-five points in systolic pressure but none in the diastolic pressure and after two days the systolic pressure resumed its preoperative level. There was no change in cardiac rate. Recovery from operation was uncomplicated.

After operation, on repeated tests the responses to pressure over the right sinus were

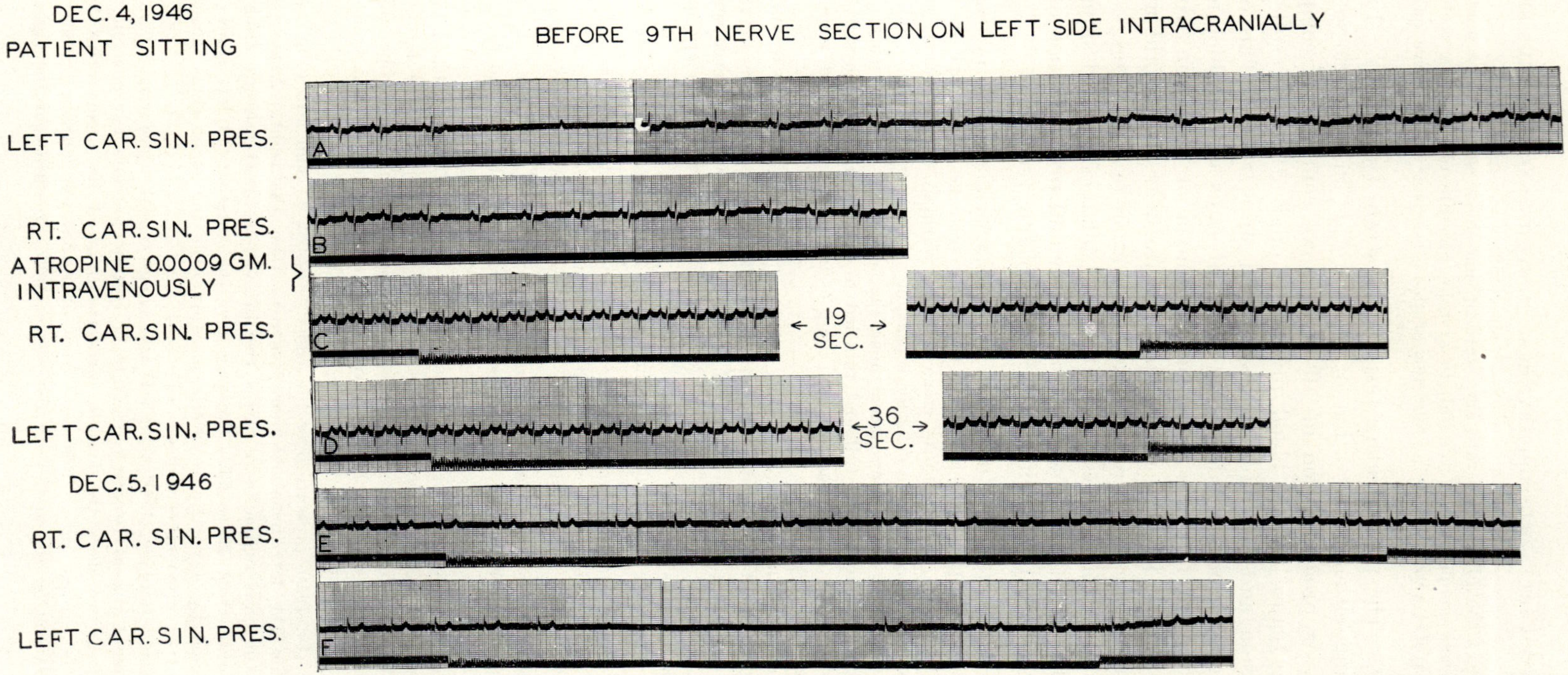

Fig. 7.—This figure as well as Figs. 8 and 9 record data relating to Case 3 (E.C.). *A* shows the effect of pressure over the left carotid sinus, and *B* of pressure over the right carotid sinus. *C* and *D* show electrocardiograms during pressure over the right and over the left carotid sinuses, respectively, after the administration of 0.0009 Gm. atropine intravenously. *E* and *F* show the effect of pressure over the left and over the right carotid sinuses, respectively, on the following day, after the atropine effect had worn off.

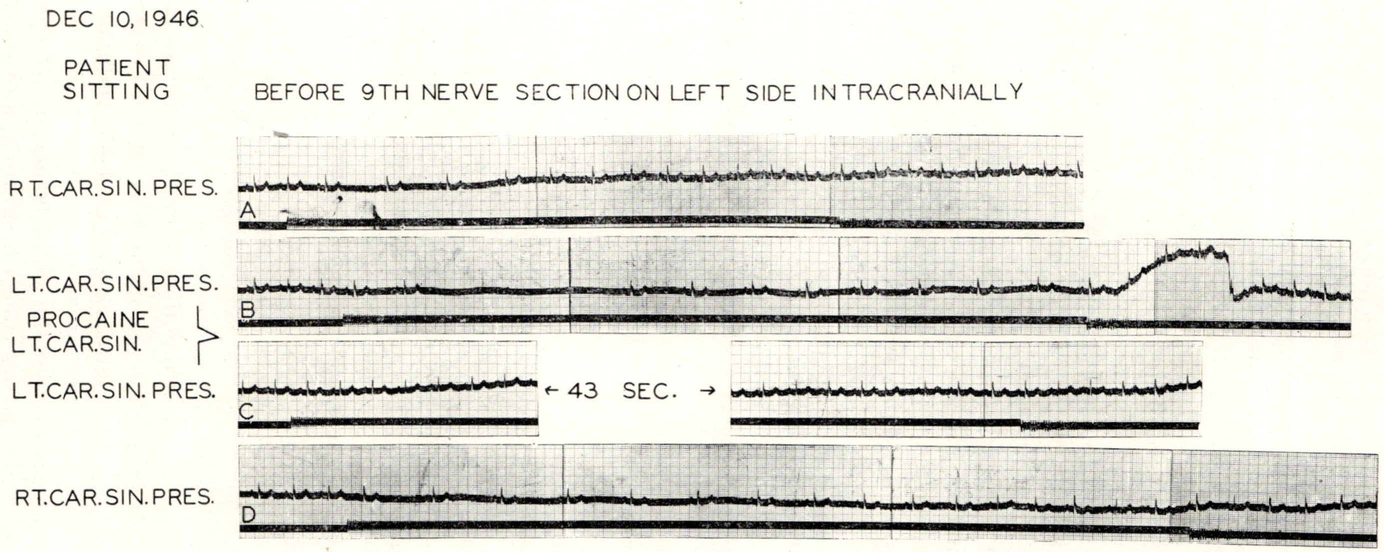

Fig. 8.—In *A* and *B* are shown the effect of pressure over the right and over the left carotid sinus, respectively, on Dec. 10, 1946, in Case 3. *C* and *D* record the effect of pressure over the left and over the right carotid sinuses after procainization of the left carotid sinus.

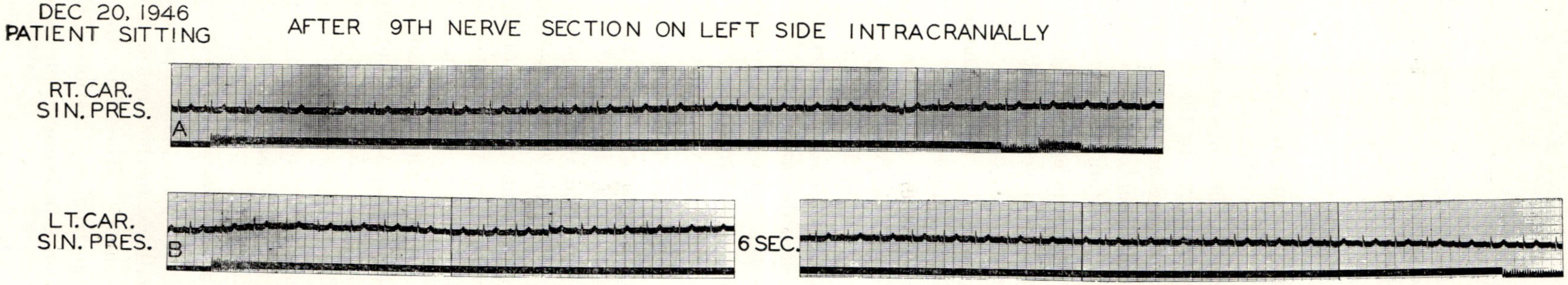

Fig. 9.—In this figure are shown observations made on Dec. 20, 1946, in Case 3 after section of the left glossopharyngeal nerve intracranially. *A* and *B* show the effect of pressure on the right and on the left carotid sinuses, respectively.

unaltered (Fig. 9, *A*) while responses to pressure over the left carotid sinus (on the side of the nerve section) (Fig. 9, *B*) were found to have been entirely abolished. In the eight months since operation there have been no spontaneous attacks of syncope.

In an effort to explore the effect of glossopharyngeal nerve section on the chemically induced component of the carotid sinus reflex the following test was made on one patient (Case 2).

Three months following intracranial division of the right glossopharyngeal nerve the findings on pressure over each carotid sinus were unaltered from those present early in the postoperative period. Pressure over the left carotid sinus caused cardiac slowing, fall in blood pressure, and dizziness, while pressure over the right sinus (on the side of the nerve section) caused no effects except slight fall in systolic pressure sometimes when the artery was occluded.

Sodium cyanide (0.35 c.c. of 2 per cent solution) was injected in the right antecubital vein and the interval until a sudden clear-cut respiratory reaction occurred was timed. This interval was twenty-two seconds and presumably corresponded to the time required for circulation from the right forearm to the carotid sinuses.

The left carotid sinus region (on the side opposite the glossopharyngeal nerve section) was injected with 25 c.c. of 1 per cent procaine. This resulted in rise in blood pressure from 180/90 to 230/120, moderate increase in cardiac rate, complete left Horner's syndrome, hoarseness, difficulty in swallowing, and marked deviation to the left of the protruded tongue. Pressure over the left carotid sinus had no effect on blood pressure, cardiac rate, or state of consciousness. In other words there was paralysis of the left carotid sinus reflex, the cervical sympathetics, and the vagus and hypoglossal nerves.

In this state of paralysis of the entire left carotid sinus mechanism and its connecting nerves, plus paralysis (by previous intracranial section) of the right glossopharyngeal nerve, the injection of sodium cyanide in the same amount and at the same site was repeated. The interval of time from injection to respiratory response was twenty-one seconds and the degree of the response was the same as that of the control injection. Under the conditions of the experiment it was not possible to determine changes accurately in cardiac rate and blood pressure, but if there were changes they were not marked.

If the site of action of sodium cyanide in producing the respiratory response is at the carotid sinus, as is maintained by Robb and Weiss,[21] this test would indicate that a large part if not all of the chemically induced portion of the carotid sinus reflex must traverse pathways other than the glossopharyngeal nerves, namely, by way of the vagus, the sympathetics, or the hypoglossal. It is likely that the carotid bodies play a part in the chemically induced reflex but for the purposes of this experiment the carotid sinus and carotid body and their interrelated nerve supply may be considered as one mechanism. Investigations on experimental animals[22] have shown that the aortic bodies are affected similarly to the carotid bodies by the stimulating effects of cyanide and other chemicals. Therefore, the respiratory response in this case could theoretically come from stimulation of the aortic bodies but the time interval of the response is more in keeping with stimulation of the carotid sinus. The matter might be settled if the same test were repeated after additional blocking of the right vagus nerve below the carotid sinus, but the bilateral vagus nerve block would be hazardous because of the resulting bilateral laryngeal nerve paralysis.

DISCUSSION

Following the stimulus of the work of Weiss and his co-workers[5] on the clinical aspects of the normal and abnormal carotid sinus reflex in man, surgical resection of the intercarotid plexus and stripping of the carotid bulb were rather widely employed in patients with hypersensitive carotid sinus reflex. Initial enthusiasm over the operation has become leavened somewhat by its failure to relieve syncope and convulsions in all cases in which it was employed. Nerves are believed to regenerate sometimes and occasional accidents to the carotid artery are known to have occurred. Obviously some cases have been poorly selected for operation and in our experience a relatively small number of patients presumed to have an abnormally sensitive carotid sinus reflex requires surgical intervention.

Although extensive investigations have been made on experimental animals of the contributions of the various nerves in the afferent arc of the carotid sinus-carotid body reflex, the experiences could not be reliably correlated to the human being. Considerable indirect evidence existed to indicate that the glossopharyngeal nerve and its branch, the "carotid sinus nerve," played a major role in this reflex although anatomic connections to the sinus of two other cranial nerves and the sympathetics have been reliably demonstrated.[7, 23] The intracranial division of the glossopharyngeal nerve in patients with the carotid sinus syndrome has positively shown that all the effects resulting from pressure on the sinus are transmitted by this nerve. Additional evidence indicates that probably the chemically induced component of the reflex is transmitted principally by nerves other than the glossopharyngeal. Since the carotid sinus syndrome appears to be largely if not wholly due to pressure stimuli, selective division of the glossopharyngeal nerve is ideally suited to those patients requiring surgery.

Because of the fact that the carotid sinus nerve joins the glossopharyngeal nerve near the base of the skull, and sometimes within the jugular foramen,[7] division of the nerve through a cervical incision is not practical. As a neurosurgical procedure, intracranial division of the glossopharyngeal nerve is relatively simple and safe and the resulting anesthesia in the glossopharynx is unnoticed by the patient. Regeneration of the nerve is impossible and an additional advantage is that the hypersensitive reflex can be interrupted in those cases of carotid body tumor, other cervical neoplasms, aneurysms, tuberculous nodes, infection, and irradiation scarring where local dissection may be precluded.

CONCLUSIONS

1. The glossopharyngeal nerve transmits the afferent impulses of the carotid sinus reflex induced by pressure on the carotid sinus.

2. Intracranial division of the glossopharyngeal nerve permanently abolishes the effects of pressure on the homolateral carotid sinus.

3. The chemically induced part of the carotid sinus reflex probably remains intact after intracranial division of the glossopharyngeal nerve.

4. As an alternative procedure to local denervation of the carotid sinus for relief of the carotid sinus syndrome, intracranial glossopharyngeal nerve section has an advantage in that the former procedure may be followed by regeneration of the nerves and possesses the hazard of damage to the carotid artery.

5. Intracranial division of the glossopharyngeal nerve can be employed in patients in whom the condition of the local tissues about the carotid sinus might make local surgery undesirable or impossible.

REFERENCES

1. Ray, B. S., and Stewart, H. J.: Observations and Surgical Aspects of the Carotid Sinus Reflex in Man, SURGERY **11**: 915-938, 1942.
2. Ray, B. S., and Stewart, H. J.: The Treatment of Hypersensitive Carotid Sinus by Glossopharyngeal Nerve Section. Transactions of the Harvey Cushing Society, Neurosurg. **1**: 338-339, 1944.
3. Heymans, C., and Rijlant, P.: Le courant d'action du nerf du sinus carotidien intact, Compt. rend. Soc. de biol. **113**: 69-73, 1933.
4. Bronk, D. W., and Stella, G.: Response to Steady Pressures of Single End Organs in Isolated Carotid Sinus, Am. J. Physiol. **110**: 708-714, 1935.
5. (a) Weiss, S., and Baker, J.: The Carotid Sinus Reflex in Health and Disease: Its Role in Causation of Fainting and Convulsions, Medicine **12**: 297-354, 1933.
   (b) Weiss, S., Capps, R. B., Jr., Ferris, E. B., Jr., and Munro, D.: Syncope and Convulsions Due to Hypersensitive Carotid Sinus Reflex; Diagnosis and Treatment, Arch. Int. Med. **58**: 407-417, 1936.
6. Boyd, J. D.: Observations on Human Carotid Sinus and Its Nerve Supply, Anat. Anz. **84**: 386-399, 1937.
7. Sheehan, D., Mulholland, J. H., and Shafiroff, B.: Surgical Anatomy of the Carotid Sinus Nerve, Anat. Rec. **8**: 431-442, 1941.
8. Ask-Upmark, E.: Carotid Sinus and Cerebral Circulation. Anatomical, Experimental, and Clinical Investigation, Including Some Observations on Rete Mirable Caroticum, Acta, psychiat. et neurol., supp. 6, pp. 1-374, 1935.
9. Hering, H. E.: Carotid Pressure Reflexes, München. med. Wchnschr. **71**: 1265-1266, 1924.
10. de Castro, F.: Ueber die Struktur und Innervation des Glomus caroticum beim Menschen und bei den Säugetieren. Anatomisch-experimentelle Untersuchungen, Ztschr. f. d. ges. Anat. **89**: 250-265, 1929.
11. Kahn, R. H.: Die Blutdruckregler, Ztschr. f. d. ges. exper. Med. **68**: 201-215, 1929.
12. Danielopolu, D., Marcu, I., Proca, G. G., and Aslan, A.: Les zones reflexogenes carotidiennes, Presse méd. **35**: 1585-1588, 1927.
13. Heymans, C., Bouckaert, J. J., and Regniers, P.: Le Sinus Carotidien, Paris, 1933, Gaston Doin & Company.
14. Wright, S.: Lecture on Recent Work on Afferent Control of Circulation in Health and Disease, Brit. M. J. **1**: 457-462, 1932.
15. (a) Code, C. F., and Dingle, W. T.: The Carotid Sinus Nerve, Proc. Staff Meet., Mayo Clin. **10**: 129-132, 1935.
   (b) Code, C. F., Dingle, W. T., and Moorhouse, V. H. K.: The Cardiovascular Carotid Sinus Reflex, Am. J. Physiol. **115**: 249-260, 1936.
16. Bucy, P. C.: Carotid Sinus Nerve in Man, Arch. Int. Med. **58**: 418-432, 1936.
17. Riley, H. A., German, W. J., Wortis, H., Herbert, C., Zahn, D., and Eichna, L.: Glossopharyngeal Neuralgia Initiating or Associated With Cardiac Arrest, Tr. Am. Neurol. A., pp. 28-29, 1942.
18. Browder, E. J.: Unpublished case observed by Ray.
19. Ray, B. S., and Stewart, H. J.: Glossopharyngeal Neuralgia: A Cause of Cardiac Arrest, Am. Heart J. (In press.)
20. Herbert, C., Zahn, D., Ryan, J., and Echlin, F.: Treatment of Carotid Sinus Sensitivity by Intracranial Section of the Glossopharyngeal Nerve, Tr. Am. Neurol. A., pp. 29-30, 1942.
21. Robb, G. P., and Weiss, S.: A Method for the Measurement of the Velocity of the Pulmonary and Peripheral Venous Blood Flow in Man, Am. Heart J. **8**: 650-670, 1933.
22. Schmidt, C. F., and Comroe, J. H., Jr.: Functions of the Carotid and Aortic Bodies, Physiol. Rev. **20**: 115-157, 1940.
23. Tchibukmacher, N. B.: Surgical Anatomy of the Carotid Sinus Nerve and Inter-Carotid Ganglion, Surg., Gynec. & Obst. **67**: 740-745, 1938.

END RESULTS IN THE TREATMENT OF PEPTIC ULCER BY POSTERIOR GASTROENTEROSTOMY

William A. Cooper, M.D., New York, N. Y.

(From the Department of Surgery of The New York Hospital and Cornell Medical College)

INTRODUCTION

IN THE forty-eight years since Doyen first performed posterior gastroenterostomy for peptic ulcer, this operation has been performed on many thousands of patients. After a period of development, the procedure came to be used with enthusiasm, and, in this country, during the period from 1910 to 1930, it was the surgical method most commonly employed for treating peptic ulcer. For a brief period the pyloroplasty (either Judd or Finney) was used in certain clinics, but it was never a serious competitor of gastroenterostomy. Up to 1930 most surgeons in this country reserved gastric resection for gastric lesions, either ulcer or cancer, although Billroth, von Haberer, and Finsterer on the continent, and Berg and Lewisohn in this country had advocated gastric resection for duodenal ulcers, particularly those in the active stage of bleeding. As the failures of gastroenterostomy became more numerous, and chronic marginal ulcers and their complications accumulated in the large clinics of this country, there was a gradual shift toward gastric resection. This change, and the conviction that gastric resection gave better results, became general during the period from 1930 to 1940. With experience, improved techniques, better pre- and postoperative care, and chemotherapy, surgeons learned to perform gastric resection with a reasonable mortality. In most clinics today gastroenterostomy is in disrepute, and has been replaced largely by the more radical procedure. The younger group of surgeons, particularly, have come to feel that gastroenterostomy is a faulty operation, and that anything short of a resection will yield a poor result. Among the more seasoned groups of surgeons are still to be found those who champion gastroenterostomy, and use it frequently. Between these two groups there is considerable controversy over the relative merits of the two procedures.

Today, the end results of a new surgical treatment for peptic ulcer, vagotomy, are being projected into this old controversy. Unless vagotomy clearly proves to be the panacea that all those interested in this field have long looked for, there is reason to believe that the evaluation of gastric operations will be further beclouded. This is particularly true if vagotomy is to be used simultaneously with gastroenterostomy or resection. It is timely, therefore, that we review our past experience and try to evaluate objectively and accurately the long-term end results of gastric operations. The purpose of this paper is not to compare the results of gastroenterostomy and gastric resection, but to give as complete and clear a picture as possible of what one can expect from the older procedure, gastroenterostomy. It is hoped that a review of our experience may give insight and perspective to those performing gastric surgery.

CLINICAL MATERIAL

In the thirteen and one-quarter year period between Oct. 1, 1932 and Dec. 31, 1945, there were 279 posterior gastroenterostomies done for peptic ulcer on the ward services of the New York Hospital. The distribution of these cases over the years is shown in Table I, which lists the number of operations done each year (Column 1), the operative deaths (Column 2), the operative survivors (Column 3), and the cumulative operative survivors (Column 4). Perusal of Column 1 shows that fewer posterior gastroenterostomies were done after 1940. This occurred in spite of a growing volume of gastric cases, for, in keeping with the popular trend, gastric resections were performed more frequently than gastroenterostomies.

METHOD OF REPORTING

The method used for reporting the end results is that which I devised in 1947.* The cases are grouped by follow-up year, irrespective of year of operation, and the poor results occurring in each follow-up year are determined. This enables us to use all of the material and to express end results in the form of a graph. Since a detailed description of this method is available in the reference, only the essentials necessary for following the text will be given in this paper. Briefly, the method is as follows:

1. The clinical material is charted first in Table I, described previously, from which we obtain figures on operative mortality and cumulative operative survivors at the end of each calendar year (Column 4).

2. The figures on cumulative operative survivors are corrected for deaths that occurred during the follow-up period by subtracting the deaths in those cases up to the follow-up year in question. This is shown in Table II, which lists the cumulative operative survivors (from Table I, Column 4), the deaths occurring in those patients up to the respective year of follow-up (Column 2),

TABLE I. LIST OF POSTERIOR GASTROENTEROSTOMIES BY CALENDAR YEAR SHOWING OPERATIVE DEATHS AND SURVIVORS

	COLUMN 1	COLUMN 2	COLUMN 3	COLUMN 4
YEAR OF OPERATION	NUMBER OF OPERATIONS	OPERATIVE DEATHS	OPERATIVE SURVIVORS	CUMULATIVE OPERATIVE SURVIVORS
1932	3	0	3	3
1933	22	2	20	23
1934	35	0	35	58
1935	24	3	21	79
1936	26	2	24	103
1937	25	0	25	128
1938	25	1	24	152
1939	19	0	19	171
1940	16	0	16	187
1941	11	0	11	198
1942	16	1	15	213
1943	32	0	32	245
1944	14	0	14	259
1945	11	0	11	270
Totals	279	9 (3.2%)	270	270 (96.8%)

*Cooper, William A.: A Method of Statistical Analysis, SURGERY 22: 367-379, 1947.

TABLE II. CORRECTION FOR DEATHS DURING FOLLOW-UP PERIOD AND CASES ACTUALLY FOLLOWED

		COLUMN 1	COLUMN 2	COLUMN 3	COLUMN 4
OPERATIVE YEAR	FOLLOW-UP YEAR	CUMULATIVE OPERATIVE SURVIVORS	DEATHS OCCURRING BEFORE F-U YEAR	CUMULATIVE NET SURVIVORS	CASES FOLLOWED EACH FOLLOW-UP YEAR
1932	14	3	1	2	2
1933	13	23	4	19	8
1934	12	58	10	48	31
1935	11	79	14	65	50
1936	10	103	16	87	67
1937	9	128	19	109	81
1938	8	152	21	131	102
1939	7	171	21	150	124
1940	6	187	19	168	143
1941	5	198	18	180	157
1942	4	213	15	198	177
1943	3	245	14	231	208
1944	2	259	8	251	237
1945	1	270	5	265	257
1946	0				

and the cumulative net survivors (Column 1 minus Column 2). *Cumulative Net Survivors* refers to the number of cases possible to follow each year after operation. The number of cases actually followed each follow-up year, irrespective of year of operation, is then obtained and recorded (Column 4). The ratio between *cumulative net survivors* and *cases actually followed* each follow-up year is converted to per cent and recorded as the follow-up curve (see Fig. 1).

3. The poor results or failures of gastroenterostomy are then determined, each failure being recorded in the follow-up year in which the case first became classified as a poor result (Table III, Column 2). In Table III, Column 1 the cases actually followed are listed (from Table II, Column 4), and the ratio of poor results to cases actually followed each follow-up year is recorded as percentage (Column 3). These percentages are accumulated (Column 4), and

TABLE III. POOR RESULTS IN FOLLOW-UP YEARS

	COLUMN 1	COLUMN 2	COLUMN 3	COLUMN 4
FOLLOW-UP YEAR	CASES FOLLOWED EACH FOLLOW-UP YEAR	POOR RESULTS	PERCENTAGE OF POOR RESULTS (COL. 2/COL. 1)	ACCUMULATED PERCENTAGE OF POOR RESULTS
14	2	0	0	25.21
13	8	0	0	25.21
12	31	1	3.2	25.21
11	50	0	0	22.01
10	67	0	0	22.01
9	81	0	0	22.01
8	102	0	0	22.01
7	124	1	0.81	22.01
6	143	0	0	21.20
5	157	4	2.54	21.20
4	177	7	3.96	18.66
3	208	4	1.92	14.70
2	237	10	4.22	12.78
1	257	22	8.56	8.56
0				

are then charted on Fig. 2, *A*, which is the failure curve. The percentage of failures or poor results is thus measured at the level of each follow-up year.

FOLLOW-UP

It is important to know what portion of the cases in the series were followed. This information is charted in Fig. 1, which shows the ratio of cases actually followed to cases that could have been followed for each year after operation.

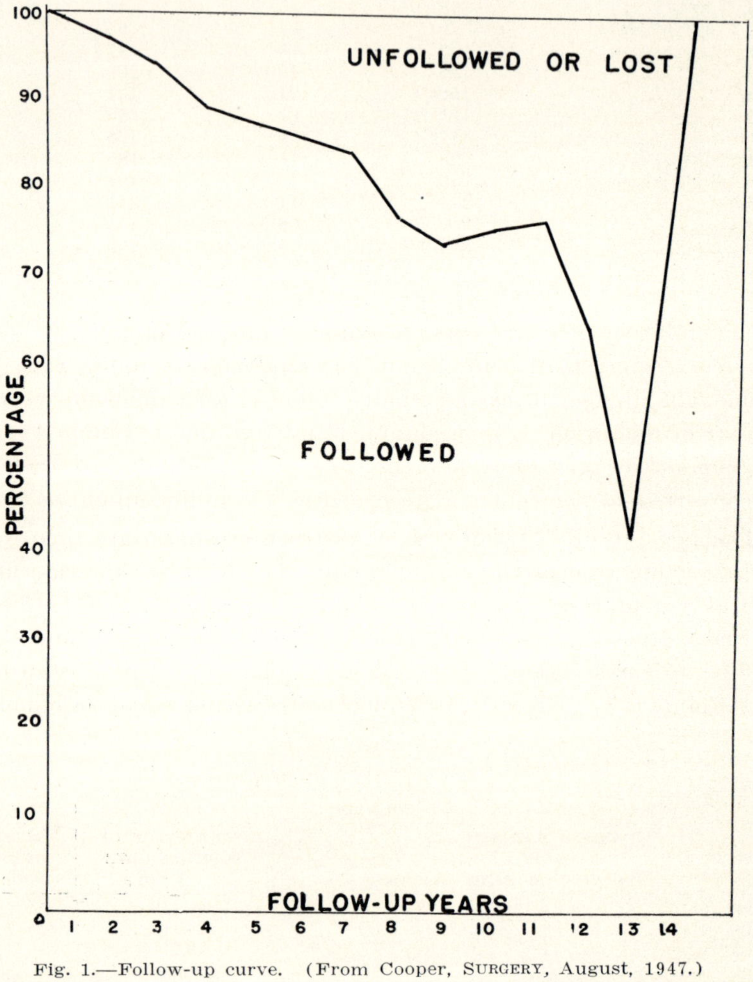

Fig. 1.—Follow-up curve. (From Cooper, SURGERY, August, 1947.)

The percentage above the line is lost, and that below the line is followed. It will be noted that the follow-up decreases from 97 per cent the first year to a low of 42 per cent in the thirteenth year. In the fourteenth year it goes up to 100 per cent, for follow-ups happened to have been carried out on the two patients who were operated upon and survived the fourteen-year period.

It is felt that a follow-up graph, or similar information, is important in any follow-up study, for it tells the reader how much of the total picture the author has been able to observe and report upon. This is particularly true if the author or the reader is to compare two groups of cases. Unless the completeness of the follow-up is similar in two groups of cases, they must be compared with caution.

ANALYSIS OF CASES

The cumulative operative survivors (Table I, Column 4) are divided into good and poor results. For the purpose of this study a poor result is defined as any patient who, at any time after gastroenterostomy, (1) must be rehospitalized for peptic ulcer either in this or any other hospital, or (2) has any evidence, either by history or examination, of bleeding from the upper gastrointestinal tract, or (3) has either clinical or x-ray evidence of a marginal ulcer. This includes all patients having many gastric complaints after gastroenterostomy. It does not include a number of patients with pain, gas, belching, or indigestion, all of a mild or transient nature. These cases are considered satisfactory results. The ratio between good and poor results at the level of each follow-up year is shown in Fig. 2, *A*, the *failure curve.* The figures for the failure curve are listed in Table III.

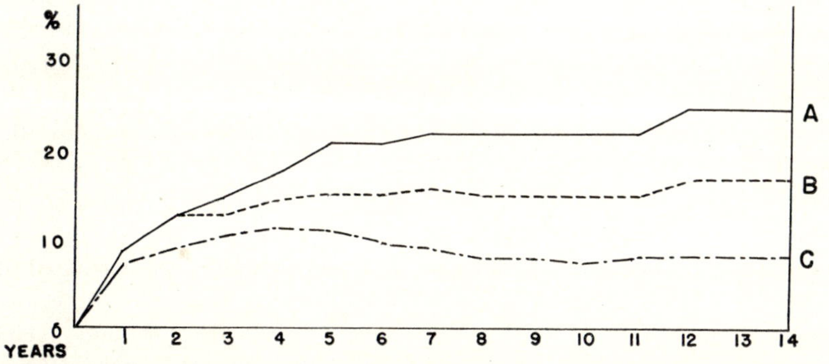

Fig. 2.—Failure curves. *A*, Failure curve; *B*, failure curve after conservative treatment; *C*, failure curve after conservative and operative treatment.

The criteria of a poor result in this study are quite rigid, for any patient having had any notable recurrence *at any time* after operation is considered as having a poor result and charted as such on the failure curve. By the fourteenth year 49 cases are recorded as poor results (Table III, column 2) on the failure curve, each case being represented by the percentage of those followed each follow-up year, irrespective of operative year. It will be noted that 47 of the 49 failures occurred by the fifth year after operation. This strongly supports the view that if a gastroenterostomy does well for five years after operation the chances of continuing to do so are excellent.

A number of the 49 poor results are now classified as good results. Thirteen cases satisfied the criteria of failure, yet subsequently the patients became well, and remain well at the time of this study, without further operative treatment. For these patients gastroenterostomy, considered from the perspective of a good many years of follow-up, has been a highly successful operation. Yet at one time during the postoperative course (within five years of operation) they were considered as having poor results. If this study confined itself to five-year end results, many of these would have to remain poor results. The obvious question that arises is how they should be catalogued now. One can take the view that these cases should not be reported as failures of gastro-enterostomy, yet all will have to concede that whether these cases are reported as good or poor depends upon the year in which the end result study is made. In view of this, I am of the opinion that the truest picture is presented by considering these cases as "once a failure, always a failure" on the primary failure curve, and correcting this pessimistic picture by a second or modified failure curve, on which the poor results that subsequently became good results under conservative treatment are subtracted. This *modified failure curve* gives a true and clear picture of the end results of gastroenterostomy over a period of years. The values on this modified curve, rather than those on the primary curve, are the ones that reflect the long-term end results of the operation.

The failure curve, modified by subtracting the cases that become good without further surgery, is given in Fig. 2, *B*. It will be noted that this curve is flatter than the primary failure curve, and that it is actually reduced slightly from the seventh to the eleventh years. On the basis of this curve we can state that the poor results of gastroenterostomy at the end of five years is 16.3 per cent, at the end of ten years is 16.0 per cent, and at the end of fourteen years is 18.5 per cent.

The constitutional nature of peptic ulcer and the tendency for ulcerations to recur after both conservative and all known operative treatments are well recognized. Therefore, another important consideration in any operation for peptic ulcer concerns the situation in which we leave the patient in regard to subsequent gastric operations that may have to be done if the primary operation fails. This is particularly true in gastroenterostomy because of the well-known tendency to form marginal or jejunal ulcers. The question that arises is how favorable (or unfavorable) is the situation of the patient in whom gastroenterostomy fails. Is his position hopeless or can he be salvaged and put in a condition to enjoy a normal life free of gastric symptoms?

To answer this question the failures of gastroenterostomy after further operative treatment (26 cases) are analyzed. The failure curve modified by both conservative and further operative treatment is given in Fig. 2, *C*. It will be noted that with the benefit of further operative treatment on the patients in whom gastroenterostomy has failed, the net failures are reduced to 8.2 per cent.

METHOD OF MODIFYING THE FAILURE CURVE

To modify the failure curve by cases that subsequently become good results we must calculate the percentage for the modified curve for each follow-up year by the formula:

Cumulative failures : modified cumulative failures :: failure curve percentage : modified failure curve percentage.

TABLE IV. FIGURES FOR MODIFYING THE FAILURE CURVE

	COLUMN 1	COLUMN 2	COLUMN 3	COLUMN 4	COLUMN 5	COLUMN 6
FOLLOW-UP YEAR	CUMULATIVE FAILURES	CUMULATIVE FAILURES MODIFIED BY CONSERVATIVE TREATMENT	PERCENTAGE ON PRIMARY FAILURE CURVE	PERCENTAGE ON FAILURE CURVE MODIFIED BY CONSERVATIVE TREATMENT	CUMULATIVE FAILURES MODIFIED BY CONSERVATIVE AND OPERATIVE TREATMENT	PERCENTAGE ON FAILURE CURVE MODIFIED BY CONSERVATIVE AND OPERATIVE TREATMENT
0						
1	22	22	8.56	8.56	20	7.79
2	32	30	12.78	12.80	24	9.57
3	36	30	14.70	12.24	24	9.80
4	43	35	18.66	15.19	27	11.70
5	47	36	21.20	16.27	24	10.82
6	47	36	21.20	16.27	22	9.94
7	48	36	22.01	16.50	21	9.63
8	48	35	22.01	16.05	18	8.26
9	48	35	22.01	16.05	18	8.26
10	48	35	22.01	16.05	17	7.79
11	48	35	22.01	16.05	17	7.79
12	49	36	25.21	18.54	16	8.24
13	49	36	25.21	18.54	16	8.24
14	49	36	25.21	18.54	16	8.24

The figures for the modified failure curves, *B* and *C*, are given by follow-up year in Table IV which lists the cumulative failures (by adding the cases from Table III, Column 2), the cumulative failures modified by conservative treatment (Column 2—by subtracting the patients who had good results without further surgery), the percentage on the primary failure curve (from Table III, Column 4), the percentage on the failure curve modified by conservative treatment (Column 4), the cumulative failures modified by conservative and operative treatment (Column 5), and the percentage on the failure curve modified by conservative and operative treatment (Column 6).

OPERATIVE MORTALITY AND END RESULTS

In a sense, the first failure of any operative procedure is a death due to operation. In considering which gastric operation to do on a given patient, the surgeon must estimate the chance of survival and the possibility of a satis-

TABLE V. ANALYSIS OF OPERATIVE DEATHS

CASE	AGE (YR.)	OPERATIVE YEAR	POSTOPERATIVE DAY OF DEATH	CAUSE OF DEATH
1. W. M.	67	1933	1st	Massive pulmonary embolus from deep veins of leg
2. N. R.	72	1933	19th	Evisceration and multiple small ulcers in gastric mucosa
3. C. F.	58	1935	4th	Peritonitis
4. E. H.	64	1935	22nd	Massive pulmonary embolus from deep veins of leg
5. M. M.	29	1935	37th	Peritonitis
6. F. M.	76	1936	7th	Bronchopneumonia
7. A. L.	69	1936	3rd	Bronchopneumonia
8. J. C.	51	1938	5th	Bronchopneumonia and cirrhosis of liver
9. C. M.	69	1942	15th	Cerebral thrombosis

factory end result. Therefore, operative mortality must be considered in any gastric operation. Operative mortality is brought into the end result picture in Fig. 3, where the various failures are charted on top of the operative mortality. Thus, we see that the failure of gastroenterostomy at the end of the follow-up period, taking operative mortality into consideration, is 28.4 per cent, that with the benefit of conservative treatment it is 21.7 per cent, and that with the benefit of further operative treatment it is 11.4 per cent. Fig. 3 brings together all of the information related to end results in the entire group of 279 gastroenterostomies done at the New York Hospital.

During the thirteen and one-quarter year period, 279 gastroenterostomies were performed with nine operative deaths, an operative mortality of 3.2 per cent. Details of the operative deaths are outlined in Table V.

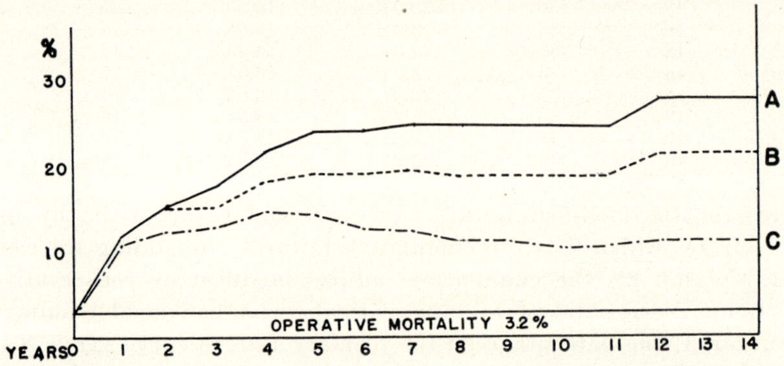

Fig. 3.—Failure curves superimposed on operative mortality. *A*, Failure curve; *B*, failure curve after conservative treatment; *C*, failure curve after conservative and operative treatment.

It will be noted that the operative deaths are fairly evenly divided into three groups: those caused by vascular accidents (Cases 1, 4, and 9); those caused by pulmonary complications (cases 6, 7, and 8); and those caused by peritonitis (Cases 3 and 5). One patient (Case 2) died of evisceration and multiple gastric erosions. With the advances in chemotherapy today it seems likely that the pulmonary and peritonitis deaths (about half of the nine deaths) could be avoided. Perusal of the operative deaths listed in Table I, Column 2 shows that there were but 2 deaths in the last 169 operations done. This evidence supports the view that gastroenterostomy can be done today with an operative mortality of not more than 2 per cent.

ANALYSIS OF POOR RESULTS

Pathology.—There were 49 patients who had unsatisfactory results at some time during the follow-up period after gastroenterostomy. The pathology in those with recurrent symptoms is listed in Table VI.

Many of the patients who eventually proved to have marginal or jejunal ulcer had x-ray findings at one time or another during the course which suggested reactivation of the original duodenal ulcer. Yet in all patients in whom the pathology was proved, except the last three listed, reoperation or repeated

TABLE VI

PATHOLOGY	NUMBER OF CASES
Marginal or jejunal ulcer	37
(2 also had gastrojejuno colic fistula, 1 also had a new gastric ulcer)	
Suspected but not proved marginal ulcer	9
Gastric ulcer (primary ulcer duodenal)	1
Gastric ulcer which persisted	1
Duodenal ulcer which persisted	1
Total	49

x-rays have proved them to have a marginal or jejunal lesion. One patient with primary duodenal ulcer had a gastric ulcer that accounted for the recurrent symptoms; one patient with primary gastric ulcer had a fatal hemorrhage three weeks after gastroenterostomy; in only 1 case in the 49 failures did the patient prove at operation to have a persistent duodenal ulcer after gastroenterostomy. Three months after the primary operation this patient had a bleeding episode for which a pylorectomy was done. The duodenal ulcer was removed, but the stoma failed to function, and was resected three weeks later. No marginal lesion was found. This patient developed a marginal ulcer at the site of the new stoma, which later perforated and was the cause of death. This patient continued to have poor results after two operative procedures since the unsuccessful gastroenterostomy. In no other case in this entire series was the pathology proved to be reactivation or persistence of the duodenal ulcer. In every other case in which the pathology was established by reoperation, the original duodenal ulcer was healed.

Clinical Symptoms.—In the 49 poor results the outstanding clinical manifestations of failure were as shown in Table VII.

TABLE VII

MANIFESTATION	NUMBER OF CASES	PER CENT
Pain only	21	42.8
Hemorrhage only	12	24.6
Pain and hemorrhage	16	32.6
Total	49	100.0

The most common recurrent symptom was pain (75.5 per cent), which was usually intermittent, boring, and relieved by food and alkalies. In most cases the pain was similar to that caused by the original ulcer except for its location. The pain in marginal ulcer is usually a bit lower and to the left of the duodenal ulcer pain, and a patient who has experienced both can often distinguish them. In only two of the patients having recurrent pain as their only symptom was marginal ulcer not proved.

Gastrointestinal hemorrhage followed pain in frequency (57.1 per cent). There were between one and five bleeding episodes after operation, and the clinical manifestations of bleeding varied from a few tarry stools to vomiting of unchanged blood with fatal shock, depending upon the severity of the hemorrhage. In 4 of the 26 patients who bled the hemorrhage was fatal, and in 8 it could be considered mild. Of the 12 who had bleeding as their only recurrent symptom, marginal ulcer was proved in 6, and suspected but not proved in 6.

This brief analysis suggests that when pain becomes a prominent clinical feature after gastroenterostomy, a diagnosis of marginal ulcer is most likely. The most significant physical finding is point tenderness localized in the region of the stoma or the marginal lesion. It is believed that point tenderness, when present, is highly significant in establishing the diagnosis. Nausea and vomiting were often present, but were inconstant, and are not considered of particular diagnostic importance.

Correlation of Symptoms Before and After Gastroenterostomy.—Practically all of the patients had some pain before operation, yet there were 12 who had hemorrhage without pain as the recurrent symptom of failure. There were 19 who had hemorrhage before gastroenterostomy, and 28 who bled after operation. Twelve of these patients had hemorrhage both before and after operation. Seven bled before operation, but not afterward, while 16 bled afterward, and not before. Pain is a more constant finding in the primary ulcers, and hemorrhage a more common occurrence in marginal ulcers, yet there is considerable overlapping of all pre- and postoperative symptoms. There is no particular correlation between primary and recurrent symptoms, nor would one expect there to be such a correlation if the new symptoms are due to a new (marginal) ulcer.

The Diagnostic Value of Roentgenology and Gastroscopy.—It is difficult to evaluate the accuracy of x-ray and fluoroscopic examinations in diagnosing marginal ulcer. The impression exists among clinicians that the method often fails to visualize the marginal or jejunal lesion, yet the clinician too is often mistaken in assuming its presence. This is particularly true of the patients with painless hemorrhage, who may have a negative examination after recovering from the bleeding episode, and who, indeed, may be found to have a normal stoma and a healed duodenal ulcer on exploration. In patients who bleed without pain, and in whom the pain is not persistent, treatment may have healed the superficial lesion before the x-ray studies were done. In this series, particularly those studied in recent years, we have found the roentgenologist quite accurate in diagnosing marginal or jejunal lesions. Although he is not always successful in demonstrating an ulcer crater, accompanying jejunitis or spasm often adds sufficient confirmatory evidence to make the diagnosis reasonably certain. The roentgenologist is not accurate in estimating the activity of the old duodenal lesions. It has been repeatedly borne out in this series that, though he demonstrated a crater in the duodenum, the crater may be healed.

Gastroscopy has not been particularly helpful in diagnosing marginal lesions. The stoma is often partially obscured by the reflux of the jejunal contents, and the overhanging margins and jejunum cannot be clearly visualized. If the stoma does appear normal from the stomach side, an ulcer on the jejunal side cannot be ruled out. Occasionally, however, a marginal lesion will be clearly seen, and visualization may clarify the clinical problem.

Factors Influencing End Results.—Since some patients do very well after gastroenterostomy, and others do equally poorly, there has been a continuous effort to discover the factors that influence this varied response. Some of the factors that have been thought to be pertinent are type of personality, age, nationality, occupation, clinical type of ulcer, and location of ulcer. Though something is known of the psyche in most of the patients in this series, the information is too superficial and spotty to be of value. It is not within the scope of this study to analyze all of the forces that may have influenced end results; age, nationality, clinical type, and location will be considered.

Results in age groups: In the days before gastroenterostomy was relegated to the category of discarded or obsolete operations, one often heard it said that the older rather than the younger age groups did better with the operation. The age distribution of the 270 operative survivors and the 49 failures of gastroenterostomy are shown in Table VIII.

TABLE VIII. AGE DISTRIBUTION OF ENTIRE SERIES AND POOR RESULTS

AGE (YR.)	ENTIRE SERIES	POOR RESULTS	PERCENTAGE OF POOR RESULTS
20-29	9	1	11.1
30-39	78	20	25.6
40-49	98	14	14.3
50-59	56	11	19.6
60-69	22	1	4.5
70-79	7	2	28.6
	Average age 45.95	Average age 44.2	

The table lends but weak support to this view, for the average age in the failures is about the same as in the entire group. In the percentages, however, there is some downward trend of failures in the older decades, except for those in their seventies, in which there are only 7 cases. The 2.7 per cent difference in those above and below 50 years reflects this trend, but the difference is not striking. A larger series might raise these figures to the level of a significant difference.

Results in nationality groups: It has been said that certain races, notably the southern Europeans and Hebrews, tend to do poorly with gastroenterostomy. In this series the racial stock of the entire series and of the failures is as shown in Table IX.

TABLE IX

RACIAL STOCK	ENTIRE SERIES (%)	POOR RESULTS (%)
Hebrews	18.3	24.4
Italians	10.5	16.3
All others	71.2	59.3
Total	100.0	100.0

Though the differences are not striking, they bear out the general impression that the Hebrews and Italians tend to do less well than the other races. There were no notable differences in the other races, so they were grouped together.

Results in clinical groups: Another factor that has been considered of prognostic significance in gastroenterostomy is the clinical type of peptic ulcer. It is frequently said that obstructing ulcers do better than bleeding ulcers. To test the accuracy of this observation, the cases in this series are divided into three clinical groups, and the failures occurring in each group are determined. These groups are those with (1) hemorrhage, (2) obstruction, and (3) pain. It should be emphasized that the division of the cases into these groups is somewhat empirical, for there is considerable overlapping of clinical symptoms. For the purpose of this analysis the groups are defined as follows:

1. Hemorrhage: Cases that have had clinical evidence of bleeding at any time during the preoperative course, regardless of the presence of pain or obstruction. This includes both the serious bleeders, with hematemesis, tarry stools, and shock, and the milder bleeders with occasional tarry stools. It does not include those patients with obstruction or pain who may have occult blood in the stools or some changed blood in the emesis.

2. Obstruction: Cases that have had any appreciable evidence of gastric retention four hours after the barium meal. The x-ray criteria are used because a history of vomiting occurred in so many patients who had no obstruction. There is very little overlapping between those with obstruction and the bleeding group described previously. If the bleeding was a prominent symptom, they were classified as such, regardless of the presence of obstruction.

3. Pain: Cases that had pain, but no bleeding or obstruction. There is great overlapping between the pain cases and the two groups just described, for most patients had pain at some time during the preoperative course.

The distribution of the 270 operative survivors and the 49 poor results is as shown in Table X.

TABLE X

CLINICAL TYPE	CASES	POOR RESULTS	% POOR RESULTS
1. Hemorrhage	76	19	25.0
2. Obstruction	124	19	15.3
3. Pain	70	11	15.7
Total	270	49	

One might postulate that the ulcer that obstructs has demonstrated the greatest tendency to heal, that the ulcer that bleeds has the least tendency to heal, and that the ulcer with persistent pain lies somewhere between these two extremes. One might, with some rationale, group those with persistent pain and those with bleeding together, for in one sense severe hemorrhage is an incident in an active ulcer that depends upon whether or not the active ulcer has eroded a large vessel. But the rate of erosion and the fibrocytic response of the tissues to ulceration must also be factors in bleeding, for all portions of the gastrointestinal tract subject to ulceration are highly vascular. The greater incidence of failures in the hemorrhage group (25 per cent), as compared with the pain and obstruction groups (15 per cent), gives credence to the postulate outlined previously. Of the various clinical factors influencing failure, it appears that bleeding is more important than age or race.

Results in gastric ulcers: So far in this analysis, all operative survivors having gastroenterostomy for ulcer have been grouped together, regardless of the location of the ulcer. The primary pathology in the operative survivors is distributed as shown in Table XI.

Though the operation has not been used extensively on gastric ulcers, the end results in the 18 patients having had gastric or gastric and duodenal ulcer are

TABLE XI

PATHOLOGY	NUMBER OF CASES
Duodenal ulcer	252
Gastric ulcer	15
Duodenal and gastric ulcer	3
Total	270

of interest. There are not enough cases to warrant construction of a separate failure curve, for only 2 of the patients failed to do well. One of these had a large penetrating ulcer high on the lesser curvature, in which the symptoms were pain and vomiting without bleeding. At operation extensive inflammation and induration were found extending up to the esophageal hiatus, and removal of the lesion would have required an extensive procedure. He also had polycythemia vera, and died of a single massive hemorrhage three weeks after gastroenterostomy. The other patient had a duodenal ulcer with almost complete obstruction, a small penetrating gastric ulcer near the angularis, and bilateral pulmonary tuberculosis. Three months after gastroenterostomy a marginal ulcer perforated and was plicated. A secondary resection was done three years later for a persistent marginal ulcer, and this patient has now been well for one year. The remaining sixteen patients (89 per cent) have done well, and the average follow-up period since operation is 5.4 years. The average duration of symptoms before operation was 4.2 years.

The gastric ulcers were all on the lesser curvature, 6 in the lower one-third, 8 in the middle one-third, and 4 in the upper one-third. In most instances, gastroenterostomy was not considered the procedure of choice, but was done because of one or more circumstances that made the surgeon feel the lesser procedure expedient. Among these were age, poor condition of the patient, and local conditions that made resection hazardous. We cannot advocate gastroenterostomy for general use in gastric ulcers, largely because of the difficulty in being certain that the lesion is benign rather than malignant, but it may be that, in these cases, the combined risk of cancer and gastroenterostomy is less than the risk of total resection. There are other clinical situations encountered in which similar reasoning may apply, and in which choice of the lesser procedure may be the wiser decision. The main point to be made from this limited experience is that a gastric ulcer may do very well with gastroenterostomy, that all is not lost if the lesion cannot be resected, and that the surgeon must carefully reflect on these things before he undertakes unwarranted risks.

RESULTS OF TREATMENT OF FAILURES

The results of treatment of the 49 patients with poor results of gastroenterostomy can be summarized as shown in Table XII.

Results of Conservative Treatment.—It should be emphasized that most of the 49 patients with failures of gastroenterostomy received conservative treatment for the symptoms they had after operation. Twenty-six of these came to further operative treatment because this conservative treatment failed, while 10 were not subjected to surgery and remained failures. The net poor results are 36 cases which are charted in Fig. 2, *B*.

TABLE XII

TREATMENT	NUMBER OF CASES	PER CENT
Conservative treatment	23	47
Good results	13	56.5
Poor results	10	43.5
Net failures after conservative treatment*	36	
Operative treatment	26	53.0
Good results	20	77
Poor results	6	23
Net failures after both conservative and operative treatment†	16	

*See Fig. 2, *B*.
†See Fig. 2, *C*.

Of the 13 patients in whom results became satisfactory after conservative treatment, 6 had proved marginal ulcers, 6 had suspected marginal ulcers, and 1 had a gastric ulcer, while the primary ulcer was in the duodenum. These results have now remained satisfactory for an average of 5.2 years.

Of the 10 patients in whom conservative treatment remained a failure, 4 continue to have intermittent pain, 2 continue to have intermittent bleeding of a milder nature, and 4 are dead; 2 died of hemorrhage and 2 died of a perforated marginal ulcer. The fact that 4 of the 10 have died of ulcer emphasizes the risk incident to the prolonged conservative treatment of recurrent symptoms after gastroenterostomy.

Results of Operative Treatment.—Of the 26 patients who submitted to one or more secondary gastric operations, results in 20 are now good and results in 6 remain poor. Analysis of the operations is shown in Table XIII.

It is seen that 36 operations were done on the 26 patients who were treated surgically, with 3 operative deaths (8.3 per cent). Just half of the 26 failures

TABLE XIII. RESULTS OF TWENTY-SIX FAILURES TREATED SURGICALLY

FIRST OPERATION AFTER POSTERIOR GASTROENTEROSTOMY			SECOND OPERATION AFTER POSTERIOR GASTROENTEROSTOMY		
NUMBER OF CASES	TYPE SECONDARY OPERATION	RESULTS	NUMBER OF CASES	TYPE SECONDARY OPERATION	RESULTS
19	Dismantling and secondary gastric resection	Good—13 Poor—5 Operative death—1	→ 1 3 →	Suture of perforated marginal ulcer	Good—1
2	Dismantling and resection of marginal ulcer	Poor—2	→ 8	Secondary gastric resection	Good—6 Poor—2
1	Dismantling and pyloroplasty	Poor—1	↗		
1	Dismantling and jejunal patch	Operative death—1			
1	Ligation of left gastric artery	Poor—1	↗		
1	Plication perforated marginal ulcer	Poor—1	↗		
1	Exploration for hemorrhage	Poor—1	→ 1	Exploration for hemorrhage	Operative death
Total 26	Net good results	13	Total 10	Net good results	7

became good results after the first secondary operation, and 7 out of 10 became good results after the second secondary operation. In all, 20 became good results, and have been so for an average of 3.4 years after one or two surgical procedures following gastroenterostomy.

There were 6 out of 26 results that remained poor. These were 3 operative deaths (see Table XIII), 1 secondary resection that still has a marginal ulcer after one secondary resection, and 2 secondary resections that have marginal ulcers after two secondary resections. 1 of these last patients died of a perforated marginal ulcer.

It would seem clear from the evidence presented that the only effective secondary operation in this series was gastric resection. Every other procedure used in this series failed, except for one perforated marginal ulcer in a patient who has remained symptom-free for two years after simple plication. In all, there were 27 secondary resections done (19 and 8, see Table XIII), with 1 operative death, a mortality of 3.7 per cent.

Out of the original 49 failures of gastroenterostomy, there were 10 results that remained poor after conservative treatment, and 6 that remained poor after further operative treatment, leaving, at the time of writing, a net of 16 failures in the entire series of 270 operative survivors.

We can say that the patient subjected to gastroenterostomy has a 96.7 per cent chance of surviving the operation (and it may be 98 to 99 per cent); that if he does survive, he has a 78 per cent chance of being well thereafter; that he has an 88 per cent chance of being well without further surgery, even though he has some further trouble; that he has a 92 per cent chance of eventually being well, even though he has to have further surgery. In short, his chances of survival and eventually being cured are about 89 per cent.

COMMENT

It is apparent from the failure curve (Fig. 2, *A*) that one can expect about 25.2 per cent of patients after gastroenterostomy to have recurrent symptoms, usually within five years of the operation, and that about one-quarter of these will eventually become well without further surgery (Fig. 2, *B*). From the pathology found in the patients in whom the operation failed, it is clear that, if the recurrent symptoms are persistent, they are, in all probability, due to a marginal ulcer rather than to reactivation or persistence of the primary ulcer. Since most of the primary ulcers in this series (all but 1 gastric and 1 duodenal ulcer) healed after gastroenterostomy, it would appear that the procedure was a very effective method of dealing with the primary lesion. It would seem that much of the talk one hears about reactivation of duodenal lesions after gastroenterostomy is fallacious. Indeed, we are led to the general conclusion that, if the gastroenterostomy functions, the primary duodenal ulcer will heal, whether it be an obstructing ulcer, penetrating ulcer, or bleeding ulcer. The only exception in this series was the case described, in which the stoma functioned poorly. The only other exceptions we have observed (not in this series, occurred late, when involvement of the stoma by the marginal ulcer led to poor function of the stoma, and consequent reactivation of the original duodenal ulcer.

Effective as gastroenterostomy may be for treating the primary ulcer, it is perfectly clear that it often fails to prevent the formation of new ulcers. A more general way of stating this is that it often fails to interrupt the ulcer diathesis. The impression exists that gastric resection is more effective than gastroenterostomy in this regard, but we must not lose sight of the fact that resection also fails in certain cases. From the analysis of the secondary operations done, it is apparent that certain patients have such a marked ulcer diathesis that they do poorly with both gastroenterostomy and resection.

Comment should be made upon the selection of cases for gastroenterostomy in this series from all of the peptic ulcer cases in this hospital requiring operation. From 1932 to 1939 the surgical treatment of choice was gastroenterostomy except for those patients with either gastric ulcer or recent hemorrhage. During that period patients, both good and poor risks, coming to surgery for ulcer had gastroenterostomy. After 1939 resections were done more frequently, and the patients selected for gastroenterostomy were largely those with obstruction and the poor risks. Included in these were patients with extensive inflammation around the lesion and those in whom one would suspect that the ulcer diathesis, or the tendency to recurrence, was strong. In general, in all patients with a history of bleeding resection was done in the later years, while only in the recent and severe bleeders were resections done in the earlier period.

The question that comes to mind is what influence the selective policy after 1939 had on the poor results of gastroenterostomy. In the 171 operative survivors up to and including 1939, there were 36, or 21 per cent, poor results. In the 99 after 1939 there were 13, or 13 per cent, poor results. The percentage of poor results each year in the earlier period varies between 8 and 30 per cent, while that in the later period varies between 0 and 19 per cent (see Table XIV). Although the two groups are not truly comparable because of the shorter follow-up period of the second group, the data tend to support the selective policy. It is evident, however, that even in selected cases gastroenterostomy often fails, and that gastric resection is a stronger, though still imperfect, tool for interrupting the tendency to form ulcers.

TABLE XIV. DISTRIBUTION OF POOR RESULTS BY YEAR OF OPERATION

OPERATIVE YEAR	NUMBER OF POOR RESULTS
1932	1
1933	4
1934	8
1935	6
1936	6
1937	2
1938	7
1939	2
1940	3
1941	1
1942	0
1943	7
1944	2
1945	0
1946	0

It is probably accurate to state that most of the surgeons in this country have come to the feeling that gastroenterostomy is an inadequate and poor operation. This view, and the teachings incident to it, are open to some question in the light of the experience in this series. Until vagotomy has been evaluated, the alternative to gastroenterostomy is usually gastric resection. Had resection been attempted on all the patients in this series, the mortality would have been high, if not formidable, particularly in the group selected for gastroenterostomy since 1939, for among them were the poor risks. A comparative evaluation of gastroenterostomy will have to await the completion of similar studies of end results in gastric resection, but the low mortality and generally favorable outlook reflected in the failure curves strongly supports the view that gastroenterostomy is a useful and often curative procedure which has a definite place in the repertory of gastric surgery. It may be that the passage of time and the accumulation of experience will show that gastroenterostomy, supplemented by vagotomy in the cases where it fails, will give the lowest mortality and the highest incidence of cures.

LATE RESULTS FOLLOWING PERFORATED PEPTIC ULCER

S. W. Moore, M.D., and Robert Hendricks, M.D., New York, N. Y.

(From the Second Surgical [Cornell] Division, Bellevue Hospital)

THE following study was undertaken to determine the end results in patients with perforated peptic ulcers operated upon in a large City Hospital. It has been stated that following suture of a perforated peptic ulcer, the ulcer heals and the patient is cured. There are those who do not agree with this statement and Harrison and Cooper[7] found that 82.5 per cent of patients continue to have symptoms.

One hundred and one patients treated on the Second Surgical (Cornell) Division of Bellevue Hospital from 1928 to 1945 for perforated peptic ulcer have been reviewed and, in particular, the follow-up results have been studied.

Sex.—As in all studies on this subject, males far outnumber female patients with perforated peptic ulcer. In this series there are 97 males and 4 females. There were 6 negroes of which 5 were males and 1 a female.

Age.—Although perforation of a peptic ulcer is reported in the newborn infant[10] and even before birth,[15] the usual age group is between 25 and 50 years. For this series the ages are as shown here:

3	13	21	27	28	8	1
10-20	21-30	31-40	41-50	51-60	61-70	71-80

It will be seen that the age group from 50 to 60 years showed most perforations, 28 in number, and over one-half (or 55) occurred between 41 and 60 years. The youngest patient was 18 and the oldest 71 years of age.

Season of Year.—Although there were more perforations in winter, the fact does not seem significant. There were 23 patients whose ulcer perforated in the fall, 33 in winter, 25 in spring, and 20 in the summer.

Preoperative Bleeding.—It has long been felt that bleeding ulcers do not perforate and that those that perforate do not bleed. Ulcers of the duodenum which perforate usually are on the anterior wall, while those which bleed tend to be on the posterior wall. Estes and Bennett[5] found that 26.9 per cent of perforations showed evidence of bleeding before operation. In this group of 101 perforations, 20 had had preoperative hemorrhage as evidenced by tarry stools or the vomiting of blood.

Chronic Symptoms.—Peptic ulcers may perforate without previous symptoms, however, White and Patterson[19] are correct in stressing the point that careful history taking usually will elicit chronic symptoms. Twenty-three of these patients are reported to have had no chronic symptoms while in the others symptoms had been present for from three months to thirty years. The duration of symptoms is given here:

Cases	13	5	8	8	5	3	10	2	2	6	0	8	3	2	1	1
Years	¼	½	1	2	3	4	5	6	7	8	9	10	15	20	26	30

Acute Symptoms.—At times it is hard to evaluate the onset of acute symptoms caused by a perforated ulcer. The large majority of patients in this series were seen within six hours of the perforation, but one patient came in to the hospital three days after the ulcer perforated.

Time of Perforation.—It is supposed that ulcers perforate most frequently after the consumption of a large meal or after indulgence in alcoholic beverages and that this may account for the higher incidence of perforations in winter. In this series, perforations occurred after eating or drinking in 14 patients, and while in bed in 27; of the latter 8 perforations occurred while the patient was in a hospital bed being treated for symptoms of ulcer. Twenty-four patients were working or walking when the perforation occurred; 9 had taken a laxative before the perforation occurred.

Site of the Ulcer.—The number of duodenal ulcers as compared with gastric ulcers which perforate varies with reports, but the duodenal ulcers usually far outnumber the gastric. Heuer[1] recorded 40 duodenal to 17 gastric, Estes and Bennett[5] 63 duodenal to 16 gastric and Harrison and Cooper[7] 51 duodenal to 6 gastric. Our series of 101 cases shows 17 in the duodenum and 84 in the stomach. Of the 84 ulcers in the stomach, 29 were classified simply as gastric, 42 as prepyloric, 9 as pyloric, and 4 as situated at the cardiac end.

Mortality.—Following operation on the 101 patients there were 18 deaths, an operative mortality of 18 per cent. The relation of mortality to length of time between perforation and operation is interesting. It was found that the mortality under six hours was 11.8; between six and twelve hours, 22.5; between twelve and forty-eight hours, 33.3; and over forty-eight hours, 50 per cent (Table I). This fact has been brought out by Dineen[16] (Table II) and also by Sallick[18] (Table III).

TABLE I. ONE HUNDRED ONE CASES OF PERFORATED PEPTIC ULCER

NUMBER OF CASES	TIME BETWEEN PERFORATION AND OPERATION (HR.)	DEATHS	PER CENT
65	Under 6	8	11.8
17	6-12	4	22.5
9	12-48	3	33.3
2	Over 48	1	50.0
8	Unknown		

This table shows the relation of mortality to length of time between perforation and operation.

TABLE II. RELATIONSHIP OF MORTALITY TO TIME OF OPERATION IN DINEEN'S SERIES (142 CASES)

NUMBER OF CASES	HOURS AFTER PERFORATION	DEATHS	MORTALITY PER CENT
94	Under 6	7	7
32	6-22	11	31
16	Over 22	13	81

TABLE III. RELATIONSHIP OF MORTALITY TO TIME OF OPERATION IN SALLICK'S SERIES (74 CASES)

NUMBER OF CASES	HOURS AFTER PERFORATION	DEATHS	MORTALITY PER CENT
49	6	1	2
13	6-12	2	15
10	12-48	3	30
2	Over 48	2	100

Type of Operation.—In this group of perforations, simple suture was carried out in 98 patients; on 2 a posterior gastroenterostomy was added to simple suture and in 1 omentum alone was used to cover the defect.

Follow-up Studies.—It is difficult to find and follow every patient who comes into a large City Hospital, as many of them have no home nor address. The longest follow-up record in this series is eleven years. In 26 patients there are no follow-up reports. We strongly suspect that in this group of unfollowed cases may be some of our best as well as some of our worst results. Of the entire series, 18 patients died and 26 were not followed; 10 were followed less than six months, 8 more than six months, 11 more than one year, 11 for two years, 5 for three years, 3 for four years, 6 for five years, 1 for six years, 1 for seven years, and 1 for eleven years.

In order to evaluate results, all patients who could be followed were seen and examined; many had x-ray examinations and also, in a large number subsequent operations gave much information. There is no standard method of presenting follow-up studies; our cases were divided into four groups, as follows:

1. Excellent result: no symptoms; able to work; x-ray evidence of healing of ulcer or no ulcer.
2. Good result: mild symptoms controlled by therapy; no loss of time from work because of ulcer; x-ray evidence of healing ulcer.
3. Fair result: symptoms fairly well controlled by therapy; some loss of time from work because of ulcer; x-ray evidence of active ulcer.
4. Poor result: symptoms not controlled by diet; able to do very little work; active ulcer by x-ray examination; repeated hospitalization; operation.

Duodenal Ulcer.—There are in the series 17 patients who had duodenal ulcers which perforated. Two of these patients died, a mortality of 12 per cent. In the surviving patients there were 4 with excellent results, none with good, 3 with fair, 6 with poor results, and 2 in whom follow-up was not possible. By combining the excellent and good results and the fair with the poor results, we have 4 satisfactory and 9 unsatisfactory results. It certainly is clear from this that simple suture of a perforated duodenal ulcer is not the ultimate solution of the problem (Table IV).

Gastric Ulcer.—In the group of gastric ulcers there were 84 perforations. Sixteen of these patients died postoperatively, an operative mortality of 19.0 per cent. In the follow-up records 9 are classified as excellent, 6 as good, 12 as fair, and 17 as poor. In 24 cases there was no follow-up. If we combine these results as in the duodenal group we find 15 which can be considered satis-

TABLE IV. PERFORATED DUODENAL ULCERS
(SEVENTEEN CASES)

RESULTS			NUMBER
Excellent	4	Satisfactory	4
Good	0		
Fair	3	Unsatisfactory	9
Poor	6		
Not followed	2		
Deaths	2		
Mortality	12.0%		

factory and 29 unsatisfactory (Table V). Again, a simple suture of a perforation of gastric ulcers leaves much to be desired. When the causes of the unsatisfactory results are studied, certain facts stand out clearly—namely, that perforation is only one complication in the life history of an ulcer which may include all the major complications such as reperforation, bleeding, obstruction, and intractable pain.

Reperforation.—The complication of reperforation occurs following each type of ulcer and also each type of operation performed. Estes and Bennett[5] found reperforation in 7 of 61 patients treated by simple suture (11 per cent). Williams[6] in 100 cases reviewed, found a secondary perforation in 3 patients after simple suture.

Royster[12] reported a gastric ulcer high on the greater curvature of the stomach in a young woman 23 years of age, which perforated five times. At the second operation, the ulcer and perforation were in the exact site of the previous perforation; however, on 3 subsequent occasions in which a perforation was diagnosed, clinically by x-ray examination because of obliteration of hepatic dullness and gas under the diaphragm, conservative treatment was carried out. This case illustrates three points: (1) that when symptoms of ulcer continue, the ulcer has failed to heal; (2) that perforation and suture do not guarantee healing, and (3) that each reperforation encounters increased resistance to infection in the abdominal cavity and a quicker walling off of the perforation.

Lysaght[13] reported a patient 26 years of age whose father died of a perforated peptic ulcer at 34 years of age. The son within a period of fifteen months suffered four perforations of an ulcer on the anterior wall of the pylorus. Each time the perforation was in the same location. Between the second and third perforations, a posterior gastroenterostomy was performed and following the fourth, a gastric resection. Three months following the resection the patient was reported to be well.

TABLE V. PERFORATED GASTRIC ULCERS
(EIGHTY-FOUR CASES)

RESULTS			NUMBER
Excellent	9	Satisfactory	15
Good	6		
Fair	12	Unsatisfactory	29
Poor	17		
Not followed	24		
Deaths	16		
Mortality	19.0%		

Herten-Greaven[11] also reported a patient 21 years of age with a gastric ulcer low on the lesser curvature which perforated three times within a period of four years. Again in this patient, each perforation appeared to be in the same location.

Henry[17] had a patient with a large recent perforation on the anterior wall of the stomach. This was closed and an anterior gastroenterostomy was performed. Following this procedure the patient had three perforations of a jejunal ulcer within a period of four years, and then, three months later a fifth perforation, this time again in the gastric ulcer. All five perforations occurred within a period of five years.

Pearse[14] in a careful review of the literature on reperforation examined reports of 4,813 cases and found 33 instances of recurrent perforation, a percentage of 0.69. The mortality for recurrent perforation was 9 per cent while that for perforated ulcers in general was 27 per cent. Pearse concluded that the incidence of reperforation is the same regardless of the type of primary procedure. However, in our series simple suture and simple suture plus gastroenterostomy were the operations most frequently used (Table VI).

TABLE VI. REPERFORATION OF PEPTIC ULCER IN PEARSE'S SERIES

OPERATION	NO.	PER CENT	REPERFORATIONS NO.	REPERFORATIONS PER CENT
Simple suture	710	67.0	24	72.0
Suture & P.G.E	281	26.6	8	24.3
All others	65	6.2	1	3.0
Mortality				
Perforated		27.0		
Reperforated		9.0		
Total				
Perforations	4813			
Reperforations	33	0.69		

In our own series of 101 patients with perforation there were, to our knowledge, 5 who suffered a second perforation, a percentage of 5.0. When only those surviving the first operation are considered, the percentage is over six, or almost ten times that found by Pearse.[14] In the group of patients with reperforation there was 1 death, a mortality of 20 per cent. This reperforation occurred six days after the first and may be considered a postoperative complication.

Bleeding.—Estes and Bennett[5] reported that in 26.8 per cent of patients with perforation in his series there was bleeding prior to the perforation. In this series the figure is 20 per cent. Following operation for perforated ulcer, 4 patients had evidence of massive hemorrhage for which additional surgery was carried out.

Obstruction.—In 6 patients a secondary operation was carried out for obstruction.

Intractable Pain.—There were 2 subsequent operations for intractable pain.

Carcinoma.—Reports concerning the possibility of ulcer developing into carcinoma vary. Williams[6] reported one secondary operation for carcinoma following a perforated ulcer. In our series there has been no evidence of cancer. It seems that gastric ulcers rarely become malignant.

Secondary Operations.—Secondary operations were carried out in 17 cases as follows:

Reperforation:	(1) Suture of perforation.
	(2) Reperforation on sixth postoperative day; died.
	(3) Suture of reperforation one year after primary suture.
	(4) Suture of reperforation.
	(5) Suture of reperforation followed later by gastric resection.
Hemorrhage:	(1) For massive hemorrhage five years later.
	(2) Gastric resection for bleeding duodenal ulcer.
	(3) Pylorectomy for bleeding ulcer.
	(4) Gastroenterostomy for bleeding ulcer.
Obstruction:	(1) Posterior gastroenterostomy for obstruction.
	(2) Anterior gastroenterostomy for obstruction.
	(3) Gastric resection for obstruction.
	(4) Gastric resection for obstruction.
	(5) Gastric resection for obstruction.
	(6) Gastric resection for obstruction.
Intractable Pain:	(1) Posterior gastroenterostomy for intractable pain.
	(2) Gastric resection for intractable pain.

It is quite clear that, although the immediate results of surgery for perforated ulcer are good, the late results, as determined by follow-up studies, are poor. This leads to the question, whether we can modify the late results by the type of operation performed at the time of the first perforation. Attempting to solve this question has led to many different procedures and various answers. In the main there are three schools of thought: (1) Those who advocate the least possible surgery and close the perforation by the simplest method; (2) those who combine closure with gastroenterostomy; and (3) those who resect the stomach and perforated ulcer at the same time.

Simple Closure of Perforation.—Many surgeons feel that these patients are poorly prepared for operation and that the simplest surgery possible is the best, in the attempt to lower the initial mortality. The perforation is closed by simple suture usually with reinforcement of the suture line by a small tab of omentum. Even though at times the pyloric opening is somewhat compromised, this group of surgeons feels that additional surgery is unnecessary. DeBakey,[3] in a collected series of 1,525 perforations closed by simple suture, found that over one-half the patients, or 65 per cent, remained symptom-free, 35 per cent continued to have symptoms, and 16.9 per cent required subsequent surgery (Table VII).

In our series of 57 patients on whom follow-ups were carried out after treatment by simple suture, there were 13 excellent, 6 good, 15 fair, and 23 poor results; or to combine them as satisfactory and unsatisfactory, there were 19 of the former and 38 of the latter. The unsatisfactory cases thus constituted 66 per cent of those followed, and 29.8 per cent of those followed have required subsequent surgery.

TABLE VII. RESULTS OF OPERATIONS IN 2670 CASES (DE BAKEY, 1940)

PROCEDURE	NUMBER	PER CENT	
Simple closure	1525		
Symptom-free		65	
With symptoms		35	
Subsequent operation			16.9
Simple closure plus gastroenterostomy	764		
Symptom-free		67	
With symptoms		33	
Subsequent operation			4
Partial gastrectomy	385		
Symptom-free		81.8	
With symptoms		18.2	

Simple Closure Plus Gastroenterostomy.—It is the opinion of others that patients with perforated ulcer operated upon within six or twelve hours are good operative risks and have only a chemical peritonitis without bacterial involvement. In addition, they feel that by simple suture the outlet of the stomach often is obstructed. With this in mind, they combine simple suture with gastroenterostomy. They point to immediate mortality figures which are no higher than those given for simple closure. They admit that gastroenterostomy is used only for good-risk patients operated upon shortly after perforation; for others a simple closure only is done. DeBakey[3] in his review of 764 collected cases of patients treated by this method found 67 per cent permanently relieved, which is the same as the percentage following simple closure. On the other hand, only 4 per cent required subsequent operation as compared to 17 per cent following simple closure (Table VII).

Gastric Resection.—European surgeons have for a long time been pioneers in the use of gastric resection for the treatment of peptic ulcer (Billroth, Polya), and as one would expect, they also have treated perforated ulcer by gastric resection with a low reported mortality rate. Again, this is in good-risk patients and shortly after perforation. DeBakey[3] in 385 collected cases found 81.8 per cent of patients treated by gastric resection to be symptom-free. Bisgard[4] in an excellent review of the literature concluded that subtotal gastric resection can be performed in the presence of diffuse soiling of the peritoneal cavity within twelve hours after perforation of ulcerated lesions of the stomach, duodenum, and jejunum in good-risk patients with a lower mortality than that obtained by simple suture. He also added that with few exceptions the resection results in permanent cure in contrast to the high incidence of recurrent ulceration following simple closure of the perforation.

CONCLUSIONS

The following conclusions have been drawn from our study. Patients with perforated ulcers should be operated upon promptly. The perforation should be closed by simple suture. When simple suture causes obstruction, it should be combined with gastroenterostomy. No drainage is employed in the abdominal wound. Patients with persistent symptoms and/or an active ulcer at the end of six months after operation, and while on adequate medical treatment, should have an additional operative procedure.

REFERENCES

1. Heuer, George J.: The Treatment of Peptic Ulcer, Philadelphia, 1944, J. B. Lippincott Company.
2. Parker, Edward F.: The Late Results in Acute Perforated Peptic Ulcer Treated by Simple Suture, SURGERY **10**: 49-63, 1941.
3. DeBakey, M.: Acute Perforated Gastroduodenal Ulceration, SURGERY **8**: 1028-1076, 1940.
4. Bisgard, J. D.: Gastric Resection for Certain Acute Perforated Lesions of Stomach and Duodenum With Diffuse Soiling of the Peritoneal Cavity, SURGERY **17**: 498-509, 1945.
5. Estes, W. L., Jr., and Bennett, B. A., Jr.: Acute Perforation in Gastroduodenal Ulceration With Special Reference to End Results, Ann. Surg. **119**: 321-341, 1944.
6. Williams, A. C.: Perforated Peptic Ulcer. A Follow-up Study of One Hundred Cases, New England J. Med. **230**: 785-790, 1944.
7. Harrison, C., and Cooper, F. W., Jr.: Immediate and Late Results of Perforation of Peptic Ulcer, Ann. Surg. **116**: 194-199, 1942.
8. Strauss, A.: Primary Gastric Resection for Perforated Gastroduodenal Ulcers, Ann. Surg. **120**: 60-65, 1944.
9. Wakely, C. P.: Late Results of Perforated Peptic Ulcer, Lancet **1**: 11-12, 1944.
10. Benhow, E. V.: Duodenal Ulcer in Newborn Infant, North Carolina M. J. **3**: 303-304, 1942.
11. Herten-Greaven: Recurrent Perforation of a Gastric Ulcer, Brit. M. J. **1**: 1070, 1923.
12. Royster, Henry P.: Five Perforations of a Peptic Ulcer, North Carolina M. J. **2**: 234-236, 1942.
13. Lysaght, A. C.: Repeated Perforation of a Peptic Ulcer, Lancet **1**: 809-810, 1937.
14. Pearse, Hermann E.: Recurrent Perforation of Peptic Ulcers, Ann. Surg. **96**: 192-199, 1932.
15. Lee, Walter E., and Wells, J. R.: Perforation in Utero of a Gastric Ulcer, Ann. Surg. **98**: 36-41, 1923.
16. Dineen, P.: Acute Perforated Ulcer of the Stomach and Duodenum, Ann. Surg. **90**: 1027-1034, 1929.
17. Henry, Charles K.: Recurrent Gastric Perforation, Surg., Gynec. & Obst. **32**: 542-543, 1921.
18. Sallick, M. A.: Late Results in Acute Perforated Peptic Ulcer Treated by Simple Closure, Ann. Surg. **104**: 853-863, 1936.
19. White, W. C., and Patterson, H. A.: Late Results of Simple Suture in Acute Perforation of Duodenal Ulcer, Ann. Surg. **94**: 242-255, 1931.

NEUROGENIC TUMORS OF THE STOMACH

JOHN P. WEST, M.D., AND GRAHAM KNOX, M.D., NEW YORK, N. Y.
(From the Surgical Service, St. Luke's Hospital)

TUMORS derived from the nerve sheath are not common in the stomach. Because of the confusion in terminology and the difference of opinion among pathologists in the interpretation of their histopathology, these tumors are variously described as neurofibromas, schwannomas, neurolemmomas, neurinomas, and perineural fibroblastomas.[1-3]

It is difficult to estimate their true incidence, for neurogenic tumors of the stomach are often confused with neoplasms derived from smooth muscle. However, Minnes and Geschickter,[4] in 1936, collected 931 reported cases of benign tumors of the stomach and classified 102, or 10.9 per cent, as neurofibromas.

A review of reported cases of tumors classified as being of nerve sheath origin and those believed to be derived from smooth muscle reveals great similarity in the clinical features, in gross appearance, and in microscopic structure.[3, 5-11]

We do not wish to enter the controversy concerning the histogenesis of these tumors.[12] Our principal objective is to emphasize two important clinical features of these lesions, first, the tendency of the gastric mucosa over the tumor to ulcerate and cause serious bleeding, and, second, the possibility of malignant transformation.

This report is concerned primarily with eight patients operated upon at St. Luke's Hospital and found to have gastric tumors of nerve sheath or smooth muscle origin. Six tumors have been classified as neurofibromas, one as a neurogenic sarcoma, and one as a leiomyoma, probably malignant (Table I). Six of the patients were admitted to the hospital because of gastrointestinal bleeding, one because of vague epigastric distress, and one because of epigastric pain which apparently was due to a duodenal ulcer. Five of the tumors were found in the cardiac portion of the stomach and three in the pyloric region. Four were removed by local excision and four by gastric resection. There were no deaths and the seven patients on whom we were able to do follow-up studies have remained well to date, two more than five years and five less than one year.

CASE REPORTS

CASE 1 (92901).— P. N., a 41-year-old man, was admitted to the hospital in April, 1932, because of a severe gastric hemorrhage. The patient gave a history of postprandial pain of five years' duration. The admission blood count showed a hemoglobin of 29 per cent and 1,440,000 red cells per cubic millimeter of blood. Roentgenograms, two weeks after admission, failed to reveal any gastric pathology, and gastric acidity was found to be normal. The patient was discharged with the clinical diagnosis of bleeding duodenal ulcer. Eighteen months later he returned to the hospital because of a second severe hemorrhage. Roentgenograms at this time showed a tumor at the pyloric end of the stomach. The tumor and the pyloric portion of the stomach were removed by a Billroth I type of gastric resection. The postoperative course was uncomplicated. Unfortunately, we were unable to maintain contact with the patient after his discharge from the hospital.

TABLE I. NEUROGENIC TUMORS OF THE STOMACH

CASE NUMBER	SEX	AGE (YR.)	CHIEF COMPLAINT	LOCATION OF TUMOR	OPERATION	DIAGNOSIS	RESULT
1	M	41	Bleeding (acute)	Pylorus	Gastric resection	Neurofibroma, ulcerated	No follow-up
2	F	46	Epigastric distress	Cardia	Local excision	Neurofibroma	Well 7 yr.
3	M	51	Pain	Pylorus	Gastric resection	Neurofibroma, ulcerated; duodenal ulcer	Well 5 yr.
4	F	64	Fatigue, bleeding (chronic)	Pylorus	Gastric resection	Neurogenic sarcoma, ulcerated	Well 1 yr.
5	M	51	Bleeding (acute)	Cardia	Gastric resection	Neurofibroma, ulcerated	Well 9 mo., no appetite
6	F	50	Bleeding (acute)	Cardia	Local excision	Neurofibroma, ulcerated	Well 6 mo.
7	F	33	Bleeding (acute)	Cardia	Local excision	Neurofibroma, ulcerated	Well 2 mo.
8	F	61	Bleeding (acute)	Cardia	Local excision	Leiomyoma, ulcerated (?) malignant	Well 2 mo.

Gross Pathology.—The excised portion of stomach was 9 cm. long on the greater curvature. Just proximal to the pylorus and partially involving it, there was a large tumor (Fig. 1) measuring 10 by 10 by 5 cm. which projected into the lumen of the stomach. The mucosa over the tumor was intact, except at the site of a deep ulcer, 2 cm. in diameter and from 1 to 3 cm. deep. The mucosal border overhung the ulcer base. The tumor was well encapsulated and was only loosely attached to the muscularis and mucosa.

Microscopic Examination.—Sections of the stomach showed portions of an ulcer with an indolent necrotic base and margins which showed only slight hyperplasia of the epithelium. There was a considerable degree of inflammation in the stroma. The base of the ulcer extended through the submucosa into the tumor mass. The tumor was fairly discrete, and consisted of spindle-shaped cells with considerable intercellular gelatinous material and a smaller amount of hyaline degeneration. The form of the cells and their spindle-shaped arrangement, with palisading nuclei and some giant nuclei, was characteristic of the perineural fibroblastomas. In some areas swollen and hypertrophied tortuous nerve trunks could be seen at the periphery of the solid tumor masses. The submucosa showed chronic infection. The muscle coat showed very little change. This tumor appeared benign.

Diagnosis.—Diagnosis was neurofibroma of the stomach with chronic ulcer.

CASE 2 (A-17476).—R. W., a 46-year-old woman, was admitted to the hospital in May, 1939, because of mid-epigastric pain of one year's duration. This pain had no relation to meals and there had been no evidence of bleeding. Roentgenograms revealed a tumor of the cardiac portion of the stomach. At operation a nonulcerated tumor, 4 by 4 by 2 cm. in size, was found in the posterior wall of the cardia of the stomach. This was excised after opening the stomach through the anterior wall. The postoperative course was uncomplicated. The patient has remained well to date, seven years.

Gross Pathology.—The tumor from the stomach wall (Fig. 2) was a rough brownish oval, 4 by 1.3 by 1 cm. Section showed a solid mass with grayish surface. There were thin fibrous bands dividing the tissue irregularly.

Microscopic Examination.—Section (Fig. 3) of the tumor showed a growth composed of edematous, vacuolated fibrillar material with rather infrequent nuclei. These were usually short with blunt ends and did not contain mitoses. They had the general appearance of fibroblasts and although there was no definite palisading, the growth had many of the characteristics of a tumor of the nerve sheath. It did not appear to be malignant.

Diagnosis.—Diagnosis was neurofibroma of the stomach.

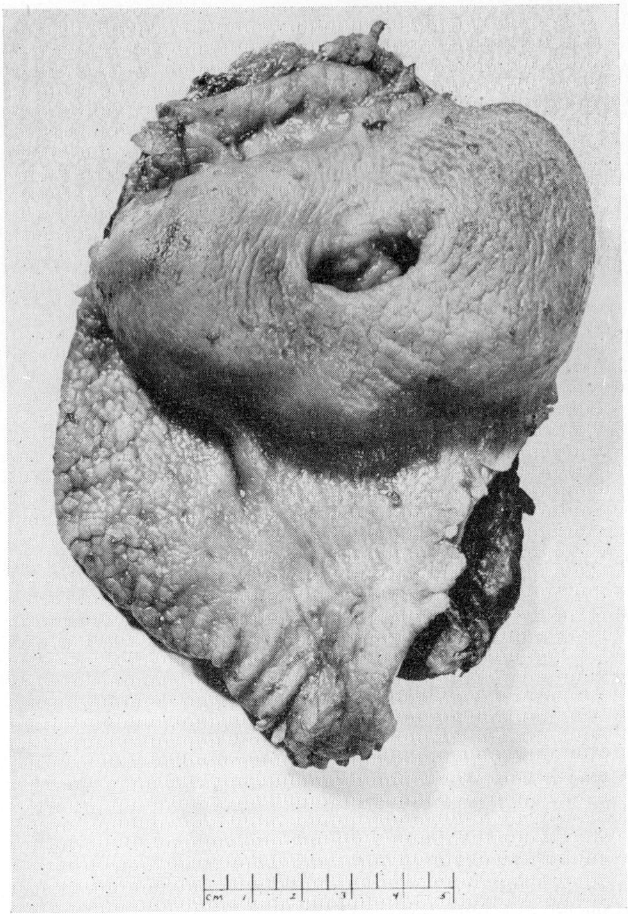

Fig. 1 (Case 1).—Neurofibroma of pyloric region of stomach showing a central area of ulceration.

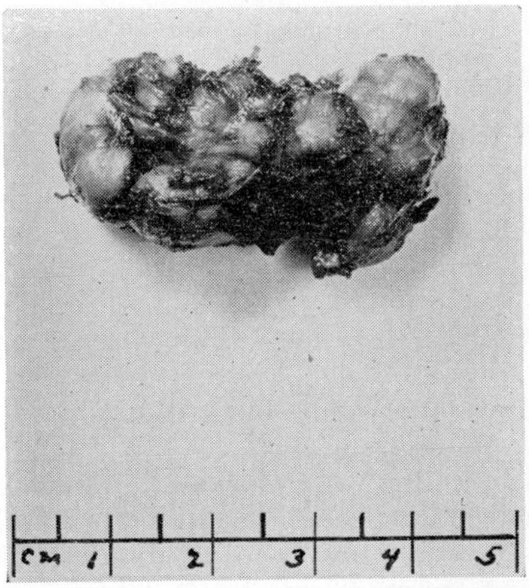

Fig. 2 (Case 2).—Neurofibroma from cardia of stomach; there is no ulceration.

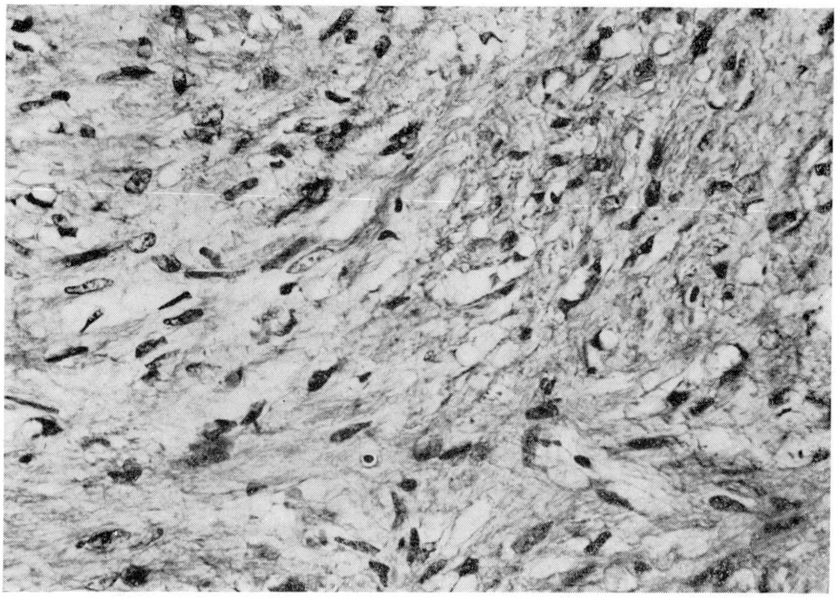

Fig. 3 (Case 2).—Section through tumor showing edematous, vacuolated fibrillar material with rather infrequent nuclei (×375).

CASE 3 (A-72054).—P. Q., a 51-year-old man, was admitted to the hospital in January, 1942, because of postprandial pain, of twenty-five years' duration, relieved by food and soda. The pain had become more severe during the six months prior to admission. There was no history of bleeding. Roentgenologic studies showed an irregularly deformed duodenal cap and gastric acidity was elevated. At operation the patient was found to have a duodenal ulcer and a freely movable tumor, 3 cm. in diameter, in the lesser curvature of the stomach near the pylorus (Fig. 4). A Polya type of gastric resection was done. The patient's postoperative course was uncomplicated and he has remained well to date, five years.

Gross Pathology.—The portion of the excised stomach measured 17 cm. in length at the greater curvature and 8 cm. at the lesser curvature. The surface was normal in appearance except at a point, 2 cm. from the pyloric end, where there was a projecting mass, 3 by 3.5 cm. in size, on the lesser curvature. The serosa over the mass was somewhat congested. On section, it appeared to lie between the muscularis and the mucosa and extended inward to the mucosa, which was ulcerated. It was firm in consistency, pale, and had a smooth cut surface.

Microscopic Examination.—Section (Fig. 5) showed a small ulcer of the chronic type with the base in the submucosa. It was covered with a large amount of fibrin. Underneath this, there was a small amount of scar tissue in which were many large bundles resembling nerve trunks with proliferation of the cells of the neurilemma. These trunks extended down through the muscle. In one area there appeared to be muscle left in the base of the ulcer but only fibrous tissue and large nerve bundles. The nodules showed a lobulated structure made up of twisted bundles in which the nuclei had a palisading arrangement. Some were vacuolated and the small rounded globules suggested mucoid degeneration. This is often seen in tumors which have originated in sheaths of Schwann. The growth appeared benign.

Diagnosis.—Diagnosis was neurofibroma of the stomach, with ulcer.

CASE 4 (A-114-909).—C. J., a 64-year-old woman, was admitted to the hospital in January, 1946, complaining of fatigue, palpitation, and epigastric distress of nine months' duration. There was no history of vomiting and the patient had not observed the color of the stools. On admission, the patient's hemoglobin was 35 per cent and the red cells were

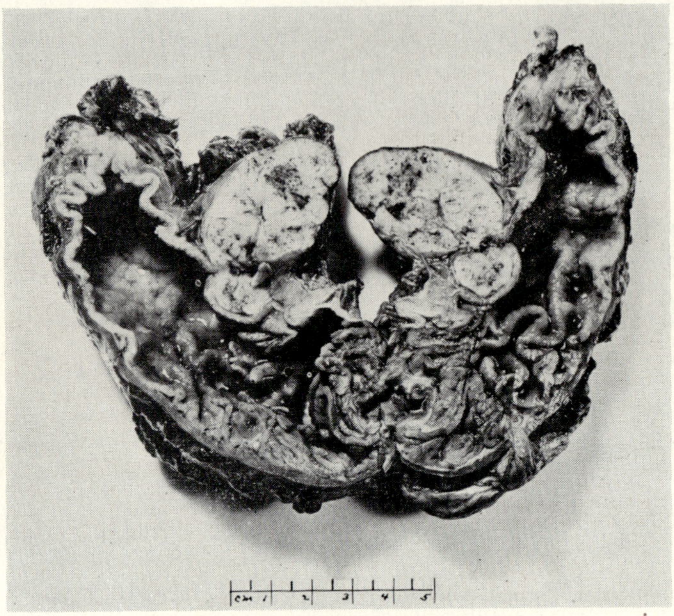

Fig. 4 (Case 3).—Neurofibroma on lesser curvature of stomach, near pylorus.

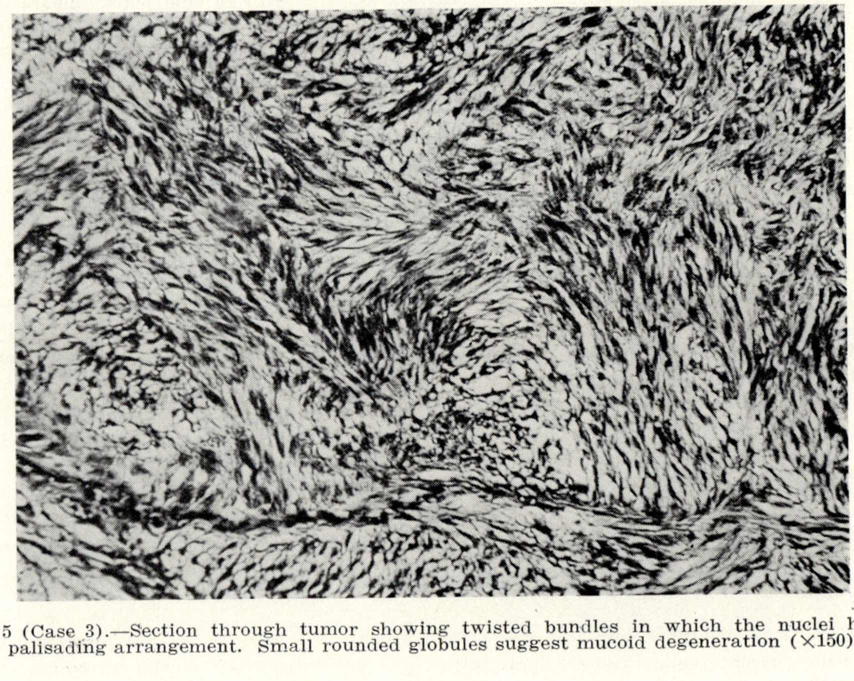

Fig. 5 (Case 3).—Section through tumor showing twisted bundles in which the nuclei have a palisading arrangement. Small rounded globules suggest mucoid degeneration (×150).

2,000,000 per cubic millimeter of blood. The stools contained blood. Roentgenogram (Fig. 6) showed a polypoid mass 5 cm. in diameter on the lesser curvature of the stomach and about 5 cm. from the pylorus. Gastric acidity was low. On Jan. 24, 1946, the ulcerated area, which appeared benign, was excised. The pathologic diagnosis, however, was neurogenic sarcoma.

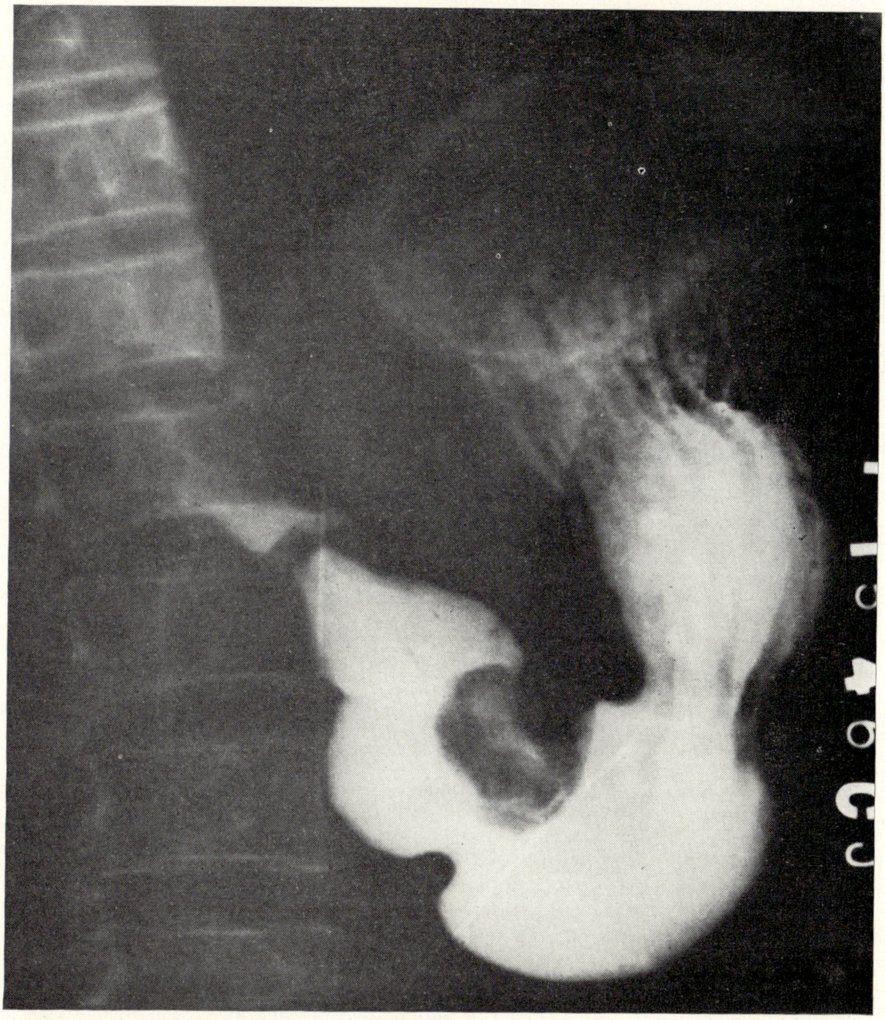

Fig. 6 (Case 4).—Roentgenogram showing tumor in prepyloric area of stomach.

Gross Pathology.—The specimen consisted of a portion of the wall of the stomach 5 by 5 by 3.5 cm. There was an ulcer, 8 mm. in diameter, on the anterior surface, toward the lesser curvature. Section through this showed a thick hypertrophied underlying muscularis.

Microscopic Examination.—Section (Fig. 7) through the base of the ulcer showed it to be composed of tumor which had apparently arisen from a nerve trunk. The growth extended up to the mucosal surface, being covered with only a very little exudate, and replaced the normal tissues down to the muscle coat. The latter was thickened by fibrosis, hypertrophy, and edema. The tumor was made up of twisted strands of spindle-shaped cells of the connective tissue type; some of them, seen in longitudinal section, were rather plump with rounded ends. The fibers were closely packed together, showed very little myxomatous degeneration, but practically no collagen. There were a few areas in which the nuclei were palisading and in these the appearance was that of a neurogenic tumor. There were a few mitotic figures and the tumor was too cellular to be regarded as benign, but it was of a type which would be unlikely to metastasize at this early stage. It is possible that it had not been entirely removed.

Diagnosis.—Diagnosis was neurogenic sarcoma of the stomach, ulcerated.

Because of this diagnosis, the patient was returned to the hospital and on March 7, 1946, a partial gastric resection was done. No tumor, gross or microscopic, was recognized in the portion of stomach removed. Convalescence was uncomplicated and the patient has remained well to date, one year.

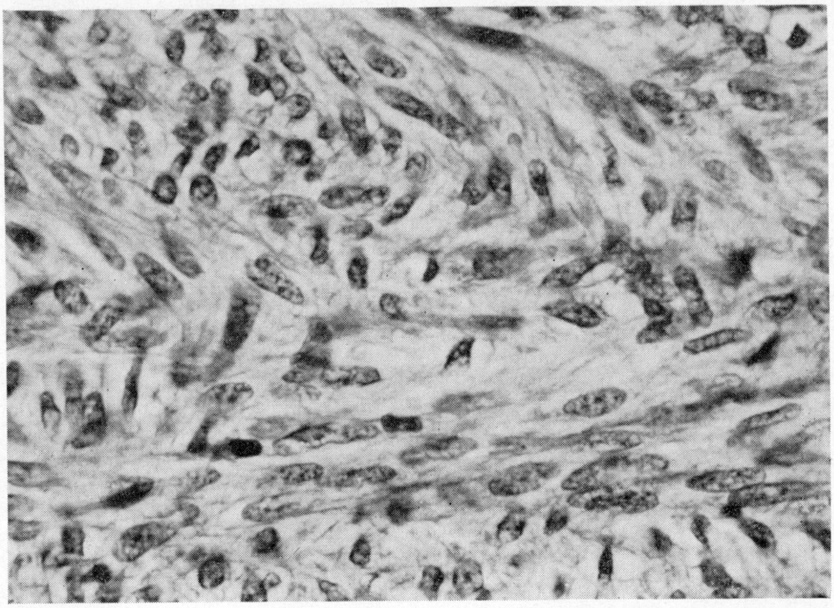

Fig. 7 (Case 4).—Neurogenic sarcoma; this tumor is very cellular with some palisading of the nuclei and a few mitotic figures (×875).

CASE 5 (A-118-493).—H. M., a 51-year-old mechanic, was admitted to the hospital in April, 1946, because of severe gastrointestinal bleeding. He had noted tarry stools for one week and the day before admission vomited a large amount of bright red blood and fainted. On admission the hemoglobin was 27 per cent and there were 1,120,000 red cells per cubic millimeter of blood. After a period of two weeks the stools were free of blood and the roentgenograms (Fig. 8) taken at this time showed an ulcer crater on the posterior wall of the stomach about 4 cm. from the esophagus. At operation, performed two months after admission, an ulcerated tumor (Fig. 9) was found in the posterior wall of the stomach near the esophagus. The tumor was removed by a high gastric resection, which left about 3 cm. of the stomach attached to the esophagus. A left subphrenic abscess developed and was drained two weeks after the resection. There was rapid improvement in the patient's condition and the course since has been fairly satisfactory, although he still has some discomfort immediately following meals. He was discharged from the hospital Aug. 20, 1946, two months after resection, in good condition and with the drainage wound healed. Nine months after operation he appeared well but had not regained his normal weight and still complained of anorexia.

Gross Pathology.—The specimen consisted of cardia and fundus of the stomach with a tumor in the posterior wall. On the greater curvature it measured 17 cm. and on the lesser

12 cm. The distal half appeared normal, but, beginning at the site of resection at the proximal end, there was a large irregular mass extending from the mucosa entirely through the wall and forming a nodular mass 6 by 8 by 6 cm. On the inner surface, the mucous membrane was stretched over the tumor, which protruded into the stomach cavity for a distance of 4 cm. In the center there was a deep ulcer 2 by 2 by 2 cm. The mucosal edges were overhanging, the base was smooth and composed only of tumor. On the serous surface the tumor protruded, forming a mass 4 by 5 by 3 cm. Section showed that the tumor was composed of firm bluish-white trabeculae, small hemorrhagic areas, and small cavities.

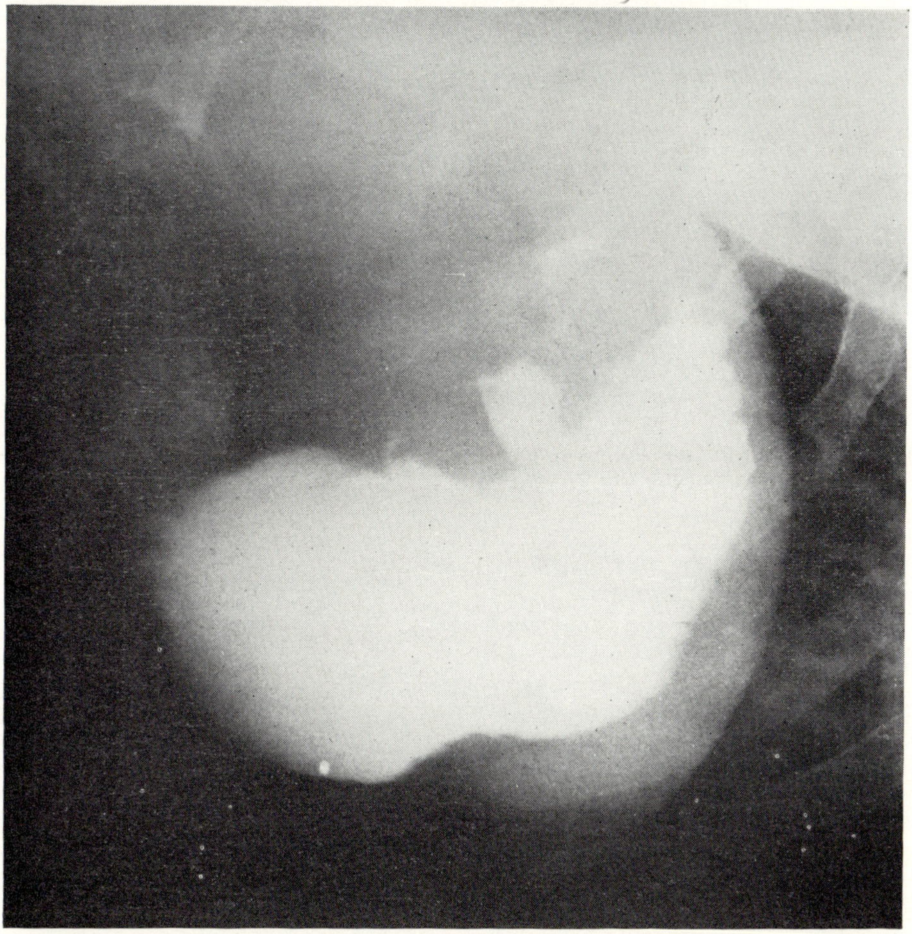

Fig. 8 (Case 5).—Roentgenogram showing a deep ulcer in the posterior wall of stomach.

Microscopic Examination.—Section (Fig. 10) through the base of the ulcer showed a necrotic area with some fibrous tissue and tumor and many thrombosed vessels. Beneath this the tumor extended to the serous surface, and showed considerable infection and edema. It was composed of large twisted bundles of spindle-shaped cells with long pointed nuclei, some of which were arranged to suggest the neurilemma. The nuclei showed frequent cross striations due to mucinous degeneration such as takes place in Schwann cells. There were numerous areas in which these mucoid inclusions had distended and enlarged the cell bodies, pushing aside the nuclei. Mitoses were not seen, although the tumor was fairly cellular and the nuclei were hyperchromatic. It would appear, however, that the growth was probably relatively benign.

Diagnosis.—Diagnosis was neurofibroma of the stomach, ulcerated.

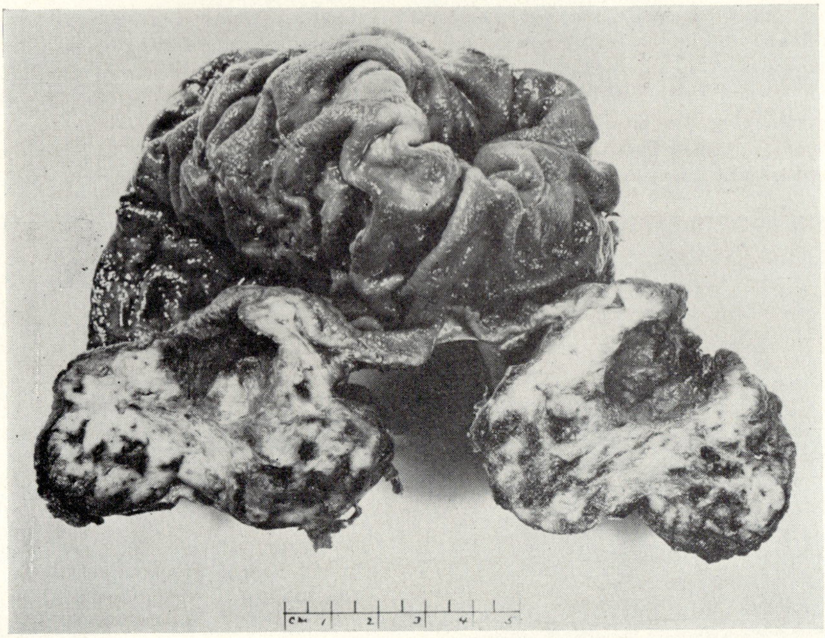

Fig. 9 (Case 5).—Neurofibroma from posterior wall of stomach showing a central area of ulceration.

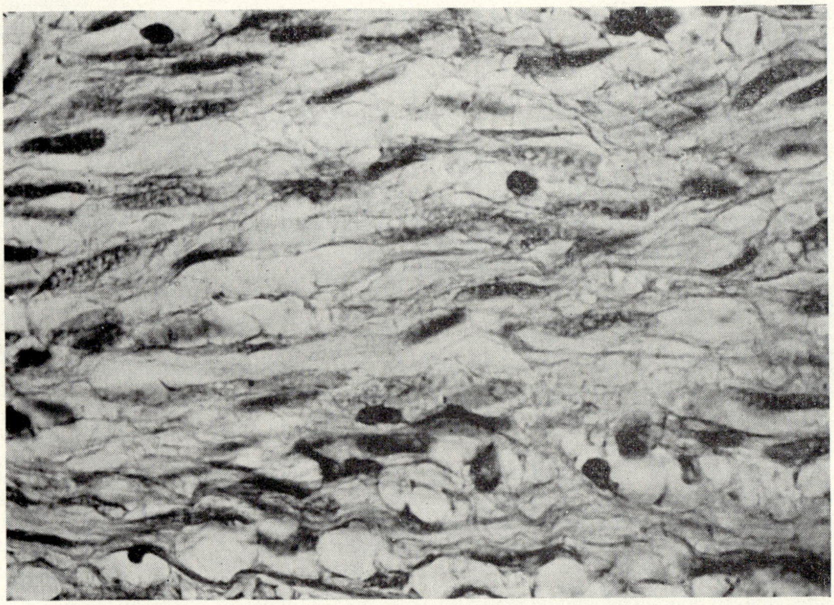

Fig. 10 (Case 5).—Section through tumor showing spindle-shaped cells with long pointed nuclei and rather marked mucinous degeneration (×875).

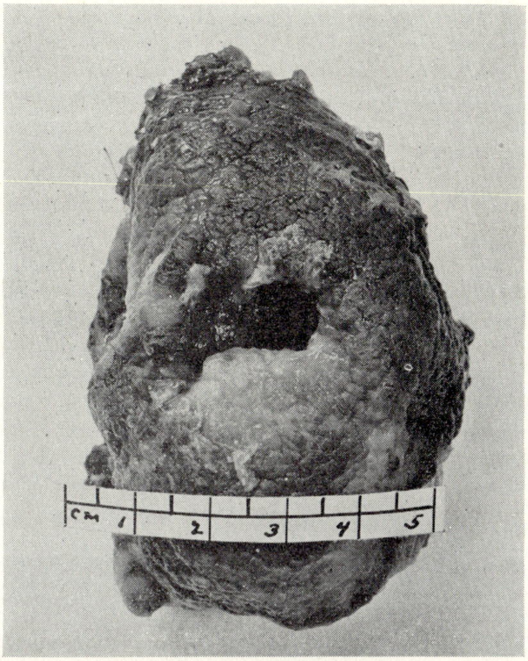

Fig. 11 (Case 6).—Neurofibroma from posterior wall of stomach showing a large central ulcer.

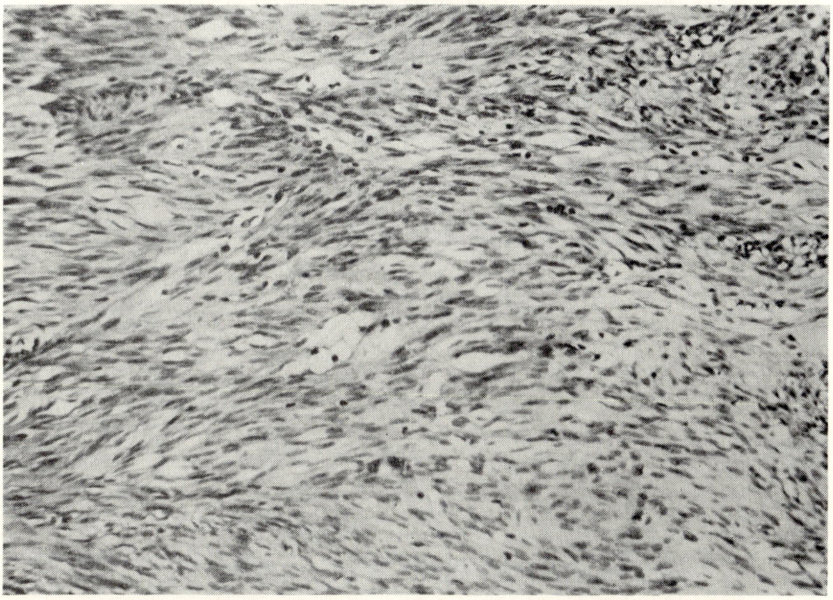

Fig. 12 (Case 6).—Section through tumor showing bundles and whorls of spindle-shaped cells with palisading nuclei (×187.5).

Case 6 (A-108-503).—H. P., a 51-year-old woman, was admitted to the hospital Oct. 8, 1946, because of severe chest pain of three hours' duration. She was known to have hypertension and on several occasions had been treated for cardiac decompensation. One week prior to admission she vomited blood and later noted black stools. On admission the blood pressure was 220/110. Hemoglobin was 76 per cent and there were 3,700,000 red cells per cubic millimeter of blood. The stools contained blood. Roentgenograms showed an ulcerated tumor of the posterior wall of the cardiac end of the stomach. On Nov. 8, one month after admission, the gastric tumor was removed by local excision. The postoperative course was satisfactory. The patient has remained well to date, four months.

Gross Pathology.—The specimen consisted of a tumor (Fig. 11) from the stomach measuring 8 cm. in length, 4½ cm. in width, and 3½ cm. in depth. One surface was covered with gastric mucosa at the center of which was an ulceration measuring 2 cm. in diameter and 2 cm. in depth, but 4 cm. at its base. The serosal surface on the opposite side of the tumor appeared smooth. On section it was noted that the tumor extended through the entire thickness of the stomach wall and was composed of firm, yellowish white tissue. The ulcer undermined the edges and was widest at the base which was covered with a necrotic slough.

Microscopic Examination.—Section (Fig. 12) through the tumor including the mucosa of the stomach showed the latter to be fairly normal, although somewhat infected. Beneath the muscularis mucosa and replacing the submucosa and muscle was a mass of tumor which was growing in the form of large bundles and whorls of spindle-shaped cells. These frequently

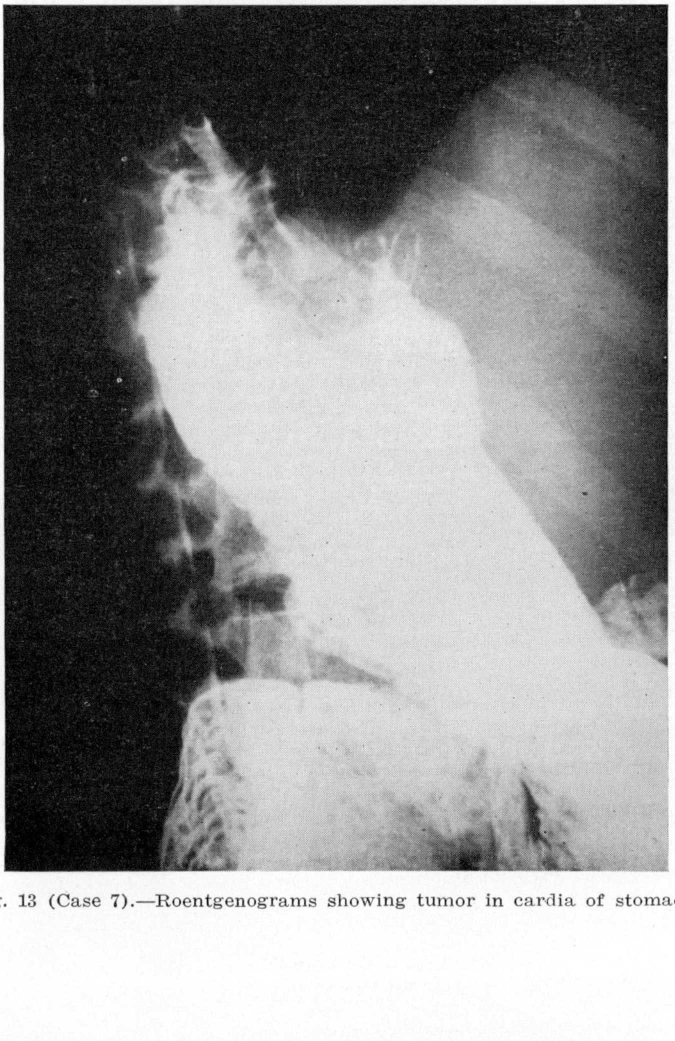

Fig. 13 (Case 7).—Roentgenograms showing tumor in cardia of stomach.

had palisading nuclei and between the nuclear areas were zones of hyaline connective tissue. This had the appearance of a tumor derived from a nerve sheath. It appeared benign.

Diagnosis.—Diagnosis was ulcerated neurofibroma.

CASE 7 (A-129-311).—R. K., a 33-year-old woman, was admitted to the hospital because of a marked secondary anemia which was first noted during pregnancy. After delivery of a normal child, the anemia became more severe and it was then noted, for the first time, that the patient's stools were tarry. Epigastric distress, not relieved by food, had been a complaint throughout most of the pregnancy. On admission the hemoglobin was 40 per cent and there were 2,590,000 red cells per cubic millimeter of blood. Gastric analysis, after histamine, showed no free hydrochloric acid and a total acidity of 29 units. The gastric fluid contained blood. Roentgenogram (Fig. 13) showed a roughly oval polypoid tumor in the cardiac end of the stomach. At operation, Feb. 11, 1947, the tumor (Fig. 14) was removed by local resection. The postoperative course was uncomplicated.

Gross Pathology.—The specimen consisted of a tumor of the stomach 4 by 3½ by 3 cm., covered on one surface with mucous membrane with a small fringe of normal gastric mucosa around it. In the center of the mucosal surface there was an ulcerated area 4 mm. in diameter and 9 mm. deep. Cross section revealed the tumor to be composed of pale firm tissue, arising in the submucosal layer and elevating the mucosa. The tumor measured 2 cm. in its thickest portion.

Microscopic Examination.—Section (Fig. 15) showed some of the mucosa of the stomach, but underneath this and occupying the submucosa was a fairly cellular tumor which was probably derived from the nerve sheath. It was growing in the form of twisted bundles of rather plump spindle-shaped cells. The nuclei contained many fine transverse lines which alternated with the globules of mucinous material, thus giving to many of the nuclei the appearance of Schwann cells. Between them there were very delicate collagenous fibrils. The tumor was infiltrated with plasma cells and lymphocytes, but mitoses were absent or extremely infrequent.

Diagnosis.—Diagnosis was neurofibroma of the stomach.

CASE 8 (A-129-257).—G. S., a 61-year-old woman, was admitted to the hospital because of anemia and tarry stools. One year before admission she vomited a large amount of blood and passed tarry stools. Roentgenographic studies made at this time were said to be negative. Following this episode the patient remained well until one month prior to admission when she noted that the stools were again tarry. She had no real epigastric pain or distress at any time. Gastric analysis, after histamine, showed 67 units of free hydrochloric acid and a total acidity of 90 units. Roentgenogram (Fig. 16) showed an hourglass tumor of the cardiac end of the stomach. At operation, on Feb. 11, 1947, the tumor was found in the posterior wall of the cardiac end of the stomach and was removed by local excision. The postoperative course was uncomplicated.

Gross Pathology.—The specimen (Fig. 17) consisted of a portion of stomach, measuring 7 by 3 by 4 cm. and containing a tumor which apparently had arisen in the submucosal layer and extended out beyond the serosa forming a spherical, polypoid, encapsulated nodule which bulged outside the stomach wall. This pedunculated portion of the tumor measured 4 by 5 by 3 cm. Section showed the tumor to be composed of lobulated pale reddish tissue which extended through the serosa to form a cystlike structure filled with degenerated tissue and blood clot. The wall of this cystic portion was 3 mm. in thickness.

Microscopic Examination.—Section (Fig. 18) through the tumor showed a growth which was composed of closely packed plump cells which appeared to anastomose with each other, but did not possess any connective tissue fibrils. The nuclei tended to be rather short and plump and a few mitoses were found. In a few areas where there had been some hemorrhage, the nuclei were much larger than elsewhere, but were multinucleated. There was a moderate amount of palisading such as is seen in neurofibromas and leiomyomas. The Bielschowsky stain showed very little connective tissue in this tumor and the morphology suggested a tumor of the smooth muscle. It is possible that the growth was already malignant and the large nuclei were an indication of active growth.

Diagnosis.—Diagnosis was leiomyoma of the stomach, possibly malignant.

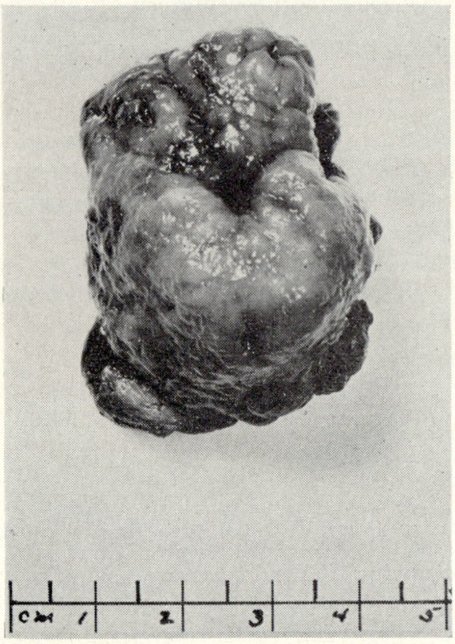

Fig. 14 (Case 7).—Neurofibroma of stomach with central ulceration.

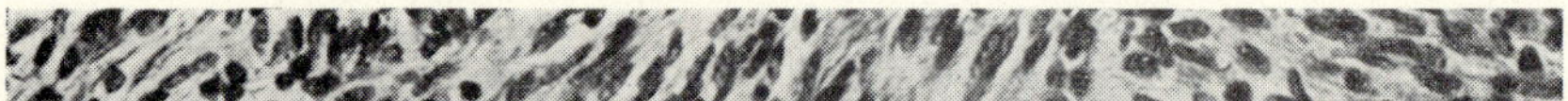

Fig. 15 (Case 7).—Section through tumor showing twisted bundles of rather plump spindle-shaped cells with palisading nuclei (×300).

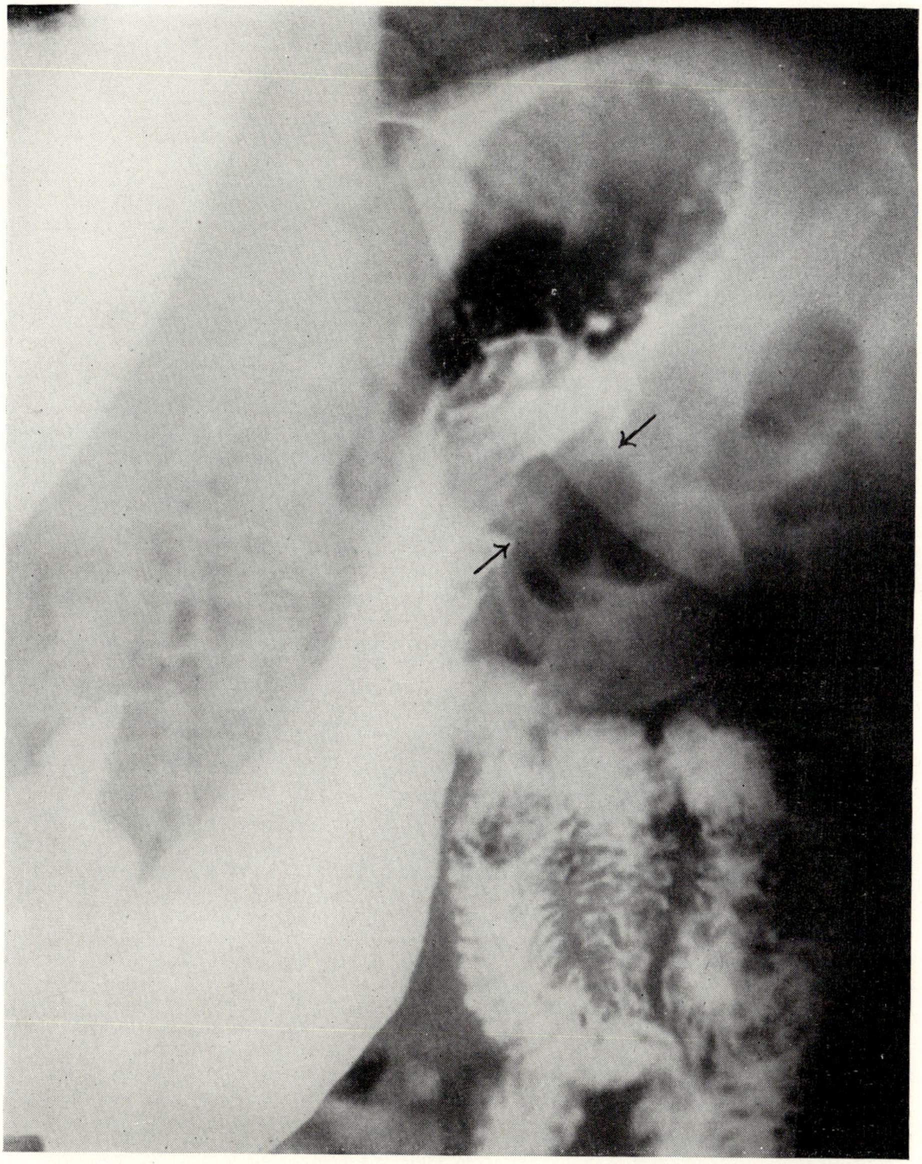

Fig. 16 (Case 8).—Roentgenograms showing an hourglass tumor of the cardia of the stomach.

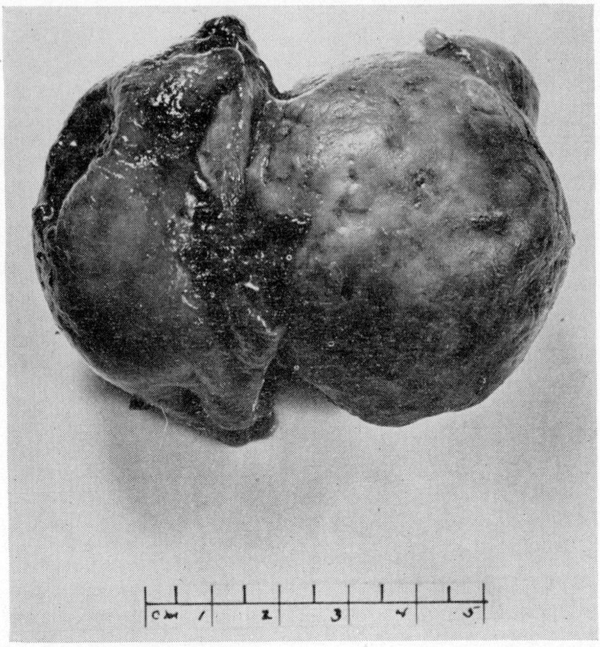

Fig. 17 (Case 8).—Leiomyoma of stomach with ulceration through the overlying mucosa.

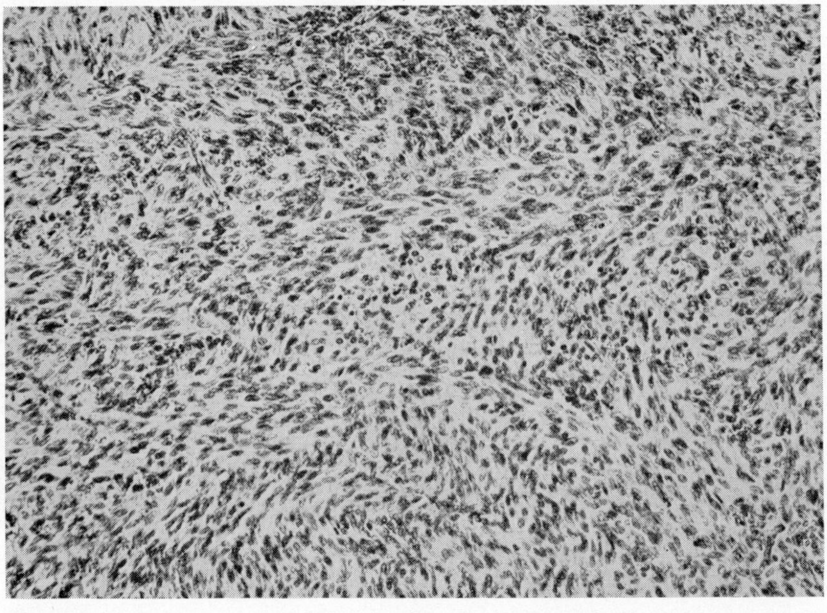

Fig. 18 (Case 8).—Section through tumor showing closely packed cells with a moderate amount of palisading and a few mitoses (×150).

DIAGNOSIS

The preoperative diagnosis of these tumors may be difficult but the following important features suggest a gastric tumor of smooth muscle or nerve sheath origin.

1. *Bleeding.*—The outstanding symptom in six of the eight patients was bleeding. This appeared to be caused by a central area of ulceration and in five cases caused a sudden severe hemorrhage. In one case the bleeding was of a chronic nature and the tumor was discovered when a search was made for the cause of the patient's secondary anemia.

2. *Pain.*—Pain was not a prominent symptom except in one man who had an active duodenal ulcer as well as tumor of the pyloric end of the stomach. All the patients, however, complained of a vague type of epigastric distress.

3. *Gastric Acidity.*—Gastric analysis was not of definite value as a diagnostic procedure. The gastric acidity, after histamine, was recorded for six of the eight patients. In two the acid values were high, in two they were low, and two were found to have normal gastric acidity.

4. *Roentgenograms.*—There was no constant diagnostic roentgen picture although the tumors usually appeared smooth in outline and often it was possible to demonstrate a central area of ulceration. A roentgen diagnosis of gastric tumor was made in seven of the eight patients.

MALIGNANT TRANSFORMATION

The possibility that these neoplasms may undergo malignant transformation is suggested by the fact that two of the eight tumors, on the basis of their microscopic appearance, were considered probably malignant. The symptoms and the gross appearance of the malignant tumors were essentially the same as those of the benign lesions.

TREATMENT

Four of the patients were treated by local excision of the tumor and four by gastric resection. There were no postoperative deaths. One patient with a benign tumor of the cardia was treated by resection of nine-tenths of the stomach. Nine months after operation this patient still has digestive complaints and has been unable to regain his preoperative weight. Because of this, and the magnitude of a gastric resection as compared with local excision, we feel that every effort should be made to determine the nature of the tumor at operation and that all benign tumors, at least those of the cardia, should be treated by local excision.

SUMMARY

1. Seven neurogenic and one smooth muscle tumor of the stomach are reported.

2. There is great similarity in the clinical features, the gross appearance, and the microscopic structure of the two types of tumors.

3. Bleeding was the chief symptom in six cases.

4. Two of the tumors appeared to have undergone malignant transformation.

5. Local excision appears to be adequate for the benign tumors.

REFERENCES

1. Smith, L. W., and Gault, E. S.: Essentials of Pathology, ed. 2, New York, 1942, D. Appleton-Century Company, Inc., pp. 328.
2. Wood, F. C.: Delafield and Prudden's Text-book of Pathology, ed. 16, Baltimore, 1936, William Wood & Company, pp. 1230.
3. Ranson, H. K., and Kay, E. B.: Abdominal Neoplasms of Neurogenic Origin, Ann. Surg. **112**: 700, 1940.
4. Minnes, J. F., and Geschickter, C. F.: Benign Tumors of the Stomach, Am. J. Cancer **28**: 136, 1936.
5. Lahey, F. H., and Colcock, Bentley P.: Diagnosis and Surgical Management of Leiomyomata and Leiomyosarcomata of the Stomach, Ann. Surg. **112**: 671, 1940.
6. Golden, T., and Stout, A. P.: Smooth Muscle Tumors of the Gastrointestinal Tract and Retroperitoneal Tissues, Surg., Gynec. & Obst. **73**: 784, 1941.
7. Cabot Case No. 21112: Spindle Cell Sarcoma of the Stomach, Probable Neurofibrosarcoma, New England J. Med. **212**: 485, 1935.
8. Cabot Case No. 23312: Neurogenic Fibrosarcoma of the Stomach, New England J. Med. **217**: 226, 1937.
9. Cabot Case No. 32061: Neurinoma of Stomach, New England J. Med. **234**: 194, 1946.
10. Cabot Case No. 32161: Neurinoma of Stomach, New England J. Med. **234**: 535, 1946.
11. Sanguily, J., and Blanco, F. L.: Gastric Schwannoma, SURGERY **17**: 328, 1945.
12. Forum: Stout, A. P., Warren, S., Ranson, H. K., and Kay, E. B., Re: Abdominal Neoplasms of Neurogenic Origin, by Ranson, H. K., and Kay, E. B., and Diagnosis and Surgical Management of Leiomyomata and Leiomyosarcomata of the Stomach, by Lahey, F. H., and Colcock, B. P., Ann. Surg. **114**: 117, 1941.

PRIMARY TUMORS OF THE JEJUNUM AND ILEUM

JOHN H. ECKEL, M.D., NEW YORK, N. Y.

PRIMARY tumors of the jejunum and ileum, though rare, are being recorded with increasing frequency. McDougal[1] stated that less than 300 cases of malignant disease have appeared in the literature up to 1944. Mayo and Nettrour[2] reported a total of 31 cases of carcinoma of the jejunum in patients seen at the Mayo Clinic prior to Feb. 1, 1937, of which only 15 could be subjected to resection and enteroenterostomy. Palliative enteroenterostomy or gastroenterostomy was carried out in 13, exploratory laparotomy in 2, and in 1 no surgical treatment was given. The operative mortality in this series was 20 per cent and the duration of life after operation 17.6 months. Shallow, Eger, and Carty[3] reported a series of 24 cases of primary malignant tumors of the jejunum and ileum encountered in the Jefferson Medical College Hospital. Of this number only 4 were found to be free of metastases. All of the jejunal lesions were resected and a primary anastomosis was performed. In the ileum 6 malignant tumors were resected with primary anastomoses; 1 lesion was exteriorized, and 3, which were not resectable, were given x-ray treatment. The operative mortality was 36 per cent and an analysis of the end results showed that 3 patients were living and well for periods of twelve, seven, and four years, respectively, after operation. Three others died of metastases after periods of fifteen, four, and three years, respectively. Fraser,[4] in presenting a series of 21 patients treated at the Western Infirmary in Glasgow, noted that 15 of this number were subjected to operation, resections being performed in 14. In the remaining patient a pelvic abscess was drained. The operative mortality was 60 per cent and of those who survived operation, none lived longer than nine years. One patient was alive three years; 3 patients, two and one-half years; and 1 patient one year after operation. Warren[5] reviewed 26 cases of malignant tumor of the small bowel from the Toronto General Hospital. Twenty-one of the tumors were situated in the jejunum or ileum. Of these patients one was well seventeen years, 1 patient eight years, and 1 patient 7 years after operation. Four patients were discharged improved, 3 died of metastases after approximately two years, 1 after one year, and 10 patients died in the hospital.

The rarity of these tumors is stressed by all authors. A review of our own experience and those of various other clinics indicates that the results of surgery compare unfavorably with those for malignancy of the large bowel. Although these tumors are manifested by a typical symptomatology, the establishment of the diagnosis is frequently delayed and a grave prognosis is the result.

Although a total of one-half million patients have been admitted to the New York Hospital since Sept. 1, 1932, the diagnosis of primary tumor of the jejunum and ileum has been histologically established in only 19 cases of which 12 were malignant and 7 benign. Of the latter group, 3 were incidental autopsy findings and were in no way related to the cause of death.

TABLE I. PRIMARY MALIGNANT TUMORS OF JEJUNUM AND ILEUM—PREOPERATIVE CLINICAL FINDINGS

Case number Name Hospital number	1 M. H. 53940	2 H. B. 197518	3 Z. B. 41932	4 L. M. 301544	5 O. M. 319274	6 J. F. 340543	7 A. A. 340797	8 R. H. 336343	9 F. W. 92595	10 J. F. 373632	11 H. R. 442280	12 S. E. 478686
Year admitted	1934	1938	1940	1941	1942	1942	1942	1942	1944	1945	1946	1947
Sex	M	M	F	M	M	M	F	M	M	F	F	M
Age (yr.)	34	42	48	44	44	50	47	52	38	62	49	36
Duration of symptoms (mo.)	6	1	12	6	4	1	12	60	8	8	12	24
Abdominal pain	+	+	+	+	+	+	+	+	+	+	+	0
Weight loss (pounds)	30	4	0	17	35	0	25	12	25	54	20	0
Vomiting	+	0	+	0	+	+	+	+	+	+	+	0
Constipation	+	+	0	0	+	0	+	+	+	0	+	0
Fatigue, weakness	+	+	+	+	+	+	+	+	+	+	+	+
Melena	+	0	0	0	0	0	0	+	+	+	0	+
Palpable abdominal mass	0	+	0	+	+	0	+	+	+	+	0	0
Occult blood in stool	+	+	0	+	0	+	0	+	0	+	+	+
R.B.C. (millions)	4.0	5.0	5.1	4.3	4.2	3.0	3.2	3.8	4.4	3.0	4.8	3.4
Hb. (Gm.)	12	13	14	12	10	6.5	9	11	14	8	13	8.5
Obstruction demonstrable by x-ray	+	+	+	+	0	+	+	0	+	0	+	+
Tumor demonstrable by x-ray	+	+	+	+	0	+	+	0	+	0	+	+

REPORT OF CASES

Primary Malignant Tumors

Age and Sex (Table I).—In this series of 12 cases, 8 were men and 4 women. The ages of the patients varied from 34 to 64 years, and the average for the group was 45.5 years. The women were slightly older than the men; their average age was 50.1 and that of the men, 42.5 years.

Symptoms (Table I).—The duration of symptoms before admission varied between one and sixty months, the average being 12.8 months. In all but one of the patients *pain* was present and usually this was the chief complaint. It was cramplike in nature in the majority of cases and was associated with varying degrees of obstruction. Not infrequently the pain, at the onset of the symptomatology, was mild and vague and was confused with the pain associated with cholecystitis or peptic ulcer. Its location was usually in the midepigastrium and the umbilical region. *Loss of weight* was a prominent symptom and only 3 patients gave no history of losing weight. The average loss in the others was 18.3 pounds and one man lost 54 pounds. *Vomiting* occurred in 9 patients. A marked degree of intestinal obstruction is the main factor in the production of vomiting, therefore, this symptom usually manifests itself late in the course of the disease. *Constipation* was recorded in 7 cases and a feeling of *fatigue* and *weakness* in all. A history of *melena,* as evidenced by tarry stools, was elicited from 6 patients.

Physical Signs (Table I).—A *palpable abdominal mass* was present in 7 of the 12 patients and some degree of *abdominal distention* associated with obstruction occurred in an equal number. One patient was admitted with symptoms and signs of *generalized peritonitis* and high obstruction of the small bowel (Case 3). *Pallor* and evidence of recent loss of weight were common findings.

Laboratory Tests (Table I).—*Anemia* was present in 8 of the 12 patients and *occult blood* in the stool was recorded in a like number. This test for blood in the feces is a very reliable aid and should be employed in all patients complaining of abdominal pain, whether cramplike or vague in nature. When there is no marked evidence of obstruction and after a period of careful observation, a roentgenologic examination should be made to ascertain whether a lesion is present. The passage of the barium as a split stream at the site of the lesion and narrowing of the lumen of the bowel are indicative of a tumor. The x-ray examination revealed a tumor in 9 of the cases. Varying degrees of obstruction, manifested by a widening of the lumen and consequent retention of barium proximal to the lesion were demonstrated in an equal number of cases.

Diagnosis.—The presence of a tumor of the small bowel can be established preoperatively by careful analysis of the symptoms, physical findings, laboratory tests, and roentgenologic examination. The history of intermittent intestinal obstruction manifested by cramplike abdominal pain and vomiting; the symptoms of anemia and presence of occult blood in the stools are highly suggestive. A small intestinal barium series establishes the diagnosis in a high percentage of cases. A careful exploration is indicated in all cases with the signs and symptoms just described. Cases 11 and 12 are examples of errors in diagnosis and are worthy of elaboration.

CASE REPORTS

CASE 11.—A 49-year-old woman entered the New York Hospital on July 5, 1946, with the history of abdominal pain of one year's duration, frequent vomiting, generalized weakness, malaise, chronic constipation, and loss of twenty pounds in weight. A cholecystectomy had been performed two months previous to this admission and the gall bladder was found to be chronically inflamed and contained gallstones. The patient's symptoms were unaltered by this procedure. Examination failed to reveal evidence of distention or a palpable mass. The stools were strongly positive for occult blood. A small intestinal barium series disclosed a tumor of the proximal jejunum, causing partial obstruction. Following adequate preparation, a laparotomy was performed on July 10, 1946, disclosing a stenosing adenocarcinoma of the jejunum, 10 cm. from the ligament of Treitz. A 16 cm. segment of jejunum, bearing the tumor, was resected and an enteroanastomosis was carried out. The patient had an uneventful recovery and has remained well to the present time.

CASE 12.—A 36-year-old man was admitted to the New York Hospital on June 13, 1947, with the history of fatigue and weakness for a period of two years. There were three admissions to another hospital—two in October, 1946, and the third in February, 1947, at which time a splenectomy was performed for presumed hemolytic anemia. Following this procedure the patient failed to improve and the blood picture remained unaltered. At the time of admission to the New York Hospital there was no history of abdominal pain, vomiting, or loss of weight. The red blood cell count was 3.4 million and the hemoglobin 8.5 Gm. The stools were strongly positive for occult blood and a small intestinal barium series showed a tumor in the proximal jejunum with slight obstruction. An exploratory laparotomy, performed on June 30, 1947, disclosed an adenocarcinoma in the proximal jejunum with extensive involvement of mesenteric lymph nodes. Resection and anastomosis were performed but there were metastases which could not be removed. The patient now feels well and the anemia has cleared.

Comment.—These two cases are examples of errors in preoperative and operative diagnosis. In both instances the initial operators apparently failed to examine the small bowel in the region of the duodenojejunal junction. Thorough exploration would have avoided the errors.

Treatment (Table II).—Resection and enteroanastomosis were performed in 8 cases out of the 12 and exploratory laparotomy in 3. One patient was not subjected to operation as there was evidence of widespread metastases and ascites. Examination of the ascitic fluid removed by paracentesis disclosed lymphoid tumor cells. This patient received intensive x-ray therapy but died six weeks after admission.

The procedure of choice is resection of the segment of bowel bearing the lesion with a wide margin of mesentery and the restoration of the continuity of the intestinal lumen by aseptic end-to-end anastomosis performed over clamps. The discrepancy between the diameters of the dilated proximal and the normal distal transected intestine can be readily corrected by placing the clamp obliquely on the latter. In the 8 patients who underwent this procedure there was no postoperative death and only one complication, a wound infection in a patient who was admitted with generalized peritonitis secondary to a perforated leiomyosarcoma of the jejunum (Case 3).

Before any operative procedure is attempted, it is essential to correct the anemia, the plasma protein deficiency, and any other fluid or electrolyte imbalance. The obstructed bowel should be decompressed by applying continuous suction to a Miller-Abbott or Levine tube.

Roentgen therapy is of no value in the postoperative management of carcinomas of the small bowel, but should be employed when the diagnosis of lymphosarcoma has been established, whether the lesion is resectable or not. Radiation therapy was used in Cases 1, 2, 4, and 8. It was also employed in the one case of carcinoid of the jejunum with extensive metastases (Case 5).

Pathology (Table II).—The tumor was situated in the jejunum in 10 and in the ileum in 2 cases, the proximal jejunum being the commonest location. Six of the lesions were adenocarcinomas, 4 lymphosarcomas, 1 a leiomyosarcoma which had perforated, and 1 a carcinoid with widespread metastases. No metastatic involvement could be demonstrated in 5 of the cases, either at operation or in the resected specimen. Of this group, one patient ultimately died of a recurrent lesion and metastases (Case 3). Intussusception was present in 2 cases.

Prognosis (Table II).—The long period of delay before a diagnosis is established results in a poor prognosis. Of the 12 patients, 5 are now living. One (Case 1) is well thirteen years following resection of multiple lymphosarcomas of the jejunum. Four (Cases 6, 7, 11, and 12) are living following resection of the jejunum for adenocarcinoma; 2 for five years, 1 for fifteen months, and 1 for three months. The latter 2 patients had metastases which could not be removed. Seven patients have died; one not subjected to operation died in the hospital of widespread metastases from a jejunal lymphosarcoma. Of the remaining 6, one died six years and seven months after resection of the jejunum for a perforated leiomyosarcoma; one lived sixteen months after exploration which disclosed a jejunal carcinoid with metastasis. Two patients (Cases 9 and 10) died eighteen and seventeen months, respectively, after resection of the jejunum for adenocarcinoma with metastases, while the remaining two died eight and four months, respectively, after exploratory laparotomy which revealed inoperable lymphosarcoma of the ileum.

Benign Tumors

The small intestine may harbor a variety of benign tumors although these are extremely rare. A review of the literature and our own cases show that lesions include leiomyomas, fibromas, submucous lipomas, lymphangiomas, hemangiomas, polyps, and carcinoids. In our series there were only 7 cases of which 3 were incidental autopsy findings apparently unrelated to the cause of death, as clinical findings referable to the tumor were not recorded in the case histories (Table III). Four of the 7 lesions were leiomyomas, 1 a lipoma, 1 a fibroma, and 1a polyp (Tables III and IV).

Four patients were admitted to the New York Hospital with symptomatic benign tumors of the jejunum. The duration of symptoms varied from three days to fifteen months and there was an equal sex incidence. An analysis of the clinical findings shows that the prevailing symptoms are similar to those of the malignant lesions and that the differentiation can only be made by the operating surgeon and the pathologist. Obstructive symptoms, melena, weakness, and loss of weight are common findings. Examination failed to disclose an abdominal mass in any of the cases. Severe intestinal hemorrhage and anemia were present in 2 patients. In 3 of the cases a roentgen examination revealed evidence of small intestinal obstruction or the presence of a tumor (Table III).

TABLE II. PRIMARY MALIGNANT TUMORS OF JEJUNUM AND ILEUM

CASE NUMBER	DATE OF OPERATION	OPERATIVE FINDINGS	OPERATIVE PROCEDURE	SURGICAL PATHOLOGY	COMPLICATIONS	OPERATIVE RESULT	X-RAY THERAPY	FOLLOW-UP
1	2/12/34	Multiple stenosing lesions of jejunum, obstruction	Resection of 42 cm. of jejunum; lateral anastomosis	Multiple lymphosarcoma of jejunum; no metastases	None	Improved	Yes	Living and well 13 yr.
2	None						Yes	Died 6 weeks after admission; autopsy verified lymphosarcoma of jejunum with widespread metastases
3	10/ 4/40	Perforated tumor of lower jejunum; obstruction; peritonitis	Resection of 10 cm. of jejunum; end-to-end anastomosis	Leiomyosarcoma of jejunum; no metastases	Wound infection	Improved	None	Apparently well for 5 yr.; died of metastases, after 6 yr. and 7 mo.
4	7/ 7/41	Inoperable tumor of ileum; extensive metastases	Exploratory laparotomy	Lymphosarcoma	None	Unimproved	Yes	Lived 8 mo.
5	1/23/42	Inoperable tumor mass; metastases	Exploratory laparotomy and biopsy	Carcinoid of jejunum with metastasis	None	Unimproved	Yes	Lived 16 mo.
6	10/28/42	Tumor proximal jejunum; obstruction, intussusception, no metastases	Resection of 22 cm. of jejunum; end-to-end anastomosis	Mucus adenocarcinoma of jejunum	None	Improved		Living 5 yr.; well to the present time

7	10/24/42	Tumor proximal jejunum; obstruction, intussusception, no metastases	Resection of 26 cm. jejunum; end-to-end anastomosis	Mucous adenocarcinoma of jejunum; no metastases	None	Improved	Yes	Living 5 yr.; well to the present time
8	12/15/42	Inoperable tumor of ileum with partial obstruction	Exploratory laparotomy	Lymphosarcoma of ileum	None	Unimproved	Yes	Lived 4 mo.
9	8/31/44	Tumor lower jejunum; obstruction, metastases	Resection of 25 cm. of jejunum; end-to-end anastomosis	Adenocarcinoma of jejunum with metastases	None	Improved	None	Lived 17 mo.
10	9/15/45	Tumor proximal jejunum; obstruction, metastases	Resection of 14 cm. of jejunum; end-to-end anastomosis	Adenocarcinoma of jejunum with metastases	None	Improved	None	Lived 18 mo.
11	7/10/46	Tumor proximal jejunum, obstruction; no metastases	Resection of 16 cm. of jejunum; end-to-end anastomosis	Adenocarcinoma of jejunum	None	Improved	None	Well 15 mo.
12	6/30/47	Tumor proximal jejunum; metastases	Resection of 20 cm. of jejunum; end-to-end anastomosis	Adenocarcinoma of jejunum with metastases	None	Improved	None	Patient felt well 3 mo. after operation

TABLE III. BENIGN TUMORS OF JEJUNUM AND ILEUM—CLINICAL FINDINGS

CASE NUMBER	1	2	3	4	5	6	7
Name	L. B.	G. B.	S. H.	W. S.	C. Y.	B. D.	C. B.
Hospital number	22831	215560	439722	117668	70263	178306	277887
Year admitted	1940	1941	1946	1947	1934	1937	1940
Sex	M	F	F	M	M	M	F
Age (yr.)	47	2½	38	52	54	3 days	62
Duration of symptoms	15 mo.	10 days	2 mo.	3 days			
Abdominal pain	0	+	+	+			
Weight loss (pounds)	20	?	10	0	Incidental autopsy finding; diagnosis, polypoid fibroma of jejunum	Incidental autopsy finding; diagnosis, submucous polyp of ileum	Incidental autopsy finding; leiomyoma of jejunum
Vomiting	0	+	0	+			
Constipation	0	+	+	+			
Fatigue, weakness	+	+	+	0			
Melena	+	0	+	0			
Palpable mass	0	0	0	0			
Occult blood in stools	+	0	+	0			
R.B.C. (millions)	3.0	4.5	2.1	4.2			
Hb. (Gm.)	7.8	13.	6	14.2			
Obstruction demonstrable by x-ray	0	+	0	+			
Tumor demonstrable by x-ray	0	0	+	0			

TABLE IV. BENIGN TUMORS OF THE JEJUNUM AND ILEUM

CASE NUMBER	PATIENT	DATE OF OPERATION	OPERATIVE FINDINGS	OPERATIVE PROCEDURE	SURGICAL PATHOLOGY	COMPLICATIONS	RESULT	FOLLOW-UP
1	L. B.	6/21/40	Tumor mass, proximal jejunum	Resection of 7 cm. jejunum; end-to-end anastomosis	Leiomyoma	None	Cured	Well since operation
2	G. B.	5/10/41	Tumor mass, jejunum; obstruction adhesions	Resection 20 cm. jejunum; side-to-side anastomosis	Leiomyoma	None	Cured	Well since operation
3	S. M.	4/10/46	Tumor mass proximal jejunum; intussusception, obstruction	Resection 17 cm. jejunum; end-to-end anastomosis	Pedunculated leiomyoma	None	Cured	Well since operation
4	W. S.	4/22/47	Tumor mass, midjejunum; obstruction, intussusception	Resection 10 cm. jejunum; end-to-end anastomosis	Submucous lipoma	None	Cured	Well since operation

Exploratory laparotomy was performed on the 4 patients admitted to the hospital with symptoms and the lesion was resected in all four. Restoration of the continuity of the bowel was accomplished by aseptic end-to-end anastomosis in 3 and side-to-side anastomosis in 1 case (Table IV). Intussusception was present in 2 cases and varying degrees of obstruction in 3 cases. The operative procedures were accomplished without complications and there were no deaths. Follow-up studies show that all patients have been completely well since operation.

SUMMARY AND CONCLUSIONS

1. The clinical findings of 19 cases of tumor of the jejunum and ileum are presented.

2. Of the 12 patients with malignant lesions, 11 were subjected to operation. Resection of the tumor with enteroanastomosis was carried out in 8 instances without a death.

3. Of the 8 patients with resectable malignant lesions, 5 still survive: 1 over thirteen years, 2 over five years, 1 less than two years, and 1 less than one year.

4. Resection of the jejunum was performed in 4 patients with benign tumor of the jejunum without complication or mortality.

5. The poor prognosis in malignant lesions of the small bowel is the result of the long interval between the onset of symptoms and surgical intervention.

6. A history of intermittent intestinal obstruction and melena and the presence of occult blood in the stool are of great diagnostic significance. The small intestinal barium series will establish the diagnosis in a high percentage of cases.

7. The importance of careful exploration, in the presence of the symptoms and signs referred to, is stressed.

REFERENCES

1. McDougal, W. J.: Carcinoma of the Small Intestine, Am. J. Surg. **66**: 119, 1944.
2. Mayo, C. W., and Nettrour, W. S.: Carcinoma of the Jejunum, Surg., Gynec. & Obst. **65**: 303, 1937.
3. Shallow, T. A., Eger, S. A., and Carty, J. B.: Primary Malignant Disease of the Small Intestine, Am. J. Surg. **69**: 372, 1945.
4. Fraser, K.: Malignant Tumors of the Small Intestine—Review of Literature and Report of 21 Cases, Brit. J. Surg. **32**: 479, 1945.
5. Warren, R. W.: Primary Malignant Tumors of the Small Bowel, Canad. M. A. J. **51**: 451, 1944.
6. Foot, N. C.: Pathology in Surgery, Philadelphia, 1945, J. B. Lippincott Company.

PENETRATING WOUND OF THE CHEST WITH DIVISION OF A BRONCHIAL ARTERY

Report of a Case

Charles M. Brane, M.D., Yonkers, N. Y.

Wounds involving the bronchial arteries with recovery apparently are rare. A review of the literature for the past twenty-eight years has failed to reveal a reported case. In the case here reported, recovery followed the division of the left bronchial artery by a shell fragment of unusual size.

Ordinarily there are three bronchial arteries, two on one side and one on the other. Two arteries on the right side and one on the left are found as commonly as the classical description of two arteries on the left side and one on the right.[1] When there are two bronchial arteries on one side, both usually take their origin from the front of the aorta, one below the other at or near the level of the fourth thoracic vertebra. A single bronchial artery on one side may arise either as a common trunk with the upper bronchial artery of the opposite side or from the first aortic intercostal artery. Occasionally bronchial arteries may arise from the internal mammary, inferior thyroid, or subclavian arteries. Hovelacque, Monod, and Evrard,[1] and Nakamura[2] have investigated the great variability of the origin and course of the bronchial arteries. In the case being reported, a left bronchial artery arose from the lateral surface of the aorta, passing directly to the posterior surface of the left bronchus.

CASE REPORT

A 28-year-old officer was admitted to an evacuation hospital, Jan. 14, 1945, two hours after being wounded in the left posterior part of the chest by a shell fragment. He showed no evidence of shock, the pulse rate being 90, and the blood pressure 128/84. Removal of the dressing revealed a wound 6 cm. long and 3 cm. wide, medial to the scapula. There was no obvious sucking or hemorrhage. Roentgenograms (Figs. 1 and 2) showed a large foreign body penetrating the left side of the chest in a posteroanterior direction, through the fifth costal interspace.

Ninety minutes after admission, nitrous oxide-ether anesthesia under positive pressure was begun. After suitable cleansing and preparation, the wound was gently explored. The outer end of the foreign body was palpated 2.5 cm. below the level of the skin, and strong pulsations synchronous with the heartbeats were transmitted through it. The foreign body was tightly wedged between the badly comminuted fifth and sixth ribs and was not manipulated for fear of starting an intrathoracic hemorrhage. A posterior thoracotomy incision was made through the eighth interspace on the left. The postero-inferior border of the upper lobe of the left lung was lacerated along its entire length with the inner end of the foreign body lodged against the lateral surface of the aorta. Five hundred cubic centimeters of clotted blood were removed from the pleural cavity, and the shell fragment was dislodged and withdrawn from its wedged position between the ribs. This was followed by profuse arterial bleeding. Digital pressure against the hilus of the lung close to the aorta controlled the bleeding but not before a loss of approximately 1,500 c.c. of blood had occurred. Replacement with cross-matched stored blood was started.

After removal of the blood by suction, the pressure was gradually released, revealing the spurting stump of what was determined to be a bronchial artery. The artery was clamped and doubly ligated with silk 1.5 cm. from its aortic origin. Its diameter was between 3 and 4 mm. No other arteries arising from the aorta and passing to the lung were noted in this area. The pleura covering the posterior surface of the hilus had been

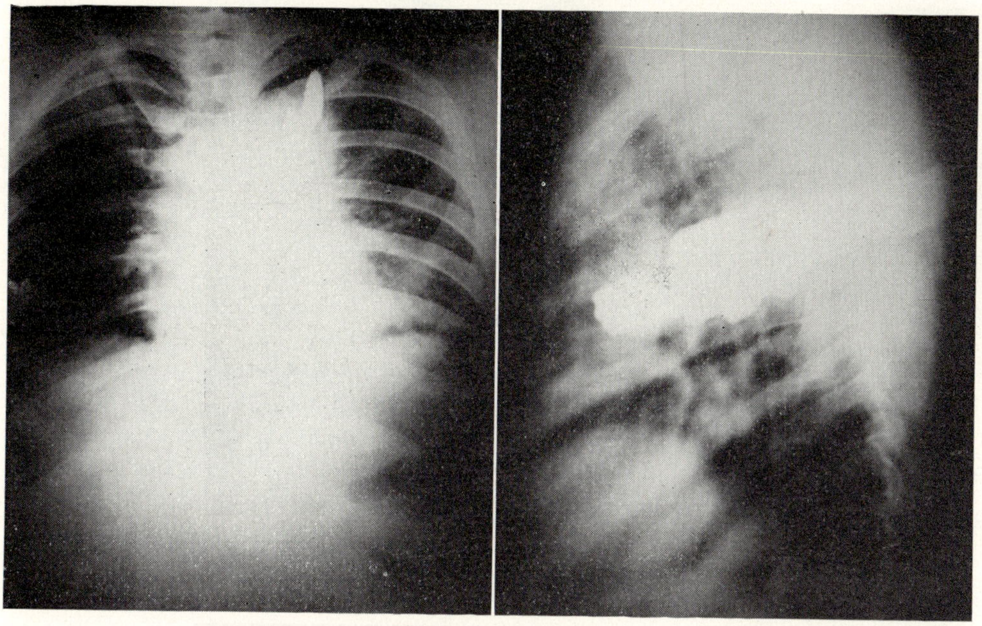

Figs. 1 and 2.—Roentgenograms, Jan. 14, 1945, showing huge size and position of shell fragment before removal.

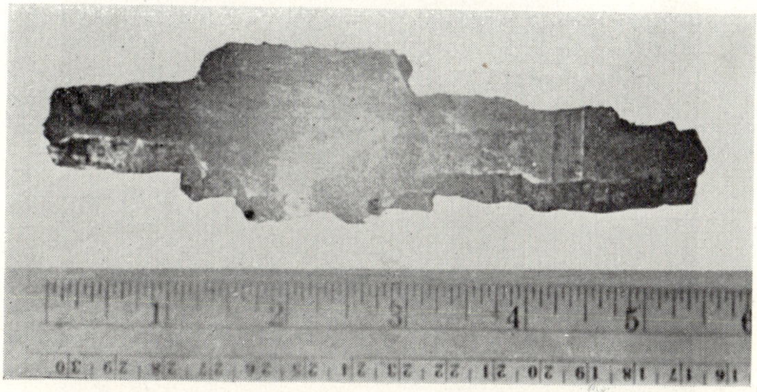

Fig. 3.—Shell fragment with scale in centimeters and inches.

lacerated so extensively by the missile that the entire width of the main bronchus close to the aorta and the inferior pulmonary vein were exposed. The badly damaged lung tissue was resected and the lung closed with mattress sutures of silk. Thirty-five thousand units of penicillin and 7 Gm. of sulfanilamide were placed in the pleural cavity and the thoracotomy incision was closed in layers with interrupted silk sutures. The wound of entrance was débrided, the ends of the fractured ribs resected, and the wound sutured. The patient's condition remained good throughout the procedure.

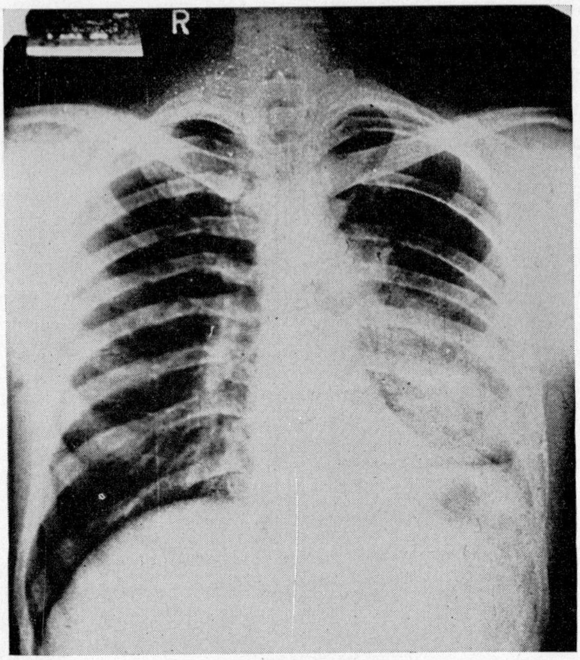

Fig. 4.—Roentgenogram, March 8, 1945, showing condition of chest approximately seven weeks after operation.

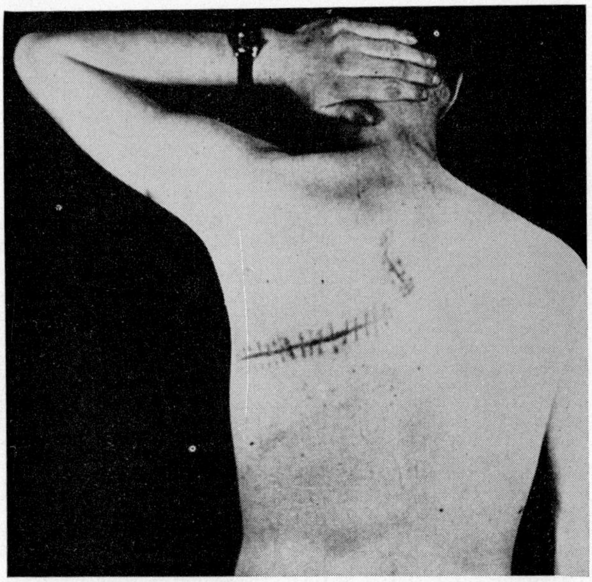

Fig. 5.—Patient, March 8, 1945. The upper scar shows the site of entry of the fragment; the surgical approach is indicated by the lower scar.

The postoperative course was uneventful. For several days there was a cough productive of small amounts of old dark blood. On the second day 700 c.c. of serosanguineous fluid were aspirated from the left pleural cavity. On the fourth day aspiration was repeated and 200 c.c. of fluid were removed. Forty thousand units of penicillin were given intramuscularly every four hours for forty-eight hours, and 1 Gm. of sulfadiazine was given by mouth every four hours for seven days. This patient made satisfactory progress toward recovery and was evacuated to a general hospital on the seventh postoperative day.

Subsequent reports from a general hospital and from the patient over a period of eight months indicated that a satisfactory recovery was made. The patient stated by letter that there was a ''lag'' of the left chest during respiration and that he has had breathlessness on moderate physical exertion. He felt well however, was able to engage in such sports as golf, swimming, and dancing, and had been returned to limited duty.

COMMENT

No evidence of necrotic change in the lung of this patient occurred. The source of the blood supply to the bronchi and lung substance may have been from another bronchial artery not seen posteriorly or, as rarely happens, from a bronchial artery passing along the anterior surface of the bronchus. It seems more probable that the blood supply was obtained through anastomoses between the bronchial arterial system above the point of division and other arteries. All recent investigators agree on the presence of a capillary anastomosis between the bronchial and pulmonary arteries, but deny the existence of a precapillary anastomosis.[3-6] An injection method in the living dog has shown the existence of gross anastomoses between the bronchial, internal mammary, intercostal, and esophageal arteries.[7] Injections of human autopsy specimens have demonstrated gross extracardiac anastomoses between the auricular branches of the coronary arteries and the bronchial arteries.[8]

SUMMARY

1. An unusual case, a wound of the chest with division of a bronchial artery, is reported.

2. A satisfactory recovery followed ligation of the artery without evidence of gangrene of the bronchi or lung substance.

REFERENCES

1. Hovelacque, A., Monod, O., and Evrard, H.: Note au sujet des arteres bronchiques, Ann d'anat. path. **13**: 129, 1936.
2. Nakamura, N.: Zur Anatomie der Bronchialarterien, Anat. Anz. **58**: 508, 1924.
3. Miller, W. S.: The Vascular Supply of the Bronchial Tree, Am. Rev. Tuberc. **12**: 87, 1925.
4. Mathes, M., Holman, E., and Reichert, F. L.: A Study of the Bronchial, Pulmonary, and Lymphatic Circulations of the Lung Under Various Pathological Conditions Experimentally Produced, J. Thoracic Surg. **1**: 339, 1932.
5. Berry, J. L.: The Relation Between Bronchial and Pulmonary Circulations in the Human Lung Investigated by Radio-opaque Injections, Quart. J. Exper. Physiol. **24**: 305, 1935.
6. Wood, D. A., and Miller, M.: The Role of the Dual Pulmonary Circulation in Various Pathologic Conditions of the Lungs, J. Thoracic Surg. **7**: 649, 1938.
7. Horine, C. F., and Warner, C. G.: Distribution of the Pulmonary and Bronchial Circulation, J. Thoracic Surg. **2**: 80, 1932.
8. Hudson, C. L., Moritz, A. R., and Wearn, J. T.: The Extra-cardiac Anastomoses of the Coronary Arteries, J. Exper. Med. **56**: 919, 1932.

RESECTION OF THE RECTUM WITH PRESERVATION OF THE ANAL SPHINCTER

William F. Nickel, Jr., M.D., New York, N. Y., and
Arthur I. Chenoweth, M.D., Birmingham, Ala.

In the past few years increasing attention has been devoted to methods by which malignant tumors of the rectosigmoid and rectum might be extirpated without sacrifice of the normal mechanism of defecation. There has been the question in the minds of many surgeons whether it were not possible to avoid the creation of a permanent abdominal colostomy and at the same time perform a resection of the tumor-bearing tissues sufficiently radical as not to compromise the patient's chance for survival. The question is a highly controversial one, and the answer can come only through the accumulation of a sufficiently large volume of cases performed by the two methods to allow comparative studies. In view of this, it seems worth while to review a series of cases in which resection of the rectum was carried out by the perineal route or by the combined abdominal and perineal routes, the anal sphincters being preserved to allow voluntary control of defecation. The present series, while not large, is presented for the purpose of supplementing existing and future series of similar cases with a view toward assessing the proper value of such procedures.

HISTORICAL

The technique utilized in this series is by no means new, nor is the idea of preserving the sphincters new. In an excellent article published in 1945, Bacon[1] reviewed "the evolution of sphincter muscle preservation and re-establishment of continuity in the operative treatment of sigmoidal and rectal cancer." Mandl[2] also, in a recent article, reviewed the history of such procedures, while reviewing his experiences with the Hochenegg[3] "pull-through" operation. It was the latter who, near the end of the nineteenth century, evolved the technique of resecting the growth-bearing segment of rectum, and invaginating the proximal divided end of sigmoid through the anus, with or without stripping of the anal mucosa.

This procedure, with slight modifications, was also performed by a number of other surgeons in the late nineteenth and early twentieth centuries.

Since 1932 Babcock[4] and his colleague Bacon[5] have been enthusiastic proponents of a procedure based upon the Hochenegg maneuver, but having an important modification. These surgeons mobilize the sigmoid and upper rectum through the abdomen, after ligation of the superior hemorrhoidal vessels, and then proceed to resect the rectum from below, leaving the external sphincter intact.

Other authors in the past few years have advocated transabdominal resection with end-to-end anastomosis. Dixon[6] in 1944 found a three-year survival rate of 58 per cent in a series of 104 patients on whom he had performed this procedure for carcinoma of the rectosigmoid. Wangensteen[7] reported that he resected the ampulla of the rectum in twenty-seven patients, using the Hochenegg procedure in some, and end-to-end anastomosis in others. Waugh and Custer[8] likewise have found it possible to perform end-to-end anastomosis through the abdomen after resection of lesions very low in the rectum.

A different approach is that recently proposed by Murray[9] who utilized the transsacral approach in performing resection with end-to-end anastomosis. He resects the fourth and fifth sacral segments and has carried out this procedure on fifteen patients with one permanent fecal fistula and perfect continence in all other cases.

Mahorner[10] reported a combined procedure, carried out on five patients. He mobilizes the bowel through an abdominal incision, then turns the patient over and resects the lesion through an oblique incision over the perirectal fossa, performing an end-to-end suture.

MATERIAL

The present study comprises a review of sixty-eight patients operated upon on the Surgical Service of New York Hospital between September, 1932, and December, 1946. The operations were performed by Dr. Heuer, or his associates, or his residents: approximately fifteen different surgeons. Follow-up studies are based upon examinations carried out in the Follow-up Clinic of the Surgical Service, where each patient was seen at intervals of six months. In only four cases was the evaluation based upon a letter or telephone conversation.

The pathologic diagnoses made on the surgical specimens were as follows: adenocarcinoma (not graded) fifty-nine; polypoid carcinoma three; adenoma malignum three; scirrhous carcinoma, carcinoma simplex, and metaplastic adenoma, one each.

OPERATIVE TECHNIQUE

The operation as performed at present is carried out as follows: through a left rectus incision the abdomen is explored. This permits the operator to assess the factors which enable him to determine whether or not preservation of the sphincter muscles is advisable.

The sigmoid is mobilized by incising the parietal peritoneum on either side of the bowel down to the reflexion of the peritoneum. The mesentery of the sigmoid is then clamped and ligated below the superior hemorrhoidal artery. We do not hesitate to divide the superior hemorrhoidal artery if its integrity prevents sufficient mobilization of the sigmoid to bring it down to the perineum. The rectum is mobilized in the hollow of the sacrum posteriorly and from the bladder anteriorly. The dissection is carried as far downward beneath the peritoneal reflexion as is possible through the abdominal incision which is then covered with several laparotomy pads. Two assistants remain at the abdominal field to complete the surgery there.

The patient is then placed in lithotomy position with the foot of the table slightly elevated, and the perineum is prepared and draped. The operator and one assistant then proceed with the perineal part of the operation.

A circular incision is made at the mucocutaneous junction around the anus and is carried vertically downward over the coccyx and lower end of the sacrum. The anus is readily dissected free from the sphincter muscles. A purse string

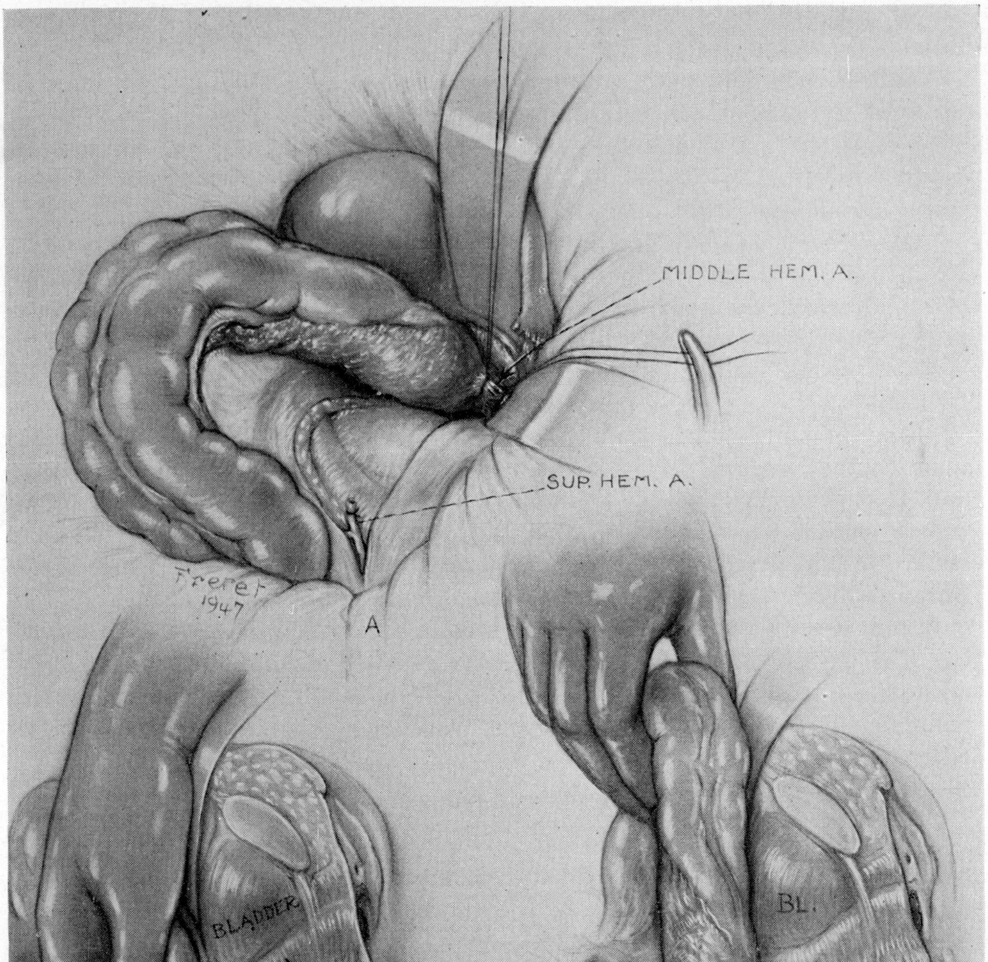

Fig. 1.—*A, B,* and *C* illustrate the abdominal portion of the operative procedure demonstrating the mobilization of the sigmoid.

of braided silk is used to occlude the anus and for traction on the rectum. The sphincter ani muscles are encircled by two silk ligatures on either side of the median raphe posteriorly and are then divided between the ligatures. These are left in place to identify the severed ends when the plastic repair is performed at the close of the procedure.

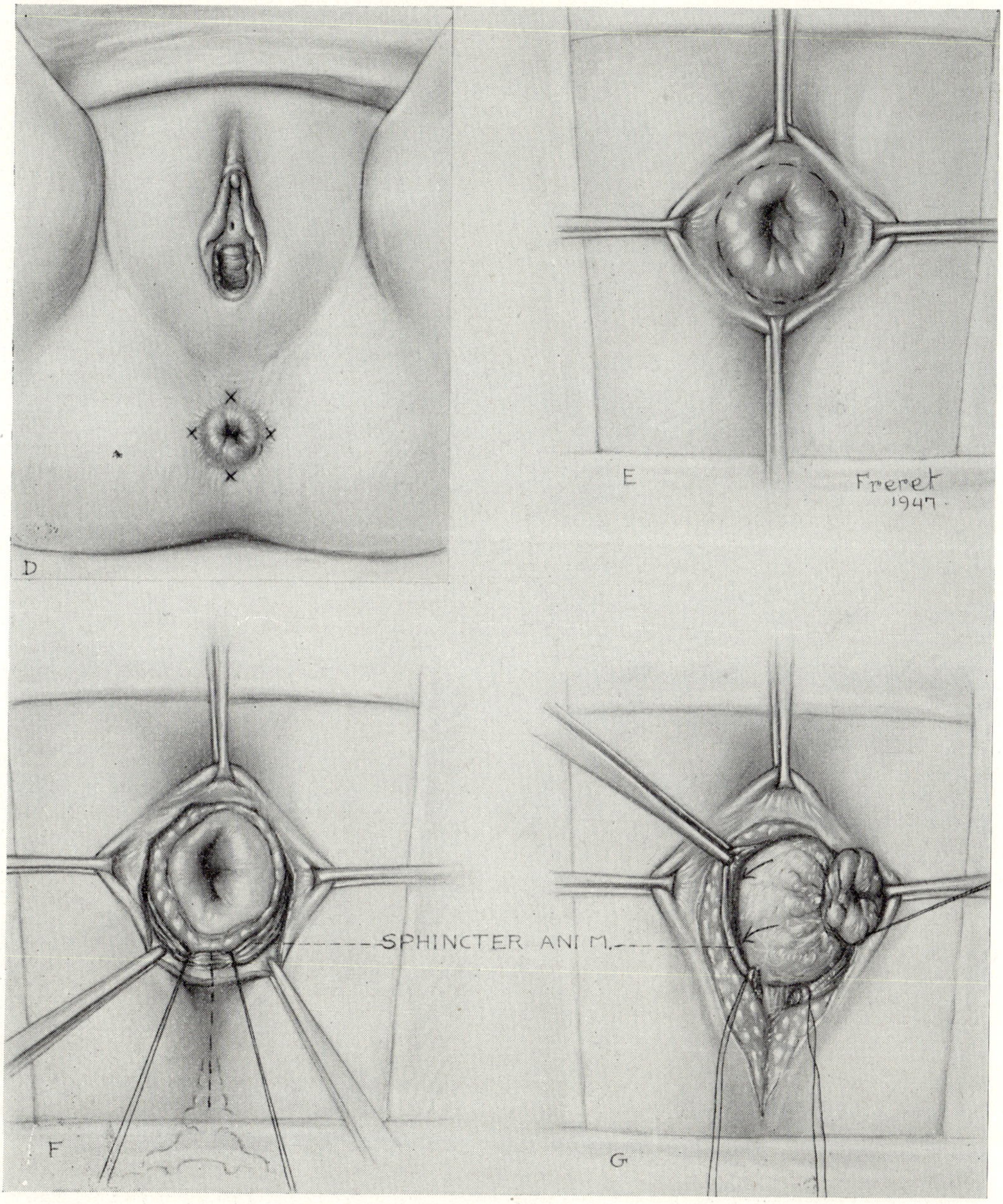

Fig. 2.—*D, E, F* and *G* illustrate the mobilization of the rectum with preservation of the sphincter ani muscles (see Fig. 3).

The vertical incision is deepened through the subcutaneous tissues. The coccygeal ligaments are divided, and if the coccyx interferes with the dissection, it is removed. Mobilization of the rectum is then carried upward until the levator ani muscles are encountered. These are divided as far laterally as the operator believes necessary. The rectum is separated from the prostate and

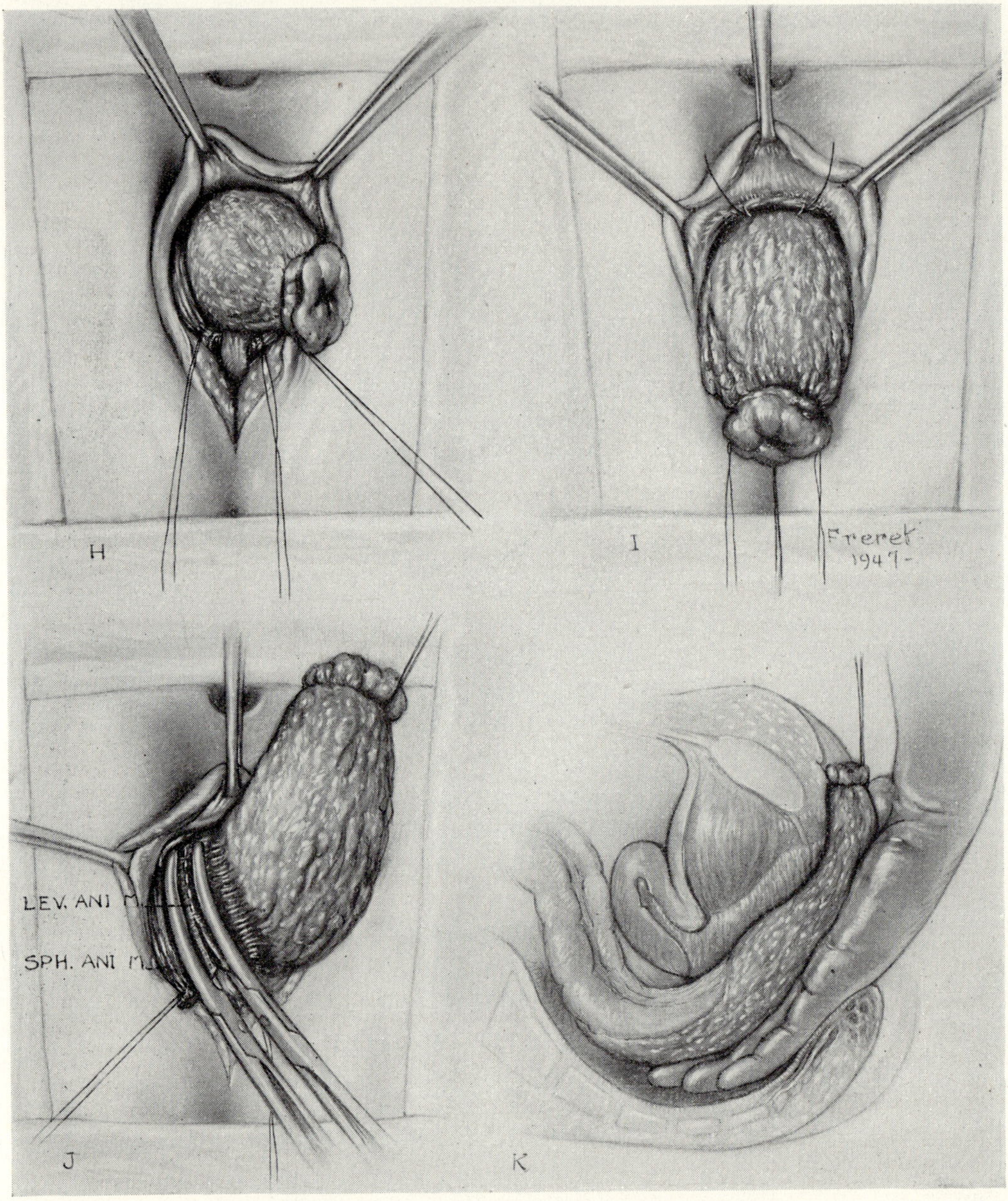

Fig. 3.—*H, I, J,* and *K* illustrate the mobilization of the rectum with preservation of the sphincter ani muscles (see Fig. 2).

seminal vesicles or vagina by blunt and sharp dissection. At this point the rectum may usually be delivered through the wound without difficulty and the sigmoid drawn down to the anal sphincters.

If sufficient tissue remains, the levator ani muscles are reapproximated to the wall of the sigmoid, as we believe that they aid in control of defecation. The ends of the divided sphincter muscles are identified by the previously

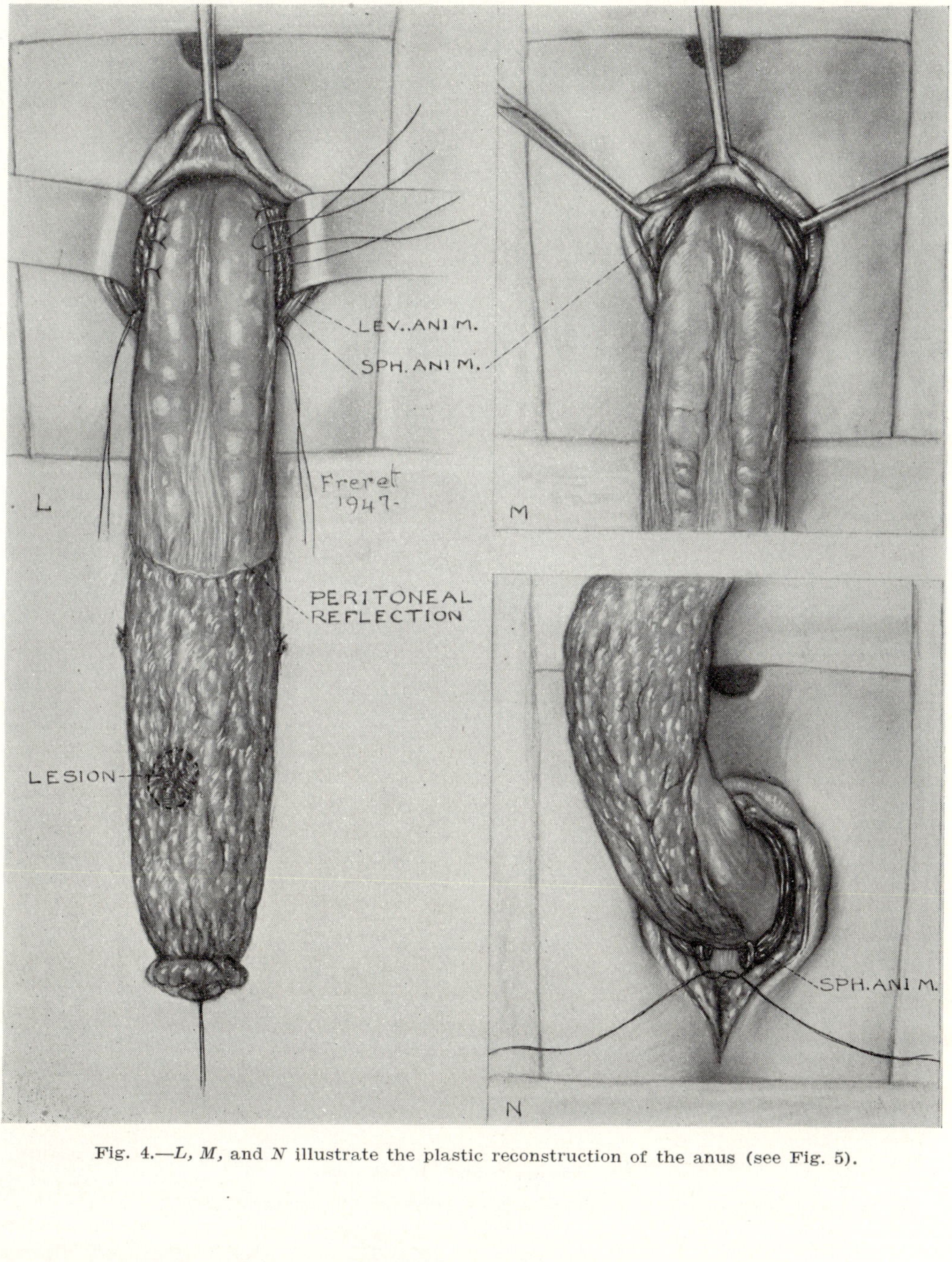

Fig. 4.—*L, M,* and *N* illustrate the plastic reconstruction of the anus (see Fig. 5).

placed silk sutures and are reapproximated around the sigmoid. One or two cigarette drains are then placed into the pelvis posterior to the bowel wall. The sigmoid is sutured to the anal skin margin and the vertical incision closed. The final step in the perineal part of the procedure is excision of the bowel flush with the skin. When it has been ascertained that the sigmoid safely reaches the anal sphincters, the two assistants at the abdominal field complete the repair of the peritoneum around the sigmoid and close the abdominal wound.

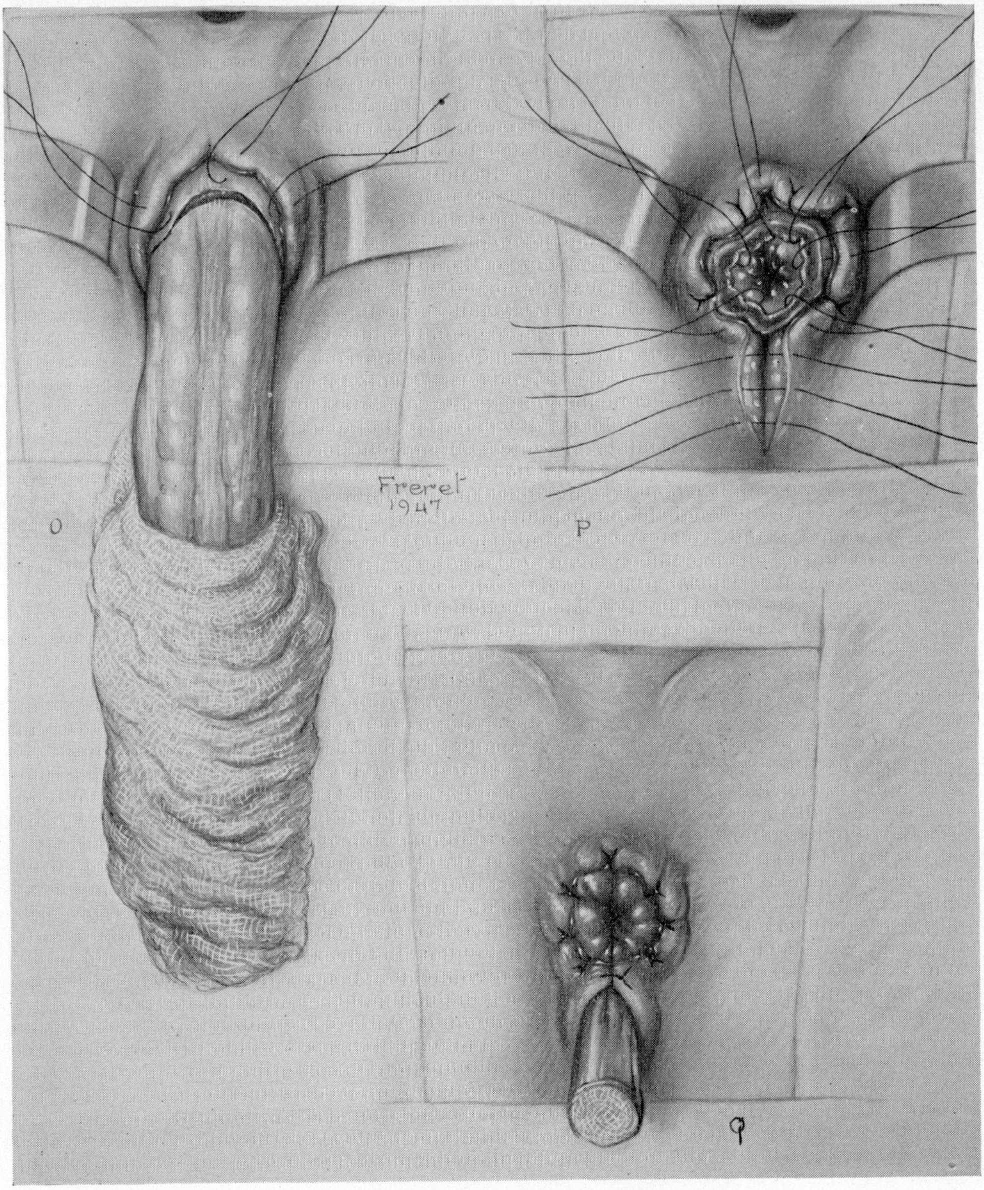

Fig. 5.—*O* and *P* illustrate the plastic reconstruction of the anus (see Fig. 4). *Q* represents the final appearance of the anus.

MORTALITY

Of sixty-eight patients operated upon, nine died in the hospital, yielding a postoperative mortality rate of 13.2 per cent. This figure, when compared to other figures published in recent years, seems excessive. For this reason it is of interest to inquire further into the deaths and to subdivide them according to years (Table I). It is significant to note that all deaths occurred prior to 1941, and that there were no deaths in the group of twenty-three patients operated upon between 1941 and 1946.

TABLE I. MORTALITY BY YEARS

	YEAR	NUMBER OF CASES	NUMBER OF DEATHS
	1932	3	0
	1933	5	0
	1934	9	4
	1935	4	0
	1936	2	0
	1937	3	0
	1938	8	2
	1939	10	2
	1940	4	1
	1941	7	0
	1942	3	0
	1943	3	0
	1944	4	0
	1945	0	0
	1946	3	0
Total	15 Years	68	9

It is of further interest to observe the causes of death and the ages of the patients (Table II). One death, that of a 39-year-old patient, should have been prevented; another patient of 50 years should not have been subjected to operation, inasmuch as he was found to have pulmonary metastases. All the others were patients in the seventh decade or older.

TABLE II. PATIENTS DYING POSTOPERATIVELY

HISTORY NO.	NAME	SEX	AGE (YR.)	CAUSE OF DEATH
22511	R. G.	F	64	Peritonitis
58822	M. G.	F	67	Gas gangrene in perineal wound
65688	J. R.	F	62	Purulent phlebitis and septicemia
69997	H. T.	M	73	Pneumonia and infarcts
79801	P. M.	M	64	Multiple abscesses, abdominal wall, buttocks
211143	L. G.	F	66	Pulmonary embolus
227038*	A. W.	M	50	Bronchopneumonia superimposed on pulmonary metastatic cancer
270596	L. F.	F	39	Hemorrhage and shock
194158	S. B.	M	74	Suicide

*This case was wrongly diagnosed as bilateral bronchiectasis prior to operation. The patient died of bronchopneumonia. At autopsy metastatic cancer of the lungs was found, obviously not a suitable case for operation.

The decline in the mortality rate reflects the improvements in preoperative preparation, methods of anesthesia, and postoperative care of surgical patients. Furthermore, our experience has run closely parallel to that of Lehman and Becker[11] who, in reviewing all surgical deaths at the University of Virginia

TABLE III

YEARS OF SURVIVAL	NUMBER OF PATIENTS UNDER CONSIDERATION	NUMBER OF PATIENTS SURVIVING	SURVIVAL RATE (%)
3	61	38	62
5	55	22	40
10	23	6	26

Hospital, found a progressive decline from 7.1 per cent in 1934, to 3.5 per cent in 1940, to 2.5 per cent in 1946. To be more specific in regard to patients in this group, there can be no doubt that increased attention to nutritional requirements, especially proteins and vitamins, is an important factor in the decline. The advent of the sulfonamide drugs and penicillin played a part, as well as an appreciation of the importance of thorough mechanical cleansing of the gastrointestinal tract before operation.

SURVIVAL RATES

In computing the survival rates in this series, we base our figures on the results in sixty-one patients, since seven patients were operated upon after 1943, or less than three years before this study was undertaken. We have, of course, not excluded the nine patients who died in the immediate postoperative period. There was a three-year survival rate of 62 per cent, a five-year rate of 40 per cent, and a ten-year rate of 26 per cent (Table III).

TABLE IV. SURVIVAL STATISTICS

YEARS OF SURVIVAL	NUMBER OF PATIENTS	PRESENT STATUS
15	1	Living without evidence of recurrence
14	1	
12	1	
11	1	
10	2	
9	1	Living without evidence of recurrence but lost to follow-up since October, 1944
8	3	1 living without evidence of recurrence 1 living with recurrence when last seen in May, 1946 1 died of metastases in 1946
7	2	1 living without recurrence 1 living with recurrence, April, 1946
6	4	3 living without recurrence, one last seen in August, 1945 1 now dead
5	6	4 no evidence of recurrence 2 now dead
4	7	All dead
3	9	6 dead 3 living without evidence of recurrence; 1 last seen in June, 1944
2	2	Both dead
1	5	All dead
Less than 1 year	7*	All dead
Postoperative death	9	
Total 61		

*Includes two patients who had purely palliative procedures.

These figures are to be compared with those recently published by Bacon, based upon records of eighty-one patients operated upon three or more years before his study. He found a three-year survival rate of 58.6 per cent and a five-year rate of 50 per cent.

Table III may be further broken down and presented in a more comprehensive form as shown in Table IV.

FUNCTIONAL RESULTS

It would be futile to go to great lengths to preserve the anal sphincters if, after their preservation, they failed to function. We have, therefore, investigated closely the functional results in this group of patients. It should be pointed out again that evaluation is based, in all except four cases, upon direct questioning and examination of the patients. We have, perhaps, been rather too strict in our assessment of these results in a sincere desire to judge for ourselves the efficacy of this technique.

Of 68 patients subjected to this procedure, 9 died in the immediate postoperative period; 10 patients either died within 1 year of operation or have been operated less than 1 year before and so are not suitable for evaluation; 5 patients developed recurrence within one year and were subjected to colostomy.

Since no information as to function is available on nine patients, there remain thirty-four cases suitable for evaluation from the standpoint of function of the reconstructed anal outlet. Results have been evaluated as follows: (1) Perfect: indicating normal control regardless of consistency of stools, no staining, and the presence of a sphincter which on examination contracts normally; (2) good: indicating control of bowels with no soilage except under unusual circumstances, such as an episode of diarrhea or following the use of a laxative —a few patients in this group have rather tight strictures, two requiring occasional dilatation; (3) fair: these patients must wear a perineal pad at all times because of unpredictable accidents; they have control of the bulk of the stool but there is a slight leak or staining on frequent occasions; for this reason they are insecure without a pad; (4) poor: in this category are carried those patients who have no control of the stools, no sphincter, and who have what amounts to a perineal colostomy.

As judged by these standards the results are: perfect, 3; good, 7; fair, 10; poor, 14; making a total of 34.

Admittedly this is a small series of patients (thirty-four) from which to draw conclusions as to function. Some value, however, stems from the fact that each has been critically examined and no evaluation made without sound basis.

DISCUSSION

In the light of our present knowledge, then, is there justification for a procedure such as this?

Lahey and Miles, to name only two of the opponents of sphincter-preservation operations, firmly believe that there is no place for such a procedure in the attack upon cancer. They base their arguments upon the assumption that no procedure in which the sphincters are preserved can be sufficiently radical. Miles, furthermore, stated that carcinoma of the rectum has three zones of spread: upward, downward, and laterally. Recent careful investigations concerning the spread of cancer of the rectum have been made by Coller, Kay, and MacIntyre,[12] by Gilchrist and David,[13] and by Glover and Waugh.[14] The findings of these several investigators are fairly uniform, and while they do not directly contradict the statements of Miles, they do serve to modify the meaning of the three zones of spread. The conclusions of these authors indicate that the primary zone of spread is upward, to the nodes of the mesosigmoid; that lesions whose lower border is 2 cm. or more above the insertion of the levator muscles do not tend to spread laterally, and that retrograde spread takes place only to a distance of 3 cm. below the lower margin of the growth, except in rare instances.

If we can assume, as a result of the findings of these investigators, that extension does not, in general, occur laterally along the levators or downward toward the skin and sphincters, there remains only the question of whether it is possible to secure a resection sufficiently high to remove involved nodes in the mesosigmoid. Certainly this cannot be accomplished entirely from below. Whether or not it can be accomplished by a combined abdominal and perineal approach is determined by several variables: (a) length and "redundancy" of sigmoid; (b) distribution of blood vessels; and (c) depth of pelvis.

It is possible, by mobilizing the decending colon and splenic flexure to provide sufficient length of colon to reach the perineum through a pelvis of any depth, provided the blood vessels do not restrict the transplantation. It has been found, contrary to earlier opinion, that it is possible to divide the superior hemorrhoidal artery and the lowest sigmoidal branch of the inferior mesenteric artery without consequent necrosis of the lower end of the sigmoid. On the other hand, in some cases even after division of these vessels the sigmoidal arcades are so short as to prevent descent of the sigmoid sufficiently far into the pelvis. These factors, therefore, can be judged only at the operating table with the abdomen open.

This procedure has a limited field of application. Our belief, based upon our experience with this series and the investigations of others, is that it is applicable only to lesions whose lower margin is at least 6 cm. above the anal orifice, and whose upper limit is at or below the peritoneal reflection. When cases are restricted within this field, favorable results may be expected. If, however, enthusiasm for the procedure influences one to stretch the indications, the value of the operation becomes lost. As to the functional results, it was noted that in fourteen patients the attempt to provide sphincteric control was a failure; possibly these patients would have been better off with an abdominal colostomy. On the other hand, all of the remaining twenty patients, even those required to wear a perineal pad, are probably better equipped to pursue their daily activities than are others with abdominal colostomies.

In conclusion, then, we believe that if cases are properly selected, the operation of abdominoperineal resection can be carried out and the anal sphincters preserved without jeopardizing the patient's chance of survival, and with a good chance of providing him with a functioning anal outlet.

REFERENCES

1. Bacon: Surg., Gynec. & Obst. **81**: 113, 1945.
2. Mandl: SURGERY **18**: 318, 1945.
3. Hochenegg: Wien. klin. Wchnschr. **2**: 515, 1889.
4. Babcock: S. Clin. N. America **12**: 1397, 1932.
5. Bacon: Am. J. Surg. **71**: 728, 1946.
6. Dixon: SURGERY **15**: 367, 1944.
7. Wangensteen: Surg., Gynec. & Obst. **81**: 1, 1945.
8. Waugh and Custer: Surg., Gynec. & Obst. **81**: 593, 1945.
9. Murray: Surg., Gynec. & Obst. **82**: 283, 1946.
10. Mahorner: Ann. Surg. **123**: 866, 1946.
11. Lehman and Becker: Ann. Surg. **125**: 515, 1947.
12. Coller, Kay, and MacIntyre: SURGERY **8**: 294, 1940.
13. Gilchrist and David: Ann. Surg. **108**: 621, 1938.
14. Glover and Waugh: Surg., Gynec. & Obst. **82**: 434, 1946.

RADICAL ONE-STAGE PANCREATICODUODENECTOMY

CHARLES G. CHILD, III, M.D., NEW YORK, N. Y.

(From the Department of Surgery of The New York Hospital and Cornell University Medical College)

DURING the twelve years which have elapsed since Allen O. Whipple and his associates[1] announced their initial success in extirpating the duodenum and the head of the pancreas, the original two-stage operation has undergone many modifications. Although the story of the development of what might be termed the present-day radical operation is a fascinating one, it has been covered adequately elsewhere and reiteration at this time does not seem particularly profitable. Because, however, numerous of the details in the operation continue to be the subject of debate, it still seems in order to report even a relatively small series of cases in which one general method of completing the operation has been rather rigidly observed. It is the purpose of this report, therefore, to review an operation which has proved satisfactory in a group of twenty-two patients operated upon at the New York Hospital during the past six years.

In November, 1943, I[2a] reported a one-stage procedure which was justly criticized by Whipple not only because drainage of the biliary tract was reestablished by means of the gall bladder, but also because this anastomosis was placed distal to that between the stomach and the jejunum. The operation was promptly changed to one in which biliary drainage was obtained by way of a choledochojejunostomy placed proximal to the gastroenterostomy. In all of these cases save five a Coffey[3] type of end-to-end pancreaticojejunostomy was performed.[2b]

In this series of twenty-two consecutive radical pancreaticoduodenectomies the operation was performed by six different surgeons, three of whom were surgical residents. For purposes of convenience these cases have been outlined in Table I. The postoperative mortality was 27 per cent.

In the course of acquiring experience with the technique of this one-stage procedure, it was found helpful to have clearly in mind a series of steps which, if followed in orderly progression, contribute materially to shortening and facilitating a procedure which is always long and arduous.

1. The abdominal cavity is entered through an upper transverse incision. Although several of these cases were operated upon quite satisfactorily through the right rectus incision, it seemed that the transverse position offered the most satisfactory exposure, particularly if the dissection needed to be carried far out on the tail of the pancreas.

2. After entering the peritoneal cavity a preliminary search is made for distant metastasis which if found constitutes a contraindication to any further procedure other than a palliative cholecystenterostomy.

TABLE I. RADICAL ONE-STAGE PANCREATICODUODENECTOMY (NEW YORK HOSPITAL, 1941-1947)

CASE NO.	INITIALS	AGE (YR.)	HIST. NO.	PRIMARY CARCINOMA	DATE OF OPERATION	PANCREATICO-JEJUNOSTOMY	RESULT
1	A. C.	62	451310	Ampulla	8/ 6/46	No	I & D Intraperitoneal abscess 8/30/46; now well 14 mo.
2	S. H.	55	363096	Ampulla	12/20/43	Yes	Dead; metastases 14 mo.
3	G. T.	46	409149	Ampulla	3/31/45	Yes	Well 2 yr., 7 mo.
4	E. M.	67	436554	Ampulla	2/27/46	No	P.O. death 13th day; pancreatic fistula, anuria
5	A. F.	46	464078	Ampulla	1/ 9/47	Yes	P.O. death 14th day; anuria
6	B. T.	65	471549	Islet cell	3/14/47	Yes	P.O. death 1st day; adm. blood sugar 19 mg. per 100 c.c.
7	J. C.	55	49256	Pancreas	4/28/41	No	P.O. death 15th day
8	S. M.	58	445401	Pancreas	5/21/46	Yes	Dead 11 mo.; presumed recurrence
9	R. F.	11	408141	Pancreas	10/ 1/46	Yes	Dead 5 mo.; recurrence
10	H. G.	54	459407	Pancreas	11/ 1/46	Yes	Well 11 mo.
11	C. F.	59	145716	Pancreas	11/ 8/46	Yes	P.O. death 30th day; spontaneous pneumothorax
12	E. F.	46	460622	Pancreas	11/12/46	Yes	Alive 12 mo.; recurrence
13	E. M. S.	62	429937	Pancreas	2/11/47	Yes	Well 6 mo.
14	N. C.	70	472383	Pancreas	4/ 1/47	No	P.O. death 5th day; division of superior mesenteric vein
15	B. M.	74	107557	Pancreas	1/23/47	Yes	Alive 10 mo.; (?) recurrence
16	M. M.	69	Memorial Hosp.	Pancreas	12/14/46	Yes	Alive 8 mo.; lost to follow-up
17	J. B.	57	311583	Duodenum	11/28/41	Yes	Dead 18 mo.; recurrence
18	W. M.	69	361219	Duodenum	7/ 3/43	Yes	Well 4 yr., 3 mo.
19	C. K.	53	380758	Duodenum	4/ 4/44	Yes	Well 3 yr., 6 mo.
20	A. O.	66	439925	Duodenum	4/11/46	No	Well 1 yr., 6 mo.
21	W. H. J. M.	65	375553	Stomach	1/ 6/44	Yes	Well 17 mo.; died, "stroke"
22	J. F.	49	273642	Ascending colon	2/25/47	Yes	Well 8 mo.

3. Attention is then directed to the common duct, the pancreas, and the duodenum. At this point the problem of the differential diagnosis between common duct stone, chronic pancreatitis, carcinoma of the pancreas, and primary tumors of the ampulla of Vater and duodenum arises. This may be extremely simple, as would be the case in promptly producing a large common duct stone, or tremendously complex, as in a patient harboring a small carcinoma little more than 1 cm. in diameter buried deeply in the head of the pancreas. Many surgeons have attempted to elucidate this difficult problem without, as yet, any simple answer becoming evident. Suffice it to state that fortunately, or unfortunately, the ease with which a positive diagnosis is made still must rest with the surgeon's skill as a gross pathologist. Yet a decision must be made. Cattell[4] has probably made the most helpful single suggestion, namely, that if

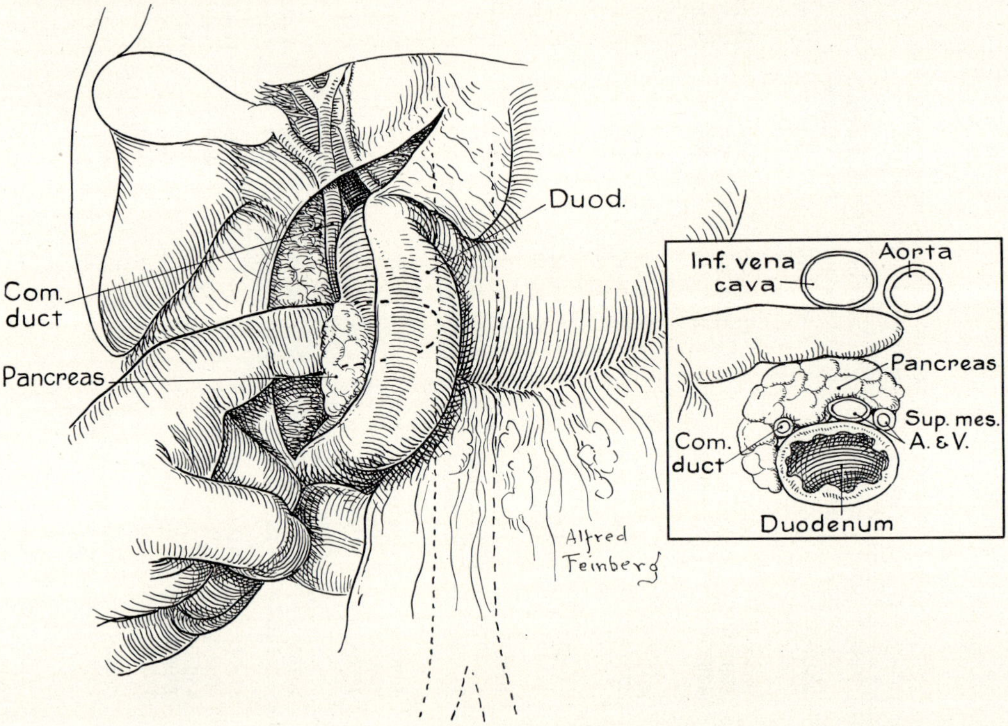

Fig. 1.—By dividing the peritoneal reflection over the duodenum as far caudad as possible, the loose areolar space between the pancreas and the deeper structures may be entered readily. At this point the presence or absence of periaortic nodes involved in metastatic cancer may be determined. If such lymphatic involvement or direct extension is identified the procedure should be abandoned at this stage.

the presence of cancer cannot with reasonable certainty be proved, a two-stage procedure should be accepted as the maneuver of choice at this time. After subsidence of the jaundice, re-exploration may then indicate whether or not a perplexing pancreatic enlargement is carcinomatous or inflammatory. If, however, there is reasonable assurance that a malignant tumor is present, the operator is justified in proceeding, with the realization that the majority of pancreatic cancers have been removed without benefit of a positive microscopic diagnosis.

At this point it might be well to note that as yet there is no complete agreement as to whether or not enlarged regional lymph nodes constitute an absolute contraindication to progressing with an otherwise operable neoplasm. It is my opinion that as long as these tumors technically permit extirpation the patient should not be denied his only chance of cure because of the presence of a few enlarged lymph nodes.

4. Having elected to proceed, the next step involves division of the right paraduodenal peritoneum from the orifice of the foramen of Winslow as far caudad as possible (Fig. 1). By careful digital dissection behind the duodenum and uncinate process of the pancreas, valid information may be obtained with regard to direct extension of the tumor to the aorta, and by palpation just beyond the tip of the uncinate process some indication may be obtained as to whether the superior mesenteric vein is grossly invaded. Should these maneuvers prove encouraging, the duodenum may be replaced and attention directed toward the next step.

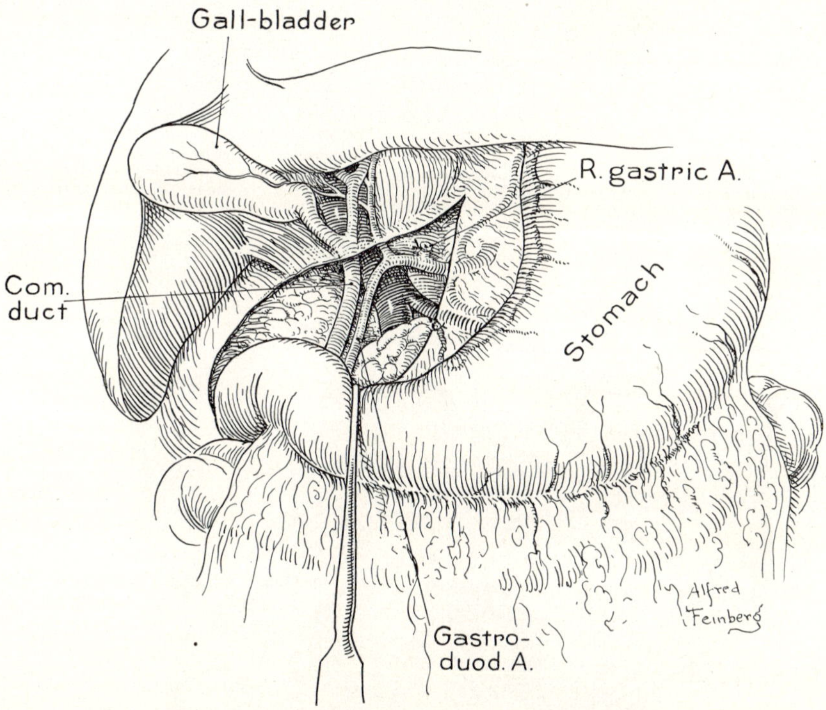

Fig. 2.—Division of the right gastric artery, the lower gastrohepatic ligament, and upper portion of the peritoneal reflection of the duodenum provides excellent exposure of the portal vein and superior aspect of the pancreas. Since many of the pancreaticoduodenal tumors tend to extend early to this area the question of operability may occasionally be decided by this exposure alone.

5. This step involves division of the right gastric artery and adjacent gastrohepatic ligament, exposing the cephalic aspect of the pancreas and ventral aspect of the superior mesenteric vein as it fuses with the splenic vein to become the portal vessel. Cautiously these structures are identified and digitally explored, again for evidences of direct invasion of the superior mesenteric vein by tumor (Fig. 2).

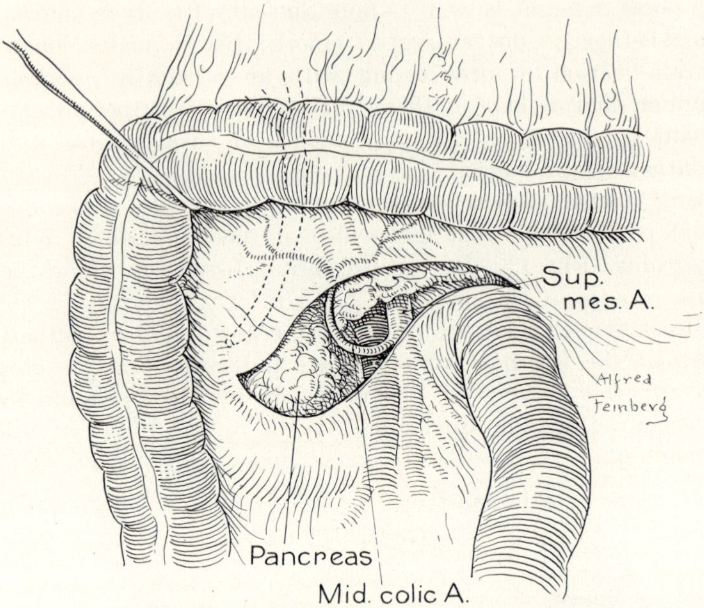

Fig. 3.—Indication as to whether or not the superior mesenteric vein is involved by direct extension of the cancer may be obtained by exploring this vessel from below. Although this can be accomplished by entering the lesser omental sac, access to this area can sometimes be more readily accomplished by dividing the base of the mesocolon transversely. Careful dissection is then helpful in delineating the inferior extension of the tumor.

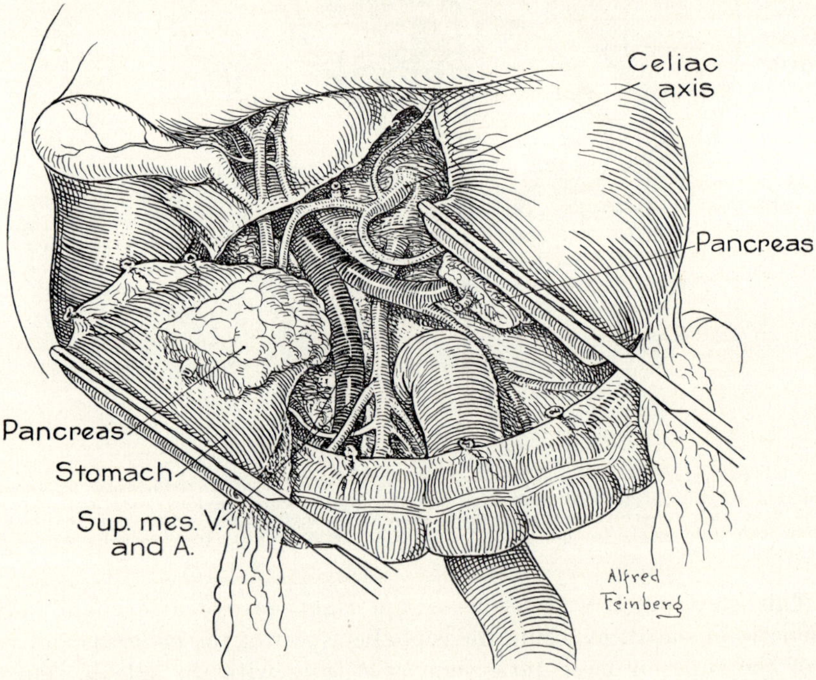

Fig 4.—Should the preceding three maneuvers have indicated that the tumor is operable, the first definitive step in resection must be taken, namely, division of the stomach and pancreas. This is accomplished at about the level of the midportion of the stomach. Dissection is then carried toward the right side of the patient, exposing the superior mesenteric vein as it lies in the groove made by the head and uncinate process of the pancreas.

6. The next step involves further investigation of the superior mesenteric vein, this time from below. This can be accomplished through the lesser omental sac, but it has seemed easier and more productive of useful information to explore the emergence of this vein from behind the pancreas by way of the mesocolon. The colon is therefore delivered into the wound and the base of the mesocolon incised transversely. Identification of the middle colic artery is relatively simple, and beyond this the border of the pancreas (Fig. 3). By palpating behind the pancreas with the right index finger above and the left below, it

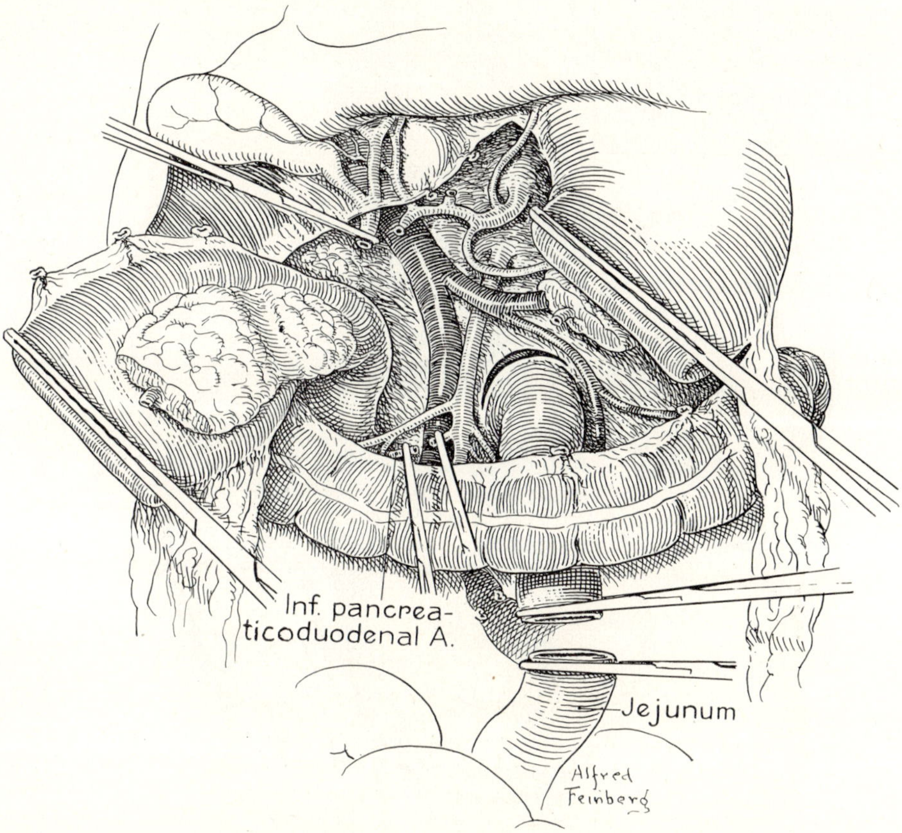

Fig. 5.—If the superior mesenteric vein can be freed successfully from the pancreas and its tumor, the resection is then completed by dividing the inferior pancreaticoduodenal artery, the jejunum, and the various structures constituting Treitz ligament. This permits the terminal duodenum and proximal jejunum to be delivered easily into the upper abdomen.

is possible to acquire reasonably accurate information as to whether or not the inaccessible middle third of the retropancreatic segment of the superior mesenteric vein is comprised by actively infiltrating neoplasm. If the operator feels unhesitatingly as a result of these two last steps that this vein, the *bete noire* of pancreatectomy, is invaded by tumor, the procedure may be readily abandoned; if there is indication that it is uninvolved, the first definitive step in the resection may be taken.

7. This step involves dividing the stomach at its mid-portion and, in the same vertical plane, traversing the pancreas, temporarily ligating the pancreatic duct. Dissection is then swept closely along the liver and splenic artery, including all the regional lymphatic beds. The specimen is allowed to fall inferiorly and to the left. As the lesser omental sac is skirted inferiorly, the immediately adjacent segments of greater omentum may be conveniently re-

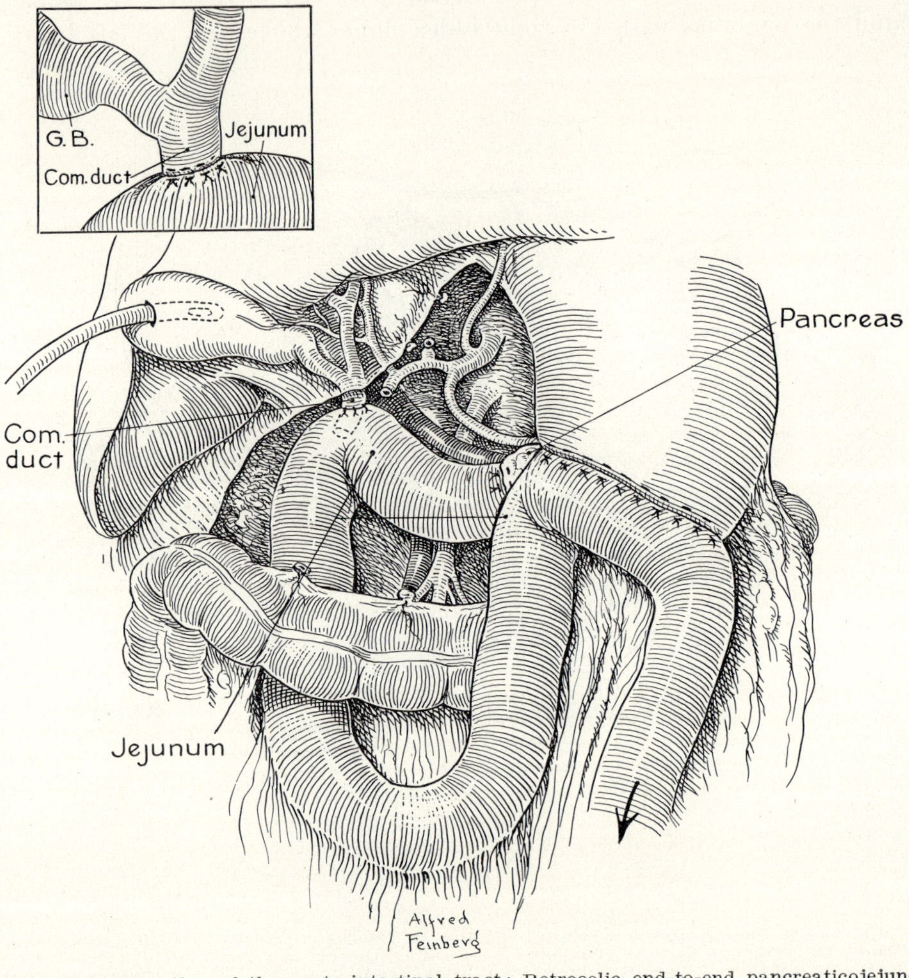

Fig. 6.—Reconstruction of the gastrointestinal tract; Retrocolic end-to-end pancreaticojejunostomy and end-to-side choledochojejunostomy; antecolic gastrojejunostomy.

moved. At this point the feasibility of dissecting free the superior mesenteric vein can be answered (Fig. 4). If this structure be hopelessly involved, retreat is still a relatively simple matter and is accomplished, first, by removing the tail of the pancreas and, second, by performing an end-to-end anastomosis between the proximal and distal halves of the stomach. If the vein can be freed the operation quickly proceeds by dividing in succession the gastroduodenal artery and the common duct.

8. As the duodenum is further mobilized, attention is directed toward accurate identification and division of the inferior pancreaticoduodenal artery as it arises from the superior mesenteric artery. Division of this vessel permits complete and ready extrication of the terminal duodenum and proximal few centimeters of the jejunum from behind the colon (Fig. 5).

9. Reconstruction of the enteric canal is accomplished by (Fig. 6):

(a) Retrocolic end-to-end pancreaticojejunostomy[2a]

(b) Retrocolic end-to-side choledochojejunostomy or simple implantation of the common duct into the jejunal lumen

(c) Antecolic long-loop isoperistaltic gastrojejunostomy

10. As safety measures, the retroperitoneal space, which it is impossible to reperitonize, is drained through a stab wound in the flank and a cholecystostomy tube is inserted through a separate stab wound just below the costal margin.

11. The wound is closed in layers, employing through-and-through No. 28 stainless steel stay sutures buried beneath the skin and interrupted No. 32 stainless steel sutures, approximating the peritoneum and various fascial planes.

12. Postoperatively the drains are withdrawn whenever the discharge becomes scant and the cholecystostomy tube is withdrawn following demonstration of the patency of the choledochojejunal anastomosis.

DISCUSSION

The initial features of this operation are the maneuvers directed toward determining, if possible, whether or not the superior mesenteric vein is compromised by tumor. It can be hoped that eventually some successful method of avoiding the necessity of preserving this structure may be devised, for it is certainly the weakest point as well as the most frustrating in the entire operative attack upon the pancreatic cancers. Indication that it may be sacrificed is to be found in a case reported by Brunschwig,[5] and in a patient (Case 14) in this series in whom post-mortem examination five days following division of the superior mesenteric vein failed to reveal any significant venous engorgement of the small bowel. In Brunschwig's case there had been a previous pelvic operation as a result of which sufficient venous collaterals may have been established; in the case in this series there was no such antecedent operation. The importance of re-establishing pancreatic drainage is twofold: first, it protects an extensive operative field from being flooded by pancreatic ferments should the ligature upon the duct fail. Second, postoperative studies of pancreatic function by means of the secretin test[6a, b] have proved conclusively in these patients that the anastomoses were patent one, two, and three years postoperatively. Secretin tests were performed in the remaining patients, and though in several there was produced a copious amount of secretion, the presence of pancreatic ferments could not be demonstrated because the specimens had unavoidably become acidified with gastric juice.

The importance of choledochojejunostomy instead of cholecystenterostomy has been well established by Whipple,[7] and a gastrojejunostomy distal to the biliary anastomosis is accepted as an important feature of the operation if troublesome ascending cholangiitis is to be avoided during both the early and late postoperative periods.

REFERENCES

1. Whipple, A. O., Parsons, W. B., and Mullins, C. R.: Ann. Surg. **102**: 763, 1935.
2. (a) Child, Charles G., III: Ann. Surg. **118**: 838, 1943.
   (b) Child, Charles G., III: Ann. Surg. **119**: 845, 1944.
3. Coffey, R. C.: Ann. Surg. **50**: 1238, 1909.
4. Cattell, R. B.: New England J. Med. **232**: 521, 1945.
5. Brunschwig, Alexander: Radical Surgery in Advanced Abdominal Cancer, Chicago, 1947, University of Chicago Press.
6. (a) Lake, Michael: J. A. M. A. **3**: 18, 1947.
   (b) Child, Charles G., III: Advances in Science, Vol. I, New York, 1947, The Interscience Publishers, Inc.
7. Whipple, A. O.: Surg., Gynec. & Obst. **82**: 623, 1946.

THE COURSE OF PEPTIC ULCERATION IN ELDERLY PERSONS

A Clinical and Anatomic Study of 122 Cases

Earl P. Lasher, Jr., M.D., Seattle, Wash.

(From the Department of Surgery, University of Washington School of Medicine)

ALTHOUGH the over-all death rates in the age decades of 55 to 64 years and 65 to 74 years declined strikingly between 1911 and 1925 and 1925 and 1935 (Table I), the number of deaths due to gastric and duodenal ulcer rose discouragingly.[1, 2] In Cowdry's *Problems of Ageing*,[3] Ivy suggested that the majority of older people with the disease acquired the lesions when young, but even when one allows for the forgetfulness and confusion of the senescent patient this assumption is not entirely justified. Within the ten years from 1937 to 1947, several authors[4-7] have reported instances of the initial appearance of peptic ulcers in the aged and, because their manifestations here are different from those in the young, diagnosis may be difficult and therapy perplexing.

Therefore, the records of the 122 patients over 50 years of age, with peptic ulcer proved by operation or autopsy, who were treated at the Harborview Hospital between Jan. 1, 1936, and Jan. 1, 1947, have been reviewed and some of the salient peculiarities of this malady in the older age groups brought forward. In this interval, excluding obstetric admission, 122,763 patients entered for treatment, and 4,988 autopsies were done, 101 of them in the present series of peptic ulcers, a post-mortem incidence of 2 per cent.

Twelve of the patients were women; seven with gastric ulcers, four with duodenal, and one with a marginal lesion.

In Table II, *A* shows the distribution of cases in the various decades, *B* the anatomic location of the ulcers according to the age groups, and *C* the average duration of symptoms in months. Supplementary to this last it is apparent that in the sixth decade 56 per cent of patients had histories of gastrointestinal troubles for less than two years, in the seventh decade 50 per cent suffered less than two years, in the eighth decade 76 per cent, and in the ninth decade 67 per cent. In the youngest group six persons denied any symptoms prior to the calamity that led to their operation or death. In patients past the age of 60 years, ten who were able to give satisfactory histories could not recall premonitory digestive disturbances.

Unfortunately, the discomforts of peptic ulceration in the older person, when present, are milder than in the younger person and an undetermined but large percentage of these people do not seek medical care until one of the major complications appears. Table III gives the incidence of these disasters in lesions of the stomach including the pylorus and the duodenum, and it is interest-

Read at a meeting of the Seattle Surgical Society, Oct. 31, 1947.

TABLE I

CHANGE IN ANNUAL DEATH RATES PER 100,000				1911 TO 1925	1925 TO 1935
All causes—white	M	Ages	55-64	-22%	- 6%
			65-74	-20%	- 2%
	F	Ages	55-64	-24%	-10%
			65-74	-21%	- 5%
				1911-1915 FROM 1931-1935	
Gastric ulcer—white	M	Ages	55-64	+54.9%	
			65-74	+26.2%	
	F	Ages	55-64	-44.2%	
			65-74	-55.3%	
				1921-1925 FROM 1931-1935	
Duodenal ulcer—white	M	Ages	55-64	+147.7%	
			65-74	+ 70.6%	
	F	Ages	55-64	No change	
			65-74	+ 50 %	

From Dublin and Lotka.[1]

TABLE II

	AGES BY DECADES			
	50-59	60-69	70-79	80-89
A				
Number of cases	52	31	29	10
B				
Gastric ulcer	24	20	8	3
Duodenal ulcer	21	9	12	6
Pyloric ulcer	5	1	6	1
Marginal ulcer	1		1	
Multiple ulcers				
Gastric	2	3	3	1
Duodenal	2	0	4	0
Both	1	1	3	0
C				
Average duration symptoms (mo.)	56.5	55.1	62.3	27
Symptoms less than 2 yr. (per cent)	56	50	76	67
Average duration symptoms gastric ulcer (mo.)	50	63	67	6.3
Symptoms less than 2 yr. gastric ulcer (per cent)	59	45	71	100

TABLE III

	AGES BY DECADES				
	50-59	60-69	70-79	80-89	TOTAL AFTER 60
DUODENAL ULCER WITH					
Perforation	13	5	6	3	14
Hemorrhage	5	4	7	2	13
Massive fatal hemorrhage	5	3	5	2	10
Obstruction	1	0	1	1	
Intractable pain	3	0	0	0	
GASTRIC ULCER WITH					
Perforation	19	8	3	1	12
Hemorrhage	5	9	7	3	19
Massive fatal hemorrhage	1	6	4	1	11
Obstruction	2	1	1	0	
Intractable pain	3	3	1	0	

ing to note that in patients past the age of 60 years hemorrhage is more common than perforation in the patients with gastric ulcers and as frequent in those with duodenal, whereas before this age perforation is seen about three times more often than bleeding.

DISCUSSION

Because this series comprises only those patients who came to operation or autopsy it does not give a true picture of the over-all incidence of complications or of the years in which the course of the disease is less violent. Between 7 and 10 per cent[8] of the population have peptic ulceration at some time of life. Before the fifth decade of life only about 22 per cent[9] of these persons develop any complication requiring operation and only 4 per cent[8] die of the disease.

In patients past 50 years of age about 20 per cent show some signs of obstruction and about 25 per cent bleed significantly.[10, 11] There is, therefore, a compounding of troubles. Complications are more common in the aged, the more serious ones are the most common, and the patients are progressively less well equipped in all respects to cope with the devastations of their illness.

Explanations of the development of the greater hazards are only tentative but require discussion because they influence the treatments to be considered.

The increased incidence of gastric ulcer over duodenal ulcer is most important be it due to failure of some stomachs to empty more rapidly as most do when a person ages,[8, 12] to circulatory lesions in the gastric mucosa,[8] or to dietary fadism or malnutrition[13] from disinterest in food. In published reports the mortality from gastric ulcer in all age groups is greater (22:1) than that from duodenal ulcer.[1] And because of the ever-present likelihood of cancer in gastric lesions the incidence of operation for them is higher.[9] Because their initial appearance is usually at a later age than duodenal ulceration the hazard of operation is greater.[14]

It is the opinion of some[15] that, in general, gastric lesions, though potentially more dangerous, respond to medical treatment better than duodenal ones and it is therefore desirable to employ all diagnostic measures available in the elderly patient to segregate the malignant from the benign lesions. In doing this the gastrointestinal series and gastroscopy performed by the experienced observer are accurate methods (about 80 per cent),[16] but the routine gastric analysis done on only one occasion is much less helpful than in the younger person. Table IV shows the average peak rise of free hydrochloric acid following either 120 c.c. of 7 per cent alcohol, histamine, or both in the thirty-five patients in whom the test was done in this study. In patients past the age of

TABLE IV

AVERAGE PEAK OF FREE HYDROCHLORIC ACID

	AGES			
	50-59	60-69	70-79	80-89
Gastric ulcer	8 cases 50.7°	8 cases 28°	6 cases 31°	1 case 0
Duodenal ulcer	7 cases 60.2°	1 case 30.2°	2 cases 28.5°	2 cases 47°

60 years there were five instances of achlorhydria, four of them in the presence of proved benign gastric ulcers, and the fifth in a 74-year-old man who had had abdominal symptoms for only four months; he subsequently died after acute perforation of a chronic duodenal ulcer.

The low average level of gastric acidity in the patients over 60 years of age might be kept in mind when therapy is considered. It is unreasonable to expect that neutralizing substances will accomplish as much in the hypochlorhydric patient as in the person secreting excessive amounts of acid. There is evidence, however, that the retention of gastric juices may be important in perpetuating peptic ulcer[17] and it has been repeatedly shown that the introduction of acid into the stomachs of elderly persons delays their emptying time significantly.[18] In this review three patients were found in whom the onset of symptoms due to peptic ulcer followed the administration of ammonium chloride used as an adjuvant in the treatment of heart failure. This is probably not coincidence and should demand discontinuation of the drug in any elderly individual manifesting digestive complaints.

Perhaps the most rational treatment of the older patients with gastric or duodenal ulcer would stress frequent highly nutritious feedings supplemented by a protein hydrolysate,[19, 20] high vitamin intake, belladonna or its equivalent to promote pyloric relaxation, and a much closer following of the individual than is customary. Many will have reached a state of indifference to the outcome of their illnesses and are reluctant to alter the habits of many years. If they and their physicians can be made to realize that an ulcer late in life is immeasurably more dangerous than in youth, the inconveniences of the therapy might be more gracefully accepted.

Although there are, as yet, no data to outline the way, criteria for surgical intervention cannot be the same for the old as for the young.[21] There is a trend toward immediate operation where massive hemorrhage appears[22] and the greater frequency of hypertension and of vascular rigidity makes resection of the bleeding area in the elderly almost obligatory. In this series twenty-one of the thirty-two patients who bled died of massive hemorrhage. It is unlikely that the operative mortality, had an aggressive attitude been taken, would have exceeded 65 per cent.

As in other studies,[23] deaths due to perforation of an ulcer in the aged increase in direct proportion to the interval between perforation and operative repair and few patients recover when the defect is not closed by suture.

It is in the group where surgical treatment may be elective that standards of evaluation are different. The tendency is to delay operation and then to do as little as one may hope will suffice. Vagotomy[24] because of its technical simplicity is alluring but, on theoretical grounds, seems a poor choice. The advantage of further reduction in gastric acidity, already low, is overbalanced by the prospect of increasing gastric retention.[25, 26] And the few operative casualties reported during vagotomy,[27] due to vagovagal reflexes or other effects on the heart and respiration, have been in the older patients.

If gastroenterostomy is combined with vagotomy a more ideal procedure is obtained but one is tempted to omit the latter step when the circulatory reserve is impaired.

Certainly both are inadequate for the control of bleeding and nothing less than gastric resection should then be chosen. With the improvements in anesthesia, and pre- and postoperative care now available in most hospitals, a more bold approach to surgical treatment should be adopted and one can reasonably anticipate better control of the ravages of peptic ulceration in the aged.

SUMMARY

1. In elderly persons death rates due to peptic ulcer are increasing. Therefore, 122 known cases in patients over 50 years of age entering Harborview Hospital in the last eleven years are reviewed.

2. Between the sixth and eighth decades of life about one-half of the patients with peptic ulcer sufficiently severe to require hospitalization gave histories of gastrointestinal symptoms of less than two years' duration. In the eighth and ninth decades over two-thirds had noticed the discomforts of their disease for less than two years.

3. Sixteen individuals had no symptoms prior to the appearance of a major complication of peptic ulceration.

4. In patients past the age of 60 hemorrhage is more common than perforation and the bleeding is often massive.

5. Peptic ulcer in the aged is not accompanied, as a rule, by gastric hyperacidity though prolonged retention of stomach secretions is not uncommon.

6. In three instances symptoms of a subsequently proved ulcer first appeared after the use of ammonium chloride in the treatment of cardiac decompensation.

7. The treatment of peptic ulcers in the elderly patient cannot be standardized until further data are available but a plea is made for the segregation of the patients with ulcers making the initial appearance in later life, for a more aggressive attitude toward surgical treatment of the complications, and for the publication of mortality statistics of elective operations by age groups.

REFERENCES

1. Dublin, L. I., and Lotka, A. J.: Twenty-Five Years of Health Progress, New York, 1937, Metropolitan Life Insurance Co., pp. 382, 531, 541.
2. Mueller-Deham, A., and Rabson, S. M.: Internal Medicine in Old Age, Baltimore, 1942, Williams & Wilkins Company, p. 219.
3. Cowdry, E. V.: Problems of Ageing, ed. 2, Baltimore, 1942, Williams & Wilkins Company, pp. 265, 270.
4. Muslow, F. W.: Peptic Ulcer of the Aged, Am. J. Digest. Dis. **8**: 112, 1947.
5. Meyer, J., and Saphir, O.: Peptic Ulcer in the Aged; A Clinical and Post-Mortem Study, Am. J. Digest. Dis. **10**: 28, 1943.
6. Boles, R. S., and Dunbar, W.: Peptic Ulcer in Old Age, Geriatrics **1**: 217, 1946.
7. Wood, M. N.: Chronic Peptic Ulcer in Ninety-Four Diabetics, Am. J. Digest. Dis. **14**: 1, 1947.
8. Bockus, H. L.: Gastroenterology, Philadelphia, 1944, W. B. Saunders Company, pp. 270, 318, 324, 331, 332, 497.
9. Eusterman, G. B., and Balfour, D. C.: The Stomach and Duodenum, Philadelphia, 1935, W. B. Saunders Company, p. 259.
10. Klingenstein, P.: Gastroduodenal Ulcer in Individuals More Than Fifty Years of Age, J. Mt. Sinai Hosp. **7**: 432, 1941.
11. Crohn, B. B.: Affections of the Stomach, Philadelphia, 1927, W. B. Saunders Company, p. 619.
12. Davies, D. T., and James, T. G. I.: Achlorhydria and Anaemia in Advancing Years, Lancet **2**: 899, 1930.

13. Weech, A. A., and Paige, B. H.: Nutritional Edema in the Dog; IV. Peptic Ulcer Produced by the Same Low Protein That Leads to Hypoproteinemia and Edema, Am. J. Path. **13**: 249, 1937.
14. Drossner, J. L., and Miller, T. G.: The Natural History and Diagnosis of Gastric Ulcer, Am. J. M. Sc. **199**: 90, 1940.
15. Palmer, W. L., Schindler, R., and Templeton, F. C. The Development and Healing of Gastric Ulcer—A Clinical, Gastroscopic, and Roentgenologic Study, Am. J. Digest. Dis. **5**: 501, 1938.
16. Heuer, G. J.: The Treatment of Peptic Ulcer, Philadelphia, 1944, J. B. Lippincott Company, p. 26.
17. Sandweiss, D. J., Sugarman, M. H., Podolsky, H. M., and Friedman, M. H. F.: Nocturnal Gastric Secretion in Duodenal Ulcer—Studies on Normal Subjects and Patients, With Their Bearing on Ulcer Management, J. A. M. A. **130**: 258, 1946.
18. Shay, H., Gershon-Cohen, J., and Fels, S. S.: Gastric Anacidity: Its Physiologic and Clinical Significance and Its Management, Am. J. Digest. Dis. **8**: 155, 1941.
19. Co Tui, F., Wright, A. M., Mulholland, J. H., Galvin, T., Barcham, I., and Gerst, G. R.: The Hyperalimentation Treatment of Peptic Ulcer With Amino Acids (Protein Hydrolysate) and Dextri-Maltose, Gastroenterology **5**: 5, 1945.
20. Hodges, H. H.: Protein Hydrolysate Therapy for Peptic Ulcer—Report on 26 Cases, Gastroenterology **8**: 476, 1946.
21. Lasher, E. P.: An Outline for the Treatment of Peptic Ulcer, Am. J. Digest. Dis. **13**: 221, 1946.
22. Holman, C.: Severe Hemorrhage in Gastric and Duodenal Ulcer: A Study of 90 Cases, Arch. Surg. **40**: 150, 1940.
23. Paletta, F. X., and Hill, W. R.: Acute Perforated Gastric and Duodenal Ulcers, SURGERY **14**: 32, 1943.
24. Dragstedt, L. R.: Vagotomy for Gastroduodenal Ulcer, Ann. Surg. **122**: 973, 1945.
25. Moore, F. D., Chapman, W. P., Schulz, M. D., and Jones, C. M.: Resection of the Vagus Nerves in Peptic Ulcer—Physiologic Effects and Clinical Results, With a Report of Two Years' Experience, J. A. M. A. **133**: 741, 1947.
26. Grimson, K. S., Baylin, G. J., Taylor, H. M., Hesser, F. H., and Rundles, R. W.: Transthoracic Vagotomy—The Effects in 57 Patients With Peptic Ulcer and the Clinical Limitations, J. A. M. A. **134**: 925, 1947.
27. Weeks, C., Ryan, B. J., and Van Hoy, J. M.: Two Deaths Associated With Supradiaphragmatic Vagotomy, J. A. M. A. **132**: 988, 1946.

TANTALUM FOIL CUFFS IN PERIPHERAL NERVE SURGERY

Eugene E. Cliffton, M.D., New Haven, Conn.

FOLLOWING World War I the general consensus of opinion was that the use of cuffs of any material to surround damaged or repaired peripheral nerves was of little value.[1-3] The common materials used had been sections of vein or artery, fresh or fixed, fascia, Cargile membrane, and various metallic materials. Just prior to World War II the new metal tantalum was developed for surgical use and it was strongly urged that it be used in peripheral nerve surgery particularly. The rationale of its use was that it was an inert metal and so would not result in reaction or adhesion formation and that if used as a smooth cuff about the nerve it would prevent ingrowth of scar tissue into the suture line or damaged nerve.[4-8]

This opinion was confirmed by short-term results with nerves, both experimental and clinical, when upon reoperation almost invariably a smooth pseudomembrane was found both outside and inside the foil.[5, 7] However, as time went on and more and more nerves were re-explored late, more cases were found in which there was dense scar tissue formation both outside and inside the foil and in many instances marked fragmentation of the foil was found.

Fortunately, sufficient foil was not available in all neurosurgical centers at all times so that we have been furnished with a control series. The present study is an attempt to judge, from one small series of cases, the relative value of the use of tantalum foil.

The two groups of cases are not exact duplicates, but they are of sufficient similarity to warrant broad deductions. The chief discrepancies are in the time interval between injury and operation, which is much greater in those nerves repaired without foil (see Tables I and II). This should favor those nerves treated with foil as it is fairly well accepted that early operation is the procedure of choice. It will also be noted that the average gap between the neuroma and glioma is greater in those nerves sutured without foil. This also should favor the group with foil according to usual opinion, which has favored suture of nerves without tension. So far as the relative numbers of each individual nerve are concerned, one may see that they are very similar, there being no great discrepancies.

Sensory nerves have not been included in the tables because the number repaired without foil so greatly outweighed the number with foil. Only those cases have been included in which there is certain knowledge that foil was or was not used. Approximately 500 questionable cases were excluded. Only cases in which sufficient time had passed for adequate follow-up have been included. This factor, in all probability, weights the statistics in favor of those patients treated without foil as they were more frequently the later cases and so a very much greater percentage has been excluded for insufficient follow-up.

Table I. Neurorrhaphies With and Without Foil

	No. cases	Av. time (mo.)*	Av. gap (cm.)†	Result (rated) 4	3	2	1	0	Ave. result	Paresthesia	Trigger point	No. patients reop.	No. patients improved‡
Brachial plexus with foil	6	1.3		0	2	3	1	0	2.2	0	0	0	0
Brachial plexus without foil	5	5.4	1.7	1	2	1	1	0	2.6	0	0	0	0
Radial with foil	19	3.2	1.0	3	12	3	1	0	2.9	0	0	0	0
Radial without foil	8	6.0	1.3	3	4	0	1	0	3.1	0	0	1	1
Median with foil	21	4.0	0.8	1	12	6	2	0	2.5	4	4	2	2
Median without foil	50	9.1	1.5	7	36	6	1	0	2.9	2	0	2	1
Ulnar with foil	56	3.5	1.1	0	9	31	15	1	1.8	7	14	8	4
Ulnar without foil	84	6.2	2.1	1	26	40	16	1	2.1	3	4	9	3
Musculocutaneous with foil	2	2.5	0	1	1	0	0	0	3.5	0	0	0	0
Musculocutaneous without foil	2	6.5	3.5	1	1	0	0	0	3.5	0	0	0	0
Sciatic with foil	14	3.9	1.6	1	1	10	2	0	2.0	0	0	2	1
Sciatic without foil	19	5.5	2.0	0	8	6	3	2	2.3	0	0	4	1
Peroneal sciatic with foil	12	2.4	0.1	2	1	7	1	1	2.1	1	0	2	0
Peroneal sciatic without foil	6	5.2	0	0	0	2	2	2	2.0	0	0	1	0
Tibial sciatic with foil	3	3.6	0	0	0	3	0	0	2.0	2	0	1	0
Tibial sciatic without foil	2	3	0.8	0	2	0	0	0	3.0	0	0	0	0
Peroneal with foil	7	2.5	0	1	1	2	1	2	1.7	0	0	3	3
Peroneal without foil	19	6.0	2.3	3	5	6	4	1	2.3	2	2	2	0
Tibial with foil	12	8.7	1.2	2	4	3	2	1	1.9	0	0	1	0
Tibial without foil	3	3.3	0	0	2	0	0	1	2.0	2	1	1	0
Total with foil	143	4.0	1.1	9	41	65	23	5	2.18	16	19	19	10
Total without foil	207	6.5	1.9	18	88	64	30	7	2.4	6	4	20	6

*Between injury and operation.
†Between neuroma and glioma.
‡After reoperation.

In the tables the return of function is recorded as follows:

4. Return of some function in all muscles innervated plus return of sensation; none necessarily normal
3. Return of some function in 50 to 75 per cent of the muscles and/or sensory area
2. Return of one element to 50 per cent of elements
1. Return of one element
0. No return of function other than Tinel's sign

P. Paresthesia in the sensory area

T. Moderate to severe trigger point

There is a total of 523 cases, of which 362 were neurorrhaphies. Of this latter number 145 nerves were wrapped in foil and 208 were not wrapped. (Of those wrapped, reoperation was deemed necessary in 21 cases or 14.4 per

TABLE II. NEUROLYSES WITH AND WITHOUT FOIL

	NO. CASES	AV. TIME (MO.)*	RESULTS (RATED) 4	3	2	1	0	AV. RESULT	PARESTHESIA	TRIGGER POINT	NO. PATIENTS REOP.	NO. PATIENTS IMPROVED†
Brachial plexus with foil	5	2.8	2	2	1	0	0	3.0	0	0	0	0
Branchial plexus without foil	3	2.0	0	1	1	0	0	2.5	0	0	0	0
Median with foil	30	3.2	7	11	10	2	0	2.7	10	7	8	6
Median without foil	24	6.2	15	9	0	0	0	3.2	2	0	0	0
Ulnar with foil	22	3.4	2	8	10	1	1	2.4	1	6	4	3
Ulnar without foil	22	8.6	8	9	3	2	0	3.0	0	0	1	1
Radial with foil	10	2.3	3	7	0	0	0	3.3	0	1	0	0
Radial without foil	9	6.7	5	3	1	0	0	3.4	0	1	1	0
Sciatic with foil	6	6.4	3	0	1	1	1	2.3	1	0	1	1
Sciatic without foil	12	7.3	2	5	4	1	0	2.6	6	1	0	0
Peroneal with foil	4	7.7	0	2	1	0	1	2.0	1	1	1	1
Peroneal without foil	6	4.6	3	2	1	0	0	3.3	0	1	0	0
Tibial with foil	3	6.3	1	1	1	0	0	3.0	0	0	0	0
Tibial without foil	4	9.7	2	1	1	0	0	3.2	0	1	0	0
Total with foil	80	4.1	16	34	23	4	3	2.5	13	15	14	11
Total without foil	79	7.1	35	30	11	3	0	3.2	8	4	2	1

*Between injury and operation.
†With reoperation.

cent. Of those not wrapped in foil, reoperation was deemed necessary in 22 or 10.5 per cent.) There is a total of 161 neurolyses, of which 83 had foil wrapping and 79 were without wrapping. (Of the 83 wrapped, 14 of them or 16.8 per cent were reoperated upon and of the 79 not wrapped only 2 of them or 2.5 per cent were reoperated upon.) The principal cause for reoperation in these patients was the presence of a trigger point.

It will be noted that the figures do not coincide with those in the tables. In the neurorrhaphies this is due to the fact that 3 patients were reoperated upon without sufficient time for follow-up, 2 in the group with foil and 1 in the group without foil. In the neurolyses it is due to the fact that 3 femoral nerves treated without foil are not included, because there were no femoral nerves with foil. None of these femoral nerves were reoperated upon.

TABLE III. RESULTS OF NEURORRHAPHIES WITH AND WITHOUT FOIL

	WITH FOIL NUMBER	PER CENT*	RATED	WITHOUT FOIL NUMBER	PER CENT*	RATED
	9	6.5	4	18	8.5	4
	41	29	3	93	45	3
	65	45	2	63	30	2
	23	16	1	31	15	1
	5	3.5	0	3	1.5	0
Total	143			208		
	16	11	Paresthesia	6	3.2	Paresthesia
	19	15	Trigger points	4	2	Trigger points

*Percentages were computed to nearest whole figure except in those below 10, when they were computed to the nearest .5 per cent.

From an observation of Table III, it will be observed that though the results favor the nerves treated without foil these are not of sufficient difference to be of real statistical significance. When one considers the number of cases with paresthesia or trigger points the figures are definitely in favor of not using foil.

Table IV. Results of Neurolyses With and Without Foil

	With Foil			Without Foil		
	Number	Per Cent*	Rated	Number	Per Cent*	Rated
	16	20	4	35	44	4
	34	24	3	30	38	3
	23	28	2	11	14	2
	4	5	1	3	4	1
	3	4	0	0	0.0	0
Total	80			79		
	15	18	Paresthesia	4	5	Paresthesia
	14	17	Trigger points	2	2.6	Trigger points

*Percentages were computed to nearest whole figure except in those below 10, when they were computed to the nearest .5 per cent.

In a review of the patients in whom reoperation was carried out it seems certain that the nerves from which foil was removed were more scarred and damaged and the operative procedure was much more difficult than in those in which the nerve was not wrapped in foil. If the foil be intact, the scarring is most dense at the edges of the foil, upper and lower, and where the horizontal edges overlap both inside and outside. At times it is very difficult to separate these edges from the nerve and they may seriously cut into the nerve. Wherever there are any cracks in the foil there will be increased scarring. In at least 3 cases the foil was fragmented and small bits were imbedded deeply in the nerve. In 2 cases the nerve was so badly chewed up that neurorrhaphy was absolutely necessary (Fig. 1, *A, B,* and *C*). In 2 cases there was severe constriction of the nerve to less than one-half of the diameter of the nerve above, and only scar tissue was present in the constricted area, no nerve fibers being seen even on microscopic examination (Fig. 2). Of those patients in whom only a neurolysis had been done there were several on whom adequate notes were present for both operations. In at least two of these cases it is certain that the damage to the nerve was minimal at the first operation when the foil was applied, whereas at the second operation there was serious scarring and neuroma formation (Fig. 3). In other cases the changes ranged from marked edema of the nerve to serious scarring, moderate neuroma formation, or partial constrictions. Strangely enough, there were no cases of definite separation of the suture line.

In the nerves reoperated upon without foil there were 3 with separation of the suture line. There were no cases of marked constriction and in those patients on whom both notes were adequate there were no instances in which the condition of the nerve had definitely degenerated between the operations.

It is of note that of the nerves with foil which were reoperated upon, 60 per cent showed improvement after the second operation and all but two lost their trigger points. Of the patients without foil who were reoperated upon, only 27 per cent showed improvement after the second operation. These figures would lead one to believe that the foil in these cases was actually a harmful element.

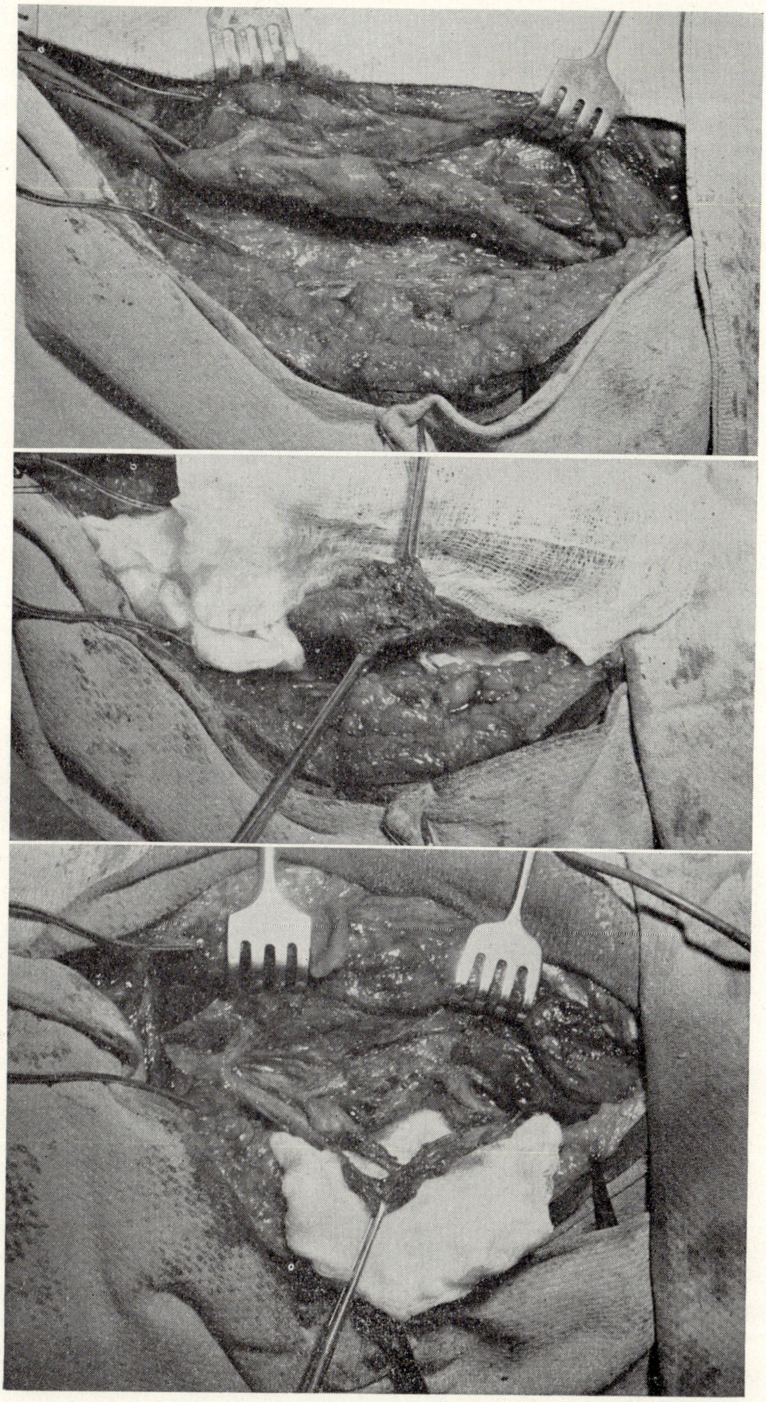

A.

B.

C.

Fig. 1.—*A*, Reoperation of sciatic nerve wrapped in foil twenty months previously; note increased size of nerve in operative area. *B*, Same nerve, beginning removal of foil; note fragmentation and marked thickening of capsule, many fragments embedded in nerve substance. *C*, Appearance of nerve after complete removal of foil; neuromas proximally on both peroneal and tibial trunks, normal trunks above and below.

Unfortunately, the reports of the operation in most instances are not complete as to details of the foil application technique. The cases with bad result may have been due to errors in technique of application. These might include (1) cracking of the foil while preparing or applying it or (2) sutures to hold the foil in place tied too tightly so as to constrict the nerve.

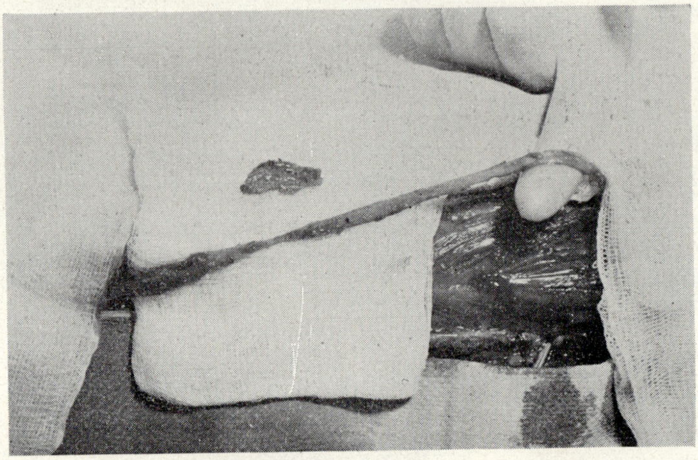

Fig. 2.—Ulnar nerve after removal of foil, eighteen months after operation, complete paralysis; note marked constriction. Pathology report revealed scar tissue only in narrowed area.

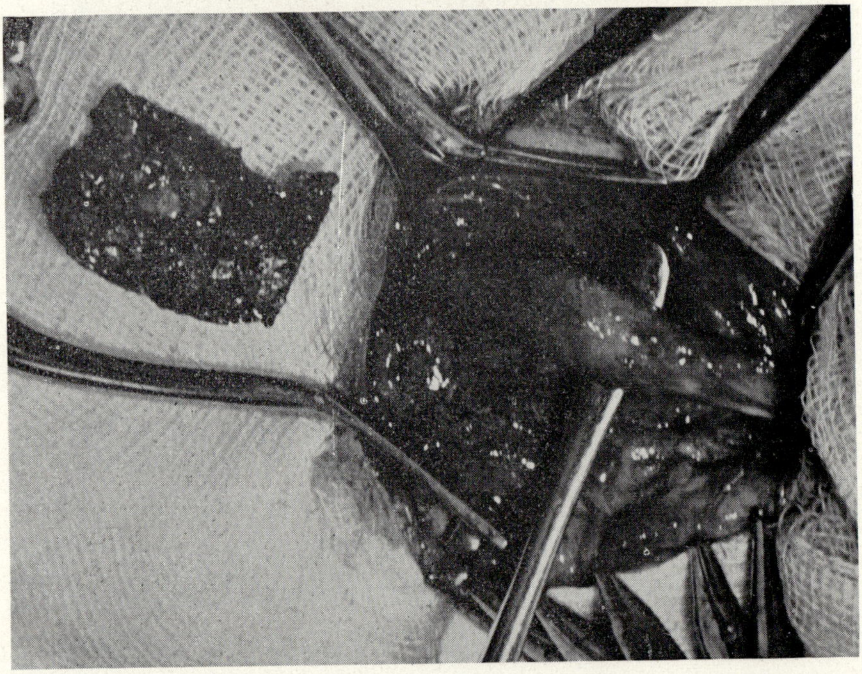

Fig. 3.—Neuroma present after removal of foil from median nerve. This was one of the nerves with adequate previous operative note which reported nerve normal in appearance. foil was applied only to prevent constriction by surrounding scar.

If tantalum foil is to be used, infinite care must be used in preparing and applying it. Perhaps the most satisfactory technique is to prepare the cuff by wrapping the piece of foil of proper size around a smooth round object slightly smaller in diameter than the nerve to be wrapped. The one edge is then drawn around the nerve and the instrument with its foil is crossed over this edge, drawn around the nerve, and then the instrument withdrawn. The roll of foil will then snap into place on the nerve firmly but not so as to constrict it. No ligatures will be necessary to hold it in place (Fig. 4). A second method to be used in neurorrhaphies, when enough room is available, is to place a formed cuff over one end of the nerve up onto the trunk and then to slip it back over the suture line when suture is completed. These methods were well illustrated by White and Hamblin.[4]

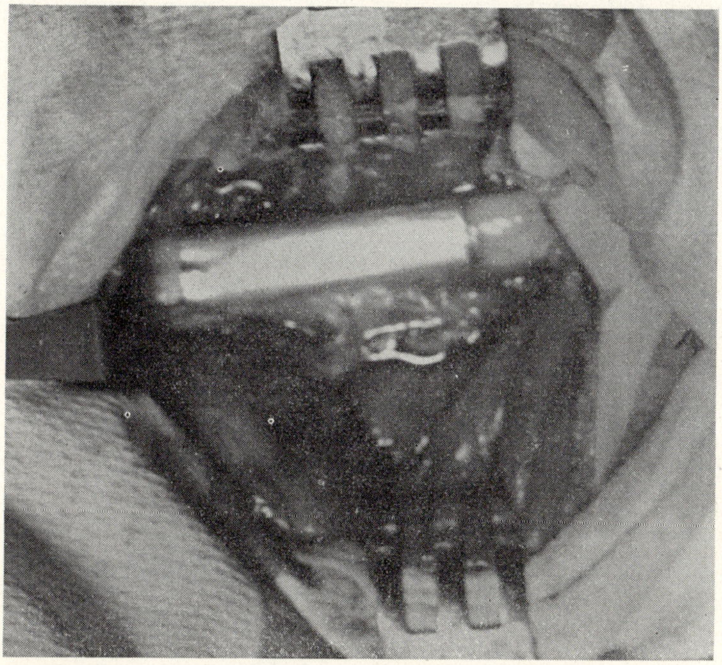

Fig. 4.—Photograph showing appearance of properly applied cuff at time of operation; note smooth contour, small depression at distal end to be elevated so as not to cause pressure.

The use of tantalum foil in two-stage procedure is unquestionably justified and of great value. If applied at the first stage procedure one finds at the second stage, if done in less than two months, a smooth pseudomembrane surrounding the foil and between the foil and the nerve. This tends to make at least temporarily a smooth sliding surface for the nerve at the suture line. The only disadvantage found has been that in some cases there is a definite tissue reaction of the nerve sheath with fairly marked edema. This type of sheath is definitely more friable than the normal sheath and sutures tend to pull out easily. Whether or not this type of nerve tends to do poorly has not been determined.

In only 3 cases was another material used for a cuff. One was a lead bone wax cover which was later removed. Two patients with use of fibrin film cuff were examined. Both showed satisfactory recovery. Another more satisfactory method of forming a cuff from the nerve sheath will be reported in a later communication.

CONCLUSIONS

1. Tantalum foil as a cuff in peripheral nerve surgery has not been proved to be of value in this particular series of cases.

   (a) Since its proper application is time consuming and the material relatively expensive, its routine use is not considered advisable.

   (b) If a satisfactory result has not been obtained or if a severe trigger point or paresthesia remain, the foil should be removed.

2. If used, foil should be applied so as to give a smooth even covering without pressure. Methods are described for reaching this ideal.

3. The use of foil in the first of two-stage procedures is considered of value.

REFERENCES

1. Stookey, Byron: Surgical and Mechanical Treatment of Peripheral Nerves, Philadelphia, 1922, W. B. Saunders Company, pp. 121-127.
2. Pollock, Lewis J., and Davis, Loyal: Peripheral Nerve Injuries, New York, 1933, Paul B. Hoeber, Inc., pp. 188-189.
3. The Medical Department of the U. S. Army in the World War, Vol. XI, pp. 968-969.
4. White, J. C., and Hamlin, H.: New Uses of Tantalum in Nerve Suture, Control of Neuroma Formation, and Prevention of Regeneration After Thoracic Sympathectomy, J. Neurosurg. 2: 402-413, 1945.
5. Weiss, P.: Tantalum Elastic Cuffs in Sutureless Reunion of Severed Nerves, J. Neurosurg. 1: 319-225, 1944.
6. Olson, C. T.: Tantalum; Place in Surgery, Indust. Med. 13: 917-920, 1944.
7. Spurling, R. G.: Symposium on War Surgery; Use of Tantalum Wire and Foil in Repair of Peripheral Nerves, S. Clin. North America 23: 1491-1504, 1943.
8. Carney, H. M.: Experimental Study With Tantalum, Proc. Soc. Exper. Biol. & Med. 51: 147-148, 1942.

TWENTY-SEVEN YEARS OF PROSTATIC SURGERY AT BELLEVUE HOSPITAL

A Study of Comparative Mortality Rates

John W. Draper, M.D., New York, N. Y.

(From the Department of Urology, Bellevue Hospital, and Cornell University Medical College)

During the past quarter century many bitter arguments have been waged concerning the relative merits of the various methods of operative treatment for benign prostatic hypertrophy. Many changes have taken place in the methods used during these years of discussion and development of new operations. It seems appropriate, therefore, at this time to rise above the smoke of battle and evaluate the progress which has been made. The study presented includes all patients with benign prostatic hypertrophy treated surgically at Bellevue Hospital between 1920 and 1946. The chief interest lies in the comparative mortality rates, for the early follow-up records were inadequate for statistical analysis.

Table I has been arranged to show the total number of patients with benign prostatic hypertrophy operated upon during each of the twenty-seven years. Figs. 1 to 5 show (1) the annual mortality rate for all operative procedures, (2) the annual mortality rate for transurethral resection, (3) the annual mortality rate for the second stage of a two-stage prostatectomy, (4) the annual mortality rate for one-stage prostatectomy, and (5) the annual mortality rate for cystotomy alone.

A study was made of the 2,221 consecutive patients treated in the twenty-seven-year period; all post-mortem reports were reviewed.

Table I, which gives the total number of operations each year, shows a gradual upward curve from 42 cases in 1920 to 153 in 1946. The increase in yearly operative cases is due to several factors, the most important of which undoubtedly is the realization by the medical profession that patients who are treated for prostatic obstruction before they are in extremis have a much better chance of surviving the surgery than those in whom surgical treatment is delayed. Another important factor has been the increasing confidence of patients in the outcome of surgery, having observed their friends relieved of their symptoms by operation.

Fig. 1 shows the annual mortality rate of all operative procedures for benign prostatic hypertrophy during the twenty-seven years studied. When it is realized that one out of every two patients subjected to operation died, as in 1922, it is easy to understand why their friends and associates failed to seek surgical relief for prostatism with any degree of hope of recovery. It is gratifying to find that the mortality rate has decreased from 50 per cent to 4.6 per cent in recent years. At this point it would seem worth while to ask how this reduction in mortality has been achieved. One has only to read the charts of 1920 to realize how great has been the improvement in the pre- and postoperative care of these patients over the years. In the early period covered by this study

TABLE I

YEAR	NUMBER OF OPERATIONS	NUMBER OF DEATHS	MORTALITY (PER CENT)
1920	42	18	42.8
1921	36	17	47.2
1922	60	31	50.2
1923	47	16	34.0
1924	49	18	36.7
1925	52	16	30.8
1926	60	18	30.0
1927	50	8	16.0
1928	51	7	13.7
1929	72	13	18.1
1930	69	16	23.2
1931	71	7	9.9
1932	66	9	13.6
1933	91	19	20.9
1934	98	19	19.4
1935	83	20	24.1
1936	89	18	20.2
1937	92	20	21.7
1938	110	12	10.9
1939	120	14	11.6
1940	121	12	9.9
1941	107	14	13.1
1942	100	24	24.0
1943	105	7	6.7
1944	123	12	9.8
1945	104	8	7.7
1946	153	7	4.6
	2,221	400	Average 18.0

the dangers of intravenous therapy were so great that it was rarely used. What parenteral fluids were given were administered subcutaneously or, occasionally, by proctoclysis. Blood transfusions were uncommon. Urotropin, methylene blue, and oil of sandalwood were the only urinary antiseptics available. The ketogenic diet and mandelic acid therapy, sulfa drugs, penicillin, and streptomycin were as yet unknown. At present a patient is seldom operated upon without the use of at least one, and often several, antibiotics. Hundreds of transfusions and thousands of other intravenous infusions are given annually, including amigen.

It is believed that the advent of the resectoscope has also aided the urologic staff in lowering the over-all operative mortality. It can be seen from Fig. 2 that the mortality rate for transurethral resection has been fairly low since the beginning of its use and in 1946, the year of our lowest over-all mortality rate, 87, or somewhat over one-half of the 153 patients operated upon for prostatic hypertrophy, had transurethral resections and with a mortality rate of only 3.4 per cent.

One very important factor in reducing the over-all annual mortality rate has been the increase in the number of the resident staff and the length of time required for training. From 1920 to 1930 much of the surgery was done by the visiting staff of urologists. In the last decade most of the surgery has been performed by the resident staff whose interest in the pre- and postoperative care of the patient has been enhanced by greater participation in the surgery done.

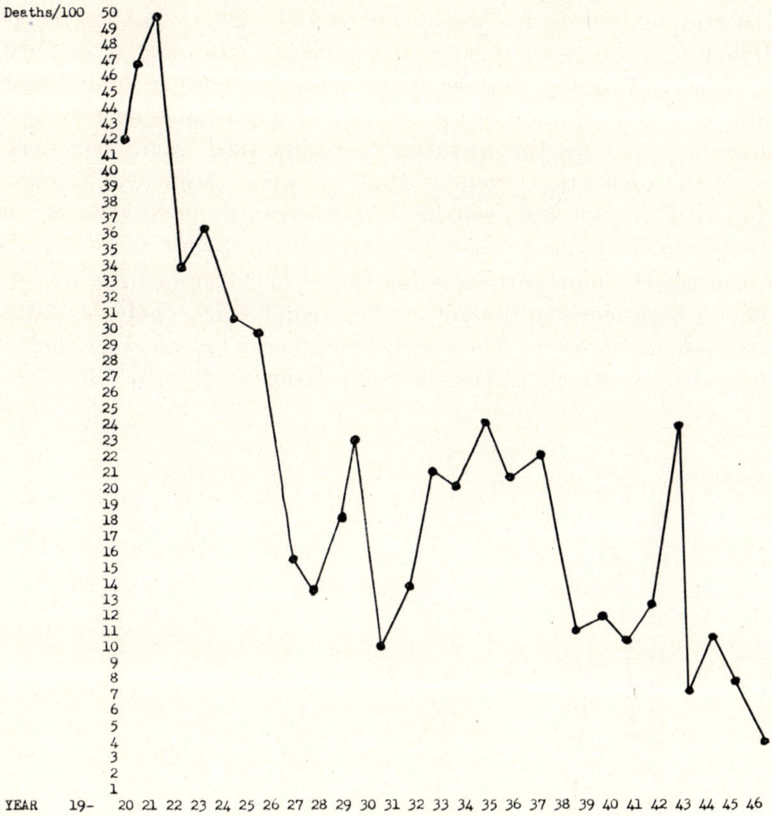

Fig. 1.—Annual mortality rate for all procedures, 1920 to 1946.

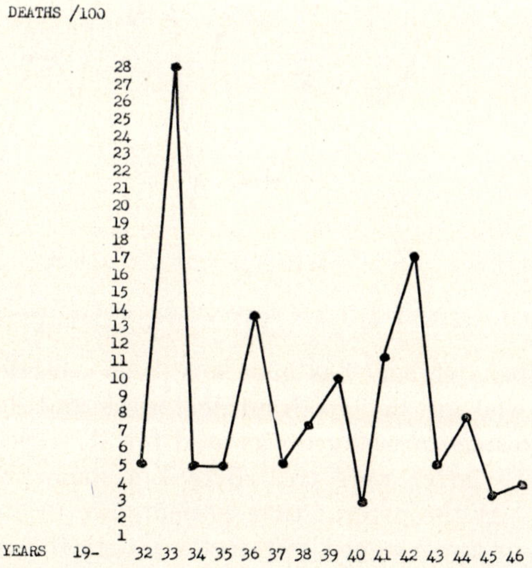

Fig. 2.—Annual mortality rate for transurethral resection, 1932 to 1946.

In 1920, of the 42 patients operated upon 11 had a cystotomy only; in 1946 the corresponding figure was 3 out of 153. This suggests the possibility that a higher percentage of seriously ill patients was treated in 1920 than in 1946. It should be noted that at Bellevue no patient is denied operation if such treatment, in the opinion of the staff, holds any hope of success, even though this practice may increase the operative mortality rate. Many comatose patients are taken to the operating rooms at Bellevue and a sufficient number of them survive to justify cystotomy even in the presence of coma when an indwelling catheter is not tolerated or for some reason catheterization is impossible.

Fig. 3 gives the mortality rate for the second stage of the two-stage prostatectomy. All patients subjected to the second stage obviously survived the cystotomy done previously. These cystotomy cases are not included in the list of cystotomies only, which makes the compilation of figures difficult.

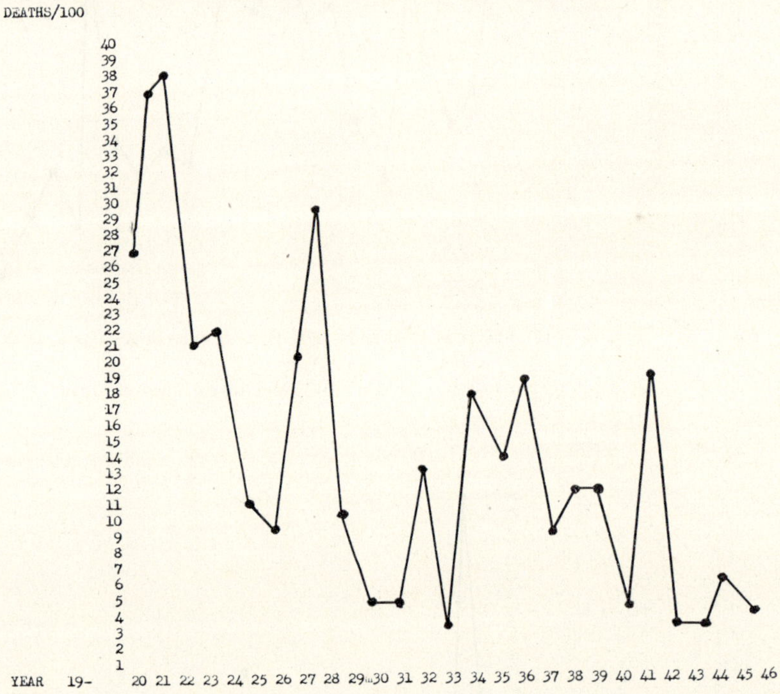

Fig. 3.—Annual mortality rate for second stage prostatectomy, 1920 to 1946.

A two-stage prostatectomy has generally been considered the operation of choice in patients who are not good surgical risks and during the early years of this report a two-stage procedure was used for all patients save those in very good condition. The latter were treated by one-stage prostatectomy or transurethral resection. At the present time patients are treated by a transurethral resection, perineal, or a one-stage prostatectomy with the exception of those with severe uremia, infection, and those with strictures.

The gradual lowering of the mortality rate for the second of a two-stage operation in the past twenty-five years cannot be attributed to great improvement in technique but must be an index of the value of the supplementary therapy.

In Fig. 4, giving the results of the one-stage suprapubic prostatectomy, it will be seen that the average twenty-seven year mortality is 13 per cent, which is lower than the mortality rate for all operative procedures.

There appears to have been considerable interest in one-stage operations from 1928 through 1931, as almost one-half of the operations were done by the one-stage method and the mortality in 1931 and 1932 was only 3 per cent—the lowest rate that has been reached by any procedure, in a significant number of cases, for benign prostatic hypertrophy at Bellevue.

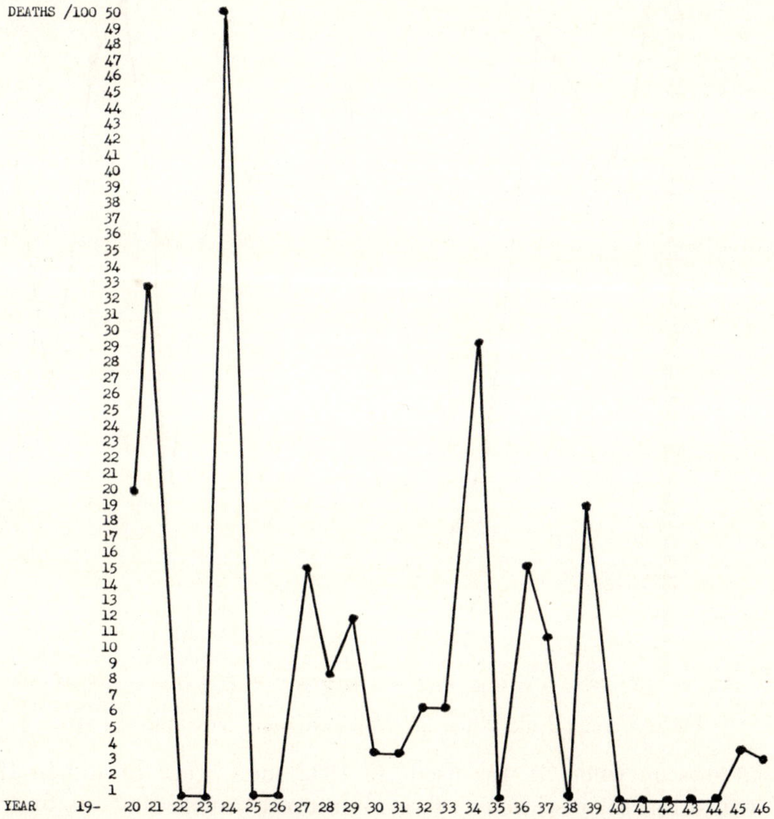

Fig. 4.—Annual mortality rate for one-stage prostatectomy, 1920 to 1946.

The recent mortality curve again shows a marked decrease for the one-stage operation, in fact, 86 consecutive one-stage prostatectomies have been done in the past seven years with only two deaths, an operative mortality of 2.3 per cent. It is worthy of comment that one of the two deaths occurred in a patient admitted to the hospital for severe bleeding from the prostate. A one-stage prostatectomy was carried out when all other means of checking the bleeding had proved unsuccessful; however, the patient died of shock from excessive loss of blood.

A review of these figures gives the impression that the merits of the one-stage procedure were proved years ago and overlooked for many years until recently.

In Fig. 2 the curve represents the mortality rate for transurethral resection which will be seen to improve as time goes on. The resectoscope became available in 1932 and since then each year has brought an increase in the num-

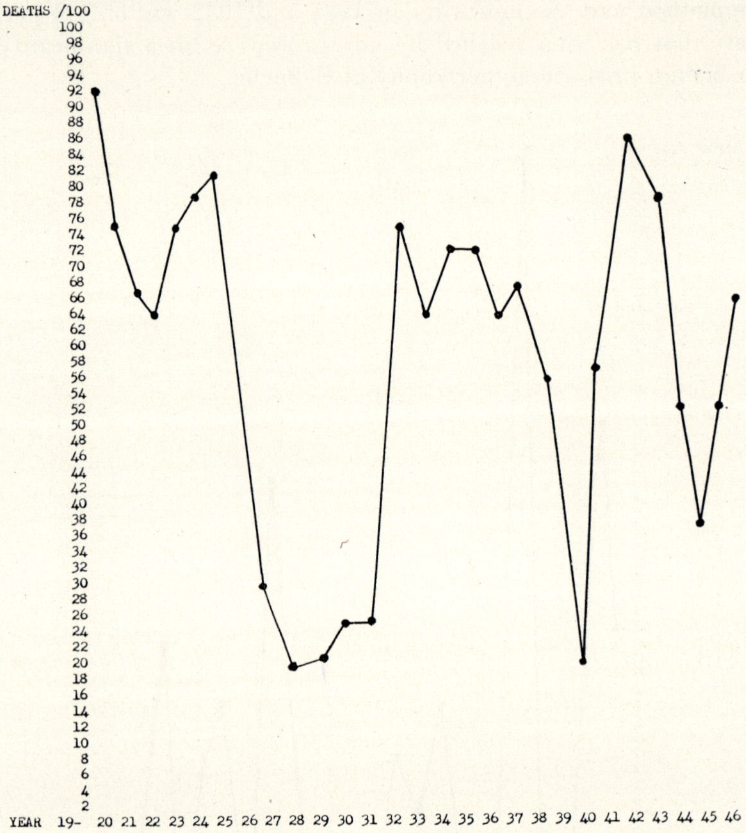

Fig. 5.—Annual mortality rate for cystotomy only, 1920 to 1946.

ber of patients on whom it was used; in 1932 there were 19 and in 1946 there were 87 transurethral resections. It is of interest to note that the first year this instrument was used the death rate was only 5 per cent, but the following year it rose abruptly to 28 per cent. This suggests that after the successful results of the first year attempts may have been made by less experienced operators to remove overlarge glands by this route. It has become the policy at Bellevue to reserve transurethral resection for glands which we anticipate will weigh less than 50 grams. This is the only limitation of its use and often patients with severe cardiac disease and elderly debilitated patients are subjected to this procedure as a matter of choice.

Prostatectomy by the perineal route has been carried out in only 81 cases during the past twenty-seven years, and 12 of the 81 were done in 1946. There has been little enthusiasm for this approach to the prostate gland and there have been years in which no perineal prostatectomies were done and in others there were only one or two. The infrequent use and unpopularity of this procedure is reflected in the mortality rate which averages 19 per cent for the twenty-seven years, an appallingly high figure.

It should be stated that 12 patients were subjected to perineal prostatectomy in 1946 by the technique advocated by Dr. Elmer Belt, without one death.

The charts and autopsy records of all patients who died after operations for benign prostatic hypertrophy during the period reviewed were studied in an effort to determine the chief cause of death. It is obvious that there are almost always several factors which contribute to the fatal outcome and it is difficult to tell which is most important. Certainly the most common cause of death in the earlier cases was infection, with uremia and hemorrhage following as the next most common causes. Since the advent of the sulfa drugs and penicillin, infection has assumed a somewhat less formidable role. However, as most of the stubborn urinary infections are caused by the gram-negative bacilli which are not controlled by penicillin and are also resistant to sulfa drugs, the urinary infection remains a serious problem. Streptomycin promises to be of material help in the treatment of these infections but we hesitate to use it except in the severely ill patients because of unfavorable side effects. Hemorrhage is a more important factor in postoperative morbidity than is generally realized. This fact is amply illustrated by a review of the autopsy findings.

CONCLUSIONS

It is obvious, from reviewing the records of Bellevue Hospital for the past twenty-seven years, that more patients are being subjected to prostatic surgery each year and a smaller percentage are dying as a result of their surgery. The over-all mortality has dropped from 40 or 50 per cent in the early twenties to 4.6 per cent in 1946. This is a most gratifying record and is attributable to the ingenuity, industry, and surgical skill of a large group of urologists who have worked during the twenty-seven years for no greater reward.

UNUSUAL COMPLICATIONS FOLLOWING RESECTION OF CARCINOMA OF THE CARDIAC END OF THE STOMACH

Report of a Case

William A. Barnes, M.D., New York, N. Y.

(From the Department of Surgery, Cornell University Medical College and The New York Hospital)

During the past several years the operation of intrathoracic esophagogastrostomy has gained wide recognition as the procedure of choice in the surgical treatment of neoplasms of the lower third of the esophagus and of the cardiac end of the stomach. More recently carcinoma of the middle third of the esophagus has been successfully removed and by drawing the stomach up to and above the arch of the aorta, intrathoracic esophagogastrostomy has been accomplished in an ever-increasing number of patients.

The purpose of this presentation is to review the course and emphasize several of the pitfalls encountered in the diagnosis and treatment of a patient with cancer of the cardiac end of the stomach.

CASE REPORT

The patient was a 51-year-old man employed in the storeroom of the New York Hospital. He was seen in the Personnel Health Service in October, 1943, complaining of poor appetite of five months' duration. He had previously been in good health save for an attack of right ureteral colic that confined him to the New York Hospital for one month. For five months the patient suffered from loss of appetite. Breakfast and dinner called forth the usual response but at lunch time delay in his work caused considerable tension and desire for food was lost. He developed fullness in the epigastrium about two hours after meals and this was relieved by belching. He lost ten pounds in the five-month period, but on his vacation during the two weeks before admission he regained six pounds and fatigue associated with increased hours of work disappeared.

Physical examination showed no pathologic changes.

It was the impression in the gastrointestinal clinic that he had a functional disorder associated with tension, but in order to rule out organic changes a gastrointestinal series was ordered. Fluoroscopic examination showed a minimal amount of cardiospasm but x-ray examination was reported as showing an apparently normal stomach and duodenum. Examination of the stool for blood gave negative results on one examination and positive on a second. Gastric analysis revealed no free hydrochloric acid even after histamine, and blood flecks were noted in the specimens. Gastroscopic examination was attempted but neither the large rubber lavage tube nor the gastroscope could be passed into the stomach and the patient was referred to the hospital.

Esophagoscopy was done and a polypoid lesion found at the distal end of the esophagus. A biopsy was made and the report of the pathologist was carcinoma of the cardiac end of the stomach. X-ray views of the chest showed no evidence of metastases but throughout the lung fields were several scattered parenchymal nodules and calcified hilar lymph nodes bilaterally.

On the eleventh day after admission, operation was done. Approximately 22 cm. of the left ninth rib were resected and the eighth rib was broken posteriorly. The visceral and parietal pleura were adherent requiring tedious dissection to approach the diaphragm and mediastinum. The esophagus was isolated and a firm lesion palpated at its junction with the stomach. An incision was made in the diaphragm and the capsule of the spleen was found to be fused to the diaphragm. This point of attack was abandoned and another opening made in the diaphragm, nearer the esophageal hiatus. Here again adhesions between what was subsequently found to be the greater omentum and the diaphragm were encountered. The cardiac portion of the stomach was densely adherent to the liver and a portion of the left lobe of the liver was resected. Numerous large firm nodes in the gastrohepatic omentum that undoubtedly contained carcinoma were also removed in the block dissection.

Division of the esophagus 4 cm. above the upper limit of the tumor and of the stomach 7 cm. from the cardia on the lesser curvature was done. After closing the stomach, it was found that anastomosis with the esophagus could be accomplished only under considerable tension. An attempt was made to isolate a loop of jejunum for the anastomosis but so dense were the intra-abdominal adhesions that small intestine was never even visualized. Accordingly the gastrohepatic omentum was further divided and the stomach sutured under tension to the chest wall. An esophagogastric anastomosis was then accomplished without tension but the tip of the stomach attached to the chest wall was cyanotic. The diaphragm was closed about the stomach and sutured high to the chest wall, relieving tension on the stomach. Two grams of sulfanilamide were sprayed about the suture line and the chest was closed with catgut and buried sutures of silver wire about the ribs.

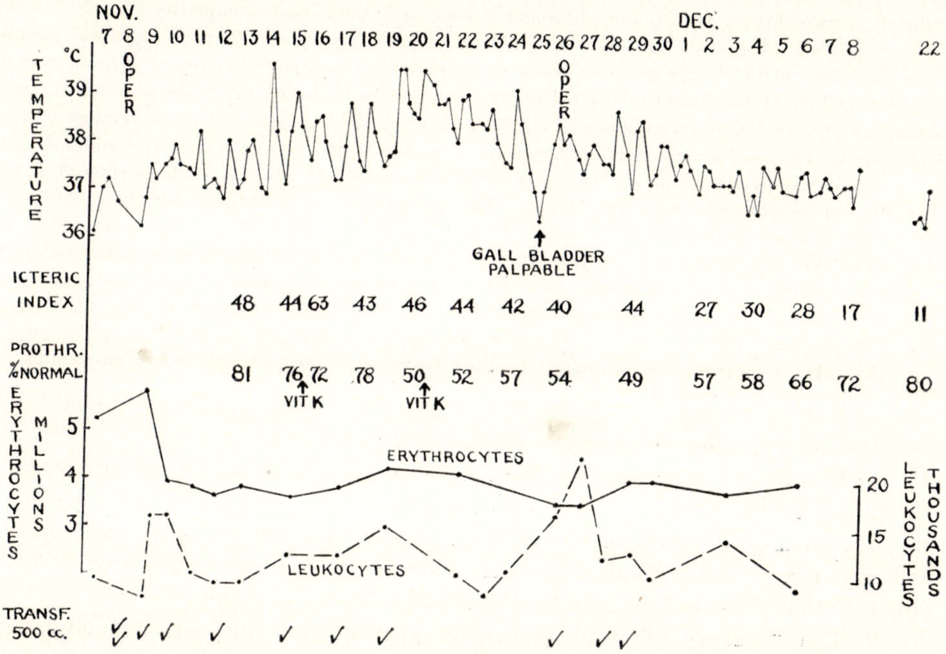

Fig. 1.

The lesion was described* as a serpiginous ulcer with stony hard margins which wandered around the cardiac end of the stomach 7 cm. and extended downward 5 cm. along the axis of the viscus. Outside the organ just beneath this ulcer there was a group of enlarged lymph nodes all massively invaded by stony hard white tumor tissue. The tumor extended up the esophagus for about 2 cm. The liver was not grossly invaded. Microscopic examination showed the tumor to be arising in the gastric mucosa where it was forming long glandular complexes composed of cylindrical cells with numerous mitotic figures. The tumor was found spreading upward in the esophagus beneath the epidermoid lining.

Findings of interest in the patient's postoperative course are recorded in Fig. 1.

The patient was placed in an oxygen tent and did well until the fifth postoperative day, when jaundice was noted. The icteric index was 48 and the prothrombin 81 per cent of normal. Sulfadiazine that had been given (2.5 Gm. twice daily) was discontinued. The patient's temperature ranged from 37 to 39.6° C. and the icteric index rose to 63 by the eighth day after operation. Roentgenograms of the chest showed a pleural effusion on the left.

A small amount of pus drained from the wound on the fourteenth day. He had no complaints until the seventeenth day when he had discomfort in the right upper quadrant of the abdomen and an enlarged tender gall bladder was felt. Bile was vomited. The icteric

*N. C. Foot, pathologist.

index remained about 40, and stools continued to be brown. On the next day a cholecystostomy was done under local anesthesia. The gall bladder was tremendously distended but not grossly acutely inflamed, although microscopic examination of a portion of its wall showed infiltration with polymorphonuclear leucocytes and necrosis. No stones were found.

Several transfusions were given. As bile continued to drain from the gall bladder, the icteric index fell and the patient improved symptomatically.

The cause of the patient's jaundice was the subject of speculation. The possibility of hepatitis with jaundice due to sulfadiazine, of which the patient received 25.5 Gm. during six days, was considered but this could not have accounted for the tremendous distention of the gall bladder and for the same reason a transfusion reaction was not considered a likely cause. Because of the considerable tension under which the stomach had to be sutured to effect the esophagogastric anastomosis it was thought that partial kinking of the common duct might have occurred with resultant obstruction. Since the patient vomited bile and continued to pass brown stools, the obstruction could not have been complete.

Study of the plasma prothrombin level showed a progressive fall from the time jaundice was observed until it began to clear about six days after the cholecystostomy. Most significant was the failure of the diminished level of prothrombin to rise even after the parenteral administration of vitamin K on two occasions (see Fig. 1). This suggested liver damage explainable on the basis of a hepatitis rather than as a result of obstruction of the common duct.

Roentgenograms taken on the forty-fourth day after the first operation showed a well-functioning esophagogastrostomy stoma. The patient was discharged two days later with the cholecystostomy wound still draining a small amount of bile. The subsequent course was favorable save for recurrence of infection in the thoracotomy wound two months after discharge at which time the buried silver wire sutures were removed. Again, one year after operation, a localized empyema with abscess of the chest wall occurred in the same region, necessitating drainage.

At the time of this communication, four years after esophagogastrostomy, the patient shows no evidence of residual disease.

Included among the points of interest in this case are:

1. Failure to diagnose accurately by x-ray examination the presence of carcinoma at the cardiac end of the stomach. It is well known that lesions in this region may be overlooked and it is only with repeated x-ray examinations and the use of additional diagnostic aids including esophagoscopy and gastroscopy that these lesions may be diagnosed at an early stage.

2. The presence of a polyserositic reaction that had all but obliterated the pleural and peritoneal cavities. This offered such technical difficulties that abandonment of attempted resection might have been considered prudent.

3. The massive involvement by carcinoma of lymph nodes in the gastrohepatic omentum and attachment of the stomach to the liver. This rendered the operability of the lesion even more doubtful, but, that it was justified is evidenced by the fact that four years after operation there is no evidence of recurrence.

4. The occurrence of jaundice five days after esophagogastrostomy. This seemed best explained on the basis of partial obstruction of the common duct by upward traction on the stomach resulting in conspicuous distention of the gall bladder, and, in addition, associated hepatitis that produced low levels of plasma prothrombin that failed to respond to vitamin K administered parenterally.

5. The recurrence of infection in the chest wall with localized empyema, as late as one year after operation. While a small segment of a silver wire stay suture remains in the chest wall the empyema apparently was not associated with this.

MALIGNANT TUMORS OF THE THYROID GLAND

Barton McSwain, M.D., and Walter Diveley, M.D., Nashville, Tenn.

(From the Department of Surgery, Vanderbilt University School of Medicine)

THIS small series of malignant tumors of the thyroid gland is being reported in order to point out the fact that such lesions are uncommon in a general hospital outside of the goiter belt and to emphasize some points in their clinical manifestations, microscopic characteristics, and treatment.

INCIDENCE

The only large series of cases which have been published in the United States literature have been from the Mayo Clinic, the Lahey Clinic, and the Cleveland Clinic, where the proportion of operations upon the thyroid gland to other operations is larger than in most of the other institutions in this country. The numbers of patients with malignant tumors of the thyroid gland operated upon, followed, and reported from these clinics are as follows: From the Mayo Clinic in 1938 by Pemberton,[19] 464 cases; from the Lahey Clinic in 1940 by Lahey and associates,[16] 231 cases; and from the Cleveland Clinic in 1941 by Portmann,[20] 147 cases. However, from the Bellevue Hospital (3,082 beds) in New York City, Rosh and Raider[21] stated in 1945 that only 64 malignant tumors of the thyroid gland had been seen in their radiation therapy department from 1924 to the time of writing of their report. From the Memorial Hospital (223 beds) in New York City Haagensen,[9] in 1931, reported 30 patients who had been treated by radiation therapy only. Coller,[1] in 1929, reported 90 patients with malignant epithelial neoplasms who had been operated upon from 1912 to 1927 in the University of Michigan Hospital (899 beds) at Ann Arbor, Mich., which is in the goiter belt. In 1947 Horn and associates[12] from the University of Pennsylvania Hospital (697 beds) reported 71 patients with thyroid carcinoma observed from 1933 until the time of writing of the report.

Over a period of twenty-two years, during which time 122,633 patients have been admitted to the Vanderbilt University Hospital (340 beds), there have been only 23 patients admitted with malignant disease of the thyroid gland. Twenty-two of these patients were operated upon and one died and was subjected to autopsy without operation upon the thyroid gland. During this same period there have been 399 patients operated upon for carcinoma of the breast. In the surgical pathology laboratory 1,168 specimens of thyroid glands have been examined, the 22 specimens of malignant tumors of the thyroid gland thus giving a percentage of 1.88 of the thyroid lesions upon which operation had been performed.

Age.—The ages of these patients ranged from 13 to 70 years (Table I).

Sex.—In this series there were 6 male and 17 female patients.

CLASSIFICATION

Malignant tumors of the thyroid gland have never been satisfactorily classified but that same statement holds true for other malignant neoplasms,

TABLE I. AGE IN YEARS OF TWENTY PATIENTS IN FOLLOW-UP STUDY

AGE (YR.)	TOTAL CASES	PATIENTS ALIVE	PATIENTS DEAD
13	1	1	0
21-30	3	2	1
31-40	4	1	3
41-50	5	4	1
51-60	4	0	4
61-70	3	1	2
Total	20	9	11

Ages of two patients with carcinoma of the thyroid seen within the past year were 58 and 59 years. Age of one patient who died in the hospital without operation upon the thyroid gland was 65 years. These three patients are not included in this table.

for example, those of bone. The tumors in this series could be placed in one of the following categories:

1. Papillary adenocarcinoma
2. Adenocarcinoma
3. Alveolar adenocarcinoma
4. Alveolar carcinoma
5. Giant-cell carcinoma
6. Squamous-cell carcinoma
7. Sarcoma

The first four types are not completely distinct, that is, they merge gradually from one morphologic type to another. They could be tabulated thus:

1. Adenocarcinoma
   (a) Papillary
   (b) Purely acinar (not papillary or alveolar)
   (c) Alveolar
2. Alveolar carcinoma

Papillary Adenocarcinoma (Figs. 1, 2, and 3).—Portions of such tumors are papillary and other portions show definite acinar formations. In some areas of the neoplasm colloid is present in the acini. The proportion of papillary areas to acinar areas varies in different tumors and in different sections of the same tumor from almost purely papillary to almost purely acinar. In one of the tumors (Fig. 2) the areas of acinar formation were minimal but, since they did exist, it was felt unnecessary to use another class, that is, papillary carcinoma.

Adenocarcinoma (Figs. 4 and 5).—Two of the tumors were true adenocarcinomas and the qualifying adjective, papillary or alveolar, was unnecessary. Both of these tumors contained areas of cells which were well enough differentiated to secrete colloid.

Alveolar Adenocarcinoma (Figs. 6, 7, 8, and 9).—The word "alveolus" is the diminutive form of the Latin word *alveus* which means tray, basin, or trough. Alveolus also means air sac of the lung (Dorland[7]). It is probably because of one of these meanings that tumors said to show cells growing in alveolar fashion are understood to be those which grow in groups separated by septa of connective tissue. Ewing[4a] stated that, "Small alveolar carcinoma is a specific

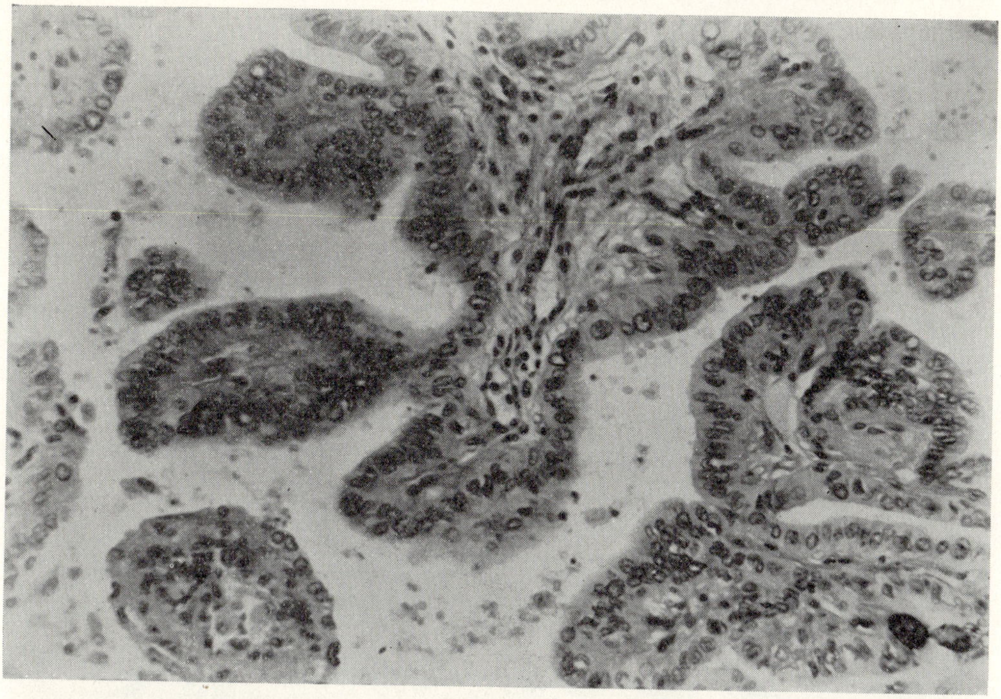

Fig. 1 (Surg. Path. No. 4915).—Papillary adenocarcinoma; this field is almost purely papillary.

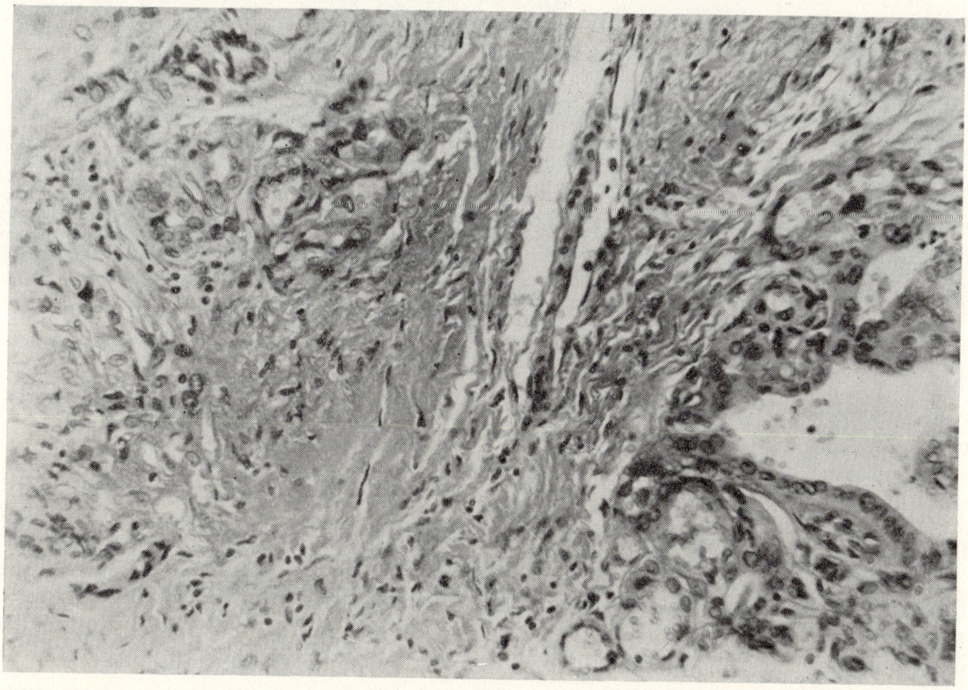

Fig. 2 (Surg. Path. No. 4915).—Papillary adenocarcinoma, same patient as Fig. 1. This field shows both papillary and glandular areas.

term which may properly designate a carcinomatous structure in which the cells appear in small groups supported by a moderate amount of connective tissue. . . . Large alveolar carcinoma equally well designates a similar structure in which the cell groups are large, but still well defined.'' This type of tumor of the thyroid shows acinar formation, but in some areas the cells are seen in groups or sheets without showing a central lumen. It is in this class that we have placed the tumors formerly classified as Hürthle cell carcinomas. There is no positive proof, as pointed out by Wilensky and Kaufman,[25] of the existence of the interfollicular thyroid cells described by Hürthle.[13] Hürthle did not describe a tumor arising from such cells but Ewing[3] in his third edition of *Neoplastic Diseases* stated that in two tumors which he had seen ''the acidophile cells might represent hypertrophic Hürthle cells of the thyroid alveoli.'' How-

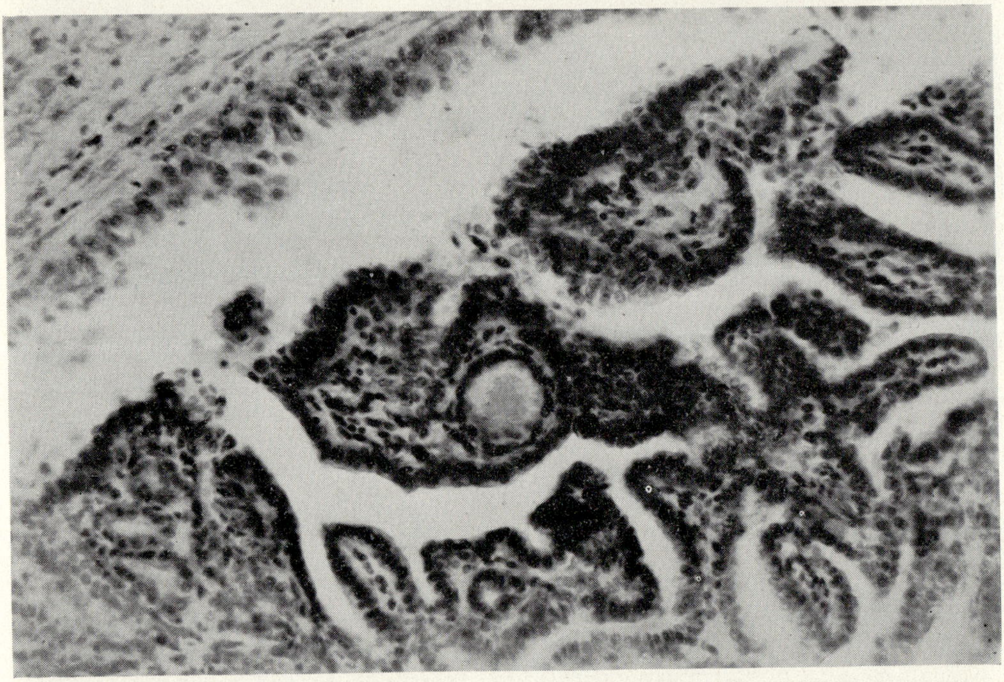

Fig. 3 (Surg. Path. No. 1511).—Papillary adenocarcinoma, an acinus containing colloid is shown.

ever, in his fourth edition[4b] he stated that, ''assumption of a special anatomical origin of this tumor is unnecessary.'' The term ''small alveolar, large cell'' *(kleinalveolare, grosszellige)* carcinoma sometimes applied to this tumor (Ewing[4b]) was originated by Langhans.[17] If these tumors are parathyroid in origin as suggested by Eisenberg and Wallerstein,[2] there should be evidence of hyperparathyroidism; such manifestations were not present in their patient and have not, to our knowledge, been reported. In addition, there is morphologic evidence (Fig. 9) that the tumor tends to reproduce the cells of the thyroid acini. Hence it seems that the term ''Hürthle cell carcinoma'' is unnecessary.

Alveolar Carcinoma (Fig. 10).—In the alveolar carcinoma the cells grow in sheets separated by connective tissue septa. No acini are present in the tumor.

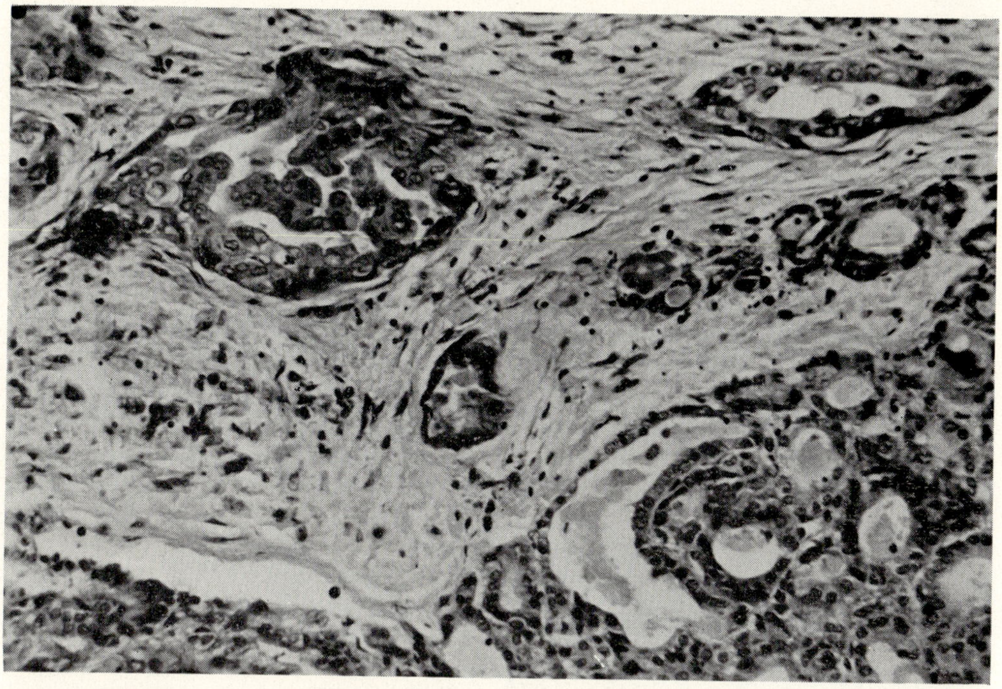

Fig. 4 (Surg. Path. No. 15536).—Adenocarcinoma.

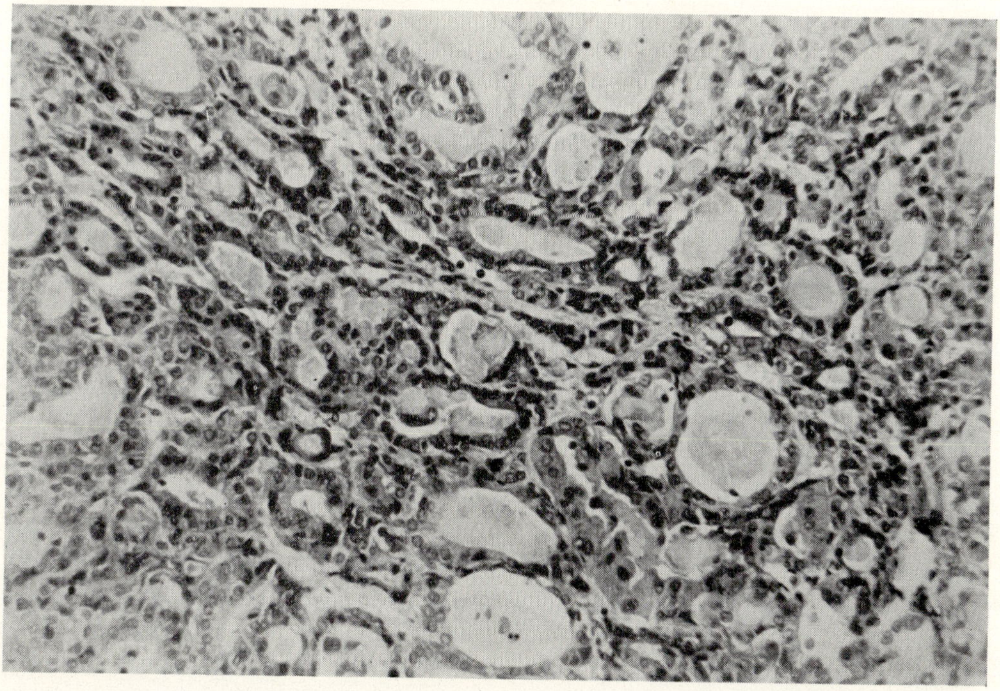

Fig. 5 (Surg. Path. No. 15536).—From same patient as Fig. 4. Areas of hyperplasia are seen; patient had preoperative treatment with Lugol's solution.

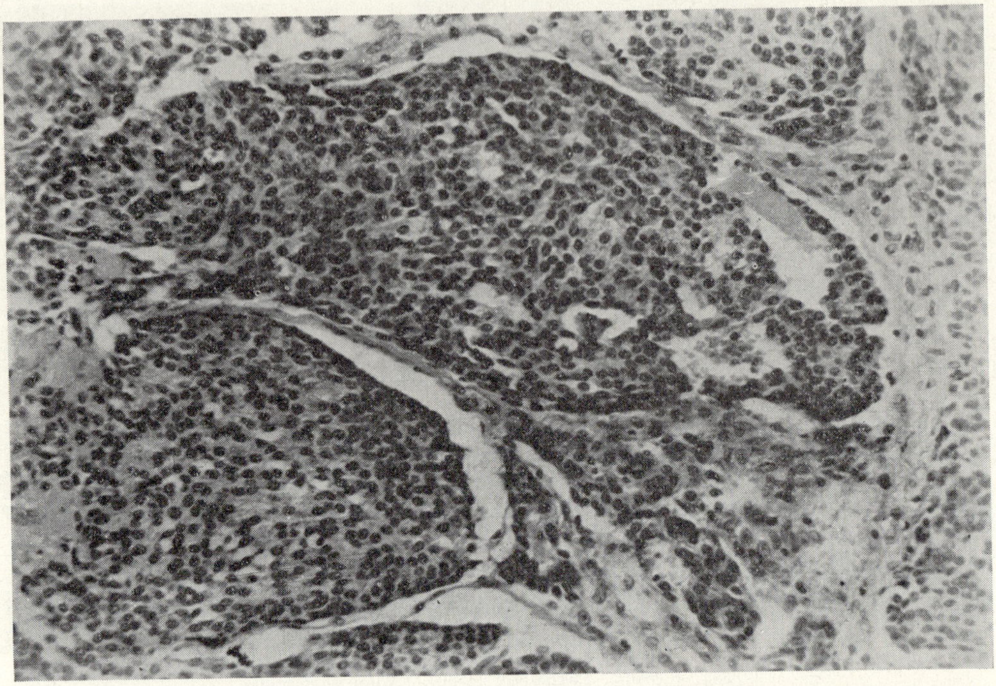

Fig. 6 (Surg. Path. No. 15930).—Alveolar adenocarcinoma. In this field most of the cells are seen in the form of sheets without glandular formation.

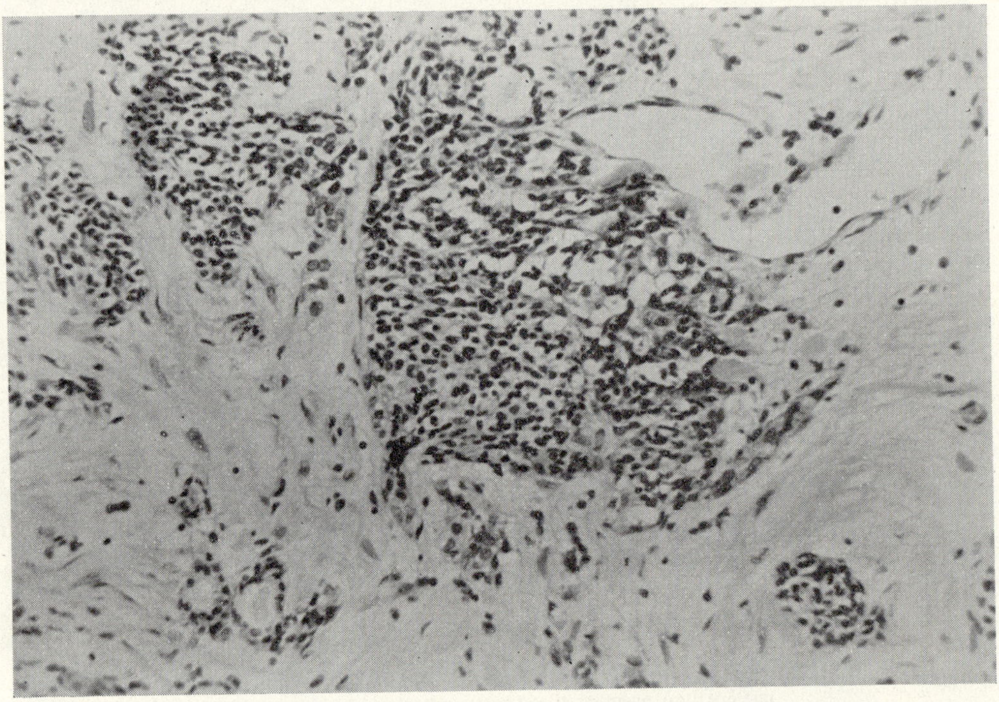

Fig. 7 (Surg. Path. No. 15930).—Alveolar adenocarcinoma, from same patient as Fig. 6. Areas of glandular formation are present as well as cells growing in alveolar fashion.

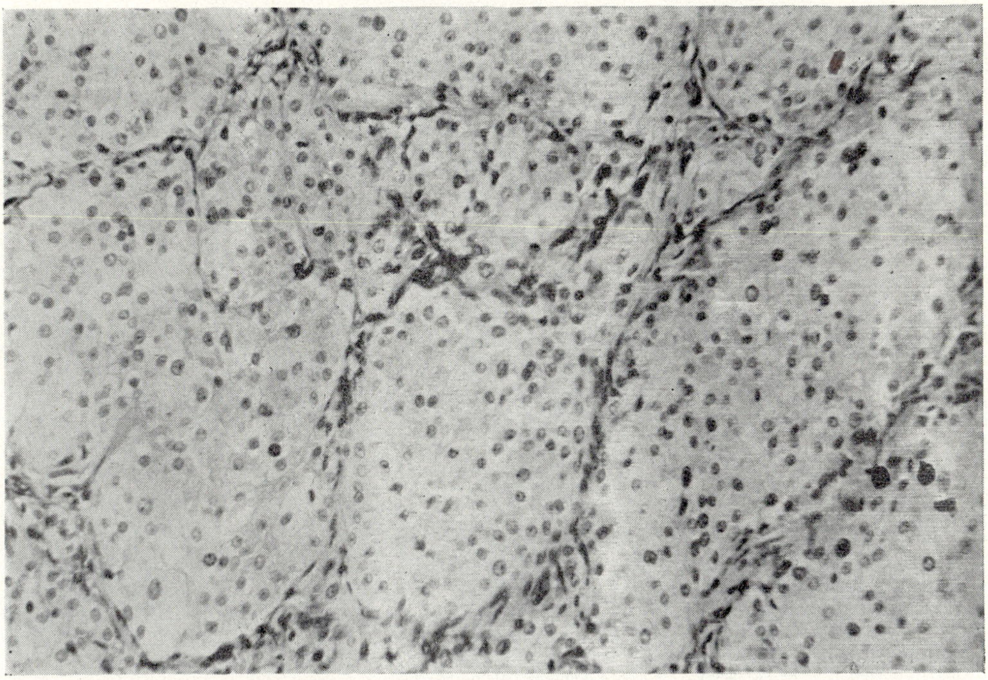

Fig. 8 (Surg. Path. No. 14435).—Alveolar adenocarcinoma. This is the type of tumor which some observers call Hürthle cell carcinoma. This field shows alveolar areas.

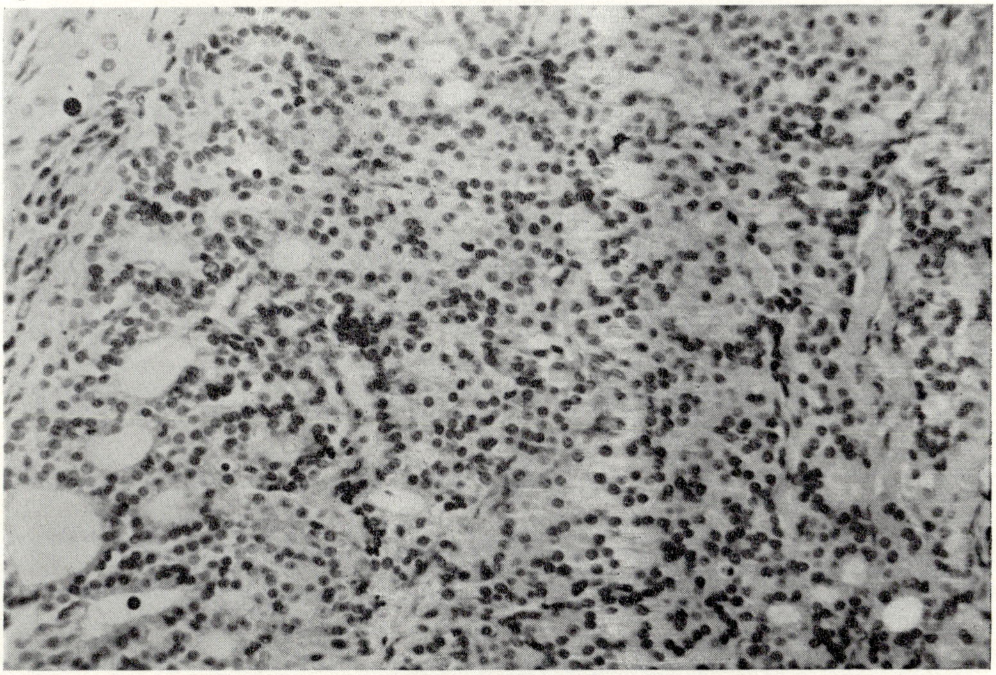

Fig. 9 (Surg. Path. No. 14435).—Alveolar adenocarcinoma, from same patient as Fig. 8. Glandular formation is shown.

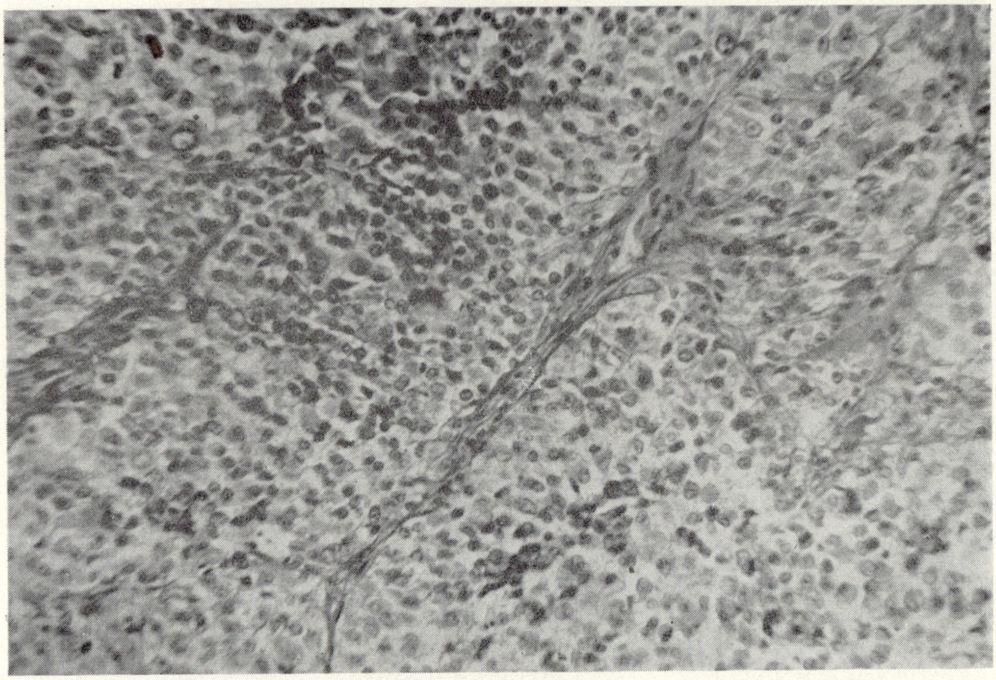

Fig. 10 (Surg. Path. No. 5226).—Alveolar carcinoma. Cells growing in sheets separated by connective tissue septa.

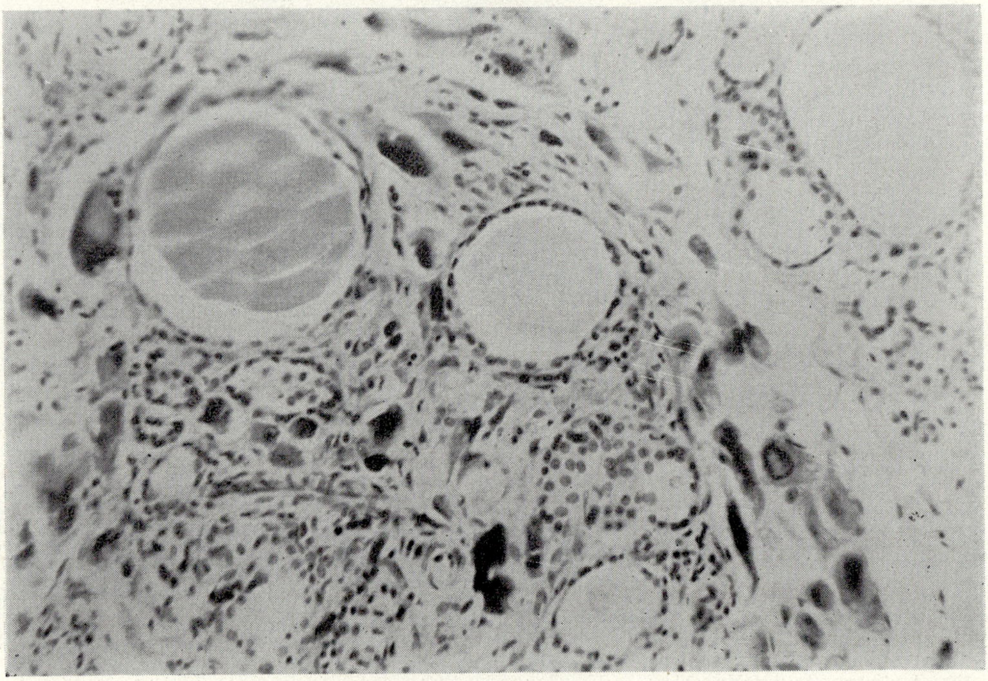

Fig. 11 (Gen. Path. No. V-47-62).—Giant-cell carcinoma.

Giant-Cell Carcinoma (Figs. 11, 12, and 13).—Giant-cell carcinoma is so poorly differentiated that the cells are hardly recognizable as having originated from thyroid epithelium. The predominating cell is the malignant tumor giant cell. This tumor has previously been called carcinoma-sarcoma but it appears to be really a carcinoma. In one such case poorly formed acini were present (Fig. 13).

Squamous-Cell Carcinoma (Fig. 14).—Squamous-cell carcinomas show the same microscopic characteristics in the thyroid as do such tumors arising in the skin. Their origin has not been definitely determined but it seems more likely to be from remnants of the thyroglossal duct (Means[18]) than from glandular thyroid tissue by metaplasia as suggested by Jaffe.[14]

Sarcoma (Fig. 15).—The single sarcoma in this series was, on the basis of morphology, a fibrosarcoma. The presence of spindle cells and connective tissue fibrils indicated that the tumor was not of epithelial origin.

COMMENT ON OTHER TERMS

There was no tumor in this series which necessitated including the class of small cell carcinoma. Although this type of tumor may exist, we agree with Graham[6] that there is a danger of applying this term to lymphosarcomas. Furthermore, the photomicrographs of some of these tumors so classified by Ewing[4c] and Foot[8] lead us to believe that they could be classified as alveolar carcinomas.

The word "scirrhous" means hard and was useful in the description of gross pathologic specimens before examination of stained sections by the microscope was possible. At the present time it seems unnecessary to use this word in the classification of thyroid carcinomas.

The term "malignant adenoma" is one which could be abolished. Adenoma means "benign epithelial tumor with gland-like structure" (Dorland[7]). Hence, this combination of words means "malignant benign epithelial tumor. . . ." It seems preferable to call the tumor a carcinoma if it is malignant. If there is evidence on examination of the gross specimen or the section of its having arisen in an adenoma, that fact may be stated parenthetically.

The occurrence in the lateral portion of the neck of the so-called lateral aberrant thyroid may be explained on an embryologic basis (Weller[24]). However, such a tumor may be a metastasis from a thyroid carcinoma. In one case in point (Figs. 6 and 7) in this series the patient was subjected to excision of the lateral mass. When this procedure was completed, the thyroid lobe on the same side of the neck was examined and found to be quite hard. There was no connection demonstrable between the lateral mass and the thyroid gland. A portion of the latter was excised and microscopic sections showed tumor tissue of the same type from both sites. The lateral mass showed lymphoid tissue around the periphery. We agree with King and Pemberton[15] that the so-called aberrant thyroids usually are lymph node metastases from thyroid carcinoma. If microscopic section reveals tissue suggestive of thyroid carcinoma, the thyroid gland should be explored. If exploration reveals tumor, lobectomy should be done or as much of the tumor as possible should be removed.

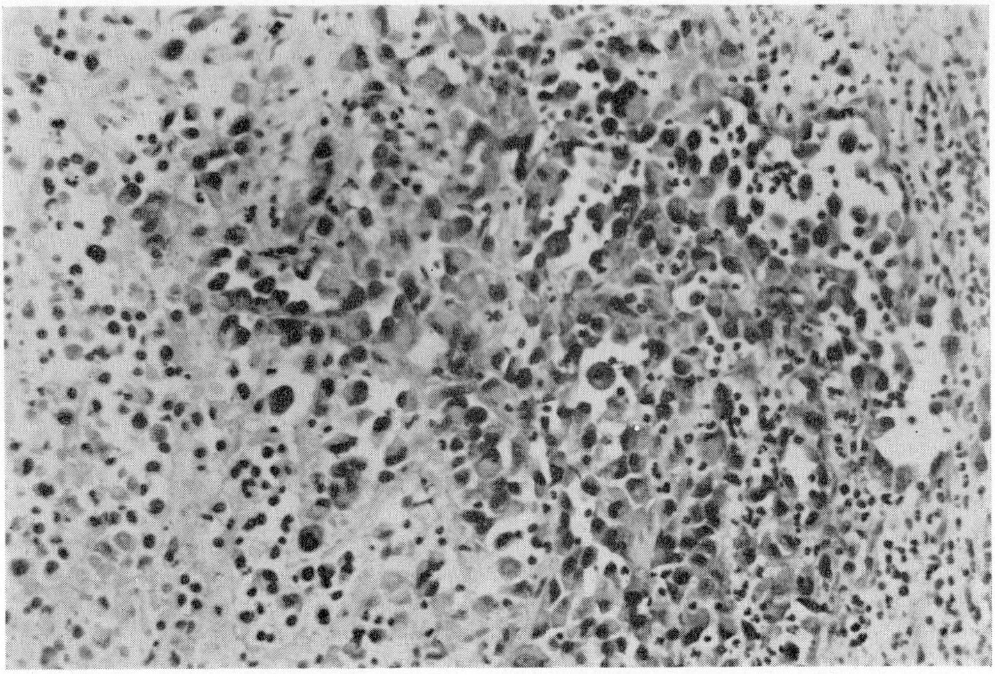

Fig. 12 (Surg. Path. No. 12039).—Giant-cell carcinoma.

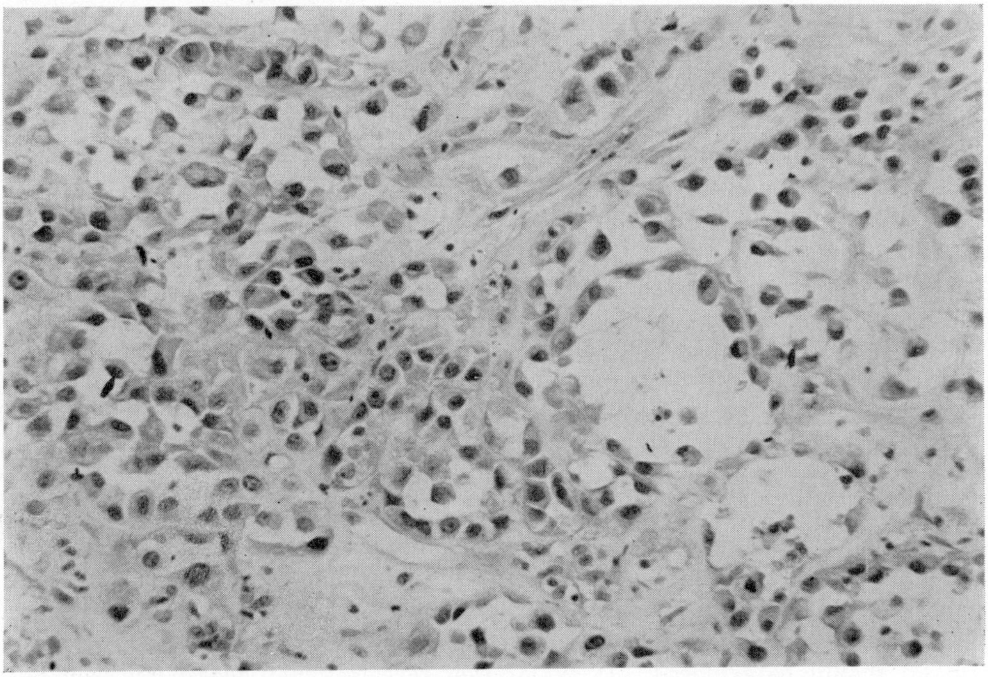

Fig. 13 (Surg. Path. No. 12039).—From same patient as Fig. 12; acinar formation.

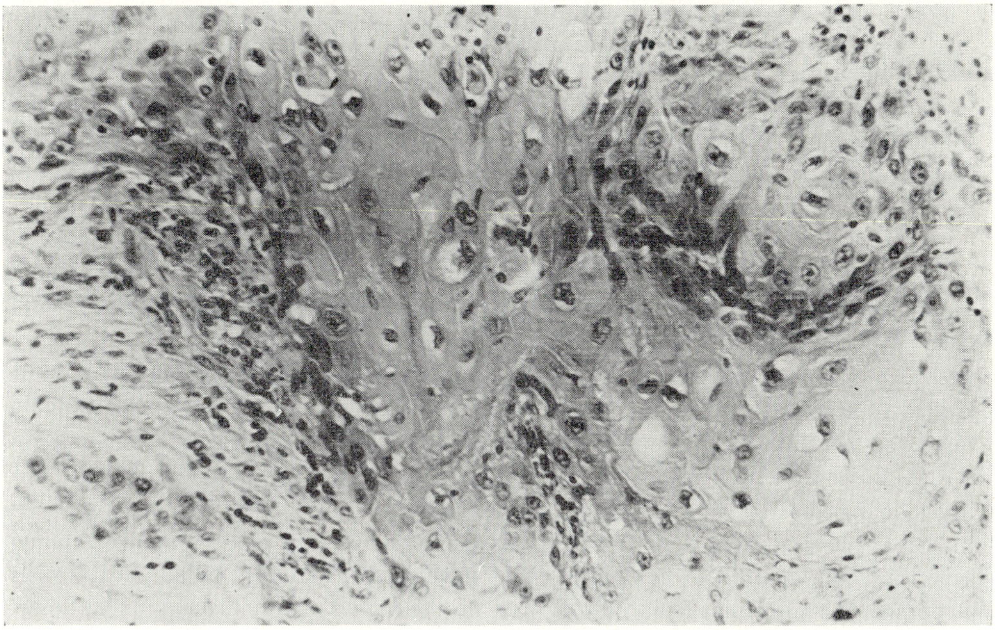

Fig. 14 (Surg. Path. No. 14761).—Squamous-cell carcinoma.

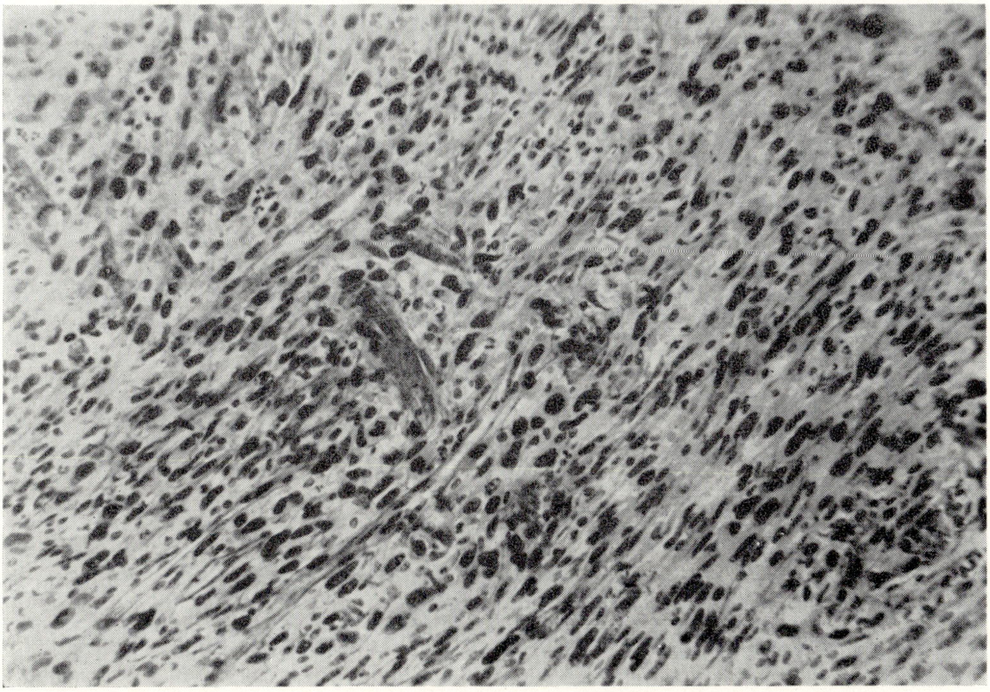

Fig. 15 (Surg. Path. No. 4613).—Fibrosarcoma.

CRITERIA OF MALIGNANCY

While actual blood vessel invasion as discussed by Graham[5] is a criterion of malignancy, its existence is extremely difficult to prove. If upon examination of the gross specimen, one finds tumor in a vein and confirms this observation upon microscopic examination, there can be no doubt that the tumor has invaded a blood vessel. However, in the literature there have apppeared photomicrographs purportedly showing blood vessel invasion which are not convincing. Tumor cells surrounded by connective tissue strands resemble neoplasm in an endothelial lined vessel. Tumor in acini which contain red blood cells may cause confusion. In 1931 Warren[23] reported thirty-two cases of adenoma with blood vessel invasion followed for two and one-half to seven years and stated that twenty-nine of the patients were living and well. It is difficult to understand how such a high survival rate is possible in such instances unless the microscopic observations are inaccurate or the importance of blood vessel invasion has been overemphasized. Means[18] stated that such microscopic findings may be artefacts due to the cutting of the section. Furthermore, Means said that, as dependable evidence of blood vessel invasion Dr. T. B. Mallory, in a personal communication, stated that he required "penetration of a vessel large enough to possess some musculature with extension of the tumor through this muscularis."

In carcinoma showing evidence of origin in adenoma, there are signs of malignancy other than blood vessel invasion. These signs are those of malignancy in carcinoma of other sites such as mitoses, lack of differentiation, variation in size, shape, and staining qualities of the cells, and the invasion of the capsule and adjacent tissues. It is quite rare for a tumor to show unquestionable blood vessel invasion without showing other criteria of malignancy.

CLINICAL MANIFESTATIONS

Chief Complaint.—In this series there were nine patients alive four to eighteen years after the diagnosis of carcinoma was made. These nine patients complained of goiter but the presence of the goiter was not the chief reason for seeking medical advice in any one of them. The chief reasons for consulting physicians were rapid increase in the size of the goiter (three patients); slow increase in the size of the goiter (two patients), along with pressure symptoms in one of these two; rupture of a mass in the neck (one patient); symptoms of hyperthyroidism (one patient); weight loss (one patient); sleepiness and, six months later, the presence of a cervical lymph node (one patient).

Duration of Goiter.—Seven of the nine surviving patients had goiters which had been present for periods varying from four to thirty years. Seven of the eleven patients who died had goiters which had been present for four to twenty-five years. The only conclusions that can be drawn from this observation are that an enlarged thyroid is more likely to be the site of carcinoma than a thyroid of normal size and that the duration of the goiter had no bearing on the prognosis.

Hyperthyroidism.—Reports in the literature give the incidence of the coexistence of cancer of the thyroid gland and manifestations of toxicity as low as 3 per cent (Herbst[11]) and as high as 50 per cent (Simpson[22]). In this series there were four patients who had elevations of the basal metabolic rate, but only two in whom the diagnosis of hyperthyroidism was not open to question. In one man (Fig. 5), the clinical manifestations of toxic goiter were typical and included fatigability, sweating, dyspnea on exertion, weight loss of twenty-five pounds in three months, tachycardia, tremor, slight exophthalmos, and a basal metabolic rate of plus 60. Lugol's solution was administered daily for thirteen days and then a subtotal thyroidectomy was done. Microscopic sections showed the characteristic findings of diffuse toxic goiter after iodine therapy and also an adenocarcinoma. In one woman (Surg. Path. No. 1511) the manifestations included nervousness, increased appetite, sweating, palpitation, weight loss of thirty-seven pounds in three years, tremor, slight exophthalmos, and basal metabolic rate of plus 57. Lugol's solution was given daily for sixteen days and then subtotal thyroidectomy was done. Microscopic sections showed an alveolar adenocarcinoma and definite hyperplasia of the remainder of the thyroid gland. In neither of these individuals was there evidence that the tumor cells had been responsible for the symptoms and signs of toxic goiter.

Hypothyroidism.—Simpson[22] stated that "hypothyroidism is practically unknown even in the most massive growths." Means[18] stated that "hypothyroidism from malignancy is in our experience practically nonexistent." In one patient in this group, a male student, the symptoms of sleepiness and inability to concentrate upon studies caused a physician to determine the basal metabolic rate which was minus 32. He was given 0.15 Gm. of thyroxin daily for six months at which time lymph nodes appeared in the posterior cervical region. As the operation consisted only of excision of a lymph node and of a small amount of thyroid gland for microscopic study, it is impossible to state the degree of destruction of functioning thyroid tissue that had occured. In the biopsy specimen no normal thyroid was present.

Consistency of the Tumors.—Physical examination of these twenty-two patients showed that twelve of the tumors were hard, eight were firm, and two were soft. Carcinoma of the thyroid is usually described as being hard, but in this small series, only slightly more than one-half of the tumors were hard.

Origin in Adenoma.—Graham[5] found that 92.4 per cent of the thyroid carcinomas which he studied arose in adenomas. In only seven of our patients did gross and microscopic studies reveal such an origin.

TREATMENT AND RESULTS

Lahey and associates[16] stated that "surgery finds its most satisfactory place, of course: first, in the prophylactic removal, while the tumor is still benign, of the discrete tumors of the thyroid gland in which malignancy may later arise." Furthermore, since the diagnosis of carcinoma in this series was not suspected before operation or even at operation, in six of the twenty-two patients being reported, excision of a single nodule is certainly justifiable because of the fact that such a nodule may already be malignant when first observed.

In the series reported by Pemberton[19] of 464 cases of thyroid cancer there were 259 five-year survivals. Lahey and co-workers[16] stated the percentages of five-year survival rate for each type of tumor but did not state the number of five-year survivals. Portmann[20] stated that 42 of 147 patients with thyroid cancer were alive and well five years after the diagnosis had been established.

Two of the patients in this series were operated upon within the past year and are not included among the twenty patients in the follow-up study. Nine of these twenty patients are alive, the survival time ranging from four to twenty years (Table II). Only one of the nine subjects has a recurrence at present.

The results in relation to the type of tumor are shown in Table III. Half of the patients who had papillary adenocarcinoma are alive, one with recurrence. Both of the individuals who had adenocarcinoma are alive and well. One-third of the patients who had alveolar adenocarcinoma are alive and well. In the single case of squamous-cell carcinoma in this series, the tumor arose in the left lobe of the thyroid and had involved the regional lymph nodes. The patient was subjected to removal of the left lobe of the thyroid gland, excision

TABLE II

SURG. PATH. NO.	TUMOR COMPLETELY REMOVED	TUMOR CONFINED TO THYROID	X-RAY TREATMENT	RESULT	INTERVAL
		Papillary Adenocarcinoma			
1511	Yes	Yes	No	Alive	18 yr.
2819	No	Yes	Yes	Dead	6½ yr.
4915	No	No	Yes	Alive	14 yr.
5326	No	No	Yes	Alive	14 yr.
11471	No	No	Yes	Dead	6 yr.
15470	No	No	Yes	Dead	2½ yr.
16926	No	No	Yes	Alive*	4 yr.
19441	No (biopsy only)	No	No	Dead	11 mo.
		Adenocarcinoma			
10996	No (biopsy only)	No	Yes	Alive	8 yr.
15536	Yes	Yes	No	Alive	5 yr.
		Alveolar Adenocarcinoma			
6047	No	No	Yes	Dead	1 yr. 10 mo.
8282	No	No	Yes	Dead	1 yr. 9 mo.
14435	Yes	Yes	No	Alive	5 yr.
15930	No	No	Yes	Alive	4 yr.
16534	Yes	No	No	Dead	2 yr. 9 mo.
17294	No	No	No	Dead	4 mo.
		Alveolar Carcinoma			
5226	No	No	Yes	Dead	3 mo.
		Giant-Cell Carcinoma			
12039	No	No	No	Dead	3 mo.
		Squamous-Cell Carcinoma			
14761	No	No	Yes	Alive	5 yr.
		Fibrosarcoma			
4613	No	No	No	Dead	1 mo.

This table shows the results in relation to the type and extent of tumor, to the completeness of its removal, and to whether or not roentgen-ray therapy was administered.

*With recurrence.

TABLE III

TYPE OF TUMOR	NUMBER OF PATIENTS		
	TOTAL	ALIVE	DEAD
Papillary adenocarcinoma	8	4	4
Adenocarcinoma	2	2	0
Alveolar adenocarcinoma	6	2	4
Alveolar carcinoma	1	0	1
Squamous-cell carcinoma	1	1	0
Giant-cell carcinoma	1	0	1
Sarcoma	1	0	1
Total	20	9	11

This table shows the results in relation to the type of tumor. Not included are a case of adenocarcinoma and one of papillary adenocarcinoma observed within the past year and a patient with giant-cell carcinoma who died without operation upon the thyroid gland.

of the lymph nodes, and roentgen-ray therapy. She is alive and without evidence of recurrence five and one-half years after operation. The patients who had alveolar carcinoma, giant-cell carcinoma, and fibrosarcoma are dead.

Of the thirteen patients in whom the diagnosis of malignant disease was made positively or tentatively before operation, four are alive and well (Table IV). One is alive with recurrence and eight are dead. The five surviving patients received postoperative x-ray therapy as did five of the eight individuals who died. Of the three patients in whom the diagnosis of malignancy was first suspected at operation, two died and one is alive and well. There were four patients in whom the diagnosis of carcinoma was not made until the microscopic section was seen. Three of these patients are alive and well. One died, but since death occurred at home, supposedly from cerebral hemorrhage, it is impossible to state whether or not the carcinoma was responsible for death. None of these four patients received roentgen-ray therapy.

TABLE IV

DIAGNOSIS OF CANCER	NUMBER OF CASES		
	TOTAL	ALIVE	DEAD
Suspected before operation	13	5	8
Suspected at operation	3	1	2
Not suspected until microscopic sections were seen	4*	3	1

*These four patients were the only ones in whom the tumor was completely removed.

The tumor was completely removed in only three of the surviving patients (Table II). Hence in six, or two-thirds, of the living patients removal of the tumor was incomplete and in one of the six only a biopsy was done. In only one of the patients who died was the tumor thought to have been completely extirpated. The four patients in whom complete removal of the tumor was done are the same four in whom the diagnosis of carcinoma was not made until the microscopic sections were seen. Two patients were seen within the past year in whom the diagnosis of carcinoma was not made until the microscopic sections were seen and were not irradiated. It is felt that if examination of the gross specimen and microscopic sections lead one to believe that all the tumor has been removed, irradiation should not be given.

Excision of recurrences, if possible, seems justified by the course of two patients in this series. One of these patients had a papillary carcinoma extending into the neck muscles and was subjected to right lobectomy and roentgen-ray therapy. Three months later a nodule to the right of the scar was excised and found to exhibit the same microscopic characteristics as the original tumor. She was given more x-ray therapy and is alive and well fourteen years after operation. The second patient had an alveolar adenocarcinoma which had not invaded the surrounding structures. A left lobectomy was done with almost complete excision of the tumor and x-ray therapy was not given. A recurrence, showing the same type of tumor, was excised four and one-half years later and although roentgen-ray therapy was not given, she is alive and well one and one-half years after excision of the recurrence.

The length of time from the establishment of the diagnosis until the death of the eleven patients is shown in Table II. This period ranged from one month to six and one-half years. The duration of life after the diagnosis of cancer was made was six years in one patient and six and one-half years in another. The average survival time of these eleven patients was twenty-five months. The survival time of the six subjects, now dead, who received roentgenologic therapy ranged from 21 to 78 months and averaged 37½ months. The period of survival of the five patients who died without roentgen-ray therapy ranged from one to twenty-four months and averaged ten months.

In this clinic at the present time the usual procedure in treatment of carcinoma of the thyroid by roentgen-ray is as follows:

Employing 20 ma. at 200 kv. with target-skin distance of 50 cm. and filtration of 0.5 mm. of copper and 1 mm. of aluminum, doses of 400 r. are given to one field per day. Two fields are employed and each is given a total of approximately 2,800 r depending upon skin tolerance.

CONCLUSIONS

1. Malignant tumors of the thyroid gland are uncommon in general hospitals outside the goiter belt.

2. As determined upon physical examination, thyroid cancers are not always hard in consistency; some are firm and some are soft.

3. A single nodule in the thyroid gland should be excised because it may be malignant at the time it is first observed.

4. Microscopic observation of tumor cells in blood vessels is not necessary for the diagnosis of carcinoma of the thyroid gland and is not always a reliable criterion of malignancy.

5. Carcinoma of the thyroid so extensive as to preclude operation other than a biopsy should not be considered hopeless inasmuch as such a patient is herein reported alive and without recurrence eight years after diagnosis and x-ray therapy.

6. Recurrent malignant nodules in the thyroid region should be removed.

7. The clinical manifestations of hypothyroidism may be present in a patient with carcinoma of the thyroid gland.

The sections of the tumors of our surviving patients were reviewed by Dr. E. W. Goodpasture, Professor of Pathology, Vanderbilt University School of Medicine, and Dr. N. C. Foot, Professor of Surgical Pathology, Cornell Medical College. They confirmed the diagnosis of carcinoma in every instance herein reported.

REFERENCES

1. Coller, F. A.: Adenoma and Cancer of the Thyroid, J. A. M. A. **92**: 457, 1929.
2. Eisenberg, A. A., and Wallerstein, H.: Hürthle Cell Tumor, Arch. Path. **13**: 716, 1932.
3. Ewing, James: Neoplastic Diseases, ed. 3, Philadelphia, 1928, W. B. Saunders Company, p. 954.
4. Ewing, James: Neoplastic Diseases, ed. 4, Philadelphia, 1940, W. B. Saunders Company, (a) p. 522, (b) p. 982, and (c) p. 983.
5. Graham, Allen: Malignant Epithelial Tumors of the Thyroid, Surg., Gynec. & Obst. **39**: 781, 1924.
6. Graham, Allen: Discussions of New Growth, Tr. Am. A. Study Goiter, p. 206, 1938.
7. Dorland, W. A. N.: The American Illustrated Medical Dictionary, ed. 17, Philadelphia, 1936, W. B. Saunders Company, p. 48.
8. Foot, N. C.: Pathology in Surgery, Philadelphia, 1945, J. B. Lippincott Company, p. 329.
9. Haagensen, C. D.: Cancer of the Thyroid: Its Radio-Sensitivity, Am. J. Cancer **15**: 2063, 1931.
10. Harper's Latin Dictionary, New York, 1907, American Book Company, p. 100.
11. Herbst, W. P., Jr.: Malignant Tumors of the Thyroid, Ann. Surg. **79**: 488, 1924.
12. Horn, R. C., Jr., Welty, R. F., Brooks, F. P., Rhoads, J. E., and Pendergrass, E. P.: Carcinoma of the Thyroid, Ann. Surg. **126**: 140, 1947.
13. Hürthle, K.: Beiträge zur Kenntniss des Secretionsvorgangs in der Schilddrüse, Arch. f. d. ges. Physiol. **56**: 1, 1894.
14. Jaffe, R. H.: Epithelial Metaplasia of the Thyroid With Special Reference to the Histogenesis of Squamous Cell Carcinoma of the Thyroid (Abstract), Am. J. Path. **13**: 671, 1937.
15. King, W. L. M., and Pemberton, J. de J.: So-Called Lateral Aberrant Thyroid Tumors, Tr. Am. A. Study Goiter, p. 177, 1941.
16. Lahey, F. H., Hare, H. F., and Warren, S.: Carcinoma of the Thyroid, Ann. Surg. **112**: 977, 1940.
17. Langhans, T.: Ueber die epithelialen Formen der malignen Struma, Arch. f. Path. Anat. u. Physiol. **189**: 69, 1907.
18. Means, J. H.: The Thyroid and Its Diseases, Philadelphia, 1937, J. B. Lippincott Company, p. 483.
19. Pemberton, J. de J.: Malignant Lesions of the Thyroid Gland, Tr. Am. A. Study Goiter, p. 154, 1938.
20. Portmann, U. V.: Experiences in the Treatment of Malignant Tumors of the Thyroid Gland, Am. J. Roentgenol. **46**: 454, 1941.
21. Rosh, Rieva, and Raider, Louis: Radiation Therapy of Carcinoma of the Thyroid, Radiology **44**: 556, 1945.
22. Simpson, W. M.: A Clinical and Pathological Study of Fifty-Five Malignant Neoplasms of the Thyroid Gland, Ann. Clin. Med. **4**: 643, 1926.
23. Warren, Shields: The Significance of Invasion of Blood Vessels in Adenomas of the Thyroid Gland, Arch. Path. **11**: 255, 1931.
24. Weller, G. L., Jr.: Development of the Thyroid, Parathyroid and Thymus Glands in Man, Contributions to Embryology **24**: 95, 1933.
25. Wilensky, Abraham O., and Kaufman, Paul A.: Hürthle Cell Tumor of the Thyroid Gland, Surg., Gynec. & Obst. **66**: 1, 1938.

ILIAC LYMPHADENOPATHY AS A CAUSE OF URETERAL OBSTRUCTION

Victor F. Marshall, M.D., and Morris Schnittman, M.D., New York, N. Y.

(From the Department of Surgery [Urology] of Cornell University Medical College, The New York Hospital, and the Department of Urology of Memorial Hospital)

Current urologic textbooks and available literature upon the subject omit entirely, or merely mention, iliac lymphadenopathy in their discussions of the various etiologic factors which may cause ureteral obstruction. In considering diagnostically the patients with ureteral obstruction most of these authors accept enlarged lymph nodes as a cause only where they are large enough to be clinically palpable or to cause displacement of regional viscera. Recently, however, five patients have been studied in whom ureteral function was found compromised by only moderately enlarged iliac lymph nodes. In reviewing these cases critically the similarity of the clinical, laboratory, and pyelographic studies led us to conclude that this type of ureteral obstruction constitutes a definite diagnostic entity.

CASE HISTORIES

Case 1 (N.Y.H. No. 253117).—M. R., a 56-year-old man, was admitted to the hospital in 1942 complaining of pain in the right flank. The general physical and routine laboratory examinations revealed no abnormality. Although the left upper urinary tract appeared normal, a right hydronephrosis was shown on intravenous pyelography. Catheters could be introduced easily up the right ureter for 9 cm., but no farther. Using the Woodruff technique a retrograde pyeloureterogram (Fig. 1) demonstrated hydronephrosis and hydroureter down to the pelvic brim (the same level as the obstruction noted by catheterization from below), where an abrupt narrowing occurred. The ureter within the pelvis appeared normal. At exploration, the ureter was freed from a mass of matted lymph nodes, some of which were three-fourths the size of a hen's egg, located over the bifurcation of the common iliac artery. The pathologic examination of several of these nodes demonstrated Hodgkin's disease, which was not preoperatively suggested by any findings. Radiotherapy proved to be only mildly effective since the patient died fourteen months later of the generalized disease.

Case 2 (N.Y.H. No. 267639).—V. G., a 49-year-old man, was admitted to the hospital in 1942 complaining of pain in the right flank and fever. Two years previously a perineal resection of the rectum for cancer had been done, but the patient had been asymptomatic until five days before admission. General physical and laboratory examinations revealed no abnormality except evidences of sepsis and a tender right kidney. Studies of the left upper urinary tract were normal, but there was nonfunction on the right by intravenous pyelography. On catheterization of the right ureter an obstruction was met at 9 cm. although there was no difficulty to this point. Because of the acute septic condition a right nephrostomy was done followed by improvement. A pyeloureterogram (Fig. 2) made by injecting the nephrostomy tube as well as the ureter from below cystoscopically revealed hydronephrosis and a dilated ureter down to the pelvic brim where an abrupt stricture was evident. The lower ureter appeared normal. The degree of dilatation had undoubtedly decreased following the nephrostomy but these abnormalities were clearly evident on the films, which unfortunately were too light for good reproduction, therefore the outline has been traced in the illustration. At exploration the ureter was found so adherent to enlarged hard nodes over the iliac artery that a section of ureter had to be removed to overcome the obstruction. The ureteral defect was bridged with a vitallium tube. Pathologic examination revealed carcinomatous metastasis, probably of rectal origin, and direct invasion of the ureteral wall from the nodes. The vitallium tube was demonstrated to be patent one month later, but at autopsy eighteen months later further cancerous growth and precipitation of urinary salts inside the metal tube had again obstructed the ureter. Except for the history regarding the rectal operation two years previously, the actual cause of this ureteral obstruction was not suggested until exploration even though the common causes of ureteral obstruction seemed excluded.

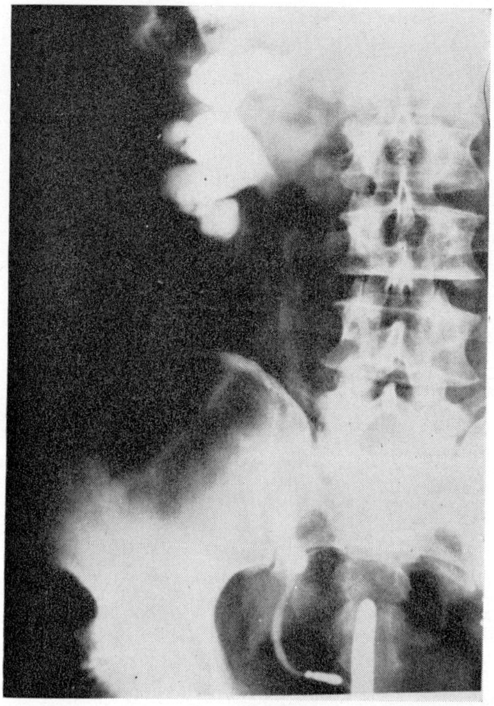

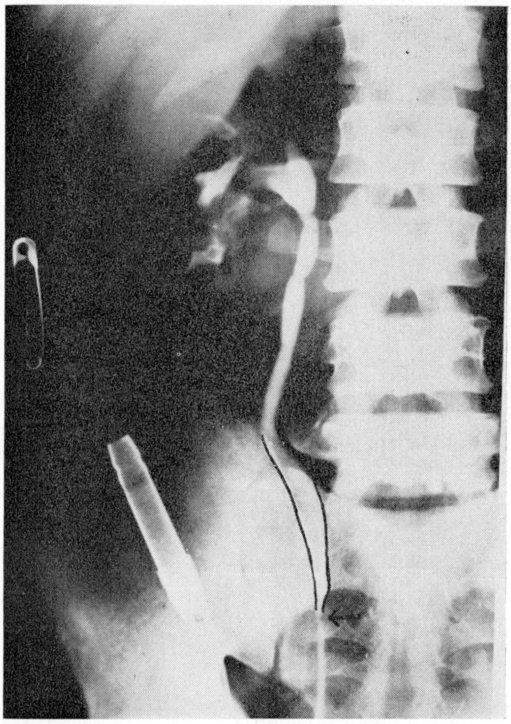

Fig. 1 (Case 1).—Woodruff pyeloureterogram demonstrating abrupt obstruction at the pelvic brim due to Hodgkin's disease.

Fig. 2 (Case 2).—Retouched pyeloureterogram showing abrupt obstruction at the pelvic brim due to iliac node metastases.

Case 3 (N. Y. H. No. 458051).—F. M., a 57-year-old man, was admitted to the hospital in 1946 complaining of pain and a persistently draining urinary fistula in the left flank. A resection of the sigmoid for carcinoma had been done two years previously. The patient remained asymptomatic until one month before admission when evidences of an acute perinephritic abscess led to incision and drainage at another hospital. The perinephritic abscess seemed related to ureteral obstruction but the urologic studies performed elsewhere failed to clarify the etiology more specifically. A barium enema showed no bowel lesion. After the patient's transfer, studies on the right upper urinary tract found it to be normal, but a left hydronephrosis with poor function was shown by intravenous pyelography. Here again, catheters met an obstruction 10 cm. from the ureteral orifice though there was no difficulty up to this level. With the Woodruff technique (Fig. 3) complete obstruction was demonstrated at the pelvic brim, but the lower ureter appeared normal. A diagnosis of ureteral obstruction due to metastatic carcinoma in the iliac nodes was made and was confirmed by exploration and biopsy. Nephrectomy was done for symptomatic relief. The characteristic findings regarding the obstruction permitted the preoperative diagnosis, though the patient would otherwise have been supposedly free of cancer.

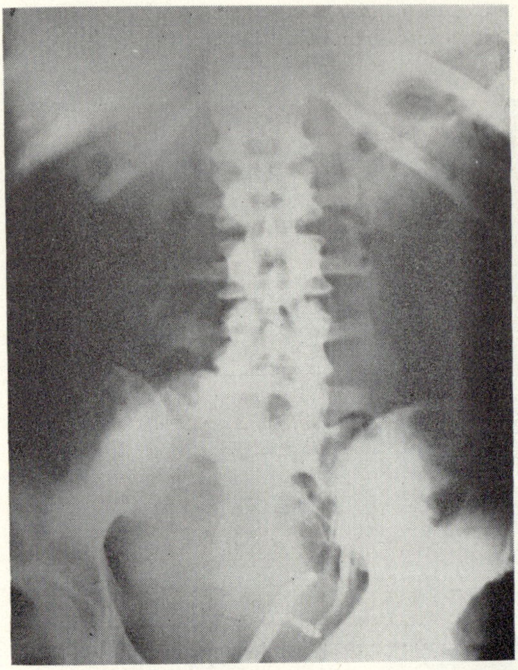

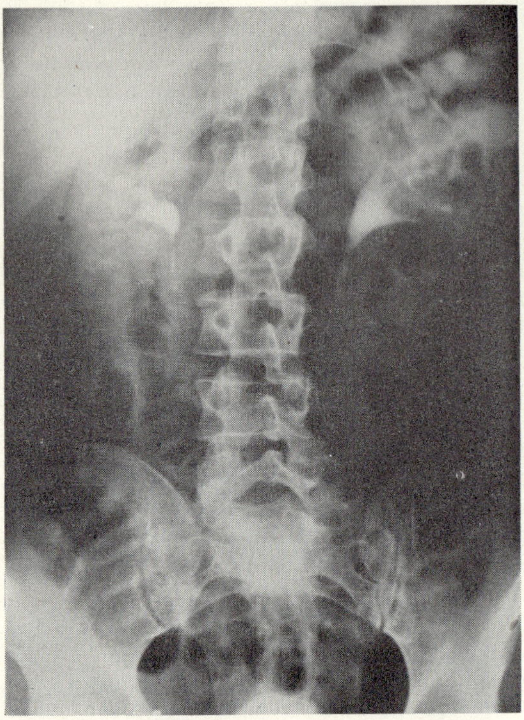

Fig. 3 (Case 3).—Ureterogram by Woodruff technique demonstrating a normal pelvic ureter obstructed at the pelvic brim by iliac lymph node metastases from carcinoma of the sigmoid.

Fig. 4 (Case 4).—Normal intravenous pyelogram eight months before onset of right flank pain.

Case 4 (M.H. No. 81751).—W. H.,* a 66-year-old man, was admitted in 1947 with a chief complaint of pain in the right flank. An abdominoperineal removal of the rectum for carcinoma had been done eight months previously, but frequently examinations thereafter had found the patient in apparently excellent condition. General physical and laboratory examinations revealed no abnormality except operative scars and the colostomy. Studies of the left upper urinary tract were normal but intravenous pyelography showed no function on the right. After much manipulation a number 4 French catheter was passed by an obstruction 9 cm. above the ureteral orifice, though various catheters could be easily introduced up to this level. The best pyeloureterogram, by the Woodruff technique (Fig. 6), revealed hydronephrosis and a dilated ureter down to the pelvic brim where there was an abrupt constriction and some angulation. The lower ureter appeared normal. A preoperative diagnosis of metastasis to the right iliac nodes was made even though there were no palpable masses or any other evidence of residual cancer. This was confirmed by exploration and removal of a ureteral segment along with the single, rather small node which was found. Pathologic examination revealed that the metastasis had directly invaded the ureteral wall from the node. An end-to-end anastomosis was done over a splinting number 6 French catheter which was removed on the twenty-second postoperative day. The patient has remained asymptomatic in regard to the right upper urinary tract, the urine became normal within one month,

*Seen with Dr. Gray Twombly.

Fig. 5.

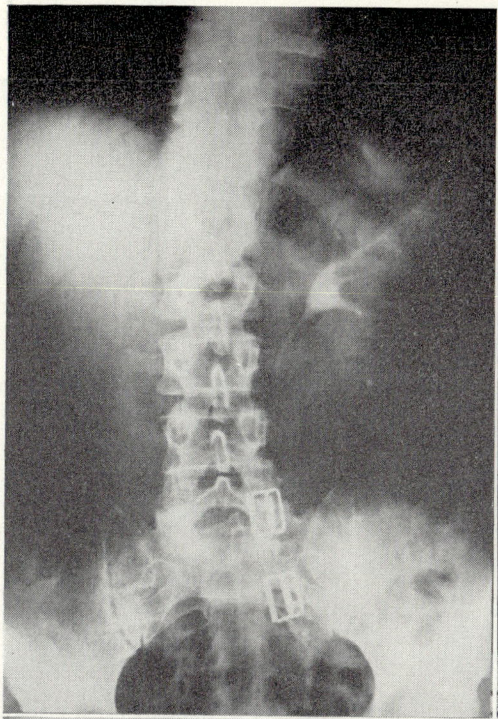

Fig. 6.

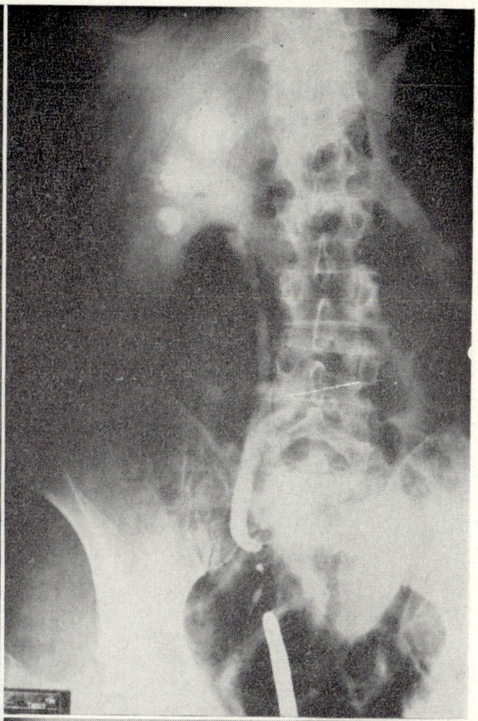

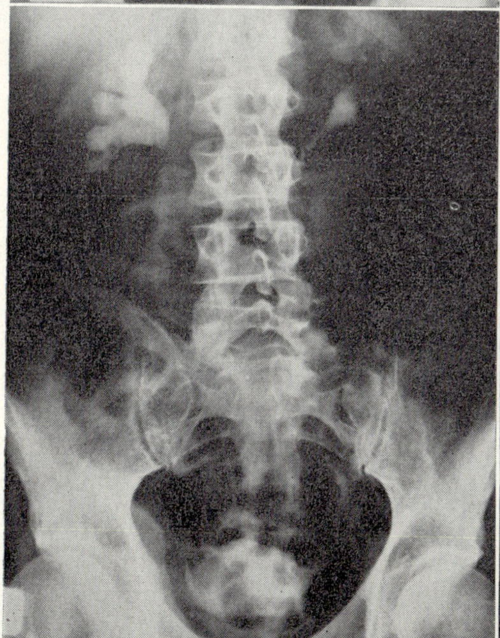

Fig. 7.

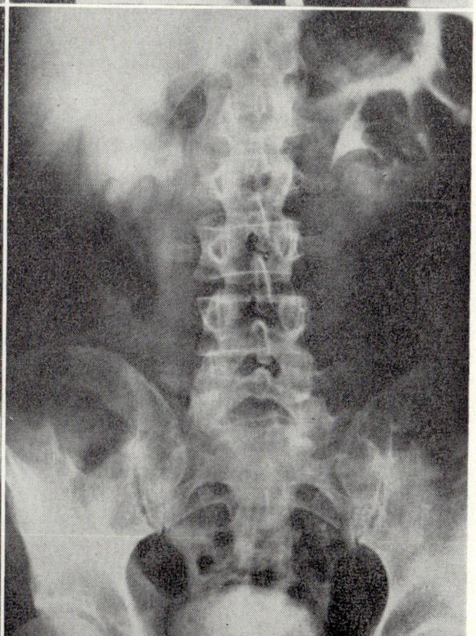

Fig. 8.

Fig. 5 (Case 4).—Intravenous pyelogram with nonfunction on the right, but an apparently normal kidney with good function on the left.

Fig. 6 (Case 4).—Woodruff pyeloureterogram revealing abrupt and limited obstruction at the pelvic brim due to iliac metastases from rectal carcinoma.

Fig. 7 (Case 4).—Intravenous pyelogram one month after ureteral resection; return of function is evident.

Fig. 8 (Case 4).—Intravenous pyelogram nearly two months after right ureteral resection; note normal left pyelogram.

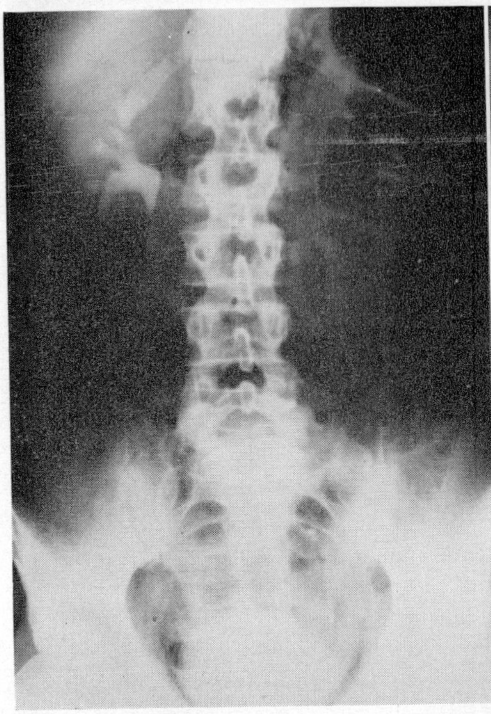

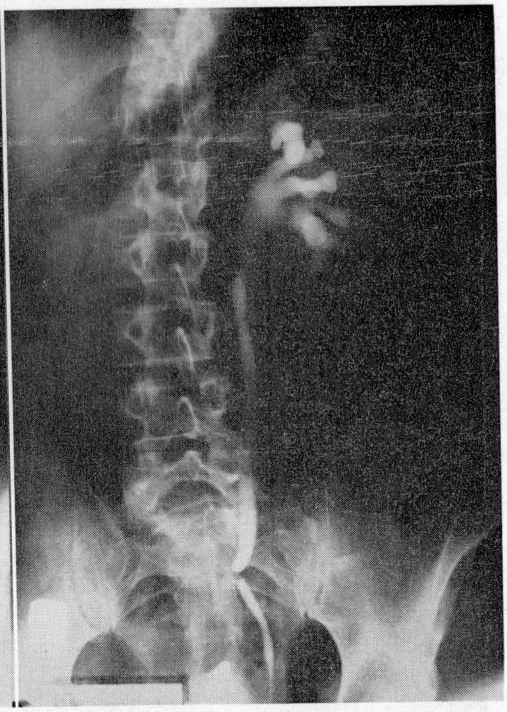

Fig. 9 (Case 4).—Intravenous pyelogram nearly four months after right ureteral resection, but demonstrating loss of function on the left.

Fig. 10 (Case 4).—Pyeloureterogram of the left side demonstrating limited area of obstruction at the pelvic brim due to metastases from rectal carcinoma.

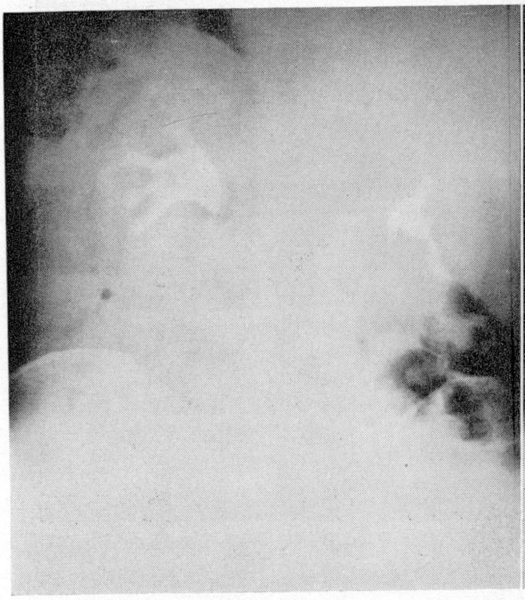

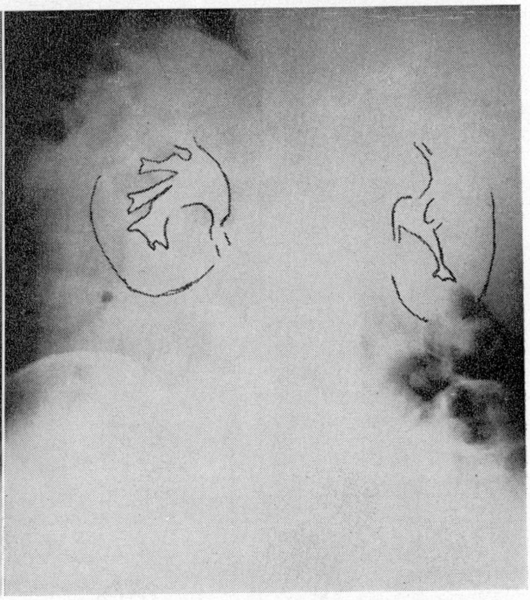

Fig. 11 (Case 4).—Intravenous pyelograms approximately five months after right ureteral resection and three weeks after left ureteral resection demonstrating bilateral function with only mild hydronephrosis.

Fig. 12 (Case 4).—Tracings of the pyelograms of Fig. 11.

and the hydronephrosis has almost disappeared (Figs. 9, 11, and 12). In fact, as will be evident later in this communication, this kidney has been able to maintain the patient satisfactorily through another operation in the absence of appreciable function of its mate. Here again, the patient was considered healthy except for recent ureteral obstruction. This obstruction was evidently not due to stone, primary ureteral neoplasm, traumatic stricture, or pregnancy, but was nearly identical to those in the preceding cases.

As if this were not enough, this patient returned three months later complaining of an exactly similar pain in the left flank of one day's duration. General physical and laboratory examinations were again of no aid in establishing the diagnosis, but the old pattern, consisting of flank pain, hydronephrosis and dilatation down to the pelvic brim, obstruction to ureteral catheters 9 cm. above the ureteral orifice, and an apparently normal lower ureter, was familiar. Almost needless to say, the diagnosis was made and confirmed. Resection of the ureter with end-to-end anastomosis was again carried out in the same manner. The final technical result could not be determined as death occurred two months later. The patient did have an episode of fever and pain in the left flank during the terminal stage of carcinomatosis. The first indication of spread of malignant disease was ureteral obstruction of the type described in the other cases.

Fortunately an intravenous pyelogram was made before the abdominoperineal operation and frequent pyelograms thereafter, so that the development, as well as the radiologic characteristics, of this case can be serially illustrated (Figs. 4 through 12).

DISCUSSION

Analysis of these cases revealed the following features common to all:

1. Flank pain without significant urinary symptoms was the presenting complaint.
2. A hydronephrotic or nonfunctioning kidney (by intravenous pyelography) was present upon the involved side.
3. The ureteral constriction was consistently present at the pelvic brim and was invariably located 9 to 10 cm. above the ureteral orifice.
4. The ureter below the point of constriction was normal.
5. The length of the constriction was never more than 3 mm., usually only 1 mm.
6. The cause of the constriction was proved in each instance to be neoplastic involvement of the iliac lymph nodes.

If these features, however, are to be accepted as diagnostic of iliac lymphadenopathy, the recognized causes of ureteral obstruction at the pelvic brim must be excluded. In general, a careful urologic survey can be relied upon to demonstrate a ureteral calculus or a primary ureteral neoplasm. A traumatic stricture should give signs and symptoms early following the injury. Pregnancy can be readily excluded. An iliac aneurysm should be recognized by its diagnostic calcification. Congenital valves, folds, and aberrant vessels causing marked obstruction are usually manifest at an early age and, rarely, at this particular level. Preoperatively the exclusion of idiopathic stricture was difficult. However, idiopathic strictures are rarely so sharply demarcated and are unlikely to present so consistently at this specific level. Furthermore, a common characteristic of this type of constriction is chronicity whereas the illness in each of the patients in this series was acute. In a reasonably complete review of the patients with tuberculous ureteritis seen in these clinics only one was discovered in whom the pyeloureterograms closely resemble those obtained in the patients in this series. In this case, however, the obstructing lesion at the pelvic brim involved several centimeters of ureter (Fig. 14).

As a result of the experience gained from these four cases, the diagnosis of ureteral obstruction due to carcinomatous metastasis in the iliac nodes was made without operation in the following case.

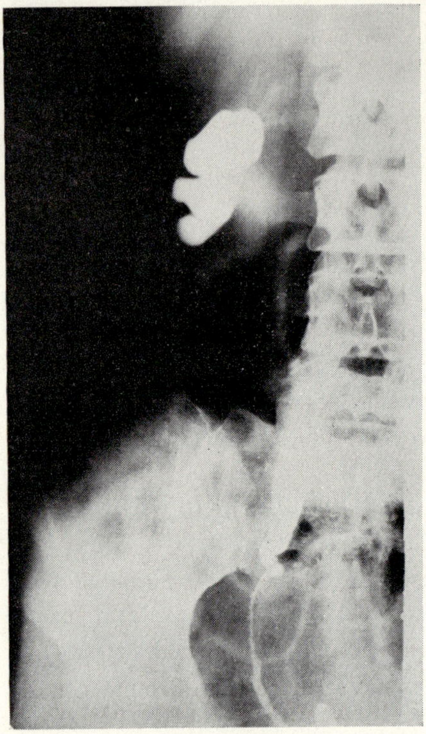

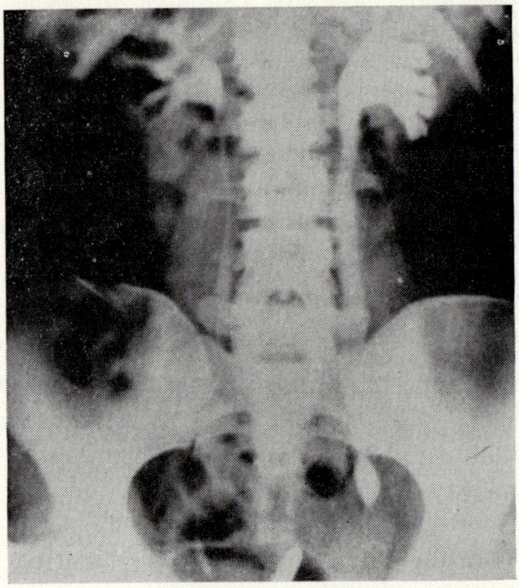

Fig. 13 (Case 5).—Pyeloureterogram showing obstruction at the pelvic brim, presumed to be due to metastases from carcinoma of cervix.

Fig. 14.—Pyeloureterogram of proved tuberculous ureteritis (left). This is similar to, but not typical of, ureteral obstruction due to iliac lymph node disease. In the first place the area of obstruction is 2 cm. below the pelvic brim and in the second place it is not sharply delimited but extends over a segment of several centimeters.

CASE REPORT

Case 5 (N.Y.H. No. 433351).—G. L.,* a 41-year-old woman, complained of pain in the right flank for six weeks. Cancer of the cervix had been treated by radiation with regression but not disappearance. The residual neoplasm seemed limited to the cervix and uterus on pelvic examination. General physical and laboratory examinations revealed no other abnormality. Studies of the left upper urinary tract were normal but a right hydronephrosis was shown by intravenous pyelograph. Ureteral catheterization met obstruction 9 cm. above the orifice though catheters were easily passed to this level. With the Woodruff technique a pyeloureterogram (Fig. 13) demonstrated hydronephrosis with a dilated ureter down to the pelvic brim where an abrupt constriction and angulation occurred. The lower ureter appeared normal. This obstruction was above the broad ligament, the pelvic ureter was normal, and there was no demonstrable extension of the cervical cancer beyond the uterus, so the obstruc-

*Seen with Dr. Norman Treves.

tion was considered due to metastases in the iliac nodes, especially as the diagnostic pattern was the same as in the previous cases. Subsequently, the right kidney became nonfunctioning by intravenous pyelography, but carcinomatosis soon appeared and the patient died. The first indication of carcinomatosis, however, was the ureteral obstruction from the iliac metastases. The subsequent course seemed to bear out the diagnosis of iliac metastases even though positive proof was lacking.

SUMMARY

Four cases have been presented in which an acute ureteral obstruction was proved to have been due to iliac lymphadenopathy. In a fifth case clinical evidence warranted the same diagnosis.

A diagnostic pattern has been described by which it is believed that this type of ureteral obstruction can be recognized even though the offending iliac nodes are not large enough to be palpated either on abdominal, pelvic, or rectal examination.

ARTERIAL AND VENOUS HYPERTENSIVE STATES BENEFITED BY SURGICAL INTERVENTION

JERE W. LORD, JR., M.D., NEW YORK, N. Y.

DURING the past ten years three surgical techniques have been developed which influence favorably a group of circulatory states exhibiting hypertension as their outstanding feature. Let us consider them in the order of the condition influenced most successfully by operative intervention.

In 1945 Crafoord and Nylin[1] and Gross and Hufnagel[2] reported independently the resection of the stenosed segment of the aorta with end-to-end anastomosis for relief of hypertension in the upper half of the body of patients suffering from coarctation of the aorta. Recently Gross[3] reported some twenty-three patients operated upon, with successful anastomosis accomplished in seventeen. Only two of the seventeen patients died. We* have operated upon three patients with coarctation of the aorta. Their case reports follow.

CASE REPORTS

CASE 1.—In a colored boy, 12 years of age, it was impossible to accomplish a resection of the stenotic area of the aorta because it arose immediately beyond the left common carotid artery. There was no left subclavian artery. The end of the left third intercostal artery was anastomosed to the side of the common carotid artery but the anastomotic opening was small and somewhat angulated. The postoperative angiocardiogram showed no evidence of function (Fig. 1). The patient showed no change one way or the other in the postoperaive follow-up of six months.

CASE 2. (K. 10255).—M. C., a 27-year-old white woman, was admitted to the New York Post-Graduate Hospital on April 21, 1947. She was referred by the physicians who made the diagnosis and advised surgical intervention. For two and one-half years the patient had known high blood pressure was present, and for several months prior to operation it had fluctuated between 270/110 and 330/160. The patient was completely asymptomatic. Preoperative angiocardiogram at the New York Hospital showed a proximal stump of aorta 1.0 cm. beyond the left subclavian artery (Fig. 2). Also the thickness of the left ventricle was 1.5 cm., 0.5 cm. beyond the normal limit. On April 26 the stenosed segment of aorta was resected and end-to-end anastomosis carried out with 00000 Deknatel silk (Fig. 3, *A*, *B*, and *C*). A lumen 8 mm. in diameter was fashioned. The postoperative convalescence was uneventful and the patient was discharged on the twenty-first day.

Fig. 4 is a chart of the patient's preoperative and postoperative blood pressure levels. It is of interest that a relatively normal blood pressure in the arms was attained only four months after operation. Preoperatively no pulsation could be felt in the abdominal aorta or in the feet although a blood pressure of 130/105 was obtainable with the stethoscope placed in the popliteal space. The postoperative blood pressure in the legs averaged 160/120 and good pulsations were present in the abdominal aorta and in the feet. Preoperatively oscillometric examination was 2.0 in the calf at 80 mm. of mercury, whereas on the eleventh postoperative day it was 2.5 and at six months it was 4.5 at 110. Teleroentgenograms showed a decrease in the transverse diameter of the heart of 1.5 cm. (Fig. 5, *A* and *B*). The patient became asymptomatic although it required three months for her to regain full strength.

*The three operations for coarctation of the aorta were carried out in conjunction with Dr. Louis R. Davidson.

CASE 3 (K11787).—F. P., a 24-year-old white married housewife, was admitted to New York Post-Graduate Hospital on June 16, 1947. She had known high blood pressure was present for four years. In February, 1947, the patient suffered a stroke from which she recovered in two weeks, leaving no residual weakness. On admission the blood pressure in the arms was 235/135 and 0/0 in the legs. Oscillometric examination in the left calf was 0.2/100. She was operated upon on June 21, 1947; the stenosed segment of aorta was resected and an end-to-end anastomosis carried out (Fig. 6, *A* and *B*). A lumen approximately 15 mm. in diameter was fashioned and the procedure was considerably easier than in Case 2 because there were 2.5 cm. of normal aorta proximal to the narrowed zone but distal to the left subclavian artery. There was a persistent tachycardia of 140 to 150 for the first five days postoperatively, but from then on the patient made an uneventful recovery.

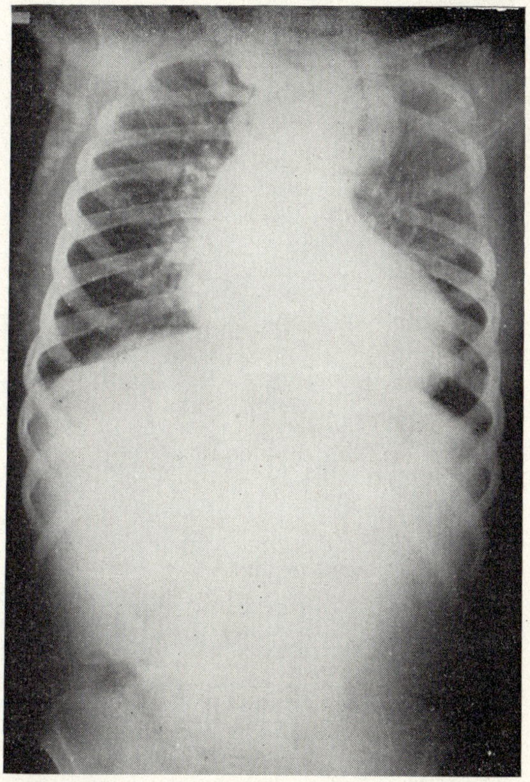

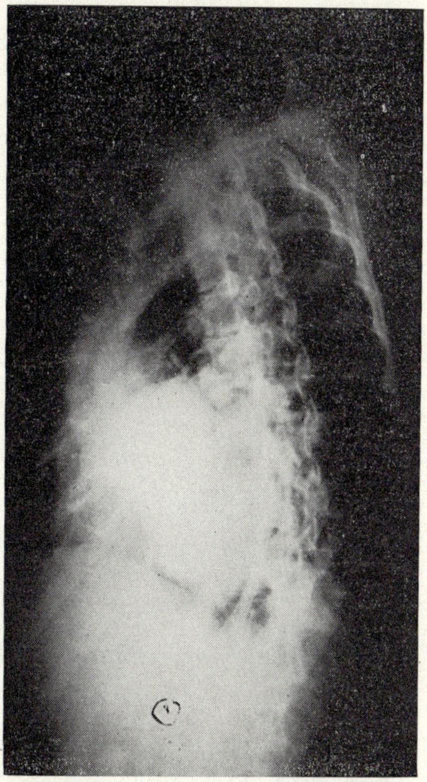

Fig. 1.—Postoperative angiocardiogram showing dilation of the left common carotid artery, absence of the left subclavian artery, and no evidence of function of the anastomosis.

Fig. 2.—Preoperative angiocardiogram showing the 1 cm. stump of the aorta distal to the left subclavian artery.

Fig. 7 is a chart of the pre- and postoperative blood pressures. The oscillometric examinations in the calf were 0.2/100 preoperatively, 3.5/110 at two months, and 6.0/100 at four months postoperatively. Pulsations in the legs absent preoperatively were normal after operation. This patient regained full strength one month after operation and has remained asymptomatic.

By way of comment the following facts seem established: (1) Reifenstein and his associates[4] analyzed 104 autopsied cases of coarctation of the aorta and found that, as a group, life was shortened (average age at death, 35 years) and complications related to the hypertension occurred in 76 per cent of the patients; (2) the operation described by Crafoord and Nylin[1] and by Gross has proved to be a long one, averaging in our hands six and one-half hours. The procedure has been well tolerated; (3) if the anastomosis is satisfactory the circulatory dynamics return to normal.

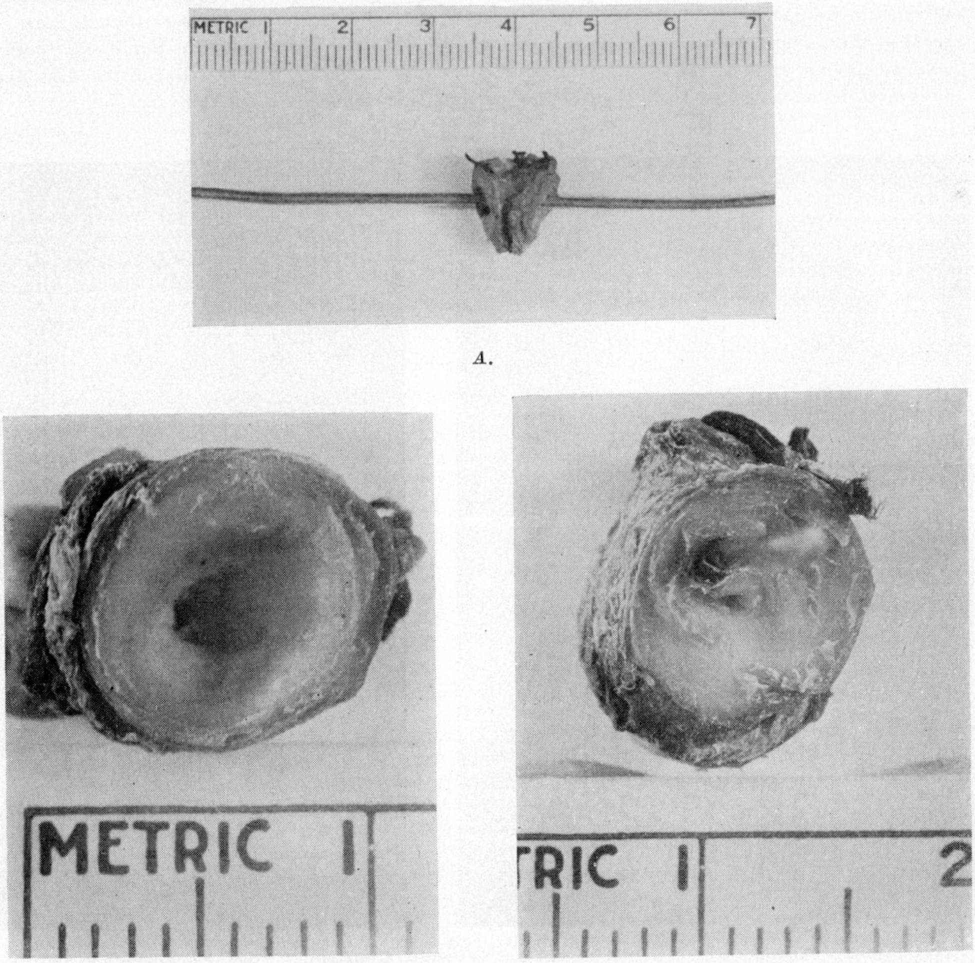

A. *B.* *C.*

Fig. 3.—*A*, Resected stenotic area of aorta capable of barely admitting a probe: *B*, view from one end; *C*, view from the other end.

The second hypertensive state favorably influenced by surgical intervention is essential and malignant arterial hypertension. Smithwick[5] is the surgeon most responsible for widespread interest in thoracolumbar sympathectomy for relief of this condition and his operation or some modification of it[6, 7, 8] is being utilized by many surgeons throughout the country. The results of my small personal series are quite similar to the larger series reported with Hinton.[9] Twenty patients have been operated upon and there have been three deaths. Two of these occurred postoperatively some four hours and three days from a coronary occlusion and cerebral thrombosis, respectively. Neither of these patients should have been operated upon as each one's hypertensive state was too far advanced to withstand the effects of operation. The first patient had experienced a coronary occlusion two years prior to operation and for one year had exhibited progressive cerebral damage evidenced by difficulty in thinking and thick, slowed speech. Autopsy revealed a fresh coronary occlusion and multiple areas of softening and scarring throughout the brain. The second patient suffered from malignant hypertension and was in congestive heart failure and mild uremia on admission. The eye grounds were 4 plus and the total count was 12 plus.

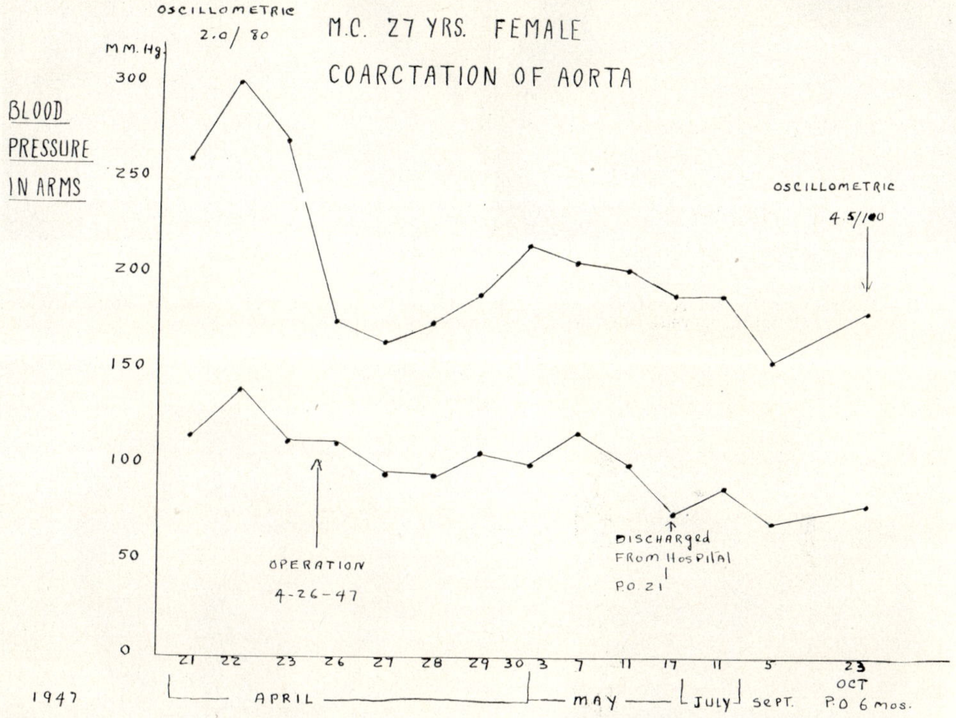

Fig. 4.—Chart showing blood pressures of one patient (Case 2) with coarctation of the aorta.

We[10] have recently reported on a set of rules which are based on an analysis of 375 patients subjected to thoracolumbar sympathectomy. The definitions and rules are shown in Tables I and II. If it were possible to apply them to the original group of patients the mortality (in hospital and for the first six months out of hospital) would have been reduced from 10 per cent to 2.5 per cent. Only twenty-five patients who withstood the operation and benefited would have been rejected. We firmly believe that the rules outlined are merely adjuncts to sound clinical judgment and are not intended to be a substitute for good judgment. Both of these hospital deaths would have been eliminated if the rules had been developed prior to their preoperative study and analysis. The third

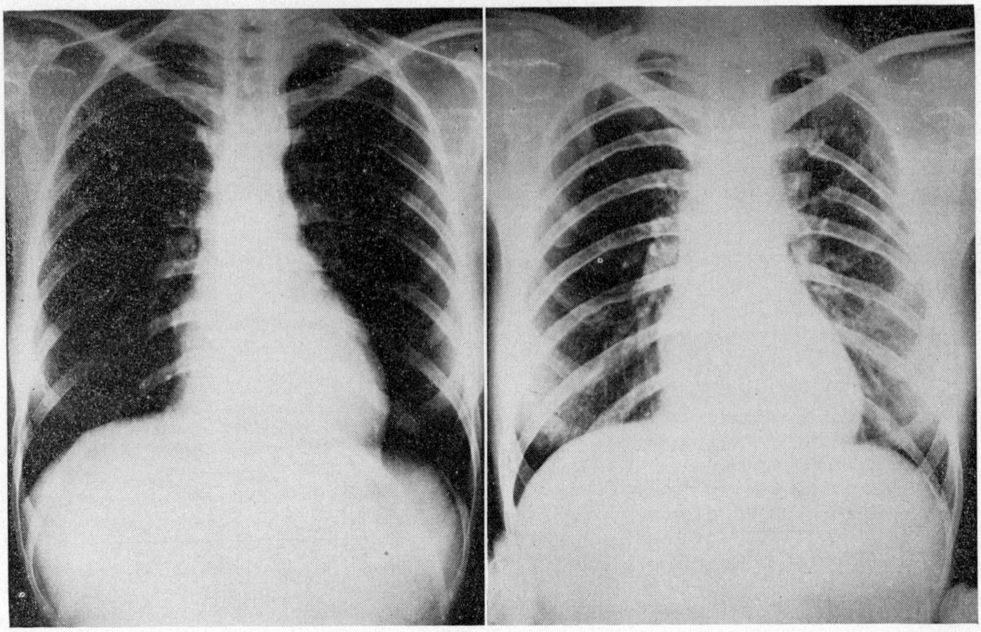

A. B.

Fig. 5.—*A*, Preoperative teleroentgenogram. *B*, Teleroentgenogram, five months postoperatively, showing decrease in transverse diameter of the heart by 1.5 cm.

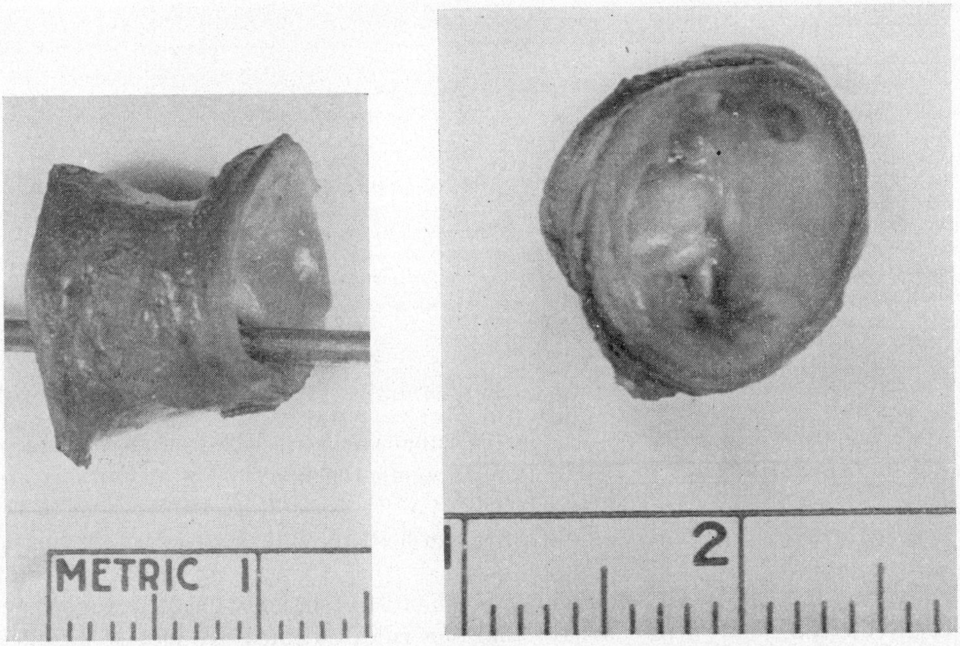

A. B.

Fig. 6.—*A*, Lateral view of resected stenotic area from Case 3. *B*, View from one end.

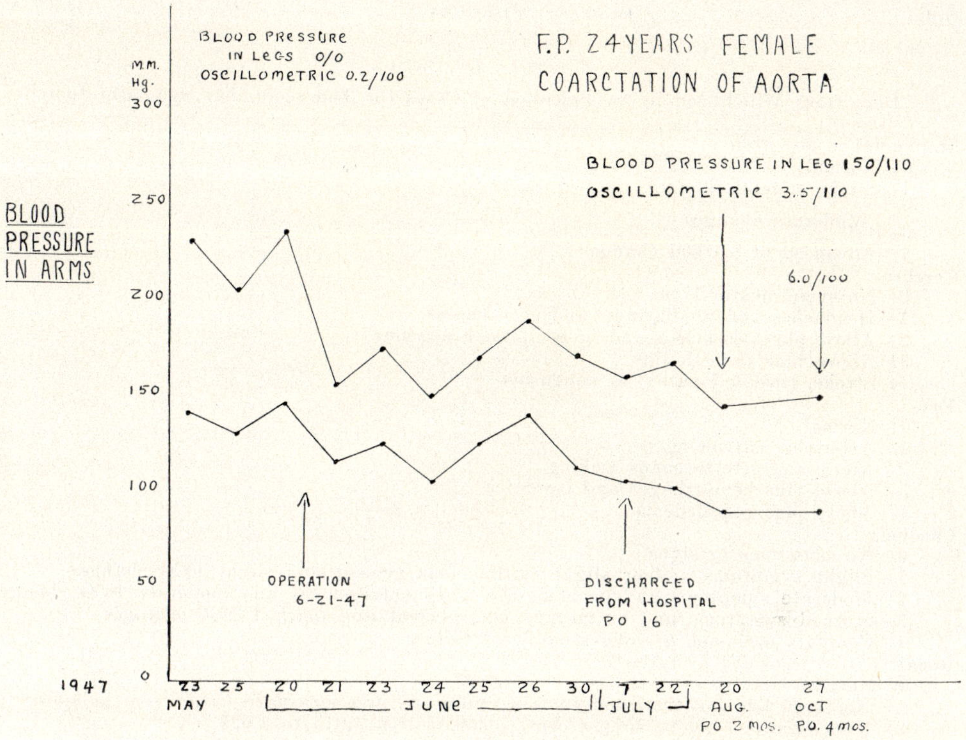

Fig. 7.—Chart showing blood pressures in coarctation of the aorta (Case 3).

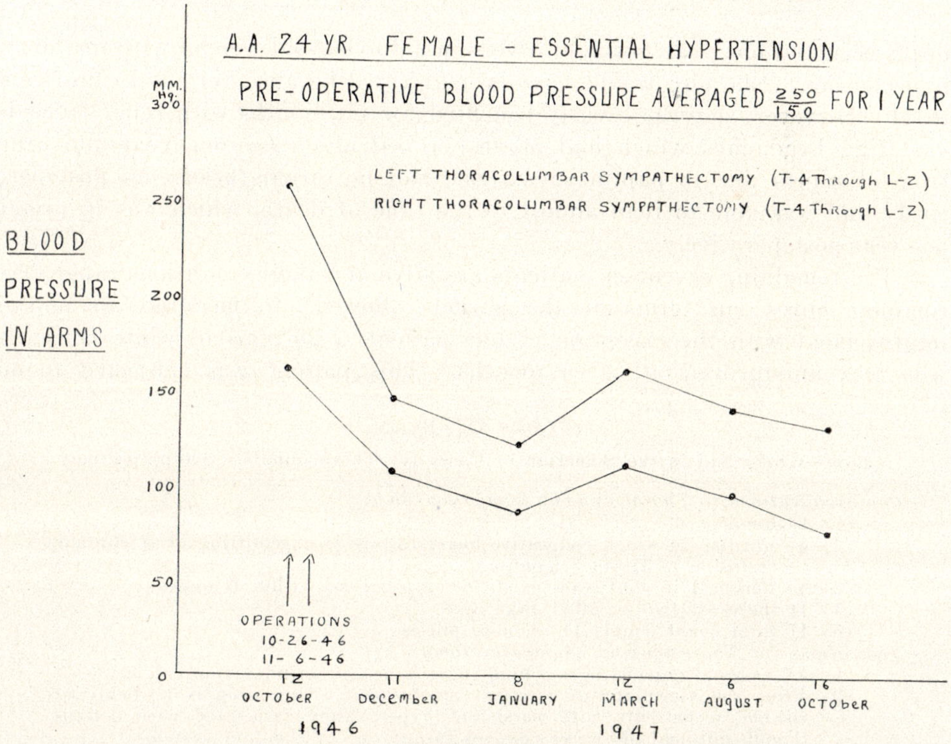

Fig. 8.—Chart showing blood pressures of patient with severe essential hypertension.

TABLE I. DEFINITIONS

Definitions Which Aid in the Selection of Cases for Thoracolumbar Sympathectomy

In general in any system:
- 0+ Normal
- 1+ Slight or mild changes
- 2+ / 3+ Moderate changes
- 4+ Advanced or marked changes

Cerebral:
- 0+ No symptoms or signs
- 1+ Headaches and/or dizziness and nervousness
- 2+ Above plus nosebleeds and/or occipital headaches
- 3+ Above plus paresthesias
- 4+ Stroke, encephalopathy, or confusion

Eyes:
- 0+ Normal
- 1+ Arteriolar narrowing
- 2+ Above and arteriovenous nicking
- 3+ Above plus hemorrhages and exudates
- 4+ Above plus papilledema

Cardiac:
- 0+ No symptoms or signs
- 1+ Slight symptoms and/or slight cardiac enlargement and slight ECG changes
- 2+ Moderate symptoms and/or moderate x-ray enlargement and moderate ECG changes
- 3+ Marked symptoms and/or marked enlargement and marked ECG changes
- 4+ Coronary occlusion or congestive heart failure

Renal:
- 0+ Normal
- 1+ Nocturia, but concentration 1.024 or more and urea clearance 75 per cent or more
- 2+ Urea clearance 40 to 75 per cent, concentration 1.015 to 1.023
- 3+ Urea clearance less than 40 per cent, concentrate less than 1.015, normal blood chemistry
- 4+ Persistent elevation of N.P.N. to 45 mg. or more and B.U.N. to 25 mg. or more.

death occurred one year postoperatively in a 43-year-old woman with malignant hypertension. She also would have been rejected because her total count came to 11. However, she was greatly benefited for six months with relief from devastating headaches which had made her bedridden for one year and relief from blindness due to papilledema. She had no serious headaches postoperatively and was able to read almost to the time of death, which was in uremia one year postoperatively.

The remaining seventeen patients are alive and their conditions range from complete cures (in terms of the period followed) to moderate or marked improvement with the exception of one patient, a 26-year-old white housewife who was unimproved at seven months. This patient was subjected to our

TABLE II. RULES

Rules Which Aid in the Selection of Cases for Thoracolumbar Sympathectomy

Contraindications to Thoracolumbar Sympathectomy:

(1) 4+ Renal
(2) 4+ Cardiac in which congestive heart failure is unremitting or if coronary occlusion is within 3 months
(3) 4+ Cerebral if confusion exists or if a stroke within 6 weeks
(4) If there are two 4+ other than eyes
(5) If total count equals 11 or more pluses

Indications for Thoracolumbar Sympathectomy:

(1) All cases are operable in which there is no contraindication rule
(2) From the viewpoint of minimal involvement: Operation is probably advisable in patients with persistent hypertension associated with definite though minimal objective changes in any one of the four systems

extensive sympathectomy but should be included in Group 4 blood pressure results; she felt unimproved subjectively. Table III shows the salient features of the twenty cases. Fig. 8 shows the blood pressure data of a 24-year-old white married college graduate. Presence of hypertension had been known for four years but for the year prior to sympathectomy it had averaged 250/150. The electrocardiogram showed marked left ventricular strain and the teleroentgenogram revealed the transverse diameter of the heart to be 1½ cm. over the

TABLE III

INITIALS	AGE (YR.)	SEX	PREPARATIVE EVALUATION	EXTENT OF OPERATION	BLOOD PRESSURE RESULT—SMITHWICK GROUP (MOST RECENT P.O. EXAM.)	DIASTOLIC BLOOD PRESSURE BELOW 100	OVER-ALL RESULT; IMPROVEMENT	SUBJECTIVE EVALUATION
M. L.	53	F	6+	T-9 to L-2 T-9 to L-2	1 (24 mo.)	Yes	Marked	Worth while
S. S.	45	F	5+	T-9 to L-2 T-9 to L-2	1 (15 mo.)	No	Moderate	Worth while
G. N.	35	F	12+ (malignant)	T-9 to L-2 T-9 to L-2	2 (24 mo.)	No	Marked	Worth while
R. H.	48	F	11+ (malignant)	T-9 to L-2 T-9 to L-2	4 (6 mo.)	No	Moderate (6 mo.) Dead 12 mo.)	Worth while Uremia
V. P.	51	F	8+	T-9 to L-2 T-9 to L-2	3 (24 mo.)	No	Moderate	Worth while
M. R.	45	F	5+	T-9 to L-2 T-9 to L-2	3 (24 mo.)	Yes	Moderate	Worth while
R. V.	33	F	8+	T-9 to L-2 T-9 to L-2	1 (24 mo.)	No	Marked	Worth while
M. K.	46	F	8+	T-6 to L-2 T-7 to L-2	3 (15 mo.)	No	Moderate	Worth while
R. J.	50	F	7+	T-5 to L-2 T-5 to L-2	4 (18 mo.)	No	Moderate	Worth while
M. F.	55	F	9+	T-7 to L-1 T-8 to L-2	2 (12 mo.)	Yes	Moderate	Worth while
S. G.	39	M	6+	T-6 to L-2 T-6 to L-2	1 (9 mo.)	Yes	Marked	Worth while
L. C.	43	F	12+ (malignant)	T-9 to L-2 T-9 to L-2			Dead P.O. 3 days	Cerebral accident
J. O.	34	M	8+	T-5 to L-2 T-6 to L-2	3 (12 mo.)	No	Moderate	Worth while
A. M.	26	F	7+	T-5 to L-2 T-4 to L-2	4 (7 mo.)	No	Unimproved	No benefit
G. S.	45	M	12+	T-6 to L-2			Died 4 hr. P.O.	Coronary occlusion
A. A.	24	F	8+	T-4 to L-2 T-4 to L-2	1 (12 mo.)	Yes	Marked	Worth while
J. T.	60	M	8+	T-10 to L-2 (1943, Sydenham Hosp.) T-3 to L-3	1 (9 mo.)	Yes	Moderate	No benefit
E. M.	39	F	4+	T-4 to L-3 T-4 to L-3	4 (6 mo.)	No	Moderate	Worth while
H. S.	48	M	9+	T-9 to L-2 T-8 to L-2	1 (2 mo.)	Yes	Markedly	Worth while
M. S.	42	F	5+	T-3 to L-3 T-3 to L-3	1 (9 mo.)	Yes	Marked	Worth while

upper limits of normal. The patient had a two-stage extensive thoracolumbar sympathectomy (from the fourth thoracic through the second lumbar ganglia inclusive) and was fully recovered in two months. She felt entirely well and had a normal blood pressure. The postoperative electrocardiogram and chest roentgenogram showed marked improvement.

It would seem that thoracolumbar sympathectomy is an operation which brings relief to many patients with hypertension. However, in the too far advanced cases it usually fails. The decision on whether or not it will ever effect so-called "permanent" cures must await the passage of another twenty years. We believe that the extensive sympathectomy (from the third or fourth thoracic through the second or third lumbar vertebrae) should be reserved for milder cases in the younger age group and the classical Smithwick sympathectomy (eighth or ninth thoracic through second or third lumbar ganglia) should be used in patients with more advanced stages of hypertension and in older patients.[11]

The third hypertensive state favorably influenced by surgical intervention is portal hypertension. This condition may be due to an intrahepatic block (cirrhosis of the liver) or to an extrahepatic block (Banti's syndrome) due to thrombosis of the portal vein or the splenic vein or to cavernomatous transformation of the portal vein. The two chief symptoms by which portal hypertension may be manifested are hemorrhage from esophageal varices and ascites. The latter is usually due to hypoalbuminemia but ascites which persists after prolonged liver therapy may be due to portal hypertension. The first successful operation for this condition was developed by Blakemore and his associates[12, 13] in 1943. Recently Blakemore[14] reported forty patients operated upon for portal hypertension with only five deaths. Linton[15] reported a series of fifteen cases with five deaths, all in patients suffering from cirrhosis of the liver. Linton had much greater success with patients of the Banti type. Follow-up in both series has shown a number of patients whose hemorrhages have ceased or have been greatly diminished in frequency and in volume. Also ascites has usually been eradicated postoperatively. Liver function on the other hand has not been significantly altered.

I have carried out anastomosis between the portal system and caval system in six patients. In three an anastomosis was made between the end of the portal vein and the side of the inferior vena cava by means of a vitallium tube. One of these patients died in the hospital on the eleventh postoperative day of an adynamic duodenal ileus due to a small infected retroduodenal hematoma. It is believed that if the anastomosis had been performed by end-to-side suture as advocated by Blalock,[16] John,[17] and Welch[18] that this patient would have survived. A severe hemorrhage occurred from a small branch of the inferior vena cava when the lower Blakemore-Crump clamp was being applied. This hemorrhage was difficult to control, led to temporary shock, and prolonged the operation one hour. In the suture method only the anterior part of the cava is obstructed and not nearly as wide a posterior dissection is necessary. At autopsy the anastomosis was patent. The patient had a typical portal cirrhosis. The second patient who died in the hospital was also suffering from portal cirrhosis and died from cholemia on the fourteenth postoperative day after getting along fairly well for ten days. Again failure may have been due to the extreme measures necessary to obtain a sufficient length of portal vein for the vitallium tube anastomosis.

The third patient was a 48-year-old white man who had portal cirrhosis and also a marked impairment of renal function bilaterally. The two-hour phenolsulfonphthalein test showed only 15 per cent excretion and the urea clearance was 45 per cent of normal. Intravenous pyelogram showed poor function bilaterally. The patient withstood the portacaval anastomosis by means of the vitallium tube very well and did not develop ascites after two paracenteses performed during the third and fourth postoperative weeks. He developed anasarca five months postoperatively and died eight months after operation in uremia. Autopsy showed the anastomosis between the end of the portal vein and the side of the inferior vena cava to be entirely patent.

Of the three patients* who had splenorenal anastomosis one improved greatly, one died five months postoperatively, and the third was in fair condition six weeks postoperatively. It is of great interest that in this small series of three cases, there were double renal veins in two of them. In the second case the two renal veins were so small (appoximately 5 mm. each in diameter) that an end-to-end anastomosis between the large splenic vein (15 mm.) was difficult and proved at autopsy to have thrombosed. This man had an obvious cirrhosis of the liver at operation but at autopsy five months postoperatively in addition to the cirrhosis the portal vein was found to be thrombosed. It was concluded that he represented a late stage of the Banti syndrome with a significant degree of cirrhosis of the liver.

In the two living patients with splenorenal conditions the operative diagnoses were portal cirrhosis although in the most recent one the preoperative diagnosis was Banti's syndrome. At operation the very high pressure of 540 mm. of water was measured in a branch of the left gastroepiploic vein and is therefore suggestive of a combined intra- and extrahepatic portal vein block.

From the experience gained in this small series of patients suffering from portal hypertension the following suggestions are made:

1. A splenorenal anastomosis is preferable to a portacaval anastomosis because it (a) is easier, (b) safer, (c) does not necessarily shunt all of the portal vein blood from the liver, and (d) eliminates the splenic artery which carries approximately 25 to 30 per cent of the blood which ordinarily must pass through the liver.

2. The anastomosis is best done by an end-to-side suture between the end of the splenic vein and the side of the left renal vein because: (a) Johns has shown this type of anastomosis remains open experimentally more frequently than the end-to-end suture and the end-to-end vitallium tube technique; (b) the left kidney is not sacrificed; (c) less length of vein is required when the suture method is employed than in the vitallium tube technique.

*I performed the complete operation in all but one of the six patients. In this one, the patient who had a splenorenal anastomosis and who died five months postoperatively, Dr. William F. Nickel carried out all of the procedure except for the anastomosis.

3. Results will improve and mortality will be lowered as the selection of cases is better delineated and as greater operative experience is gained.

SUMMARY

Three types of arterial and venous hypertensive states are now benefited to some degree by surgical intervention.

1. Coarctation of the aorta may be completely relieved by resection of the stenotic area and end-to-end anastomosis of the aorta.

2. Essential and malignant arterial hypertensive cases will to a significant degree be favorably altered by thoracolumbar sympathectomy.

3. Portal hypertension may be partially relieved with improvement in a fair percentage of cases by an anastomosis between the portal system and caval system of veins.

REFERENCES

1. Crafoord, C., and Nylin, J.: Congenital Coarctation of Aorta and Its Surgical Treatment, J. Thoracic Surg. **14**: 347-361, 1945.
2. Gross, R. E., and Hufnagel, C. A.: Coarctation of Aorta; Experimental Studies Regarding Its Surgical Correction, New England J. Med. **233**: 287, 1945.
3. Gross, R. E.: Personal communication.
4. Reifenstein, G. H., Levine, S. A., and Gross, R. E.: Coarctation of the Aorta, a Review of 104 Autopsied Cases of the "Adult Type," 2 Years of Age or Older, Am. Heart J. **33**: 146, 1947.
5. Smithwick, R. H.: A Technique for Splanchnic Resection for Hypertension, SURGERY **7**: 1-8, 1940.
6. Grimson, K. S.: Total Thoracic and Partial to Total Lumbar Sympathectomy and Celiac Ganglionectomy in Treatment of Hypertension, Ann. Surg. **114**: 753, 1941.
7. Hinton, J. W., and Lord, J. W., Jr.: Operative Technique of Thoracolumbar Sympathectomy, Surg., Gynec. & Obst. **83**: 643, 1946.
8. Poppen, J. L.: Extensive Combined Thoracolumbar Sympathectomy in Hypertension, Surg., Gynec. & Obst. **84**: 117, 1947.
9. Hinton, J. W., and Lord, J. W., Jr.: Thoracolumbar Sympathectomy in the Treatment of Advanced Essential Hypertension, New York State J. Med. **46**: 1223, 1946.
10. Hinton, J. W., and Lord, J. W., Jr.: The Selection of Patients for Thoracolumbar Sympathectomy, Description of a Set of Rules for the Elimination of Failures and Fatalities, Ann. Surg. (In press.)
11. Hinton, J. W., and Lord, J. W., Jr.: The Surgical Treatment of Essential Hypertension, A Comparison of the Results of the Classical Smithwick Operation and the Extensive Thoracolumbar Sympathectomy, S. Clin. North America. (In press.)
12. Blakemore, A. H., and Lord, J. W., Jr.: Technic of Using Vitallium Tubes in Establishing Portacaval Shunts for Portal Hypertension, Ann. Surg. **122**: 476, 1945.
13. Whipple, A. O.: Problem of Portal Hypertension in Relation to Hepatosplenopathies, Ann. Surg. **122**: 449, 1945.
14. Blakemore, A. H.: Paper read at the Forum on Fundamental Surgical Problems, American Colleges of Surgeons, Sept. 11, 1947.
15. Linton, R. R.: Paper read at the Forum on Fundamental Surgical Problems, American College of Surgeons, Sept. 11, 1947.
16. Blalock, A.: The Use of Shunt or By-pass Operation in the Treatment of Certain Circulatory Disorders, Including Portal Hypertension and Pulmonic Stenosis, Ann. Surg. **125**: 129, 1947.
17. Johns, T. N. P.: A Comparison of Suture and Nonsuture Methods for the Anastomosis of Veins, Surg., Gynec. & Obst. **84**: 939, 1947.
18. Welch, C. S.: A Technique for Portacaval Anastomosis (Eck Fistula), Surg., Gynec. Obst. **84**: 492, 1947.

THE RISK OF SURGERY IN HEART DISEASE

DONALD R. MORRISON, M.D., WEST HARTFORD, CONN.

(From the Department of Surgery of The New York Hospital and Cornell University Medical College)

THE problem of heart disease in surgical patients is one of ever-increasing interest and importance. Our population is becoming older as each decade passes and consequently the incidence of arteriosclerotic heart disease is on the increase. At the same time these older people become more susceptible to the various diseases requiring surgical treatment, such as cancer, prostatism, and the complications of peptic ulcer. In a similar fashion the improved treatment of rheumatic fever and syphilis has brought about a higher survival rate in these diseases, which again exposes increasing numbers of people to the necessity of surgical treatment in the presence of their already damaged hearts.

It seems pertinent then, to examine our experience with heart disease in the surgical patient with the idea of determining the operative risk in these cases and the various factors contributing to it.

This report is based on the detailed analysis of a group of 478 inpatients with heart disease who were subjected to 701 operations, comprising our total experience in this field during the ten-year period 1933 to 1943. Patients with minor procedures performed in the outpatient department were excluded from this study. No selection was exercised except that certain cases in which the diagnosis of heart disease was equivocal were excluded. Three etiologic types of heart disease are considered, namely rheumatic, arterio- sclerotic, and syphilitic, and each of these is further considered under its respective anatomic, physiologic, and functional aspects. The *Criteria for the Classification and Diagnosis of Heart Disease,* published by The New York Tuberculosis and Health Association (Heart Committee) and approved by the American Heart Association has been used as a basic guide.

The medical literature for the past twenty years does not abound with studies of this subject[1-31] and none of them has pursued a uniform set of standards for the diagnosis and classification of the cases of heart disease which they include. The difficulty of obtaining a large enough number of cases in any one series to be statistically significant is well known. The only hope of providing conclusions which approach the truth probably lies in combining the experience of several hospitals and this is a faint hope indeed if uniform standards are not adhered to. It is to be hoped that others interested in this subject may approve this set of standards and assemble their experience in a similar way, thus providing the very essence of statistical accuracy which is "numbers." No claim of statistical infallibility is made for many percentage figures in this study. The standard error of the difference is more than one-half the actual difference in most instances. It is hoped that the addition of more cases from this or other institutions will ultimately strengthen the significance of all these figures.

RHEUMATIC HEART DISEASE

The requirements for inclusion in the rheumatic heart disease group of cases are those recommended by the American Heart Association: (1) a history of any of the manifestations of rheumatic fever (polyarthritis, chorea, muscle or joint pains, subcutaneous nodules) and (2) evidence of a characteristic structural lesion of the heart (carditis, cardiac valvular disease, adherent pericardium).

There were 150 patients answering these requirements and they were subjected to 189 operations. There were 7 deaths in the immediate postoperative period, a mortality of 3.7 per cent.* In addition there were 7 cardiorespiratory complications, a rate of 3.7 per cent. These complications are potential mortalities and should be calculated as a definite part of the operative risk. For this reason the term "risk rate" has been used in this work and is simply the sum of the mortality and complication rates (Table I).

TABLE I. "RISK RATE" IN PATIENTS WITH HEART DISEASE

	RHEUMATIC	ARTERIO-SCLEROTIC	SYPHILITIC	TOTAL
Number of patients	150	311	17	478
Number of operations	189	485	27	701
Number of deaths	7	72	3	82
Mortality rate	3.7%	14.8%	11.1%	11.6%
Number of complications	7	21	3	31
Complication rate	3.7%	4.3%	11.1%	4.4%
Risk rate	7.4%	19.1%	22.2%	16%

A comparison of the mortality rates in certain groups of operations on patients with heart disease with our general mortality for the same type of case is of interest. In this series of patients with rheumatic heart disease there were 18 thyroidectomies for toxic goiter and 6 for nontoxic goiter. One death occurred (in a patient with nontoxic goiter) from atelectasis, a mortality rate of 4.2 per cent. Our general mortality for thyroidectomy is 1.4 per cent. There were 16 appendectomies for acute appendicitis, 16 for chronic appendicitis, and 1 appendectomy with drainage for acute appendicitis with perforation. Two deaths occurred in this group. One patient had chronic appendicitis and died suddenly of unknown cause. The other had acute appendicitis with perforation and died on the fifth postoperatice day of heart failure. This was a mortality of 6.1 per cent. Our general mortality is 0.9 per cent among all cases of appendicitis. Of the other common operations there were 10 cholecystectomies, 14 hernioplasties, and 15 operations for hemorrhoids and fistulas in ano, all without a death.

The thought has been repeatedly expressed that the heart that is able to carry out its function in everyday life will add no risk to any surgery which may be contemplated. In the rheumatic group this aphorism is true; for the mean functional classification (see Table II) was significantly higher in the mortality group than it was in the complicated and uncomplicated group. In

*The mortality and complication rates are uniformly calculated on the basis of the number of operations rather than the number of patients. Where a patient has undergone more than one operation it is considered that he submits to a new risk each time.

TABLE II. INFLUENCE OF CARDIAC FUNCTION, AGE AND OPERATING TIME ON THE SURGICAL "RISK RATE" IN PATIENTS WITH RHEUMATIC HEART DISEASE

	MEAN FUNCTIONAL CLASSIFICATION	MEAN AGE (YR.)	MEAN OPERATING TIME (MIN.)
No complications	1.4	30	70
Complications	2.1	39	93
Died	2.6	43	63

Mean Functional Classification

Class I. Patients with cardiac disease and *no limitation of physical activity;* ordinary physical activity does not cause discomfort

Class II. Patients with cardiac disease and *slight limitation of physical activity;* they are comfortable at rest but on ordinary physical exertion experience discomfort in the form of undue fatigue, palpitation, dyspnea, or anginal pain

Class III. Patients with cardiac disease and *marked limitation of physical activity;* they are comfortable at rest but the above symptoms are caused by less than ordinary activity

Class IV. Patients with cardiac disease who are *unable to carry on any physical activity without discomfort;* symptoms of cardiac insufficiency or of the anginal syndrome are present, even at rest

addition, 57 per cent of the mortality group were patients from Class III or Class IV, while only 6.3 per cent of the uncomplicated group were from Class III. There were no patients in Class IV who survived operation without complication. This is evidence of the importance of classifying this type of heart disease on a functional basis. As will be seen later, the mortality rate in other types of heart disease bears no such consistent relation to the functional classification.

Concerning age, reference to Table II will support the view that the older rheumatic patients present an increased risk for surgery. In the mortality and complication groups there were only two patients under 33 years of age. Those who died were all over 33 years.

It has been repeatedly said and written that rapidity in the performance of the surgical procedure is of the utmost importance in the treatment of surgical patients with heart disease. That any relationship exists between speed in operating and good results cannot be shown in this series (Table II). If anything, it would seem that one should be even more meticulous in dealing with cardiac patients. The anesthesiologist, who can administer high concentrations of oxygen and even breathe for the patient if necessary, is very well equipped to handle faltering hearts. That a rapid and easy convalescence is the important factor is borne out by the fact that the mortality of surgery on cardiac patients rarely occurs in the operating room. Sudden death, associated with surgery, is much more common among noncardiac patients than it is among those with a cardiac complication.

There were 19 patients (22 operations) with auricular fibrillation in the rheumatic group. Of these, 4 died and 4 had postoperative cardiorespiratory complications (Table III). From another aspect, auricular fibrillation was present in 57 per cent of the mortality group, in 57 per cent of the complication group, and in 8 per cent of the uncomplicated group. The increased risk of surgery in patients with fibrillating rheumatic hearts is obvious and the inference of delaying elective surgery and attempting to restore a normal sinus rhythm is equally clear.

Cardiac enlargement was present in 75 patients who were subjected to 108 operations. There were 7 deaths, a rate of 6.5 per cent, and 6 complications, a rate of 5.6 per cent (Table III). From another point of view, cardiac enlargement was present in 100 per cent of the mortality group, in 86 per cent of the group with complications, and in only 54 per cent of uncomplicated cases. These data suggest that an enlarged heart may increase the risk of surgery in rheumatic heart disease, although it is not as striking a factor as auricular fibrillation.

Mitral stenosis was diagnosed in 108 patients who underwent 147 operations. There were 7 deaths and 6 complications, rates of 4.8 per cent and 4.1 per cent, respectively (Table III). Mitral stenosis was present in 100 per cent of the mortality group, in 86 per cent of the complication group, and in 71 per cent of the uncomplicated group. Here again is a factor which appears to increase the operative risk, albeit to a lesser extent than those previously recorded.

The combined presence of auricular fibrillation, enlarged heart, and mitral stenosis produces a risk rate which is not the sum of the rates for each factor but rather a reflection of the rate of the most important one, that is auricular fibrillation. The same thing can be said for the combination of enlarged heart and mitral stenosis (Table III).

Concerning the combined presence of aortic and mitral lesions, there seems to be no significant increase in the risk rate. There were 35 such cases (41 operations) with 2 deaths and 1 complication for rates of 4.9 per cent and 2.4 per cent, respectively (Table III).

TABLE III. INFLUENCE OF VARIOUS FACTORS ON THE RISK OF SURGERY IN PATIENTS WITH RHEUMATIC HEART DISEASE

	(1) AURICULAR FIBRILLATION	(2) CARDIAC ENLARGEMENT	(3) MITRAL STENOSIS	(4) COMBINATION OF 1, 2 & 3	(5) COMBINATION OF 2 & 3	(6) AORTIC PLUS MITRAL LESION
Number of operations	22	108	147	20	98	41
Number of deaths	4	7	7	4	7	2
Mortality rate	18.1%	6.5%	4.8%	20%	7.1%	4.9%
Number of complications	4	6	6	4	5	1
Complication rate	18.1%	5.6%	4.1%	20%	5.1%	2.4%
Risk rate	36.2%	12.1%	8.9%	40%	12.2%	7.3%

To summarize, the risk of surgery appears to be enhanced in rheumatic patients by auricular fibrillation, cardiac enlargement, mitral stenosis, age, and a high functional classification. No relationship to risk could be demonstrated for operating time or the combined presence of aortic and mitral lesions.

ARTERIOSCLEROTIC HEART DISEASE

For inclusion in this group of cases it has been required that the patient present signs or symptoms of cardiac abnormality (for example, enlarged heart, previous episode of failure, previous coronary occlusion, anginal attacks, abnormal dyspnea, orthopnea, etc.) without a history of rheumatic fever, syphilis, or thyroid disease, and supported by at least one characteristic clinical finding (for example cardiac enlargement shown by x-ray examination, electrocardiographic changes, or congestive heart failure. Post-mortem evidence of coronary sclerosis, definite electrocardiographic findings (for example, inverted T waves, diphasic T waves, or auricular fibrillation or flutter and heart block in the absence of other etiologic possibilities) have been accepted as proof of the disease without requiring any symptoms. People with symptoms of heart disease and no other more specific findings of cardiac arteriosclerosis were not included.

Three hundred eleven patients were found to answer these requirements and they were subjected to 485 operations. There were 72 deaths and 21 postoperative cardiorespiratory complications for rates of 14.8 per cent and 4.3 per cent, respectively (Table I). Of these arteriosclerotic patients, 19 per cent failed to survive operation without complication.

TABLE IV. COMPARISON OF GENERAL MORTALITY RATES WITH MORTALITY RATES IN ARTERIOSCLEROTIC HEART DISEASE

OPERATION	GENERAL MORTALITY RATE		ARTERIOSCLEROTIC MORTALITY RATE	
	PER CENT	NUMBER OF OPERATIONS	PER CENT	NUMBER OF OPERATIONS
Thyroidectomy	1.4	1650	8	25
Biliary	2.6	1931	8.3	24
Hernioplasty	0.57	2615	3.1	32
Amputation	6.7	313	30	20
Incision and drainage of abscess	2	1290	13.6	22
Excision of carbuncle	6	167	50	6
Colostomy	15	348	20	15
Transurethral prostatectomy	3.9 (7.5%)	412	10 (19%)	50
Suprapubic prostatectomy	8.1 (7.5%)	272	39 (19%)	23
Perineal prostatectomy	1.5 (7.5%)	68	11.8 (19%)	17
Suprapubic cystostomy	32 (7.5%)	71	23 (19%)	35

In Table IV the mortality rates in arteriosclerotic heart disease are compared with our general mortality rate for the same type of operation. The rather high mortality rates in the common operations for prostatism are worthy of note.

A comparison of Table V with Table II will show two interesting differences between patients with arteriosclerotic heart disease and those with rheumatic heart disease. In the first place the arteriosclerotic heart may be doing its everyday work quite well only to fail under the stresses of surgery, while the rheumatic heart producing few or no symptoms adds no risk under these circumstances. In the second place older arteriosclerotic patients do not appear

TABLE V. INFLUENCE OF CARDIAC FUNCTION, AGE, AND OPERATING TIME ON THE SURGICAL "RISK RATE" IN ARTERIOSCLEROTIC HEART DISEASE

	MEAN FUNCTIONAL CLASSIFICATION	MEAN AGE (YR.)	MEAN OPERATING TIME (MIN.)
Uncomplicated	1.8	63	80
Complicated	1.6	59	75
Died	1.9	65	71

to present any increased risk for surgery, whereas patients with rheumatic heart disease in the older age groups are definitely poorer risks. Table V shows only one similarity to Table II, that is, no relationship between operating time and the results of surgery could be demonstrated.

Among the arteriosclerotic group there were 62 patients with auricular fibrillation, 6 with auricular flutter, and 1 with nodal rhythm. These patients presented the highest mortality and complication rates, as shown in Table VI.

TABLE VI. INFLUENCE OF VARIOUS FACTORS ON THE RISK OF SURGERY IN PATIENTS WITH ARTERIOSCLEROTIC HEART DISEASE

	ABNORMAL RHYTHM	CARDIAC ENLARGEMENT	HEART BLOCK	PREVIOUS CORONARY OCCLUSION	HISTORY OF ANGINA
Number of operations	87	315	105	37	58
Number of deaths	16	40	13	3	5
Mortality rate	18.4%	12.7%	12.4%	8.1%	8.6%
Number of complications	9	11	8	1	1
Complication rate	10.4%	3.5%	7.6%	2.7%	1.7%
Risk rate	28.8%	16.2%	20%	10.8%	10.3%

Cardiac enlargement was present in 196 patients who had 315 operations. The majority of these patients had this diagnosis confirmed by x-ray examination. The mortality and complication rates are shown in Table VI.

There were 65 patients with heart block in this series of arteriosclerotic heart disease and they included the following varieties: left bundle branch block (discordant) 6; left bundle branch block (concordant), 6; right ventricular block, 21; Intraventricular block, 11; left intraventricular block, 2; bundle branch block (wide S wave), 3; incomplete block (P-R/0.28 – 0.39), 2; bundle branch block, 1; 2:1 block, 1; prolonged P–R interval, 10; prolonged Q–R–S (.11), 1.

The mortality and complication rates are shown in Table VI.

Definite historical or post-mortem evidence of a previous coronary occlusion was obtained in 25 patients who were subjected to 37 operations. Three deaths occurred in this group, a rate of 8.1 per cent. One patient died of a second coronary occlusion, one of heart failure and pneumonia, and one after a prolonged period of fever and tachycardia without adequate explanation. The single complication was a coronary occlusion which the patient survived (Table VI).

A history of angina of effort was elicited in 41 patients who underwent 58 operations. There were 5 mortalities, a rate of 8.6 per cent. One patient had an episode of heart failure after the first operation and finally died of uremia after a second operation. Heart failure and pulmonary infarction accounted for the death of 2 patients, and 2 others had fresh coronary occlusions, confirmed at autopsy. The single patient with a complication in this group suffered a pulmonary infarction.

If elevation of the blood pressure was a factor increasing the risk of surgery one would expect that hypertension would be present to a greater degree in the mortality and complication groups than in the uncomplicated group. That it is not a factor can be seen from Table VII. The percentage of patients in which hypertension was recorded is about the same in the three groups.*

TABLE VII. INFLUENCE OF HYPERTENSION ON THE RISK OF SURGERY IN PATIENTS WITH ARTERIOSCLEROTIC HEART DISEASE

BLOOD PRESSURE	DEATHS		COMPLICATIONS		UNCOMPLICATED CASES	
	PERCENTAGE	NUMBER OF CASES	PERCENTAGE	NUMBER OF CASES	PERCENTAGE	NUMBER OF CASES
150/ 90	48.5	35/72	57.2	12/21	57.7	126/218
200/100	13.9	10/72	4.8	1/21	12.4	27/218

In an effort to find some danger line of renal function for patients with arteriosclerotic heart disease, various combinations of the blood urea nitrogen, phenolsulfonphthalein and albumin excretion rates were tested against these 311 patients. The combination showing the greatest difference between the mortality group and the uncomplicated cases was a blood urea nitrogen of 20 or more, or a phenolsulfonphthalein of 50 or less, or, albuminuria of 2+ or more. This criterion of renal function was answered by 45 per cent of the deaths, 26 per cent of the complications, and only 11 per cent of the uncomplicated cases. Stated in another way, 41 per cent of the deaths and complications had one or more of these evidences of poor renal function as against 11 per cent for the uncomplicated group.

In summary, patients with arteriosclerotic heart disease show a mortality rate four times that of rheumatic heart disease. In this disease, the heart which is doing a satisfactory day-to-day job cannot be depended upon to withstand surgery. Abnormalities of rhythm and poor kidney function appear to enhance the surgical risk. No definitely increased risk could be demonstrated for patients with cardiac enlargement, heart block, previous coronary occlusion, angina pectoris, or hypertension. No relationship could be established between the risk of surgery and the patient's age or the time consumed in performing the surgical procedure.

SYPHILITIC HEART DISEASE

Our experience in the surgical treatment of patients with syphilitic heart disease has been very limited. There were 17 patients who had 27 operations. All of these except 2 had a 4 plus Wassermann reaction and a widened aorta confirmed by x-ray examination. Of these 2 one had a 4 plus Wassermann reaction, but no roentgenogram was taken. However, syphilitic aortitis was proved at post-mortem examination. The other had a negative Wassermann reaction, but did have a wide aorta on x-ray examination plus tabes dorsalis and a neurogenic bladder. Nearly all of the patients in this group had other signs of syphilitic heart disease.

There were 3 deaths and 3 cardiorespiratory complications for identical mortality and complication rates of 11.1 per cent.

*During the period covered by this study 165 operations were performed for the relief of essential hypertension with 5 deaths, for a mortality rate of 3 per cent.

The mean functional classification for the uncomplicated group was 1.4, for the group with complications 2.0, and for those who died 1.3. In the same order the mean age in years was 60, 61, and 60, and the mean operating time in minutes 56, 70, and 72 (Table VIII).

There were 5 patients with angina, 1 of whom died and 2 of whom had postoperative complications.

TABLE VIII. INFLUENCE OF CARDIAC FUNCTION, AGE, AND OPERATING TIME ON THE SURGICAL "RISK RATE" IN SYPHILITIC HEART DISEASE

	MEAN FUNCTIONAL CLASSIFICATION	MEAN AGE (YR.)	MEAN OPERATING TIME (MIN.)
Uncomplicated	1.4	60	56
Complicated	2.0	61	70
Died	1.3	60	72

There were 3 cases of heart block with 2 complications.

There were 2 patients with combined heart block and angina and they both went into congestive heart failure during the postoperative period but survived.

There were no sudden deaths during any of the 27 operative procedures.

Seven of the 14 survivors were dead within two years.

The mortality and complication rates which we experienced in this series for various anesthetic agents are detailed in Table IX. The only two sets of figures which are of statistical significance, as determined by calculation of the standard error, are the rates for local and spinal anesthesia. This significance is probably vitiated by the weighting of the local anesthesia group with operations of relatively minor severity. A comparison of spinal with all types of inhalation anesthesia barely misses falling into numerical significance and in this group the weighting of prolonged and serious operations would be in the reverse direction.

It is probably safe to say that local anesthesia should be used when feasible and that spinal should be avoided if possible. It should be emphasized, however,

TABLE IX. ANESTHESIA—INFLUENCE OF CHOICE OF ANESTHESIA ON THE RISK OF SURGERY IN RHEUMATIC, ARTERIOSCLEROTIC, AND SYPHILITIC HEART DISEASE

	OPERATIONS		DEATHS		COMPLICATIONS		RISK RATE
	NUMBER	PER CENT	NUMBER	PER CENT	NUMBER	PER CENT	
Local	277	39.6	26	8.9	9	3.2	12.1
Spinal	150	21.4	26	17.3	7	4.7	22.0
Caudal	21	3.0	1	4.8	0	0	4.8
Open ether	99	14.1	14	14.2	3	3.2	17.4
Nitrous oxide oxygen and ether	58	8.3	6	10.3	1	1.7	12.0
Cyclopropane	32	4.6	1	3.1	5	15.6	18.7
Ethylene	9	1.2	2	22.2	0	0	22.2
Ethylene and ether	14	2.0	0	0	1	7.1	7.1
Nitrous oxide and oxygen	10	1.4	3	30.0	1	10.0	40.0
Local plus general	10	1.4	3	30.0	1	10.0	40.0
Avertin	14	2.0	0	0	3	21.4	21.4
Rectal ether	7	1.0	0	0	0	0	0
All inhalation anesthesias	232	33.1	29	12.5	12	5.2	17.7

that the reported differences, even if significant, are small. No evidence has been found in this series to refute the general rule that the choice of the anesthetist is more important than the choice of the anesthetic agent.

Table X presents the causes of deaths and the type of complications. In 45 per cent of the 82 deaths in this study there were post-mortem examinations.

TABLE X. CAUSES OF DEATHS AND NATURE OF COMPLICATIONS AMONG 478 PATIENTS WITH HEART DISEASE WHO UNDERWENT 701 OPERATIONS

	RHEUMATIC HEART DISEASE	ARTERIOSCLEROTIC HEART DISEASE	SYPHILITIC HEART DISEASE
	Deaths		
Atelectasis	1		
Mycotic brain abscess	1		
Pneumonia	2	14	1
Unknown	1	4	
Heart failure	1	23	
Arterial embolus	1	1	
Brain contusion		1	
Pulmonary embolus		5	
Cerebral hemorrhage		2	
Vascular collapse		4	
Peritonitis		3	
Dissecting aneurysm		2	
Coronary occlusion		9	
Liver necrosis		1	
Carcinomatosis		1	
Agranulocytosis		1	
Thyroid crisis		1	
Mesenteric thrombosis			1
Cirrhosis			1
	Complications		
Heart failure	5	6	2
Pneumonia		2	1
Coronary occlusion		5	
Auricular tachycardia		1	
Pulmonary embolus	1	3	
Vascular collapse		1	
Auricular fibrillation		3	
Arterial embolus	1		

CONCLUSIONS

1. The risk of surgery in rheumatic heart disease is not great. What risks there are seem to center in certain types of patients with rheumatic heart disease, namely, those over 33 years of age, those with fibrillation, and those with a high functional classification.

2. The risk of surgery in arteriosclerotic heart disease is considerably greater and seems to be centered in the etiologic diagnosis. It does not appear to be significantly modified by the various anatomic, physiologic, or functional factors except that disorders of cardiac rhythm and poor renal function produced higher "risk rates" in our experience.

3. The risk of surgery in syphilitic heart disease cannot be accurately determined in the small number of cases available. However, the evidence suggests that the risk is less than in arteriosclerotic heart disease but greater than in rheumatic heart disease. The presence of angina and/or heart block adds to the risk of surgery in patients with syphilitic heart disease.

4. No single anesthetic agent is definitely superior for patients with heart disease. However, it seems that local anesthesia should be used if feasible and spinal anesthesia avoided if possible.

REFERENCES

1. Boas, E. P.: Operation and the Cardiac Patient, J. Mt. Sinai Hosp. **4**: 275-278, 1937.
2. Brumm, H. J., and Willius, F. A.: The Surgical Risk in Patients With Coronary Disease, J. A. M. A. **112**: 2377-2380, 1939.
3. Butler, S., Feeney, N., and Levine, S. A.: The Patient With Heart Disease as a Surgical Risk, J. A. M. A. **95**: 85-91, 1930.
4. Casper, W. T.: Wisconsin M. J. **39**: 935-937, 1940.
5. Colwell, A. H.: Cardiac Patients as Surgical Risks, Pennsylvania M. J. **37**: 568-572, 1934.
6. Farnum, W. B.: Cardiac Disorders in Surgical Patients, S. Clin. North America **16**: 843-851, 1936.
7. Grindlay, J. H.: Cardiac Decompensation in Relation to Various Surgical Procedures, Proc. Staff Meet., Mayo Clin. **15**: 121-127, 1940.
8. Hamilton, B. E.: The Chronic Cardiac as a Surgical Risk, S. Clin. North America **6**: 621, 1926.
9. Hamilton, B. E.: Congestive Heart Failure and Angina Pectoris in Surgical Patients, S. Clin. North America **6**: 637-650, 1926.
10. Herrmann, G., and Herrmann, L. G.: Cardiac Disorders in Surgical Patients, Texas State J. Med. **30**: 183-191, 1934.
11. Hickman, J., Livingstone, H., and Davies, M. E.: Surgical and Anesthetic Risk in Cardiac Disease, Arch. Surg. **31**: 917-936, 1935.
12. Hnat, F.: The Common Forms of Heart Disease in Relation to Surgery, Delaware State M. J. **11**: 162-166, 1939.
13. Hunt, V. C.: The Cardiovascular System in Relation to Surgery, Southwestern Med. **20**: 163-167, 1936.
14. MacErlean, D. A.: The Heart in Disease, Irish J. M. Sc., pp. 644-653, 1934.
15. Marvin, H. M.: The Heart During Anesthesia and Operative Procedures, New England J. Med. **199**: 547-551, 1928.
16. Master, A. M., Dack, S., and Jaffe, H. L.: Postoperative Coronary Artery Occlusion, J. A. M. A. **110**: 1415-1418, 1938.
17. Maxwell, R. W.: Heart Disease Complicated by Surgery, J. Missouri M. A. **36**: 335-337, 1939.
18. Maynard, E. P., Jr.: The Cardiac and Pulmonary Complications of Genito-Urinary Surgery, Brooklyn Hosp. J. **3**: 133-139, 1941.
19. McQuiston, J. S., and Allen, E. V.: The Relationship of Arterial Hypertension to Surgical Risk, Am. J. Surg. **21**: 72-77, 1933.
20. McQuiston, J. S.: The Relationship of Arterial Hypotension to Surgical Risk, Proc. Staff Meet., Mayo Clin. **8**: 614-616, 1933.
21. McQuiston, J. S.: The Relationship of Arterial Hypotension to Surgical Risk, J. Iowa M. Soc. **25**: 331-333, 1935.
22. Patek, A. J.: The Heart in Surgery, Wisconsin M. J. **34**: 386-390, 1935.
23. Poindexter, C. A.: Evaluation of the Cardiac Status of the Surgical Patient, M. Clin. North America **22**: 1505-1511, 1938.
24. Purks, W. K.: The Cause of Death of Patients With Organic Heart Disease Subjected to Surgical Operation, Ann. Int. Med. **7**: 885-894, 1934.
25. Roberts, S. R.: The Relation of the Heart to Surgery, South. Surgeon **4**: 85-100, 1935.
26. Rodman, J. S., and Leaman, Wm. S.: The Surgical Risk, Ann. Surg. **103**: 13, 1936.
27. Rubin, I. C., and Davids, A. M.: Hypertension Associating Uterine Fibroids: Considered From Viewpoint of Etiological Connection and Surgical Risk, J. Mt. Sinai Hosp. **8**: 987-990, 1942.
28. Senturia, H. R.: Relationship of Arterial Hypertension to Surgical Risk in Breast Cancer, J. Missouri M. A. **38**: 22-24, 1941.
29. Sprague, H. B.: The Heart in Surgery, Surg., Gynec. & Obst. **49**: 54-58, 1929.
30. Stalker, W. K.: The Cardiac Aspect of Surgical Risk, Proc. Staff Meet., Mayo Clin. **11**: 625-629, 1936.
31. Willius, F. H.: A Talk on Surgical Procedures in the Presence of Cardiac Disease, Proc. Staff. Meet., Mayo Clin. **13**: 174-176, 1938.

ESOPHAGOGASTROSTOMY IN THE TREATMENT OF CARDIOSPASM

Dan C. Gill, M.D., and Charles G. Child, III, M.D., New York, N. Y.
(From the Department of Surgery of The New York Hospital and Cornell University Medical College)

Periodically during the past thirty years dissatisfaction with the nonoperative methods of treating patients with cardiospasm has found expression in the development of various surgical measures directed toward relief of the constriction at the gastric cardia. Until recently, however, none of these methods has received any very enthusiastic reception, doubtless due to the high mortality which was expected to follow any operative procedure involving open esophagotomy; fatal postoperative infections were too frequently the rule. With the development of chemotherapy it has become evident that the esophagus can be attacked surgically with far greater confidence than ever before. Furthermore, as the operations for cancer of the esophagus and the gastric cardia have been developed, surgeons have discovered that esophageal surgery can be undertaken with relative safety and that this organ per se is not the formidable structure it was once considered. For these two reasons, therefore, it might have been anticipated that the question of how to deal surgically with patients with intractable cardiospasm would again be brought into focus. Because reported cases in which the patient has been operated upon are relatively rare, and because the results obtained in eight patients in this clinic have been gratifying, there has seemed ample justification for reporting even this relatively small series.

Benign nonorganic obstruction of the esophagus at the gastric cardia is a clinical syndrome which was first recognized by Willis in the seventeenth century. Since its original description, this disease entity is one to which a bewildering variety of terms has been applied and one in which no definite etiologic agent has as yet been defined. In all probability the obstruction is due to organic factors which are intrinsic in the cardia and to its autonomic nerve supply. Also, it seems certain that all the individuals with cardiospasm present varying degrees of emotional instability and that frequently their symptoms bear an almost direct relationship to periods of stress and tension.

Although a great many of these patients can be carried along with reasonable success by explaining to them the nature of their difficulty and by means of peroral dilatation, every large clinic presents a group of these individuals in whom such conservative measures fail. These unfortunates, as they wander from doctor to doctor over long periods of time without obtaining any permanent improvement, progressively develop a tortuous, elongated, and dilated esophagus. Finally, the obstruction fails to respond more than temporarily to any form of conservative treatment. It is those patients who are finally considered subjects for direct operative intervention.

The various types of surgical procedures which have been advocated have been so completely and competently reviewed by Ochsner and DeBakey[1] in their excellent review that there is no need for repetition here. In seven cases in this series of eight, the obstruction at the gastric cardia has been overcome by means of an esophagogastrostomy devised by Grondahl[2] as a modification of Heyrovsky's[3] original procedure. In principle this operation is entirely comparable to the Finney[4] gastroduodenostomy which at one time enjoyed wide popularity as a cure for pyloric obstruction. In one patient (Case 6) the gastric cardia was generously incised in its longitudinal axis. By closing this incision transversely the constriction was corrected. Figs. 1 to 6 demonstrate diagrammatically these two types of operative procedure.

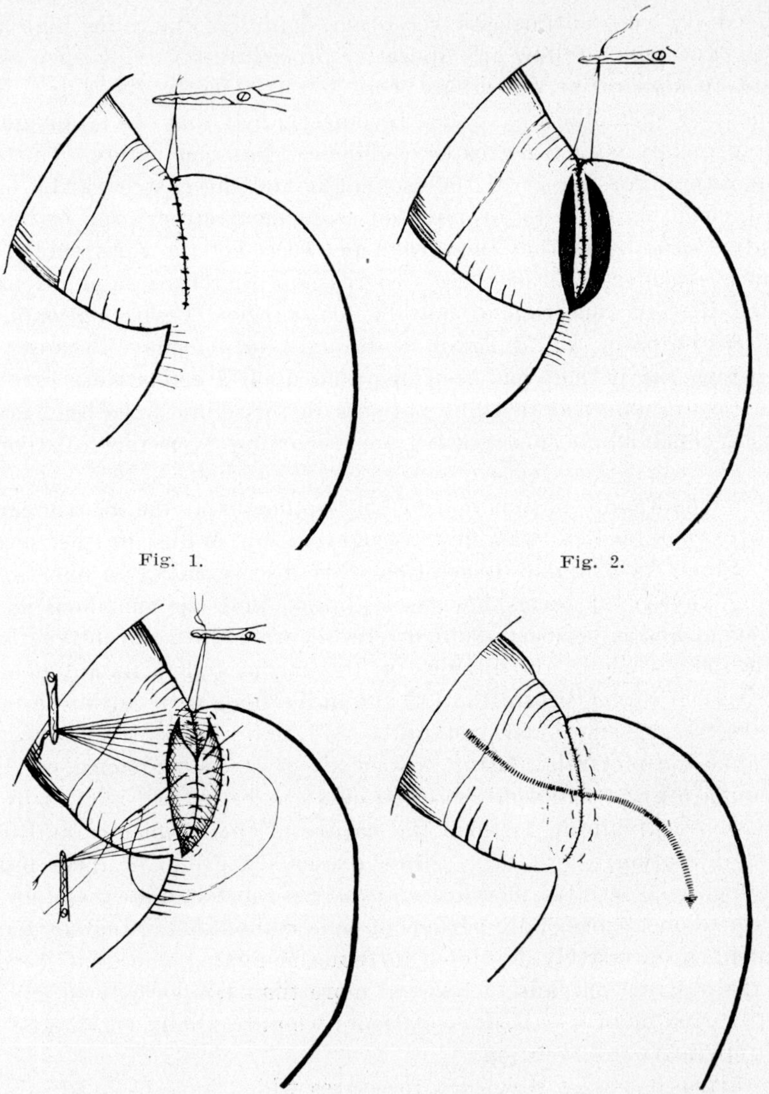

Fig. 1. Fig. 2.

Fig. 3. Fig. 4.

Figs. 1, 2, 3, and 4.—Diagrammatic representation of the successive steps employed in performing the esophagogastrostomy in Cases 1, 2, 3, 4, 5, 7, and 8. This closely resembles the well-known Finney pyloroplasty.

In two of these nine operations the lower esophagus and gastric cardia were approached transabdominally; in five the operation was performed transthoracically; in one patient (Case 2) requiring a second operation the first was done through the abdomen, while at the second, access to the area was obtained through the chest. All nine operations were performed without a death and with only one significant postoperative complication; the first patient in this series developed an empyema after transthoracic esophagogastrostomy. Following suitable thoracotomy for drainage, this girl improved rapidly and is now well save for a small pleural fistula. In view of the seriousness of this complication when it occurs, and the ease with which the esophageal-gastric

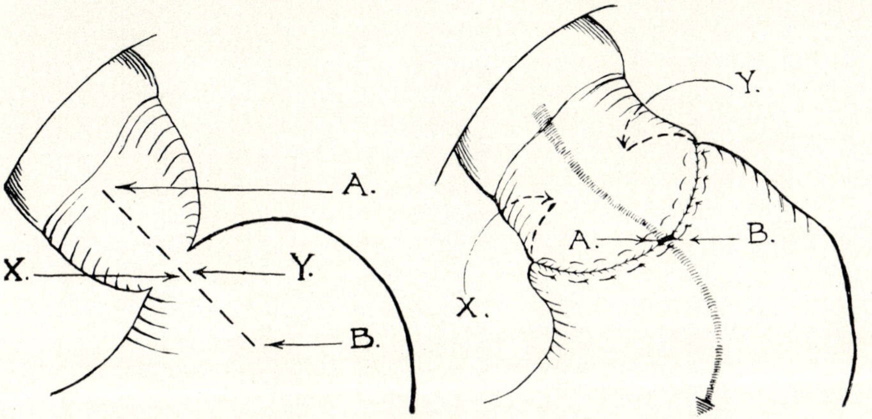

Figs. 5 and 6.—Diagrammatic representation of the method employed in relieving the esophagogastric constriction in Case 6. The principle involved is that of opening a tubular structure longitudinally and closing it transversely, thereby eliminating a diaphragm-like constriction.

junction was approached from below the diaphragm in three instances, we favor the transabdominal approach. In all of the patients in this series chemotherapy was employed in the early postoperative period. The significant facts in each of these cases are outlined in Table I. Abbreviated case reports are presented, together with unretouched reproductions of the pre- and postoperative roentgenograms.

CASE REPORTS

CASE 1 (N. Y. H. No. 388704).—C. D., a 28-year-old married woman, was first seen at this hospital in September, 1944, approximately two years after the onset of the chief complaint of difficulty in swallowing. At this time roentgenograms of the esophagus failed to reveal any definite obstruction or dilatation, but there was a suggestion of constriction at the cardiac orifice of the stomach. Esophagoscopy failed to reveal any apparent organic stricture, but a biopsy taken from the lower third demonstrated on microscopic examination a mild degree of leucoplakia. Following the initial visit this patient attended the general medical and psychiatric clinics without improvement until June, 1947, about three years later, or five years after the onset of the complaints. At this time esophagograms revealed marked dilatation of the esophagus with constriction at the cardiac orifice of the stomach. Psychiatric consultation early in the course of the disease yielded the impression that "the patient seems fairly well adjusted."

Since it was felt that this patient had been given adequate opportunity to recover under a conservative regime and had not only failed to improve but had become progressively worse, she was admitted for surgical treatment. She had not been subjected to instrumental

TABLE I

								Follow-up			Postoperative Roentgenograms	
No.	N. Y. H. Hist. No.	Sex	Age (Yr.)	Duration of Symptoms	Weight Loss (Pounds)	Dilatation of Esophagus	Date of Operation	Duration	Symptoms	Weight Gain (Pounds)	Dilatation of Esophagus	Function of Anastomosis
1	388704	F	28	5 yr.	None	None (1944) Marked (1947)	6/20/47	6 mo.	Mild dysphagia under tension	10	None	Excellent
2	345435	M	19	2 yr.	30	Moderate (1942)	6/11/43	7 mo.	Severe cardiospasm	None	Marked	Failure
			20	2 yr. 7 mo.		Marked (1943)	2/23/44	4 yr.	Mild substernal fullness after eating	None	Minimal	Excellent
3	167879	M	51	30 yr.	None	Marked (1941, 1945, 1947)	4/18/47	6 mo.	Mild; no nocturnal regurgitation	None	None	Excellent
4	206158	F	51	4 yr.	None	Minimal	8/21/47	3 mo.	Mild	None	None	Excellent
5	466970	F	25	6 yr.	15	Moderate	1/29/47	10 mo.	None	17	None	Excellent
6	483521	M	34	5 yr.	20	Marked	7/30/47	3 mo.	Dysphagia under tension	15	Moderate	Excellent
7	467001	F	24	5 yr.	30	Moderate	3/ 5/47	8 mo.	None	30	None	Excellent
8	404150	F	59	19 yr.	67	Enormous (1945)	2/ 7/45	3 yr.	Unchanged	See Case Report	Marked	Excellent

dilatation in any form during the course of the conservative management. On June 20, 1947, an esophagogastrostomy was performed transthoracically. The postoperative course was complicated by the development of an empyema necessitating drainage. Six months postoperatively, the patient was still well. She stated that she had gained ten pounds in weight and was completely free of the most significant preoperative complaint, namely, that of

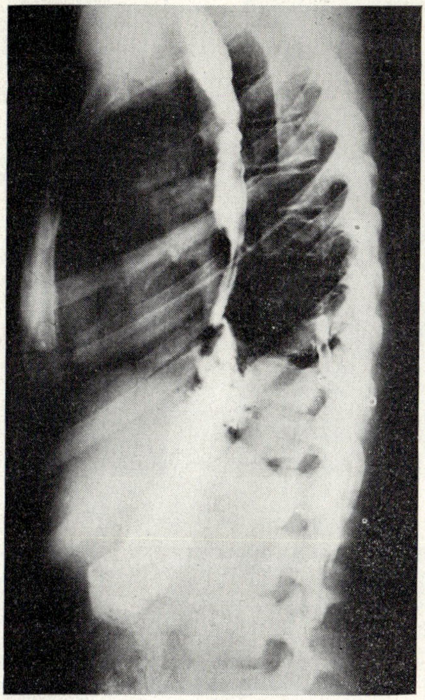

Fig. 7 (Case 1).—Postoperative film demonstrating excellent function of the esophagogastrostomy. A small tube remains in the empyema sinus tract. (Preoperative films lost in this case.)

nocturnal regurgitation, which was most distressing in that the pillow was constantly soiled by foul esophageal contents. It is of particular interest that even today when the patient is subjected to emotional tension the subjective symptoms reappear without, however, any of the preoperative objective phenomena such as vomiting and regurgitation. Postoperative x-ray examination revealed excellent correction of the defect at the gastric cardia without dilatation of the esophagus. The passage of barium from the esophagus into the stomach was entirely free.

CASE 2 (N. Y. H. No. 345435).—R. B., 19-year-old man was first admitted to the hospital in December, 1942, with a two-year history of difficulty in swallowing. The onset then was gradual but, once started, progression was unremitting so that on admission liquids constituted the only food that the patient was able to take by mouth. He had lost thirty pounds in weight. X-ray examination revealed dilatation of the esophagus terminating in a smooth conical constriction. Esophagoscopy was negative save for a tightly closed gastric orifice which was readily dilated to admit a 9 mm. Jackson esophagoscope. During the course of the following six months this patient was treated conservatively without benefit. Bouginage was employed without sustained improvement. Psychiatric consultation yielded the following impression: ''The writer was unable to work out any definite psychogenic factors. . . . However, the patient appears to be one of the rather dull intellectual level who has displayed psychoneurotic reactions.''

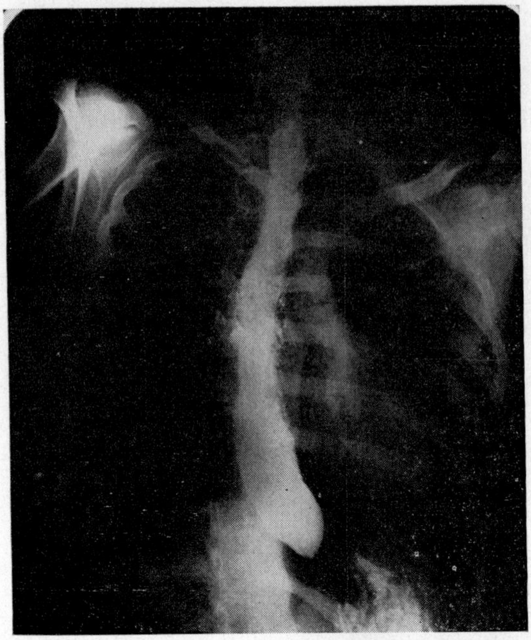

A.

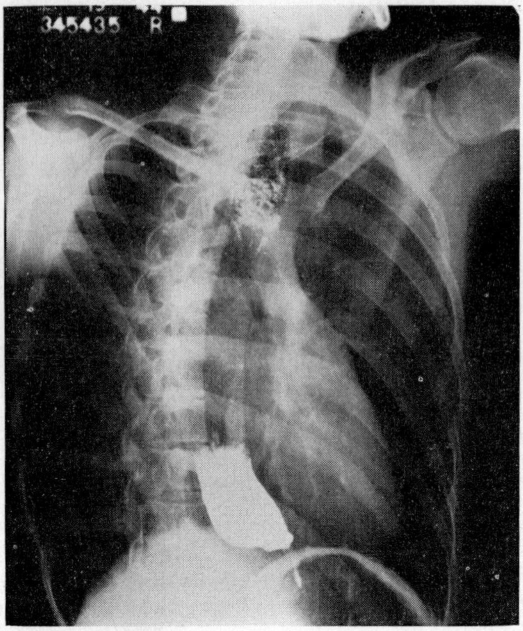

B.

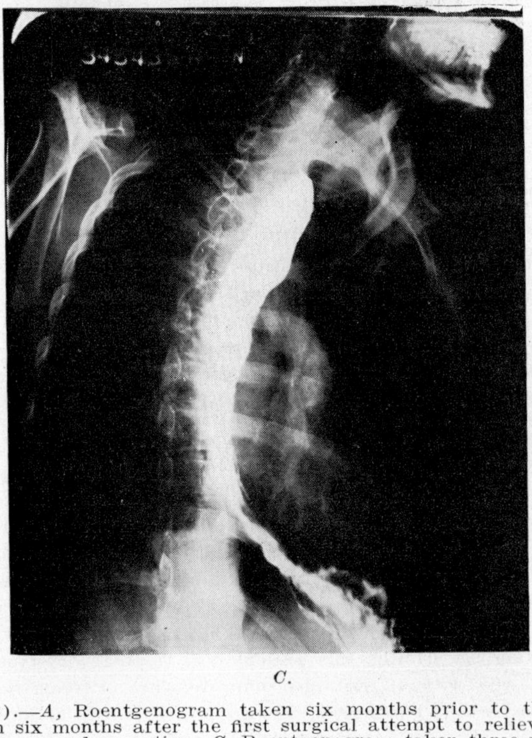

C.

Fig. 8 (Case 2).—*A*, Roentgenogram taken six months prior to the first operation. *B*, Roentgenogram taken six months after the first surgical attempt to relieve the obstruction and one month prior to the second operation. *C*, Roentgenogram taken three years after the second operation. This demonstrates excellent function of the anastomosis between the stomach and esophagus.

On June 11, 1943, an esophagogastrostomy was performed through an upper abdominal incision. The patient's immediate postoperative course was uneventful but he failed to obtain any improvement in symptoms.

After approximately seven months of ineffectual dilatations, exploration was again done (February, 1944), this time through the left side of the thorax. Upon exposing the site of the previous operative procedure, an area of constriction was found which had apparently not been released at the initial operation. This lay just at the upper border of the previous anastomosis. Again an esophagogastrostomy was undertaken, carefully including the persistent area of stricture. The immediate postoperative course was gratifying and repeated esophagograms revealed a normal esophagus with excellent function at the cardiac end of the stomach.

Four years after the operative procedures, although x-ray studies persistently failed to indicate any obstruction in the distal esophagus, the patient intermittently complained of substernal fullness on eating. Rarely has he vomited. Through all of the treatment and over a period of five years, the patient's weight remained constant; he has not regained the initial weight loss of thirty pounds.

CASE 3 (N. Y. H. No. 167879).—E. P., a 51-year-old man, was admitted to the hospital in April, 1947, with a thirty-year history of difficulty in swallowing. In June, 1941, x-ray pictures revealed marked dilatation of the esophagus with cardiospasm and evidence of a healed duodenal ulcer. During the course of the next six years he was treated conservatively but without bouginage. He failed to improve subjectively though he did not lose weight.

On April 18, 1947, an esophagogastrostomy was performed transabdominally. Because of the presence of a duodenal ulcer both vagi were divided. The immediate postoperative course was unremarkable and postoperative roentgenograms revealed a definite decrease in the size of the esophagus and excellent function of the cardioplasty. The patient, however, failed to gain weight and although he still has numerous vague complaints such as ''nervousness'' and ''constipation,'' these are no longer associated with dysphagia. Furthermore, he states that he is completely free of the most significant preoperative symptom, that of nocturnal regurgitation which invariably appeared upon lying down.

CASE 4 (N. Y. H. No. 206158).—E. B., a 51-year-old woman, might be characterized as one of those patients who presents a ''lifetime'' history of one complaint or another. The operations included an appendectomy, a hysterectomy, an exploratory celiotomy without significant findings, and a repair of an umbilical hernia. For some four years prior to admission she complained persistently of nausea and vomiting. In the first esophagograms, taken, in 1944, findings were negative. Beginning in 1946, esophagograms began to reveal variable degrees of cardiospasm without dilatation of the esophagus. In 1947 esophagograms revealed cardiospasm with esophagitis. Esophagoscopy at this time revealed marked inflammatory reaction at the lower end of the esophagus. This was confirmed on microscopic examination of a biopsy of the mucosa taken just above the cardiac sphincter.

Aug. 21, 1947, an esophagogastrostomy was performed transthoracically. At this time findings in the esophagus were negative save for a smooth area of constriction at the cardiac orifice of the stomach. The postoperative course was unremarkable and esophageal fluoroscopy has failed to reveal any evidence of obstruction. She is symptom-free.

CASE 5 (N. Y. H. No. 466970).—V. A., a 25-year-old woman, was admitted to the hospital in January, 1947, with a six-year history of dysphagia. Following the initial symptoms she was treated medically and dilatation was carried out frequently. The dysphagia increased steadily. Even while under treatment she began losing weight and vomited after almost every meal. Preoperative x-ray pictures revealed a moderately dilated esophagus terminating in a smooth, conical constriction. There was no filling of the stomach after two hours.

On January 29, 1947, an esophagogastrostomy was performed transthoracically. The patient's postoperatvie course was unremarkable.

Six months postoperatively she was without symptoms and the anastomosis between the esophagus and stomach functioned well. She has gained seventeen pounds in weight.

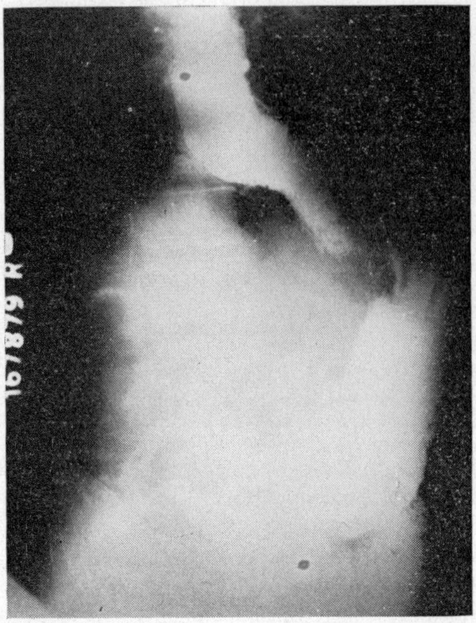

A.

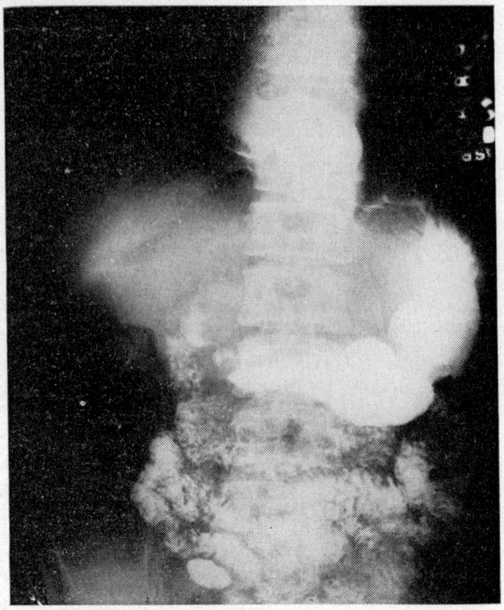

B.

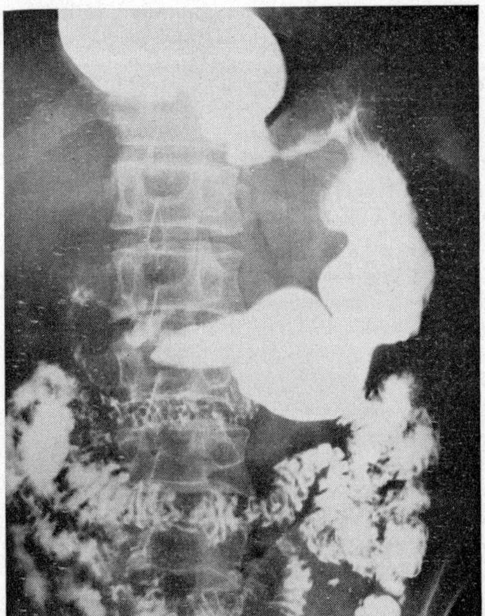

C.

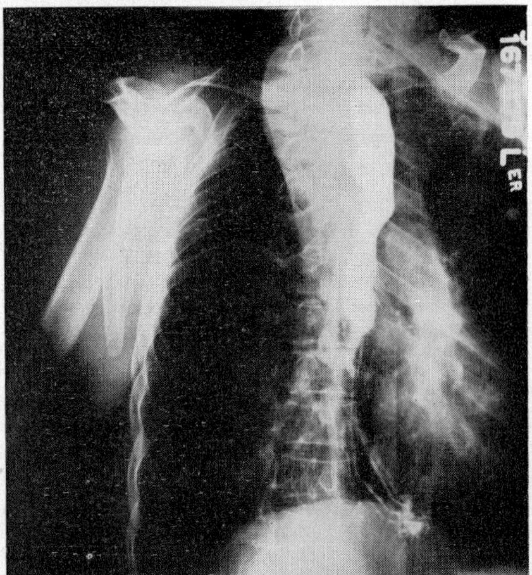

D.

Fig. 9 (Case 3).—*A, B,* and *C,* Preoperative esophagograms taken in 1941, 1945, and 1947. These are of interest in that they clearly demonstrate the progressive enlargement of the esophagus which all too frequently is permitted to take place.

D, Postoperative esophagogram revealing excellent function of the esophagogastric anastomosis. This view taken but one month after operation demonstrates remarkable decrease in the diameter of the esophagus.

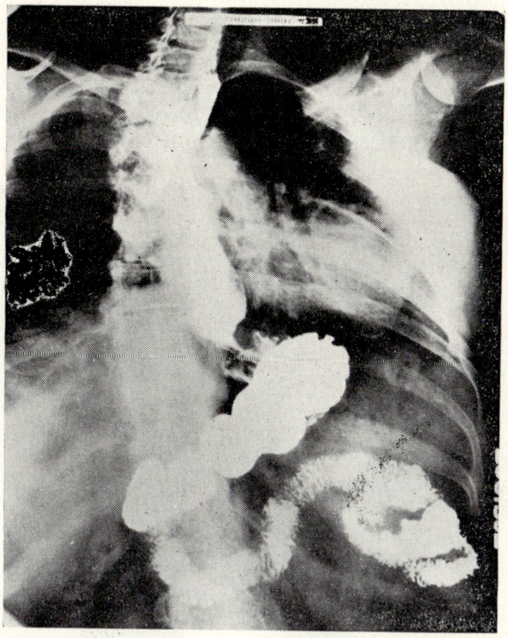

Fig. 10 (Case 4).—Preoperative esophagogram. Postoperative fluoroscopy of the esophagus revealed excellent function with the barium passing promptly into the stomach.

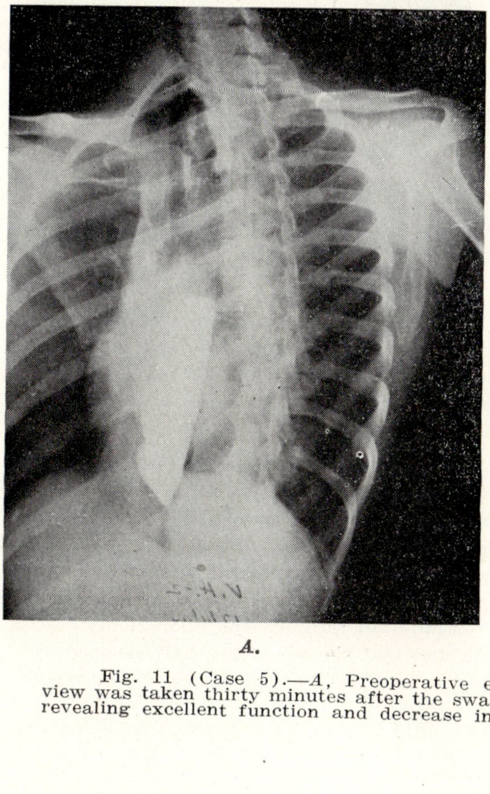

A.

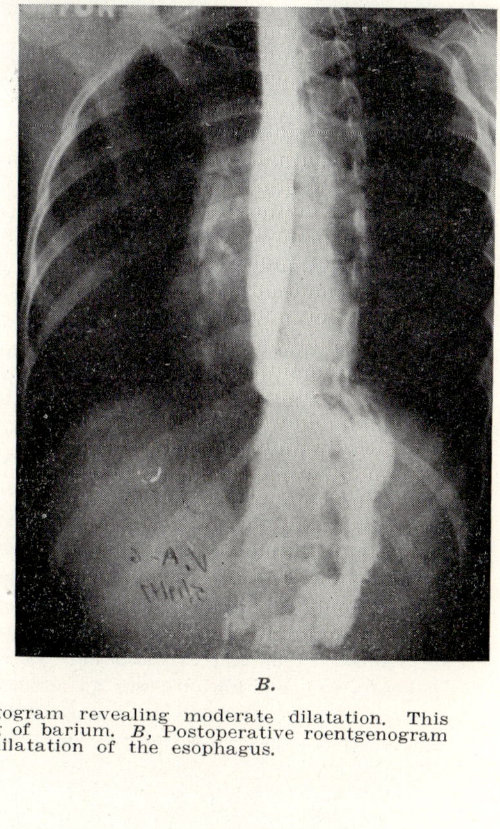

B.

Fig. 11 (Case 5).—*A*, Preoperative esophagogram revealing moderate dilatation. This view was taken thirty minutes after the swallowing of barium. *B*, Postoperative roentgenogram revealing excellent function and decrease in the dilatation of the esophagus.

Case 6 (N. Y. H. No. 483521).—E. W., a 34-year-old man was admitted to the hospital in July, 1947, with a five-year history of progressive inability to swallow. Shortly after the onset of symptoms a diagnosis of cardiospasm was made and he was treated by bouginage and formal psychotherapy. Following each series of dilatations he would remain well a month or so and then the difficulty would return. Repeated esophagograms over this period revealed steadily increasing dilatation of the esophagus.

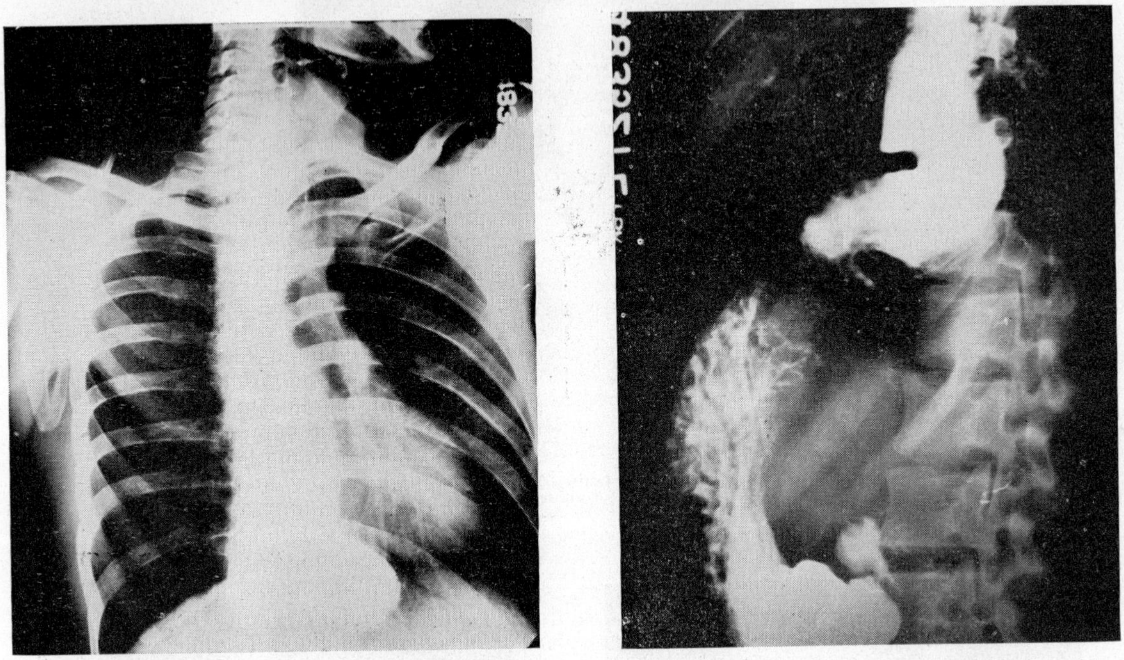

A. B.

Fig. 12 (Case 6).—*A*, Preoperative roentgenogram of the esophagus revealing dilatation and tortuosity without passage of barium into the stomach for a period of forty-five minutes. *B*, Postoperative study demonstrating prompt emptying of the esophagus. This view was taken three months after operation and there is as yet little decrease in the size and deformity of the esophagus.

July 30, 1947, the cardiac end of the stomach was explored transabdominally and a smooth stricture at the cardiac orifice identified. A 6 cm. longitudinal incision was made through the anterior esophageal and gastric walls. This was then closed transversely.

The postoperative course was unremarkable, the patient being discharged from the hospital on the twelfth day after operation, taking a general diet without difficulty.

Three months postoperatively he was without complaint, having gained fifteen pounds in weight. Esophageal fluoroscopy reveals prompt passage of barium from the esophagus into the stomach and roentgenograms demonstrate an adequately functioning esophagogastric junction.

Case 7 (N. Y. H. No. 467001).—J. D., a 24-year-old woman, was admitted to the hospital in February, 1947, with a five-year history of substernal burning and inability to swallow. During this period she received adequate medical attention including several dilatations of the gastric cardia and a long period of self-bouginage. In spite of this she became progressively worse and esophagograms on admission revealed moderate dilatation of the esophagus and cardiospasm. Psychiatric consultation afforded the opinion that the patient's primary difficulty was an anxiety hysteria and that she would probably respond to prolonged psychotherapy in a psychiatric hospital. In spite of this opinion, operative intervention seemed to be the procedure of choice.

On March 5, 1947, an esophagogastrostomy was performed transthoracically. The postoperative course was uneventful and she was discharged thirteen days after operation.

Her course has been most gratifying. She has gained thirty pounds in weight and esophagograms reveal excellent function of the esophagogastrostomy without dilatation of the esophagus.

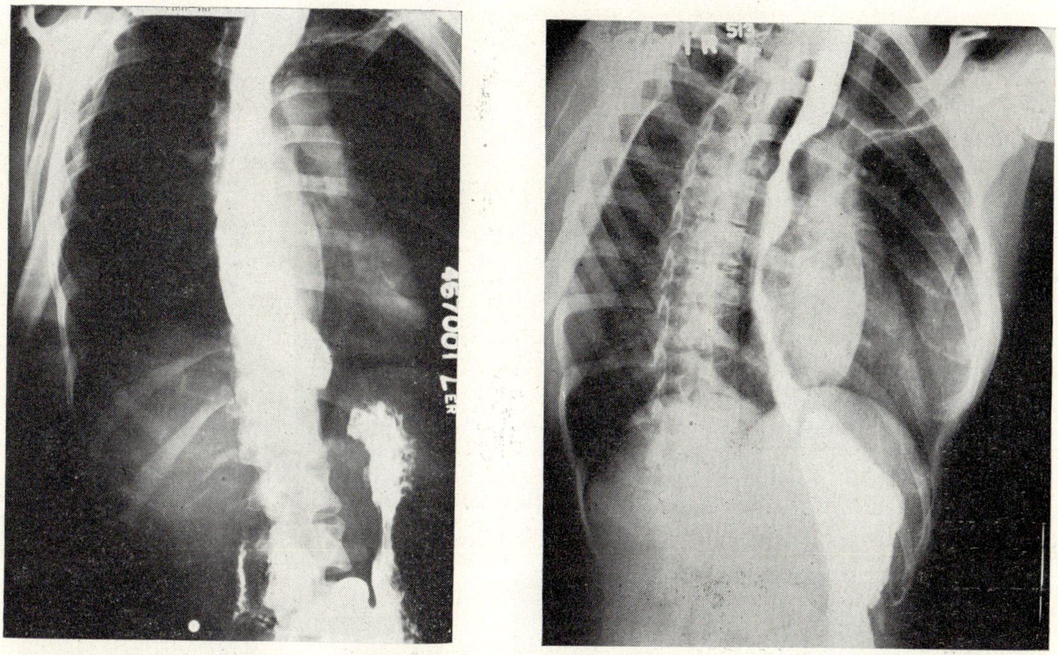

A. *B.*

Fig. 13 (Case 7).—*A*, Preoperative esophagogram. *B*, Postoperative esophagogram.

CASE 8 (N. Y. H. No. 404150).—H. C., a 59-year-old woman, entered the hospital in January, 1945, with a nineteen-year history of difficulty in swallowing. She was studied at the onset of the disease and a diagnosis of cardiospasm was made. Dilatations were unsuccessful and she secured no further definitive therapy until eight months prior to admission, when a gastrostomy was performed for feeding purposes. Over the period of nineteen years she lost a total of sixty-seven pounds, thirty of which she gained back following the initiation of gastric feedings. Because she was dissatisfied with the gastrostomy she entered the hospital for any operation which might permit her to eat normally. X-ray pictures taken at the time of admission revealed cardiospasm with extensive dilatation of the esophagus.

On Feb. 7, 1945, an esophagogastrostomy was performed transthoracically. The immediate postoperative course was uneventful, the patient leaving the hospital on the twenty-seventh day after operation. The gastrostomy closed spontaneously.

During the course of the next two years or so follow-up was carried out on this patient at regular intervals and there were two outstanding features worthy of note. First, esophagograms revealed that even though there was rapid passage of barium from the esophagus into the stomach, there was but slight decrease in the preoperative degree of dilatation; and second, that the patient's symptoms were relatively unchanged. She still vomits occasionally and has lost approximately twenty pounds since the operation.

RESULTS

Each of the patients save one was interviewed from six months to two years postoperatively. Several interesting facts appeared. First, most of the patients

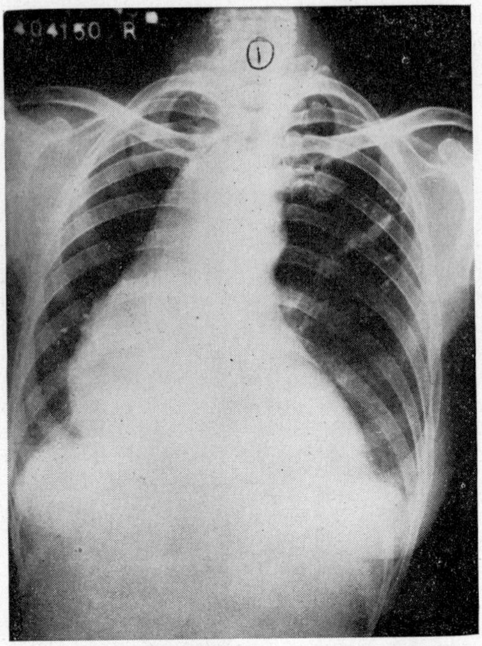

A.

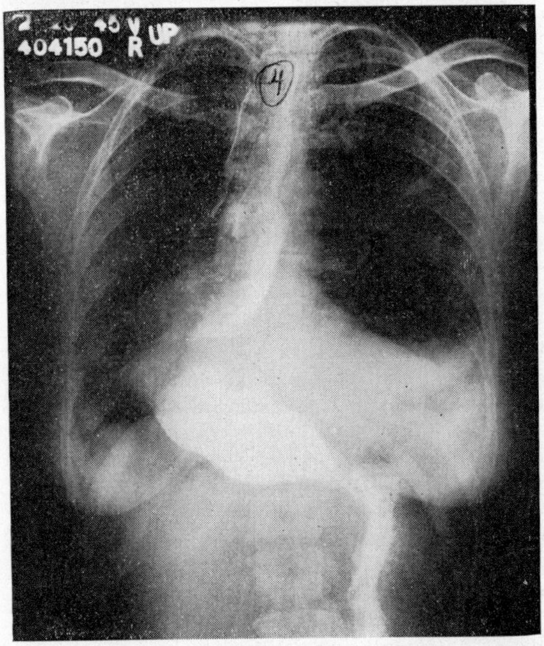

B.

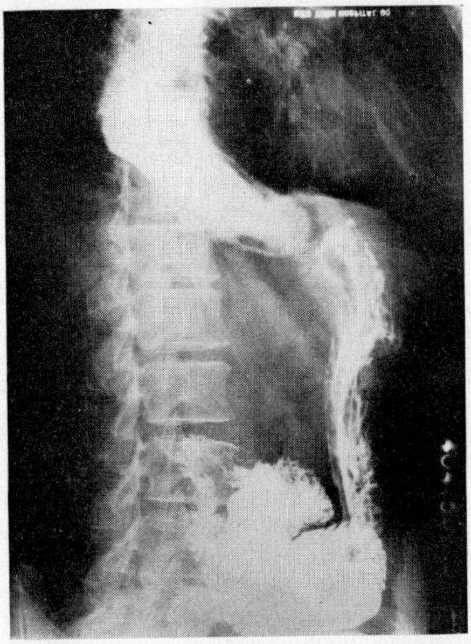

C.

Fig. 14 (Case 8).—*A* and *B*, Preoperative esophagograms revealing marked dilatation and deformity. *C*, Esophagogram two years after operation demonstrating excellent function and a decrease in the diameter but little change in the so-called sigmoid deformity.

have continued to have some untoward symptoms referable either to swallowing or to the upper gastrointestinal tract. For the most part these have been vague but have tended to become intensified during periods of emotional stress. In all instances the patients volunteered that they had been much improved by operation, and in none of those in whom nocturnal regurgitation had been present preoperatively did this distressing problem present itself postoperatively. Second, in all instances final postoperative roentgenography demonstrated excellent function of the esophagogastrostomy, the barium sulfate meal passing without hesitation from the esophagus into the stomach. We are at a loss to explain the persistence of symptoms in the face of such definite evidence of excellent function other than to suggest that possibly the syndrome of cardiospasm affects the entire esophagus and not merely its diaphragmatic orifice.

Excluding the problem of symptomatology, these patients have been improved in other respects. In five out of the eight patients there has been a very appreciable gain in weight, varying from two and one-half to thirty pounds. Three, however, have failed to gain weight, and in one patient (Case 2) none of the preoperative weight loss of thirty pounds was regained in spite of satisfactory function at the gastric cardia. In the seven patients in whom the esophagus was dilated and elongated there has been return to normal in five cases, moderate shrinkage in one, and practically no change in one. This last patient (Case 8) was 59 years of age and demonstrated an enormous esophageal dilatation which had probably been developing for some fifteen to twenty years. Certainly of real economic significance is the fact that all of these patients have been saved expensive and time-consuming office or clinic visits for repeated and ineffectual treatments.

It is concluded, therefore, from reviewing this series of eight patients, that the safety with which esophagogastrostomy can be performed today entitles the procedure to a definite place in the treatment of cardiospasm. Furthermore, it would seem reasonable to accept the general principle that in many instances this type of definitive therapy should be recommended earlier than it has been heretofore. By reserving surgical intervention for only intractable cases, a large group of patients is forced to put up with a certainly unpleasant, if not actually dangerous, train of events much longer than there is any need. Also, where the dilatation has been allowed to persist for many years (as in Case 8), the surgical result cannot be expected to be as satisfactory as it apparently is in those patients in whom operation is performed reasonably early after the onset of symptoms. Seemingly such an overstretched organ loses its power to return to normal and its very dilatation and elongation persist to become as much a basis for symptoms as was the original cardiospasm.

REFERENCES

1. Ochsner, Alton, and DeBakey, Michael: Arch. Surg. **41**: 1146, 1940.
2. Grondahl, N. B.: Nord. Kir. for. forhandl. **11**: 236, 1916.
3. Heyrovsky, H.: Arch. f. klin. Chir. **100**: 703, 1912-13.
4. Finney, J. M. T.: Tr. Am. S. A. **20**: 165, 1902.

EVALUATION OF SKIN GRAFTING IN THE TECHNIQUE OF RADICAL MASTECTOMY IN RELATION TO FUNCTION OF THE ARM

CHARLES G. NEUMANN, M.D., AND HERBERT CONWAY, M.D., NEW YORK, N. Y.

(From the Department of Surgery of The New York Hospital and Cornell University Medical College)

WHILE the primary purpose of radical mastectomy is the cure of mammary carcinoma it is also of importance that satisfactory function of the arm be maintained. This accessory aim is all the more important in view of the high percentage of cases of carcinoma of the breast which are cured by radical mastectomy. The purpose of this report is to present data giving information on the quality of function of the arm in patients who have been treated for breast cancer by radical mastectomy with simple closure of the wound and by radical mastectomy with closure by skin graft. Closure after radical mastectomy by free skin graft was first employed because the removal of a margin of skin sufficient to guard against the probability of local recurrence left a defect so large that primary suture often was not possible. However, closure by skin graft has been advocated by those who feel that extremely wide excision of skin and subcutaneous tissue is the best protection against regional recurrence. Also, the examination of patients after operation has given information which shows that the use of a primary graft in the closure of the wound of radical mastectomy results in the preservation of full function of the arm in a high percentage of cases. In this study patients have been examined postoperatively and records have been analyzed closely in an attempt to determine the actual role played by the additional step of skin grafting after radical mastectomy. Data which point out the value of the skin graft in relation to final function of the arm are presented herein.

The basis of the clinical study are 389 patients on whom radical mastectomy was performed on the surgical service of The New York Hospital from Sept. 1, 1932, to Dec. 31, 1946. Of this number, thirteen are excluded because of death soon after operation or because mastectomy had been done as a palliative operation for advanced disease. Bilateral mastectomy was done in eight cases. Thus it has been possible to study the effect of type of operation upon the function of the arm in 384 cases. The patients were examined at the time of their semiannual visits to the surgical follow-up clinic of The New York Hospital.

Operative surgery in these cases was done by twenty-five different surgeons, most of whom served as resident surgeon at the time. The basic steps of radical mastectomy followed the technique of Halsted.[1, 2] These steps may be enumerated: (1) preliminary biopsy with microscopic examination (frozen section) to ascertain the nature of the tumor; (2) preparation of the skin of the thigh as the donor site for a thick-split graft of skin; (3) use of a circular or elliptical incision about the tumor at a distance of at least 5 cm. from its palpable margins, regardless of which quadrant of the breast is involved; (4) extension of the incision from its central ellipse, superiorly to the middle or lateral third of the clavicle and inferiorly to the costal margin; (5) reflection of flaps of skin (with a small amount of subcutaneous tissue) superiorly to the clavicle, medially to the midsternum, inferiorly to the fascia of the rectus muscle, and laterally to the border of the latissimus dorsi muscle and to the insertion of the pectoralis major muscle, thus exposing the axilla; (6) detachment of the pectoralis major and minor muscles and their fasciae from their origins on the chest wall and their insertions into the humerus and the coracoid process; (7) complete dissection of the axillary vein thus permitting removal of all of the contents of the axilla including lymphatic vessels and glands, adipose and areolar tissue; (8) removal of breast, axillary contents, and pectoralis major and minor muscles en masse; (9) reconstruction of a *high* axilla by obliteration of dead space and suture of the upper and outer cutaneous flap to the chest wall immediately posterior and inferior to the axillary vein; (10) suture of the margins of the cutaneous flaps superior to, medial to, and inferior to a central defect on the chest wall; suture is effected without undue tension while the arm is held in abduction at an angle of ninety degrees; (11) application of a thick-split skin graft to the residual open wound on the chest wall, and (12) application of a suitable dressing to maintain pressure upon the graft and the flaps and to immobilize the arm in slight abduction.

ANALYSIS OF DATA

Of the 384 cases the records of which were reviewed for this analysis, the data were sufficiently complete in 308 to permit their inclusion in this report on evaluation of the use of a skin graft in radical mastectomy as a step in arrival at the goal of tumor cure with good function of the arm.

The results regarding function of the arm have been classified as follows: (1) poor (motion limited to less than 90 degrees abduction); (2) good (motion in the range of greater than 90 degrees of abduction, but less than 160 degrees); and (3) excellent (motion greater than 160 degrees of abduction and for all practical purposes as free as in the opposite extremity). In addition to range of abduction, certain other considerations, such as the degree of freedom from pain or motion and the degree of retention of power in the shoulder joint should, perhaps, be given great weight but these have not been considered separately, partly owing to lack of satisfactory follow-up information.

The methods which surgeons had utilized for closure of the wounds are classified as follows: (1) closure without graft; (2) use of a small graft for closure (less than 60 sq. cm. in area); (3) use of a large graft for closure (greater than 60 sq. cm. in area); and (4) use of a graft the size of which was not recorded.

In 95 of the 308 patients closure was without a graft and of these, 22, or 23 per cent, had poor function of the arm. Closure with a small graft was used in 131 and of these only 19, or 14.5 per cent, had a poor functional result. Fifty-nine closures were with a large graft and in 16, or 27 per cent, results were poor. Twenty-three closures were with a graft of indeterminate size and of these 3, or 13 per cent, had poor function. Although the size of the graft was not given

TABLE I. RADICAL MASTECTOMY (308 CASES)
Evaluation of Function of Arm in Relation to Use of Thick-Split Skin Graft

	CLOSURE WITHOUT GRAFT		CLOSURE WITH SMALL GRAFT		CLOSURE WITH LARGE GRAFT		CLOSURE WITH GRAFT OF UNKNOWN SIZE		TOTALS	
	NO.	PER CENT	NO.	PER CENT	NO.	PER CENT	NO.	PER CENT	NO.	PER CENT
Poor function	22	23	19	14.5	16	27	3	13	60	19
Good function	48	51	55	42	21	36	10	43.5	134	44
Excellent function	25	26	57	43.5	22	37	10	43.5	114	37
Number of cases	95		131		59		23		308 cases	

for these 23 cases, it may be presumed that the grafts were small rather than large for otherwise the surgeons would have been constrained to comment more accurately concerning the exact size of the graft employed. This conjecture seems to be borne out in the close parallelism of the results following the use of small grafts and the results after use of grafts of indeterminate size (Table I).

The postoperative treatment of radical mastectomy often included radiation therapy. Because of the erythema, inflammation, and fibrosis which such therapy may induce in the soft tissues of the chest wall and axilla, it is of interest to compare the functional results in patients who were given radiation with those who had not been so treated. Of 285 cases in which both the functional results and the size of graft are known, 150 patients were treated postoperatively by x-ray therapy. Of these 36, or 24 per cent, had a poor functional result. One hundred and thirty-five did not receive x-ray therapy and of these only 21, or 16 per cent, had a poor result (Table II). From these percentages, it appears that the use of x-ray postoperatively increases the probability of poor function of the arm.

Further analysis shows that x-ray therapy was associated with a higher percentage of poor functional results whether or not the wound was closed with a graft. Of the 95 wounds closed without a graft, x-ray therapy was used in 47 and there were poor functional results in 15, or 32 per cent. X-ray therapy was not used in 48 and of these there were poor results in only 7, or

TABLE II. RADICAL MASTECTOMY (285 CASES)
Evaluation of Function of the Arm in Relation to Use of Thick-Split Skin Graft and Postoperative X-ray Therapy

	CLOSURE WITHOUT GRAFT		CLOSURE WITH SMALL GRAFT		CLOSURE WITH LARGE GRAFT		TOTALS	
	NO.	PER CENT	NO.	PER CENT	NO.	PER CENT	NO.	PER CENT
Postoperative x-ray therapy								
Poor results	15	32	10	15	11	29	36	24
Good results	19	40	29	45	16	42	64	43
Excellent results	13	28	26	40	11	29	50	33
Total	47		65		38		150	
No x-ray therapy							21	16
Poor results	7	15	9	14	5	24	60	44
Good results	29	60	26	39	5	24	54	40
Excellent results	12	25	31	47	11	52	135	
Total	48		66		21		285	
Grand total	95		131		59			

15 per cent. Of the 131 wounds closed with a small graft x-ray therapy was used in 65 and of these there were poor results in 10, or 15 per cent. X-ray therapy was not used in 66 and there were poor functional results in 9, or 14 per cent. Of the 59 wounds closed with a large graft, x-ray therapy was used in 38 and of these there were poor results in 11, or 29 per cent. X-ray therapy was not used in 21, and of these there were poor results in 5 or 24 per cent.

Since x-ray therapy and closure of the wound without grafting both adversely affect the percentage of good functional results, it might be expected that their combined use would lead to the highest incidence of poor functional results. This is borne out in the analysis. Thirty-two per cent of patients whose wounds were closed without grafting and who then received x-ray therapy had poor function of the arm, whereas only 15 per cent of patients whose wounds were closed with a small graft and who did not receive x-ray therapy had poor results. The reporting of fewer good functional results following x-ray therapy is not advanced as an argument for the discontinuation of this treatment since it has been shown that the percentage of five-year cures can be improved with postoperative x-ray therapy.[3]

The development of edema of the arm following radical mastectomy is a factor which influences the function of the arm. For 287 cases, information as to the amount of edema as well as the functional result is available.

The patients were divided into three groups: (1) without edema; (2) with moderate edema (less than 2 cm. increase in circumference as compared with the unoperated side), and (3) with marked edema (more than 2 cm. increase in circumference). Of the 129 patients without edema, 17, or 13.5 per cent, had poor function; of the 124 patients with moderate edema, 21, or 17 per cent, had poor function; of the 34 patients with marked edema, 12, or 35 per cent, had poor function (Table III). Although it was apparent from the follow-up notes that edema of the arm did not in itself lead to poor function, it does appear that a considerably higher percentage of patients with edema had poor function. It has already been demonstrated that postoperative infection, either of the mastcetomy wound or of the extremity, is an important cause of edema.[4] It may be that lessened activity of the extremity which accompanies poor function is a contributory influence.

Because the operation of radical mastectomy, whether accompanied by grafting or not, usually is associated with a period of postoperative immobilization, the patient's age might be expected to influence the end result. For evalua-

TABLE III. RADICAL MASTECTOMY (287 CASES)
Relation of Swelling of Arm to Function of Arm

	POOR FUNCTION		GOOD FUNCTION		EXCELLENT FUNCTION		TOTALS
	NO.	PER CENT	NO.	PER CENT	NO.	PER CENT	
No swelling	17	13.5	58	45	54	42	129
Moderate swelling	21	17	58	47	45	36	124
Marked swelling	12	35	11	32.5	11	32.5	34
Total	50		127		110		287

tion of this factor the patients were divided into groups: (1) age 21 to 35 years; (2) age 36 to 50 years; (3) age 51 to 65 years; and (4) age 66 years or older.

TABLE IV. RADICAL MASTECTOMY (300 CASES)
Relation of Age of Patient to Function of the Arm

	POOR FUNCTION		GOOD FUNCTION		EXCELLENT FUNCTION		TOTALS
	NO.	PER CENT	NO.	PER CENT	NO.	PER CENT	
21 to 35 yr.	3	16	5	26	11	58	19
36 to 50 yr.	30	19.5	66	43	58	37.5	154
51 to 65 yr.	19	18	57	54	29	28	105
66 plus yr.	6	27	9	41	7	32	22
Totals	58		137		105		300

As can be seen in Table IV the percentage of poor results is greater in the advanced age decades. In the youngest group, there is 16 per cent of poor results, whereas in the oldest age group, there is 27 per cent.

DISCUSSION

It is apparent from a study of the patients included in this report that excision of a wide margin of skin, followed by reconstruction of a high axilla, approximation of cutaneous margins without undue tension, and the application of a thick-split skin graft to the residual defect is rewarded by good or excellent function of the arm in a high percentage of cases. In fact, the percentage of patients who exhibited full function of the arm after such operative care was nearly twice that of the patients treated by simple closure of the wound. It is true that a small tumor may be excised with a wide margin of adjacent skin still leaving enough skin for closure of the cutaneous margins without tension, as the arm is held in the position of right angle abduction. In other cases closure without much tension can be effected by bringing the arm nearer the side. Again, closure can be effected without a graft simply by the use of especially strong suture material to bring and hold the cutaneous margins in approximation. In each of these three methods of closure the horizontal elasticity of the skin lateral to the line of closure is utilized to help effect the closure. This skin has great elasticity, but it seems unwise, if one wishes to maintain full range of motion of the arm, not to preserve all of it for the purpose for which it was originally intended. Axillary skin and subcutaneous tissue are naturally abundant in order to provide for abduction and elevation of the arm.

The skin of the anterior axillary fold, as well as the skin of the anterior chest wall, has a remarkable degree of elasticity which comes into use during abduction. The reconstruction of the high axilla as recommended by Halsted shifts the lateral cutaneous flap to the area of the axilla where a small amount of elasticity has maximal degree of usefulness. Some of the elasticity of this lateral flap is utilized to effect closure about the axillary vein in the reconstruction of the high axilla.

These two considerations, then, the stretching of skin medially to close the defect of the anterior portion of the chest wall and the stretching of the skin of the anterior axillary fold superiorly to reconstruct a high axilla, make use of contiguous skin for repair of a surgical defect and thus serve to limit the amount of elasticity remaining for use when the arm is abducted. The suggestion is offered that the arm be placed at an angle of abduction slightly greater than 90 degrees and in external rotation before attempt is made to suture the cutaneous flaps. Then such portions of the margins of the wound as come together without tension may be approximated. Residual defect on the thoracic cage then may be covered by the application of a thick-split skin graft, after suture of the margins of the wound to the thoracic wall. This latter step is recommended because, unless it is carried out, the skin graft will undergo some contraction and no gain will be obtained from having placed a large graft. The graft should be cut large enough so that it can be approximated to the margins of the defect without tension.

It is believed that this method of closure assures that the axilla and the region of the anterior axillary fold will be covered by sufficient skin and subcutaneous tissue to allow full range of motion of the arm. It is as easy to obtain a relatively large graft as it is to obtain a smaller one. The thigh affords a generous donor site from which grafts of skin measuring 4 by 7 inches may be cut with regularity if a dermatome is applied so that the long dimension of the graft is in the horizontal rather than the longitudinal direction of the thigh. Because the graft is applied to relatively immobile external intercostal musculature and costal periosteum, the graft cannot, of itself, play any important role in the amount of elasticity of regional tissue preserved for abduction. Its usefulness lies in the manner in which it permits the operator to preserve all or most of the elasticity of the skin of the lateral chest wall and anterior axillary fold for abduction of the arm. It is important to preserve such mobility for the younger patient because, if he is cured of carcinoma, longevity is anticipated. Attention to this point also is important for the patients in the advanced decades of life because any diminution of cutaneous elasticity may be expected to reflect itself in further impairment of function owing to the problem of restoration of motion in joints which are immobilized temporarily in older people.

The thickness of split skin employed for the graft deserves consideration. A thick graft is preferable but a thin graft is acceptable since the thoracic wall is exposed to minimal trauma in adults. It is unquestionably important to secure a complete "take" of the graft. Failure of a portion of the graft is followed by infection, a causative factor in the development of edema of the arm. Areas of granulation tissue which undergo contracture before epithelization can undo partially the good functional result that may be expected after every precaution has been taken to supply the axilla with all the skin necessary for complete motion of the shoulder joint. Should any considerable portion of graft fail to grow, it is believed wise to apply a secondary graft as soon as the area can be prepared rather than to wait for epithelium to grow in from the margins of the secondary wound.

It is true that patients whose function of the arm is poor after mastectomy usually do not complain of this handicap. Attention to the problem of function of the arm is favored rather as something which the surgeon can offer the patient in addition to cure of the carcinoma.

SUMMARY

Function of the arm following radical mastectomy for carcinoma of the breast has been reviewed in 308 cases. The technique of the radical amputation of Halsted was followed in each case but there was variation in the type of closure. In 95 cases the wounds were closed by linear suture, without the use of a skin graft. In 131 cases a small skin graft was used, and in 59 cases a large skin graft was employed to cover the residual defect on the chest wall. Closure with a small graft was followed by full function of the arm in the highest percentage of cases. The use of postoperative x-ray therapy (regardless of type of closure of the wound) was associated with an increased percentage of patients who showed poor function of the arm. Other significant factors such as postoperative edema of the arm and the age of the patient have been taken into consideration in evaluation of the function of the arm after radical mastectomy. Data are listed which indicate that the closure of the wound of radical mastectomy by thick-split graft of skin is rewarded by full function of the arm in a higher percentage of cases than when simple linear closure is used. By the use of a thick-split skin graft, the elasticity of the lateral cutaneous flap, which normally allows for the full abduction of the arm, may be preserved. Thick-split skin grafts have been found to afford adequate protection for the thoracic wall. The use of a skin graft in the closure of the wound of radical mastectomy is viewed as an operative step which allows the preservation of full function of the arm in a group of patients who have good probability of cure of carcinoma.

REFERENCES

1. Halsted, W. S.: The Results of Operations for the Cure of Cancer of the Breast Performed at the Johns Hopkins Hospital From June, 1889, to January, 1894, Ann. Surg. **20**: 497-555, 1894.
2. Halsted, W. S.: The Results of Radical Operations for the Cure of Cancer of the Breast, Tr. Am. S. A. **25**: 61, 1907.
3. Pfahler, G. E., and Keefer, G. P.: The Object, the Value and the Technique of Preoperative and Postoperative X-ray Treatment in Carcinoma of the Breast, Surg., Gynec. & Obst. **85**: 35, 1947.
4. Holman, C., McSwain, B., and Beal, J. M.: Swelling of the Upper Extremity Following Radical Mastectomy, SURGERY **15**: 757-765, 1944.

CONSERVATIVE TREATMENT OF FRACTURES OF THE TIBIAL CONDYLES

BERNARD MAISEL, M.D., AND NELSON W. CORNELL, M.D., NEW YORK, N. Y.

(From the Surgical Department of The New York Hospital and Cornell University Medical College)

FRACTURES of the proximal end of the tibia extending into the joint are generally produced by either direct blows against the medial or lateral aspects of the knee or by forces directed along the shafts of the tibia or femur as in falling on the almost extended knee. Associated with this type injury, particularly following a direct blow to the knee, there may be varying degrees of disruption or of stretching of the collateral and cruciate ligaments. These fractures generally involve one but may involve both condyles with a variable degree of comminution or impaction of the bony fragments. The bony fragments may be displaced toward the medial or lateral aspect of the tibia or may be pushed down the shaft.

Because of concern that anything short of careful replacement of the fragments would likely produce a traumatic arthritis or osteochondritis dissecans, treatment of this injury most often has been directed toward as careful replacement as was possible of the fragments to re-establish a flat tibial table. The generally accepted methods for re-establishing the continuity of the tibial table include nonoperative compression manipulation by cabinetmaker's clamps, or operative replacement of the fragments and fixation of the fragments by means of screws, iron stove bolts, or grafted bony shelves.

In the case of the markedly debilitated adult, in the aged, or in a patient suffering with systemic contraindications to the vigorous pursuit of repositioning the tibial condyle fragments, a more conservative type of therapy seemed advisable. The cases reported here occurred in elderly women who either because of the extent and seriousness of their injuries or because of other contraindications to operative therapy were treated by immobilization of the affected limb on a posterior plaster splint extending from the toes to the upper thigh. By placing the thigh and lower leg in normal alignment the knee was maintained in a normal position for four weeks. During the first week it was necessary to tap the knee joint for bloody fluid to relieve the local discomfort. At the end of one month the patient was fitted with a pelvic weight-bearing walking caliper articulated at the knee and by this means weight-bearing was begun and continued for two months. At this time physiotherapy in the form of thermobridge, diathermy, and controlled active and passive motion was administered once per week. During the fourth month following the injury gradual weight-bearing without the walking caliper was permitted if there was x-ray evidence of bony union of the fracture. If x-ray evidence of bony union was lacking, the caliper support was continued and free weight-bearing permitted only after there was definite evidence of a healed fracture.

CASE REPORTS

Case 1.—E. K., a woman, aged 55 years, was admitted to the surgical service of the New York Hospital soon after having been struck by the bumper of an automobile. She was unable to bear weight on the left leg and complained bitterly of pain along the lateral aspect of the left knee. There was moderate distention of the joint by fluid and there were contusions about the knee. There was no evidence of injury of the collateral or cruciate ligaments. There were striking osteoarthritic changes in the hands and left knee. An x-ray examination revealed a markedly comminuted impacted fracture of the lateral condyle of the left tibia with approximately ½ cm. of downward and lateral displacement of the fragments. The anterior portion of the lateral table was considerably more depressed than the posterior.

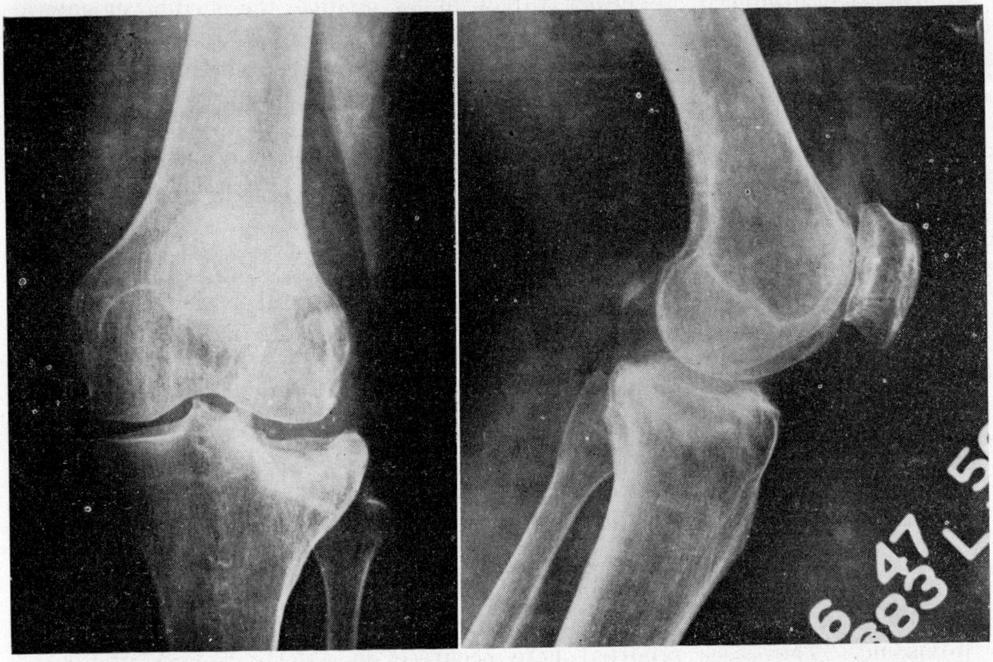

Fig. 1.—X-ray views taken two years after injury revealed a healed fracture of the lateral condyle of the left tibia with depression of this table level. The joint interval in the lateral half was increased due to the depression of the tibial table but the level of the femoral condyles was maintained and the alignment of the tibial and femoral shafts showed only slight varus deformity.

Because of the patient's rather poor general condition, the presence of osteoarthritis of several joints, and her own objection to operative treatment of the fracture, the right leg was immobilized in a posterior plaster splint extending from the toes to the upper thigh. One month after this period of immobilization a pelvic weight-bearing walking caliper, articulated at the knee, was fitted and the patient mobilized during the succeeding nine weeks with the assistance of crutches and later a cane. During this time weekly physiotherapy was provided and this included infrared, gentle massage, and flexion-extension movements of the knee. Four months after the injury the x-ray picture revealed healing of the tibial fracture with adequate callus formation. The position of the tibial table fragments remained unchanged. The walking caliper was discarded at this time and weight-bearing gradually developed during the succeeding months. Six months after injury the patient walked up and down stairs without pain or evident weakness.

At this time, two years after the injury, there was slight varus deformity of the knee. The knee could be actively and passively flexed to 90 degrees and extended to 180 degrees without discomfort. The patient walked about without a limp and experienced no discomfort upon climbing or descending stairs. Cold, damp weather produced slight stiffness of the knee without pain or swelling. An x-ray view (Fig. 1) revealed a healed fracture of the lateral condyle of the left tibia with depression of this table level. The joint interval in the lateral half was increased due to the depression of the tibial table, but the level of the femoral condyles was maintained and the alignment of the tibial and femoral shafts showed only slight varus deformity. There was moderate osteoporosis of the tibia and femur.

CASE 2.—A. L., a woman aged 62 years, was admitted to the surgical service of the New York Hospital soon after having slipped from the top rung of a six-foot ladder, landing on her feet. She was unable to bear weight on the right leg and complained of pain along the medial aspect of this knee. There was a fracture of the right radius. There was no evidence of injury of the collateral or cruciate ligaments or of the articular cartilages.

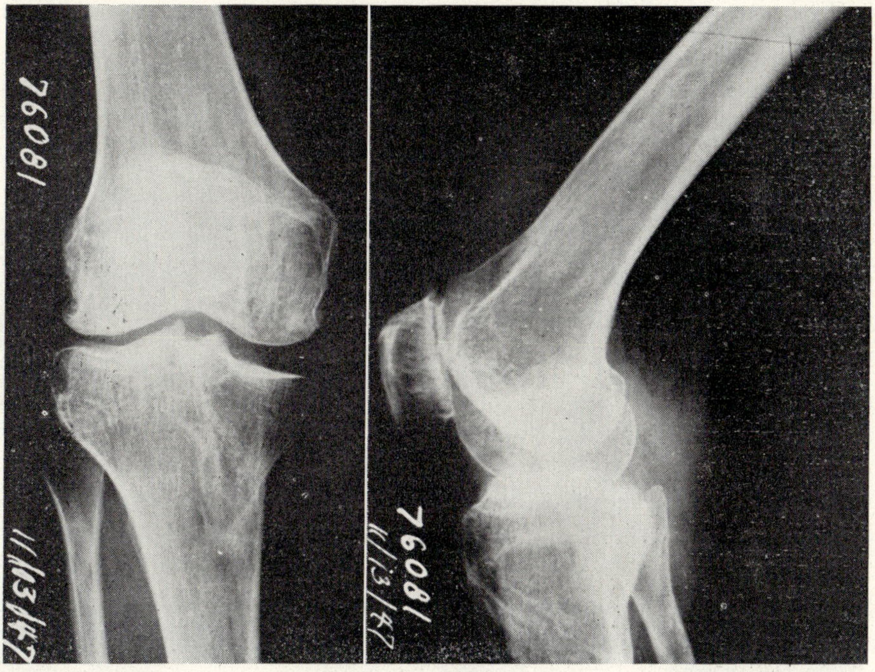

Fig. 2.—X-ray examination of the right knee performed 3½ years after injury disclosed a healed fracture of the medial condyle with distal displacement of this part of the tibial articulating table. The joint interval on the medial half was increased due to depression of the tibial table. However, the level of the femoral condyles was maintained and the alignment of the tibial and femoral shafts showed only slight varus deformity.

A right nephrectomy for hydronephrosis had been done fourteen years before the accident.

The x-ray examination of the time of admission disclosed a comminuted fracture of the medial condyle of the right tibia. There was lateral and distal displacement of the fragments with moderate varus deformity.

Two days after admission 70 c.c. of bloody fluid were aspirated from the knee joint effecting marked relief of the local discomfort. Because of the nephrectomy and poor general condition the limb was immobilized on a posterior plaster splint extending from the toes to the midthigh. Six weeks later because this patient could not afford a walking caliper a skin type plaster cast was applied to the right leg from the upper thigh to the toes incorporating in the cast a walking iron. Employing crutches minimal weight-bearing was permitted on the right leg during the succeeding eight weeks.

Three months after injury x-ray examination showed healing of the fracture of the medial condyle of the right tibia with callus formation and obliteration of the fracture line. There was some depression of the medial table and minimal varus deformity of the knee. There was moderate osteoporosis of the visible portions of the femur and tibia. A course of physiotherapy including thermobridge, diathermy, medium massage, and active and passive exercise of the knee was administered twice weekly during the next month and weekly during the fifth month after injury. Six months after injury the patient was able to walk without discomfort or limitation of motion. Slight swelling of the knee occurred during cold damp weather particularly after a full day of walking.

At this time, three and one-half years following the injury, there was slight varus deformity of the knee. The knee could be actively and passively extended to 180 degrees and flexed to 90 degrees without discomfort. She walked with a slightly perceptible limp and there was slight discomfort in climbing or descending stairs. Occasionally, during a hurried attempt to board a bus, as she stepped up, the knee seemed weak and she was obliged to grasp the safety rail. There was no swelling of the knee despite an active life. An x-ray view (Fig. 2) of the right knee disclosed a healed fracture of the medial condyle with distal displacement of this part of the tibial articulating table. The joint interval on the medial half was increased due to the depression of this portion of the tibial table. However, the level of the femoral condyles was maintained and the alignment of the tibial and femoral shafts showed only slight varus deformity.

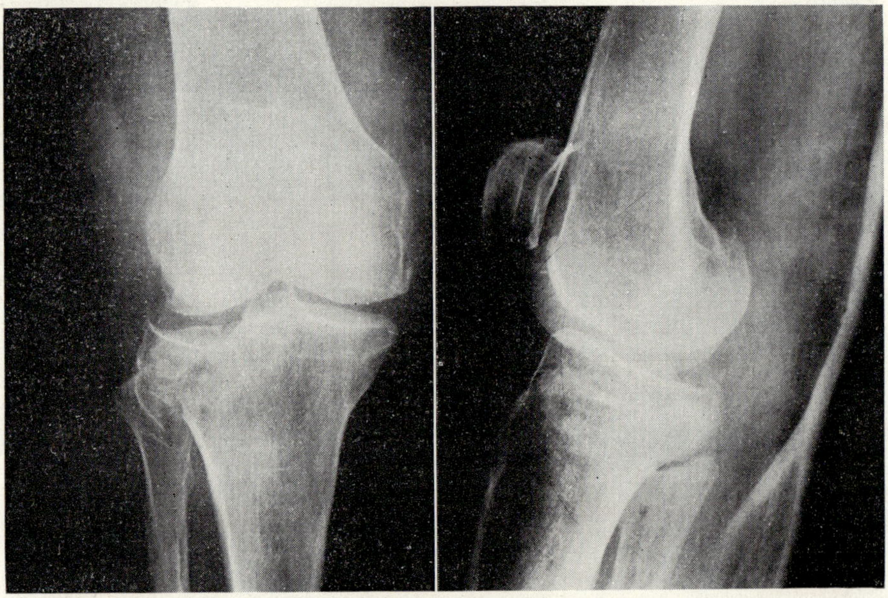

Fig. 3.—X-ray examination of the right knee at the time of admission revealed a comminuted impacted fracture involving the lateral tibial condyle with moderate lateral and distal displacement of the fragments.

Case 3.—H. C., a woman aged 67 years, was admitted to the surgical service of the New York Hospital soon after having been struck by the bumper of a taxicab. She was in profound shock. In addition to the fracture of the lateral condyle of the right tibia and weakness of the medial collateral ligaments of the right knee, there were multiple fractures of the pelvis and a compound, markedly, comminuted fracture of the left tibia and fibula.

An x-ray view (Fig. 3) of the right knee revealed a comminuted, impacted fracture involving the lateral tibial condyle, with moderate lateral and distal displacement of the fragments.

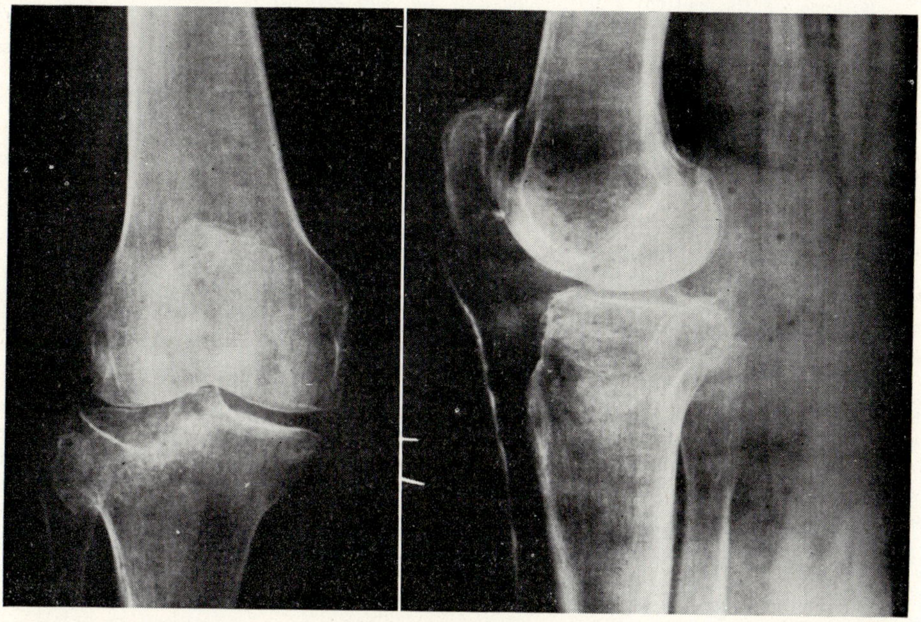

Fig. 4.—This x-ray picture taken four months following the injury disclosed a healing fracture of the lateral portion of the left tibial table with adequate callus formation. The position of the fragments remained unchanged. There was moderate osteoporosis of the visible portions of the tibia and femur.

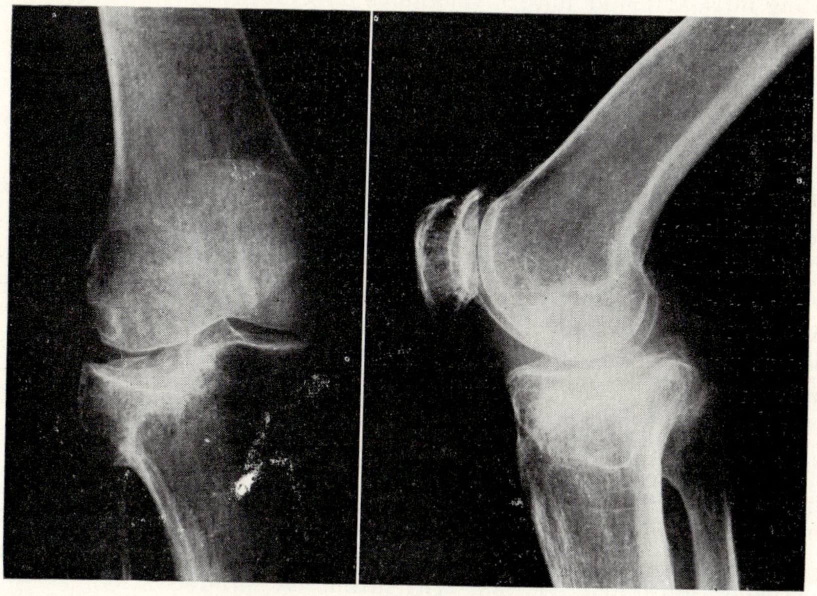

Fig. 5.—Roentgenograms of the right knee taken 1½ years after the injury showed a healed fracture of the lateral condyle of the tibia with distal displacement of this part of the articulating table. The joint interval in the lateral half of the joint was increased due to the depression of the tibial table. The lateral femoral condyle was slightly below the level of the medial condyle and suggested a minimal varus deformity. The alignment of the tibial and femoral shafts showed minimal varus deformity.

Because of the patient's poor condition and the multiple injuries, the right leg was immobilized in a posterior plaster splint extending from the upper thigh to the toes. Five weeks after admission, although she was confined to bed, physiotherapy, including massage and flexion-extension movements were carried out daily by the patient, who was an experienced masseuse. Four months after admission (see Fig. 4), when there was x-ray evidence of bony union of the fractures, weight-bearing was begun.

At this time, one and one-half years following the injury, there was slight varus deformity of the right knee. The knee could be actively and passively flexed to 90 degrees and extended to 180 degrees without discomfort. The patient walked with a slightly perceptible limp that seemed due to the slight deformity of the right knee and the partly stiffened left ankle. There was no discomfort or weakness upon climbing or descending stairs. Only slight swelling of the right knee, which was not painful, occurred in cold, damp weather. Except for the slight varus deformity of the right knee, at this time, there was no evidence of injury of the collateral or internal ligaments of the right knee.

An x-ray picture (Fig. 5) showed a healed fracture of the lateral condyle of the tibia with distal displacement of this half of the articulating table. The joint interval of the lateral half of the joint was increased due to the depression of the tibial table. The lateral femoral condyle was slightly below the level of the medial condyle and therefore suggested minimal varus deformity. The alignment of the tibial and femoral shafts showed minimal varus deformity.

DISCUSSION

Fractures extending through the tibial articular cartilage and the subjacent cancellous bony table of the tibia healed by means of fibrocartilage growing from the tibial bone through the fracture fissures into the joint.[1, 2, 3, 4] In the group of young patients this healing mechanism is often vigorous and in healing intra-articular fibrocartilaginous irregularities may occur in the tibial table surface producing pain and limitation of motion. In this group of patients irregularities in the cancellous bony surface with protruding bony elements as a result of poor position of a tibial condyle fracture may heal producing intra-articular bony spurs that may be painful and usually limit the range of motion. Fairly marked degrees of valgus or varus deformity of the knee may result from irregularities in the development of tibial cancellous bone and fibrocartilage reconstituting the articular surface.

In the young patient who has sustained injury to the tibial condyle, since subsequent vigorous use of the joint is generally contemplated, it is desirable that the fragments of a fracture of the tibial condyle be replaced to as normal position as possible to reduce the size of fracture fissures and bony prominences. Operative care is usually employed since the fragments of the injured condyle may have to be maintained by screws, bolts, or a built-up subcondylar bony shelf.

In the older patient the cancellous bone is softer, osteoporotic and following injury may be demineralized. The irregularities of the surface fragments of the fractured tibial condyle tend to be demineralized rather than to form tough bony spurs that may extend into the joint. In this group of patients the production of fibrocartilage that will ultimately produce union of the tibial condyle fragments and fill defects in the tibial articular surface is not vigorous.

One of us (N. W. C.) has had an opportunity to study cases of this last type in which exploration was done for the correction of internal ligamentous derangements or the removal of a torn semilunar cartilage, several months after treatment of a fracture of the tibial condyle. The tibial articular surface was covered with a smooth, gray, shiny layer of fibrocartilage (Fig. 6). This fibrocartilage had grown from the tibial cancellous bone through the fissures in the fractured condyle to fill the defects in the tibial cartilaginous articular surface.

During the period of healing of these fractures, if the body weight transmitted through the femoral condyle above the fractured portion of the tibial table has not been permitted to impinge on the tibial table, the regenerating fibrocartilage will extend over the surface of the injured portion of the table effecting a flat surface (Fig. 6).

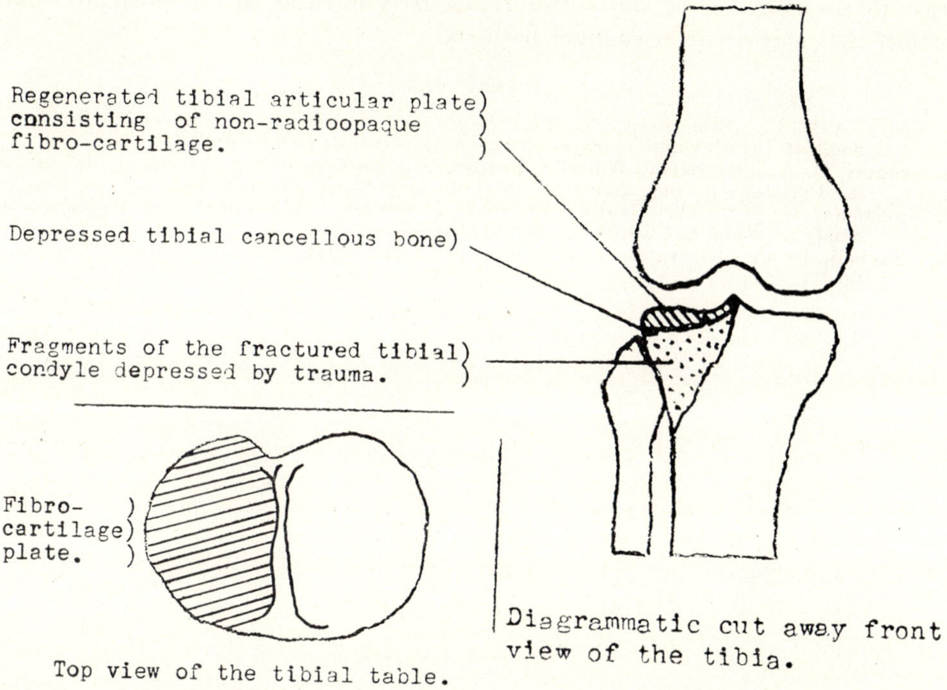

Fig. 6.—The fibrocartilage that proliferated from the tibial cancellous bone to produce union of the fracture of the tibial condyle may extend over the surface of the injured portion of the tibial table to produce a level articulating surface.

This newly formed articular surface cannot be visualized in x-rays since it rarely contains bony elements. One can readily infer its presence, for the alignment of the femoral condyles is normal and the alignment of the femoral and tibial shafts shows no valgus or varus deformity.

The roentgenologist generally reports widening of the joint space on the side of the old injury to the tibial condyle. This apparent widening of the joint space as seen in the roentgenograms (Figs. 1, 2, and 5) represents an increase in the width of the nonradiopaque tissue present between the cancellous bony surfaces of the femoral condyle and the re-established tibial condyle. Fibrocartilaginous tissue in these joints has re-established the tibial articular surface at a level that is recognized as normal if x-ray views of the injured and uninjured knee are compared.

SUMMARY AND CONCLUSIONS

The successful nonoperative treatment of fractures of the tibial condyles was accomplished by initial immobilization of the limb in a plaster splint and subsequent use of ischial weight-bearing walking caliper or walking type cast for ambulation. The relatively flat continuity of the tibial articular surface in the older patient can be re-established without intra-articular bony spurs and soft tissue irregularities in the joint surface by fibrocartilage growing from the tibial cancellous bone through the fissures in the fractured portion of the injured tibial condyle. This type healing of the tibial table fractures is in contrast to the bony spurs and softer tissue irregularities in the tibial articular surface that may occur in younger patients.

REFERENCES

1. Fisher, A. G. T.: Some Researches Into the Physiological Principles Underlying the Treatment of Injuries and Diseases of the Articulations, Lancet **2**: 541, 1923.
2. Bennett, G. A., and Bauer, Walter: Further Studies Concerning the Repair of Articular Cartilage in Dog Joints, J. Bone & Joint Surg. **17**: 141, 1935.
3. Haldeman, K. O.: The Healing of Joint Fractures. A Clinical and Experimental Study, J. Bone & Joint Surg. **20**: 912, 1938.
4. Campbell, W. C.: Operative Orthopedics, St. Louis, 1942, The C. V. Mosby Company, pp. 44, 45.

THE USE OF SODIUM TETRADECYL SULFATE IN THE SCLEROSING TREATMENT OF VARICOSE VEINS

An Experimental and Clinical Study

James A. Dingwall, M.D., David T. W. Lin, M.D., and
James A. Lyon, M.D., New York, N. Y.

(From the Department of Surgery of The New York Hospital and Cornell University Medical College)

SCLEROTHERAPY in the treatment of varicose veins has become a routine and successful method of dealing with this condition in suitable ambulatory patients. The results have been good and serious complications have been few owing to careful selection and good technique. Due, however, to subjective symptoms of pain and cramps all too often encountered when employing strong hypertonic solutions of crystalloids such as sodium and calcium chlorides and sugar, attention was directed to the soap solutions. These drugs, such as sodium morrhuate, sodium ricinoleate, sodium psylliate, monoethanolamine oleate, and others have largely supplanted the crystalloids in popularity. The soap solutions are better tolerated but distressing allergic manifestations of troublesome and occasionally serious nature have frequently been met with. Further there is evidence that recanalization detracts from the effectiveness of these solutions. Consequently, it seemed desirable to try another agent which might be less allergically toxic and at the same time more thrombogenic* even while less irritating and painful. Such a drug was described by Reiner[1] and was made available to us for study.† In his paper this author described the injection of sodium tetradecyl sulfate, a synthetic anionic detergent, into the tail veins of mice. Concurrently, sodium ricinoleate and sodium morrhuate were used as controls. It was found that sodium tetradecyl sulfate was a more potent sclerosing agent and produced less tissue reaction than the commonly employed soap solutions.

EXPERIMENTAL USE

1. Healthy mongrel dogs of either sex were selected and the major vein of all four extremities was injected with 3 c.c. of sodium tetradecyl sulfate in 1 per cent, 3 per cent and 5 per cent solutions. The method used was the "empty-vein" technique of McPheeter and Anderson.[2] Forty veins were injected and excised at the end of five days for microscopic examination. It was readily concluded that the solutions were effective in causing good thrombosis in the large majority of veins. There were some failures where the 1 per cent solution was used and instances of local irritation and reaction when the 5 per cent solution was employed. Since there was no apparent histologic difference in the obliteration effect between the 3 per cent and 5 per cent solution it was concluded that the former would be more satisfactory for clinical trials. There was no sloughing from inadvertent perivenous infiltration nor was there any evidence of a systemic reaction in any animal.

2. Intradermal wheals were raised on the backs of both dogs and rabbits using 0.4 and 0.2 c.c., respectively. Sodium tetradecyl sulfate, sodium

*The question of whether thrombosis is necessary for satisfactory sclerotherapy has long been discussed. There are some who feel that coaption of vein intima with fibrosis is necessary for satisfactory obliteration; that true sclerosis is not obtained by thrombus formation followed by organization. At the present this question is being studied in our laboratory and will be the subject of a separate communication.

†Supplied by Wallace & Tiernan Products, Inc., as Sotradecol.

morrhuate, and sodium ricinoleate were compared and although sloughing occurred in every instance the areas with their surrounding zone of inflammation were 50 to 80 per cent smaller with the test drug than with the soap solution controls.

3. Four series of five dogs each were chosen for study. The first group was fasted until the serum protein determination in every instance was 4.8 or below. Their veins were then injected as in Experiment 1 with 3 per cent sodium tetradecyl sulfate, 5 per cent sodium morrhuate, and 5 per cent sodium ricinoleate. The veins were sectioned at the end of seven days and all showed satisfactory obliteration.

In the second and third series the animals were fed 50 mg. of dicumarol daily until the prothrombin time was elevated to levels of from 50 to 140 seconds. (Normal levels in all dogs ranged from 8 to 11 seconds.) In all these animals the bleeding and clotting time was markedly elevated. Hemorrhagic tendencies were controlled by vitamin K but not until forty-eight hours after injection of the sclerosing drugs. The same sclerotics were again compared and, in addition, monoethanolamine oleate was used. There was a 50 per cent over-all failure of thrombosis which appeared in no way dependent on which sclerotic was used or to what relative level the prothrombin time was increased.

A final group was run as in the second and third series again employing dicumarol to prolong the prothrombin time. In these animals, however, sodium tetradecyl sulfate was used in 5 per cent concentration instead of 3 per cent. In this group the test drug gave an effective incidence of obliteration more than twice that of the other drugs both in number and degree. Still, however, there were random failures with sodium tetradecyl sulfate, even when one vein in the same animal showed complete success. These and other experiments using sclerotics in animals with depressed serum protein and in heparinized and dicumarolized dogs have been done and data concerning the effect of thrombogenic agents on the clotting mechanism will be reported separately since these are not considered within the scope of this paper.

CLINICAL USE

Reports on the use of sodium tetradecyl sulfate in the treatment of patients have been made by Cooper[3] and Hirschman,[4] who have concluded that this drug is more satisfactory in obliterating varicose veins; in accomplishing the desired end it causes less painful local reaction with a minimal risk of serious systemic complications than the commonly employed soap solutions. We have used this drug in approximately 200 injections using 66 patients from our varicose vein

TABLE I

			NUMBER
Obliteration			
Excellent			34
Good			8
Questionable			2
	NONE	MILD	SEVERE
Side Effects (Local)			
Pain	35	8	1
Irritation	42	2	0
Slough	40	3	1
Disability	43	1	0
Systemic reaction	39	4	1

clinic. In one-half of the patients it was the first time they had received sclerotherapy and the remainder had received injections with monoethanolamine oleate. Approximately 10 per cent of this half were chosen because they had encountered severe local reactions with pain and inflammation or had suffered allergic systemic reactions. Criteria in judging results were those commonly accepted in this type of therapy, namely, the extent and permanency of obliteration per injection, associated with the absence of undesirable local and systemic reaction. These may be quickly seen in Table I which includes only forty-four patients on whom adequate follow-up study was possible.

In 75 per cent of the injections the 3 per cent solution was used with a 1 per cent solution being employed in the remainder. Generally the weaker strength was given in subsequent therapy if a patient was noted to have any untoward side effects. In these cases, however, the 1 per cent solution seemed to have adequate thrombogenic potency and distressing pain following its use was uniformly absent. Where feasible, it was our practice to select the lowest available vein of the extremity which had a proved communication with the varicosed segments above either in the lesser or greater saphenous chains. A hypodermic needle was inserted, then the leg was elevated and milked of stagnant blood. A tourniquet was placed high on the thigh and the solution was given in amounts ranging from 1 to 5 c.c. The leg was left elevated with the tourniquet in place for ten minutes. In this fashion, particularly when larger amounts were injected, the resulting segment of thrombosed vein frequently measured as much as 40 and averaged 10 to 20 cm. There was no apparent correlation between painful reactions and the amount of solution which was injected. In no case was there any sudden or serious anaphylactic reaction. The systemic reactions noted consisted of slight fever and chills for a short time, generally noticeable about twenty-four hours after treatment. No reaction was considered severe enough to warrant discontinuation of therapy save in one patient.

It was particularly gratifying to note that the group of patients selected for treatment after having difficulty with sodium monolate were particularly free of untoward symptoms when the treatment was resumed using sodium tetradecyl sulfate.

SUMMARY

The results in experimental and clinical trials using sodium tetradecyl sulfate as a sclerosing agent in the treatment of varicose veins point out distinct advantages for this agent over the more commonly used soap solutions. Animal experiments show it to be a more potent thrombogenic drug and its use in patients has been confirmative. Further, the relative absence of side effects such as pain, redness, swelling, temporary disability and distressing systemic reactions appears to warrant its continued use rather than the widely employed soap solution.

REFERENCES

1. Reiner, L.: The Activity of Anionic Surface Active Compounds in Producing Vascular Obliteration, Proc. Soc. Exper. Biol. & Med. 62: 49, 1946.
2. McPheeters, H. O., and Anderson, J. K.: Injection Treatment of Varicose Veins and Hemorrhoids, ed. 2, Philadelphia, 1943, F. A. Davis Company.
3. Cooper, W. M.: Clinical Evaluation of Sotradecol, A Sodium Alkyl Sulfate Solution, in the Injection Therapy of Varicose Veins, Surg., Gynec. & Obst. 83: 647, 1946.
4. Hirschman, S. R.: Sclerosing Therapy of Varicose Veins With Sotradecol (Sodium Tetradecyl Sulfate), New York State J. Med. 47: 1367, 1947.

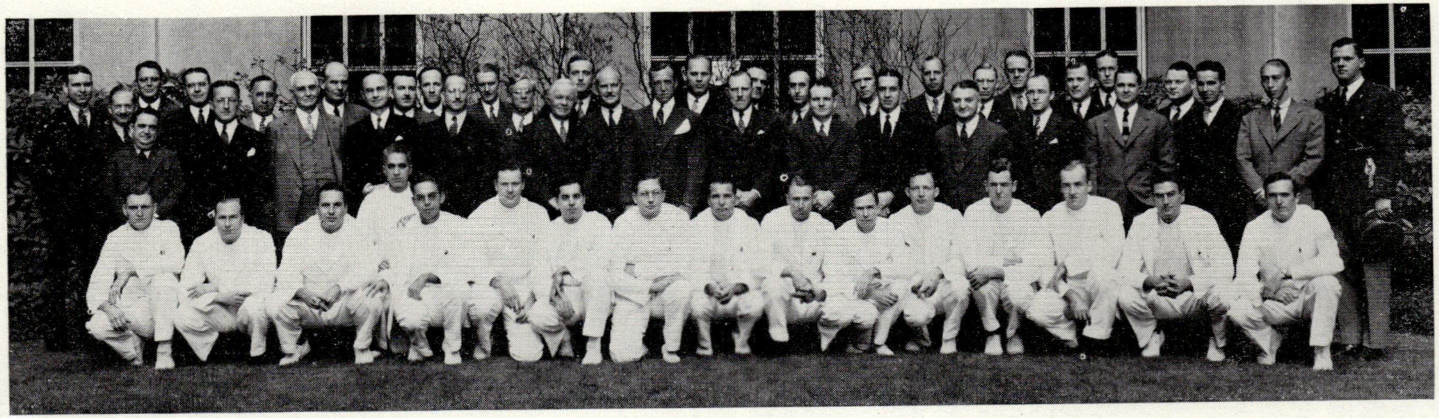

SOME MEMBERS OF DR. HEUER'S STAFF WHO ASSEMBLED FOR A DAY'S PROGRAM AND DINNER IN HIS HONOR AT THE NEW YORK HOSPITAL, NOVEMBER 8, 1941

Standing, back row: Benjamin Hoopes, John Draper, Ralph Bowers, Paul Sutton, James Doster, Herbert Conway, Frank Glenn, Robert Allison, Earl Ferguson, S. W. Moore, Cuyler Hauch, John Eckel, Cranston Holman, E. A. Kindel, Lester Huested, Lloyd Johnston, John West, George Eaton, Paul Hill.

Standing, second row: Joseph Heiman, Walter Reese, William Andrus, John Caldwell, Plato Schwartz, Max Zinninger, Henry Poer, Dr. Heuer, N. C. Foot, B. N. Carter, Beverly Douglas, Merton Griswold, Bronson Ray, Andrew Marchetti, Joseph Kauer, William Sandusky, Edward Douglas, William Cooper, Martin Healy.

Front row: Russell Hooker, James Dingwall, Carl Schmidlapp, Harold Genvert, William Quinn, Charles Neill, William Barnes, Gardner Child, Cooper Person, William Nickel, Arthur Chenoweth, Earl Lasher, Charles Chandler, Donald Morrison, Jere Lord, Eugene Cliffton.

Members of Dr. Heuer's staff not appearing in the picture include: Joseph Artusio, Harold Auerhan, Henry Babers, David Barton, John Beal, Glenn Bell, C. Bidgood, Courtney Bishop, James Boyd, Floyd Bragdon, Charles Brane, Richard Bullard, Sam Burnett, Arthur Console, Malcolm Cook, William Daniel, Armin Darmstaetter, James Davis, Robert Deans, Joseph Donnelly, Howard Dunbar, George Dunlop, Edwin Drew, Warren Eberhart, Adrian Ehler, Basil Faussett, Miles Fellows, Charles Findlay, Joseph Freiberg, Harry Fry, Scott Gardner, Richard Gates, Dan Gill, John Goode, Philip Gordy, John Gratiot, James Green, J. P. Grimes, Vincent Gorman, Glen Harman, Berton Hogle, Henry Hollenberg, George Holswade, Gustavus Humphreys, Francis Jackson, Cedric Jimerson, Charles Jones, Edward Keefer, Lee Kendall, Charles Kirby, George Knapp, Edmund Laird, David Lim-Yuen, Frances Lovejoy, George Lyford, Andrew McBride, Fred McLellan, Barton McSwain, David MacFarland, William Mahoney, Bernard Maisel, Victor Marshall, Guy Maynard, Stephen Meigher, M. C. Menard, H. L. Mikesell, Charles Neumann, Henry O'Brien, John Ogilvie, Earl O'Neill, Ward O'Sullivan, Herbert Parsons, Oliver Purnell, Francis Reinus, Ed Rose, John Schmidt, Morris Schnittman, Trimble Sharber, David Speer, Jean Stevenson, Harmon Truax, Preston Weadon, Willet Whitmore, Roscoe Wilcox, John Willoughby, Joseph Wilson.

SURGERY

VOL. 23 APRIL, 1948 No. 4

Original Communications

THE CHANGING STATUS OF SURGICAL CARE

I. S. RAVDIN, M.D., PHILADELPHIA, PA.

(From the Harrison Department of Surgical Research Schools of Medicine, University of Pennsylvania and the Surgical Clinic of the Hospital of the University of Pennsylvania)

I HAVE the most pleasant memories of my first visit to Rochester when as a very young surgeon I was told by the late John B. Deaver to take a vacation by visiting certain surgical clinics. Shortly after my arrival at the Clinic I met Dr. Judd, and I followed him closely for a week.

I saw him as a skillful surgeon. I saw him as a teacher interested in young men, offering sound advice from a life full of rare experiences. I remember well his taking me to a Wednesday evening staff meeting where I was shown a tragic accident which occurred during a supravaginal hysterectomy, and I well remember his admonition to me later, "Such tragedies happen to all surgeons—rarely to the prepared surgeon, but all too frequently to those who are not so well prepared." His terminal illness occurred, I believe, while he was on his way to Philadelphia to lecture.

With the acceptance of the antiseptic and later the aseptic discipline in surgery, "areas which previously had been denied the most intrepid of surgical adventurers were opened to all surgeons." Thus in the latter part of the nineteenth century and the early part of the present century emphasis was placed chiefly upon the technical aspects of surgery. The surgery of the body cavities took on a new birth, but the morbidity and mortality of many operative procedures, both old and new, were still high. This was in part due to the lack of knowledge by many surgeons of the normal physiology of the areas being subjected to operation and to an even greater ignorance of the deviations from the normal which occurs during disease. The responsibility for these circumstances was not solely the surgeon's. The frontiers of operative effort were extending so rapidly that physiologic and biochemical knowledge could not keep pace with them.

The Judd Lecture, given at the University of Minnesota, April, 1947.
Received for publication, Aug. 12, 1947.

I am reminded of an incident that occurred at a meeting of the British Physiological Society at Edinburgh in 1927. A symposium on the spleen was being held under the chairmanship of Sir Edward Sharpey-Shaefer. I sat next to Lord Moynihan for two hours while he became more and more restless. Finally after Professor Tait had discussed certain aspects of the spleen of fish Moynihan arose and said, "I have listened patiently for several hours but I have heard nothing that will help me in the care of patients with splenic disease." Sir Edward answered, "You must have further patience. Eventually we will be able to help you; perhaps what has been related this morning will be of help when it is better understood."

The high mortality which followed operations for thoracic empyema in the army camps during the influenza epidemic of World War I provides an excellent example of the failure of surgeons to use existing physiologic knowledge. In a few camps young surgeons, possibly as the result of superior physiologic training and possibly because of a lack of surgical skill, used interrib puncture instead of the traditional operation of rib resection. They placed the tube draining the thorax under water in some instances and in others applied suction to it. The methods which they used prevented pneumothorax and mediastinal shift. In these camps the mortality was relatively low; in others it was shockingly high.

It remained for Evarts Graham and his co-workers on the Empyema Commission to correlate physiologic, bacteriologic and pathologic knowledge to the immediate problem and a new era in thoracic surgery was opened. DuBois made the first careful studies on the nutrition of these patients and demonstrated how important it was that adequate nutrition be maintained during the period of recovery and convalescence.

George Crile had for some years been interested in certain phases of shock, in anesthesia, and in some of the problems of hyperthyroidism. He had tried to make surgeons realize that it was their responsibility to become more deeply interested in the problems with which they daily came in contact. It is true that his observations were not always correct nor his deductions always sound, but he stimulated an untold amount of research by clinicians and scientists which has been of immense value. Crile more than any other American surgeon of his time talked of improving pre- and postoperative care.

The "elder statesmen" at Rochester, of whom Dr. Judd was one, early realized the effect which scientific effort would have on the practice of medicine and surgery. Kendall, Mann, Rosenow, and many others were brought to the Clinic, not to engage in clinical medicine or surgery, but to expand the existing knowledge of the pathologic physiology of disease. Judd became a master surgeon because of his ability to utilize such contributions, as they became available, in the therapy of many surgical disorders. One only need read the contributions to surgical literature of which he was a joint author to be assured that he provided the incentive for many young men to study further the problems which they were daily meeting at the operating table and at the bedside.

It was during the period of the early twenties that one could recognize a more concerted effort by surgeons to reduce the morbidity and mortality of contemporary surgical operations by the introduction of improved methods of preoperative preparation and postoperative care. As the physiologist and the biochemist developed new techniques for investigation, they made a new body of information available. The surgeons, who could understand such knowledge, began here and there to apply it to the problems daily being met in the surgical clinic.

Such a change has had a profound influence on surgery. The borders of surgical effort were more widely extended. Many diseases which were not amenable to cure by medical therapy became subjected to surgical therapy and while cure has not always been attained a great measure of relief from suffering has been afforded. The morbidity and mortality of many of the newer, and most of the older, operations were greatly reduced. The surgeon began to be less afraid of becoming too scientific, and the pure scientist came to realize that the fundamental observations from the laboratory were more apt to find successful clinical application through the efforts of thoroughly trained young clinicians. A mutual respect and understanding arose between them.

As one reviews these early efforts in improving care and in extending the technical aspects of surgery, one might well gain the impression that surgeons are inclined to be faddists rather than critical scientists. We have gone through various eras in care and in technique. Intravenous therapy was slow in being adopted, but once it was we nearly forgot that the gastrointestinal tract was designed for a specific function and should be used whenever possible. Many surgeons did, and some still do, repair all inguinal hernias in the same way, or do every cholecystectomy or gastrectomy or thyroidectomy alike. Surgeons too frequently have become so concerned with methods that they have forgotten the importance of principles and the variable reaction of patients to disease. Too great emphasis has often been placed upon limited aspects of disease and upon certain specific aspects of care instead of realizing the interrelationships of many biologic processes.

In spite of these excesses I believe that a healthy process of development has taken place and that each phase of this development has added greatly to the knowledge of disease and to the safety of anesthesia and operation. Empiricism in pre- and postoperative care and in operative technique has become less evident although it has not disappeared, while sound clinical investigation has come to play an ever-increasing role in therapy in its broadest sense.

The Development of Surgery.—Harvey Cushing's intimate knowledge of cerebrospinal and endocrine physiology led to the development of neurosurgery as a special field of surgical endeavor, and he will always be looked upon as the first genius of this specialty. He insisted on painstaking histories of patients. He did not tolerate the divorce of the hand from the mind. A surgeon was to him an internist and something more.

The neurosurgeon must be a neuroanatomist, neurophysiologist, neuropathologist, and neurologist. Cushing stimulated an untold amount of basic and applied research, and he was respected by clinicians and scientists the world over. He won for neurosurgery a place which it had never before attained, and he and his disciples were responsible for a complete change in the surgical approach to many neurologic disorders.

Willy Meyer and Howard Lillienthal were among those who early espoused the cause of a surgical attack on certain intrathoracic diseases. The development of the negative pressure chamber was an attempt to meet the physiologic disturbances associated with intrathoracic exploration. It remained for Evarts Graham, John Alexander, Edward Churchill, and others to make the surgery of intrathoracic and intrapulmonary suppuration and benign and malignant tumors as safe as much of the intra-abdominal surgery. The surgery of pulmonary tuberculosis has provided new hope to sufferers from what previously was considered a purely medical disorder. And yet it may well be that streptomycin or some other chemotherapeutic or antibiotic agent may again return this disease to the category of nonsurgical diseases.

The brilliant work of Alfred Blalock who with Helen Taussig has provided a solution for the tetralogy of Fallot, of Robert Gross and Clarence Crafoord in the therapy of aortic coarctation, and of Reginald Smithwick in the surgical therapy of essential hypertension provides further evidence of the changing status of surgical care. The symptoms of many peripheral vascular lesions can now be relieved by sympathectomy. Embolectomy is today so common that a successful operation causes little comment. Already some men are devoting their entire effort to the problems presented by vascular disease.

D. W. Gordon Murray, at a recent meeting of the American Surgical Association, reported that when an area of experimentally induced cardiac infarction was excised before relaxation, dilatation, and paradoxical pulsation of the heart had taken place, cardiac failure and ventricular fibrillation did not occur, while death occurred in all control animals. We shall not convince our cardiologic confreres that this procedure deserves immediate clinical application, but Murray's concept bears testimony to the constantly widening interest by surgeons in what for years have been considered medical problems. And who would be so bold as to deny that before another decade has passed the outlook of coronary disease which claims so high a toll of our profession may in part be amenable to surgery.

For nearly two decades there has been general agreement that the best therapy for a gastric or duodenal ulcer, once a medical program failed to give relief, is a radical resection of the stomach and the ulcer-bearing portion of the duodenum if the ulcer is in that part of the bowel. It is, in my opinion, still the best operation for a gastric ulcer. The rediscovery by Dragstedt of the effect of vagus resection on total gastric secretion and hydrochloric acid production is another example of a physiologic approach to one of the most important characteristics of the peptic ulcer. An abundance of free acid induces chronicity of the ulcer, and is an important factor in the pain associated with the disorder. The etiology of these lesions is not yet clear although, as a result of the work done by Wangensteen and his associates, we know a great deal more than we did two decades ago. All are agreed, however, that an abundance of free hydrochloric acid plays an important part in the life history of these lesions.

Vagal neurectomy will not supplant radical gastric resection even for duodenal ulcer, but it provides a rational approach for the correction of one aspect of the pathologic physiology of this widespread disorder.

Many years ago Pasteur remarked, "Fate favors the prepared mind."

Those who have broadened and are broadening the horizon of surgical effort have had the necessary spirit of investigation in their fields of special interest. While in the main the fundamental work has been done by men in the basic sciences, a worth-while portion of it has come from the laboratories of surgical research.

The direction of surgical therapy must be more and more toward less destructive operations if lesser procedures can be found which will correct the pathologic physiology of a given disease. But until such methods are found, we must in certain instances move in an even more radical direction. Bold surgeons are now doing large operations for small tumors, and the end results of operation for many malignant tumors are showing definite improvement.

It is not possible to review all of the changes that have taken place and are taking place in operative effort, for they cover nearly the entire field of surgery. This is the result of many forces, some of which I have already referred to. It is the result of the greater responsibilities afforded young men of vision, who with modern training and an appreciation of the relationships between research and practice, have not been tied down by the dogma and empiricism of the so-called golden age of surgery. It is the result of improvements in anesthesia and anesthetization and in pre- and postoperative care.

Anesthesia.—Anesthesia, as we know it today, has contributed much to the maintenance of physiologic balance in patients during operation and in the postoperative period. Adequate working conditions for the surgeon are provided without the severe depression of body function which formerly was so common. Tissue damage secondary to anoxia is minimized by support of the circulation and inhalation of adequate concentrations of oxygen. The acidosis of deep ether anesthesia is recognized and avoided. Relaxation of the abdominal wall is secured, not by prolonged narcotic poisoning, but with spinal anesthesia or general anesthesia supplemented with a curare-like substance. The physician anesthetist no longer strives for a reduction in anesthetic mortality—this he has largely achieved. The goal now is a reduction in morbidity, a lowered incidence of postoperative nausea and vomiting, of atelectasis and pneumonia, of malaise and psychic depression. The anesthetist is moving in the direction of techniques which will accomplish these purposes to an even greater extent.

Preoperative Preparation and Postoperative Care.—The surgeon now recognizes that expert preoperative preparation and postoperative care are essential parts of surgical therapeutics. The operation remains, and probably always will remain, the most dramatic part of the surgeon's work, but a successful operation now means a well patient. The surgeon, as contrasted with the operator, is better equipped critically to evaluate the newer adjuncts to surgical therapy to the end that patients previously denied operation will receive it and that the morbidity and mortality of many operations will constantly decrease and the end results constantly improve. I can do no more than briefly review some of these concepts which have had and are having a profound influence in altering the status of surgical care.

Gastrointestinal Intubation.—The report of Wangensteen and Paine in 1933[1] on the use of gastric suction drainage marked a milestone in the care of patients requiring major abdominal surgery, in the therapy of acute intestinal obstruction, and in the control of fluid and electrolyte balance. Suction drainage is now utilized in every clinic to keep the stomach empty before operation, transforming what previously was a cesspool into an empty and clean viscus. Radical gastric resections can be done and the remaining gastric segment kept empty in the period immediately following operation. This practice has led to a substantial reduction in the morbidity and mortality of gastric operations. Acute gastric dilatation has now become a rarity in our clinics.

The development of the Miller-Abbott tube and its use by Johnston and Abbott[2] in acute intestinal obstruction unassociated with gangrene was a further step in gastrointestinal intubation. Wangensteen and Paine[1] had previously reported the use of short tube intubation in acute obstruction. There can be no doubt that in their hands and in others the use of suction drainage resulted in a substantial reduction in the mortality of this condition. In the best of clinics the mortality of acute intestinal obstruction prior to intubation was approximately 40 per cent. With the use of short tube intubation Wangensteen[3] reported a mortality of 17.1 per cent. Abbott and Johnston[4] reported a mortality of 9.3 per cent with the use of the Miller-Abbott tube, while with the same tube Whipple[5] and Leigh, Nelson, and Swenson[6] reported a mortality of 2.8 and 5.9 per cent, respectively.

Intubation has made it possible to maintain more accurately the fluid and electrolyte balance. With its use the pathologic effects of intestinal distention can be overcome, thus improving the general and local circulation and reducing the effects of distention upon respiration. It has made possible single stage resections of the right half of the colon, thus reducing the hazards of two or more operations. It has permitted the surgeon to take the poor-risk patient, dehydrated, distended, and in peripheral vascular collapse, and rehabilitate him to the extent that operation can be done with safety. It has proved to be one of the great aids to the abdominal surgeon.

It has stimulated an unbelievable amount of research and still more remains to be done. For many years we have spoken of paralytic ileus in association with diffuse peritoneal infection and yet in the presence of this condition I have seen the Miller-Abbott tube pass freely through the small bowel. Surely this could not take place if the bowel were paralyzed in the traditional sense.

Peripheral Vascular Collapse.—In 1918 Frank Mann[7] wrote of shock as follows: "A review of the results obtained in the extensive amount of work that has been done on the problem of shock, both experimentally and clinically, makes the point I have repeatedly emphasized particularly clear, namely, that the condition the surgeon calls shock may be due to a variety of causes. The variation in the primary etiologic factor in a condition in which identical clinical symptoms occur is probably the cause of the more or less contradictory conclusions arrived at by investigators, both experimentally and clinically."

In the intervening years a great deal of work has been done in this important field, and the advent of World War II stimulated further intensive research. It is now time that we attempt to reorient ourselves in regard to this condition. Recent carefully controlled investigations have cast doubt upon the concept that there is a generalized increase in capillary permeability in regions remote from trauma or even following severe hemorrhage.

Cournand and his associates[8] have shown that the essential finding in clinical shock in man is an inadequate venous return of blood to the heart with diminished cardiac output. A reduction in the circulating blood volume is, in most instances, responsible for these changes. In severe states of peripheral vascular collapse in man the blood volume may be reduced as much as 40 per cent or more. It is a curious circumstance that in the collapse of the circulation associated with some abdominal injuries and in severe infections the reduction in the effective blood volume may be much less than this.

Investigators and clinicians have long been baffled by the fact that with effective therapy some patients achieve homeostasis fairly promptly while others fail to do so. The work of Frank, Seligman, and Fine[9] has shed new light on this circumstance. They have concluded that "advanced shock constitutes a state of progressive deterioration which is not amenable to the types of therapy now available, probably because fundamental biochemical changes have developed as a result of a prolonged deficiency of capillary blood flow. These changes may result from changes predominately involving one vital organ, such as the liver, or from widespread cellular damage." Recently these authors have obtained further evidence which implicates the liver as the conditioning organ in the development of irreversible shock.[10]

The late stage of peripheral vascular collapse, so-called irreversible shock, cannot be overcome by restoration of, or even an increase over, the original blood volume. But surgeons now know that the irreversible stage of shock can be prevented by early and vigorous therapy directed toward maintenance of an adequate blood volume.

In the search for blood substitutes Wangensteen and his associates turned to bovine plasma. While the use of this material did not prove practical, it was helpful as a pilot experiment. Edwin Cohn fractionated human plasma and isolated a group of substances of great value to clinical medicine and surgery.

Two general statements can be made on the basis of the military experience with infusion fluids. First, while plasma or albumin solutions may be used as a stopgap in hemorrhagic shock, patients need whole blood to put them in shape for surgical procedures and to speed convalescence. Second, while concentrated serum albumin is effective in well-hydrated patients, it is relatively ineffective in dehydrated persons, such as desert troops. The military experience further emphasized the necessity of adequate volume therapy in shock. If a patient has lost 40 per cent of the effective blood volume, too much should not be expected from therapy which provides but 10 per cent of that lost. Lives can be and are being saved every day by adequate replacement therapy. For effective replacement one must determine the blood volume, and this is now being done daily in many of our hospitals.

To reduce the disastrous effects of irreversible shock we must rapidly and continuously replace a depleted circulatory volume, and we must just as effectively prevent overwhelming sepsis. In replacement therapy either plasma, gelatin, albumin, or whole blood should be used, and these will be found to be effective if the hypotension has been of short duration. Once significant metabolic changes have occurred in important viscera as the result of prolonged hypotension there is no therapy which today offers any hope of reversing the end stages of peripheral vascular collapse.

Chemotherapy.—In few fields of therapeutics has such progress been made as in the control of bacterial infections. For some years some progress had been made in our knowledge of infections and their control, but the contributions to the chemotherapy of bacterial infections during the past decade have had a profound influence on surgical care. The ability of the sulfonamides, penicillin, and streptomycin to check the spread of invasive infection is of enormous importance to surgeons. While our knowledge of the mechanism by which they act is still far from complete, thousands of patients throughout the world are deriving benefit from these substances which limit the ability of bacteria to survive in the tissues of the body.

Anderson,[11] working in our laboratories in 1934, after studies on the control of infections in wounds concluded that the major factor in the failure to control infection was the presence of necrotic tissue. He found that once the necrotic tissue was removed local surface infection was unimportant in the healing of a wound, for the wounds then proceeded to heal according to the Carrel-du Nöuy[12] formula. The brilliant work of Churchill[13] in formulating the reparative program in surgery in the Mediterranean Theater of Operations, which was of such great value to our injured troops, provided clinical substantiation of Anderson's carefully conducted experiments.

In the many thousands of battle casualties coming under the direct and immediate care of the 20th General Hospital, not a single patient succumbed to invasive streptococcic infections. Some died from peritonitis, some from meningitis, and others from gas gangrene, but the experiences of World War I, where thousands died from a spreading hemolytic streptococcic infection, were not repeated in World War II. While chemotherapy does not supplant the sound surgical practice of débridement, it serves as an important adjunct to this method of therapeutics.

Erysipelas is now so rare that we seldom find a patient with this disease to show students. Mastoiditis and thoracic empyema are fast becoming as rare. The bacterial population of the intestinal tract can be materially reduced prior to bowel resection by the use of certain sulfonamides and to an even greater extent by streptomycin.

The unfavorable course of experimental and even human peritonitis can be favorably influenced by sulfonamide, penicillin, and streptomycin therapy in spite of the fact that many of the pathogenic organisms found in peritonitis are not readily susceptible to these substances. It may well be that with the substantial reduction in organisms resulting from specific therapy the defense mechanisms within the abdomen, including the ability to mobilize large numbers of phagocytes, are sufficiently effective to overcome the residual infection. In the management of peritonitis the maintenance of the fluid and electrolyte balance, the relief of distention, and the use of chemotherapy all play an important part.

The dramatic control of these and many other serious infections by chemotherapy may well discourage investigators from attempting to solve fundamental problems related to infection. All serious acute infections and many chronic ones are associated with profound disturbances in normal physiologic function. We must know more about these.

Paul Cannon's[14] work on antibody production and phagocyte formation in protein deficiency is an example of such disturbance. The fact that many serious infections can now be prevented and others controlled must not deter investigation in this important field.

Thrombosis and Embolism.—Venous thrombosis and pulmonary embolism have long offered a tantalizing challenge to the medical profession. Kirby[15] in a recent article stated the following facts:

> Important recent concepts which are rapidly gaining acceptance are the following:
>
> 1. Venous thromboses of clinical importance, including those which cause pulmonary embolism, usually originate in the veins of the lower extremities, principally in veins below the knee.
>
> 2. Venous thrombosis and pulmonary embolism occur as commonly in the "medical" diseases as they do following surgical operations.
>
> 3. Venous thrombosis in the lower extremities of middle-aged and elderly persons confined to bed is a frequent occurrence, being found in about 50 per cent of such persons dying from all causes.
>
> 4. Acute thrombophlebitis and phlebothrombosis, or bland thrombus formation, are distinctly different pathological and clinical entities. In acute thrombophlebitis, which is readily recognized clinically by a marked inflammatory reaction and vasospasm, thrombi are usually firmly adherent to the walls of the involved veins. In phlebothrombosis, which often has minimal clinical symptoms and signs, or may not be recognized clinically, the thrombus is so loosely attached to the vein wall that it may be easily dislodged, with resulting pulmonary embolism.

At the Hospital of the University of Pennsylvania the incidence of fatal embolism has been about 1 in every 1,200 operations. Pulmonary embolism is responsible for about 5 per cent of all postoperative deaths.

In general, three measures are being used to reduce the incidence of fatal embolism. Early rising or ambulation has been advanced as a prophylactic measure against thrombosis and embolism. Van Jascke,[16] Zava,[17] Leithauser,[18] and others have made remarkable claims for early ambulation as a means of reducing the incidence of phlebothrombosis and of fatal embolism. In our clinic the data are not nearly so striking. During the past eighteen months early rising has been practiced nearly routinely, and the incidence of phlebothrombosis has not been greatly affected.

John Homans[19] was the first to advocate ligation as a means of preventing fatal embolism. The usual site of ligation is the superficial femoral vein or the profunda femoris. Numerous authors have advocated ligation of the inferior vena cava in the presence of thromboembolism. Allen[20] instituted the practice of prophylactic bilateral ligation before major abdominal operations, and he is convinced that this is a safe and lifesaving procedure.

It would be difficult to determine the number of prophylactic ligations that are now being done in surgical clinics in this country each month. It is even more difficult to justify the widespread use of the procedure on the basis of available statistical data. We have used it in several hundred patients as a prophylactic measure and following the development of phlebothrombosis of thromboembolism, and we are sure that some lives have been saved. It is, however, not entirely a harmless operation, for some of our patients have a residual edema which is troublesome, and others have developed skin changes which are at times most annoying if not alarming.

Heparin and dicumarol have been advocated for use as prophylaxis on the theory that it is increased coagulability of the blood that is responsible for venous thrombosis. Allen[20] has been a strong advocate of dicumarol therapy while Murray and Best[21] and Crafoord and Jorpes[22] have just as strongly supported heparin therapy.

It is an unfortunate circumstance that the advocates of one method of therapy are so positive that their method is the correct one. I am still unconvinced that in any one method we have the answer to this problem. If we were universally to reduce sedation before and after operation, if we were to bind the lower extremities from the time of admission of a patient until the time of discharge, perhaps we could reduce the incidence of phlebothrombosis and thus the incidence of thromboembolism.

Until significant data are available to prove the value of one method over another we are reducing sedation, binding the legs, and practicing early rising. When thrombosis appears, we have found it advisable to use heparin and dicumarol in certain cases and to ligate the veins in others. With such a program the incidence of fatal embolism has been materially below the previous fifteen-year average, but it must be stated that a longer experience will be necessary before data which are statistically significant are available.

Nutrition.—In few fields of pre- and postoperative care have such advances been made as in the field of nutrition. For years clinicians have believed that the nutritive state bore some vague relationship to resistance, but the complexity of this relationship is not yet solved. Varco[23] recently provided the best discussion I have seen of this important subject.

In the field of the vitamins alone great gaps in our knowledge are being filled. The administration of glucose by the intravenous routes demands an increased intake of thiamine, riboflavin, and niacin, and the administration of protein hydrolysates requires additional riboflavin because this substance is concerned with the utilization of certain amino acids.

Vitamin K has revolutionized the care of the jaundiced patient, and hemorrhage is no longer the major cause of death following operation. We have within a few short years nearly forgotten the anxiety which previously attended operations on the jaundiced patient.

Prolonged malnutrition leads to a reduction in the protein stores of the body and in the production of hypoproteinemia, the latter being a ready, although not always reliable, index of the extent to which the reserve stores of body protein have become depleted. The pattern is not always the same, as has been shown by the studies made by Keys and his associates[24] here at Minnesota.

When a protein deficiency exists with a severe anemia, the protein stores will be more rapidly replenished if the anemia is overcome by vigorous transfusions of blood, as suggested by George Whipple.[25] If this is not done ingested protein and minerals will be utilized first to overcome the anemia. The use of blood transfusions, in addition to adequate diet, when anemia and protein deficiency coexist, as they so frequently do, is thus placed on a sound clinical basis.

Injury, as well as disease, is frequently attended by prolonged periods of excessive nitrogen loss, and anesthesia and the very nature of the operation may impose a further drain upon an already depleted nutritional system. To what hazards are such patients exposed?

Cannon and his associates[26] have found that protein deficiency in the experimental animal is associated with a lowered activity of the antibody-producing mechanism and that the restoration of the depleted protein reserves results in the restoration of the normal capacity for antibody production. The data which they have collected strongly suggest that in the presence of a severe protein deficiency the "ability to acquire resistance quickly or to mobilize a specific immune mechanism effectively may also be impaired." In severe inanition the cellular tissues which supply phagocytes in large number undergo atrophy, and under such "circumstances the leukocytic tissues tend to revert to myeloblastic levels." Such tissues are not advantageously prepared to cope with acute infection by the liberation of adult phagocytes regardless of the amount of specific antibody which may be present. Protein depletion and malnutrition in this sense provide the circumstance where two of the most important biologic factors assisting in the control of infection are impaired.

As early as 1921 Whipple and Davis[27] showed that hypoproteinema conditioned the onset of shock following tissue injury. Ravdin, McNamee, Kamholz, and Rhoads[28] demonstrated that hypoproteinemia greatly increased the susceptibility to shock which resulted from hemorrhage.

Every surgeon of experience has observed how readily patients who are in a poor nutritional state develop peripheral circulatory collapse following anesthesia and operation. The reduced blood volume of these patients does not permit further great fluid loss before shock becomes evident.

The relationship of nutrition to wound healing is beyond question. In 1926 Wolbach and Howe[29] demonstrated that the specific important agent in the development of the intercellular cement substance was vitamin C. Later Lanman and Ingalls[30] showed that the tensile strength of healing wounds in guinea pigs was lowered in the presence of a C deficiency, and these findings were soon confirmed by Taffel and Harvey.[31]

In 1938 Thompson, Ravdin, and Frank[32] reported that in dogs suffering from a severe protein deficiency the healing of abdominal wounds was greatly delayed and wound infection and dehiscence were greatly increased. These observations made on experimental animals have since been confirmed by numerous investigators in man.

Donald Munro[33] first demonstrated the relationship of a protein deficiency to the failure of decubitus ulcers to heal, and his observations have been confirmed by Mulholland and his associates.[34] Every medical officer serving in general hospitals in this country during World War II became convinced that adequate nutrition was the most important factor in obtaining healing in such lesions.

Malnutrition, especially a severe protein deficiency, retards the laying down of callus in healing fractures. It plays a role in the healing of peptic ulcers. The exaggerated edema which occurs in the hypoproteinemic patient following operations on the gastrointestinal tract may so seriously retard normal function as to suggest a technical defect of the anastomosis. Malnutrition will accentuate many of the symptoms of hyperthyroidism, and the hyperthyroid patient who fails to gain weight in the preoperative period presents a more serious surgical hazard than does the patient who comes to operation with replenished body storehouses.

The value of a diet adequate in protein and carbohydrate, in vitamins and in total calories, in the preparation of patients with serious liver injury or fatty infiltration is now recognized by all surgeons.

The prolonged use of liquid and soft diets is an anachronism, and yet the traditional caution of our profession permits them to be used long after the period when a diet adequate in composition and in total calories would facilitate recovery and provide the building stones for more rapid and secure wound healing. Madden and his associates[35] have recently published important data from man in this regard. They found that of the two routes for supplying exogenous protein, the oral route was preferable. The intravenous route was valuable when oral intake was impossible or inadvisable. A pure amino acid mixture and a protein hydrolysate were not utilized as well parenterally as orally and neither was so well utilized orally as the natural food proteins.

These data are in agreement with those of Koop and associates,[36] who found that a positive nitrogen balance could be obtained in postoperative patients by the oral intake of 0.3 Gm. of nitrogen and 30 calories per kilogram of body weight per day, but that when intravenous therapy was utilized in such patients, the nitrogen intake had to be nearly doubled and the total calories increased by more than 30 per cent before a positive nitrogen balance was obtained. Intravenous therapy unless necessary is, therefore, extravagant and wasteful.

It is an unfortunate circumstance that the various nutrients have been considered all to frequently as independent entities. One group of workers is vitamin conscious, another protein conscious, and so on. It has been our experience, and I am sure it is the experience of others, that most patients suffering from a pronounced deficiency of nutrition have a complex deficiency.

We have passed through the carbohydrate era, the vitamin era, and are now in the protein era. Perhaps intensive interest in a special field has been helpful from the standpoint of clinical investigation, but the continuation of such limited interest retards rational therapy.

The best way to restore good nutrition is to feed the patient by mouth a diet adequate in carbohydrate, protein, and fat—a diet which contains the necessary vitamins and minerals. Only when the oral or orojejunal route is not available or when supplementation is necessary should parenteral therapy be employed.

Early Ambulation.—In 1899 Emil Ries of Chicago[37] advocated "some radical changes in aftertreatment of celiotomy cases," but the surgical profession as a group has continued to favor prolonged rest in bed as essential to recovery. During the past five or six years early ambulation has been receiving more widespread use. We had the opportunity to see it practiced in an extreme form in the Chinese Section of the 20th General Hospital. It was difficult to keep these patients in bed under any circumstances. They required less morphine than American patients, less cathartics, less frequent catheterization after operation, and infinitely less nursing care, and yet the mortality in both sections of the hospital was nearly identical. The convalescence of the Chinese patients was so rapid that we were amazed.

It is a bit startling to many visitors to see our patients who have had major operations walking around within so few hours after operation. Only the very obese, those with severe cardiac conditions, and those with serious infection are permitted the traditional form of bed care. The physiologic and psychologic advantages of this program are numerous.

Early ambulation facilitates the earlier restoration of a positive nitrogen balance. It prevents the rapid deterioration of musculoskeletal tone. It improves the circulation. Nursing care is reduced because fewer enemas are necessary. Finally, the psychologic effects of early rising are incalculable. Once out of bed the patient becomes convinced that the surgeon "knows he is progressing normally toward recovery."

Prolonged bed rest encourages a vicious cycle; inactivity results in prolongation of the time necessary for the return of normal function, an extension of the period of intravenous therapy, and prolonged periods of a negative nitrogen balance. These we are sure of, but there is no need to discuss this subject further when so many of the fundamental studies on convalescence and rehabilitation were made by Keys and his associates at this school. The greatest fear of early rising has been that it may interfere with wound healing and thus increase the incidence of wound disruption. It has not done this in the Arabs, according to Paul Harrison, and our experience with the Chinese is in accord with his. Evidence is already available, in fact, that early rising may facilitate the healing of clean wounds.

CONCLUSIONS

The passing years have brought a change in the concept of surgical care. Surgery is emerging from the narrow circle of the barber surgeons and from the belief that the great individual surgical technicians of the nineteenth and early twentieth century had given us the Golden Age of Surgery. The passing years have shown that teams of surgeons working as a group, each interested in science as a whole, but each becoming proficient in a special field, can do more to advance the borders of knowledge than can the individualist however skillful he may be.

Such a change in concept has resulted in an ever-increasing extension of surgical therapy to a wide variety of previously nearly hopeless disorders. It has led to a more radical approach to certain lesions and a more physiologic approach to others. It has led to a constantly decreasing morbidity and mortality of nearly all operations, and it has led to extensions in our knowledge of normal function and of the abnormalities which disease imposes upon normal function.

The surgeon of today is better equipped by training to evaluate the newer aids to therapy and to apply them. He appreciates the advantages of the newer anesthetics and their adjuncts and the value of trained medical personnel in administering them.

I repeat that the operation will probably always remain the most dramatic part of surgical therapeutics, but a successful operation now means a well patient who is restored to a useful place in society. The status of surgical therapy has changed and will continue to change to the end that patients previously denied operation will receive it and that the morbidity and mortality of operations will continue to decrease further and the end results continue to improve.

The science of surgery is in its infancy; even the art of surgery which Baron Boger 147 years ago said had reached the greatest heights to which it could ever attain is still to be expanded. If surgery is to remain a dynamic force in the medical sciences, it must constantly change as new knowledge becomes available. Surgeons, as well as all those who live and work in the field of experimental pathology, must be eager and willing to accept such changes. It was because of his facility to adjust so easily to the changing concepts of care that Judd was one of the distinguished surgeons of our time.

REFERENCES

1. Wangensteen, O. H., and Paine, J. R.: J. A. M. A. **101**: 1532, 1933.
2. Johnston, C. G., and Abbott, W. O.: Surg., Gynec. & Obst. **66**: 691, 1938.
3. Wangensteen, O. H.: Intestinal Obstruction, ed. 2, Springfield, Ill., 1942, Charles C Thomas, Publisher.
4. Abbott, W. O., and Johnston, C. G.: Surg., Gynec. & Obst. **66**: 691, 1938.
5. Whipple, O. H.: SURGERY **8**: 289, 1940.
6. Leigh, O. C., Jr., Nelson, J. A., and Swenson, P. C.: Ann. Surg. **111**: 186, 1940.
7. Mann, F.: J. A. M. A. **71**: 1184, 1918.
8. Cournand, A., Riley, R. L., Bradley, S. E., Breed, E. S., Noble, R. P., Lauson, H. D., Gregersen, M. I., and Richards, D. W.: SURGERY **13**: 964, 1943.
9. Frank, H. A., Seligman, A. M., and Fine, J.: J. Clin. Invest. **24**: 435, 1945.
10. Frank, H. A.: Personal Communication.
11. Anderson, D. P.: Ann. Surg. **108**: 918, 1938.
12. Carrel, A., and du Nöuy, P. L.: J. Exper. Med. **34**: 339, 1921.
13. Churchill, E. D.: Tr. Am. S. A. **62**: 268, 1944.
14. Cannon, P. R.: J. A. M. A. **128**: 360, 1945.
15. Kirby, C. K.: S Clin. North America, 1389-1403, 1946.
16. Van Jascke, R. T.: Chirurg **9**: 274, 1937.

17. Zava, L.: Policlinico (sez. prat.) **47**: 865, 1940.
18. Leithauser, D. J.: Arch. Surg. **47**: 203, 1943.
19. Homans, John: New England J. Med. **211**: 993, 1934.
20. Allen, A. W.: Bull. New York Acad. Med. **22**: 169, 1946.
21. Murray, G. D. W., and Best, C. H.: Ann. Surg. **108**: 163, 1938.
22. Crafoord, C., and Jorpes, E.: J. A. M. A. **116**: 2831, 1941.
23. Varco, R. L.: SURGERY **19**: 303, 1946.
24. Keys, A., Taylor, H. L., Mickelsen, O., and Henschel, A.: Science **103**: 669, 1946.
25. Whipple, G.: Am. J. M. Sc. **203**: 477, 1942.
26. Cannon, P. R., Chase, W. E., and Wissler, R. W.: J. Immunol. **47**: 133, 1943.
27. Whipple, G. H., and Davis, N. C.: Arch. Int. Med. **27**: 679, 1921.
28. Ravdin, I. S., McNamee, H. G., Kamholz, J. H., and Rhoads, J. E.: Arch. Surg. **48**: 491, 1944.
29. Wolbach, S. B., and Howe, P. R.: Arch. Path. & Lab. Med. **1**: 1, 1926.
30. Lanman, T. H., and Ingalls, T. H.: Ann. Surg. **105**: 616, 1937.
31. Taffel, M., and Harvey, S. C.: Proc. Soc. Exper. Biol. & Med. **38**: 518, 1938.
32. Thompson, W. D., Ravdin, I. S., and Frank, I. L.: Arch. Surg. **36**: 500, 1938.
33. Munro, Donald: Personal Communication.
34. Mulholland, J. J., Co Tui, Wright, A. M., and Vinci, V. J.: Ann. Surg. **117**: 512, 1943.
35. Madden, S. C., and others: Surg., Gynec. & Obst. **82**: 131, 1946.
36. Koop, C. E., Riegel, C., Grigger, R. P., and Barnes, M. T.: Surg., Gynec. & Obst. **84**: 1065, 1947.
37. Ries, Emil: J. A. M. A. **33**: 454, 1899.

THE PATHOGENESIS OF DIASTOLIC HYPERTENSION

PETER HEINBECKER, M.D.,* ST. LOUIS, MO.

(From the Department of Surgery, Washington University School of Medicine, and Barnes Hospital)

INTRODUCTION

IN THIS paper physiologic knowledge pertinent to an understanding of kidney homeostasis is presented. In addition, a concept of the pathogenesis of diastolic hypertension is offered which has evolved from such knowledge and from studies of Cushing's syndrome. Previously evidence has been advanced to show that this syndrome may result from atrophic changes in the hypothalamic nuclei or their compression by increased intraventricular pressure with a resultant depression of the neural hypophysis, without the presence of tumors of the hypophysis, of the adrenal, of the thymus, or of the ovary (Heinbecker[1]). Diastolic hypertension with circulatory characteristics indistinguishable from those observed in persons with essential hypertension invariably exists in persons with the syndrome.

It is postulated now that functional influences in the central nervous system, particularly in the frontal lobes of the cerebral cortex, in those constitutionally susceptible may be of sufficient degree to depress the hypothalamic nuclei which control the neural hypophysis, to initiate changes in the glandular hypophysis, and thereby in other endocrine glands to cause the diastolic hypertension called "essential" with characteristics similar to those observed in persons with Cushing's syndrome, but without the development of all the other stigmas of the syndrome.

The anatomic basis for such influences on the hypothalamus is well established. On depression of the functional activity of its nuclei there results a diminution in the secretion of the neural hypophysis. One consequence of this is to cause a stimulation of the eosinophile cells of the glandular hypophysis, which have been shown to exercise a trophic effect on the heart, the renal tubules, and the adrenal gland. Another effect is to sensitize the blood vessels to the constricting action of epinephrine, of desoxycorticosterone, and of renin. Overaction of the desoxycorticosterone fraction of the adrenal cortical hormone effects a constriction of the efferent glomerular arterioles of the kidney and thereby leads to the release of renin. The combined action of all three substances here as in Cushing's syndrome is believed responsible principally for generalized arteriolar narrowing and the development of diastolic hypertension.

The sympathetic nervous system and epinephrine are considered to act in a manner which is qualitatively somewhat similar to the aforementioned, but their action is regarded as periodic and temporary to meet emergency bodily requirements (Heinbecker[2]).

Read at the thirty-third annual session of the American College of Surgeons, Sept. 11, 1947, New York, N. Y.

*Recipient of a grant-in-aid of research from the Commonwealth Fund.

THE SECRETION OF THE NEURAL HYPOPHYSIS AND ITS CONTROL

The secretion of the neural hypophysis is entirely under neurogenic control since denervation of the secretory cell-containing tissue results in complete cessation of secretion (Heinbecker, White, and Rolf[3]). Fibers to the neural hypophysis arise in two hypothalamic nuclei, the supraoptic and the paraventricular. All cells of the supraoptic nucleus send their fibers to the neural hypophysis, 70 to 80 per cent to the infundibular process, the remainder to the infundibulum. The inferior rostral portion of the paraventricular nucleus, representing 30 to 40 per cent of its cell content, sends fibers to the median eminence, few if any being distributed to the posterior lobe (Rasmussen,[4] Heinbecker and White[5]). The cells in the superior caudal portion of the nucleus

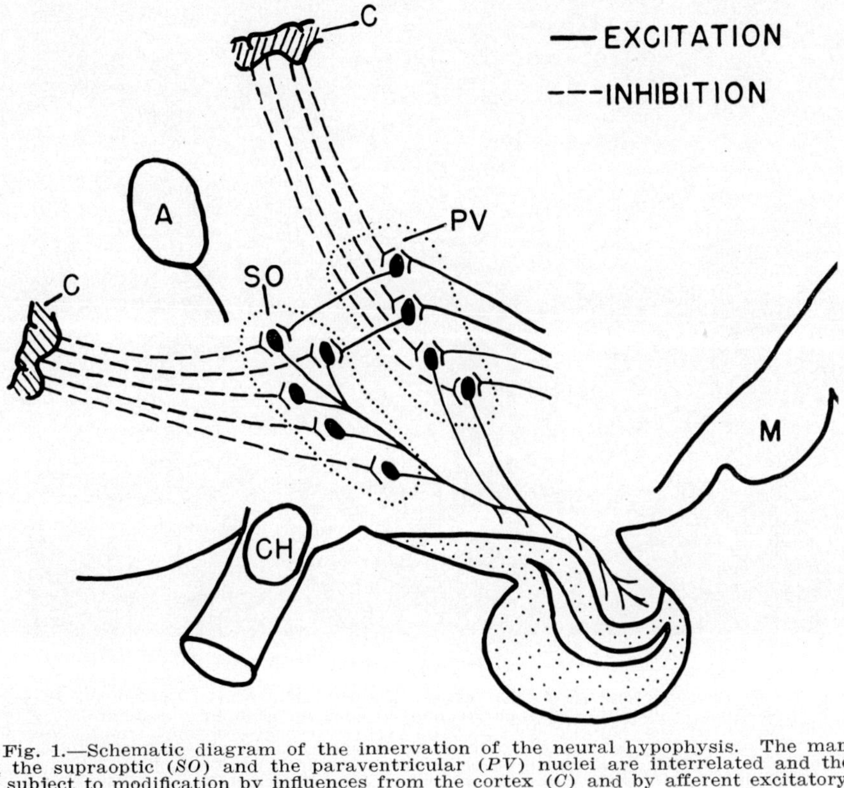

Fig. 1.—Schematic diagram of the innervation of the neural hypophysis. The manner in which the supraoptic (*SO*) and the paraventricular (*PV*) nuclei are interrelated and their activity subject to modification by influences from the cortex (*C*) and by afferent excitatory fibers to the paraventricular nucleus are indicated.

apparently send their fibers rostrally, not caudally, because following a puncture wound caudal to the stalk, between it and the mammillary bodies, the cells of the paraventricular nuclei do not show retrograde degeneration. When a lesion is made through the paraventricular nucleus the cells rostral to it degenerate. A lesion caudal to the paraventricular nuclei does not result in diabetes insipidus. This evidence supports the interpretation that fibers reaching the superior caudal portions of the paraventricular nucleus from below are afferent to the nucleus and exert an excitatory influence. Greving[6] has shown that the paraventricular nucleus is connected with the supraoptic nucleus by a chain of small cell groups and by a fiber tract, presumably affording a mechanism for influences on the supraoptic nucleus by the paraventricular nucleus. The manner in which the supraoptic and paraventricular nuclei are interrelated and under influence from other parts of the nervous system is schematically shown in Fig. 1.

EFFECT OF SECRETION OF NEUROHYPOPHYSIS ON THE GLANDULAR HYPOPHYSIS

In dogs it has been shown repeatedly (Heinbecker[7]) that total denervation of the neural hypophysis results within three to five months in a complete loss of basophile cells, leaving only eosinophile and chromophobe cells (Fig. 2). It has been shown also that a lesion in the hypothalamus caudal to the stalk, so

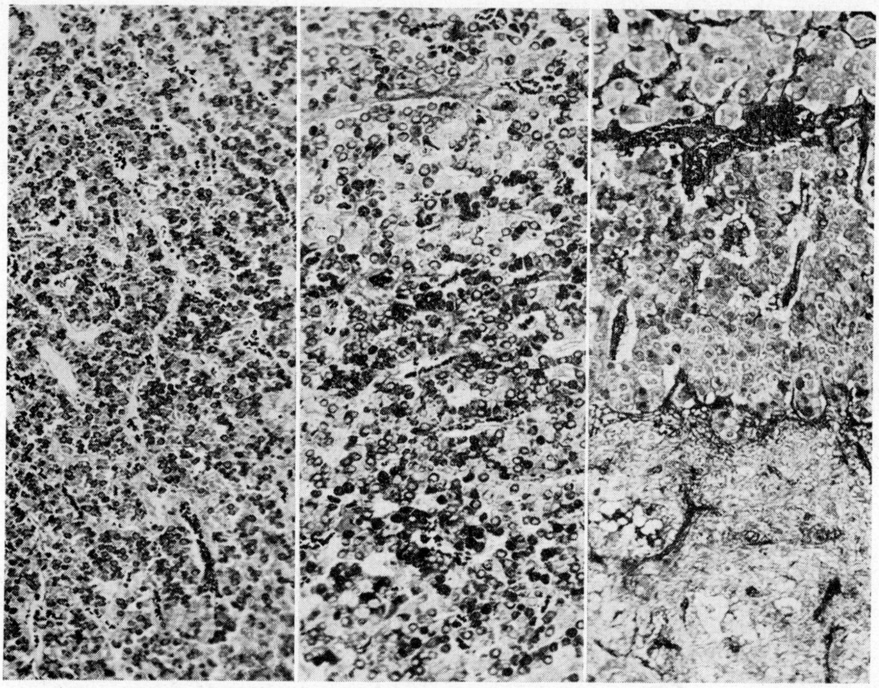

A. B. C.

Fig. 2.—*A*, Photomicrograph (×135) of the anterior lobe of the hypophysis of puncture dog, type 1, showing eosinophiles and chromophobes with no basophiles remaining. *B*, Photomicrograph (×135) of the anterior lobe of the hypophysis of a normal female control dog. *C*, Photomicrograph (×135) of anterior lobe of hypophysis of dog six months after adrenalectomy. Dog maintained on four implanted pellets of desoxycorticosterone of 125 mg. each. Note the large basophile cells, many chromophobe cells, and a marked decrease in the number of eosinophile cells.

placed as to interrupt fibers caudal to the paired paraventricular nucleus, decreases the number and lessens the density of the granules in the nuclei of the remaining basophile cells. The eosinophile and chromophobe cells remain cytologically normal. The exogenous administration of 40 units of Pituitrin and 5 units of Pitressin tannate in oil daily for thirty days has resulted in an increase in basophile cells of the glandular hypophysis (Heinbecker[8]).

TARGET ORGANS OF HYPOPHYSIAL EOSINOPHILE HORMONE

Examination of the endocrine glands of female dogs whose neural hypophysis has been denervated reveals that the adrenal gland and the corpus luteum do not atrophy. In male dogs the adrenal gland, the prostate, and the interstitial cells of the testis do not atrophy. In both the thyroid gland fails to develop colloid normally and the germ cells do not mature, due presumably to the absence of the basophile cells. It has been shown by us that in such dogs the kidney and the adrenal remaining after unilateral nephrectomy or adrenalectomy will hypertrophy to a normal or near normal degree (Heinbecker[9]).

EXPERIMENTAL PRODUCTION OF EOSINOPHILE CELL PREPONDERANCE WITH OVERACTION

Eosinophile cell preponderance has been produced experimentally in the dog in a number of ways (Fig. 3). It has been produced by total or partial denervation of the neurohypophysis. It has been produced also by the production of partial asphyxia of one adrenal gland according to the method described

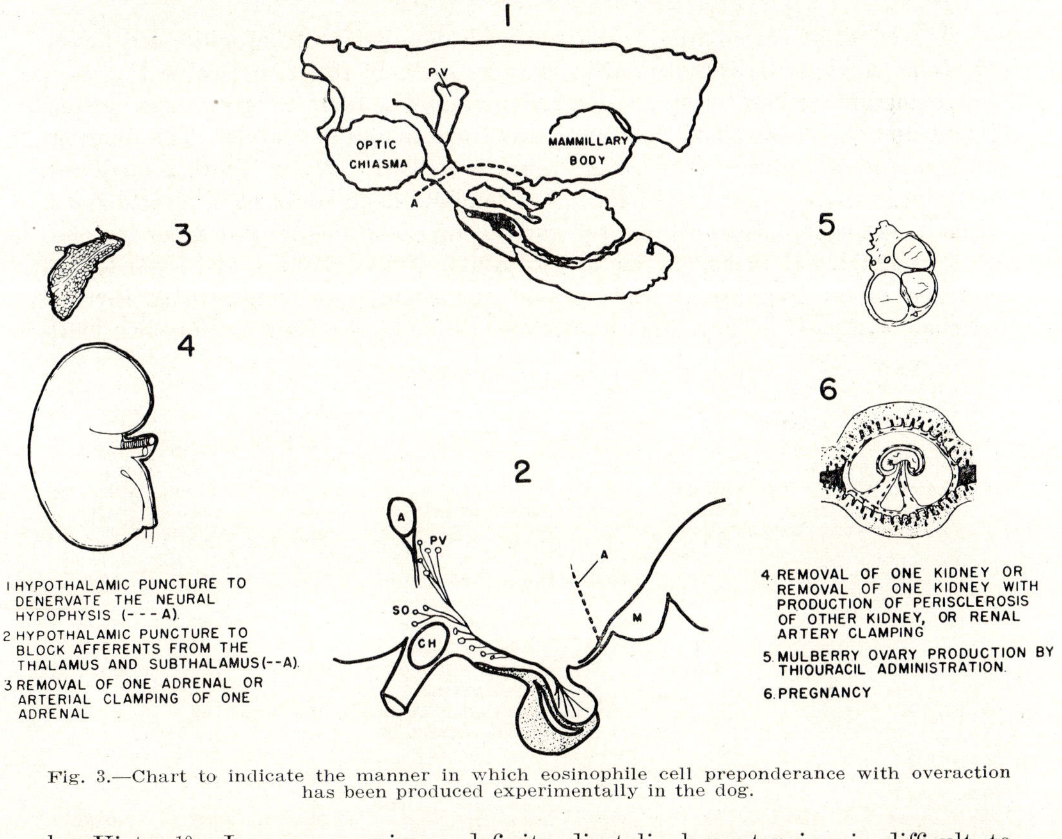

Fig. 3.—Chart to indicate the manner in which eosinophile cell preponderance with overaction has been produced experimentally in the dog.

by Victor.[10] In our experience definite diastolic hypertension is difficult to produce with any degree of regularity by this method. In two of three dogs the rise in mean pressure recorded through direct arterial puncture was 15 mm. Hg and in a third 30 mm. Hg. In the latter dog, serially cut 5 micron sections of the glandular hypophysis three months after the operation showed a definite eosinophile cell preponderance. In other experiments eosinophile cell preponderance was produced by wrapping a kidney in silk, the remaining kidney being removed. The change in the cytology of the hypophysis was evident five to eight weeks after the renal wrapping. In four female dogs it was found after the administration of thiouracil 4 mg. daily for six months. In such animals there occurred mulberry ovaries. The corpora lutea were highly vascularized and showed large actively secreting cells. The hypophyses of such female dogs revealed an increase in basophile cells such as are found after thyroidectomy, but also many more large, highly granular eosinophile cells than were found in the hypophyses of the male dogs after similar drug administration. The hypophysis of dogs examined during gestation shows a marked preponderance of eosinophile cells.

EFFECT OF EOSINOPHILE CELL PREPONDERANCE ASSOCIATED WITH BASOPHILE DEPRESSION ON BODILY FUNCTIONS OF DOGS WITH THE NEURAL HYPOPHYSIS DENERVATED

The effect of eosinophile overaction with depression of basophile cell in the glandular hypophysis is reflected in changes in body function (Table I). In a dog so modified, there occurs a marked increase in body weight. The cardiac output and the renal blood flow are maintained at normal levels. The diodrast thulium and the inulin diodrast ratio are increased. There occurs a moderate elevation in the mean arterial pressure, a fourfold decrease in insulin sensitivity, an increase in the plasma cholesterol, and a decrease in the percentage of lymphocytes in the blood to as low as 12 per cent. These changes are regarded as evidence of an increase in function of the eosinophile cell-adrenal cortical hormone complex. They are similar to changes resulting in persons with

TABLE I. RESULTS ON PUNCTURE DOG, TYPE 1

DATE	MEAN BLOOD PRESSURE (MM. PER HG.)	WEIGHT (KG.)	AVERAGE URINE OUTPUT PER DAY (C.C.)	HORMONE ADMINISTRATION	D CLEARANCE (C.C. PER MIN. PER M^2)	I CLEARANCE (C.C. PER MIN.)	D TM (MG. I PER MIN. PER M^2)
12/30/40 Preop.		14		None	250	82	13.4
10/13/41 237 days P.O.		25.7	5500	None	251	85	13.3
5/14/42		34	6500	8 days anterior lobe extract	458	128	27.22
5/21/42		34.5		15 days anterior lobe extract	332	116	26.5
9/29/42		37	7000	8 days adrenal cortical extract, 8 c.c. per day	460	140	21.3
1/ 8/43 686 days P.O.		36.2	5600	None	462	129	18.6
3/26/43	136	38	5500	None	306	100	28.96
3/ 6/44		35.9	4900	None	338	86	25.67
3/31/44		37	4000	8 days adrenal cortical extract, 8 c.c. per day	411	105	27.86
11/23/45 4 yr. 9 mo. P.O.		43.5	4800	None	261	110	23.44
12/ 7/45	140	43.5	4800	9 days doca, 4 mg. per day	268	110	25.3
12/20/45	160	43.5	5900	9 days doca, 12 mg. per day	240	163	26.1

Cushing's syndrome, whether due to an adrenal cortical tumor or to hypothalamic nuclear depression through atrophy or increased intracranial pressure (Heinbecker[11]).

In contrast a marked decrease of eosinophile cells in the hypophysis is associated with weight loss and a low blood pressure (Fig. 2).

SENSITIZATION TO EPINEPHRINE, TO RENIN, AND TO DESOXYCORTICOSTERONE

It has been found that a loss of the secretion of the neural hypophysis produces other effects which are significant in the problem of the pathogenesis of diastolic hypertension. These are a sensitization to epinephrine, to renin, and to desoxycorticosterone.

Sensitization to Epinephrine.—The evidence in support of the sensitization to epinephrine has been previously reported (Heinbecker[12]). The sensitization is considered to be due primarily to a decrease in the secretion of the neural hypophysis.

Sensitization to Renin.—Three groups of dogs are reported upon. In one group thirty were totally hypophysectomized, in another six were simply hypophysectomized (median eminence not removed), and in the third, five were punctured (type 1, Fig. 4). Attempts were made to wrap one kidney in the dogs of each group. It was found that such a procedure invariably resulted in death from shock within twenty-four to seventy-two hours of the dogs of the totally hypophysectomized and the puncture groups when marked diabetes insipidus was present. In the dogs which died there was no evidence of marked nitrogen retention, the highest recorded being 66 mg. per cent. The dogs recovered completely from the anesthetic and for twelve to twenty-four hours were apparently normal, eating and drinking. It was after this that they developed the symptoms of shock. There was no evidence of hypoglycemia or of adrenal cortical deficiency as evidenced by changes in the serum sodium and the serum potassium. The blood pressure fluctuated widely from slightly hypotensive values at the beginning to final low values such as are seen in shock. The state of shock was brought about chiefly by marked loss of plasma and of red blood cells into the walls of the gastrointestinal tract. There was always much free blood within the lumen of the bowel. The regions of most marked swelling and hemorrhage were the stomach, the duodenum, the jejunum, the lower ileum, and the first portions of the large intestine. The skeletal muscles often were dry and bloodless. Petechial hemorrhages were present in the brain, in the pancreas, in the liver, and in the lungs. The kidneys were grossly and microscopically intact, except for some enlargement of the wrapped kidney. These findings are identical with those which follow the clamping of both renal arteries so markedly as to result in rapid death of the animal (Goldblatt[13]). Dogs simply hypophysectomized stood the procedure of wrapping a kidney with some degree of depression, but after recovery the remaining kidney could be removed safely. Such dogs then went on to develop hypertension and in six to nine months uremia and death. The fact that simply hypophysectomized dogs permit the kidney wrapping indicates that it was not the loss of the glandular hypophysis which led to the sensitization to renin in the totally hypophysectomized dogs

Removal of one kidney could be successfully carried out in all three types of dog, indicating that the substance leading to the shock was released from the wrapped kidney.

From these experiments it is concluded that marked loss of the secretion of the neural hypophysis sensitizes a dog to a substance released from a wrapped kidney. Loss of the anterior lobe per se does not sensitize the dog to this substance. Kohlstadt, Helmer, and Page[14] and other investigators have demonstrated that, following the wrapping of a kidney, the substance released can be identified as renin. There seems no a priori reason to doubt that it also was the substance released in our dogs. The amount released from the wrapping of a

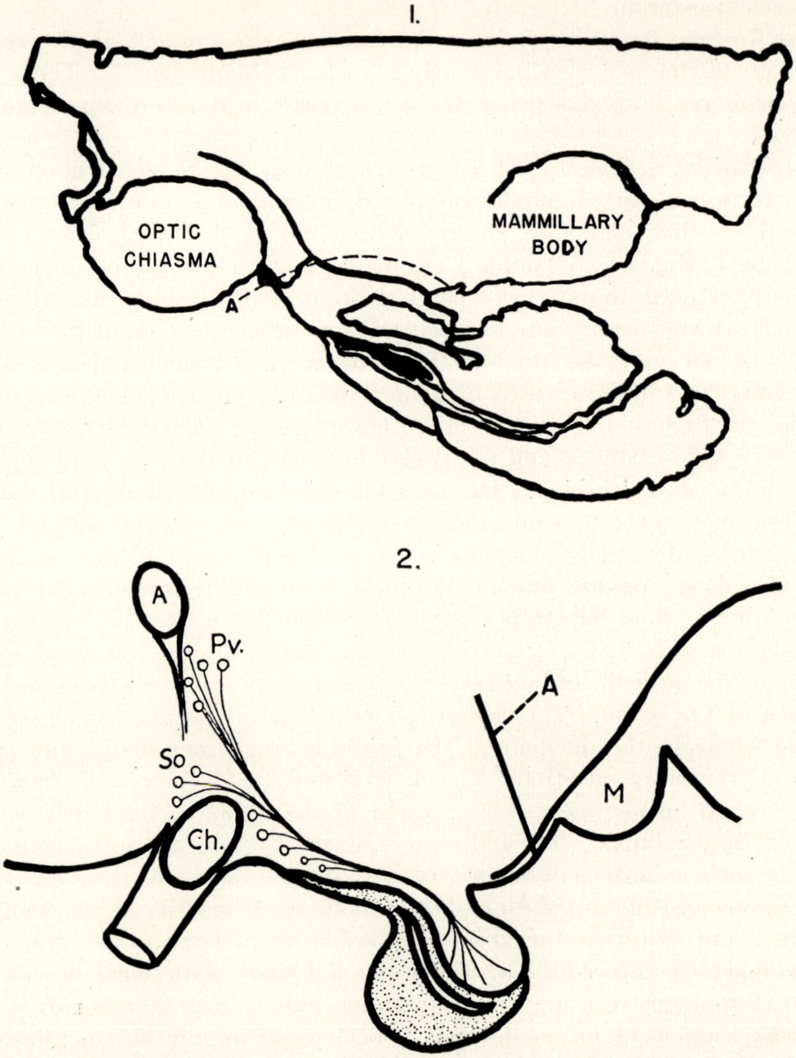

Fig. 4.—*1,* Diagram to indicate the site of the lesion (*A*) whereby the neural division of the hypophysis is severed from the supraoptic and the paraventricular nuclei. A dog so prepared is referred to as a puncture dog, type 1. *2,* Diagram to indicate the site of the lesion (*A*) for severing fibers afferent to the paired paraventricular nucleus. Such a dog is referred to as a puncture dog, type 2.

single kidney within twenty-four to seventy-two hours with the remaining kidney normal is assumed to be similar to that released when one kidney is wrapped in a normal dog, in which it is not sufficient to precipitate any untoward symptoms. The fact that death follows the procedure in dogs when the secretion of the neural hypophysis is lacking is interpreted as indicating that it is the absence of this secretion which sensitizes to renin.

Sensitization to Desoxycorticosterone.—It has been observed repeatedly in man and shown in the dog (White, Heinbecker, and Rolf[15]) that adrenal cortical deficiency results in an increased responsiveness of the blood vessels to the vasoconstricting action of desoxycorticosterone. Investigation in the dog with the neural hypophysis denervated but with the glandular hypophysis left intact reveals an increased sensitivity to the constricting action of desoxycorticosterone on the efferent glomerular arterioles as indicated by an increased filtration fraction greater than is customarily exhibited by normal dogs (Table II).

TABLE II. EFFECT OF NEURAL HYPOPHYSIAL DENERVATION (PUNCTURE TYPE 1) ON SENSITIVITY TO DESOXYCORTICOSTERONE AS INDICATED BY ALTERATION IN THE FILTRATION FRACTION*

REMARKS	D OR PAH CLEARANCE (C.C. PER MIN. PER M^2)	INULIN PLASMA CLEARANCE (C.C. PER MIN. PER M^2)	FILTRATION FRACTION
Dog K35			
Normal	279	87	.31
4 pellets (125 mg. each) desoxycorticosterone implanted 14 days previously	262	83.3	.32
6 mg. Doca per day for 6 days	270	90.9	.34
No extract for two days			
6 mg. Doca, 150 units Preloban per day for 5 days	345	120.7	.35
Dog X27			
127 days after puncture	237	73.3	.31
10 mg. Doca per day for 7 days	283	117.5	.42
Dog K18			
Normal	250	82	.32
4 yr. 9 mo. after puncture operation; no extract	261	110	.42
Doca, 4 mg. per day for 9 days	268	110	.41
Doca, 10 mg. per day for 9 days	240	163	.68

*Results of D or PAH and I clearances after the administration of desoxycorticosterone to a normal and to two puncture dogs, type 1.

EFFECT OF GLANDULAR HYPOPHYSIS ON CARDIAC OUTPUT AND RENAL TUBULAR FUNCTION

In other experiments (White, Heinbecker and Rolf[16]) it has been shown that in the dog hypophysectomy results in a marked decrease in cardiac output which is manifested within one week and may reach 50 per cent in four to six weeks. At this time the decrease in basal metabolic rate averages 30 per cent. The administration of exogenous anterior pituitary extract can be made to restore to normal or above the cardiac output of hypophysectomized dogs.

From the results of these experiments, it is concluded that the decrease in renal blood flow following hypophysectomy is to be attributed to a decrease in cardiac output rather than to any specific influences on the kidney blood vessels. Such a decrease in cardiac output does not occur in the dog with the neural hypophysis denervated and in which all basophiles in the glandular hypophysis disappear. This is reflected in the maintained renal blood flow in the dogs. From such evidence it is concluded that it is the loss of eosinophiles which is responsible essentially for the decrease in cardiac output following hypophysectomy.

After hypophysectomy the decrease in the capacity of the renal tubules to transport diodrast at high plasma levels always has been found greater than the decrease in renal plasma flow (Heinbecker, White, and Rolf[17]). It is held, therefore, that the eosinophile cells of the hypophysis exercise a direct trophic influence on renal tubular function.

EFFECT OF EXOGENOUS DESOXYCORTICOSTERONE AND OF RENIN ON URINE EXTRACT

In this laboratory, large doses of desoxycorticosterone (6 to 10 mg. daily) have been administered to totally hypophysectomized dogs with a resultant increase in urine output. Similar experiments in which even larger doses were administered to normal dogs with similar results had previously been reported by Ragan and associates[18] and by Mulinos and co-workers.[19] Such experimental results support the view that this hormone has certain effects which are antagonistic to those of the secretion of the neural hypophysis.

Experiments to show the effect of relatively large doses of intravenously administered exogenous renin on the blood pressure and the urine output of rabbits have been reported by Pickering and Prinzmetal.[20] These investigations have demonstrated adequately that a substance extracted from the kidney which has pressor effects and which is considered by them to be renin, also has a diuretic effect in the unanesthetized rabbit. The threshold for the pressor effect is considerably lower than the threshold for diuresis. The chloride content of the urine during the diuretic phase rises toward that of plasma. These investigators attribute the diuretic action of renin to an inhibition of the reabsorption of water, of sodium, and of chloride by the renal tubule cells.

THE EFFECT OF EPINEPHRINE, OF DESOXYCORTICOSTERONE, AND OF RENIN ON THE DYNAMICS OF RENAL BLOOD FLOW

The effect of exogenous epinephrine on renal blood flow has been studied by Smith.[21] He has demonstrated that in lesser concentrations it causes a narrowing of the efferent glomerular arterioles and in stronger concentration a significant decrease in renal blood flow, which is interpreted as indicating also a narrowing of the afferent glomerular arterioles.

The effect of exogenous desoxycorticosterone on renal circulation in the normal and in the dog with the neural hypophysis denervated has been investigated in this laboratory. A first effect is a narrowing of the efferent glomerular arterioles; then in higher concentrations there presumably is also some narrowing of the afferent arterioles as evidenced by a slight diminution in the circulation through the kidney as a whole. With the narrowing of the afferent arterioles there occurs a significant rise in systemic mean arterial pressure.

The effect of exogenous renin on blood flow through the kidney has been studied among others by Corcoran, Kohlstadt, and Page,[22] and by Goldring, Chasis, Ranges, and Smith.[23] Its ultimate effect is similar to that of epinephrine and of desoxycorticosterone.

RENIN IN RELATION TO HYPERTENSION

That diastolic hypertension may arise from factors primary in the kidney has been established by Tigerstedt and Bergman,[24] by Goldblatt and associates,[25] and by Braun-Menendez and co-workers.[26] It is not deemed necessary to review in detail the renin mechanism for hypertension, as this has been done recently by others (Pickering[27a]). The conclusion may be accepted that the kidney under conditions of altered hemodynamics releases renin, which working on a globulin substrate results in the production of a pressor substance, angiotonin, or hypertension. The circulation in animals made hypertensive by renin is similar in many respects to the circulation in persons with essential hypertension.

On the basis of evidence submitted in this report and that of other investigators in this field, it is believed that the factors responsible for the release of renin are those which cause a decrease in the amount of effective renal tubular tissue. This may result from a narrowing of the glomerular arterioles or of the larger arteries to the kidney or of both. The final effect is the lessening of the circulation to the renal tubules considered to be the source of renin. Known factors capable of modifying the dynamics of the renal circulation in this manner are the vasomotor nerves, epinephrine, and the desoxycorticosterone fraction of the adrenal cortical hormone. In addition to such nervous and humoral influences, there develop in man occlusive changes in the walls of the renal blood vessels themselves both in response to the hypertension and because of metabolic disturbances initiated by the very endocrine imbalances responsible for the functional arteriolar narrowing.

The decrease in effective renal tubular tissue may be brought about also by removal of one kidney. Following this, there results a preponderance and stimulation of the eosinophile cells of the glandular hypophysis and an enlargement of the adrenal glands. A similar change in the cytology of the glandular hypophysis follows the wrapping of one kidney with silk, the other being left intact. There occurs early also a definite hypertrophy of the unwrapped kidney and even of the wrapped kidney if the silk is loose enough to permit the expansion (Heinbecker[27b]). Inasmuch as it has been established that the wrapping of a kidney leads to the release of renin, it is assumed that the stimulation of the hypophysial eosinophile cells is due to the direct or indirect action of renin. Other things being unchanged, the overaction of the eosinophile-adrenal cortical hormone complex undoubtedly would cause some increase in cardiac output, and thus of general blood flow. Because the hypertrophy is confined essentially to the remaining unwrapped kidney, it follows that this kidney must receive a greater than normal fraction of the total cardiac output during its period of developing hypertrophy. Because a similar degree of hypertrophy does not occur in the absence of the glandular hypophysis and because the glandular hypophysis does not exert its influence on the kidney circulation in the absence of adrenal cortical hormone, it is postulated that the combined action of an eosinophile cell-desoxycorticosterone-renin hormone complex is to increase the blood supply of the remaining kidney to permit its hypertrophy. When the normal amount of renal tubular tissue has been restored, the release of renin ceases.

PROGESTERONE AND DIASTOLIC HYPERTENSION

Structurally, progesterone is related closely to desoxycorticosterone. Its hormonal similarity has been established in various ways. Thus, Gaunt and Hays[28] showed that its administration aids in keeping adrenalectomized ferrets alive. McKeown and Spurrell[29] proved the life of adrenalectomized rats is prolonged in pregnancy. Thorn and Engel[30] have shown that sodium retention and a slight decrease in urine output follow its administration.

Progesterone renders the uterine musculature insensitive to Pituitrin (Reynolds and Allen[31]). This accounts for the failure of the uterus of the pregnant rabbit to respond to Pituitrin (Knaus[32]). It suggests that the eosinophile cell preponderance in the hypophysis of pregnancy may result from such insensitivity to Pituitrin because the absence of Pituitrin has been shown to result in eosinophile cell preponderance and a loss of basophile cells in the dog. The adrenal hypertrophy associated with pregnancy could be attributed to such eosinophile cell preponderance because of the trophic relationship of these cells to the adrenal cortex.

In the case of Cushing's syndrome associated with an ovarian tumor reported by Norris,[33] it is assumed that the hormone secreted by the tumor was progesterone rather than estrogen because Zondek[34] has shown that large amounts of estrogenic substances depress the eosinophile but not the basophile cells. In the case reported by Norris the eosinophile cells were normal, whereas the basophile cells showed degranulation as in all other cases of Cushing's syndrome. The patient in Norris' case exhibited diastolic hypertension and arteriosclerosis.

It would be anticipated, then, that in pregnancy progesterone might exert an influence similar to that of desoxycorticosterone on the blood vessels.* Sensitization to progesterone would be expected to follow from its neutralizing influence on the secretion of the neural hypophysis.

DIASTOLIC HYPERTENSION IN PERSONS EXHIBITING CUSHING'S SYNDROME

Evidence has been presented (Heinbecker,[35, 36]) that the primary cause of Cushing's syndrome may be (1) an adrenal cortical tumor, (2) a tumor of the ovary, or (3) a tumor of the thymus. In a group of cases without any primary tumor it has been shown (4) that the initiating cause may be a depression of the paraventricular nuclei of the hypothalamus and, to a lesser degree, of other hypothalamic nuclei, particularly the supraoptic. This depression was due in five cases to an actual atrophy of the nuclear cells but in one instance was shown to be functional because recovery occurred on release of an increased intraventricular pressure on removal of a meningioma at the foramen magnum. In

*It has been reported by M. L. Goldman and H. A. Schroeder in the Federation Proceedings of the American Physiological Society, March, 1948, that the intravenous injection of 5 mg. of progesterone in 2.5 c.c. of propylene glycol in persons with essential hypertension was followed by an elevation in blood pressure.

the five cases in which atrophy of the nuclei was found, the flattened ependymal lining of enlarged ventricles indicated that pressure could have been responsible for the atrophic changes. In two early recent cases of Cushing's syndrome the intraventricular pressure was measured and found to be twice the normal. These observations suggest the possibility that an alteration in the hemodynamics of the intraventricular circulation in the tela choroidea similar to that involving the vessels of the face might be responsible for the increased intraventricular pressure.

All primary causes invariably lead to a degranulation or hyalinization of the basophile cells of the hypophysis as described by Crooke.[37] Evidence was presented to support the interpretation that when the primary cause is a tumor, its secretion may directly or indirectly have the capacity to neutralize the effectiveness of the secretion of the neural hypophysis. This brings about the same depression of the maturation of basophile cells with stimulation of eosinophile cell maturation as does a decrease of the secretion of the neural hypophysis when due to a depression of the function of hypothalamic nuclei which control its secretion. The signs and symptoms of Cushing's syndrome are such as to indicate that in this disease process the eosinophile cells are polyvalent in their trophic influence, as the adrenal cortical function is altered in relation to salt and water balance, and to metabolic and to androgenic functions. Diastolic hypertension with circulatory characteristics similar to those exhibited by persons with essential hypertension invariably develops. Arteriosclerosis indistinguishable in its nature and distribution from that seen in persons with essential hypertension also occurs. In cases of Cushing's syndrome not associated with primary tumors, the overaction of the eosinophiles is responsible for the initiation of changes leading to hypertension primarily through its stimulation of the adrenal cortex. In persons whose blood vessels, because of constitutional factors, are sensitized to the constricting action of its desoxycorticosterone fraction, generalized arteriolar narrowing as well as constriction of the efferent glomerular arterioles is effected. Constriction of the latter arterioles would be expected to result in the release of renin. On the basis of our experimental findings, such persons would be sensitized to renin, to desoxycorticosterone, and to epinephrine to the degree to which the secretion of the neural hypophysis is decreased or rendered ineffective. The overaction of the metabolic fraction of the adrenal cortical hormone, because of its influence on the metabolism of neutral fat and cholesterol, presumably leads to the infiltration of the walls of the arterioles with these substances and thereby to the development of arteriosclerosis, which makes the hypertension permanent (Heinbecker, White, and Rolf[38]).

A schematic diagram of the mechanism of development of the endocrine disturbances which lead to diastolic hypertension in Cushing's syndrome when the primary lesion is a depression of the hypothalamic nuclei is shown in Fig. 5.

DISCUSSION

Experimental and clinicopathologic evidence has been presented which now will be utilized to outline a homeostatic mechanism of which the kidney is the focus (Fig. 6). The mechanism involves the interaction of the nervous system and the endocrine glands on the kidney. Its function is to maintain the adequacy of kidney filtration and kidney tubular function. This is accomplished whenever necessary by narrowing the caliber of the extrarenal and the efferent glomerular arterioles with a concomitant stimulation of the heart to maintain the cardiac output within the normal range. Direct stimulation of renal tubular cells also is involved. Pathologic processes in the nervous system, in the endocrine glands, and in the kidney may disturb the quantitative relationships of the

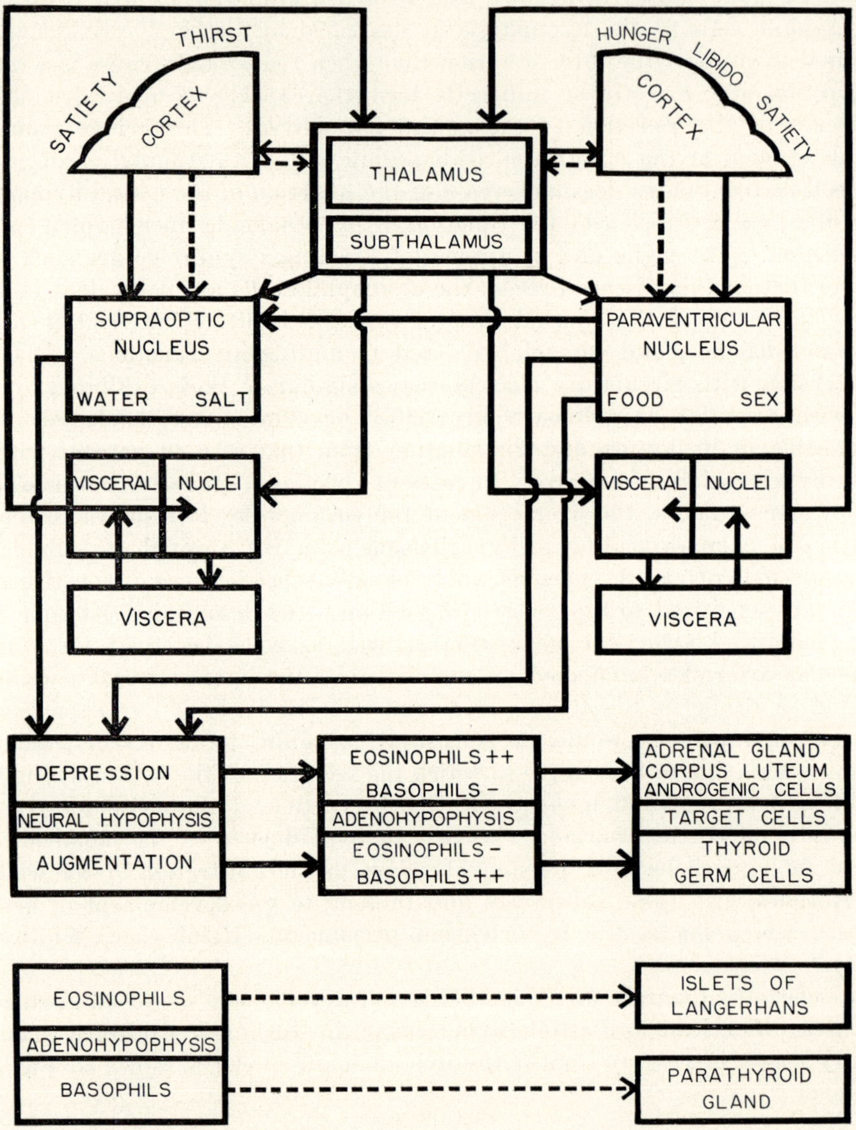

Fig. 5.—Diagram to indicate nervous system and glandular interrelationships in the production of Cushing's syndrome due to a primary lesion in the hypothalamus. (——→ excitatory, - - - -→ inhibitory influences.)

mechanism to result in diastolic hypertension. Depending upon which of the primary components of the mechanism the pathologic process involves, the associated signs and symptoms may vary. Whenever much derangement causes renal tubular inadequacy the secretion of renin is invoked to compensate by the induction of diastolic hypertension. It is assumed that in constitutionally susceptible persons the mechanism may be deranged through functional influences

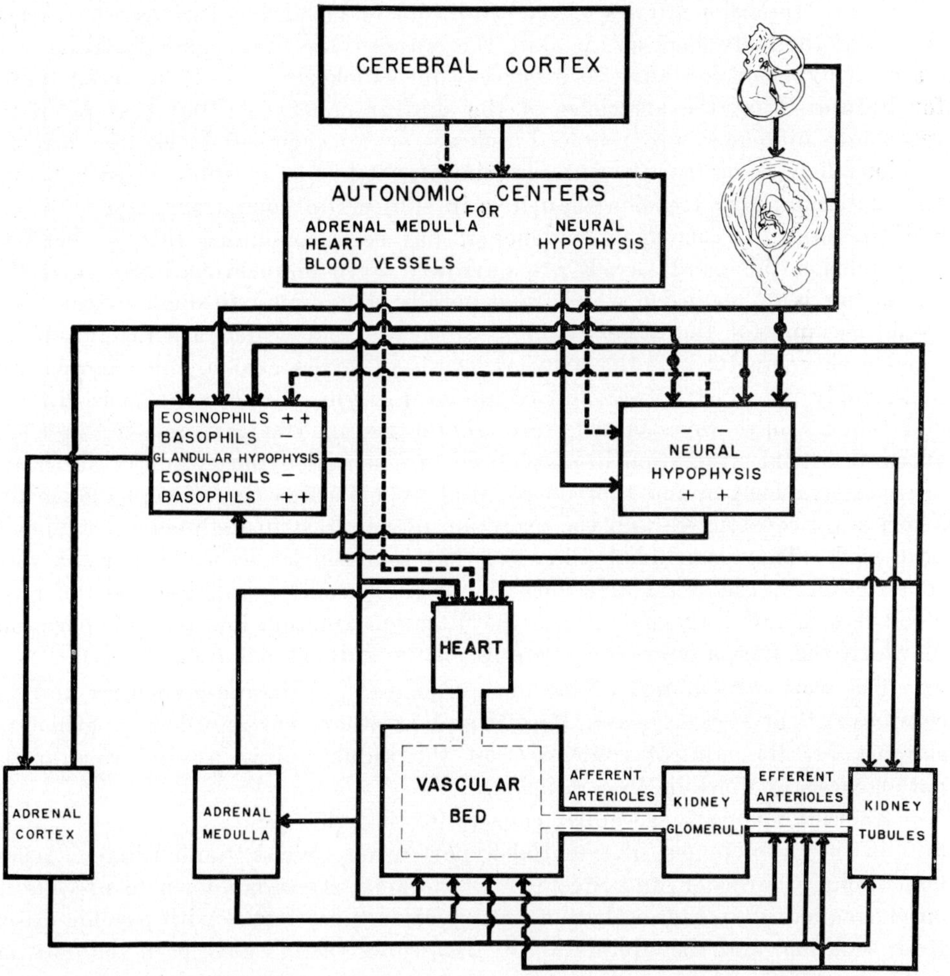

Fig. 6.—Schematic diagram to indicate the manner in which kidney function may be modified through nervous and endocrine influences. Straight ——— lines indicate excitatory, broken _ _ _ _ lines inhibitory influences; dotted straight .—.—.—. lines indicate neutralization of one influence by another. A decrease in the amount of or a depression of the functional influence of the secretion of the neural hypophysis together with other influences from the adrenal cortex, from renin and from progesterone, leads to overaction of the eosinophile cells of the glandular hypophysis. The existence of a differential susceptibility of the afferent and the efferent glomerular arterioles to vasoconstrictor influences affords a mechanism for modifying filtration by the glomeruli and by alterations in blood pressure to control the blood flow to the renal tubules whereby the adequacy of kidney function is maintained.

The excess release of a vasoconstrictor substance from the adrenal cortex, from the adrenal medulla, of renin from the kidney, or of progesterone from the ovary and placenta may lead to diastolic hypertension. In persons exhibiting Cushing's syndrome, destruction of the nuclei of the hypothalamus which are trophic to the neural hypophysis results in glandular imbalance which leads to hypertension. It is postulated that a functional depression of these nuclei by influences from the central nervous system leads, in those constitutionally susceptible, to similar glandular imbalances and to essential hypertension.

not associated with cytologically demonstrable changes in the nervous component to cause renal tubular inadequacy. Under such conditions the hypertension necessary to overcome it is spoken of as essential.*

Studies of the circulation in essential hypertension have shown that the raised arterial pressure is not due to an increased cardiac output or to increased blood viscosity, for these have been measured and found normal. It is recognized that diastolic hypertension is due to narrowing of the small arteries and arterioles. Intensive studies of the conditions of blood flow through the various tissues of the body such as the skin, the muscles, the brain, and the kidneys in essential hypertension have been carried out (Pickering[39]). It has been found, for instance, that the arterioles of the skin are narrowed, but that when the vasomotor influences are removed reflexly or by chemical block, the increase in blood flow is no greater but sometimes a little less in subjects with benign and malignant hypertension than it is in subjects of comparable age with normal pressures. From such evidence it has been concluded that in essential hypertension the hand vessels are narrowed by a nonnervous agent, and this narrowing is of an order which, if generally distributed throughout the body, would account for the hypertension. Since the skin vessels are rarely and inconsiderably involved in the arteriosclerosis of hypertension, the narrowing is presumably not of structural but of humoral origin. Goldring, Chasis, Ranges, and Smith[40] have investigated, through the use of Diodrast and inulin clearances, the renal circulation in sixty cases of essential hypertension of all grades of severity. They found that in essential hypertension the efferent glomerular arteries are constricted, and the excretion of Diodrast in high concentrations is decreased. They concluded, likewise, that in essential hypertension the vasoconstriction in the renal arterioles is not nervous in origin because the renal blood flow is not increased, nor is the filtration fraction lowered by operations in which the sympathetic nerve supply to the kidneys has been divided.

The work of Goldblatt and his associates,[41] of Braun-Menendez and his co-workers,[42] of Corcoran and Page,[43] and of others has afforded experimental support for the clinical evidence that the kidney plays a vital role in the pathogenesis of diastolic hypertension.

Another generally accepted concept is that the nervous system is important in the development of essential hypertension (Weiss,[44] and Binger, Ackerman, Cohn, Schroeder, and Steele[45]). Emotional stress is known to precede its onset frequently and exacerbations commonly are associated with psychic crises. Rest, sedation, and the elimination of disturbing factors have been the most effective measures in its medical treatment. However, as stated by Binger and his associates, in the present state of our knowledge, methods are not available to test the question of causation in the dynamic interrelationship of psyche and soma. It is also to be admitted that not all who exhibit diastolic hypertension give a recognizable evidence of psychic complex and not all who do have some

*Simultaneously with the presentation of this paper at the meeting of the American College of Surgeons in New York in September, 1947, it was learned that a sensitization of the blood vessels of patients exhibiting essential hypertension to the vasoconstricting action of desoxycorticosterone has been demonstrated by George A. Perera and David W. Blood (Ann. Int. Med. 27: 401, 1947). This is considered crucial support of the concept of the mechanism of the pathogenesis of essential hypertension herein presented.

psychic disturbance develop hypertension. Psychic influences have been shown to cause efferent glomerular arteriolar narrowing, and even to decrease the total renal blood flow of man (Smith[46]). Such effects have been observed by us repeatedly in the dog. An invariable and striking effect of the disturbing conditions has been to decrease Diodrast excretion. This depression of tubular function is regarded as a stimulus for the further release of renin now considered to be produced by the renal tubules (Friedman and Kaplan[47]).

It has been observed repeatedly that when a group of individuals is subjected to disquieting environmental influences such as are encountered in war, diastolic hypertension will develop in some but not in others, just as emotionally instable rats will develop diastolic hypertension when subjected to prolonged nervous strain such as is caused by noisy blasts, whereas rats of similar breed but emotionally stable will not develop hypertension (Farris, Yeakel, and Medoff[48]). An analogous experiment in effect has been carried out for man on the African Negro when transported to America and on the Chinese rural dweller when transferred to an urban environment. In both groups a constitutional tendency to develop diastolic hypertension has been revealed in some but not in others. The tendency is genetically linked, as shown by its hereditary transmission. The emphasis on the concept that hyperdynamic responsiveness of blood vessels is significant in the pathogenesis of hypertension is supported by the evidence of its constant presence in persons exhibiting Cushing's syndrome. The dusky plethoric appearance of the face and neck which distinguishes them must be attributed to such property in the blood vessels of the face and neck. Similarly, the exhibition of cutis marmorata indicates its existence in the blood vessels of the extremities.

Experimental evidence also attests to the importance of the adrenal cortex in the maintenance of blood pressure and in the development of experimental renal hypertension (Goldblatt[49]) and in persons with Cushing's syndrome (Heinbecker[50]).

It appears obvious then that any tenable concept of the pathogenesis of essential hypertension must assign essential roles to the nervous system, to the kidneys, and to the glands of internal secretion, particularly the adrenal cortex. Here as in all other regulatory phenomena in which the endocrine glands and the nervous system are involved, two factors play a role—one neurogenic and rapid in its action like the constrictor nerves, the other slower, humoral in nature, but functionally similar in its effects.

The concept of the pathogenesis of essential hypertension offered is that nervous influences, primarily from the frontal lobes, effect a functional depression of the supraoptic and paraventricular nuclei of the hypothalamus. Such depression may become organic as well if the intraventricular pressure becomes sufficiently elevated to exert actual pressure on the nuclei as it may in the malignant phase. The depression results in a decrease of the secretion of the neural hypophysis because of which the eosinophile cells of the glandular hypophysis become preponderant and are stimulated to overaction. The basophile cells are depressed. In persons with essential hypertension the stimulation of the eosinophiles and depression of the basophiles are presumably functional, as no obvious organic changes have been recorded (Rasmussen[51a, b]). This change in the glandular hypophysis is the result of humoral action, not of nervous influences. Overaction of the eosinophile cells increases their output of adrenotropic hormone. One effect of the overaction of the adrenal cortex is to constrict the efferent glomerular arterioles of the kidney which in turn results in a release of renin. The combined influences of the hypophysial, of the adrenal cortical, and renal hormones also result in a constriction of the extrarenal blood vessels and in a maintained cardiac output, thereby causing diastolic hypertension. The processes involved are of a low order of intensity in most instances, as indicated by the fact that about fifteen to thirty years are required for essential hypertension to become well established. Doubtless a lesser concentration of the humors can be effective because the depression of the neural hypophysis sensitizes the blood vessels to the constrictive action of the desoxycorticosterone fraction of the adrenal cortical hormone, to epinephrine, and to renin. In addition, persons developing essential hypertension are considered constitutionally susceptible to the depression of both their hypothalamic nuclei by nervous influences and their blood vessels to the constrictive action of the hormones concerned in the development of hypertension. This is postulated because not all persons with diabetes insipidus develop essential hypertension. It might be expected that persons with diabetes insipidus would develop diastolic hypertension because of the marked depression of the secretion of the neural hypophysis which exists invariably. An analysis from the records of thirteen consecutive recent patients with diabetes insipidus admitted to Barnes Hospital reveals that in five of the thirteen a diastolic pressure of over 100 mm. of mercury was recorded. This is a much higher incidence of elevated diastolic pressure than occurs in persons generally. It is postulated that others with diabetes insipidus who do not develop hypertension do not have sufficient constitutional susceptibility of the blood vessels to vasoconstrictor hormones. In some persons with diabetes insipidus, injury to the glandular hypophysis is present also. Any such deficiency would diminish its adrenotropic influence and in this way militate against the development of essential hypertension.

The overaction of the eosinophile-adrenal cortical hormone complex is responsible for the excessive infiltration of neutral fats and of cholesterol into the walls of the blood vessels. This is considered of primary significance in the development of arteriosclerosis. It is the development of such sclerosis which makes the hypertension permanent.

Hypertension is regarded as the reaction of the body to any inadequacy of renal tubular function. It is part of the mechanism for compensating, with increased blood flow, the inadequacy of the renal tubules. Renin is regarded as the substance released by the kidney tubules, which not only constricts vessels outside the kidney directly, but also stimulates the eosinophiles of the glandular hypophysis, thereby increasing the cardiac output and renal tubular function. Slight excess of desoxycorticosterone, of renin, and of epinephrine causes constriction of the efferent glomerular arterioles, but the failure of the blood vessels to the renal tubules themselves to be damaged by an excess of renin in experimental renal hypertension permits the interpretation that they are not similarly affected.

In pregnancy the preponderance of eosinophile cells is regarded as the result of the inactivation of the secretion of the neural hypophysis by progesterone. The eosinophile cell overaction here as elsewhere stimulates the adrenal glands and in those emotionally and constitutionally susceptible would be expected to result in sufficient constriction of the efferent glomerular arterioles to release renin. As in essential hypertension, the combined action of these three hormones on vessels sensitized by depression of the neural hypophysis is regarded as primarily responsible for the initiation of the diastolic hypertension.

In support of the concept is the frequent association of obesity (Terry[52]), of hypercholesterolemia (Westphal[53]), of decreased sugar tolerance (Joslin[54]), of accelerated ageing and of the menopause (Alvarez and Zimmermann[55]) with the existence of essential hypertension. In the experimental animal, eosinophile adrenal overaction has been shown to be associated with obesity, with hypercholesterolemia, with a decreased insulin sensitivity, and with a failure of the ovarian follicles or of the spermatogonia to maturate (Heinbecker[56]). In Cushing's syndrome in which the mechanism for the development of hypertension seems similar to that postulated for essential hypertension, obesity, hypercholesterolemia, decreased insulin sensitivity, marked acceleration of the ageing processes, and depression of gonadal function are constant features (Heinbecker[57]). In persons with essential hypertension these signs often are not pronounced; they even may be absent. Such variations are attributed to differences in organ susceptibility to the common influences which impinge on them.

SUMMARY

Experimental evidence pertinent to the problem of pathogenesis of diastolic hypertension is reviewed.

Denervation of the neural hypophysis in the dog results in a loss of basophile cells and a preponderance with overaction of eosinophile cells in the glandular hypophysis.

With marked depression of the secretion of the neural hypophysis in the dog a normal cardiac output is maintained, the insulin-Diodrast clearance ratio increases, and a moderate elevation in mean arterial pressure develops.

Eosinophile cell preponderance and overaction in the dog also develop when the nervous pathways from the thalamus and subthalamus to the paraventricular and supraoptic nuclei are interrupted, when asphyxia in one adrenal gland is produced by ligation of a portion of its arterial supply, when a diminution in the amount of effective renal tubular tissue is produced by removal of one kidney with the wrapping of the remaining kidney in silk, when mulberry-like ovaries are produced by the prolonged administration of thiouracil, and when pregnancy occurs. Since several of these associated conditions result in development of diastolic hypertension, their common factor of eosinophile overaction is considered to be significant as a causative factor in the development of hypertension.

The eosinophile cells of the glandular hypophysis are trophic to the adrenal gland, to the renal tubules, and to the interstitial tissue of the gonads.

Loss or depression of the secretion of the neural hypophysis results in a sensitization of the blood vessels to epinephrine, to desoxycorticosterone, and to renin. Under the conditions where depression of the neural hypophysis causes and induces increased output of the latter two of these hormones, the blood vessels are also sensitized to overaction and hypertension results.

In persons exhibiting Cushing's syndrome primarily because of an atrophy of the paraventricular and supraoptic nuclei or because of depression by a raised intraventricular pressure, a decrease in the secretion of the neural hypophysis results in a hyalinization of the basophile cells and a preponderance with overaction of the eosinophile cells. Among the effects invariably produced are diastolic hypertension and arteriosclerosis. These effects are considered to result from a narrowing of the extrarenal blood vessels and of the efferent glomerular arterioles. Because of the latter action, renin is released. It is the combined action of these hormones in persons whose neural hypophysis is depressed and whose blood vessels are, therefore, sensitized to the constrictive action of these hormones that hypertension is attributed. There appears also to be a constitutional susceptibility in addition.

Overaction of the eosinophile cell-adrenal cortical hormone complex results in an increased formation and storage of neutral fat and of cholesterol. This is considered of primary significance in the development of arteriosclerosis.

Hypertension is regarded as the reaction of the body to any inadequacy of renal tubular function. It is part of the mechanism for compensating with increased blood flow the deficiency of the renal tubular mass. Renin is regarded as the substance released by the kidney tubules which not only constricts vessels outside the kidney directly, but also stimulates the eosinophile cells of the glandular hypophysis and thereby increases the cardiac output and renal tubular function. In combination with the desoxycorticosterone fraction of the adrenal cortical hormone it leads to extrarenal vascular constriction, but without constricting the blood vessels to the renal tubules themselves.

In persons with essential hypertension, the depression of the neural hypophysis is regarded as, first, functional because of nervous influences, particularly from the frontal lobes; later, particularly in the malignant phase, it is regarded as organic as well, because of the increased intraventricular pressure acting on the cells of the supraoptic and the paraventricular nuclei.

Constitutional susceptibility, both of the nervous system to the depression of the hypothalamic nuclei and of the blood vessels to the constricting action of the hormones responsible for the extrarenal vasoconstriction, is postulated for persons with essential hypertension.

In persons with essential hypertension, the depression of the basophile cells and the stimulation of the eosinophiles presumably are functional, as obvious structural alterations have not been demonstrated.

In pregnancy, the eosinophile cell preponderance is regarded as the result of the inactivation of the secretion of the neural hypophysis by progesterone. The eosinophile overaction here, as elsewhere, stimulates the adrenal glands and in those individuals who are emotionally and constitutionally susceptible it would be expected to result in sufficient constriction of the efferent glomerular arterioles to release renin. As in essential hypertension, the combined action of these three hormones together with that of progesterone on vessels sensitized by depression of the neural hypophysis is regarded as primarily responsible for the initiation of diastolic hypertension.

Evidence to support the concept of the pathogenesis of essential hypertension herein presented is sought in the accepted importance of emotional influences in its development. The frequent association of obesity, of premature ageing, of decreased insulin sensitivity, and of increased intracranial pressure, particularly in later stages of essential hypertension, is considered to support the probability of the hypothesis presented. The fact that the characteristics of the circulation in essential hypertension are similar to those which exist in the hypertension associated with Cushing's syndrome where such a mechanism has been established is regarded as supporting its probability.

In essential hypertension the sympathetic nervous system and epinephrine are regarded as mechanisms for rapid homeostatic adjustments of the renal circulation, but they are not considered of primary importance in the pathogenesis of such hypertension.

The concept affords a mechanism for explaining the prevailing earlier and wider incidence of hypertension and arteriosclerosis in response to the stress and strain of modern existence.

REFERENCES

1. Heinbecker, Peter: Cushing's Syndrome, Ann. Surg. **124**: 252-261, 1946.
2. Heinbecker, Peter: Factors Limiting Surgery for Essential Hypertension, Ann. Surg. **126**: 535-544, 1947.
3. Heinbecker, P., White, H. L., and Rolf, D.: The Essential Lesion in Experimental Diabetes Insipidus, Endocrinology **40**: 104-113, 1947.
4. Rasmussen, A. T.: Effects of Hypophysectomy and Hypophysial Stalk Resection on Hypothalamic Nuclei of Animals and Man, A. Research Nerv. & Ment. Dis., Proc. **20**: 245-269, 1940.
5. Heinbecker, P., and White, H. L.: Hypothalamico-Hypophysial System and Its Relation to Water Balance in the Dog, Am. J. Physiol. **133**: 582-593, 1941.
6. Greving, R.: Makroskopische Anatomie und Histologie des vegetativen Nervensystems. Bumke und Foerster, Handbuch Neurologische, vol. 1, Berlin, 1935, Julius Springer, pp. 810-886.
7. Heinbecker, Peter: The Pathogenesis of Cushing's Syndrome, Medicine **23**: 225-247, 1944.
8. Heinbecker, Peter: Unpublished data.
9. Heinbecker, Peter: Unpublished data.
10. Victor, J.: Hypertension Produced in Dogs by Unilateral Ligation of Periadrenal Blood Vessels and Tissue, Proc. Soc. Exper. Biol. & Med. **60**: 332-334, 1945.
11. Heinbecker, Peter: 1944, loc. cit.
12. Heinbecker, Peter: Studies on the Sensitivity of Smooth Musculature to Exogenous Epinephrine, Am. J. Physiol. **118**: 276-284, 1937.
13. Goldblatt, H.: Experimental Hypertension Induced by Renal Ischemia, Harvey Lecture, Bull. New York Acad. Med. **14**: 523-553, 1938.
14. Kohlstadt, K. G., Helmer, O. M., and Page, I. H.: Activation of Renin by Blood Colloids, Proc. Soc. Exper. Biol. & Med. **39**: 214-215, 1938.
15. White, H. L., Heinbecker, P., and Rolf, D.: Some Endocrine Influences on Renal Function and Cardiac Output, Am. J. Physiol. **149**: 404-417, 1947.
16. White, H. L., Heinbecker, P., and Rolf, D.: 1947, loc. cit.
17. Heinbecker, P., White, H. L., and Rolf, D.: Effects of Hypophysectomy on Some Renal Functions, Proc. Soc. Exper. Biol. & Med. **45**: 44-47, 1941.
18. Ragan, C., Ferrabee, J. W., Phyfe, P., Atchley, D. W., and Loeb, R. F.: A Syndrome of Polydipsia and Polyuria Induced in Normal Animals by Desoxycorticosterone Acetate, Am. J. Physiol. **131**: 73-78, 1940.
19. Mulinos, M. G., Spingarn, C. L., and Lojkin, M. E.: Desoxycorticosterone and Diabetes Insipidus-like Condition, Am. J. Physiol. **135**: 102-112, 1941.
20. Pickering, G. W., and Prinzmetal, M.: Effect of Renin on Urine Formation, J. Physiol. **98**: 314-335, 1940.
21. Smith, H. W.: Studies in the Physiology of the Kidney, Lawrence, Kansas, 1939, Univ. of Kansas, Univ. Extension Division.

22. Corcoran, A. C., Kohlstadt, K. G., and Page, I. H.: Changes of Arterial Blood Pressure and Renal Hypodynamics by Injection of Angiotonin in Human Beings, Proc. Soc. Exper. Biol. & Med. **46**: 244-248, 1941.
23. Goldring, W., Chasis, H., Ranges, H. A., and Smith, H. W.: Effective Renal Blood Flow in Subjects With Essential Hypertension, J. Clin. Investigation **20**: 637-653, 1941.
24. Tigerstedt, R., and Bergman, P. G.: Niere und Kreislauf, Skandinav. Arch. f. Physiol. **8**: 223-271, 1898.
25. Goldblatt, H., Lynch, J., Hanzol, R. F., and Summerville, W. W.: Studies on Experimental Hypertension; Production of Persistent Elevation of Systolic Blood Pressure by Means of Renal Ischemia, J. Exper. Med. **59**: 347-379, 1934.
26. Braun-Menendez, E., Fasciolo, J. C., Leloir, L. F., Munoz, J. M., and Taquini, A. C.: Renal Hypertension, Springfield, Ill., 1946, Charles C Thomas, Publisher.
27. (a) Pickering, G. W.: The Circulatoin in Arterial Hypertension, Brit. M. J. **2**: 1-4, 31-34, 1943.
(b) Heinbecker, Peter: Unpublished data.
28. Gaunt, R., and Hays, H. W.: The Life-Maintaining Effects of Crystalline Progesterone in Adrenalectomized Ferrets, Science **88**: 576-577, 1938.
29. McKeown, T., and Spurrell, W. R.: The Results of Adrenalectomy in the Pregnant Albino Rat, J. Physiol. **98**: 255-262, 1940.
30. Thorn, G. W., and Engel, L. L.: The Effect of Sex Hormones on the Renal Excretion of Electrolytes, J. Exper. Med. **68**: 299-312, 1938.
31. Reynolds, S. R. M., and Allen, W. M.: Physiology of the Corpus Luteum, Am. J. Obst. & Gynec. **30**: 309-318, 1935.
32. Knaus, H.: Experimentelle Untersuchungen zur Physiologie und Pharmakologie der Uterusmuskulatur in der Schwangerschaft, Arch. f. exper. Path. u. Pharmakol. **124**: 152-184, 1927.
33. Norris, E. H.: Arrhenoblastoma, Am. J. Cancer **32**: 1-29, 1938.
34. Zondek, B.: Clinical and Experimental Investigations on the Genital Functions and Their Hormonal Regulation, Baltimore, 1941, Williams & Wilkins Company.
35. Heinbecker, P.: 1944, loc. cit.
36. Heinbecker, P. : 1946, loc. cit.
37. Crooke, A. C.: Change in Basophil Cells of Pituitary Gland Common to Conditions Which Exhibit Syndrome Attributed to Basophil Adenoma, J. Path. & Bact. **41**: 339-349, 1935.
38. Heinbecker, P., White, H. L., and Rolf, D.: Experimental Obesity in the Dog, Am. J. Physiol. **141**: 549-565, 1944.
39. Pickering, G. W.: The Peripheral Resistance in Persistent Arterial Hypertension, Clin. Sc. **2**: 209-235, 1935.
40. Goldring, W., Chasis, H., Ranges, H. A., and Smith, H. W.: 1941, loc. cit.
41. Goldblatt, H., Lynch, J., and Hanzol, R. F.: 1934, loc. cit.
42. Braun-Menendez, E., and others, 1946, loc. cit.
43. Corcoran, A. C., and Page, I. H.: Renal Aspects of Experimental and Clinical Hypertension, J. Lab. & Clin. Med. **26**: 1713, 1941.
44. Weiss, Edward (Philadelphia): Psychosomatic Aspects of Hypertension, J. A. M. A. **120**: 1081-1086, 1942.
45. Binger, C. A. L., Ackerman, N. W., Cohn, A. E., Schroeder, H. A., and Steele, J. M.: Personality in Arterial Hypertension. Psychosomatic Medicine Monographs, New York, 1945, Am. Soc. for Research in Psychosom. Probl., Inc.
46. Smith, H. W.: The Physiology of the Kidney, London, 1937, Oxford University Press.
47. Friedman, M., and Kaplan, A.: Studies Concerning the Site of Renin Formation in the Kidney, J. Exper. Med. **77**: 65-70, 1943.
48. Farris, Edmond J., Yeakel, E. H., and Medoff, H. S.: Development of Hypertension in Emotional Gray Norway Rats After Air Blasting, Am. J. Physiol. **144**: 331-333, 1945.
49. Goldblatt, H.: The Renal Origin of Hypertension, Physiol. Rev. **27**: 120-165, 1947.
50. Heinbecker, P.: 1946, loc. cit.
51. (a) Rasmussen, A. T.: 1940, loc. cit.
(b) Rasmussen, A. T.: The Relation of the Basophilic Cells of the Human Hypophysis to Blood Pressure, Endocrinology **20**: 673-678, 1936.
52. Terry, A. H., Jr.: Obesity and Hypertension, J. A. M. A. **81**: 1283-1284, 1923.
53. Westphal, K.: Pathogenesis of Essential Arterial Hypertension; Paradoxical Vascular Reaction Following Compression in Arterial Hypertension, Ztschr. f. klin. Med. **101**: 545-557, 1925.
54. Joslin, Elliott P., and others: Treatment of Diabetes Mellitus, ed. 3, Philadelphia, 1923, Lea & Febiger, p. 578.
55. Alvarez, W. C., and Zimmermann, A.: Blood Pressure in Women as Influenced by Sexual Organs, Arch. Int. Med. **37**: 597-636, 1926.
56. Heinbecker, P.: 1946, loc. cit.
57. Heinbecker, P.: 1944, loc. cit.

INDICATIONS FOR SYMPATHECTOMY IN THE TREATMENT OF HYPERTENSION

THOMAS FINDLEY, M.D., NEW ORLEANS, LA.

(From the Departments of Medicine, Tulane University School of Medicine and the Ochsner Clinic)

ANY internist who has the privilege of studying a large number of patients with hypertension before and after sympathectomy must be impressed by certain facts—that the operation has not yet been placed on a rational basis; that it seldom, if ever, produces manometric cure; that it is often followed by spectacular amelioration of symptoms; that the results are apt to be temporary; and finally that this treatment is violent. Until these points are properly appreciated and the limitations of sympathectomy thus recognized, the indications for surgical intervention will remain confused in the minds of many.

Since the cause of essential hypertension is unknown, all therapy is empirical. The one known basic fact is that elevation of blood pressure is due to increased peripheral resistance, but there is as yet no agreement as to whether the arteriolar constriction is of humoral or nervous origin. If the surgeon believes the former explanation to be true, he must show that sympathectomy modifies the endocrine system in an appropriate manner; if he accepts the latter view, he justifies the operation more easily in his own mind.

There are, of course, many factors in the normal organism which play upon smooth muscle in such a way as to increase its tonus. Fig. 1 is a naive representation of the fact that clinical hypertension does not occur until the sum of these vasoconstrictor influences exceeds a certain but unknown threshold. The illustrated sizes of the various fragments, however, are in no way to be interpretated as a quantitative expression of their relative importance, for our present knowledge is much too meager to permit any such assumption; it is obvious also that each patient will present his own individual pattern. If it is recalled that hypertension is not a disease but a symptom, it is worth while to speculate concerning the manner in which sympathectomy can be expected to modify or abolish each of these vasoconstrictor forces.

Surgical measures are certainly incapable of modifying the genetic influences which make one person's blood vessels more responsive than another's to a given set of stimuli. Primary vascular disease is represented because there is as yet no definite assurance that at least some cases of clinical hypertension may not be initiated by obliterative arterial disease in strategic locations; whatever the sequence may be, sympathectomy is surely an unsatisfactory remedy for arteriosclerosis. One surgeon[24] justifies sympathectomy on the grounds that it improves renal blood flow despite the facts that the renal circulation is autonomously regulated in normal man,[28] that renal ischemia is inconstantly present

---

Read at the thirty-third annual session of the American College of Surgeons, Sept. 11, 1947, New York, N. Y.

in hypertension,[23] and that sympathectomy does not increase the renal clearances of certain test materials.[3, 9, 10, 31]

The relationship between renal disease and sympathectomy cannot be lightly dismissed, however, since there is now reason to believe that chronic overproduction of the renal enzyme (renin) may lead to a persistent nonrenal (neurogenic ?) type of hypertension.[21] These experimental findings are in harmony with the clinical experience that nephrectomy is usually not successful in relieving long-standing hypertension associated with unilateral renal disease[2] and that sympathectomy is often surprisingly helpful in cases of chronic bilateral renal disease.[1, 5, 19, 29] The inference has been made that even in "renal" hypertension, the nervous system is sufficiently disturbed to justify sympathectomy. This operation is said by some to be helpful because it decreases peripheral resistance by paralyzing a large portion of the vascular bed. However, the evidence offered in support of this contention needs critical examination.

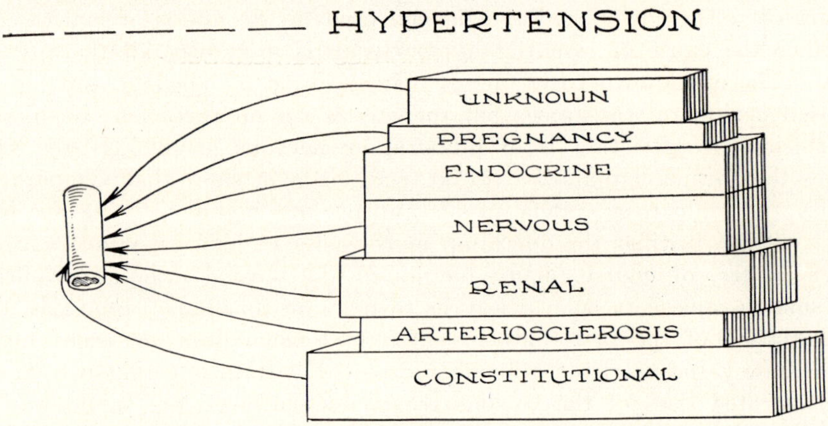

Fig. 1.—Hypertension is the summation of many vasoconstrictor forces.

The existence of neurogenic clinical hypertension has often been postulated[6, 11, 18, 22] but the data can be interpreted in other ways. It may be that as some persons grow older and their cerebral neurons atrophy, the blood pressure may rise because of lack of cerebral inhibition,[7] but such individuals are commonly thought to be unsuitable for operation because of age and arteriosclerosis. There appears to be no good evidence, however, that presenile essential hypertension is ever due to overactivity of the sympathetic nervous system and there is much persuasive evidence that it is not.[25, 26, 30]

Any enlargement of the vascular bed which follows sympathectomy is probably temporary because of the capacity of the peripheral vasomotor apparatus to regain its former tone and size. In our experience with about 100 hypertensive patients who have been subjected to bilateral splanchnicectomy and excision of both sympathetic chains from the fourth or fifth thoracic through the second lumbar ganglia we[20] have yet to see anything resembling a "cure" and have invariably found that the blood pressure slowly rises postoperatively to or somewhat below the preoperative level. This recrudescence of hypertension is not due to an increase in blood volume[4] and we believe it is due to the autonomous action of peripheral arterioles. Postural hypotension is the only phenomenon which we can clearly attribute to vascular denervation and, as shown in Fig. 2, this disappeared within one year in the vast majority of our cases. We, therefore, look upon postural hypotension as an undesirable surgical complication rather than an asset and believe that such reduction in blood pressure as may persist after sympathectomy is due to vascular relaxation from causes other than denervation of the splanchnic bed and legs. Denervation of the splanchnic bed may, it is true, abolish certain visceral reflexes in a helpful manner and extensive sympathectomy may to a certain extent protect peripheral vessels from fluctuation in vasomotor tone, but these effects are of themselves too minor to justify radical surgical procedures. It is difficult to accept radical sympathectomy as a form of treatment for what appears to be a humoral disease.

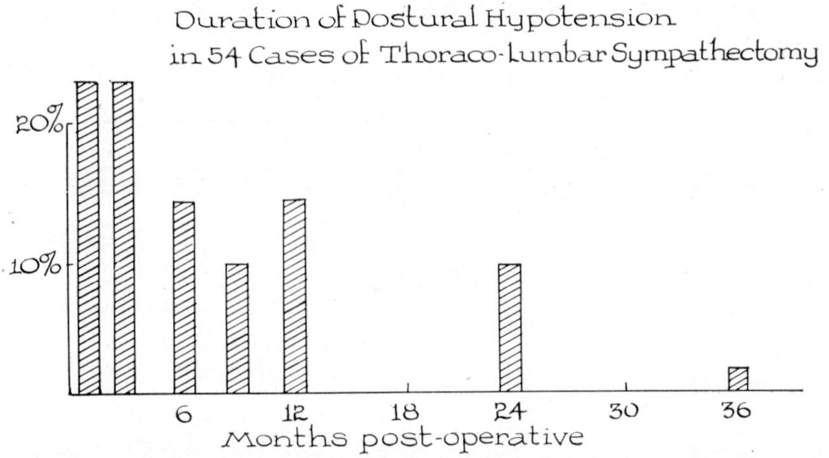

Fig. 2.—Postural hypotension is a temporary postsympathectomy response.

Since the weight of present evidence is in favor of a humoral origin of hypertension, the possibility should be considered that sympathectomy is able to modify the chemical composition of the blood in some favorable manner. Heinbecker's[12-15] highly original observations led him to conclude that hypofunction of the neurohypophysis sensitizes blood vessels to a variety of pressor substances such as renin, epinephrine, and progesterone. If confirmed by others, this view is of great theoretical and practical importance because it offers an explanation of the pathogenesis of hypertension and suggests that sympathectomy induces vascular relaxation by diminishing the activity of the adrenal medulla. From the surgical standpoint this theory is perhaps compromised by evidence that epinephrine output is not abolished by adrenal denervation,[16] but even diminished secretion should be helpful since epinephrine is a substance with definite analeptic and vasoconstrictor properties. It may also regulate the activity of the adrenal cortex,[17] a gland currently suspected of playing an important role in the etiology of hypertension.

Further speculation at this time would be unprofitable but our experience with the surgical treatment of hypertension is such as to incline us toward the view that sympathectomy relieves symptoms and occasionally lowers blood pressure through some humoral mechanism rather than by denervation of peripheral arterioles. If this be true, then the operation should be regarded as palliative rather than curative and extensive sympathectomy would be unphysiologic. In common with other observers we have noted a high incidence of symptomatic relief after sympathectomy and we agree that there is no correlation between the degree of subjective improvement and the postoperative blood pressure levels. This has led some to conclude that the clinical improvement is due entirely to suggestion. This point of view may be correct but it implies, first, that nearly

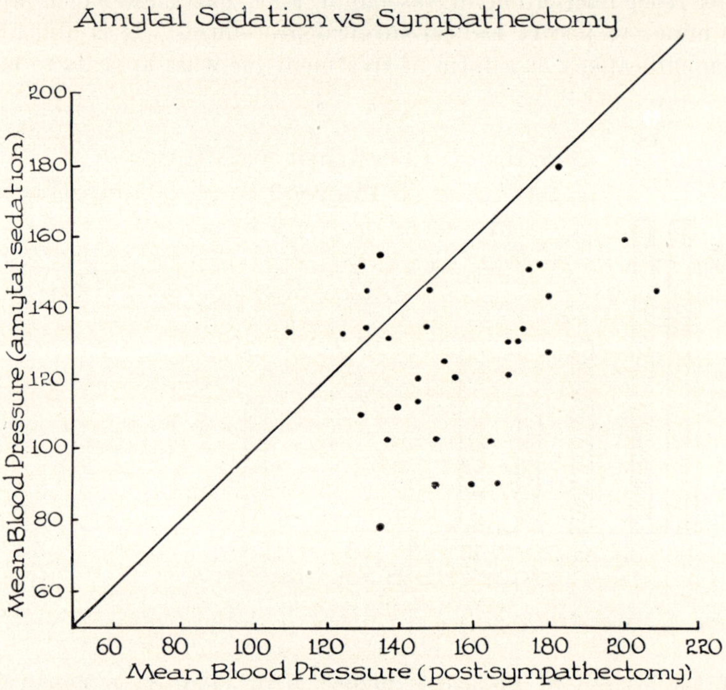

Fig. 3.—Lack of correlation between the sodium amytal sedation test and the postoperative results.

every patient with symptomatic hypertension is psychoneurotic and, second, that this is a special kind of psychoneurosis in that it responds instantly and with more or less permanence to one treatment. Most psychoneuroses, of course, yield only, if at all, to firm and continued pressure. It is difficult to persuade anyone in close contact with a large number of sympathectomized hypertensive patients that the surgeon has performed only a psychotherapeutic act. In our experience it has been rare to find a patient who is not glad he has had the operation and we have seen no comparable results accomplished by standard psychiatric methods. We are convinced that sympathectomy performs some useful physiologic function in some patients. At the moment it appears possible that adrenal denervation is the essential feature but the additional effect of cardiac denervation is worthy of study.

Patients should, therefore, not be selected for operation solely on the basis of tests which measure only blood pressure fluctuations. Certainly such procedures as the cold pressor test, the amytal sedation test, splanchnic block, and the induction of high spinal anesthesia have proved notoriously unreliable as gauges of postsympathectomy results. Fig. 3 illustrates our experience with the sodium amytal test; little correlation is seen between the lowest mean blood pressure reading obtained by heavy sedation and the mean pressure six to twelve months after thoracolumbar sympathectomy. Usually the amytal test gave falsely optimistic results, although the few cases above the line ran in the opposite direction. We have had no experience with high caudal anesthesia as recommended by Russek, Southworth, and Zohman[27] but doubt, on theoretical grounds, that it will prove to be more accurate. Disappointments will be fewer if the operation is reserved for those with disabling symptoms and early malignant hypertension, but the manometric results will, of course, be better if the patient also has a labile blood pressure. It also seems reasonable to try a low sodium regimen first,[8] but we have had little success with it thus far.

CONCLUSIONS

At the time of this communication, therefore, we make the following suggestions regarding the selection of patients for sympathectomy:

(1) That less reliance be placed upon prediction tests which measure the response of blood pressure to sedation or to anesthetization of the nervous system,

(2) that the operation be reserved for those with severe symptoms but no gross impairment of cerebral, cardiac, or renal function,

(3) that the operation not be done on young individuals with mild asymptomatic hypertension because of the possibility of nerve regeneration,

(4) that sympathectomy may profitably be done on patients over 50 years of age, provided other requirements are met, and

(5) that patients be told that sympathectomy offers palliation and not cure.

REFERENCES

1. Ayman, D., and Goldshine, A. D.: New England J. Med. **229**: 797, 1943.
2. Barker, N. W., and Braasch, W. F.: Internat. Abstr. Surg., 1947; Surg., Gynec. & Obst. **84**: 299, 1947.
3. Corcoran, A. C., and Page, I. H.: Arch. Surg. **42**: 1072, 1941.
4. Davis, W. D., Jr., and Mayerson, H. S.: Unpublished data.
5. de Takats, G., and Fowler, E. F.: SURGERY **21**: 773, 1947.
6. Dock, W.: Am. J. Physiol. **130**: 1, 1940.
7. Dock, W.: New York State J. Med. **45**: 93, 1945.
8. Dock, W.: Rocky Mountain M. J. **44**: 372, 1947.
9. Findley, T., Clinton, E., and Edwards, J. C.: SURGERY **12**: 64, 1942.
10. Goldring, W., and Chasis, H.: Hypertension and Hypertensive Disease, London, 1944, Commonwealth Fund, p. 157.
11. Gregory, R., Levine, H., and Lindley, E. L.: Texas Rep. Biol. & Med. **2**: 121, 1944.
12. Heinbecker, P.: Medicine **23**: 225, 1944.
13. Heinbecker, P.: Ann. Surg. **124**: 252, 1946.
14. Heinbecker, P.: Ann. Surg. **126**: 535, 1947.
15. Heinbecker, P.: SURGERY **23**: 618, 1948.
16. Kobro, M.: Acta med. Scandinav. **126**: 97, 1946.

17. Long, C. N. H., and Fry, E. G.: Proc. Soc. Exper. Biol. & Med. **59**: 67, 1945.
18. Medoff, H. S.: Am. J. Physiol. **143**: 300, 1945.
19. Nesbit, R. M., and Plumb, R. T.: J. Urol. **57**: 116, 1947.
20. Ochsner, A., and Findley, T.: Unpublished data.
21. Miner, R. W.: Experimental Hypertension, New York, 1946, New York Academy of Sciences, p. 153.
22. Page, I. H.: New York State J. Med. **44**: 2686, 1944.
23. Page, I. H., and Corcoran, A. C.: Arterial Hypertension, Chicago, 1945, The Year Book Publishers, Inc., p. 249.
24. Peet, M. M.: New England J. Med. **236**: 270, 1947.
25. Pickering, G. W.: Clin. Sc. 2: 209, 1936.
26. Prinzmetal, M., and Wilson, R.: J. Clin. Investigation **15**: 63, 1936.
27. Russek, H. I., Southworth, J. L., and Zohman, B. L.: J. A. M. A. **130**: 927, 1946.
28. Smith, H. W.: J. Clin. Investigation **18**: 319, 1939.
29. Smithwick, R. H.: Arch. Surg. **49**: 180, 1944.
30. Stead, E. A., Jr., and Kunkel, P.: J. Clin. Investigation **19**: 25, 1940.
31. Talbott, J. H., and others: J. Clin. Investigation **22**: 387, 1943.

GUNSHOT WOUNDS INVOLVING THE ABDOMINAL AORTA

A Report of Two Cases

C. E. Holzer, Jr., M.D., Cincinnati, Ohio

(From the Department of Surgery, College of Medicine, University of Cincinnati and the Cincinnati General Hospital)

PENETRATING wounds involving the aorta which permit the victim to survive for a sufficient time for surgical care are exceedingly few, and instances of successful treatment of such wounds have been reported rarely. Dshanelidze,[1] Blalock,[2] and Elkin[3] have each reported successful suture of a stab wound of the ascending portion of the thoracic aorta. The latter two authors reported wounds which had been caused by ice picks and were only tiny perforations. Wildegans[4] in 1926 reported a case in which a 1 cm. stab wound of the abdominal aorta was successfully repaired. Dubinskiy[5] in 1944 sutured a 0.3 cm. shrapnel wound of the abdominal aorta followed by recovery of the patient. In a comprehensive review of the literature no instance of the survival of a patient after the repair of a direct bullet injury of the abdominal aorta has been found.

It has been my unique experience to encounter and treat successfully in a period of eight months two patients with gunshot wounds of the abdominal aorta. In the first instance a vitallium tube was utilized to maintain the continuity of the vessel, while in the second direct suture was possible. The first case is believed to be the only one in which a vitallium tube has been placed in the human aorta with a successful result.

CASE REPORTS

Case 1 (No. 209392).—C. J., a 26-year-old Negro woman, was brought to the hospital at 7:40 P.M. on Dec. 28, 1945, forty minutes after having been shot in the abdomen with a 32 caliber revolver. She was in severe shock, pulseless, with a blood pressure too low to record, but was conscious and complaining of abdominal pain. She was moderately obese but normal except for the findings related to the injury. Respiratory rate was 30 and cardiac rate 100 per minute. Over the left rectus muscle, midway between the umbilicus and the xiphoid process, was a bullet wound .5 cm. in diameter. There was no wound of exit. The abdominal wall was splinted and diffusely tender. Peristaltic sounds were absent and a fluid wave was demonstrable. Rectal examination was unremarkable. A neurologic examination was not performed but it was noted that the patient was able to move all extremities.

A Levine tube was passed into the stomach and a small amount of fresh blood was aspirated. Urinalysis was negative for blood. After the intravenous administration of 1000 c.c. of plasma the blood pressure rose to 100/70 and the condition was greatly improved. Roentgenologic survey of the body showed a bullet adjacent to the neck of the left femur (Fig. 1).

Under endotracheal cyclopropane and ether anesthesia a long left rectus incision was made, with a transverse extension to the right. Approximately 500 c.c. of fresh blood were evacuated from the peritoneal cavity, but no persistent bleeding was observed. Exploration of the abdominal viscera revealed that the bullet had passed through the anterior wall of

Received for publication, June 23, 1947.

the stomach near the pylorus, through the posteroinferior wall of the first portion of the duodenum, and through the head of the pancreas into the retroperitoneal area. There was a large retroperitoneal hematoma around the head of the pancreas and at the base of the transverse mesocolon. The gastric and duodenal perforations were closed with silk mattress sutures.

In order to explore the retroperitoneal hematoma the operator divided the lateral peritoneal attachments of the second and third portions of the duodenum and the hepatic flexure of the colon and retracted these structures toward the midline. As the hematoma was being cleared away, there was a tremendous spurt of blood from the depths of the operative area. Digital pressure was applied immediately to check the hemorrhage. Palpation revealed that the blood was coming from a wound in the aorta. With the hemorrhage controlled by

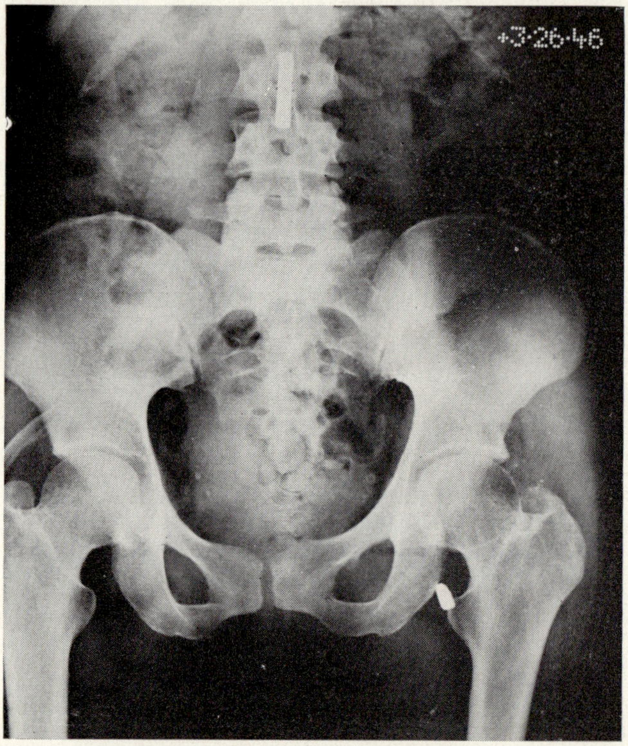

Fig. 1.—Roentgenogram three months after injury showing bullet in relation to neck of left femur and tube in aorta overlying the third lumbar vertebra.

digital pressure on the wound, the aorta was mobilized and strips of cotton tape were passed around it and twisted down. The field was then cleared of blood revealing a perforation through the aorta 5 mm. in diameter extending in an anteroposterior direction (Fig. 2). By palpation it was established that the wound lay 6 cm. above the aortic bifurcation, presumably below the origin of the inferior mesenteric artery. The edges of the wounds were ragged and there was considerable loss of substance in the damaged segment. An unsuccessful attempt was made to close the perforations with silk sutures. Ligation of the vessel was deemed inadvisable because of the possibility of secondary hemorrhage or gangrene of the lower extremities. It was therefore decided to attempt re-establishment of the continuity of the aorta by means of a vitallium tube. Although the largest tube available was only 5 mm. in diameter, it was felt that a lumen of this size would permit adequate blood flow to the lower extremities until collateral flow could be established. The anterior bullet wound was enlarged slightly and the tube slipped into the lumen of the aorta. A silk ligature had been attached to the tab in the middle of the tube in order to control it. A heavy braided silk ligature was then tied around the aorta and the tube on either side of the damaged area. Because of the possibility that these ties might cut through, a strip of ¼ inch cotton tape was tied down flatly on each side of the pair of silk ligatures (Fig. 3). When the tourniquets were released, no leakage occurred, and palpation revealed fairly strong pulsations in the common iliac arteries. No further injuries were found upon completion of abdominal exploration. Cigarette drains were placed in the retroperitoneal tissues in both lumbar areas and brought out through a stab wound in each flank. The abdominal incision was closed using through-and-through steel wire stay sutures. The skin was closed with fine cotton sutures.

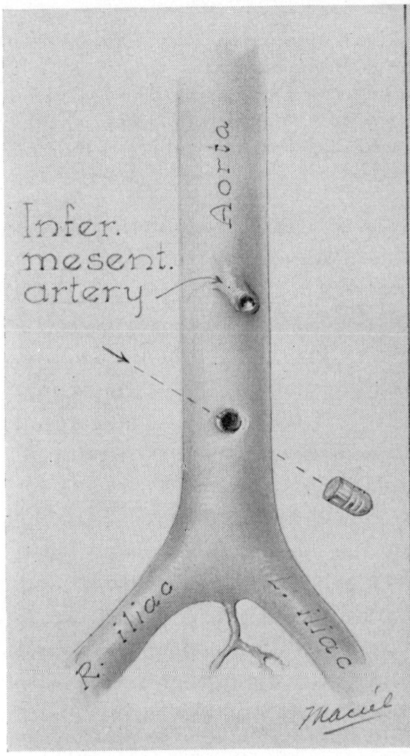

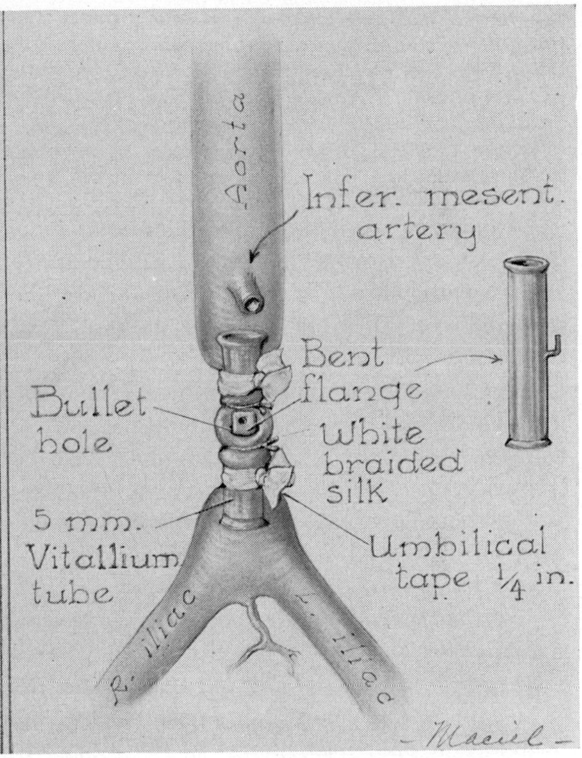

Fig. 2.—Diagram showing the course of the bullet and the location of the wound.
Fig. 3.—Drawing showing method of fixation of the tube within the lumen of the aorta.

During the procedure the patient's blood pressure never fell below 90/50, 1000 c.c. of plasma and 2500 c.c. of whole blood having been given.

The postoperative course was uncomplicated except for a transfusion reaction on the sixth day. Continuous gastric suction was maintained for two and one-half days, following which the Levine tube was removed and progressive feedings started. Sulfadiazine was given for eight days and penicillin for twenty-five days. The incision healed per primam.

In an attempt to prevent thrombosis at the site of repair and in the lower extremities, administration of dicoumarin was begun on the third day. A total of 650 mg. was given in the next twelve days, maintaining the prothrombin time between 30 and 38 seconds, the normal control being 15 seconds.

On the first day after operation it was noticed that the right calf was tender and enlarged. There was a complete foot drop on the right and 50 per cent reduction in the power of plantar flexion of the ankle. There was anesthesia over the entire foot in the distribution of the fifth lumbar and first sacral nerve roots. Both feet were warm and both femoral pulses were palpable though diminished in volume. The weakness and anesthesia were interpreted as evidence of direct injury to the nerve roots. During the forty-one days of her stay in the hospital there was gradual improvement of muscle power and diminution of the area of anesthesia. The femoral pulses did not change and on several occasions faint pulsations in both dorsalis pedis arteries were felt. Oscillometric readings on the lower extremities indicated that the pulsations were diminished about 75 per cent.

Following discharge from the hospital she gradually regained strength and returned to her household duties. Examination seventeen months after operation revealed no change in blood pressure or in the size of the heart. She could walk briskly a hundred yards without difficulty. The femoral pulses were still palpable and had not changed in volume. A roentgenogram of the abdomen revealed the vitallium tube in its original position. At no time has it been possible to obtain blood pressure recordings on the lower extremities.

As a result of partial paralysis and atrophy of the anterior tibial muscles on the right, an equinus deformity developed along with flexion contractures of the toes. Nine months after the original operation a tenotomy of the tendon of Achilles and an arthrodesis of the interphalangeal joint of the right great toe were performed to correct the deformity.

Comment.—An injury to the abdominal aorta should be suspected when a large retroperitoneal hematoma is encountered during the exploration of a wounded abdomen. It is our firm conviction that such a hematoma should be explored regardless of whether or not it is increasing. Before the surgeon enters upon the exploration of such a hematoma, however, he should be prepared to manage a damaged aorta or vena cava by having available the proper instruments and adequate amounts of whole blood for immediate and rapid transfusion. Reluctance to disturb a retroperitoneal hematoma may result in the subsequent death of the patient from secondary hemorrhage.

Although it may seem perfectly obvious it should be emphasized that the most effective and safest method for controlling the immediate gush of blood from a large vessel is digital pressure. I have seen at least two patients become exsanguinated while the surgeon made frenzied attempts to grasp with a clamp a torn vessel completely obscured by a pool of blood. With the damaged vessel compressed beneath the fingers, the operator may thoroughly and carefully clean the field, accurately determine the site and nature of the injury, and formulate a plan for repair.

The method of management must of course vary according to the nature of the wound. In the previously reported successful cases and in my second case simple suture was the method of choice. This is certainly the ideal mode of management of such a wound because it restores continuity of the vessel with a minimum of trauma and decreases the danger of intravascular thrombosis. In the case described, however, because of loss of substance and extensive damage to the wall of the vessel, simple suture of the perforations was not possible. Three methods of management were considerd. Ligation was rejected because of the danger of gangrene of the lower extremities or hemorrhage due to cutting through of the ligatures. Elkin[6] in 1940 collected twenty-four cases of ligation of the abdominal aorta and added one of his own. In only ten of these cases was ligation complete and only seven of the patients survived the operation. No case of successful ligation of the aorta for traumatic injury has been found in the literature.

The second possible method, and the ideal one in this case, resection of the damaged segment with end-to-end anastomosis, would perhaps have been feasible in the hands of a surgeon experienced in the technique and under ideal conditions. However, because of the precarious condition of the patient and because of the operator's lack of experience in the anastomosis of blood vessels this procedure was deemed too hazardous and time consuming to be attempted.

The third method, repair of the vessel by means of a vitallium tube, seemed to offer the best hope of success and certainly was the most simple in the case reported. Tuffier[7] in 1915 described a method of blood vessel anastomosis using a paraffin-coated silver tube. Blakemore and Lord[8] have devised a nonsuture method of blood vessel anastomosis employing vitallium tubes lined with a segment of vein. This work suggested the mode of management of the case described. It would have been desirable to have used a tube of larger caliber than 5 mm. had such been available. At the time of operation it was fully expected that the tube would sooner or later be occluded by a thrombus inasmuch as no intimal lining was provided. This has not, however, been the case as far as can be determined. It is likely that the increase in velocity of flow through the tube due to the diminution in the lumen of the vessel accounts for the lack of coagulation.

Although desirable, determinations of the pressure in the femoral arteries were not made because of lack of the appropriate apparatus and because of fear of damaging the vessels and producing thrombosis. There is, however, convincing evidence that the pressure in the arterial system distal to the tube is considerably less than that above the tube. The femoral pulse volume is greatly decreased and the dorsalis pedis pulses are only occasionally palpable. Oscillometric readings show pulsations which are much smaller than normal.

CASE 2 (No. 45171).—W. B., a 28-year-old white man, was brought to the hospital on Aug. 8, 1946, thirty minutes after having been shot with a 22 caliber rifle. The bullet passed through the soft tissue medial to the distal end of the left humerus and entered the chest through the left tenth rib interspace in the posterior axillary line. He was in moderately severe shock as evidenced by a blood pressure of 80/40 and a cold, clammy, ashen skin. Physical examination of the chest corroborated by roentgenograms, revealed no signs of pneumothorax, hemothorax, or pulmonary trauma. The abdomen was full, doughy, diffusely tender, and moderately rigid. The urine was grossly bloody. Roentgenograms showed the bullet in the pelvis.

Blood and plasma transfusion was started through a cannula in the right saphenous vein and the patient was prepared for operation. Despite rapid administration of 1500 c.c. of plasma and whole blood his condition failed to improve and the blood pressure began to fall. Increasing distention of the abdomen indicated rapid intraperitoneal hemorrhage. Therefore, under drop ether anesthesia the abdomen was opened by means of a long left rectus incision. A large amount of blood was encountered in the peritoneal cavity. After evacuation of most of the blood the origin of the hemorrhage was discovered to be in the gastrohepatic omentum where the main trunk of the left gastric artery had been severed. The distal cut end of the vessel was spurting vigorously. This was clamped and ligated with medium silk.

Exploration of the abdomen then revealed the bullet lying free in the cul-de-sac of Douglas. There was no injury to any portion of the gastrointestinal tract. A large retroperitoneal hematoma was discovered behind the splenic flexure of the colon. In order to expose the hematoma the parietal attachments of the splenic flexure were divided and the colon was mobilized medially by blunt dissection. The fascia of Gerota, distended with blood, was incised and the kidney palpated. Its entire upper one-third was shot away and there was active bleeding from the cut surface. Nephrectomy was done, the renal vessels and ureter being divided and ligated with double ligatures of braided silk.

Although this procedure served to control all bleeding the operator proceeded to explore the wound in the gastrohepatic ligament for the other end of the left gastric artery. During the search for the proximal end of the vessel there was a spurt of blood from deep in the retroperitoneal area. Digital pressure was applied and the area carefully exposed. A 1 cm. longitudinal rent was found in the anterior wall of the abdominal aorta. No other bleeding point could be found. It was postulated that the left gastric artery had in this case a separate origin from the aorta and that the bullet had passed through the junction of the artery with the aorta. The margins of the rent were grasped and approximated by means of Babcock intestinal forceps, while the wound was closed with a continuous locked suture of 00000 silk and several interrupted sutures of the same material. No leakage occurred from the aorta after release of the clamp.

The left kidney bed was drained by means of four lengths of Penrose tubing brought out through a stab wound in the left flank. The abdominal incision was closed with buried vertical figure-of-eight mattress sutures of No. 34 steel wire, and the skin was closed with fine silk.

At the end of the procedure the patient's blood pressure was 120/80 and his condition greatly improved. He received 2500 c.c. of whole blood and 750 c.c. of plasma during the operation, which lasted two hours and twenty minutes.

Postoperatively he was treated with penicillin, Wangensteen suction, and parenteral fluids. There was a marked oliguria and hemoglobinuria for two days, during which time the blood nonprotein nitrogen rose to 132 mg. per cent and periorbital edema appeared. This was attributed to a hemolytic transfusion reaction at the time of operation, and 0.6 molar sodium lactate was given, bringing the urinary pH from 5 to 7. By the fourth day the output was adequate and the azotemia subsided. Subsequent course was uneventful; the wound healed per primam, and he was discharged on the eighteenth day.

When seen nine months after the operation he was well and showed no sign of circulatory disturbance in the lower extremities. Blood pressure was 130/90. There was no mass or bruit over the upper abdomen.

Comment.—This case presented a much less difficult and complicated problem than did the first. The wound was tangential and consisted only of a small slit which was easily repaired. The importance of exploration of retroperitoneal hematomas is again illustrated. Failure to discover and repair injuries to retroperitoneal structures accounts for a large proportion of the preventable mortality in traumatic abdominal injuries.

DISCUSSION

Wounds of the aorta are found to be not necessarily fatal. Numerous cases have been reported in which persons have survived for varying periods of time up to ten years following aortic injuries.[9-30]

The survival of these patients has been attributed to three factors:

1. That the wound was small and became sealed by blood clot during the period of primary hemorrhagic shock.

2. That the injured portion of the aorta was in such a position that the surrounding tissues, together with the escaping blood, served as a tamponade.
3. That an acute arteriovenous fistula was formed allowing the return to the systemic circulation of much of the blood lost from the aorta.

The survival of both of the patients in my cases until the time of operation, which in each case was at least two hours after the injury, can be attributed to sealing of the wounds by blood clot and tamponade by blood extravasated into the retroperitoneal tissues.

Despite the fact that some patients survive injuries of the aorta, it should again be emphasized that failure to explore retroperitoneal hematomas is hazardous and may result in fatality from missed injuries to retroperitoneal viscera. It is also to be emphasized that anatomic reconstruction of an injured vessel is the desirable goal. This was accomplished in one of our cases while in the other, because of the circumstances, restoration of continuity with a vitallium tube was elected and proved successful.

SUMMARY

1. Two cases are reported in which a bullet wound of the abdominal aorta has been successfully repaired.

2. A review of the literature discloses only five previous instances of the successful repair of an aortic perforation.

3. Direct suture is the method of choice for repair of the aorta.

4. In one of my cases a nonsuture method utilizing a vitallium tube met with success when suture was not feasible.

5. The importance of exploration of retroperitoneal hematomas is emphasized.

REFERENCES

1. Dshanelidze, I. I.: Cited by Blalock.[2]
2. Blalock, A.: Successful Suture of a Wound of the Ascending Aorta, J.A.M.A. **103**: 1617-1618, 1934.
3. Elkin, D. C.: The Diagnosis and Treatment of Cardiac Trauma, Ann. Surg. **114**: 169-185, 1941.
4. Wildegans, Hans: Verletzungen der Aorta, Deutsche med. Wchnschr. **52**: 1810-1812, 1926.
5. Dubinskiy, M. D.: Sluckai shva bryushnoi aorti, Khirurgiya **4**: 71, 1944.
6. Elkin, D. C.: Aneurysm of the Abdominal Aorta, Ann. Surg. **112**: 895, 1940.
7. Tuffier: Intubation arteriélle substitutée à certaines ligatures immédiates des gros vaisseaux blessés, Presse méd. **23**: 416, 1915.
8. Blakemore, A. H., and Lord, J. W.: A Nonsuture Method of Blood Vessel Anastomosis, Ann. Surg. **121**: 435, 1945.
9. Heil: Beobachtung einer Verwundung der Art. Aorta ascendens, welche durch die Natur geheilt worden ist, Ztschr. f. d. Staatsarzneik. **33**: 458-460, 1837.
10. Bindemann: Eine Schussverletzung der Aorta abdominalis, Berl. klin. Wchnschr. **24**: 826-827, 1887.
11. Perthes, G.: Schussverletzung der Arteria Pulmonalis und Aorta, Beitr. z. klin. Chir. **19**: 414, 1897.
12. Hankel, Ernst: Stichverletzung der Aorta, traumatisches Aneurysma, Tod 17 Tage nach der Verletzung durch Erstickung, Deutsche Arch. f. klin. Med. **64**: 140-145, 1899.
13. Brentano: Schussverletzung der Aorta, Verhandl. d. deutsch. Gesellsch. f. Chir. **33**: 92-94, 1904.
14. Kratter: Cited by Oberhelman, H. A., and LeCount, E. R.: Peace Time Bullet Wounds of the Abdomen, Arch. Surg. **32**: 373-412, 1936.

15. Berg: Nicht tödliche Schussverletzung der Aorta, Ztschr. f. Med. Beamte **21:** 389-393, 1908.
16. Tegeler: Schussverletzung der Aorta mit eingeheilter Kugel in der Herzklappe, München. med. Wchnschr. **56:** 1740, 1909.
17. Momm: Cited by Oberhelman and LeCount.[14]
18. Minkowski: Schussverletzung der Aorta thoracica, Jahresb. d. schles. Gesellsch. f. vaterl. Kult. **38:** 38-39, 1917.
19. Hulst: Aneurysma spurium aortae abdominalis nach Schussverletzung, Vrtljschr. f. gerichtl. Med. **59:** 108, 1920.
20. Bonnet, Paul: Plaie de l'aorte abdominale pare balle: considérations sur les lésions anatomiques dans leurs rapports possibles avec l'hémostase spontanée, Gaz. d. hôp. **93:** 725-727, 1920.
21. Oesterlein, O.: Traumatic Aneurysm of Abdominal Aorta, Aerztl. Sachverst.-Ztg. **32:** 324-327, 1926.
22. LaRoque, G. Paul: Penetrating Bullet Wound of the Thoracic Aorta Followed by Lodgement of the Bullet in the Femoral Artery, Ann. Surg. **83:** 827-830, 1926.
23. Lubenau: Beitrag zur Ueberlebungsdauer und Handlungsfähigkeit nach tödlicher Verletzung der Aorta ascendens, Ztschr. f. Med.-Beamte **40:** 251-254, 1927.
24. Nissen, R.: Aneurysma des Aortenbogens nach Schussverletzung, Deutsche Ztschr. f. Chir. **211:** 262-265, 1928.
25. Mennyey, G.: Wounds of Aorta, With Varying Periods of Survival of Patient, Arch. di antropol. crim. **52:** 185-202, 1932.
26. Edmundson, K.: Transfixion of Aorta (by Arrow), Brit. J. Surg. **23:** 869-870, 1936.
27. Tesăr, J.: Knife Wound of Abdominal Aorta With Fatal Outcome After 11 Days, Časop. lék. česk. **76:** 1495-1497, 1937.
28. Kornblith, B. A.: Gunshot Wound Through the Abdominal Aorta, Ann. Surg. **113:** 637-640, 1941.
29. Pemberton, J., Seefeld, P. H., and Barker, N. W.: Traumatic Arteriovenous Fistula Involving the Abdominal Aorta and the Inferior Vena Cava, Ann. Surg. **123:** 580-589, 1946.
30. Storck, A. H.: Case Report, Ann. Surg. **123:** 607, 1946.

WAR WOUNDS OF THE RECTUM AND ANAL SPHINCTER

William S. McCune, M.D., Washington, D. C.

(From the Department of Surgery, George Washington University School of Medicine)

During World War II Walter Reed General Hospital was designated as a center for the treatment of wounds involving the rectum and anal sphincter. Harvey B. Stone, civilian consultant in surgery, had direct supervision over the treatment of these patients, made frequent visits to the hospital, examined practically all of the cases, and performed many of the operations personally. The Army is greatly indebted to Stone for thought and energy which he spent to give each man the best possible result in the repair of the injury. Following is an account of the classification, methods of treatment, and results obtained in this group of patients under his direction.

MATERIAL

Forty-one patients with wounds of the rectum and anal sphincter were treated. All except one of the wounds were due to enemy inflicted gunshot wounds, the majority caused by shell fragments or machine gun fire. All patients were between 20 and 36 years of age. In most instances no definitive treatment for sphincter incontinence or external rectal fistula had been given prior to transfer of the patient to this hospital, though in many instances skin grafts, secondary wound closures, and recto-urethral fistula repairs had been performed. One patient had had two previous attempted closures of a large external rectal fistula. The average lapse of time between receiving the wound and the first definitive treatment in this hospital was ten months. This length of time is explained by the fact that most cases were complicated by other injuries which received treatment priority. These included eleven rectovesical or urethral fistulas and numerous instances of sciatic nerve injury, perforations of the colon and small bowel, and compound fractures of pelvic bones. All patients had had débridement of the wounds and most of them a temporary sigmoid colostomy at the time of injury. Most of them had had local application of sulfanilamide crystals and shock treatment in the form of plasma and blood transfusions.

PRELIMINARY TREATMENT AND CLASSIFICATION

On admission each patient was carefully examined, proctoscopy was carried out, the case was discussed, and the injury classified. He was then placed on a regime of sphincter and gluteal muscle exercises and re-examined at weekly intervals for a period of about four weeks before any operative treatment was carried out. This was done because of the striking results which followed these exercises, alone, in many instances. By this routine eleven patients regained adequate sphincter control without operation and the colostomies were closed with satisfactory outcome. The remaining thirty cases fell into five groups: (1) high rectal fistulas not involving the anal sphincter; (2) wounds of the anal sphincter in which part of the muscle was replaced by scar, but the remainder functioned satisfactorily; (3) complete destruction of the sphincter, but

Received for publication, July 14, 1947.

with good perianal tissues and good gluteal muscle function (this group included injuries of the nerve supply of the sphincter, as those which occurred in sacral wounds); (4) complete destruction of the sphincter with additional loss of perianal tissues; (5) complete loss of sphincter, lower rectum, perianal tissues, and gluteal muscles, with extensive scar formation. (By the term "sphincter" is meant the entire muscular mechanism for voluntary control of bowel movements and it includes both the external and internal muscles.)

GENERAL OPERATIVE ROUTINE

All patients were given sulfasuxidine, 5 Gm. every eight hours by mouth and 2 Gm. daily into the lower loop of the colostomy for five days before operation; rectal and colostomy saline enemas were given until clear the night before operation. Except for high rectal fistulas all operations were performed in lithotomy position because that seemed to give better exposure than the prone or jackknife positions. Because of the extensive scarring the difficulty in finding torn ends of sphincter muscle and the danger of breaking into old recto-urethral fistulas, etc., we became thoroughly impressed with the fact that the general surgical principles of good light, adequate exposure, and hemostasis are essential for success in this work.

In determining the end result of treatment several factors were considered. Objectively the result was judged largely by the degree of sphincter function which was detectable on examination and the patient's ability to control liquid and solid bowel movements. Of equal importance, however, was found to be the patient's subjective satisfaction in his result. Many patients who had relatively little sphincter control were able, with the aid of a low residue diet and an occasional low enema, to lead normal economic lives and were well satisfied, while others, with better control, complained bitterly of occasional accidents.

High Rectal Fistulas.—Four patients with external rectal fistulas, above the anal sphincter, were admitted. One extended from the rectum, one inch above the sphincter, backward, around the coccyx to end in a granulating area on the skin. Another (Fig. 1) extended from a wound of entrance just to the right of the sacrum inward to the rectosigmoid junction. These slowly healed completely after thorough curettement of granulation tissue and the rongeuring away of sequestrated bone from the coccyx and sacrum. In the two remaining patients the coccyx and lower sacrum had previously been removed, the fistulas extending straight out from the rectum below the amputated stump of sacrum. These fistulas were closed by a method demonstrated by R. F. Bowers. With the patient in a prone position the external opening of the fistula was excised by a midline elliptical incision. Dense scar tissue was then carefully dissected completely away from the rectal wall for a distance of at least 1½ inches from the fistulous opening on all sides. Bone was rongeured away from the sacral stump until the fistula was quite free. Its edges were then excised and the fistula was closed by a running 00 chromic suture reinforced by interrupted serosal sutures. Large well-vascularized flaps of muscle and subcutaneous tissue were dissected out as far laterally as possible until they could be united in the midline to close dead space. The skin was closed with silk, leaving a stab wound drain well away from the old fistulous tract. The wounds healed by primary intention in both cases. In one the fistula has now remained closed for six months since closure of the colostomy. In the other the colostomy was closed in August, 1946, but the fistula reopened in October and it was necessary to reopen the colostomy. The fistula has now entirely closed again spontaneously.

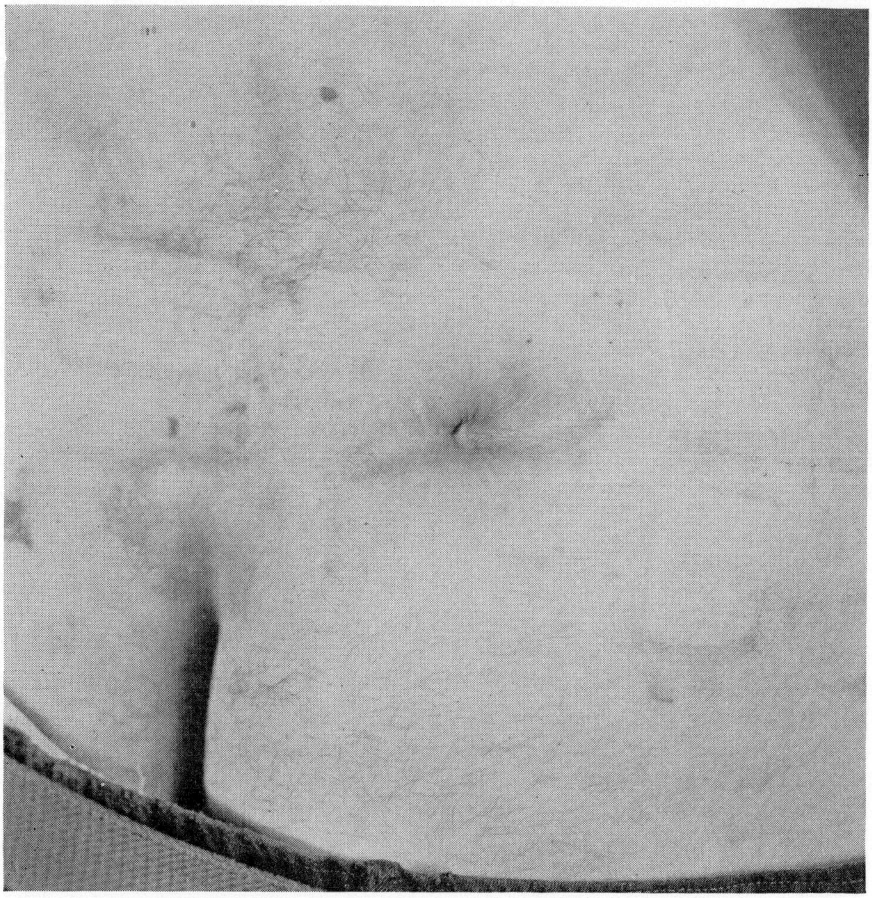

Fig. 1.—High rectal wound resulting in external fecal fistula.

CASE 1.--A 36-year-old private first class of the Infantry was admitted to Walter Reed General Hospital on May 13, 1945. He had been well until Nov. 22, 1944. On that date near Luxemburg he was wounded by enemy machine gun fire which resulted in a wound of the left upper arm with fracture of the left humerus and a gunshot wound in the left hip, the bullet traversing the upper rectum and having its wound of exit through the lower part of the sacrum. He received medical aid six hours after injury and was taken to a battalion aid station, from which he was transferred to the evacuation hospital, arriving on Nov. 22, 1944. There it was found that the sigmoid colon had likewise been perforated. On Nov. 23, 1944, under gas-oxygen anesthesia, closure of the perforation of the rectosigmoid was performed, a Penrose drain placed in the pelvis, and colostomy performed. The wounds gradually healed. He was then sent through air evacuation to the Zone of Interior.

In April, 1945, he began to complain of pain in the left hip and was finally placed in traction with an x-ray diagnosis of osteoarthritis of the left hip. Meanwhile a high rectal fistula had developed in the gunshot wound of exit. An attempt at closure had been made but had not been successful.

Physical examination on admission to Walter Reed General Hospital revealed a markedly emaciated patient lying in bed in a body cast. There was a midline incisional scar and a left-sided double-barreled colostomy functioning well. There was a deep wound over the coccygeal area; it was draining purulent exudate. The anus and rectum appeared normal on inspection. On a digital examination the anal sphincter was normal but there was found to be a direct communication through the coccygeal wound into the rectum. A probe passed through this wound, which was approximately 1 cm. in diameter, could be seen with a proctoscope in the upper rectum.

The rectum was irrigated daily with saline solution and a penicillin pack placed in the external opening of the fistula, but the fistula failed to heal. On Jan. 28, 1946, therefore, under general anesthesia with the patient in a prone position an incision was made excising the fistulous tract, carried down through dense scar tissue to the rectum itself. What appeared to be the third and fourth segments of the sacrum were removed in order to allow better exposure of the fistula. There was dense scar entirely around the opening in the bowel and this was excised. Gluteal muscles and the origins of the sacrospinalis muscles were then carefully dissected backward retaining their blood supply as much as possible until sufficiently large flaps of muscle were formed to cover the defect. The fistula itself was closed by a purse-string suture. With heavy catgut sutures the muscle flaps were imbricated over the defect and the wounds closed tightly except for one cigarette drain.

The postoperative convalescence was uneventful. On Feb. 20, 1946, the wound had apparently completely healed. The patient was walking with the aid of crutches, the left hip being almost entirely ankylosed. In August, 1946, the colostomy was closed by intraperitoneal end-to-end anastomosis. The postoperative course was satisfactory and when last seen the patient was about to be discharged from the Army.

Destruction of Part of Anal Sphincter.—Eleven of the forty-one cases fell into the group with part of the anal sphincter destroyed and were treated surgically. Operative treatment consisted of four steps, all performed as a single procedure (Fig. 2). (1) In lithotomy position an incision was made at or just outside the mucocutaneous border of the anus and usually extended entirely around the anus. Sometimes only one-half of the anal circumference was necessary. The mucous membrane was dissected proximally for 1½ to 2 inches to a point well above the scarred area so that after excision of the scar the mucous membrane could be pulled down and resutured to the skin covering the defect. (2) The scar tissue was excised from the sphincter muscle, skin, and mucous membrane. (3) The ends of the anal sphincter were then carefully dissected out far enough back to allow them to be crossed over, sutured together with several mattress catgut sutures, and anchored to the perianal tissues. (4) The mucous membrane was drawn down and sutured back to the skin with carefully placed interrupted silk sutures. In large defects a small rubber drain was sometimes placed through a stab wound outside the sphincter for a period of forty-eight hours. Postoperatively, hot sitz baths were begun on the fourth or fifth day and the skin sutures removed on the eighth day.

In general, the final results in this group were good. Six of the eleven patients had good sphincter power, could hold liquid or solid bowel movements, and were well satisfied. Three had fairly good sphincter power and could control water for a short time, solid bowel movements indefinitely. One of these was somewhat dissatisfied with the result. Of the remaining two both had severe injuries. One developed slight sphincter power postoperatively and because of the scarred distortion of the anal canal was able to control solid bowel movements to his own satisfaction. The last of the eleven (Case 3, Fig. 3) entered

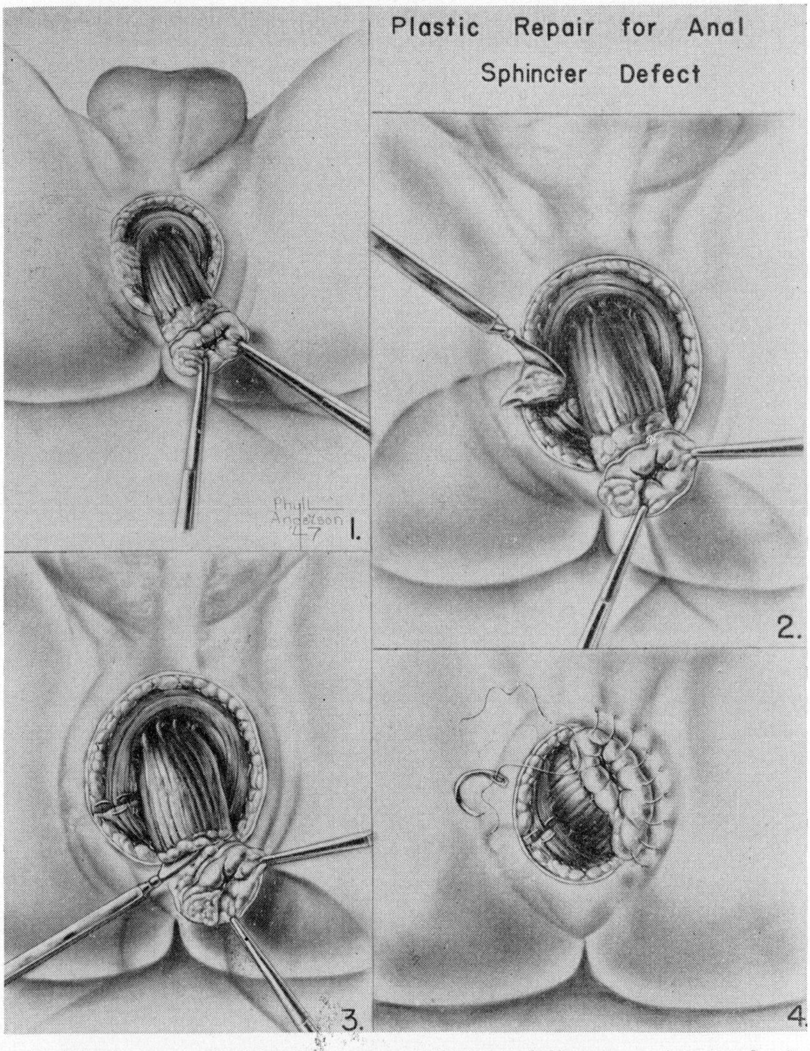

Fig. 2.—*1,* A circular incision has been made around the mucocutaneous border of the anus and the mucous membrane of the rectum dissected upward for a distance of about 1½ inches. Mucous membrane, including scarred area, is drawn downward. *2,* Scar is excised from exposed anal sphincter. *3,* Sphincter muscle has been repaired. Rectal mucous membrane is cut across above scarred area. *4,* Remaining mucous membrane is sutured to skin to cover repaired sphincter.

this hospital with a four square inch defect in the posterior wall of the rectum and an old rectourethral fistula. The rectal defect was closed as a first step. At a later stage an attempt was made to find sufficient muscle to form an adequate sphincter with only partial success. In this procedure the old rectourethral fistula was inadvertently reopened. At a third stage a Young-Stone plastic repair of the urethral fistula was performed and scar tissue excised. This was successful. He now has slight sphincter control and has a good anus without excessive scarring. The colostomy has not yet been closed.

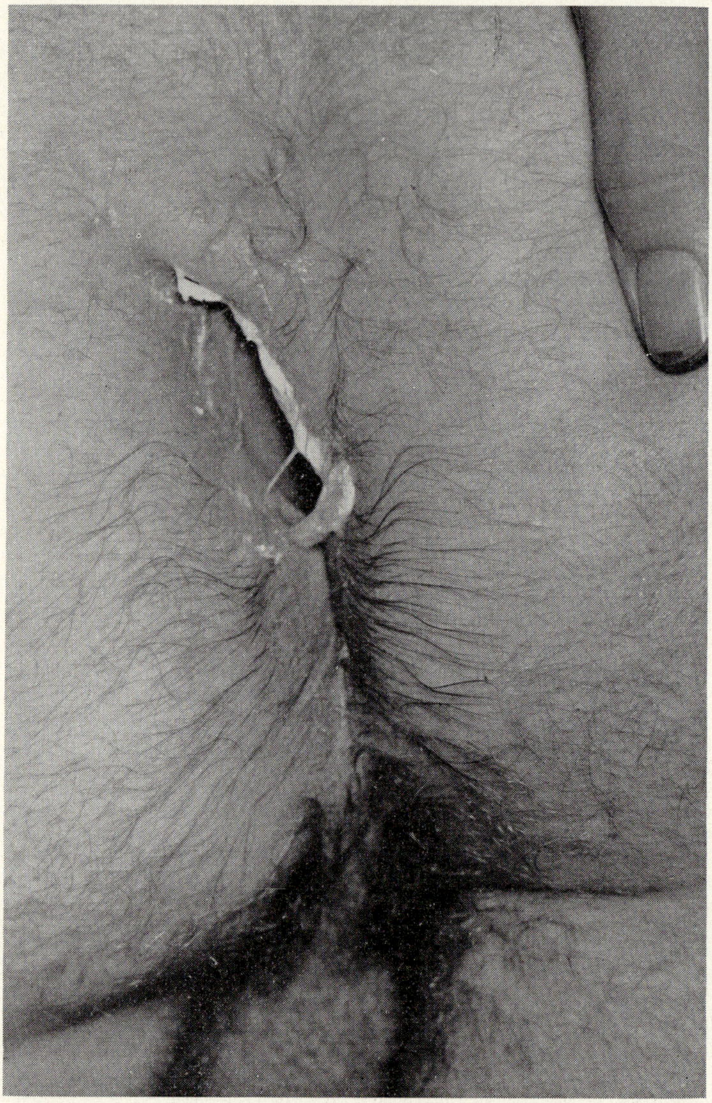

Fig. 3.—Wound causing complete destruction of posterior wall of the rectum and almost the entire anal sphincter.

CASE 2.—A 24-year-old corporal of the Engineers, with three years and two months service, was admitted to Walter Reed General Hospital on March 2, 1945. He had been well until Aug. 17, 1944. On that date, while in action against the enemy, near Chartrez, France, he was severely wounded by a shell fragment which produced a penetrating wound of the right buttock on its medial surface, involving the rectum, bladder, terminal ileum, and jejunum.

On the date of injury a laparotomy was performed at an evacuation hospital with resection of twelve inches of mid-ileum and six inches of the lower jejunum with end-to-end anastomosis, repair of the bladder wound, and performance of a lower sigmoid colostomy. Wounds of entrance and exit were débrided. His condition gradually improved and he was transferred through a series of hospitals, arriving at this hospital for definitive care.

Physical examination on admission revealed a left sigmoid colostomy functioning well. There was considerable scarring about the rectum but all wounds were healed. There was a scar on the right side of the rectum which distorted the anal canal. The anal sphincter function was fairly good but was interfered with by this scar. Water injected into the distal loop of the colostomy passed through the rectum and the patient was unable to control it. He was able to partially control barium solution injected into the lower loop of the colostomy. He was given a regime of sphincter muscle strengthening exercises without appreciable improvement in his condition.

On April 7, 1945, under transacral-caudal anesthesia, plication of the rectal sphincter and plastic to the anus were performed. The postoperative course was uneventful and on Aug. 3, 1945, examination showed good sphincter power, no drainage from the rectum, and a well-healed scar. A small amount of scarring was palpable in the upper third of the anus on the right side. Water placed into the lower loop of the colostomy could be held indefinitely. On Aug. 13, 1945, under spinal anesthesia, an intraperitoneal closure of the left sigmoid colostomy was performed. On Aug. 22, 1945, examination showed continued improvement in the function of the sphincter muscle and on Sept. 19, 1945, the patient was discharged from the service.

Case 3.—On Feb. 23, 1945, on Luzon, Philippine Islands, this Infantry soldier was wounded by machine gun fire sustaining two wounds, one in the right thigh near the groin and the other in the left thigh near the lateral surface. Both of these wounds made their exits through the rectum. He was operated upon that day, a colostomy performed, and the wounds débrided. He was then evacuated through a chain of hospitals, arriving at Walter Reed General Hospital for definitive care.

Physical examination on admission to this hospital was essentially negative with exception of the rectum and perineal area. There was a large open defect lying between the tip of the coccyx and the anterior border of the anal sphincter through which the anterior wall of the rectum was exposed over an area of about two inches in diameter (Fig. 3). The posterior wall of the rectum was entirely absent to that extent. No sphincter action whatever was demonstrable. A urethral fistula which had been present previously was healed. The colostomy was functioning well.

The wound was treated by daily wet dressings. Examination on Oct. 20, 1945, showed a clean wound with no sinus or fistula and it was felt that some degree of movement of the sphincter could be detected. The large defect in the posterior rectal ampulla appeared to be unchanged. In November, 1945, under satisfactory spinal anesthesia, the edges of the large defect were excised with the removal of a large amount of scar tissue. The rectum was then carefully freed from the overlying tissues entirely around the defect to a sufficient degree so that the rectum could be closed and the skin closed over the defect leaving only a small opening for the anus. This wound healed well.

In February, 1946, an attempt was made to restore anal sphincter function. Scarring was so dense, however, that although the sphincter muscle was found and could be brought around the anus, it was impossible to free the mucous membrane sufficiently to bring it outside the newly formed anus to prevent further scar formation. In dissecting free the scar tissue anteriorly the old urethral fistula was inadvertently broken into. A urethral catheter was placed in the urethra and the patient returned to the ward. Postoperative convalescence was somewhat stormy because of the development of cystitis. However, the anal sphincter thus formed functioned satisfactorily and a definite degree of contraction was discernible. Water placed in the lower loop of the colostomy could only be slowed and could not be definitely stopped by the new sphincter. The posterior drainage on removal of the catheter decreased to only a few cubic centimeters a day and the wound slowly healed.

In November, 1946, another attempt at dissection of mucous membrane of the rectum upward was made successfully, the urethral fistula was closed, and a satisfactory anus resulted. There is now some detectable sphincter function. The colostomy has not yet been closed. A fascial sling plastic procedure is being considered to provide more effective sphincter function.

Complete Sphincter Loss With Good Perianal Tissues.—Patients with no sphincter action but good gluteal muscle action if not complicated by excessive scar or stricture formation were found to be suitable candidates for the Stone

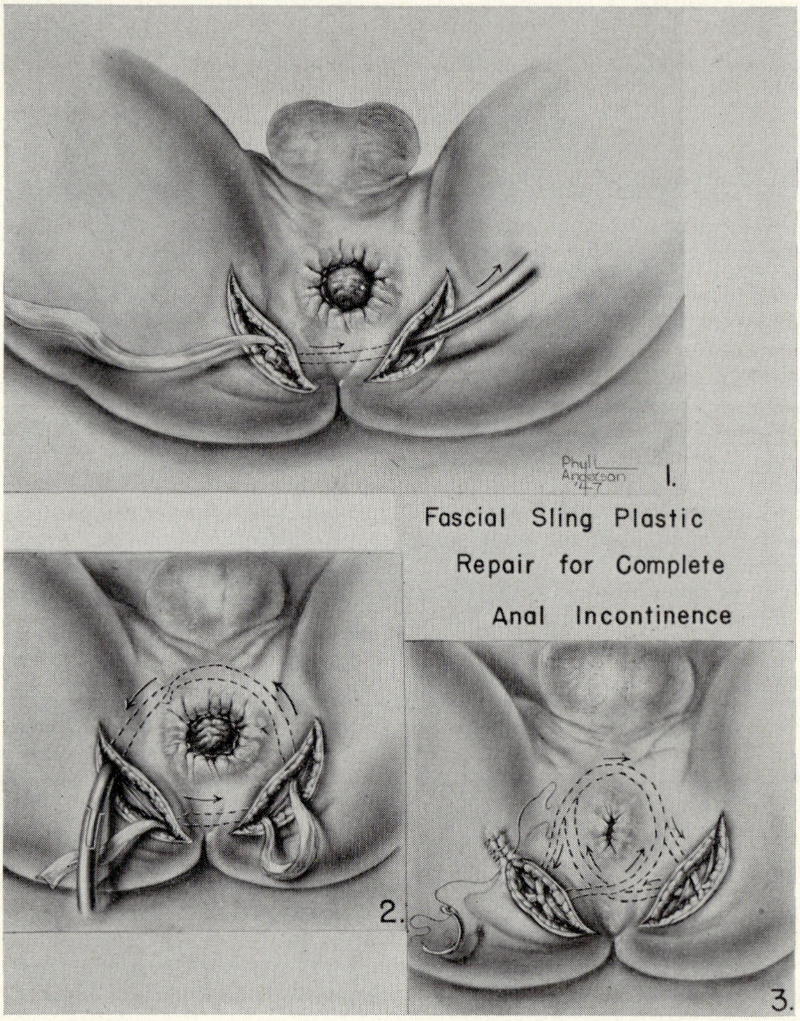

Fig. 4.—*1,* Short incisions have been made on each side of anus posteriorly, exposing lower edge of gluteus maximus muscle. A strip of ox fascia is pulled through posterior subcutaneous tunnel from one incision to the other. *2,* End of the strip is drawn back through anterior subcutaneous tunnel, passed through a portion of gluteus muscle, and tied to the distal end of the same strip, forming a sling around one side of the anus. *3,* Beginning at the opposite incision a second strip of fascia is passed in the opposite direction and tied in a similar way completing the circle. The skin is closed with silk.

type of fascial plastic operation.* These cases were difficult problems at best. Although the operation did not insure good sphincter function in all instances it often made the difference between total incontinence and sufficient control for a reasonably normal life. The Stone fascial repair was performed nine times in eight patients, one repeat operation being necessitated by sloughing out of the first strip of fascia. With the patient in lithotomy position (Fig. 4) 3 cm. incisions were made posterolateral to the anus on each side. These were carried down to the medial border of the gluteus maximus muscle. By blunt dissection with a curved Kelly clamp a tunnel was made in the subcutaneous tissues around the anus anteriorly connecting the two lateral incisions. A similar tunnel was made posteriorly. Care had to be exercised not to make these tunnels too close to the mucous membrane of the rectum or to the skin for fear of the fascial strips sloughing through. Anteriorly there was danger of breaking into old recto-urethral fistulas. When the tunnels had been completed a strip of ox fascia was slipped through the anterior tunnel from left to right, then the end returned through the posterior tunnel from right to left. A similar strip was placed beginning from the right side. Thus a double noose purse string was formed. Each loop was passed through a large bite of gluteus maximus muscle and tied tightly enough to produce a definite sphincter effect but not tightly enough to slough through the mucous membrane of the rectum. Careful aseptic technique was essential. Penicillin in oil, 300,000 units daily, was given for seven days postoperatively. Fascia lata has been used in some cases by Stone, but he has reported ox fascia to be equally effective.

CASE 4.—A 23-year-old private of the Armored Force had been well until Aug. 31, 1944. On that date, while on reconnaissance duty, he was captured by the enemy in France. Some time later Americans appeared and this soldier and the men with whom he had been captured were shot in the back by pistol fire by the Germans. He was hit by two bullets. One penetrating the right buttock posteriorly made its exit anterior to the tuberosity of the ischium. The other struck him in the perineum, anus, scrotum, and rectum, resulting in avulsion of the left testis and severe injury to the perineum, anus, and rectum with perforation of the posterior urethra and rectum. He was taken to a field hospital and on Sept. 1, 1944, a colostomy, suprapubic cystotomy, laparotomy, left orchidectomy, and débridement of the perineum were performed. He was transferred to a general hospital in England where it became evident that there was a recto-urethral and rectoperineal fistula. He arrived by transfer at the Walter Reed General Hospital April 24, 1945.

Examination on admission revealed a functioning double loop colostomy, suprapubic cystotomy, and a perineal scar with a 1 cm. fistulous tract opening from which purulent fluid could be expressed. There was some anal sphincter tone posteriorly and considerable stenosis of the anal orifice. He developed nephrolithiasis which was treated conservatively until August 21, when a left pyelotomy and nephrolithotomy were performed. On Jan. 29, 1946, a Young-Stone repair of the recto-urethral fistula was performed. The patient was transferred to the General Surgical Service.

Examination on transfer revealed a tight fibrous band at the mucocutaneous border of the rectum, considerable fibrotic scarring of the anal canal, and slight weak anterior sphincter action. Because of the fact that this sphincter action was nearly absent it seemed improbable that any sphincter could be successfully brought around the anal canal to function satisfactorily. Therefore, since the gluteal function was good, it was felt that a fascial strip plastic

*Stone, H. B., and McLanahan, S.: Results With Fascia Plastic Operation for Anal Incontinence, Ann. Surg. **114**: 73-77, 1941.

operation would be feasible. On Feb. 21, 1946, this was done under sacral anesthesia. The postoperative course was satisfactory and on the seventh postoperative day there was some definite sphincter action on contraction of the gluteus maximus muscles. The sigmoid colostomy was closed. Sufficient sphincter action was present for control of liquid and solid bowel movements.

CASE 5.—A corporal of the Infantry was admitted to the Walter Reed Hospital on March 10, 1945, because of a lacerated wound of the anus and rectum. He had been well until June 16, 1944. On that day near St. Lo, France, he was wounded by enemy machine gun fire sustaining a severe lacerated injury of the right and left buttocks and perineum with penetration of the anus, rectum, and membranous urethra and a fracture of the left ischial tuberosity. These injuries were followed by a chronic perineal-urethral fistula. He received emergency treatment in the form of débridement of wounds, suprapubic cystotomy, and later a sigmoid colostomy on June 17, 1944, at an evacuation hospital. He was evacuated to the United States on Nov. 2, 1944, and transferred to Walter Reed General Hospital.

On admission examination revealed considerable scarring of the anal canal with a very hard ridge of scar tissue posteriorly and a softer, thinner narrow ridge of scar tissue anteriorly. The examining finger could be inserted only about 1½ to 2 cm. into the anus because of the dense scarring. The urinary fistula had closed. On April 1, 1945, examination revealed very little sphincter control and since no sphincter muscle could be felt it was decided that a fascial sling operation should be performed. On July 7, 1945, this was done. Examination on Aug. 2, 1945, still showed considerable scarring but a very slight constriction of the canal was produced when the patient tightened the gluteus maximus muscles. On Sept. 2, 1945, examination showed fair anal constricting power and it was decided that the colostomy should be closed and at the same time the rectum dilated to two fingers at operation. The colostomy was closed under spinal anesthesia as an end-to-end intraperitoneal anastomosis and the rectum dilated. Postoperatively he was able to control solid bowel movements fairly satisfactorily, liquid movements only partially. He was discharged from the service on a certificate of disability.

Complete Sphincter Loss With Damage to Perirectal Tissues.—The group with complete sphincter loss with daamge to perirectal tissues was similar to the preceding one except for the fact that damage to perianal tissues made a preliminary plastic operation necessary before fascial strips could be introduced with safety. There was only one patient of this type in whom the coccyx had been removed and nothing remained over the posterior aspect of the rectum except skin. Through a midline posterior incision flaps of subcutaneous tissue were mobilized laterally and brought together in the midline between rectum and skin. At a later operation fascial strips were successfully placed around the anus.

CASE 6.—A 26-year-old Infantry soldier had been well until June 1, 1944. On that date while in action in Italy he was wounded by shell fragments in the area posterior to the rectum. A left sigmoid colostomy was performed. A urinary fistula later developed from the urethra into the rectum. On admission to the Walter Reed General Hospital the wound had healed entirely. He had good gluteal muscle function but no function of the anal sphincter whatsoever. After admission to Walter Reed Hospital a Davis-Stone repair of the urethral fistula was performed. When the patient was transferred from the urologic to the general surgical section his only complaint was complete paralysis of the anal sphincter due apparently to interference of the nerve supply of the sphincter because of the shell fragment wound. As a result of this wound examination on May 15, 1945, revealed only a thin scar posteriorly between the rectal mucosa and the skin. No sphincter action was discernible and it was felt that this patient would require a fascial strip operation to produce sphincter action. It was believed, however, that first excision of the scar posterior to the anus should be performed with the bringing of a fat and fascia layer between the skin and the rectal mucosa. On July 28, 1945, under satisfactory inhalation anesthesia, the old scar was excised, and subcutaneous tissue and fascia were interposed between skin and rectum. The skin was closed with interrupted silk sutures. This procedure healed well but because there was no return in sphincter function, on March 12, 1946, under satisfactory spinal anesthesia, a Stone type of ox fascia sling plastic sphincter was performed. The wound healed satisfactorily and on April 1, 1946, the patient was able to hold water for about two minutes when the latter was placed in the lower loop of the colostomy. When last seen the colostomy had not yet been closed.

Two of the eight patients in whom fascial plastic operations were performed had good or fairly good postoperative sphincter power, were able to control liquid as well as solid bowel movements, and were classified as having good results. Five had some contractile power and of these one could hold water for a short time and two were unable to hold water but could control solid bowel movements. The other two had not been tested in the ability to control water but could control solid bowel movements. The one remaining patient had no contractile power at all and could not control water or liquid bowel movements. This patient had only slight gluteal function on one side and none on the other. Due to scarring and obliquity of the anal canal, however, he rarely soiled himself and having been very much depressed when he entered this hospital was truly happy over the final result. All but two of the eight patients in this group were satisfied with their repairs.

TABLE I. RESULTS OF TREATMENT IN SPHINCTER INJURIES

TYPE OF TREATMENT	NUMBER OF CASES	SPHINCTER ACTION			HOLD WATER	HOLD FECES	PATIENT SATISFIED
		GOOD	FAIR	POOR			
Sphincter exercise only	11	10	1	0	11	11	10
Sphincter repair	10	6	2	2	7	9	9
Fascial sling plastic	8	2	5	1	3	8	6
Excision of scar and pull-through	1	0	0	1	0	1	Fairly

Complete Sphincter Loss With Extensive Scarring and Loss of Gluteal Function.—The patients with complete sphincter loss with extensive scarring and loss of gluteal function, the most severely wounded of all, comprised the group for which no satisfactory sphincter repair could be devised. Repairs of the preceding types were attempted but without success. The question then arose as to the type of treatment which would best enable these patients to lead relatively normal lives. This varied somewhat with the opinions of the surgeons and the wishes of the patients. Of the seven who fell within this category the first four were treated by converting their loop colostomies into end abdominal colostomies and resecting the remainder of the sigmoid and the scarred rectum by a Miles abdominoperineal resection. This rid the patients of a mucous seeping uncontrollable perineal colostomy. Because of the slight possibility that in the future some method might be devised of giving such patients a satisfactory perineal anus, three were treated conservatively. In one a pull-through perineal operation was performed with excision of the scarred area of the rectum and production of a perineal colostomy. In the remaining two no perineal surgery was performed. One of these was discharged with the loop sigmoid colostomy untouched. The other had the abdominal colostomy closed producing a perineal colostomy. In all such patients regular bowel habits, a low residue diet, and occasional low saline enemas were found to contribute materially to the management of the colostomies, whether perineal or abdominal.

The four patients with abdominoperineal resections and one with an open loop colostomy accepted the abdominal colostomies well. The two patients discharged with perineal colostomies were, on the whole, disappointed and may require abdominoperineal resections at a later date.

Case 7.—This private in the Infantry was wounded in action by shell fragments in Italy during the fall of 1944, sustaining a severe lacerated wound of the perineum and anal region with loss of muscle from both buttocks, exposing the sacrum and fracturing the tip of the sacrum. The lower rectum and anus were traversed by the fragments and the patient was admitted to an evacuation hospital in shock. The wound was débrided, he was given large amounts of blood and plasma intravenously, and a left sigmoid colostomy was performed. After a long period of convalescence he was transferred through several general hospitals, finally arriving at Walter Reed General Hospital in July, 1945.

Examination on admission revealed extensive scarring over the dorsum of the sacrum, in both buttocks and in the anal region. The sacrum had been covered by a skin graft which was very thin. No function of either gluteus maximus muscle was discernible and there was so much scarring of the anal region that not even a probe could be admitted into the rectum. He was seen in consultation and it was felt because of the absence of any contractile power either of the gluteus maximus muscle on either side or of the sphincter and the loss of the lower part of the rectum that an abdominoperineal resection of the lower sigmoid and rectum should be performed. Consequently, after preparing the patient with sulfasuxidine an abdominoperineal resection of the rectosigmoid was performed in August, 1945. The entire lower rectum was found to be replaced by scar tissue and the rectum was removed with considerable difficulty without injury to the urethra. An end colostomy in the left lower quadrant was performed. The wound healed satisfactorily and quite quickly and the left sigmoid colostomy functioned well. The only complaint of the patient was thinned-out tissue over the sacrum. He preferred, however, to have no further surgical operations at the time and was discharged from the Army.

CONCLUSION

The classification and treatment of these forty-one rectal war wounds and the evaluation of the results of the various operative procedures employed has convinced us of several facts: (1) sphincter muscle exercises are of great value in improving anal sphincter power; (2) the best operative results are usually obtained in those cases in which torn muscle ends can be approximated, even though not perfectly; (3) the Stone fascial plastic operation has a definite place in the treatment of such patients if the sphincter ends cannot be found. This operation has given enough control to restore many men to fairly normal lives; (4) when no repair of sphincter power can be devised an abdominoperineal resection is probably the procedure of choice. It must be remembered, however, that this precludes any later repair based upon future developments in rectal surgery.

A CANNULA FOR PANCREATIC FISTULA

A Device for Permitting Complete Periodic Experimental Collection of Pancreatic Juice

Ivan D. Baronofsky, Ph.D., M.D.,* Minneapolis, Minn.

(From the Department of Surgery, University of Minnesota)

THE study of pancreatic function in disease of the upper gastrointestinal tract has led to various experimental approaches to complete pancreatic fistulas in the surgical laboratory. It is evident from reviewing the literature that the preparation of permanent pancreatic fistula in a dog is a procedure that requires great patience on the part of the surgeon and diligent postoperative care. Those of us willing to undertake the care of such a preparation must remember Elman and McCaughan's classical observation that total drainage of pancreatic juice to the exterior resulted in the death of dogs in seven or eight days. This was true only if the entire output of the external secretion was excluded from the intestine.

In our laboratory, during the course of various studies on the etiology and treatment of peptic ulcer, it became necessary to prepare total pancreatic fistulas. It is the purpose of this paper to present a method by which such a preparation may be attempted and which lends itself to more prolonged experiments with a minimum of care and expense.

TYPES OF PANCREATIC FISTULAS THAT HAVE BEEN PROPOSED

Pavlov[2] described a fistula similar to Heidenhain,[3] in which an oval piece of duodenal wall bearing the orifice of the main duct is dissected out and transplanted into a slit on the abdominal wall. The opening of the bowel is then closed and the duodenum maintained against the anterior abdominal wall by temporary suspension sutures. In his classical description, Pavlov told of the use of rooms in which the floors are covered with sawdust and sand on which the animals may lie, allowing the pancreatic juice to be absorbed and thus preventing digestion of the skin by this juice. These fistulas are not complete, for in the dog the smaller pancreatic duct is important functionally, and in fact empties in association with the common bile duct.

Methods which make use of cannulas leading from the pancreatic duct to the anterior abdominal wall have been proposed by Bernard,[4] Ludwig,[5] and Fodera.[6] These preparations, however, allow for the escape of only part of the juice; moreover, the cannulas fall out.

Lattes,[7] in 1912, proposed a technique similar to Pavlov's. The ducts are brought out through the muscular walls. When the muscles contract, the secretions can thus be held back when not in use. In order to use this type of fistula,

---

The researches upon which this presentation is based were supported by the Robert A. Cooper Fund for Surgical Research, the Dr. and Mrs. Harry B. Zimmerman Fund for Experimental Surgical Research, and the Dr. Berenice Moriarity Fund.

Received for publication, June 10, 1947.

*National Cancer Trainee.

a cannula is inserted periodically. However, it is to be noted that the ampulla behind the external opening soon becomes dilated, as are the other ducts.

Frouin[8] attempted to bring the duodenum into the anterior abdominal wall. When sufficient fixation occurs, the duct is transplanted to the skin. Intestinal obstruction results, in addition to intestinal fistulas.

In 1922, Inlow[9] presented a method in which the duodenum is brought subcutaneously; the ducts are finally severed at a subsequent operation and brought externally. An attempt is made to sever all other small vessels and ducts immediately around the main duct. He employed an incision which is curved away from the duct; it was Inlow's contention that this maneuver will prevent obstruction and cicatrization as occurred in Frouin's experiments.

Elman and McCaughan[10] used the method of major pancreatic duct intubation, very much after the method of Rous and McMaster.[11] In their method, the minor pancreatic duct is cut and avulsed. The major duct is then cannulated, and the end attached to a long catheter. This tube is brought out through the flank and connected to a glass T tube, at one end of which a sterile rubber balloon is attached. The other end of the glass tube is used for emptying the balloon of its contents daily. Stringent aseptic precautions are necessary and therefore all joints are covered with gauze soaked in 5 per cent phenol. Again the problem of the cannula slipping out is presented.

More recently, Dragstedt, Montgomery, and Ellis[12] described a method which lends itself to more prolonged experiments. This method consists of transforming that portion of the duodenum with the pancreatic ducts emptying into it, into a closed loop. This duodenal sac is then cannulated by means of a gold-plated cannula which is led to the outside and carefully wrapped in omentum. The common duct is transplanted and the stomach is joined to the lower duodenum by means of a gastroduodenostomy. The total pancreatic juice is then collected in sterile rubber bags. The entire pancreatic secretion is thus lost to the outside at all times. These animals must be cared for rather intensively. Intravenous feeding or return of the pancreatic juice orally must be accomplished, otherwise the dogs will succumb.

In 1940, Bolydreff and Thompson[13] described a method of preparing a pancreatic fistula in which a glass cannula is placed directly into the major pancreatic duct transduodenally. A rubber catheter, which is attached to the glass cannula on the one end and a string on the other, can be brought in and out of the duodenum via a duodenal fistula which is prepared simultaneously. Thus, when the dog is not in use the pancreatic juice is within the intestine. The glass cannulas generally slip out and this may terminate an experiment.

A PERMANENT CANNULA METHOD FOR PANCREATIC FISTULA

In trying to evaluate the various types of pancreatic fistulas, it was decided that the type of fistula proposed by Dragstedt, Montgomery, and Ellis, in which the duodenum containing all the pancreatic ducts was used as a conduit, was the best in principle. However, since this type of procedure allowed for a continuous external loss of secretions to meet this objection, a new type of cannula was devised, which would allow for external collection of pancreatic juice when necessary, and at other times would allow for drainage into the distal intestine, thus preventing the fatal effect of total loss of pancreatic juice. The cannula, itself, as used in our laboratory, was constructed of stainless steel.* (Fig. 1.)

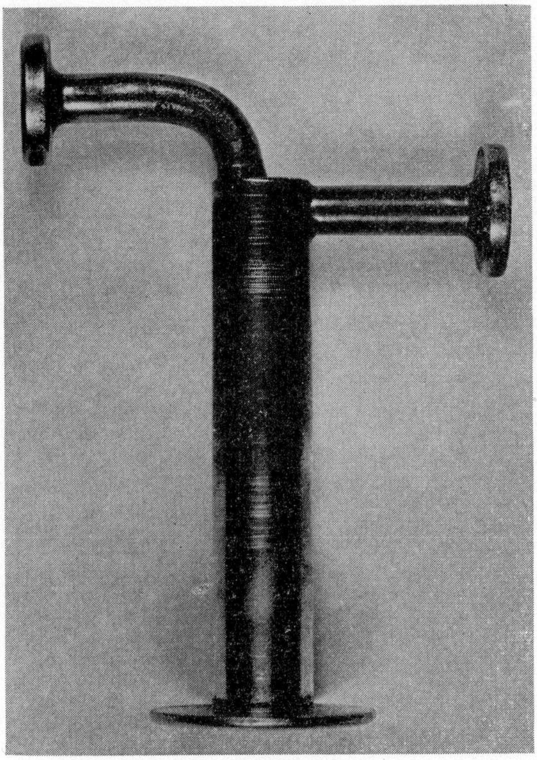

Fig. 1.—Permanent pancreatic cannula, constructed of stainless steel (full size).

Its use is best described by a diagrammatic sketch (Figs. 2 and 3). The common duct is carefully isolated as it enters the duodenum and is ligated and cut. The proximal end is then either transplanted to the stomach or intestine or ligated permanently, and an external biliary fistula is created by inserting a mushroom catheter into the gall bladder and bringing it out through a separate stab wound. The duodenum is then cut across about 2 cm. distal to the pylorus, and again just below the entrance to the lower pancreatic duct. The proximal end of the duodenal sac is then inverted and closed, while one flange of the cannula is placed in the other end. A purse-string type of inversion is then made to secure this in place. This latter procedure is then repeated, with the distal flange being placed and secured into the distal segment of duodenum, which is continuous with the intestinal tract. The continuity of the gastro-intestinal tract is then re-established by an aseptic end-to-side anastomosis of stomach to duodenum distal to this flange. Omentum is carefully wrapped

*By Mr. John Phelan of the Scientific Apparatus Division of the University of Minnesota.

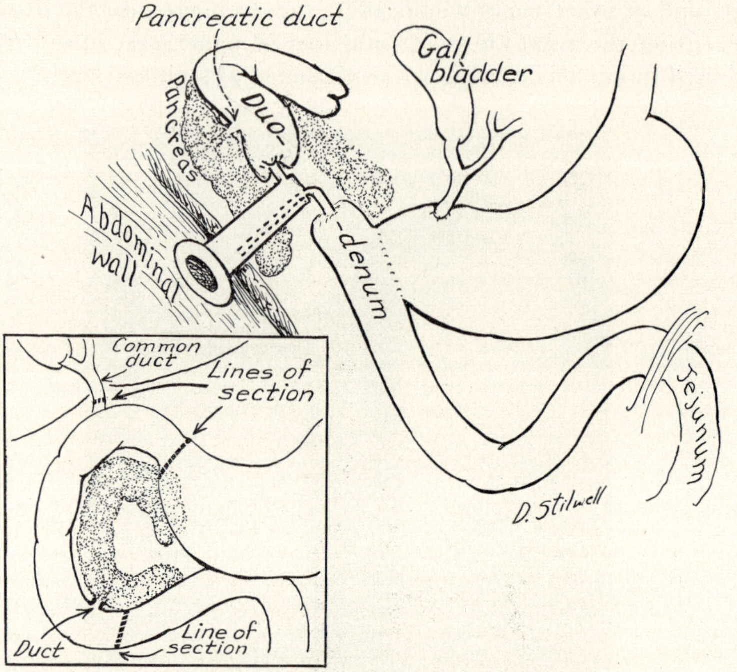

Fig. 2.—Small inset shows the lines of section of the duodenum and commonn bile duct. The common duct is carefully isolated as it enters the duodenum and is ligated and cut. The proximal end is transplanted to the stomach or duodenum. The duodenum is then cut across about 2 cm. distal to the pylorus, and again just below the entrance of the lower pancreatic duct.

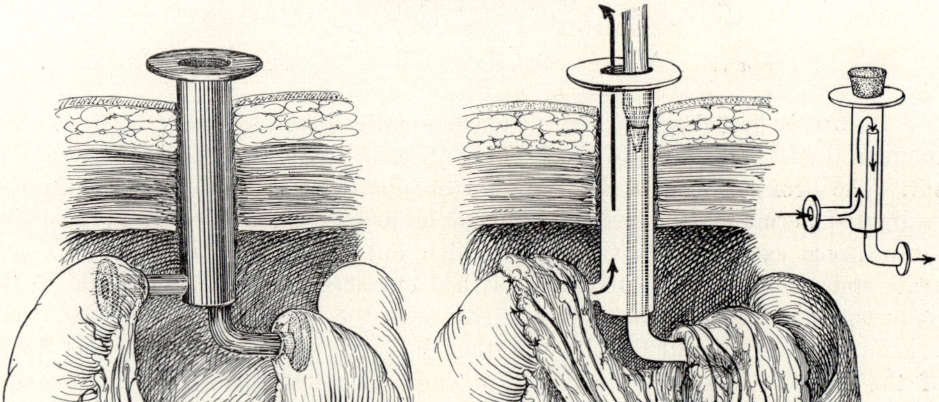

Fig. 3.—The method of placement of the pancreatic cannula. Left, placement of flanges into both proximal and distal portions of the duodenum. Purse-string types of inversions are used to secure this in place. Omentum is carefully wrapped around the metal cannula and this is then led to the outside through a stab wound. Right, direction of flow of pancreatic juice when preparation is being used. Small inset shows direction of flow of pancreatic juice when the animal is not actively employed in an experiment.

around the metal cannula and this is then led to the outside through a stab wound. The duodenal sac is fixed to the parietal peritoneum around the stab wound with a few sutures.

When in use, a small wooden plug is inserted into the inner opening within the cannula. This will prevent any reflux of juice from the intestinal tract proper. When not in use, a rubber stopper is inserted into the main cannula opening. This stopper is about 2 mm. thick and is flush with the external opening. This will prevent the animal from pulling it out and will allow for flow of pancreatic juice into the intestinal tract.

This preparation has been used in four animals with good results. Two of the animals were sacrificed after four months. Post-mortem examination showed the omentum had securely fixed the entire apparatus to the anterior abdominal wall with no leakage around it. One animal died of peritonitis due to leakage at the duodenal entrance of the cannula. The last animal had had an extensive gastric resection (95 per cent), a total biliary fistula, and a complete pancreatic fistula. This animal died after four months because of an accidental introduction into the intestinal tract of concentrated hydrochloric acid. All of the animals were fed normally with kennel ration and table scraps without the use of intravenous or subcutaneous feeding. Supplementary vitamins or bile salts were added to the diet as was deemed necessary.

SUMMARY

A method of total pancreatic fistula preparation is presented. This procedure offers the use of a metal T-shaped cannula which will allow for the selective removal of pancreatic juice, and the automatic return to the intestinal tract of this fluid when the animal is not actively employed in an experiment. The care of animals with pancreatic fistulas is much simplified by this procedure.

REFERENCES

1. Elman, R., and McCaughan, J. M.: Fatal Effect of Complete Loss of Pancreatic Juice, Proc. Soc. Exper. Biol. & Med. 24: 99, 1926.
2. Pavlov, I. P.: The Work of the Digestive Glands, second English edition, Philadelphia, 1910, J. B. Lippincott Company, pp. 4-10.
3. Heidenhain Quoted in Pavlov.[2]
4. Bernard Quoted in Pavlov.[2]
5. Ludwig Quoted in Pavlov.[2]
6. Fodera, Ph.: Permanente Pankreasfistel. Untersuchungun zur Naturlehre der Menschen und der Tiere, 1896, p. 16, 79.
7. Lattes, L.: Eines Methode Zur Herstellung Kontinenter Pankreasdauerfisteln, Ztschr. f. Biol. Techn. W. Method. 2: 366, 1912.
8. Frouin, A.: Nouvelle technique de la fistule pancreatique permanente. Presentation d'animaux et de pieces, Compt. rend. Soc. de biol. 74: 1283, 1913.
9. Inlow, Wm. DeP.: A Technique for the Establishment of a Permanent Pancreatic Fistula With the Secretion of Inactive Proteolytic Ferment, J. Lab. & Clin. Med. 7: 86, 1922.
10. Elman, R., and McCaughan, J. M.: Collection of Entire External Secretion of Pancreas Under Sterile Conditions and Fatal Effect of Total Loss of Pancreatic Juice, J. Exper. Med. 45: 561-570, 1927.
11. Rous, P., and McMaster, P. D.: Method for Permanent Sterile Drainage of Intra-abdominal Ducts as Applied to Common Duct, J. Exper. Med. 37: 11, 1923.
12. Dragstedt, L. R., Montgomery, M. L., and Ellis, J. C.: New Type of Pancreatic Fistula, Proc. Soc. Exper. Biol. & Med. 28: 109, 1930.
13. Boldyreff, W. N., and Thompson, O. E.: A New Type of Permanent Pancreatic Fistula, Permitting the Regulation of the Outflow of the Secretion, Tohoku J. Exper. Med. 38: 581, 1940.

VERRUCOUS CARCINOMA OF THE ORAL CAVITY

LAUREN V. ACKERMAN, M.D., COLUMBIA, MO.

(From the Department of Pathology, The Ellis Fischel State Cancer Hospital)

DURING the past seven years, we have noted a variety of squamous carcinoma whose behavior is unique and which has a typical clinical course with characteristic gross and microscopic findings. We have designated this type of squamous carcinoma as verrucous carcinoma and feel it should be separated from other epidermoid carcinomas for, even when extensive, with proper treatment the prognosis is excellent.

We have seen 31 patients; 26 were men and 5 were women. The majority of these patients were rather aged, the average age being 67 years (25 were over 60 years of age, and 13 of these were over 70). There was only one patient under 57 years. This patient was a woman of 41 years, with a lesion of the buccal mucosa; case history revealed that she was a tobacco chewer.

Tobacco chewing was probably a most important factor in the etiology of these lesions. Eleven of the 18 patients with lesions of the buccal mucosa were inveterate tobacco chewers. Seven of these patients also had lesions associated with leucoplakia. Friedell and Rosenthal* reported 8 patients with buccal mucosal and lower gingival lesions of verrucoid character in which tobacco chewing was thought to be an important etiologic factor. Over one-half of the patients reported here had poorly fitting dentures, poor oral hygiene, and carious and jagged teeth.

The lesions were distributed as follows: 18 were of the buccal mucosa; 8 of the lower gingiva; 1 of the upper gingiva; 2 of the hard palate; 1 of the tongue, and 1 of the tonsil. It was difficult to estimate clinically the duration of these lesions, but often they had been present for considerably over one year, and growth was relatively indolent.

As the lesions gradually increased in size to extend over a fairly large area, the patients not too infrequently complained of pain and difficulty in mastication, but there was seldom any bleeding. When the tumor arose in the region of the buccal mucosa, it tended to extend into the buccal gingival gutter. As it extended in surface area, it also locally invaded contiguous structures. It may grow into the cheek, even ulcerate on its surface (Fig. 1), may grow out to form a mass beneath the mandible (Fig. 2), and even grow from within the oral cavity to implicate the buccal commissure (Fig. 3). As the verrucous carcinoma frequently arises on the lower alveolus or extends into the buccal gingival gutter, it grows into the soft tissues overlying the mandible and quickly becomes fixed to the periosteum. With increased growth plus infection, it gradually destroys periosteum and directly invades and even destroys a considerable portion of the mandible (Figs. 4 and 5). Because of concomitant

Received for publication, June 21, 1947.

*Friedell, H. L., and Rosenthal, L. M.: The Etiologic Role of Chewing Tobacco in Cancer of the Mouth, J. A. M. A. 116: 2130-2135, 1941.

infection, the draining lymph nodes (particularly submental and submaxillary) frequently become enlarged and are invariably tender. This enlargement often leads to an erroneous diagnosis of metastatic carcinoma. The papillary lesions present a characteristic, somewhat pebbly, mammillated surface. The tumor may be relatviely soft, but with coexisting infection induration becomes prominent.

When these lesions are surgically resected, filmy leucoplakia may be found associated with them and invariably the often extensive lesion is piled up in rugal folds with deep cleftlike spaces between them (Figs. 6, 7, 8, and 9). If the tumor is cut into, it is often seen extending in the deeper tissues, and when deeply invasive it is associated with considerable infection.

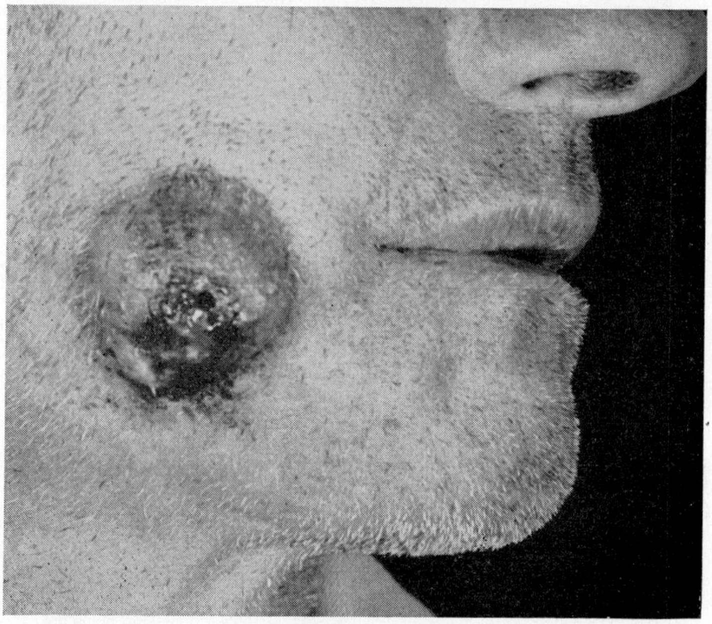

Fig. 1.—Verrucous carcinoma of buccal mucosa invading skin of cheek.

Microscopically there is often a rather rough transition between somewhat atrophic epithelium and the process. The first change noted is a piling up of keratin on the surface, with beginning downgrowth of fingers of epithelium (Fig. 10). As the process continues, club-shaped fingers of hyperplastic epithelium gradually push rather than infiltrate their way into the deeper tissues (Fig. 11). It should be emphasized that this epithelium is well differentiated and that the basement membrane remains intact. With further growth, the pattern becomes somewhat more complicated as more of the surface becomes involved. Cleftlike spaces with degenerating keratin project rather deeply. As the epithelium grows, the central portion of the fingers becomes well differentiated and finally undergoes cystic degeneration (Fig. 12). There is a wall of inflammatory tissue which is coexistent with the lesion and is present beyond it. This inflammation is made up of connective tissue, plasma cells, mononuclears, and, rarely, focal abscesses. The tumor gradually extends, but its invasion of other structures is probably considerably influenced by the presence of the accompanying inflammatory process. The local invasive qualities are prominent and any contiguous structure such as cheek, soft tissues in the submaxillary area, mandible, or antrum can be invaded. However, it is unique that

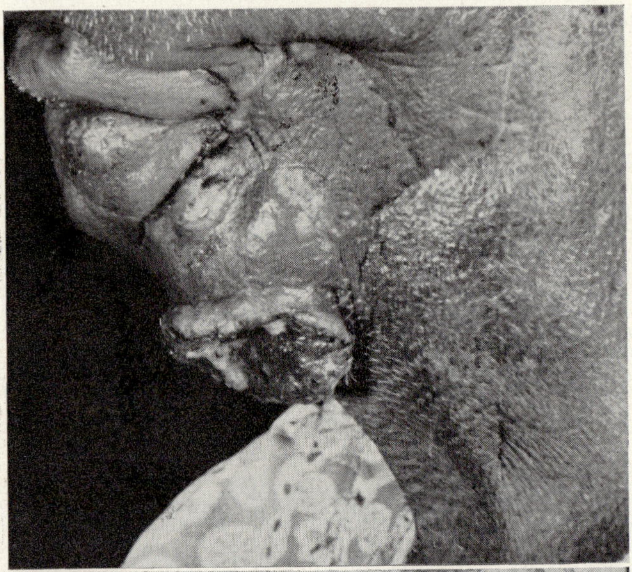

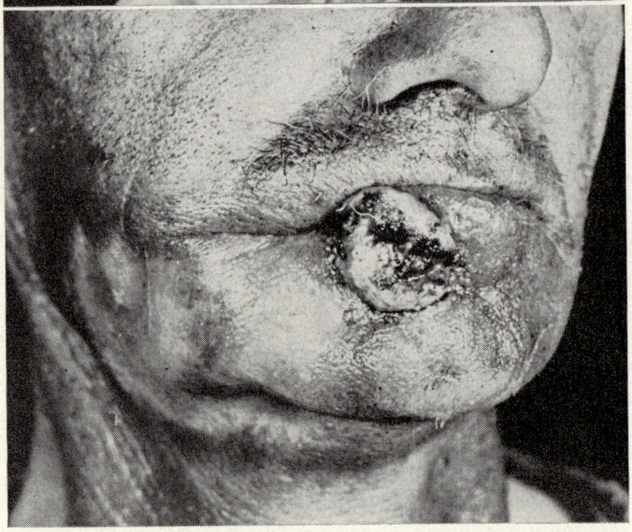

Fig. 2.—Local recurrence following partial mandibular resection. (The only case of such recurrence. This patient had been treated previously by irradiation.)

Fig. 3.—Verrucous carcinoma extending from within the oral cavity to implicate the buccal commissure.

although the tumor may grow in the immediate proximity of lymph nodes, it invariably grows around them rather than metastasizing to them. Although in 10 instances the extensiveness of the tumor necessitated partial or complete mandibular resection with upper neck node dissection, in only one patient was a regional node involved by direct extension and in only one other patient recently seen was a single high metastatic node implicated. In no instance have distant metastases appeared.

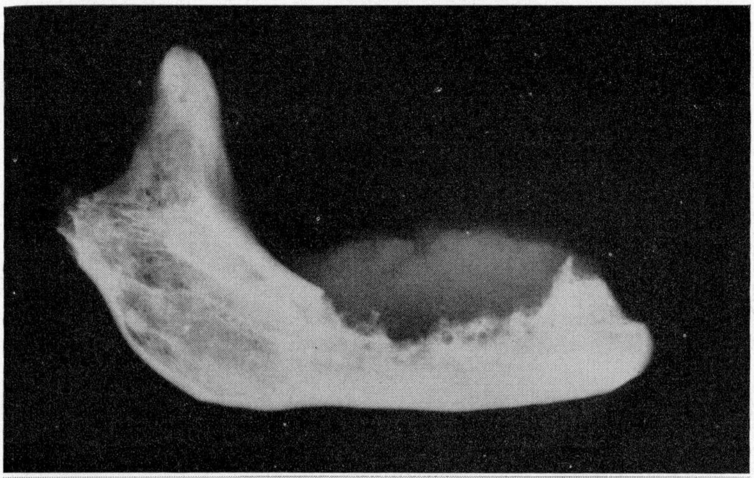

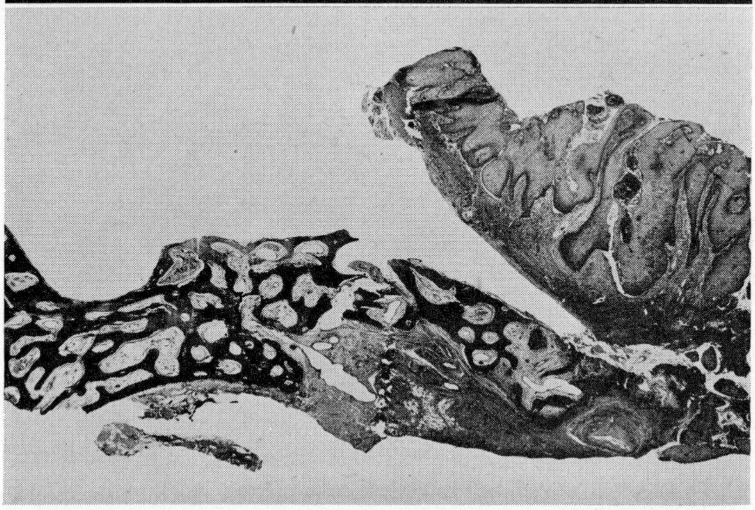

Fig. 4.—Extensive secondary destruction of the mandible.
Fig. 5.—Replacement of the mandible by verrucous carcinoma (very low power).

Friedell and Rosenthal reported 8 cases which apparently fall into this group, for the lesions described by them occurred in aged men on the buccal mucosa and lower gingiva. The lesions were described as papillary verrucoid in character and, although often extensive, only one out of 8 metastasized. They were treated by irradiation and this was immediately successful in controlling the disease. However, the longest follow-up was two years, and most of the other surviving patients had been followed six months or less.

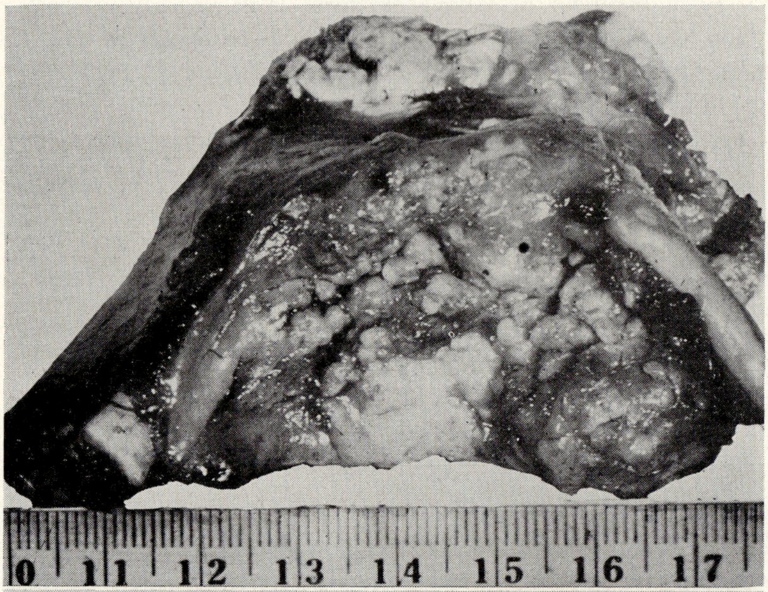

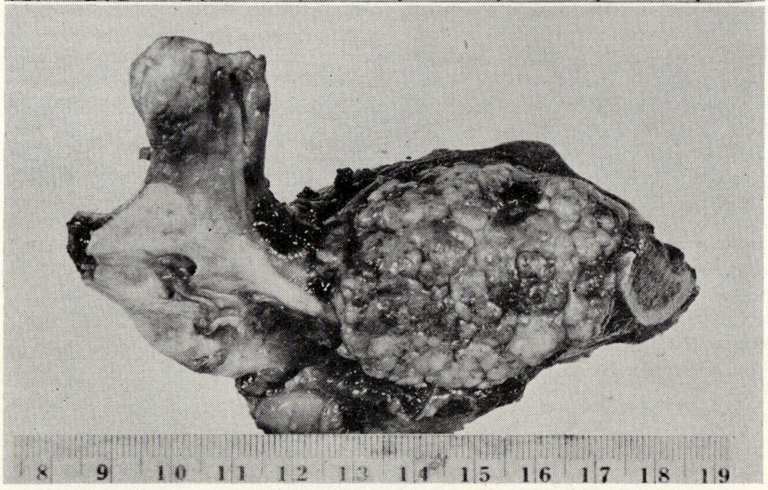

Fig. 6.—Photograph of gross specimen of verrucous carcinoma; note papillary character and associated leucoplakia.

Fig. 7.—Photograph of gross specimen; typical pebbly verrucous carcinoma.

The biopsy material from this neoplasm is often confusing. Superficial biopies are often taken and a positive diagnosis of carcinoma cannot be made. Even with thin deep biopsies, which are recommended, diagnosis may be difficult because of the intact basement membrane and the well-differentiated nature of the growth. However, after the characteristic pathologic pattern is recognized, even early lesions can be diagnosed and proper treatment instituted without delay.

These verrucous carcinomas of the oral cavity have been treated by a variety of methods:

Radiation Alone.—Seven patients were treated by radiation alone. In all of these, the lesion was rather superficial. Two died, both of pneumonia, one five months after therapy and the other eight months after. One patient had a

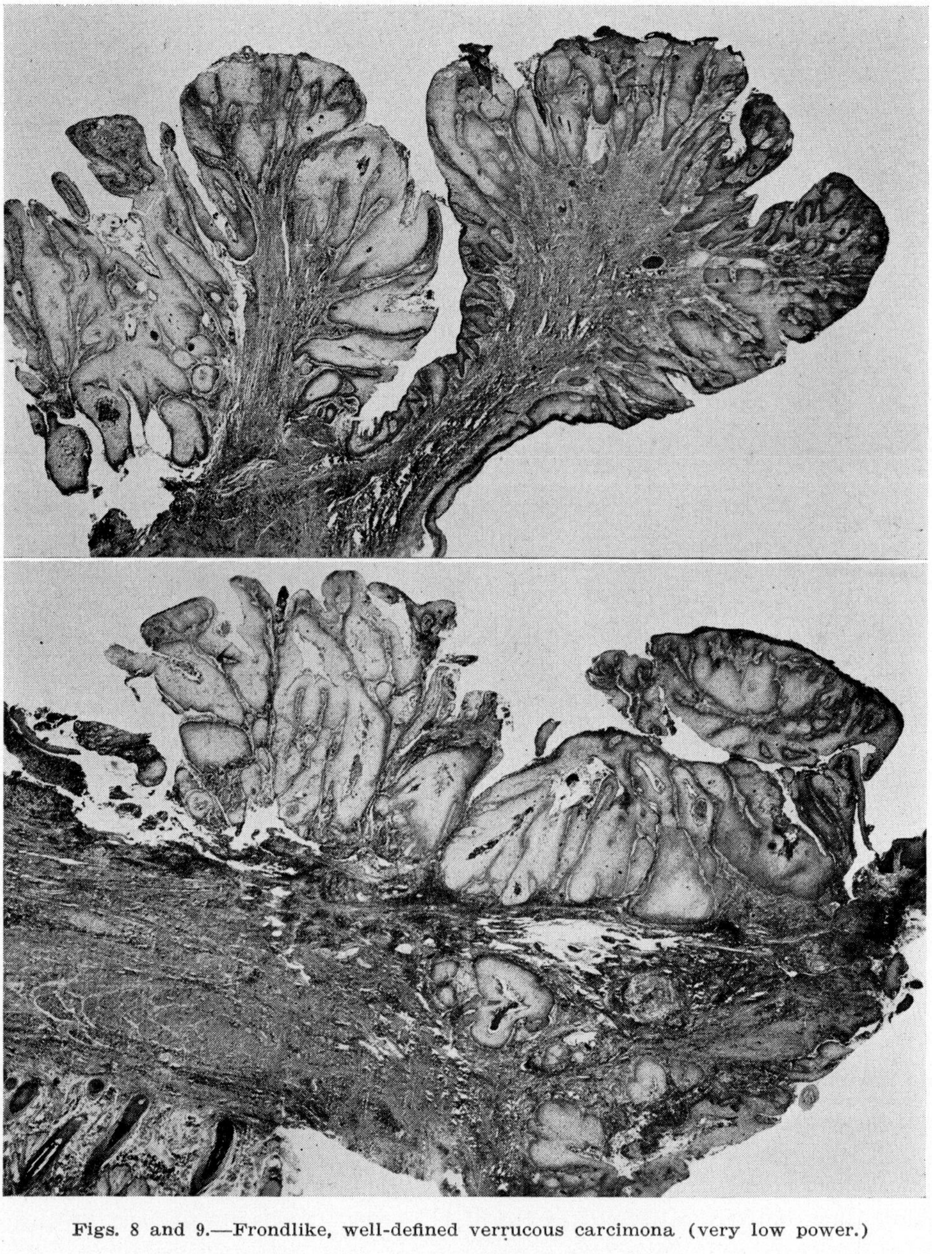

Figs. 8 and 9.—Frondlike, well-defined verrucous carcimona (very low power.)

recurrence after forty-two months, and the rest are living without disease after forty-one- forty-six, seventy-four, and eighty-six months, respectively, at the time of this communication.

Radiation Followed by Surgery.—In 7 instances, radiation was given and then recurrence necessitated surgery. Following irradiation, one patient had recurrence (outside the irradiated field) and then had surgery. This patient then developed five local recurrences (over a period of 2.5 years) just outside the surgical field. Each recurrence was treated successfully. Three of the 7 patients have died, but none of disease. Four are living without disease six, fifty-two, fifty-three, and sixty months. In 3 instances it was necessary to resect the mandible.

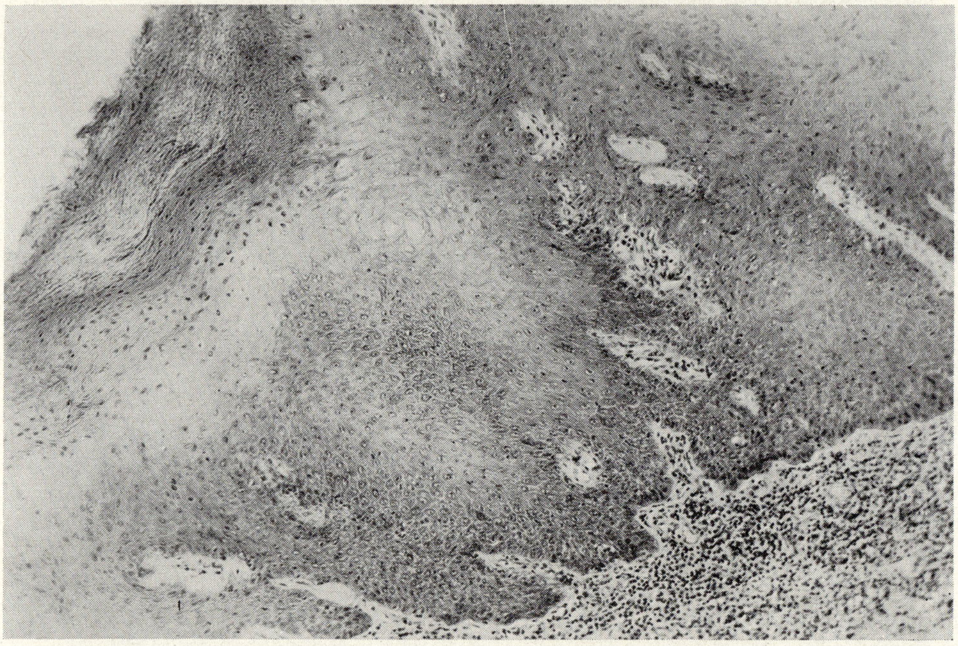

Fig. 10.—Point of transition between atrophic epithelium and beginning verrucous carcinoma (low power).

Local Excision.—Nine patients had local excision only; these patients are living four, six, nine, nine, twenty-six, thirty-one, and thirty-six months, respectively. One, at the end of twenty-four months, developed a local recurrence; another, at the end of eight months, died of intercurrent disease.

Excision Plus Mandibular Resection and Upper Neck Dissection.—One of these 8 patients died at eighteen months of intercurrent disease, but 7 are living fourteen, twenty-five, twenty-five, thirty-six, thirty-nine, forty-six, and forty-nine months, respectively.

There were 11 mandibular resections in all; 3 of these resections followed recurrence after irradiation. Roentgenologic examination revealed invasion every time that it was present (4 out of 11); when it was not present, because of inflammatory attachment to periosteum together with pressure, there was marginal erosion. In only one instance was an erroneous diagnosis of invasion made. This was a patient in whom irradiation had been done previously, and

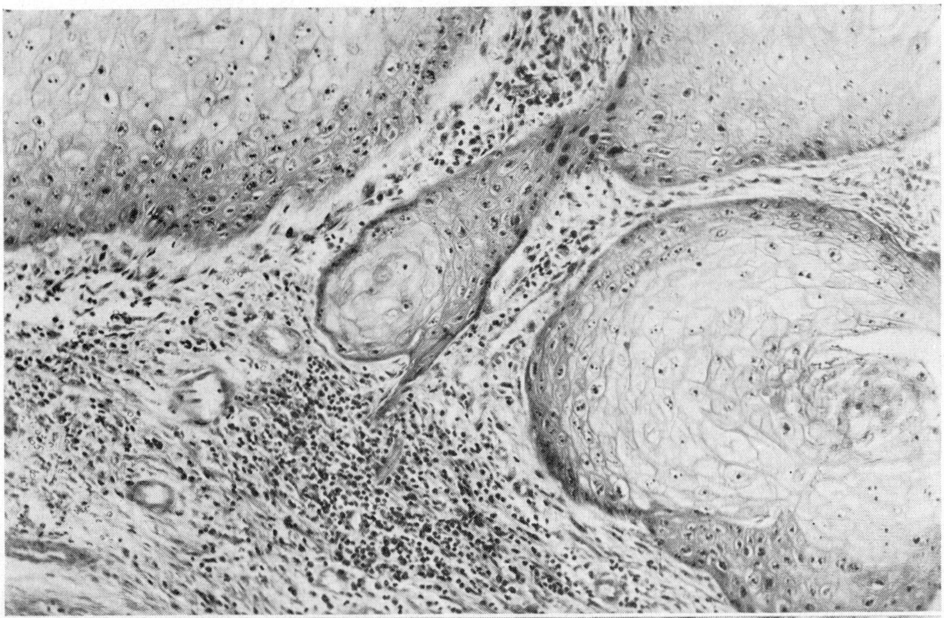

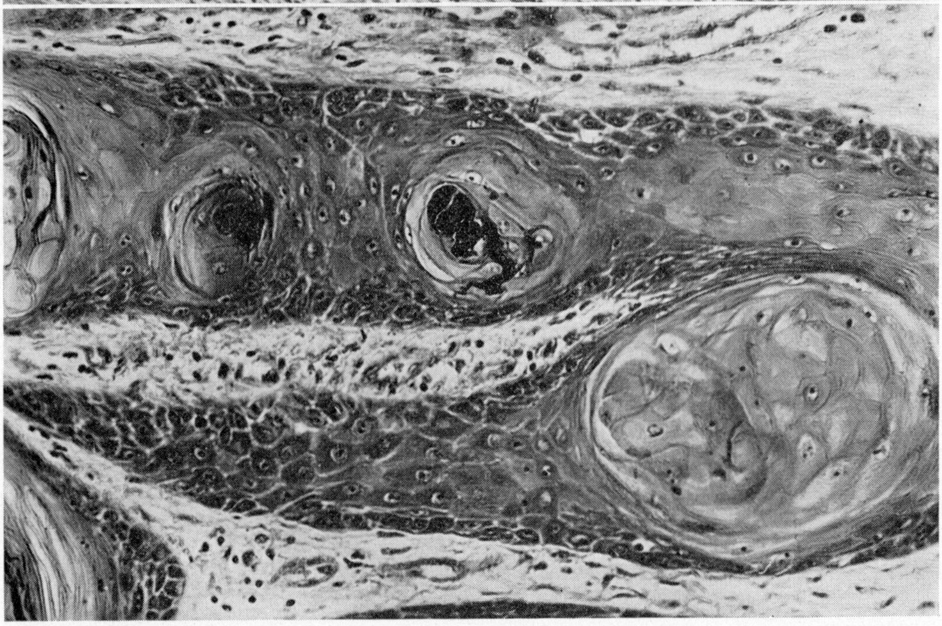

Fig. 11.—Actively growing edge of verrucous carcinoma, basement membrane is intact and inflammatory reaction is prominent (moderate enlargement).

Fig. 12.—Cystic changes and clublike fingers of well-defined epithelium (moderate enlargement).

the destructive changes in the mandible were a combination of radiation plus infection. In only one instance did a local recurrence appear after mandibular resection.

Radiation as a method of therapy is apparently successful in the relatively small, superficial lesions, but if the lesion has any size, then the chances of recurrence apparently increase, the recurrences often appearing just outside the irradiated field. In 14 patients treated by irradiation, 8 had recurrences. We have recently had two lesions too extensive for surgery, in which roentgen therapy gave excellent palliation. The cause for recurrence is unknown, but certainly there must be a predisposition of the epithelium over a wide area to become malignant. Inadequate local excision will also result in recurrence. One patient, for instance, had 5 recurrences, and there was local recurrence in 2 other instances after excision alone. If the lesion is extensive and is treated by irradiation, then it may recur, and surgery becomes somewhat more difficult. Of the group treated by primary mandibular resection, not one patient developed a local recurrence nor was there any operative mortality. Resection, therefore, seems to be the method of choice when the lesion is at all extensive. It is difficult to determine by roentgenologic examination how extensive the invasive process is, and more radical rather than conservative procedures are indicated.

SUMMARY

A type of squamous carcinoma of the oral cavity, designated as verrucous carcinoma, has been described. This lesion occurs predominantly in aged men, most commonly on the buccal mucosa and lower gingiva. Tobacco chewing may be of etiologic significance. Slowly growing, well differentiated, verrucous in character, and often extensive, this neoplasm tends to invade local structures (mandible, soft tissues, antrum). No distant metastases occurred in the group reported, and local metastases were rare. Local recurrence is common with inadequately treated patients. Radiation is successful in controlling small superficial lesions. For extensive lesions, radical surgery is indicated and often when fixation or invasion of bone is present, mandibular resection with upper neck dissection is justified.

A HIP NAIL COUNTERBORE

G. J. Curry, M.D., Flint, Mich.

(From the Section for Surgery of Trauma, Hurley Hospital)

SURGEONS selecting internal fixation for intertrochanteric femoral fractures frequently use the Smith-Petersen nail with a Thornton plate attachment. In many cases more comminution is found at operation than was disclosed by the x-ray film. This refers especially to the fracture lines occurring on the lateral surface. During the process of nail insertion, it has been the experience of many to find an advance in the comminution already present or the production of additional fracture lines. These accidents obviously cause variable degrees of interference with the security of nail fixation.

For the past two years I have used a counterbore (Fig. 1) with most satisfactory results. Its diameter corresponds to that of the Smith-Petersen nail, and enough of the femoral cortex is removed to produce a "set" for the nail. Inasmuch as the nail is inserted in a slanting projection, more of the

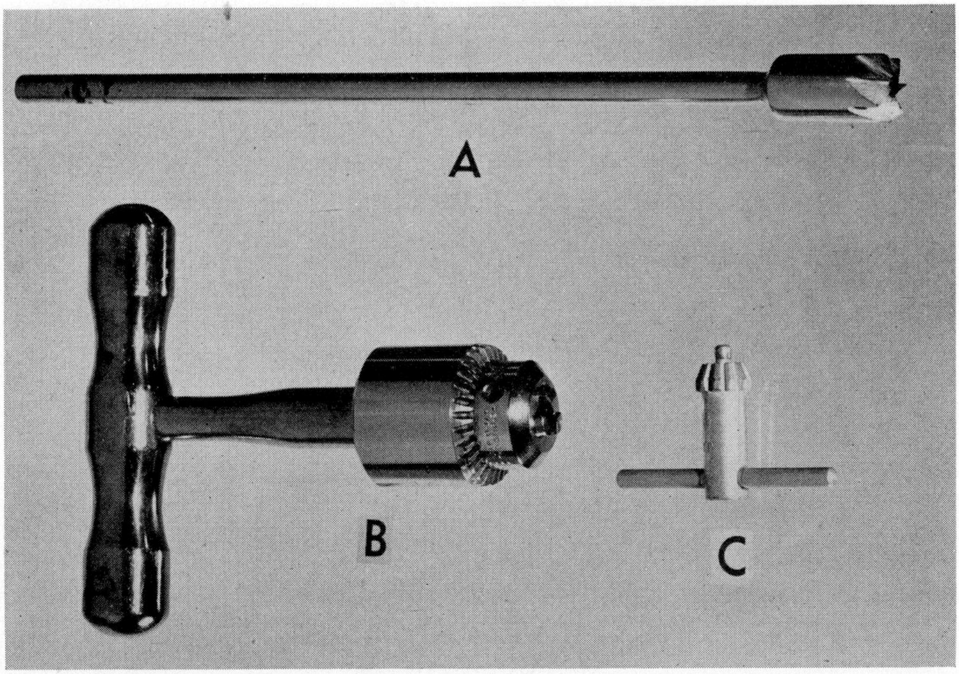

Fig. 1.—*A*, Photgraph of counterbore; *B*, handle; *C*, chuck used for fixation of the counterbore to the handle.

Received for publication, June 18, 1947.

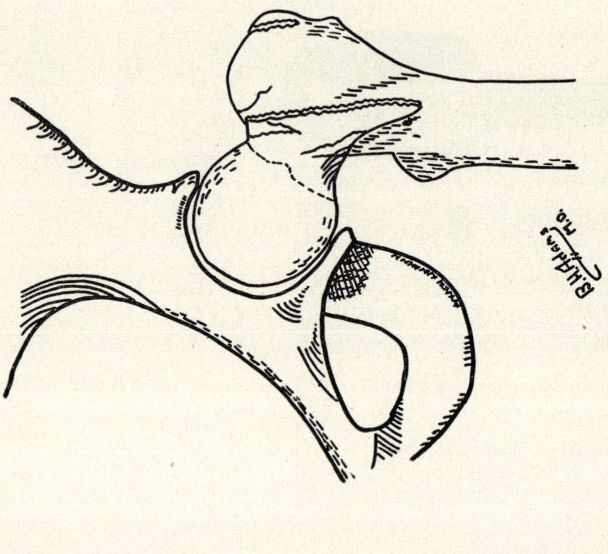

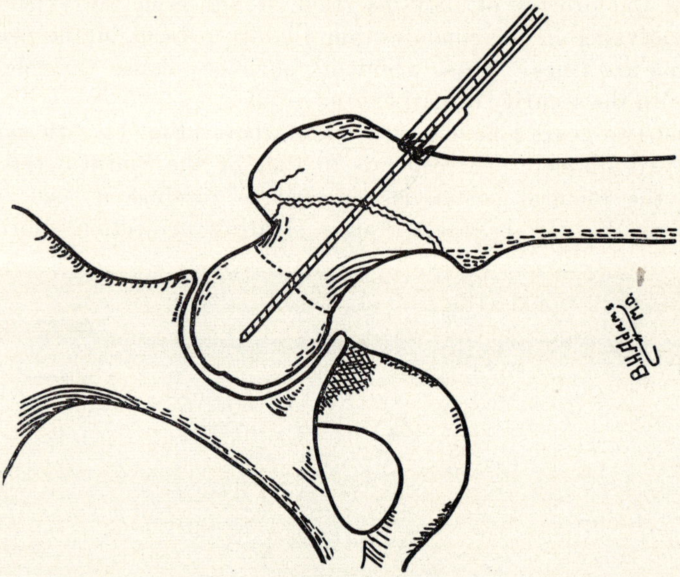

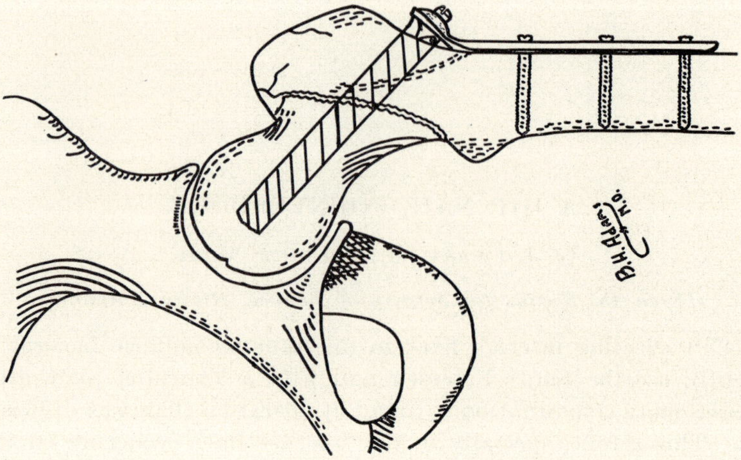

Fig. 2.—Drawing of an intertrochanteric fracture with comminution and varus deformity.
Fig. 3.—Drawing showing depth of penetration by the counterbore which has been threaded over the guide pin.
Fig. 4.—Drawing showing fracture reduction and fixation by the use of a Smith-Petersen nail and Thornton plate.

cortex in the inferior portion should be removed. It is advised that complete penetration here be accomplished (Fig. 3). A partial removal superiorly will obviously follow. The head of the Smith-Petersen nail protrudes far enough to be attached to the Thornton plate.

The trial period covered its use in fifty cases. The constant finding was the elimination of additional trauma to the trochanteric cortex.

Erratum

On page 150 of the January, 1948, issue of the JOURNAL, in the article "The Problem of Parenteral Nitrogen Administration in Surgical Patients" by Arnold J. Kremen, one reference is incomplete. It should read: 123a. Clark, J. H., Nelson, W., Lyons, C., Mayerson, H. S., and DeCamp, P.: Chronic Shock: The Problem of Reduced Blood Volume in the Chronically Ill Patient (in three parts), Ann. Surg. **125**: 218-247, 1947.

Case Reports

AN UNUSUALLY LARGE MYXOSARCOMATOUS TUMOR OF THE SUBMAXILLARY GLAND

N. Frederick Hicken, M.D., Vernon L. Stevenson, M.D., and
John H. Carlquist, M.D., Salt Lake City, Utah

(From the Department of Surgery, University of Utah Medical School and Latter Day Saints Hospital)

IT IS most unusual, in these days of modern medicine, to encounter such a large deforming neoplasm of the face as the one characterized in the accompanying photographs (Fig. 1). Forty-six years were required for this pathologic curiosity to develop. During this period the patient consulted many physicians but it was their conflicting advice as to the therapeutic management which resulted in her bewildering procrastination. Why should there be so much confusion in the minds of the men of our profession as to the correct method of handling these tantalizing tumors? Surely this case demonstrates the fact that even benign neoplasms of the submaxillary gland can and do undergo malignant transition if they are given sufficient time in which to make the change.

CASE REPORT

Mrs. C. B., a 66-year-old housewife of Bohemian birth, was admitted to the Latter Day Saints Hospital, on Sept. 18, 1942, because of a ''lump in the neck.'' She insisted that the tumor first appeared forty-six years previously, in the region of the right submaxillary gland. At that time she was told by a physician that the ''lump'' represented a swollen lymph gland originating from an ulcerated tooth. The mass had persisted, however, even after the offending tooth was removed. Seven years before admission, when the patient was 58 years of age, the ''lump began to grow,'' particularly during the eighteen months prior to admission.

Interestingly, the presenting complaints were all related to the size, weight, and position of the tumor. She was constantly annoyed by the dull aching pain along the right side of the head and face, which could be effectively relieved by manually supporting the weight of the tumor. When working, she wore a scarf, which passed in a hammock-like fashion beneath the tumor and was tied on top of the head to sustain the weight of the mass. Her concern was that the ''lump is so big that it is always getting in my way.'' One day she snagged the lower pole of the pendulous tumor on the hook of a screen door, producing such a deep laceration that an alarming hemorrhage resulted. On another occasion she was putting wood in the stove and the protruding mass came in contact with the stove, thereby producing an extensive third degree burn. Deglutition was becoming painful and difficult, and pressure on the trachea caused considerable respiratory embarrassment. She was compelled to sleep on the right side in such a position that the entire weight of the tumor could be supported by an extra pillow. She insisted that she had never had a sick day in her life and could do more work than most young women.

Received for publication, July 14, 1947.

During the past five years she had consulted many different physicians and they all advised her to "leave this cancerous growth alone as you will die if anyone attempts to remove it." So persuasive were these arguments that her own son, a very competent physician, and her two daughters, both of whom are registered nurses, could not persuade their mother to submit to surgery. The only reason she finally consented to have an operation was because the neoplastic mass began to undergo discoloration and she thought it was "abscessed."

The only abnormal findings on physical examination were related to the football-sized tumor which occupied the entire right cervicofacial area. Its exact size and location can best be ascertained by consulting the accompanying photographs (Fig. 1). The pendulous tumor was bosselated, firm, and not tender. It was so intimately attached to the deep structures of the neck that any attempt to manipulate the neoplasm resulted in a compressive occlusion of the trachea. The overlying skin was taut, thin, and had a peculiar bluish discoloration as if covering a huge hemangioma. No portion of the right parotid could be identified because the mass completely covered this area. The facial nerve, however, was still functioning. The

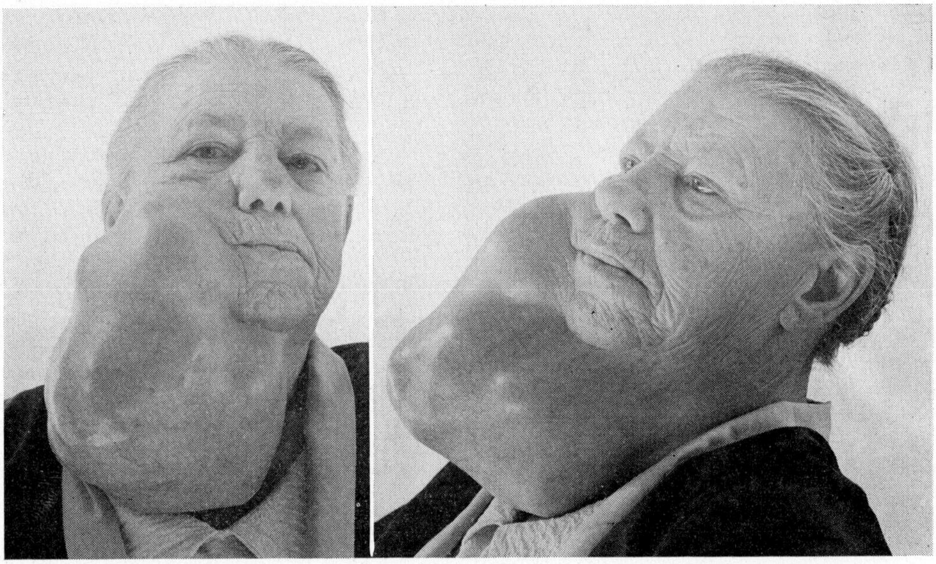

A. B.

Fig. 1.—*A*, Front view of a patient with a myxosarcomatous tumor arising in the right submaxillary gland. The excised tumor weighed 2,450 Gm. *B*, Lateral view of the same patient.

expanding tumor had pushed the floor of the mouth upward so that the tongue was resting against the hard palate. The mucous membrane of the oral cavity was intact. The left submaxillary and sublingual glands appeared to be normal. Endoscopic studies demonstrated a rotation and compression of the trachea but without evidence of actual infiltration. The vocal cords exhibited their normal range of motion. X-ray studies of the lungs, skull, the vertebrae failed to show metastatic invasion. On the presumptive diagnosis of a "mixed tumor of the right submaxillary gland," surgical intervention was advised.

At operation, because of the pronounced compression and distortion of the trachea, it was felt that cyclopropane should be administered by the endotracheal method. The tumor mass was exposed by a transverse skin incision. It was surprising to see the ease with which the encapsulated tumor was separated from the parotid gland and other cervicofacial structures. The tumor had not invaded the trachea but merely compressed it. When the dissection had been carried down to the right submaxillary fossa it was found that the neoplasm had invaded fascial planes along the floor of the mouth. Neoplastic extensions had invested the sheath and outer coatings of the carotid vessels. In spite of this widespread dissemination an extensive block dissection of the right side of the neck was carried out. Care was taken not to enter the oral cavity, therefore, Wharton's duct was ligated and divided near its mucosal orifice. Closure was accomplished with ease and the patient made a pleasing recovery.

The excised tumor measured 19.5 by 20 by 18 cm. and weighed 2450 Gm. The skin was smooth and freely movable over the tumorous mass and in several small areas it presented a bluish discoloration suggestive of underlying hemorrhage. The remaining two-thirds of the tumor was covered by a well-defined but lobulated capsule. Sections through the neoplasm revealed a yellowish white, soft or gelatinoid tissue with scattered areas of hemorrhage and necrosis. The tissue presented a relatively uniform appearance throughout.

Microscopically the tumor possessed an extremely loose, myxomatous stroma, containing stellate or spindle cells. The cellularity varied throughout the sections; in some areas, the tumor was quite acellular, and in others numerous cells were seen. In the cellular zones the mitotic figures were numerous and the cells radiated out from the vessels, producing a peritheliomatous appearance. The excessive vascularity of the tumor was due to the presence of numerous, large, dilated venous sinuses. Deposits of degenerating blood pigments within the cells evidenced previous hemorrhagic episodes. There were no gland structures or epithelial cells present so the origin of the tumor could not be determined histologically. The clinical course supplemented by the histologic findings indicated that this was a slowly growing myxosarcomatous tumor which originated in the right submaxillary gland.

An intense course of x-ray irradiation was given to the right submaxillary area, the right side of the neck, and the mediastinal zone.

About eleven months after the primary operation the patient observed a recurrent nodule in the right submaxillary area. The tumor grew rapidly but produced no discomfort. Three months later a second nodule appeared beneath the lobe of the right ear. Both of these neoplasms grew rapidly and further irradiation was advised against until the tumors had been excised.

The second admission was Nov. 10, 1944, twenty-five months after the first operation, when she was readmitted for excision of the recurrent nodules. The lemon-sized mass lying beneath the lobe of the right ear was easily excised, in fact, it seemed to be well encapsulated. The companion tumor in the right submaxillary fossa, however, had completely surrounded and invaded the larynx, trachea, and the carotid vessels. Technically it was impossible to excise all of the spreading neoplasm, therefore, only the main mass of the tumor was removed with the cautery. The wound was closed and the patient was discharged from the hospital one week later.

It was reported that the specimens consisted of four pieces of tissue varying from 4 to 6 cm. in length. These fragments were irregular in size and shape and presented a homogeneous gelatinous consistency. Microscopically the stroma presented a loose, edematous stroma. The basic cell was rather fat, plump, and hyperchromatic. Mitosis was rather frequent, much more so than in the specimen which had been removed twenty-five months previously. The morphology and clinical course was consistent with diagnosis of a recurrent myxosarcomatous tumor of the right submaxillary gland.

The residual tumorous tissue continued to grow and additional x-ray therapy was given to the right pre-auricular area and to the right submental zone.

In spite of the additional irritation the tumor grew rapidly. It invaded the floor of the mouth, pushing the tongue so firmly against the hard palate, that both speech and deglutition became impossible. Direct infiltration of the trachea so obstructed the air passage that breathing was most laborious. Complete motor and sensory paralysis of the lower extremities occurred when the neoplastic process destroyed the second and third lumbar vertebrae, thereby exerting pressure on the spinal cord. Nausea and vomiting, associated with a persistent headache, announced the presence of cerebral metastasis. This impression was further confirmed by the development of a bilateral optic atrophy associated with paralysis of the external ocular muscles, all secondary to direct metastasis to the brain and the concomitant increase in intracranial pressure. She died, forty-nine months after the primary operation. Autopsy studies were not made because the patient died in a small town where such facilities were unavailable. The clinical course, however, left no doubt that death was due to a generalized metastasis of the malignant tumor which had its origin in the right submaxillary gland.

DISCUSSION

If one reads the voluminous literature which has been published during the past thirty years on the subject of "mixed tumors of the salivary glands," he emerges from such a study in a state of abject confusion. Pathologists cannot agree on the origin, the histologic classification, or even the course these perplexing tumors will follow. For example, Hertzler,[4] in his excellent monograph on *Tumors of the Neck*, stated, "I have yet to see a tumor of the submaxillary or sublingual salivary glands invade the surrounding tissues or recur after its removal." This leads one to believe that these mixed tumors are relatively benign. On the other hand, Blair, Moore, and Byar[1] reported eight neoplasms of the submaxillary glands of which 50 per cent were definitely malignant. Wood[7] and Ewing[3] both maintained that these mixed tumors are potentially malignant, undergoing both carcinomatous and sarcomatous transitions.

The management of these tantalizing tumors likewise presents conflicting views. Hertzler insisted that "these mixed tumors of the submaxillary gland are well encapsulated, therefore, they can be removed safely by enucleation without sacrificing the submaxillary gland itself." Patey[6] believed it to be unwise to leave the submaxillary gland behind even though the mixed tumor can be easily enucleated. He pointed out that these tumors have a multicentric origin and that many of the so-called recurrences do not represent a recurrence of the excised tumor but a similar growth arising in part of the gland that was not disturbed by the primary operation. He, therefore, felt it wise to remove the submaxillary gland and its invested neoplasm, even though the tumor presents clinical and histologic evidence of benignancy.

After studying eighty-one cases of primary and recurrent malignancies of the submaxillary glands, Dockerty and Mayo[2] condemned all forms of conservative therapy. In dealing with a "mixed tumor," they insisted that the parent submaxillary gland and the tumor should be removed en masse. If an immediate examination of the excised tissues confirms the diagnosis of benignancy then nothing further need be done. If, however, the tumor mass shows evidence of malignancy, specimen of regional tissues are removed and given to the pathologist. If histologic studies indicate that the neoplastic process has spread beyond the confines of the submaxillary gland they believe that a radical unilateral dissection of the neck should be done. Likewise, if the primary submaxillary tumor is anaplastic, even though there is no evidence of local invasion they resort to a radical block dissection of the neck. We agree with this concept.

Unfortunately many "mixed tumors" have spread to important regional structures before the patients submit to surgery.[5] Technically, it is impossible to excise the infiltrative process once it has invaded the trachea, hypopharynx, or carotid sheath. In such instances one can excise the main mass of neoplastic tissue and then rely on the inhibitive influences of irradiation to further delay the inevitable extension. While irradiation is seldom curative it often retards the growth of the infiltrative process.[5]

SUMMARY

Mixed tumors of the submaxillary gland may originate as benign tumors but they most certainly possess potentialities of malignant transition. In our case it required forty-six years for the evolution of this malignant change. Histologically the excised tumor represented areas of "mixed tumor formation," and in others there were anaplastic zones showing definite myxosarcomatous changes. During the first fifty-five years of its development the tumor presented all the signs of being a benign growth, but during the last two years it exhibited clinical characteristics of malignancy. Rapid growth, recurrence after excision, and metastasis to the brain, lungs, vertebrae, and skull, combined with infiltration of the trachea, carotid sheath, hypopharyngeal structures, and the gland on the opposite side of the neck most certainly stamped the tumor as being malignant.

Conservatism, such as simple enucleation of a benign mixed tumor of the submaxillary gland, is to be condemned. The submaxillary gland and the growing neoplasm should be removed en masse. If histologic studies of the excised specimen demonstrate malignant changes, then a block dissection of the neck is indicated. This is particularly true if the neoplastic process has spread beyond the confines of the capsule of the submaxillary gland. Experience dictates that such a plan greatly minimizes the incidence of recurrence.

REFERENCES

1. Blair, V. P.: Moore, S., and Byar, L. T.: Cancer of the Face and Mouth, St. Louis, 1941, The C. V. Mosby Company.
2. Dockerty, M. B., and Mayo, C. W.: Primary Tumors of the Submaxillary Gland With Special Reference to Mixed Tumors, Surg., Gynec. & Obst. **74**: 1033-1045, 1942.
3. Ewing, J.: Neoplastic Diseases: A Treatise on Tumors, ed. 4, Philadelphia, 1940, W. B. Saunders Company.
4. Hertzler, A. E.: Surgical Pathology of the Diseases of the Neck, Philadelphia, 1937, J. B. Lippincott Company.
5. McFarland, J.: Mixed Tumors of the Salivary Glands, Surg., Gynec. & Obst. **63**: 457-468, 1936.
6. Patey, D. H.: The Mixed Tumors of the Salivary Glands, Brit. J. Surg. **18**: 241-258, 1930.
7. Wood, F. C.: Mixed Tumors of the Salivary Glands, Ann. Surg. **39**: 57-67, 1930.

Recent Advances in Surgery

Conducted by Alfred Blalock, M.D.

INTRAVENOUS CLOTTING

An Analysis of Five Hundred Cases Observed in Army Personnel at the Vascular Centers

LeRoy J. Kleinsasser, M.D.,* Dallas, Texas

During their period of operation, 502 instances of intravenous clotting were observed in Army personnel at the vascular centers at DeWitt General Hospital, Ashford General Hospital, and Mayo General Hospital. These figures, however, cannot be assumed to be representative of the incidence of this condition in the entire United States Army. All patients with intravascular clotting were not treated at the vascular centers, which received only complicated cases, recurrent cases, and cases in which ordinary methods of therapy did not achieve results. The assessment of these cases as an over-all picture of intravascular clotting within these limitations is valid, but conclusions must be drawn with due regard to the background.

Care was taken to exclude from the series all cases of thrombophlebitis migrans, which presents a special problem in relation to Buerger's disease and which should, of course, be considered as a possibility in any case of superficial thrombophlebitis.

Intravenous clotting falls into two categories, thrombophlebitis and phlebothrombosis. Thrombophlebitis, because it is an inflammatory process, gives rise to more or less severe reactions, but is usually simple to diagnose and is seldom complicated by pulmonary embolism. Phlebothrombosis, because it is a bland, quiet, non-inflammatory process, gives rise to few or no symptoms in the early stages, is frequently difficult to detect, is not infrequently followed by pulmonary embolism, and therefore is a potentially fatal lesion. The importance of differentiating between the two types of intravascular clotting has been repeatedly emphasized by Ochsner and DeBakey.[145, 147-149]

Not all instances of phlebothrombosis result in pulmonary embolism, nor do all pulmonary embolisms terminate fatally, but that the danger is real is indicated by both the reported incidence and the case fatality rate. The reported necropsy incidence of embolism varies from 1 per cent to almost 12 per cent[18, 50, 55, 84, 85, 116, 181] and the reported case fatality rate from 2.5 to 5 per cent.[84, 85, 116] The risk, furthermore, is not limited to either medical or surgical conditions. The report by Hunter and his associates[84] of eleven deaths from pulmonary embolism in 200 necropsied cases, is typical in its distribution: Five deaths occurred in medical and six in surgical cases.

*Diplomate American Board of Surgery; formerly Major, Army of the United States.

The incidence, the potential death rate, and the disabling end results of intravenous clotting thus make it a problem of serious concern to both physicians and surgeons in its immediate and its future implications. That statement is as applicable to military medicine as it is to civilian medicine.

INCIDENCE

Sex and Race.—Four hundred ninety-six of the 502 patients with intravenous clotting observed at the vascular centers in the Zone of the Interior during World War II (98.8 per cent) were white. This is a disproportionately high incidence, although the nonwhite elements of the United States Army at no time numbered more than 12 per cent.

From the standpoint of sex the figures are heavily weighted. The 27 women in the 502 cases (5.4 per cent) were nurses and WACs.

Reports in the literature are not in complete agreement as to the sex incidence of intravascular clotting. Matas[115] in a study based on reports from leading American and European clinics, found the incidence after operation practically the same for both sexes, as did Hunter and his associates[85] in 351 cases of deep venous thrombosis. Allen and his associates[2] and Fine and co-workers[66] reported a much higher incidence in men, and Veal and Hussey,[192] in a personal series of 84 cases, reported that 55 cases occurred in men against 29 in women, a disproportion which perhaps can be explained by the fact that most of their cases represented propagating thromboses requiring surgical treatment. Barker and his associates[13] reported that in acute thrombophlebitis as observed at the Mayo Clinic the ratio of women to men was 3:2. Both thrombosis and embolism were relatively more frequent in women, but fatal embolism was more frequent in men. McCartney's[116] figures suggest a somewhat opposite trend. In 689 cases of intravascular clotting which occurred in 25,771 necropsies, the incidence in men was 9.1 per cent and in women 11.2 per cent, while the proportion of fatal embolisms was 2.2 and 3.3 per cent, respectively. Post-partal cases are not included in the calculations.

Age.—From the standpoint of age the figures are also heavily weighted, most of the patients being between the ages of 20 and 39 years, because that age group included the great majority of all military personnel. In the 189 cases of intravascular clotting observed at DeWitt General Hospital, for instance, 54.6 per cent of the patients were between 20 and 29 years of age, and 41.1 per cent between 40 and 49 years. The average age was 26.8 years, although the age range for the whole series was 19 to 59 years.

Although the figures are weighted, the relative youth of the patients in this series of cases is worthy of comment, since thrombosis and embolism are generally regarded as complications of advancing age. Any type of peripheral venous thrombosis is most unusual in the first two decades of life, and all available statistics show the greatest frequency, as well as an increasing frequency, over 40 years of age.[34, 53]

McCartney,[116] for instance, in 25,771 necropsies, found the incidence of thromboembolism highest in the sixth and seventh decades. Eighty-one per cent of the patients in Stich's[184] series were over 40 years of age, 66 per cent over

60 years, and 20 per cent over 70 years. Fifty per cent of Miller and Rogers'[121] patients were over 50 years of age. Seventy per cent of Veal and Hussey's[192] 84 patients with deep venous thrombosis of the lower extremity were over 40 years of age, and more than 80 per cent of Allen, Linton, and Donaldson's[2] 367 patients were in this age group. Culp,[38] in a study of 38 instances of embolism in 4,070 deaths after operation, found that 62.5 per cent were in persons over 60 years of age, although only 41.2 per cent of all patients in the series were in this age group.

The age incidence is naturally related to other factors. Ewald,[65] the average age of whose patients was 26.8 years, stated that intravenous clotting occurred in young persons only in the presence of circulatory disturbances. Since slowing of the blood stream has been established as an important cause of intravascular clotting, it would be expected that the incidence would increase with age, since the circulation time slows with age. Koch[91] reported the circulation time to average 18 seconds between the ages of 15 and 19 years, 21 seconds between the ages of 30 and 40 years, and 23 seconds at 70 years. He also reported that it was longer at all ages after operation and in patients with circulatory disturbances. These considerations are not applicable to any of the 502 patients in the Army series, although indirect proof of their validity is found in the impressive reduction in the incidence of thrombosis and embolism achieved whenever preoperative measures to prevent and correct circulatory disturbances[69, 93, 174, 187, 197] are instituted.

PREDISPOSING AND PRECIPITATING FACTORS

Predisposing and precipitating factors are charted in Fig. 1. Though the fact is frequently overlooked, a large number of cases of intravascular clotting occur in the absence of any obvious causes. The proportion of spontaneous cases in the Army series was 27.1 per cent, and in 20 of the 84 cases reported by Veal and Hussey[192] there was no apparent cause; in 4 of their 20 cases the thrombosis originated in superficial varicosities and extended to the deep venous system. A detailed discussion of this group of cases would not be profitable, since it would entail analyses of individual cases from the standpoint of posture, hydration, varicosities, smoking habits, obesity, foci of infection, anemia and other blood dyscrasias, and similar considerations.[146] It must be emphasized that intravascular thrombosis is not only a surgical but a medical problem as well.[26]

In addition to the 136 cases of apparently spontaneous origin in the 502 cases of intravascular clotting which make up the Army series, the vascular lesion may be classified as traumatic in 183 cases (36.5 per cent), postoperative in 71 (14.1 per cent), and associated with previous illness in 92 (18.3 per cent). In the remaining 20 cases (4.0 per cent) miscellaneous causes seemed responsible.

Direct trauma to the blood vessels, such as may occur in fractures, sprains, and gunshot and stab wounds, is an obvious cause of intravascular clotting. Injuries of this kind are often associated with tearing, stretching, or crushing of regional vessels, and in other instances, though the vessel itself may not be directly implicated, the thrombus may originate at the site of injury and propagate itself from there. In the Army series, 109 of the 183 cases of traumatic origin (Fig. 2) followed local injury, chiefly direct contusions and lacerations of the tissues of the extremities, and 10 followed fractures. That fractures frequently predispose to intravascular clotting is shown in numerous reports from the literature. In 12 of the 15 instances of pulmonary embolism following trauma reported by McCartney[117] in a total of 73 cases of pulmonary embolism the patients had sustained fractures of the lower extremities and were confined to bed, and Potts,[162] who reported 5 cases of thrombophlebitis in 95 fractures of the lower extremity, considered the complication at least partially due to immobilization.

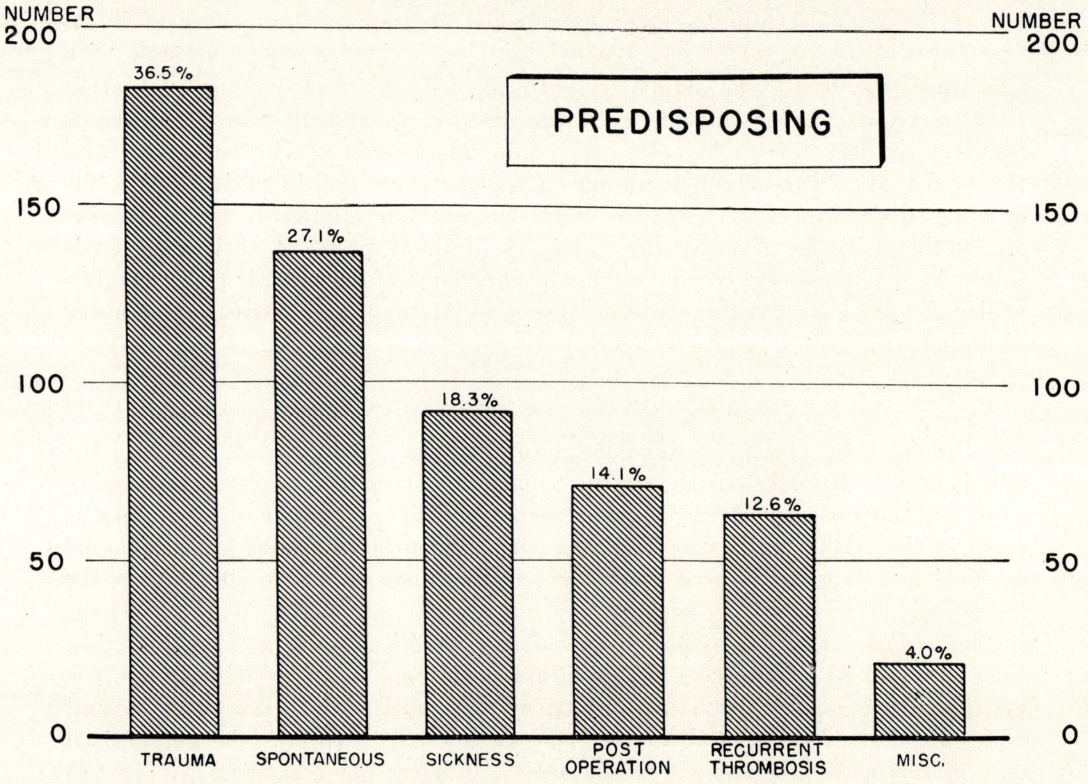

Fig. 1.

Ochsner and DeBakey,[150] who emphasized trauma as an important factor in intravascular clotting, also attempted to explain why clotting does not occur more frequently following extensive injury to an extremity. Trauma of equal severity elsewhere in the body, they pointed out, would produce blood changes (increased viscosity, hyperglobulinemia, hyperproteinemia, increased fibrinogen, antitryptic power, peptidase and calcium and decreased carbon dioxide combining power of the plasma),[148] sufficient to be considered as factors in the production of thrombosis. Other changes under these circumstances, including an increase in the formed elements of the blood and increased coagulability,[148, 208, 209] would also favor the production of thrombosis. The immobilization of an extremity in a cast would therefore seem to produce an ideal situation for the development of intravascular clotting. The lesion does not develop more frequently, according to Ochsner and DeBakey,[148] for two reasons, the youth of the patients who most frequently sustain fractures, and the vasodilating effect of choline and the increased heat of the part. It is quite possible that intravenous thrombosis subsequent to trauma is the result of injury to the vascular endothelium, with resultant acute thrombophlebitis, as distinguished from phlebothrombosis, in which the manifestations and mechanism of production are quite different.

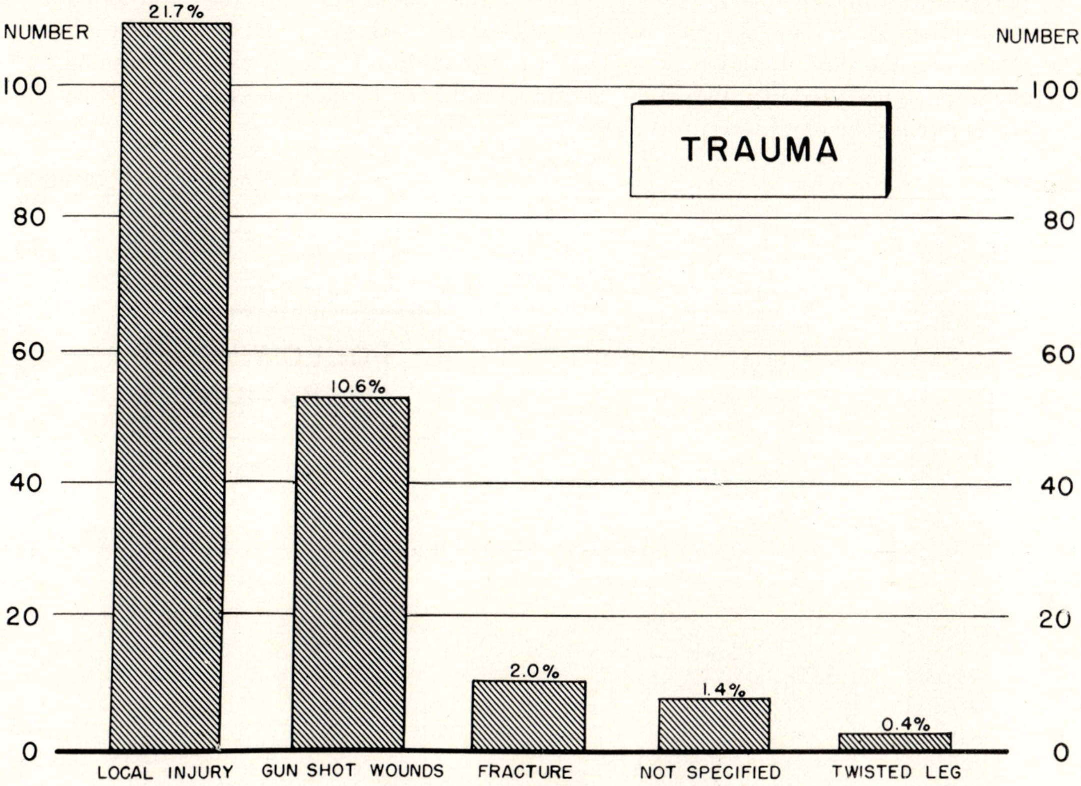

Fig. 2.

The importance of operative trauma (Fig. 3) in the production of intravenous clotting is supported by many observations.[21, 59, 61, 62, 71, 93, 107, 134] In the 71 cases in this category in the Army series the lesion followed appendectomy in 30 and hernioplasty in 10, but the figures are not particularly significant, since these are the two most frequent noncombat-connected operations performed in military hospitals.

Of the numerous reasons why the postoperative state predisposes to intravenous clotting, three are most important: (1) slowing of the blood stream, which is most marked in prolonged operations and which is associated with diminished cardiac action and lowered blood pressure; (2) injury of the endothelium; and (3) changes in the composition of the blood. Changes in the composition of the blood affect the prothrombin time, clotting time, calcium time, sedimentation rate, and platelet count. The blood platelet count rises on the fourth day after operation, reaches a maximum on the twelfth day, and does not revert to normal until the twenty-first day. According to Wright[208, 209] the platelets also become sticky, their adhesiveness increasing as they increase in numbers; the change is in the thrombocytes rather than in the serum. Newburger,[139] on the other hand, has pointed out that thrombosis may occur before the fourth postoperative day. Lambret and Driessens[100] reported a postoperative rise in polypeptides of the blood, reaching a maximum about the fifth day and being proportionate to the severity of the procedure. Mason[114] and Takaura's[188] studies on the part of tissue extracts in the production of blood clotting implied the importance of sharp dissection, gentle handling of tissues, and absolute hemostasis during the operative procedure.

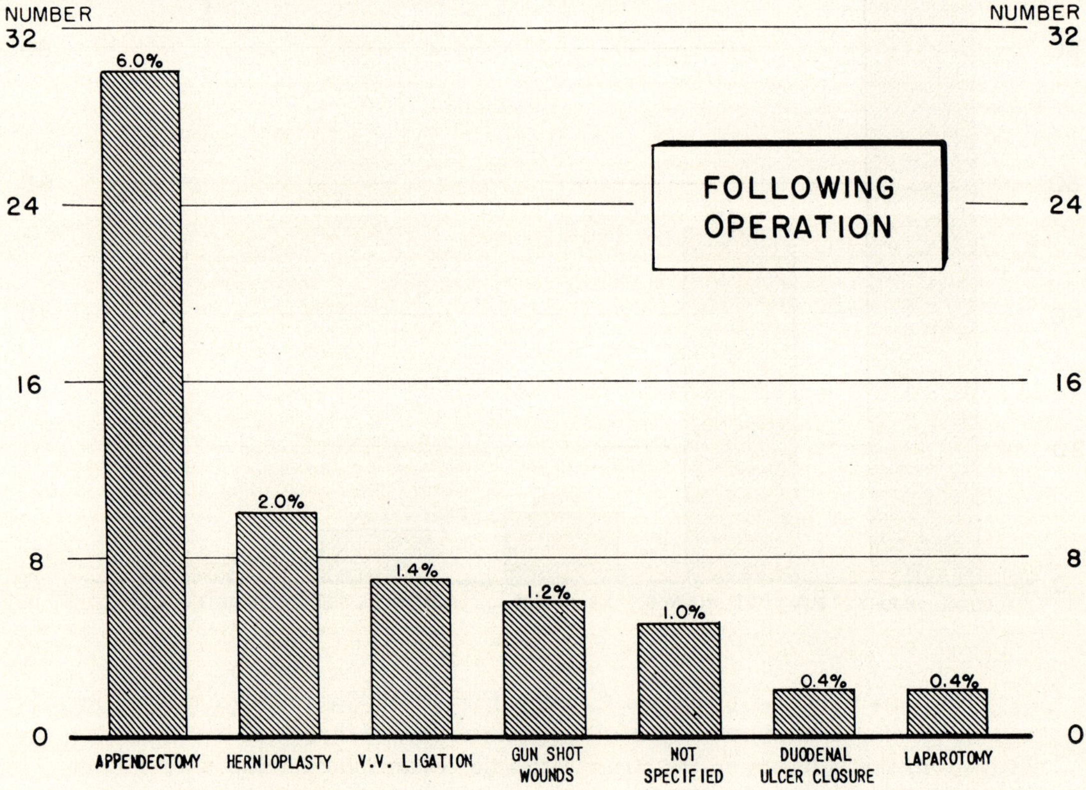

Fig. 3.

Of the various types of illness (see Fig. 4) which preceded 92 cases of intravenous clotting in the Army series, pneumonia accounted for 24 cases. Others, including myself,[90] have emphasized the importance of pneumonia as a predecessor of pulmonary embolism. White[206] has emphasized another important point, that the increasing accuracy in the diagnosis of pulmonary emboli has

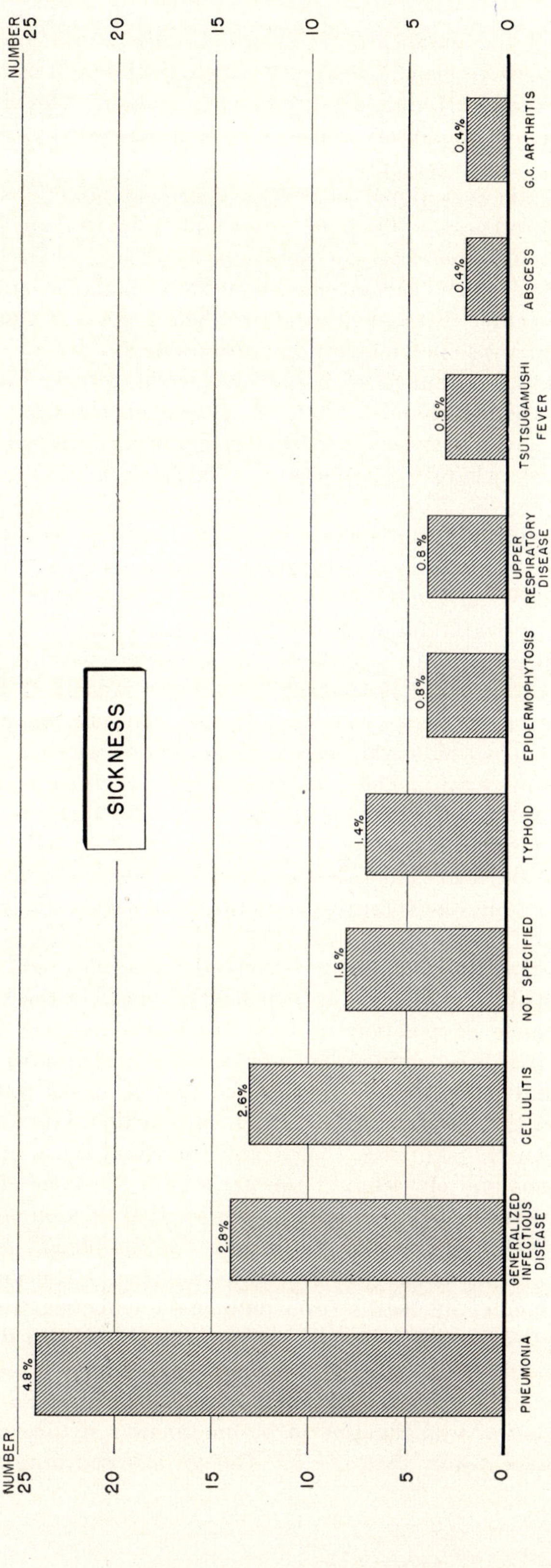
SICKNESS
NUMBER
25
20
15
10
5
0
PNEUMONIA
4.8%
GENERALIZED INFECTIOUS DISEASE
2.8%
CELLULITIS
2.6%
NOT SPECIFIED
1.6%
TYPHOID
1.4%
EPIDERMOPHYTOSIS
0.8%
UPPER RESPIRATORY DISEASE
0.8%
TSUTSUGAMUSHI FEVER
0.6%
ABSCESS
0.4%
G.C. ARTHRITIS
0.4%

Fig. 4.

materially reduced the number of cases which once would have been listed as pneumonia or congestive heart failure but which, in the light of the newer knowledge, are now correctly attributed to pulmonary emboli. The absence of preceding cardiac disease in the Army series, which is noteworthy, is probably to be attributed to the youth of the patients.

Certain systemic infections, as well as localized infections, are frequently associated with thrombosis. Typhoid fever and influenza are important examples. Rather unusual preceding conditions in the Army series include tsutsugamushi fever, jungle ulcer, poison oak, insect bite, malaria, and other illnesses contracted in the course of tropical warfare. The 2 cases of gonorrheal arthritis which preceded intravascular clotting are also unusual.

The presumption is that thrombophlebitis which follows illness is caused by blood changes, vascular changes, and the effects of infection and circulatory retardation. An obvious cause is the localization of an infection in the intima of a peripheral vessel, where it produces raw surfaces on which platelets can be deposited.

It is well established that merely keeping a patient recumbent in bed predisposes to venous thrombosis.[54] Hunter and his associates,[85] in 351 necropsies performed on middle-aged and elderly patients who had spent various periods of time in bed before death, found thrombi of various durations present in more than one-half. Hunter and co-workers,[84] in a comparative study of two series consisting of 200 necropsied cases each, found thromboses of leg veins present in 59 per cent of the patients who were in bed, without exercise, as compared with 44 per cent in patients who were ambulatory or who had exercised within forty-eight hours of death. They emphasized that the common denominator of phlebothrombosis and pulmonary embolism is confinement to bed because recumbency favors mechanical venous obstruction and affects adversely the efficient return of blood to the heart from the deep veins of the extremities, which depends on the circulation time, the compressive action of muscles, and negative pressure in the abdomen and thorax.

Luckhardt, Alpert, and Smith[110] observed that reflex inhibition of respiration will temporarily obstruct the return flow of blood to the heart and emphasized the importance of position in bed. Fowler's position is generally condemned because it causes compression of the veins and retardation of the blood flow.[178] Smith and Allen,[180] who emphasized that the most important influence on the circulation time was the skin temperature of the extremities (the velocity being slowed when the skin was cooled and increased when it was warm), observed that exercise and elevation of the parts have the same effect on the circulation time as warmth. Friedlander[77] showed that flexion of the thigh with elevation of the extremity favors the return flow of blood. Of importance in connection with posture is the observation of Simpson[178] concerning the striking increase in the number of deaths from pulmonary embolism among elderly persons who during the London blitz had sat for long hours with the legs dependent and with the pressure of the edge of the chair, particularly the crossbar of a deck chair, against the popliteal space and the back of the thigh.

Early ambulation was thought to be one answer in preventing thrombosis and has many advocates.[32, 170, 180, 197, 212] Coley[35] stressed in a study of operative cases in 30 hospitals in the 8th Service Command that no patient allowed up out of bed within seventy-two hours had detectable intravenous clotting or embolism. In any event early activity in bed is desirable.[23, 160, 169, 170, 195, 207] The significance of such exercise has been repeatedly emphasized.[14, 21, 119, 145, 147-149, 161-163, 176, 186, 201, 205]

Recurrent Intravascular Clotting.—Sixty-three of the 502 patients in the Army series (12.6 per cent) had had previous episodes of thrombophlebitis. This is a consideration of great importance. No cases in this series were fatal, but the advice of Barker and his associates[13] concerning the careful management before

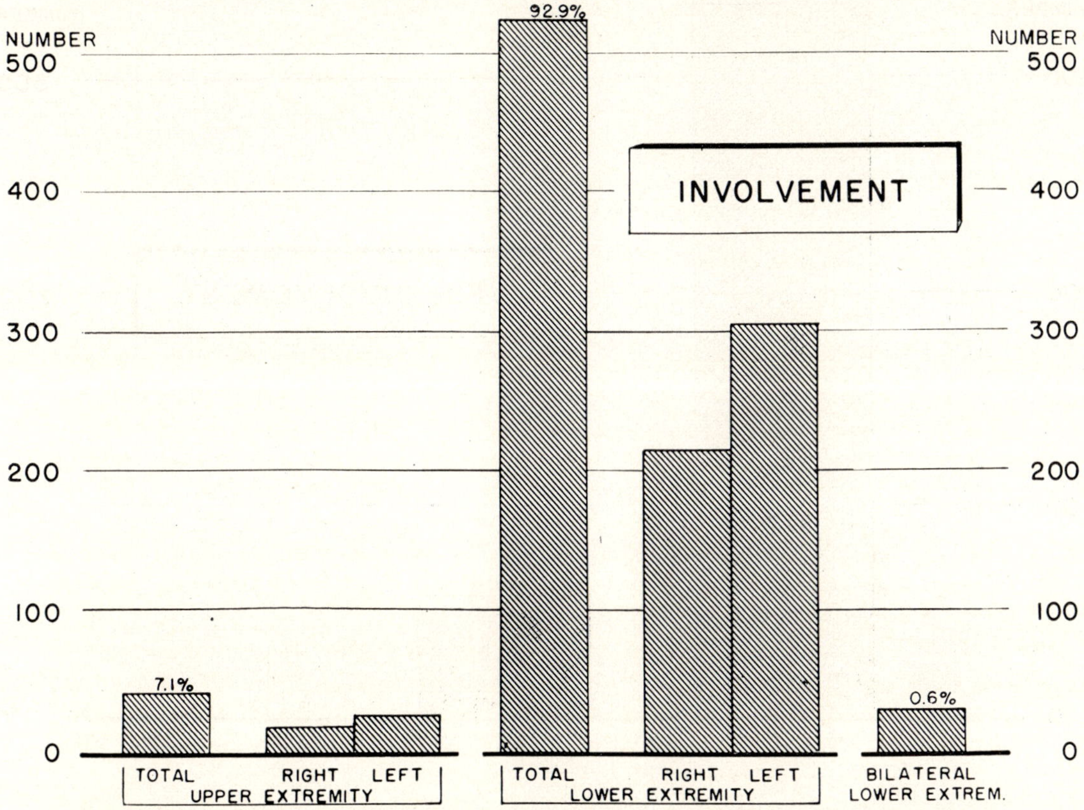

Fig. 5.

operation of patients with residual findings of previous thrombophlebitis is emphasized by the figures they report: Of 46 patients in their series who gave a history of thrombophlebitis less than one year before operation, 31 developed pulmonary embolisms, and almost one-half of the group died.

Miscellaneous Causes.—In the 20 cases of intravascular clotting of miscellaneous origin in the Army series, 7 were associated with some form of strenuous effort, such as hiking, carrying packs, throwing baseballs, and other athletic endeavors.

The remaining 13 cases were associated with varicose veins, which in one instance had been injected. The importance of this cause of intravascular clotting has been repeatedly stressed.[11, 65, 68, 146, 163, 192] The existence of varicosities favors venous stasis, which is an important factor in thrombosis. For this reason, varicosities must be corrected preoperatively or treated by compression bandages during the operative and postoperative period. Compression bandages have been shown to be effective postoperatively in reducing the incidence of thrombophlebitis even in the absence of varicosities.[68] The thrombosis usually begins in the superficial veins and extends to the deeper veins.

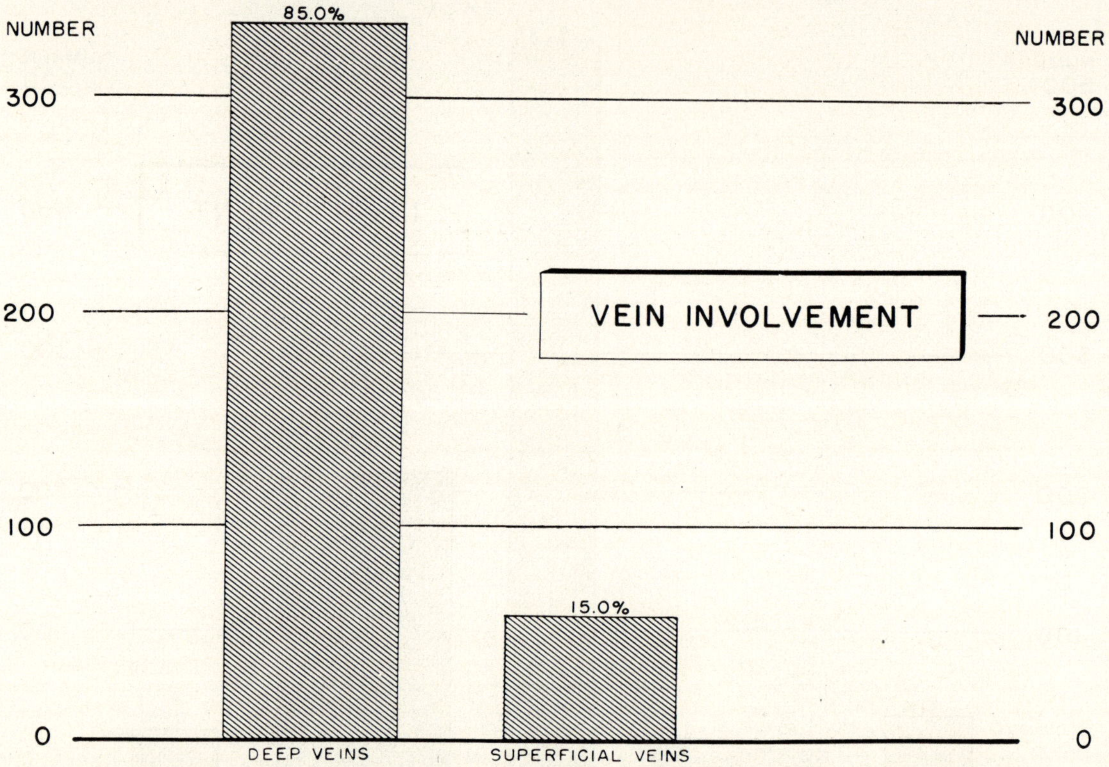

Fig. 6.

Site of Lesion.—The 502 patients with intravascular clotting in the Army series presented the lesion in 563 different sites. The lower extremity (Fig. 5). was involved more than thirteen times more often than the upper and the involvement in 29 instances was bilateral. The superior vena cava was the site of involvement in 3 instances.

In the 394 cases in the Army series in which this information was available (Fig. 6), the superficial veins were involved 59 times and the deep veins 335 times. In both the upper and the lower extremities the left side was more frequently involved than the right. The discrepancy may not be significant, but can be explained by the more marked circulatory retardation on this side, which is due to anatomic considerations: The right iliac artery crosses, and compresses in the crossing, the left iliac vein, while the presence of the sigmoid and rectosigmoid on the left side may also play a part in the production of stasis in the common iliac vein.

There has been considerable discussion concerning the site of origin of thrombosis and embolism. Virchow,[196] who in 1846 published the first correctly interpreted instances of embolism, was of the opinion that the clot obstructing the pulmonary artery came from the pelvis or the lower extremities. Aschoff's[6] theory of thrombosis postulates the origin of fatal emboli in the femoral and iliac veins, but more recent observations are to the effect that many thromboses begin in the veins of the legs and feet.[13, 43, 70, 84, 85, 116, 138, 154, 166, 172] Neumann[138] described two clinical types of thrombosis, based on the site of origin, (1) a benign variety beginning in the veins of the legs and characterized by increased frequency with age, slow progression, and a tendency toward multiple but nonfatal emboli, and (2) a malignant variety, originating in the plantar veins and characterized by rapidly progressive thrombosis, occurrence in younger persons without increasing frequency with age, and a tendency toward the development of fulminating fatal pulmonary emboli.

SUPERIOR VENA CAVAL THROMBOSIS

The 3 instances of intravascular clotting in the superior vena cava observed in the vascular centers in the Zone of the Interior during World War II represent an unusual condition. Any variety of vena caval obstruction is rare; in 1933 Ehrlich, Ballon, and Graham[63] could find only 309 cases in the world literature. Obstruction due to thrombosis is even rarer; in 1936, Ochsner and Dixon[153] could find only 120 cases in the world literature, to which they added two personally observed cases. According to Zambellini[211] the first two reported cases of superior vena caval thrombosis were by Bartolino and Hunter.

In 95 of the cases collected by Ochsner and Dixon in which details of sex and race were given, there were 64 males and 92 white persons. The average age in 82 cases in which the age was stated was 43.6 years and the range was 9 to 74 years. In 13 cases the cause was either not stated or could not be determined. In 44 cases the condition followed phlebitis, in 35 external compression, and in 28 mediastinitis. All 3 of the Army cases were of spontaneous origin.

The clinical manifestations of thrombotic obstruction of the vena cava are the result of stasis in the tributaries draining into this vessel and are chiefly limited to the upper half of the body. Edema, the principal sign, is the result of stasis, deficient drainage, and transudation of fluid. The venous pressure is elevated, due to the obstruction and the necessity for spontaneous short-circuiting of the flow of blood. Edema of the eyelids is early and frequent, though often not conspicuous because collaterals develop early and because in the upright position drainage is good. It may extend to the face, particularly if the patient is recumbent for any length of time. Cyanosis of the face, especially of the lips and lobes of the ears, is a prominent feature in many cases and may be explained chiefly on the basis of anoxemia.[153] Other symptoms and signs include dyspnea,[203] cough, headache, vertigo, somnolence,[203] prominence of the eyes,[63] disturbances of vision, tinnitus, deafness, epistaxis,[63] hemoptysis, dysphagia, paresthesia, and psychotic manifestations. Pleural effusions,[20] increased cerebrospinal fluid pressure, and varicosities are frequent. Venous hypertension in the upper extremities combined with normal venous pressure in the lower extremities is pathognomonic of the condition if it appears in association with edema and cyanosis of the face, neck, and upper extremities aggravated by recumbency.

The two principal types of vena caval obstruction, according to Carlson,[33] occur above and below the azygos vein. In the former type the azygos vein and its tributaries form the chief venous trunk for the return blood flow and the lower abdominal veins are relatively unimportant. In the latter type the superficial and deep abdominal plexuses are of greater importance and the return blood flow must be through the inferior vena cava. According to Wagner,[199] if dilated dorsothoracic superficial veins are present, the obstruction can be presumed to be below the azygos vein. Demonstrable collateral veins and other manifestations of superior vena caval obstruction are aggravated by exercise.

Clinical manifestations are dependent upon and directly proportionate to the rapidity with which thrombotic lesions form and collateral circulation develops. They are relatively few when the lesions develop slowly and an adequate collateral circulation has time to develop.

Treatment should, as far as possible, be based upon correction of the etiologic factor. Venesection[63, 153] may be helpful and mediastinotomy has been advocated[63, 153, 179] as a decompressive measure to permit recanalized vessels to function. The prognosis depends upon the rate at which the thrombosis forms and its extent, the rate at which the collateral circulation develops, and the adequacy of the collateral circulation. In the 120 cases collected by Ochsner and Dixon[153] from the world literature there were 85 deaths, or 75.9 per cent.

The 3 instances of vena caval thrombosis in the Army series illustrate most of the considerations described. The following history is typical.

CASE REPORT

A white man, 26 years of age, was first observed in the course of routine examination after induction for a minor illness. He had markedly dilated and tortuous superficial veins of both upper extremities and spider-web varicosities of the chest and axilla. In reply to specific questioning he stated that he suffered from fullness of the face and swelling beneath the eyes when he was straining and doing heavy work, as well as when he first awoke in the morning; at this time the lower eyelids felt full and puffy. He had himself noted the venous anomalies on the chest, axilla, and arms, and he thought that when the weather was warm there was possible swelling of the hands and fingers. He had completed basic training without difficulty, but for the past sixteen months had noted some shortness of breath when he was very active.

A phlebogram with diodrast disclosed marked dilatation of the veins in the chest, axilla, and upper arms. The spider-web varicosities observed clinically were found to extend bilaterally into the axillae and around the posterior shoulder regions, and dilated, tortuous veins extended downward toward the abdomen. In view of the moderate symptoms and signs no treatment was advised.

AXILLARY THROMBOSIS

Of 40 cases of thrombosis of the veins of the upper extremity (7.1 per cent), 28 (70 per cent) occurred in the axillary veins and the majority occurred on the left side (58.6 per cent). Of the axillary thromboses, the right arm was affected in 71.4 per cent and the left in 28.6 per cent. In 7 cases of axillary thrombosis which I observed[90] at a single vascular center, the age range was from 20 to 37 years. The causes in these cases included climbing a rope, throwing rocks, twisting a propeller, carrying a bucket, and playing tennis. In one case there was no obvious cause. In other cases in the series and in cases reported in the literature the causes included grinding spark plugs, washing clothes, pulling up in bed, restraining a horse, swinging a golf club, pitching a baseball, lifting various heavy weights, and putting books on a shelf.[88] Evidently some sort of strain is necessary for its production.

The cases in this series followed the usual pattern. The onset varied from acute to gradual swelling. As a rule, pain was followed within several hours or several days by swelling and cyanosis. In the early stages arterial spasm was evident, and the hand was cold, blue, and edematous in many instances. In all cases the diagnosis was confirmed by phlebography, which showed the typical pattern of obstruction of the axillary vein.

Several theories have been advanced to explain axillary thrombosis. Von Schrotter,[198] who first described the condition in 1884, maintained that stretching of the vein caused a localized reaction which took the form of thrombosis. Cadenat[31] stated that the respiratory effort associated with strain distended the vein and produced a change in the intima which led to thrombosis. Lowenstein[109] contended that the position of abduction distended the vein and permitted pressure by the costocoracoid ligament and subclavian muscle. Gould and Patey[72] were of the same opinion and demonstrated, in addition, a valve at the level of the subclavius muscle which ruptures following pressure by the muscle on the axillary vein. Veal and McFetridge,[194] from studies on the cadaver, postulated compression of the vein below the head of the humerus against the subscapularis muscle. All of these theories are probably valid, but none explains the quiet type of thrombosis, which occurs without apparent cause. It may be that the thrombosis which develops during sleep is caused by prolonged compression of the vein induced by the position of the arm, particularly when it is elevated over the head or folded under the body. This position results in obstruction of the venous flow and reduction of the oxygen content of the blood, with changes in the intima which lead to thrombosis.[190]

The early arterial spasm present in axillary thrombosis is best treated by stellate ganglion block, repeated until pain and edema subside. In the 7 cases observed at the DeWitt General Hospital Vascular Center[90] this method was employed, in combination with extreme elevation of the extremity. The anterior approach for stellate ganglion block was used exclusively because of its ease of performance and the facility with which it can be taught.[151] If the method is employed early, it should prevent the lymphedema, which is the most disabling feature of this condition. As edema subsides, there is increased prominence of the superficial veins about the shoulder. The patients at DeWitt General Hospital, who were all seen late, showed no impressive change after repeated sympathetic blocks.

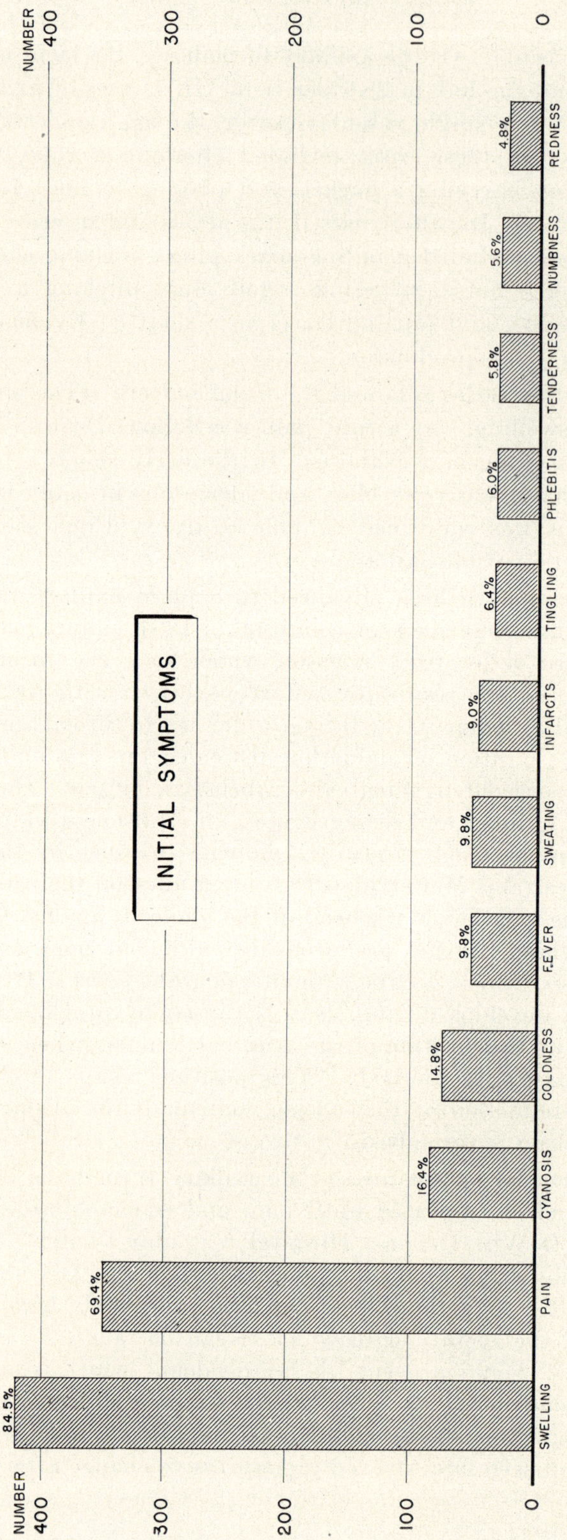
INITIAL SYMPTOMS
NUMBER
400
300
200
100
0
SWELLING 84.5%
PAIN 69.4%
CYANOSIS 16.4%
COLDNESS 14.8%
FEVER 9.8%
SWEATING 9.8%
INFARCTS 9.0%
TINGLING 6.4%
PHLEBITIS 6.0%
TENDERNESS 5.8%
NUMBNESS 5.6%
REDNESS 4.8%

Fig. 7.

CLINICAL PICTURE

The clinical picture is charted in Figs. 7 and 8. Swelling, which was present in 424 (84.5 per cent) of the 502 cases of intravascular clotting observed at the Army vascular centers, was the most prominent of the group of early symptoms, though it appeared first in only 140 cases (28 per cent). Pain, which was among the initial symptoms in 347 cases, was the first symptom in 174 (34.8 per cent). Cyanosis, which was among the initial symptoms in 82 cases, was the first symptom in only 5 cases. Coldness, which was among the initial symptoms in 74 cases, was not a first symptom in any case. Initial symptoms were always more marked in thrombophlebitis, because of its inflammatory character, and were slow and insidious in phlebothrombosis.

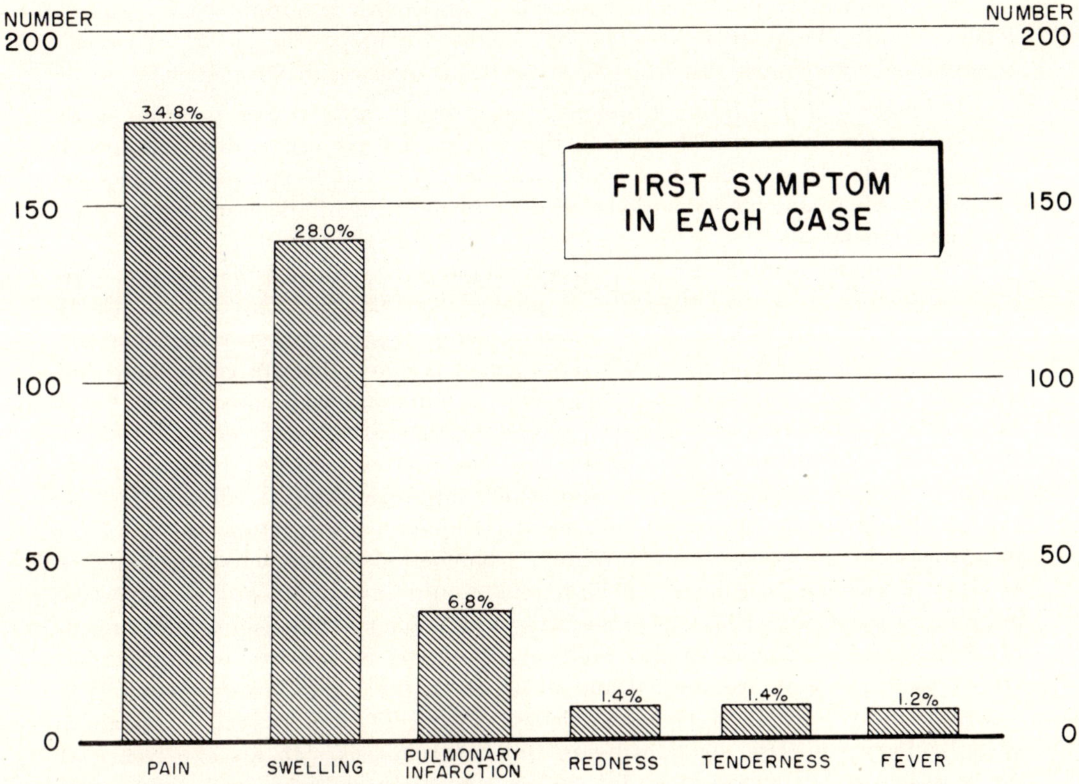

Fig. 8.

The origin of swelling, which is the most persistent and most disabling complication of intravenous clotting, is still a matter of considerable discussion. Originally the edema of thrombophlebitis was explained as due to increased venous pressure resulting from an obstructing thrombus. This factor probably does play a part in its production, but not as large a part in thrombophlebitis as in phlebothrombosis.

In thrombophlebitis not only the vein wall but also the perivenous tissues are involved in the inflammatory process. The surrounding reaction results in lymphangitis,[83, 84, 89, 94] which results in turn in fibrinous exudation into the perivascular spaces. The clinical manifestation of accumulated exudation is edema. Recently it has been shown clinically[145, 147, 149] as well as experimentally[42] that edema in thrombophlebitis is secondary to severe arterial or peripheral reflex vasospasm originating in the affected segment. In severe cases vasospasm results in ischemia and explains the pallor of the skin which has long been recognized as a prominent feature in phlegmasia alba dolens. Loss of pulsation[156] in the affected blood supply also plays a part in the production of edema, which is increased because of stagnation, and the presence of which itself prevents absorption of the collected fluid. This hypothesis, as will be pointed out later, is supported by the excellent results obtained in many instances by lumbar sympathetic block.

That pain is to be explained by reflex vasospasm is supported by the excellent results frequently secured by lumbar sympathetic block. Cyanosis is explained by venous stasis due to obstruction, with resulting anoxemia.

Pulmonary Infarction.—Pulmonary infarction, which was present as an introductory symptom in 34 cases in this series (6.8 per cent), deserves special consideration. It was the presenting symptom in 41 per cent of the cases reported by Allen and his co-workers[2] and in 19 per cent of the cases reported by Veal and Hussey.[192]

The dangerous character of phlebothrombosis is evident from the fact that it is frequently unsuspected until this potentially fatal accident occurs. Early detection is difficult unless the condition is being constantly suspected. The significance of this problem is emphasized when it is noted that statistics show that 2.5 to 5 per cent of deaths are attributable to pulmonary embolism.[84, 85, 116] If the pulmonic process is not properly diagnosed, the patient may continue to have showers of pulmonary emboli, which are regarded as manifestations of pneumonia[80, 81, 206] or cardiac disease[14] and which may eventually terminate fatally, though this is not an inevitable end result. Pulmonary infarction was not fatal in any case in the Army series. White[206] commented on the increasing number of cases in his own experience which he once would have diagnosed as congestive heart failure but which he now recognizes as pulmonary embolism originating in phlebothrombosis, though cardiac disease, of course, is a possible complication. Of 75 cases which White studied and in which cardiac disease was a possibility, it was actually present in 47 cases; the remaining 28 cases were true instances of pulmonary embolism originating in phlebothrombosis. In his experience at the Massachusetts General Hospital, 70 per cent of the patients with pulmonary embolism of nonsurgical origin had symptomless clotting insidious in onset and situated in the deep veins.

Thrombosis begins in the deep veins of the leg and foot and may propagate and go on to embolism before it gives rise to marked clinical manifestations. It is necessary, if it is to be detected before complicating embolism occurs, that the possibility be borne constantly in mind. It should always be recollected as a possible development after operation, though the incidence is small, varying from 0.02 to approximately 1 per cent.[13, 75, 207] Detection is a matter of constant watchfulness. It involves repeated palpation of the extremities, the taking and recording of serial comparative measurements, and repeated observations of the pulse rate, temperature, and respiration.[2, 48, 111, 142] Electrocardiography[8, 12, 39, 118, 126] may be very useful but opinions differ as to the value of phlebography.[2, 15, 56-58, 60, 66, 67, 90, 106, 112, 152, 174] I studied the serial phlebograms made in 110 cases of intravascular clotting at the DeWitt General Hospital Vascular Center[90] and concluded that they were of no value so far as early detection of phlebothrombosis was concerned and also of no value in identifying its location, even when the occurrence of pulmonary embolism had directed attention to its existence. My conclusion was that alert recollection of the possible occurrence of the condition is of far more value than any laboratory method.

The differential diagnosis of pulmonary embolism is frequently possible on the basis of periodic attacks of faintness, dyspnea, prostration, unexplained fever, leucocytosis, and sometimes jaundice. The diagnosis of massive pulmonary embolism, in which the patient goes into shock and dies within a few minutes, seldom presents difficulties. In patients who survive, atelectasis, pneumonia, and pleuritic effusions are secondary results. Roentgenologic diagnosis is disappointing except in the case of wedge-shaped infarctions.[74] Suspicion of the possibility of embolism and constant, close observation are the key to successful diagnosis, as I[90] pointed out in a study of 9 nonfatal cases of pulmonary embolism observed in Army personnel.

Once pulmonary infarction has directed attention to the existence of intravascular clotting, it is urgent that measures be taken to prevent its recurrence, since recurrence is a real possibility. Ziak,[213] for instance, pointed out that 70 per cent of patients who die from pulmonary embolism have had previous attacks of pulmonary infarction, and Graves,[73] in a study of 194 cases, found that while 140 patients had had only a single attack, some had had as many as 8. In 4 instances multiple emboli were not discovered until autopsy.

Not more than 20 to 25 per cent of all pulmonary emboli are immediately fatal. According to Ziak[213] at least 60 per cent of the patients live from one hour to several days. In only 45 of 154 fatal cases in Graves'[73] series did death occur within one hour or less. The remaining patients survived for at least one day, and some for longer periods of time, so that active treatment might have availed. DeTakats and Fowler[49] have also emphasized the fact that in most instances of embolism there is time for treatment, first during the actual episode, then for the prevention of other attacks, which are increasingly dangerous as their number increases. Approximately one-fifth to one-fourth of these emboli are fatal at the onset.

TREATMENT BEFORE ARRIVAL AT A VASCULAR CENTER

Treatment of the 502 patients in this series before their arrival at the vascular centers (Fig. 9) varied from bed rest in 228 cases, elevation in 141 (28.2 per cent), heat (28 per cent), sympathetic ganglion block (20 per cent), posterior tibial nerve block, typhoid, periarterial sympathectomy, and caudal anesthesia to sympathectomy in 10. The rationale of many of the methods utilized is obvious. Bed rest is employed because symptoms are increased with activity

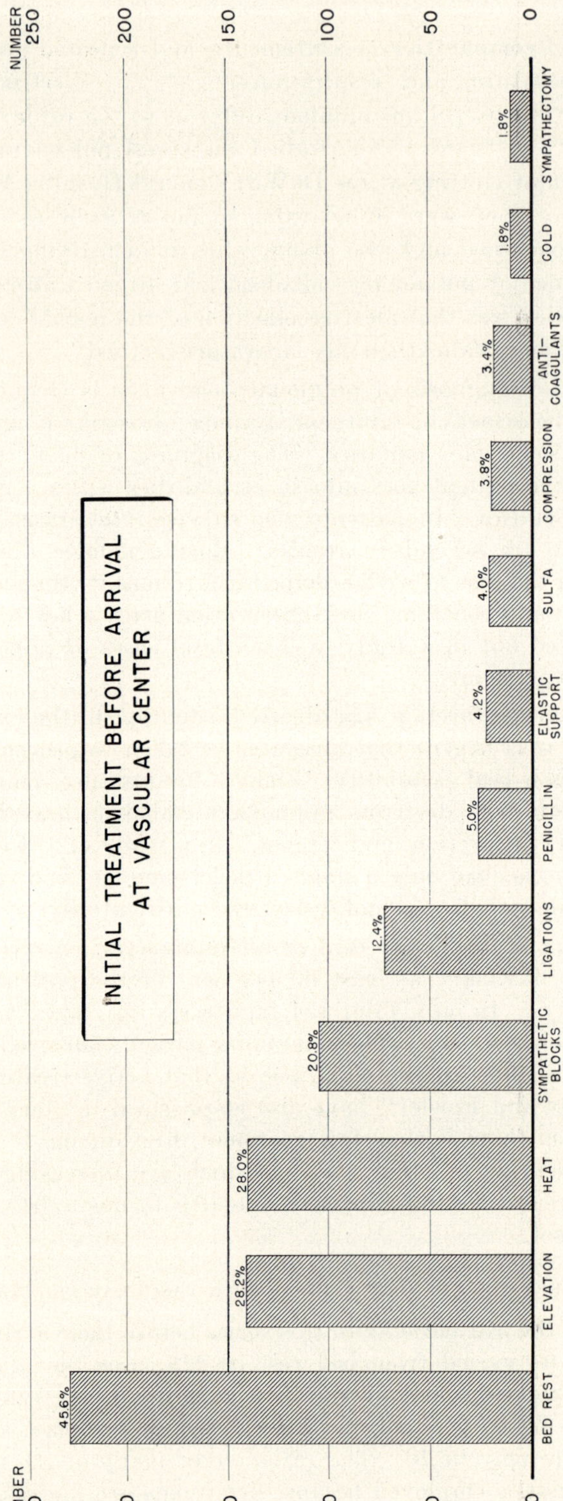
INITIAL TREATMENT BEFORE ARRIVAL
AT VASCULAR CENTER
NUMBER
250
200
150
100
50
0
BED REST
ELEVATION
HEAT
SYMPATHETIC BLOCKS
LIGATIONS
PENICILLIN
ELASTIC SUPPORT
SULFA
COMPRESSION
ANTI-COAGULANTS
COLD
SYMPATHECTOMY
45.6%
28.2%
28.0%
20.8%
12.4%
5.0%
4.2%
4.0%
3.8%
3.4%
1.8%
1.8%

Fig. 9.

and the edema becomes more severe. Elevation of the limb enhances the return flow of blood and thus prevents edema. The rest are attempts to assure vasodilatation in some form and are most effective in acute thrombophlebitis because of the improvement produced in arteriolar pulsations and the resulting decrease in edema. The rationale of the objective has frequently been explained by Ochsner and DeBakey:[145, 147-149] The symptoms of thrombophlebitis are due to vasospasm, which affects venules as well as arterioles, and the methods to increase vasodilatation are therefore logical. Treatment is directed to the correction of the spasm which is not only arteriolar but also of the venule.[42] It has been shown[98, 103, 144] that postoperatively there is a peripheral vasoconstriction. In addition there is retardation of the circulation.[180] Once the thrombophlebitis has occurred treatment of vasospasm must be started.

SYMPATHECTOMY AND SYMPATHETIC BLOCK

In the Army series of 502 cases of intravenous clotting, sympathetic ganglion block had been done in 104 cases (20.8 per cent) before the patients arrived at vascular centers (Fig. 9), and it was done at the centers in 80 (16 per cent) additional cases (Fig. 12). The technique of stellate and of lumbar sympathetic block has been described elsewhere. I now prefer to use a single site for the injection, the second or third lumbar sympathetic ganglion. The results seem as good as when three sites are used, and the procedure is much less objectionable to the patient.

Results of sympathetic block vary. According to Ochsner and DeBakey,[144] who base their remarks on personal experience, complete relief can be expected within four days or less in 50 per cent of all cases and within five to eight days in another 30 per cent. Two-thirds of the patients can be discharged from the hospital within four to eight days after treatment is begun, and another 23 per cent within ten to twelve days. A follow-up study of their patients, covering six months to two years, revealed no recurrence of edema in any instance.

In 58 patients with deep femoral phlebitis treated by sympathetic block at Mayo General Hospital Vascular Center, relief of pain was accomplished in 21 cases and relief of pain and edema in 11. In 19 cases pain was not relieved. In 2 cases there was marked relief of vasospasm and in 2 cyanosis, sweating, pain, and edema were relieved. Permanent relief of edema was secured in 1 case. In 34 patients with deep thrombophlebitis observed at the DeWitt General Hospital Vascular Center,[90] all of whom were in the chronic stage, with durations varying from two months to twenty-four years, edema was an impressive and disabling sequel. Ten patients had been treated in the acute stage by lumbar sympathetic block, with dramatic relief from pain, but edema had not been effected, and it was greatly increased by dependency and activity. Generally speaking, sympathetic block is likely to be effective in the acute stage of intravascular clotting, when edema has not yet become fixed as a result of fibrosis and consequent lymphatic destruction, but is much less effective in the chronic stage, when these effects are evident. In 16 cases of chronic thrombophlebitis which I have studied,[90] improvement in the color of the affected extremity was observed after lumbar sympathetic block, but there was no change in the degree of edema, and discomfort was also unaffected. The results in this small series seem to bear out the contention that while early treatment of vasospasm by sympathetic block frequently achieves brilliant results, edema will be permanently controlled only when the patient begins and continues to practice elevation of the part and to use an elastic support.

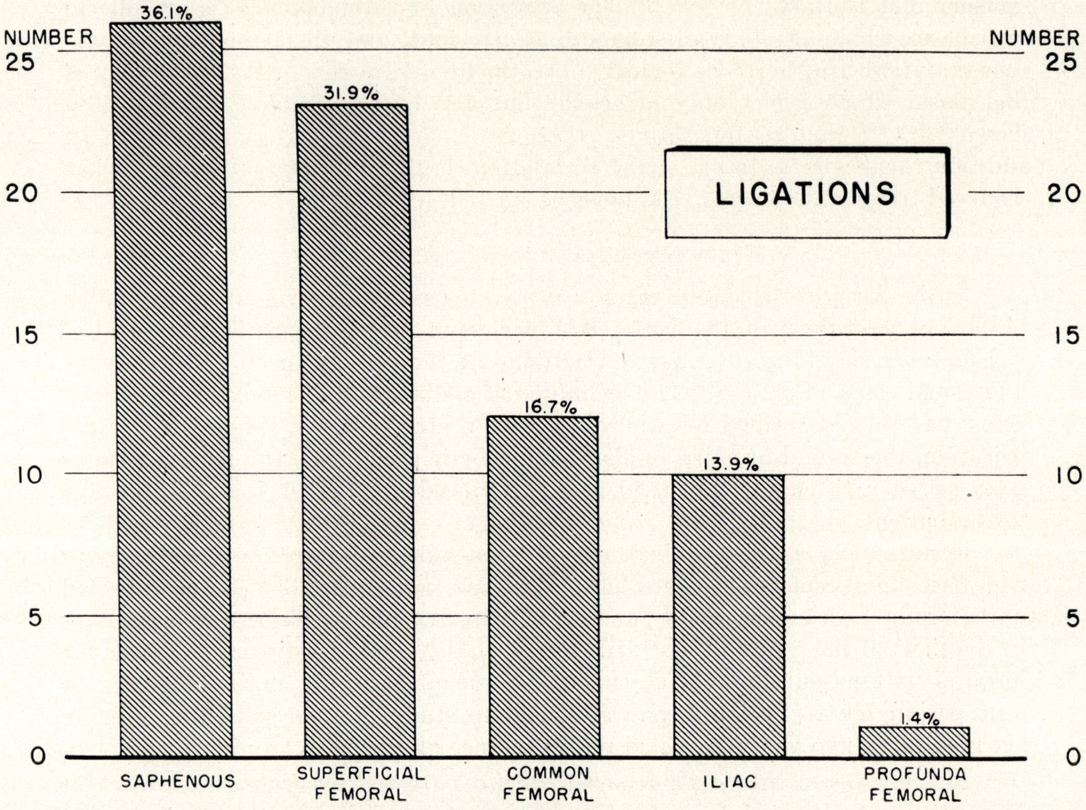

Fig. 10.

Lumbar sympathectomy was done in 15 cases of thrombosis of the deep veins on the indication of persistent pain, cold feet, sweating, and cyanosis. The effect on edema was not remarkable, though there was improvement in the patients' complaints of pain. In 1 instance of deep thrombophlebitis with edema which I observed, sympathectomy produced dramatic immediate relief from discomfort, but had no prolonged beneficial effect. The objective of sympathectomy is to achieve a permanent vasodilatation, but it is not indicated routinely and it should be done for the residuals of intravenous clotting only if a causalgic type of discomfort, excessive hyperhidrosis, and marked cyanosis are relieved by preliminary testing with lumbar sympathetic block.

VENOUS LIGATION

The venous ligations done in 72 cases (12.4 per cent) before the patients arrived at the vascular centers (Figs. 9 and 10), and done in one case at a center, chiefly represent attempts to prevent propagation of quiet venous thromboses and the development of pulmonary emboli.[213]

Once the diagnosis of phlebothrombosis or thromboembolism is made, or even suspected, immediate measures to control it are essential, in the form of venous ligation proximal to the thrombosis, anticoagulant therapy, or both. It is essential that ligation be done above the site of the thrombosis. If the clot is definitely limited to the leg, it may be safe to ligate the superficial femoral vein distal to the profunda branch, but if there is any evidence of propagation, ligation must be done proximal to it. One is impressed by the frequent efforts reported to preserve the femoris profunda, but the attempt is not safe[67]; the site of the thrombosis may be in this very vein, and the patient may die of embolism if it is not tied off.[78] Frykholm[70] has shown that an independent thrombosis frequently originates in the veins of the deep muscles of the thigh and enters the common femoral vein by way of the profunda branches.

Homans[78] advocated ligation of the iliac vein because, for anatomic reasons, a better collateral circulation is available. If bilateral ligation of the femoral vein seems necessary, as many authorities believe when the site of the thrombosis cannot definitely be determined, he advocated ligation of the inferior vena cava. The first ligation of the inferior vena cava by Kocher[92] in 1883 and the second by Billroth[19] in 1885 were both done in error. The first successful deliberate ligation was reported by Bottini[24] in 1893. In 1937 Krotoski[96] was able to collect 48 cases from the literature, and Collins, Jones, and Nelson[36] have shown that the procedure is feasible and successful in a large proportion of cases. Since then many reports concerning the advisability of inferior vena caval ligation have been described in the literature.[124, 189, 193]

Fine and Sears[67] advised ligation of the common femoral vein because of the danger of embolism from the profunda vein when it was spared by ligation of the superficial femoral vein. In their opinion the iliac vein should be explored whenever there is clinical evidence of high thrombosis. If division of the femoral vein is done below the head of the thrombus, thrombectomy is necessary.[97, 101, 102, 146] In some clinics, since the site of the thrombosis in the lower extremity is difficult to determine, bilateral femoral vein ligation is being done.[1-3, 67, 79, 204]

Buxton and Coller[29] performed femoral vein ligation in 24 patients with deep phlebitis varying in duration from two months to thirty years. Most of the patients desired treatment because of chronic, recurrent ulceration about the ankle. A smaller number suffered from swelling, pain, and easy fatigue. Superficial varices were ligated before ligation of the femoral vein. These observers attempted to exclude patients with arteriosclerosis from femoral vein ligation, and did not perform the operation in patients more than 55 years of age. Results were disappointing when ligation was performed in the absence of stasis ulceration, but when ulcers were present there was a high incidence of healing, as well as marked relief of pain, although some lesions later recurred. One death followed complicating arterial disease and thrombosis. One patient required incision and drainage of a residual abdominal abscess four months after ligation of the femoral vein. Following the second operation, acute arterial embolism of

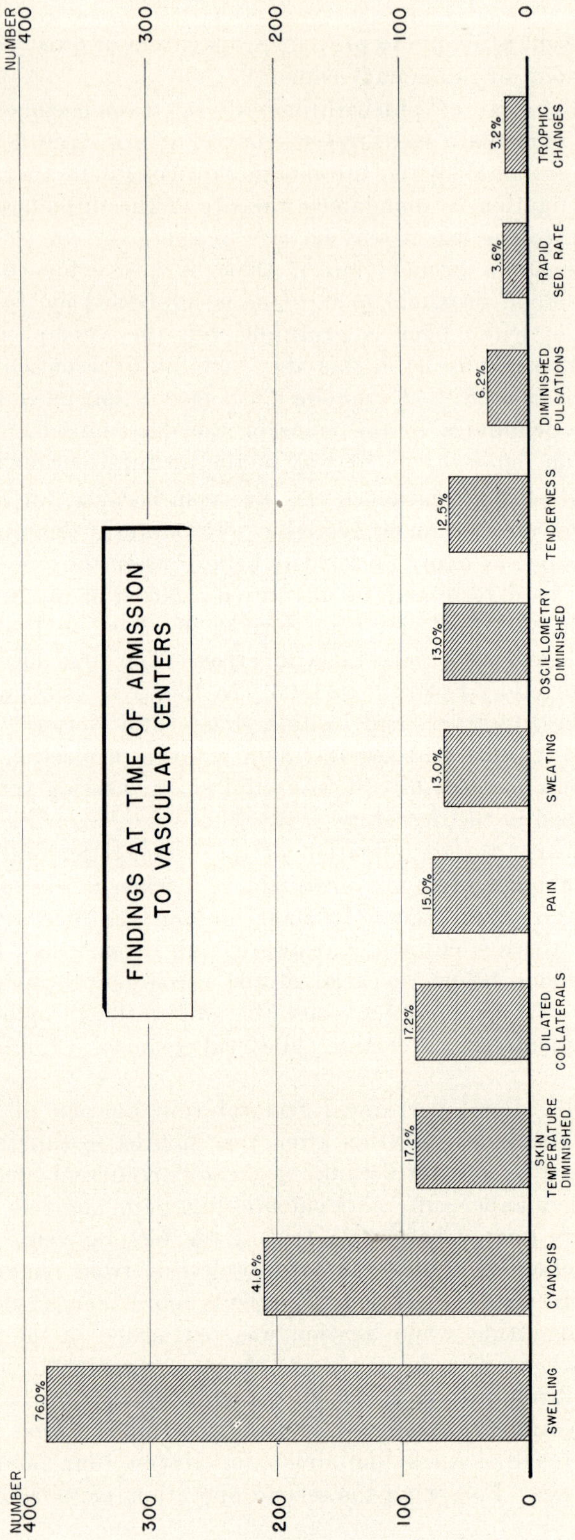
FINDINGS AT TIME OF ADMISSION
TO VASCULAR CENTERS
NUMBER
400
300
200
100
0
76.0%
SWELLING
41.6%
CYANOSIS
17.2%
SKIN
TEMPERATURE
DIMINISHED
17.2%
DILATED
COLLATERALS
15.0%
PAIN
13.0%
SWEATING
13.0%
OSCILLOMETRY
DIMINISHED
12.5%
TENDERNESS
6.2%
DIMINISHED
PULSATIONS
3.6%
RAPID
SED. RATE
3.2%
TROPHIC
CHANGES

Fig. 11.

the popliteal artery developed and amputation of the leg was necessary. One patient had more edema following femoral ligation than before. The collateral circulation became prominent and edema continued to increase until ligation of the vena cava was carried out, after which improvement was observed.

The details just presented suggest that treatment of deep phlebitis by ligation of the femoral vein is not entirely satisfactory. Certainly the method has not obtained general acceptance. The operation seems to have been performed first by Kraussold[95] for pyemia following infection of an amputation wound. In the majority of reported cases since that time the indications were acute processes such as suppurative thrombophlebitis, direct trauma to the vein, and phlebothrombosis. Homans felt it reasonable to assume that an old, sclerosed, canalized femoral or external iliac vein is better divided. Buxton and his co-workers[29, 30] explain the rationale on the basis that in thrombophlebitis there is destruction of the function of the valve. As a result, when the patient stands erect, blood pours down a valveless vein and returning blood must take, in part, collateral valved pathways which, when the phlebitic process is extensive, may themselves be in part incompetent. They endeavored to rectify the destroyed valvular system in the femoral vein by ligation of a portion of the femoroiliac system. The plan does not seem entirely rational, since division of the vein removes the remaining channel, while ligation and division of the varicose veins remove the only remaining pathways. The "persistent or increased swelling of the leg and thigh after operation," which the writers mention as a complication which has produced considerable concern, would seem almost inevitable under the circumstances. This point was also emphasized by Dennis,[44] who reported a case of femoral vein ligation for thrombophlebitis followed by pulmonary infarction and thrombosis in the opposite extremity. Dennis urged care in femoral vein ligation, in respect to destruction of the collateral veins left. I feel strongly that when femoral vein ligation is done, the collateral veins should be preserved, as they can be with the exercise of a little care.

Northway and Buxton[140] reported 10 instances of ligation of the inferior vena cava, 3 for multiple recent pulmonary emboli (in 1 instance associated with chronically recurrent edema and ulceration of the leg), 4 for chronic edema and ulceration, 2 for pain and edema, and 1 for epigastric pain associated with phlebothrombosis. Transection was done in 1 case. In the others the technique consisted of retroperitoneal exposure and ligation in continuity. Compression bandages were used after operation, and edema of the extremities was thus controlled after ambulation was begun. These writers were of the opinion that normal venous pressure cannot be expected in less than twelve months after operation.

Northway and Greenway[141] demonstrated on unembalmed cadavers the vascular alterations which follow this procedure. They ligated the superior vena cava at its entrance into the heart and removed the inferior vena cava from the region of the renal vein superiorly. The whole system was then irrigated by means of a cannula inserted into the femoral vein via the saphenous vein, in order to remove as much clotted blood as possible. The inferior vena cava was clamped just above the bifurcation and just below the renal veins; irrigation was again carried out to cleanse the collateral system. Finally, a thin suspension of red lead was forced into the system under pressure for one minute, after which the cannula was removed and the saphenous vein was ligated. Roentgenologic studies and dissection of the injected venous channels showed that the collateral vessels were amply able to take over the functions of the ligated vena cava, which readily filled above the obstruction.

If the thrombosis is in the pelvic veins, Collins and his associates[36] were of the opinion that the uterine and ovarian veins should be ligated as well as the vena cava.

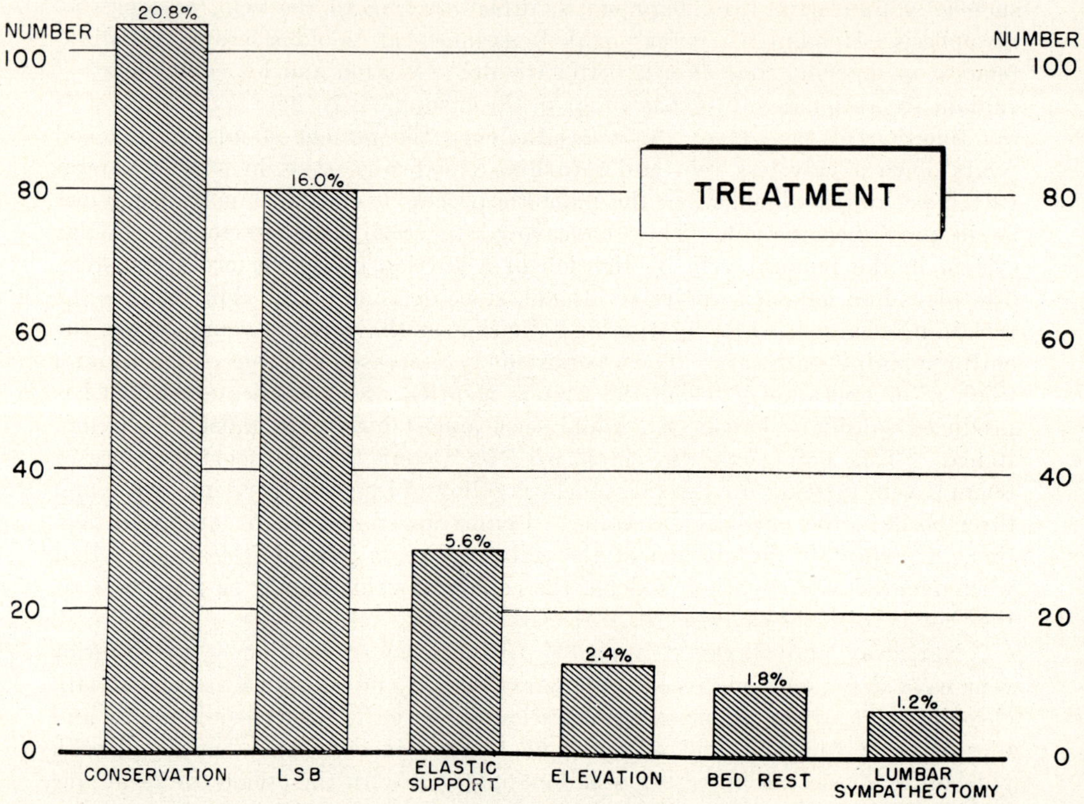

Fig. 12.

Veal and Hussey,[192] who observed 3 deaths from massive pulmonary embolism in cases of acute iliofemoral thrombophlebitis in which a new clot was engrafted on the old, expressed the opinion that there is danger of embolism in all cases of venous thrombosis for as long as four months afterward. Their preference is to perform venous ligation distal to the saphenous vein. In 45 cases they ligated one femoral vein, in 6 cases both, in 6 cases the external iliac, in 6 cases the inferior vena cava, and in 29 the common iliac. Despite their best efforts, there were 9 instances of embolism after ligation in the 45 cases in which ligation was performed before embolism was evident, but there was no further episode of pulmonary embolism in the 39 cases in which ligation was done after at least one episode of this kind.

Deep venous ligation was done in 72 (12.4 per cent) of the 502 cases of intravascular clotting which make up the Army series. It is noteworthy that in 21 instances of pulmonary embolism observed at the Mayo General Hospital, ligation had been done in only 5 cases; the remaining 16 patients recovered completely without specific therapy. Twelve patients of the 27 at the DeWitt General Hospital in whom venous ligation was done had pulmonary infarction prior to the operation but none developed it afterward, which suggests that adequate venous ligation is usually sufficient to prevent pulmonary infarction. Although many observers feel that ligation of the common femoral vein or ligation at a higher level is the method of choice in phlebothrombosis of the lower extremity, the majority of ligations in the Army series were done in the saphenous and the superficial femoral veins. No ligations of the vena cava were reported.

ANTICOAGULANT THERAPY

Anticoagulant therapy, in the form of dicoumarin, heparin, or both, was used in 17 cases in this series (3.4 per cent) with no untoward results. Theoretically, this prophylactic measure seems indicated in patients in whom there is a thrombosing tendency. Practically, the identification of such patients is difficult, though there has been renewed interest in the problem since the advent of anticoagulants.

When I[90] studied the bleeding and clotting times by the Lee and White method in 65 cases of intravascular clotting, I found no changes in the acute stage. Prothrombin time determinations also showed no variations from normal. Determinations on diluted plasma seem to detect a tendency toward increased clotting.[25] The latter method, however, requires a skilled laboratory technique. Estimation of the erythrocytic sedimentation rate has been used as an index of activity. DeTakats[46] found the response to heparin of patients with excessive coagulability of the blood to be strikingly diminished and recommended the use of the decreased heparin tolerance as a diagnostic test. However, in a study of 7 cases of intravenous clotting, I[90] was unable to confirm this and concluded that a better diagnostic aid was supplied by the erythrocytic sedimentation rate than by the heparin tolerance test.

DeTakats[46] stated that clotting factors have been known to exist in the postoperative state and in the presence of any kind of intravascular clotting. He supplied evidence that drugs like Prostigmine[47] or sulfur compounds[45] seemed to decrease the increased clotting factors. When there was an abnormal response,[45-47] it could be corrected by heparin, dicumarol, sulfur compounds, or prostigmine. In these cases, he uses anticoagulant therapy.

Although numerous observers have advised caution in the use of anticoagulants, there is considerable evidence of their value[4, 5, 22, 27, 40, 87, 99, 214] and, when they are properly used, of their safety. Dicumarol is favored, for it is less expensive than heparin. Reich and his associates[167] used it prophylactically in 102 surgical patients and Butsch and Stewart[27] used it in 23 male patients after hernioplasty. No patient developed either thrombosis or embolism, but 2 patients in the hernioplasty group developed hematomas in the wound.

Barker and his associates[12] gave dicumarol to 1,000 surgical patients in the immediate postoperative period. In patients with a history of thrombophlebitis or pulmonary embolism following previous surgery, and in cases in which abdominal hysterectomy or certain other operations were performed, the drug was begun approximately twenty-four hours after operation. They attempted to keep the prothrombin time between thirty-five and sixty seconds (against a normal of nineteen to twenty-two seconds) during the period in which intravascular thrombosis might develop. In the first 374 cases which these observers reported, pulmonary infarction developed in 1 case in which the prothrombin time was twenty-six seconds and thrombophlebitis in 1 case in which the prothrombin time was thirty-five seconds and in 1 in which it was forty-five seconds. Moderate or severe bleeding, with 2 exceptions, occurred only when the prothrombin time was above sixty seconds.

That anticoagulant therapy is not free from risk is evident in a number of reports in the literature. Evans,[64] who used dicumarol, heparin, or both in 56 cases of intravascular clotting, reported hemorrhagic phenomena in 8 cases and 2 deaths from bleeding, and Shlevin and Lederer[177] reported a death from uncontrollable hemorrhage after dicumarol therapy.

Yahr,[210] in an effort to evaluate dicumarol, treated 67 cases of thrombophlebitis by a uniform method. His series was divided as follows:

Eleven cases of superficial phlebitis: Wet boric acid dressings were applied locally. Pain was controlled by the administration of papaverine as necessary. The total average dose of dicumarol was 1,000 mg. During a follow-up period ranging from six to ten months there had been no recurrences.

Twenty-seven cases of deep phlebitis: The extremity was elevated and an icecap was applied at the point of maximum tenderness. When the patient was allowed out of bed, an elastic support was applied. Dicumarol was used in all cases. There were no instances of pulmonary embolism in the group.

Nine cases of superficial and deep thrombophlebitis: Treatment consisted of elevation of the extremity, wet dressings, papaverine, and dicumarol.

Ten cases of pulmonary embolism, in 8 of which the condition was postoperative: In 3 cases there were 2 episodes. Treatment consisted of sedation and dicumarol. No further episodes occurred.

In the whole group intravascular clotting developed after operation in 37 cases and either before or after delivery in 22. In the remaining cases the etiology was unknown. Yahr felt that in respect to length of treatment, lack of complications, absence of emboli, and wide margin of safety, dicumarol was a very satisfactory agent in the management of intravascular clotting.

Ochsner,[142] among others,[10, 41] has emphasized that the principal use of anticoagulants is prophylactic, and that when once thrombosis has occurred, this type of therapy has no effect on the lesion itself and merely serves to prevent propagation. Numerous successful cases have been reported. Reich and his associates[167] used dicumarol successfully in the treatment of 33 venous thromboses and 9 pulmonary embolisms which occurred in 2,591 surgical and obstetrical cases. Heparin was employed for the first twenty-four to forty-eight hours, since dicumarol does not become effective for this length of time. At the end of this period it was discontinued. Bauer[16, 17] used heparin in the treatment of thrombosis, and Priestly and Barker[164] used it in the treatment of 63 patients who developed thrombosis and embolism after operation and concluded that its proper use in patients in whom pulmonary embolism is not promptly fatal should prevent about one-third of the deaths which now occur from this condition. Other favorable reports were made by Wasserman and Stats[202] and by Pfeiffer and Sain.[158] Murray and his associates,[127-135] who have considerable clinical experience with heparin, reported a striking decrease in the incidence of postoperative embolism and in deaths from it following the use of this agent at the Toronto General Hospital, where originally over 10 per cent of all deaths were due to this complication, and where pulmonary emboli were found in 20 per cent of all post-mortem examinations.

Bancroft[9] expressed the opinion that the use of anticoagulants alone is not sufficient to protect patients against embolism. He reported 12 patients treated by heparin and thrombectomy, in 3 of whom simultaneous thrombectomies were performed on both iliac veins. There were 2 deaths in the series, 1 from thrombosis and 1 from postoperative renal insufficiency, and 1 patient later developed an embolism. It is well to emphasize that these drugs are more effective if used together.[168, 200]

EDEMA

The presence of edema in 380 of the 502 cases of intravascular clotting observed at the Army vascular centers is indicative of the importance of this complication. It is highly significant, furthermore, that it followed all types of initial therapy, including sympathetic block, sympathectomy, anticoagulant therapy, and venous ligation, and that it occurred regardless of whether the original condition was phlebothrombosis or thrombophlebitis.

It must be agreed, as already pointed out, that in acute thrombophlebitis, some measure to induce vasodilatation is necessary, and that if the pain is severe, a direct approach, such as is accomplished by regional sympathetic ganglion block, is effective. If phlebothrombosis is present, anticoagulant therapy or venous ligation, alone or in combination, should be employed, for the condition may give rise to an embolism which may be fatal. Anticoagulant therapy will preserve the collateral circulation, wholly or in part, and will prevent a marked degree of edema later, but the important consideration is the prevention of extension of the thrombus. Elevation of the extremity and the use of supporting bandages whenever the extremity is dependent will also have a favorable effect in the prevention of edema.

CONCLUSION

Intravenous clotting is far reaching in its complications and sequelae. It may result in persistent disabling edema or even death. A compiled series of 502 cases seen at the three vascular centers in the Army has been reviewed. Only 12 per cent presented no sequelae and 37.8 per cent were partially disabled (Fig. 13). The greatest offender was swelling. Chronic lymphedema is a serious problem and is not to be regarded lightly. I believe that a proper evaluation of different types of treatment will relegate them to their proper spheres regardless of the enthusiasm of their proponents. It must be agreed that once acute thrombophlebitis ensues some form of vasodilatation is necessary. This will not always prevent the residuals of edema in a significant number of cases. If the condition is one of phlebothrombosis, adequate therapy to prevent embolism and propagation of the thrombosis are imperative. Even though the patient's life has been spared, the consequences of the venous obstruction are serious. I am firmly convinced that the major ingredient of any form of therapy

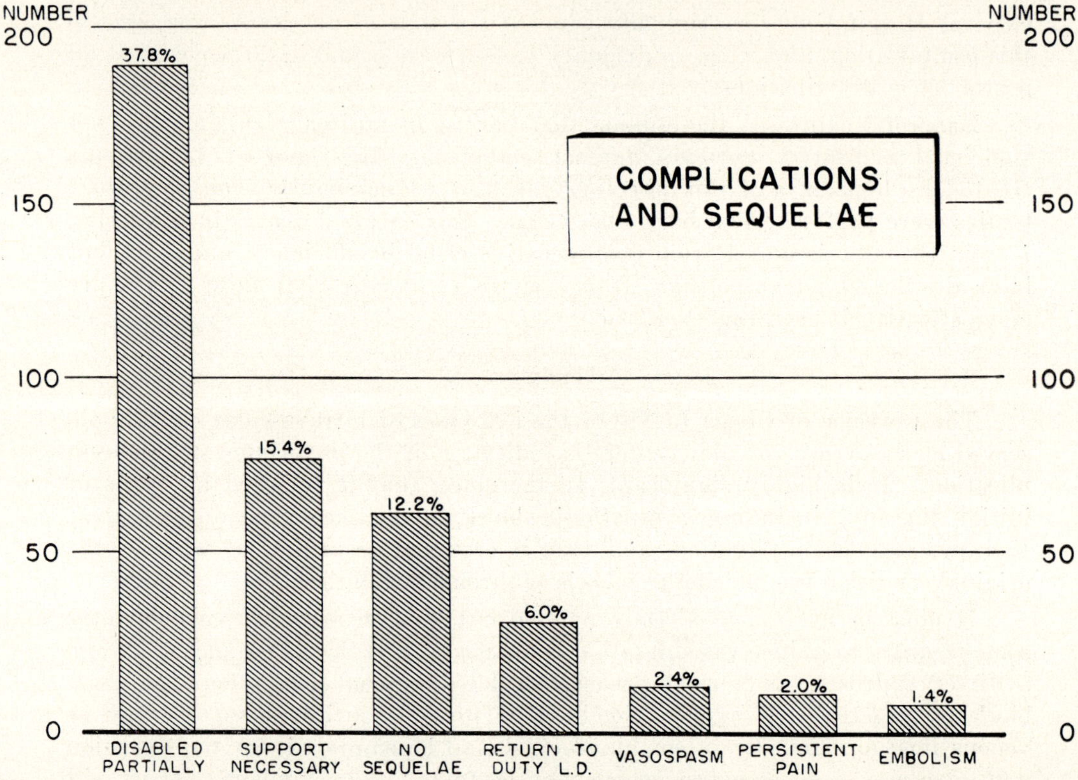

Fig. 13.

is the prevention of further thrombosis blocking an increasing number of collaterals. Obviously the end result regarding the edema will depend on the number of collaterals that are spared. The only means of prevention of propagation of the thrombus is by anticoagulant therapy and I am convinced that this should be started as soon as intravenous thrombus is evident regardless if other modes of therapy are chosen. This is not as applicable to acute thrombophlebitis as it is to phlebothrombosis. The golden period of treatment of lymphedema is immediate. This can be aided further by elevation at any time there is even the slightest suggestion of edema and the use of supportive bandages any time the extremity is dependent.

REFERENCES

1. Allen, A. W.: Interruption of the Deep Veins of the Lower Extremities in the Prevention and Treatment of Thrombosis and Embolism, Surg., Gynec. & Obst. **84**: 520-527, 1947.
2. Allen, A. W., Linton, R. R., and Donaldson, G. A.: Thrombosis and Embolism, Review of 202 Patients Treated by Femoral Vein Interruption, Ann. Surg. **118**: 728-740, 1943.
3. Allen, A. W., Linton, R. R., and Donaldson, G. A.: Venous Thrombosis and Pulmonary Embolism, J. A. M. A. **133**: 1268-1274, 1947.
4. Allen, E. V., Barker, N. W., and Waugh, J. M.: A Preparation From Spoiled Sweet Clover (3.3′-Methylene-Bis (4-Hydroxycoumarin)) Which Prolongs Coagulation and Prothrombin Time of the Blood: A Clinical Study, J. A. M. A. **120**: 1009-1015, 1942.
5. Allen, E. V.: The Clinical Use of Anticoagulants, Report of Treatment With Dicoumarol in 1686 Postoperative Cases, J. A. M. A. **134**: 323-329, 1947.
6. Aschoff, L.: Ueber Thrombose und Embolie, Wien. klin. Wchnschr. **51**: 1277-1282, 1938. Aschoff, L.: Thrombosis: Lectures on Pathology, New York, 1924, Paul B. Hoeber, Inc.
7. Aycock, T. B., and Hendrick, J. W.: The Problem of Venous Thrombosis, J. A. M. A. **133**: 1259-1263, 1947.
8. Baker, E. C., and Miller, F. A.: Further Experiences With Venography, Radiology **43**: 129-134, 1944.
9. Bancroft, F. W.: Proximal Ligation and Thromboectomy for Phlebothrombosis of the Femoral and Iliac Veins, Ann. Surg. **121**: 175-184, 1945.
10. Barker, N. W., Allen, E. V., and Waugh, J. M.: Use of Dicoumarol in the Prevention of Postoperative Thrombophlebitis and Pulmonary Embolism, Proc. Staff Meet., Mayo Clin. **18**: 102-107, 1943.
11. Barker, N. W., and Counseller, V. S.: Prevention and Treatment of Postoperative Thrombophlebitis, Am. J. Obst. & Gynec. **37**: 644-653, 1939.
12. Barker, N. W., Cromer, H. E., Hurn, M., and Waugh, J. M.: The Use of Dicoumarol in the Prevention of Postoperative Thrombosis and Embolisms With Special Reference to the Dosage and Safe Administration, SURGERY **17**: 207-218, 1945.
13. Barker, N. W., Nygaard, K. K., Walters, W., and Priestly, J. T.: A Statistical Study of Postoperative Venous Thrombosis and Pulmonary Embolism, Proc. Staff Meet., Mayo Clin. **15**: 769-773, 1940; **16**: 17-21, 33-37, 1941.
14. Barnes, A. R.: Pulmonary Embolism, J. A. M. A. **109**: 1347-1353, 1937.
15. Bauer, G.: A Venographic Study of Thromboembolic Problems, Acta chir. Scandinav. (Supp.) **84**: 1, 1940.
16. Bauer, G.: Heparin as a Therapeutic Against Thrombosis; Results of One Year's Treatment at Mariestad Hospital, Acta chir. Scandinav. **86**: 267-286, 1942; J. A. M. A. **120**: 1166, 1942.
17. Bauer, G.: Heparin Therapy in Acute Deep Venous Thrombosis, J. A. M. A. **131**: 196-203, 1946.
18. Belt, T. H.: Thrombosis and Pulmonary Embolism, Am. J. Path. **10**: 129-144, 1934.
19. Billroth, cited by Pfaff, O. G.: Ligation of Inferior Vena Cava, Am. J. Obst. & Gynec. **11**: 660-663, 1926.
20. Bittman, R. B.: Thymoma and Exploratory Thoracotomy, S. Clin. North America **112**: 1265, 1932.
21. Blair, B., in discussion of Glynn, E. E.: Pulmonary Embolism and Primary Pulmonary Thrombosis, J. Obst. & Gynaec., Brit. Emp. **31**: 521, 1924.
22. Bollman, J. L., and Preston, F. W.: Effects of Experimental Administration of Dicoumarin, J. A. M. A. **120**: 1021, 1942.
23. Boldt, H. J.: The Management of Laparotomy Patients and Their Modified Treatment, N. York M. J. **85**: 145-153, 1907.
24. Bottini, cited by Costa, G.: Arch. ital. di chir. **4**: 339-388, 1921.[140]
25. Brambel, C. E., and Loher, F. F.: Significance of Variations of Prothrombin Activity of Diluted Plasma, Proc. Soc. Exper. Biol. & Med. **53**: 218, 1943.
26. Burke, M.: Thrombosis: A Medical Problem, Am. J. M. Sc. **196**: 796-814, 1938.
27. Butsch, W. L., and Stewart, J. D.: Administration of Discoumarin Compound for Prophylaxis of Postoperative Thrombosis and Embolism, Arch. Surg. **45**: 551, 1942.
28. Butt, H. R., Allen, E. V., and Bollman, J. L.: A Preparation From Spoiled Sweet Clover Which Prolongs Coagulation and Prothrombin Time of the Blood; Preliminary Reports of Experimental and Clinical Studies, Proc. Staff Meet., Mayo Clin. **16**: 388-395, 1941.
29. Buxton, R. W., and Coller, F. A.: Surgical Treatment of Long-Standing Deep Phlebitis of the Leg—A Supplementary Report, SURGERY **18**: 663-669, 1945.
30. Buxton, R. W., Farris, J. J., Moyer, C. A., and Coller, F. A.: Surgical Treatment of Long-Standing Deep Phlebitis of Leg, A Preliminary Report, SURGERY **15**: 749-756, 1944.

31. Cadenat, F. M.: Les thrombophlebitis des membre supérieùre, Paris méd. **35**: 253-259, 1920.
32. Campeanu: Cited by Zava.[212]
33. Carlson, H. A.: Superior Vena Cava Obstruction, Proc. Soc. Exper. Biol. & Med. **30**: 293, 1932-3.
Idem: Obstruction of the Superior Vena Cava: An Experimental Study, Arch. Surg. **29**: 669, 1934.
34. Chiasserini, A.: Cause e meccanismi delle postoperatorie, Cong. Soc. internat. de chir., Rap. **1**: 3, 377, 1929-1930.
35. Coley, B. L.: Incidence of Phlebothrombosis and Embolism in Thirty Hospitals in the Eighth Service Command. Meeting of the Surgical and Orthopedic Consultants of the Service Commands, Surg., Gynec. & Obst., 10-11, 1944.
36. Collins, C. G., Jones, J. R., and Nelson, E. W.: Surgical Treatment of Pelvic Thrombophlebitis: Ligation of Inferior Vena Cava and Ovarian Veins: Preliminary Report, New Orleans M. & S. J. **95**: 324-329, 1943.
37. Copley, A. L., and Stefko, P. L.: Coagulation Thrombi in Segments of Artery and Vein in Dogs and the Genesis of Thromboembolism, Surg., Gynec. & Obst. **84**: 451-459, 1947.
38. Culp, O. S.: Postoperative Venous Thrombosis and Pulmonary Embolism: Analysis of Thirty-eight Cases, Bull. Johns Hopkins Hosp. **67**: 1-24, 1940.
39. Currens, J.: Electrocardiogram in Pulmonary Embolism, Proc. Staff Meet., Mayo Clin. **17**: 502-509, 1942.
40. D'Alessandro, A. J.: Heparin: Its Properties and Clinical Use, Collective Review, Internat. Abstr. Surg. **74**: 62-69, 1942.
41. DeBakey, M.: Dicoumarin and Prophylactic Anticoagulants in Intravascular Thrombosis, SURGERY **13**: 456-459, 1943.
42. DeBakey, M., Burch, G. E., and Ochsner, A.: Effect of Chemical Irritation of Venous Segment on Peripheral Pulse Volume, Proc. Soc. Exper. Biol. & Med. **41**: 585-590, 1939.
43. Deneche, K.: München. med. Wchnschr. **76**: 1912, 1929, cited by McCartney.[116]
44. Dennis, C.: Disaster Following Femoral Vein Ligation for Thrombophlebitis; Relief by Fasciotomy; Clinical Case of Renal Impairment Following Crush Injury, SURGERY **17**: 264-269, 1945.
45. DeTakats, G.: The Effect of Sulfur Compounds on Blood Clotting, SURGERY **14**: 661, 1943.
46. DeTakats, G.: Heparin Tolerance. A Test of the Clotting Mechanism, Surg., Gynec. & Obst. **77**: 31, 1943.
47. DeTakats, G.: The Nervous Regulation of the Clotting Mechanism, Arch. Surg. **48**: 105, 1944.
48. DeTakats, G.: Postoperative Thrombosis and Embolism, Illinois M. J. **79**: 25-32, 1941.
49. DeTakats, G., and Fowler, E. F.: The Problem of Thrombo-Embolism, SURGERY **17**: 153-177, 1945.
50. DeTakats, G., and Jeser, J. H.: Pulmonary Embolism; Suggestions for Its Diagnosis, Prevention, and Management, J. A. M. A. **114**: 1415, 1940.
51. DeTakats, G., Mayne, A., and Peterson, W. F.: The Meterologic Factor in Pulmonary Embolism, SURGERY **7**: 819-827, 1940.
52. DeTakats, G., Trump, R. A., and Silbert, N. C.: The Effect of Digitalis on Blood Clotting, J. A. M. A. **125**: 840, 1944.
53. deTorres, M.: Phlébites et embolies consécutives aux opérations gynécologiques, Progrès méd., 1609, 1934; Phlebitis and Embolism Following Gynecologic Operations, J. A. M. A. **103**: 1865, 1934.
54. Dock, W.: The Use and Abuse of Bedrest: Conferences of Therapy New York Hospital, New York State J. Med. **44**: 724-730, 1940.
55. Domrich, H.: Deutsche Ztschr. f. Chir. **222**: 20, 1930, cited by McCartney.[116]
56. Domrich, H.: Phlebegraphic directe: conception, technique, premiers resultants, J. Int. de chir. **6**: 625, 1938.
57. dos Santos, J. C.: Phlebographie d'uns veins cave inferieuse suturee, J. d'urol **39**: 588, 1933.
58. dos Santos, J. C.: Spasme vieneux du bras après injection intraartérielle: action de l'infiltration du ganglion étoilé: contrôle phlébographique avant et après l'infiltration, Rev. de chir., Paris **76**: 308-314, 1938.
59. Dougal, D.: The Etiology of Thrombosis and Embolism, J. Obst. & Gynaec. Brit. Emp. **45**: 425-450, 1938.
60. Dougherty, J., and Homans, J.: Venography, A Clinical Study, Surg., Gynec. & Obst. **71**: 697-702, 1940.
61. Duval, P., and Binet, L.: Essai Expérimental sur la pathogénie de certaines complications post-opératoires, Mem. Acad. de chir. **62**: 181-192, 1936.[146]

62. Duval, P., Roux, J. C., and Goiffon, R.: Essai sur l'intoxication par les polypeptides, Presse méd. 42: 1785-1787, 1934.[146]
63. Ehrlich, W., Ballon, H. C., and Graham, E. A.: Superior Vena Caval Obstruction With a Consideration of the Possible Relief of Symptoms by Mediastinal Decompression, J. Thoracic Surg. 3: 352, 1933.
64. Evans, J. A.: Dicoumarol Therapy in Thrombotic Emergencies, New England J. Med. 230: 131-135, 1944.
65. Ewald, C.: Therapie der Thrombophlebitis und der Thromboembolie, Wien. klin. Wchnschr. 50: 377, 1937.
66. Fine, J., Frank, H. A., and Starr, A.: Recent Experiences With Thrombophlebitis of the Lower Extremity and Pulmonary Embolism, Ann. Surg. 116: 574-595, 1942.
67. Fine, J., and Sears, J. B.: The Prophylaxis of Pulmonary Embolism by Division of the Femoral Vein, Ann. Surg. 114: 801-812, 1941.
68. Flörcken, H.: Aussprache über die Behandlung der Venenthrombose bei drohender oder bestehender Embolie, Med. Klin. 36: 244, 1940.[146]
69. Frauendorfer: Cited by Müller-Meernach.[125]
70. Frykholm, R.: Pathogenesis and Mechanical Prophylaxis of Venous Thrombosis, Surg., Gynec. & Obst. 71: 307-312, 1940.
71. Gordon-Watson, C.: In discussion of Lockhart-Mummery.[107]
72. Gould, E. P., and Patey, D. H.: Primary Thrombosis of the Axillary Vein, Brit. J. Surg. 16: 208-213, 1928.
73. Graves, W. N.: Pulmonary Embolism. A Statistical Review of Cases From 1929 Through 1938, Surg., Gynec. & Obst. 70: 958-963, 1940.
74. Hampton, A. O., and Castleman, B.: Correlation of Postmortem Chest Teleroentgenograms With Autopsy Findings, Am. J. Roentgenol. 43: 305, 1940.
75. Heard, J. E.: Papers Mayo Clinic and Mayo Staff 2: 419, 1923.
76. Henderson, E. F.: Fatal Pulmonary Embolism: A Statistical Review, Arch. Surg. 15: 231, 1927.
77. Homans, J.: Circulatory Diseases of the Extremity, New York, 1939, The Macmillan Company.
78. Homans, J.: Exploration and Division of the Femoral and Iliac Veins in the Treatment of Thrombophlebitis of the Legs, New England J. Med. 224: 179-186, 1941.
79. Homans, J.: Deep Quiet Venous Thrombosis in the Lower Limb, Preferred Levels for Interruption of Veins: Iliac Section or Ligation, Surg., Gynec. & Obst. 79: 70-82, 1944.
80. Homans, J.: Diseases of the Veins, Venous Thrombosis and Pulmonary Embolism, New England J. Med. 231: 51-60, 1944.
81. Homans, J.: Pulmonary Embolism Due to Quiet Venous Thrombosis and Simulating Cardiac and Pulmonary Disease, New England J. Med. 229: 309, 1943.
82. Homans, J.: Venous Thrombosis and Pulmonary Embolism, New England J. Med. 236: 196, 1947.
83. Homans, J., and Zollinger, R.: Experimental Thrombophlebitis, Arch. Surg. 18: 992, 1929.
84. Hunter, W. C., Krygier, J. J., Kennedy, J. C., and Sneeden, V. D.: Etiology and Prevention of Thrombosis of the Deep Leg Veins: Study of Four Hundred Cases, SURGERY 17: 178-190, 1945.
85. Hunter, W. C., Sneeden, V. D., Robertson, T. D., and Snyder, G. A. C.: Thrombosis of the Deep Veins of the Legs; Its Clinical Significance as Exemplified in Three Hundred and Fifty-one Autopsies, Arch. Int. Med. 68: 1-17, 1941.
86. Jensen, D. R.: The Problem of Thrombophlebitis, Ann. Surg. 121: 314-327, 1945.
87. Jorpes, J. E.: Anticoagulant Therapy in Thrombosis, Surg., Gynec. & Obst. 84: 677-681, 1947.
88. Kaplan, T.: Thrombosis of the Axillary Vein, SURGERY 12: 184-191, 1942.
89. Karsner, H. T.: Human Pathology, Philadelphia, 1926, J. B. Lippincott Company.
90. Kleinsasser, L. R. J.: The Present Concept of Phlebothrombosis, Thrombophlebitis, and Pulmonary Embolism, California & West. Med. 64: 18-29, 1946.
91. Koch, Cited by Müller, A.: Die Thrombophlebitis und ihre Behandlung mit Komprimierendem Gehverband, Med. Klin. 33: 793-797, 1937.[146]
92. Kocher, cited by Pfaff, O. G.: Am. J. Obst. & Gynec. 11: 660-663, 1926.
93. Koenig: Cited by Müller-Meernach.[125]
94. Koester: Inaugural Dissertations, Bonn, 1870, cited by Ochsner.[142]
95. Kraussold, H.: Ueber eine operative Methode zur Bekämpfung beginnender Pyaemie, Arch. f. klin. Chir. 22: 965-973, 1878.[146]
96. Krotoski, J.: Zur Venenunterbindung bzw.-exstirpation bei der puerperalen Allgemeininfektion von chirurgischen Standpunkt, Chirurg 9: 425-439, 1937.[146]
97. Kulenkampff, D.: Die Verhütung schwerer oder tödlicher Embolien durch Ausräumung der V. iliaca, Zentralbl. f. Chir. 62: 1258, 1938.

98. Kvale, cited by Ward, C. E., and Horton, B. T.: Postoperative Thrombophlebitis of Inferior Vena Cava in Child, Proc. Staff Meet., Mayo Clin. **12**: 811-814, 1937.
99. Lam, C.: Heparin Administration, Methods and Results in Thirty Cases, Ann. Surg. **114**: 205-211, 1941.
100. Lambret, O., and Driessens, J.: L'hyperpolypeptidémie secondaire aux opérations chirurgicales, Compt. rend. Soc. de biol. **104**: 567-568, 1930.[146]
101. Lange, K.: Beitrag zur operativen Behandlung der blanden Venenthrombose, Zentralbl. f. Chir. **65**: 2422-2425, 1938.
102. Läwen, A.: Arteriospasmus bei akuter massiver Thrombose der V. femoralis, Zentralbl. f. Chir. **61**: 1681-1685, 1934.
103. Leriche, R.: Des moyens de rédiure au minimum la maladie postopératoire; de l'operation sous rayons infra rougees, Rev. de Chir. Paris **74**: 99-108, 1936.[142]
104. Leriche, R.: The Prognosis and Treatment of Large Emboli of the Pulmonary Artery, Lyon chir. **41**: 257, 1946. Internat. Abstract Surg. (Surg., Gynec. & Obst. **84**: 382, 1947.
105. Leriche, R., and Kunlin, J.: Traitement immédiat des phlébites post-opératoires par l'infiltration novocaïnique du sympathique lombaire, Presse méd. **42**: 1481, 1934.
106. Lesser, A., and Danelius, G.: Venography: Its Value in the Diagnosis and Management of Venous Disturbances of the Lower Extremities, Ann. Surg. **119**: 903, 1944.
107. Lockhart-Mummery, P.: Discussion on Postoperative Pulmonary Embolism, Brit. M. J. 2: 850-857, 1924.
108. Loewe, L., and Hirsch, E.: Heparin in the Treatment of Thromboembolic Disease, J. A. M. A. **133**: 1263-1268, 1947.
109. Lowenstein, P. S.: Thrombosis of the Axillary Vein: An Anatomic Study, J. A. M. A. **82**: 854-857, 1924.
110. Luckhardt, A. B., Alpert, R., and Smith, S.: Hemodynamic and Respiratory Changes Following Manipulation and Traction of the Gastrohepatic Ligament, Science **76**: 545, 1932.
111. Mahler, cited by Kulenkampff, D.: Die Verhütung schwerer oder todlicher Embolien durch Ausräumung der V. iliaca, Zentralbl. f. Chir. **62**: 1258, 1938.
112. Mahorner, H.: Method for Obtaining Venograms of the Veins of the Extremities, Surg., Gynec. & Obst. **76**: 41-42, 1943.
113. Martland, H. S.: Static or Spontaneous Thrombosis of Veins of Lower Extremity and Pelvis, and Fatal Pulmonary Embolism Following Trauma and Surgical Operations, S. Clin. North America **21**: 383-407, 1941.
114. Mason, E. C.: Blood Coagulation: The Production and Prevention of Experimental Thrombosis and Pulmonary Embolism, Surg., Gynec. & Obst. **39**: 421-428, 1924.
115. Matas, R.: Postoperative Thromboses and Pulmonary Embolism Before and After Lister, Donald C. Balfour Lecture in Surgery, Univ. Toronto M. Bull. **10**: 1, 1932.
116. McCartney, J. S.: Postoperative Pulmonary Embolism, SURGERY **17**: 191-206, 1945.
117. McCartney, J. S.: Pulmonary Embolism: A Report of Seventy-three Cases, Arch. Path. **3**: 921-927, 1927.
118. McGinn, S., and White, P. D.: Acute Cor Pulmonale Resulting From Pulmonary Embolism, J. A. M. A. **104**: 1473-1480, 1935.
119. McPheeters, H. O.: Femoro-iliac Thrombosis and Thrombophlebitis, Minnesota Med. **21**: 200-223, 1938.
120. Meade, W. H., and Ochsner, A.: Spool Cotton as Suture Material, J. A. M. A. **113**: 2230, 1939.
121. Miller, R. H., and Rogers, H.: Embolism and Phlebitis, J. A. M. A. **93**: 1452, 1929.
122. Moran, T. J.: Pulmonary Embolism in Nonsurgical Patients With Prostatic Thrombosis, Am. J. Clin. Path. **17**: 205-208, 1947.
123. Morton, J. J., Mahoney, E. B., and Mider, G. B.: An Evaluation of Pulmonary Embolism Following Intravascular Venous Thrombosis, Ann. Surg. **125**: 590-600, 1947.
124. Moses, W. R.: Ligation of the Inferior Vena Cava or Iliac Veins, New England J. Med. **235**: 2, 1946.
125. Müller-Meernach, O.: Zur Frage der Prophylaxe der postoperativen Thrombose und Embolie, München. med. Wchnschr. **83**: 1880, 1936; **84**: 1169, 1937.
126. Murnaghan, D., McGinn, S., and White, P. D.: Pulmonary Embolism With and Without Acute Cor Pulmonale, With Especial Reference to Electrocardiogram, Am. Heart J. **25**: 573-597, 1943.
127. Murray, G.: Heparin in Thrombosis and Blood Vessel Surgery, Surg., Gynec. & Obst. **72**: 340-344, 1941.
128. Murray, G.: Heparin in Surgical Treatment of Blood Vessels, Arch. Surg. **40**: 307-325, 1940.
129. Murray, G.: Aortic Embolectomy, Surg., Gynec. & Obst. **77**: 157-162, 1943.
130. Murray, G.: Anticoagulants in Venous Thrombosis and the Prevention of Pulmonary Embolism, Surg., Gynec. & Obst. **84**: 665-669, 1947.

131. Murray, G., and Best, C. H.: The Use of Heparin in Thrombosis, Ann. Surg. **108**: 163-177, 1938.
132. Murray, G., and Best, C. H.: Heparin and Thrombosis: The Present Situation, J. A. M. A. **110**: 118-119, 1938.
133. Murray, G., and MacKenzie, R.: The Effect of Heparin on Portal Thrombosis: Its Use in Mesenteric Thrombosis and Following Splenectomy, Canad. M. A. J. **41**: 38-40, 1939.
134. Murray, G., and MacKenzie, R.: Postoperative Thrombosis and Embolism, Am. J. Surg. **57**: 414-428, 1942.
135. Murray, D. W. G., Jaques, L. B., Perrett, T. S., and Best, C. H.: Heparin and Vascular Occlusion, Canad. M. A. J. **35**: 621-622, 1936.
136. Nelson, E. W., Jones, J. R., and Collins, C. G.: Pelvic Thrombophlebitis, A Study of the Etiologic Factors From a Statistical Standpoint, New Orleans M. & S. J. **95**: 375-381, 1943.
137. Neuhof, H., and Seley, G. P.: Acute Suppurative Phlebitis Complicated by Septicemia, SURGERY **21**: 831-842, 1947.
138. Neumann, R.: Centers of Origin and Formation of Development of Thrombosis of the Leg, Virchows Arch. f. path. Anat. **301**: 708-735, 1938.
139. Newburger, B.: Early Postoperative Walking; II. Collective Review, SURGERY **14**: 142-154, 1943.
140. Northway, R. O., and Buxton, R. W.: Ligation of the Inferior Vena Cava, SURGERY **18**: 85-94, 1945.
141. Northway, R. O., and Greenway, G. D.: Vena Cava and Its Collateral Circulation, Univ. Hosp. Bull., Ann. Arbor **10**: 67-69, 1944.
142. Ochsner, A.: Intravenous Clotting, SURGERY **17**: 240-259, 1945.
143. Ochsner, A.: The Use of Vasodilatation in the Treatment of Venous Thrombosis, Surg., Gynec. & Obst. **84**: 659-664, 15, 1947.
144. Ochsner, A., and DeBakey, M.: Rational Therapy on Vascular Thrombosis, New Orleans M. & S. J. **94**: 173-178, 1941.
145. Ochsner, A., and DeBakey, M.: The Role of Vasospasm in Thrombophlebitis and Its Treatment by Novocain Block of the Sympathetics, Tri-State M. J. **13**: 2654, 1941.
146. Ochsner, A., and DeBakey, M.: Therapeutic Consideration of Thrombophlebitis and Phlebothrombosis, New England J. Med. **225**: 207, 1941.
147. Ochsner, A., and DeBakey, M.: Therapy of Phlebothrombosis and Thrombophlebitis, Arch. Surg. **40**: 268, 1940.
148. Ochsner, A., and DeBakey, M.: Thrombophlebitis and Phlebothrombosis, South. Surgeon **8**: 269-290, 1939.
149. Ochsner, A., and DeBakey, M.: Thrombophlebitis, The Role of Vasospasm in the Production of the Clinical Manifestations, J. A. M. A. **114**: 117, 1940.
150. Ochsner, A., and DeBakey, M.: The Significance of Phlebothrombosis and Thrombophlebitis in Orthopedic Surgery, J. Bone & Joint Surg. **23**: 788-794, 1941.
151. Ochsner, A., and DeBakey, M.: Treatment of Thrombophlebitis by Novocaine Block of Sympathetics, SURGERY **5**: 491, 1939.
152. Ochsner, A., DeBakey, M., and Schroeder, G.: The Significance of Phlebography in Thrombophlebitis and Phlebothrombosis, J. A. M. A. **123**: 738, 1943.
153. Ochsner, A., and Dixon, J. L.: Superior Vena Cava Thrombosis, Review of the Literature and Report of Cases of Traumatic and Infectious Origin, J. Thoracic Surg. **5**: 641, 1936.
154. Olow, J.: Sur en detail concernant le diagnostic de la thrombose crurale, Acta obst. et gynec. Scandinav. **10**: 159-162, 1930.
155. Ophuls, W., and Dobson, L., cited by Rosenthal, S. R.: Thrombosis and Fatal Pulmonary Embolism, Arch. Path. **14**: 215, 1932.
156. Parsons, R. J., and McMaster, P. D.: The Effect of Pulse Upon the Formation and Flow of Lymph, J. Exper. Med. **68**: 353, 1938.
McMaster, P. D., and Parsons, R. J.: The Effect of the Pulse on the Spread of Substances Through Tissues, J. Exper. Med. **68**: 377, 1938.
157. Pendergrass, E. P., Chamberlain, G. W., Godfrey, E. W., and Burdick, E. D.: A Survey of Deaths and Unfavorable Sequelae Following the Administration of Contrast Media, Am. J. Roentgenol. **48**: 741, 1942.
158. Pfeiffer, D. B., and Sain, F. D.: Heparin and Dicumarol; Collective Review, Internat. Abstr. Surg. **78**: 109-119, 1944 (Surg., Gynec. & Obst.).
159. Pilcher, R. S.: Slowly Fatal Pulmonary Embolism, Lancet **2**: 942, 1938.
160. Pool, E. H.: Systematic Exercises in Postoperative Treatment, J. A. M. A. **60**: 1202-1204, 1913.
161. Portis, B., and Roth, H. A.: Prophylaxis and Treatment of Postoperative Thrombosis, S. Clin. North America **16**: 287-290, 1936.
162. Potts, W. J.: Pulmonary Embolism, Ann. Surg. **111**: 554-563, 1940.

163. Potts, W. J., and Smith, S.: Pulmonary Embolism: An Experimental Study of Variations in the Volume Blood Flow in the Inferior Vena Cava of the Dog, Arch. Surg. **42**: 661-664, 1941.

164. Priestly, I. T., and Barker, N. W.: Postoperative Thrombosis and Embolism: Their Treatment With Heparin, Surg., Gynec. & Obst. **75**: 193, 1942.

165. Putnoky, J., and Farkas, K.: Vergleichende pathologisch-histologische Untersuchung des Herzmuskels bei 1009 Obduktionen, unter besonderer Beachtung der Fälle von Thrombosen und Embolien. Virchows Arch. f. path. Anat. **287**: 400, 1932. Cited by Ochsner.[142]

166. Putzer, R.: Die Wadenvenen Thrombose in ihrer Beziehung Zur Architektur der Wade, Arch. f. Gynäk. **169**: 444-452, 1939.

167. Reich, C., Yahr, M. D., Eggers, C., and Lipkin, R.: Dicoumarol in the Prevention of Postoperative Thrombosis and Pulmonary Embolism, SURGERY **18**: 238-243, 1945.

168. Rhoads, J. E., Walker, J. J., and Panzer, L.: Control of Blood Coagulability With Coumarin and Other Drugs; Use of Basal Doses of Dicoumarol With Intramuscular Injections of Heparin for Sustained Anticoagulant Effect, Northwest Med. **42**: 182, 1943.

169. Richardson, M. H.: On Certain Unavoidable Calamities Following Surgical Operations, Boston M. & S. J. **151**: 583-588, 1904.

170. Ries, E.: Some Radical Changes in the After Treatment of Celiotomy Cases, J. A. M. A. **33**: 454-456, 1899.

171. Robertson, H.: A Clinical Study of Pulmonary Embolism, Am. J. Surg. **41**: 3-21, 1938.

172. Roessle, R.: On the Significance and Origin of Venous Thrombosis of the Lower Legs, Virchows Arch. f. path. Anat. **300**: 180-189, 1937.

173. Schnitzler, O.: Beitrag zur Verhutung der postoperativen Thrombose und Embolie durch Sympatol, Fortschr. d. Therap. **12**: 712-718, 1936.

174. Sgalitzer, M., and Kollert, V.: Kontrast austellung der Venen in Roentgen bilde, Klin. Wchnschr. **10**: 1659, 1931.

175. Shapiro, S., and Sherwin, B.: Studies in Thrombo-Embolization; II. Observations on the Use of Dicoumarol, Am. J. M. Sc. **205**: 206, 1943.

176. Shaw, W. F., and Richards, C. E.: Postoperative Exercises as Prevention of Embolism, J. Obst. & Gynaec. Brit. Emp. **45**: 451-455, 1938.

177. Shlevin, E. L., and Lederer, M.: Uncontrollable Hemorrhage After Dicoumarol Therapy With Autopsy Findings, Ann. Int. Med. **21**: 332-342, 1944.

178. Simpson, K.: Shelter Deaths From Pulmonary Embolism, Lancet **2**: 744, 1940.

179. Skillern, P. J., Jr.: On Aneurysmal Obstruction of Vena Cava Superior With Special Reference to the Caval Syndrome, International Clin. (27th S.) **1**: 75, 1917.

180. Smith, L. A., and Allen, E. V.: Vascular Clinics XIV Studies on the Rate of Venous Blood Flow; Physiologic Studies and Relation to Postoperative Venous Thrombosis and Pulmonary Embolism, Proc. Staff Meet., Mayo Clin. **16**: 53-57, 1941.

181. Snell, A. N.: Relation of Obesity to Fatal Postoperative Pulmonary Embolism, Arch. Surg. **15**: 237, 1927.

182. Sproul, E. E.: Carcinoma and Venous Thrombosis: The Frequency of Association of Carcinoma in the Body or Tail of the Pancreas With Multiple Venous Thrombosis, Am. J. Cancer **34**: 566-585, 1938.

183. Squier, R.: Management of Postpartum Phlebitis, S. Clin. North America **17**: 33-40, 1937.

184. Stich: Annual Session of the German Surgical Society, J. A. M. A. **105**: 525, 1935.

185. Stowers, J. M., and Grossman, M. E.: Thrombosis of the Inferior Vena Cava, Technique of Its Demonstration, Lancet, 868-870, 1946.

186. Storz, H.: Klinik der Thrombose und Embolie, Klin. Wchnschr. **17**: 257-260, 1938.[70]

187. Sylvan, F.: Vorbeugung und Heilung der Thrombose durch Heilgymnastik, Fortschr. d. Therap. **15**: 20-25, 1939.

188. Takaura, G.: Experimentelle Untersuchung über die Aetiologie der Thrombose, Arch. f. klin. Chir. **188**: 138-151, 1937.[146]

189. Thiebaut, B. R., and Ward, C. S.: Ligation of the Inferior Vena Cava in Thromboembolism, Surg., Gynec. & Obst. **84**: 385-401, 1947.

190. Veal, J. R.: Thrombosis of the Axillary and Subclavian Veins, Am. J. M. Sc. **200**: 27-29, 1940.

191. Veal, J. R.: The Prevention of Pulmonary Complications Following Thigh Amputations by High Ligation of the Femoral Vein, J. A. M. A. **121**: 240-244, 1943.

192. Veal, J. R., and Hussey, H. H.: Surgery of Deep Venous Thrombosis of the Lower Extremity, SURGERY **17**: 218-231, 1945.

193. Veal, J. R., Hussey, H. H., and Barnes, E.: Ligation of the Inferior Vena Cava in Thrombosis of the Deep Veins of the Lower Extremities, Surg., Gynec. & Obst. **84**: 605-610, 1947.

194. Veal, J. R., and McFetridge, E. M.: Primary Thrombosis of the Axillary Vein, Arch. Surg. **31**: 271-289, 1935.

195. Victor, J. A.: Clinical Considerations of Thrombosis and Embolism, Ann. Surg. **82**: 193-198, 1925.
196. Virchow, R.: Beitr. Z. Exper. Path. U. Phys. H. 2: 1, 1846. Cited by McCartney.[116]
197. Von Jaschke, R. T.: Neuere Erfahrungen im Kampf gegen die postoperative Thromboembolie, Chirurg **9**: 274-278, 1937.[146]
198. Von Schrotter, in Nothnagel: Handbuch der Pathologie und Therapie, Vienna, 1901, Alfred Holder, 15/13:533. Cited by Kaplan.[88]
199. Wagner, K.: Symptomatology of Stenosis With Occlusion of Lumen of Superior Vena Cava, Polska gaz. lek. **11**: 61, 81, 1932.[153]
200. Walker, J., and Rhoads, J. E.: Effect of Dicoumarol on Susceptibility to Action of Heparin, SURGERY **15**: 859-865, 1944.
201. Wangensteen, O. H.: The Therapeutic Problem in Bowel Obstructions, Springfield, Ill., 1937, Charles C Thomas, p. 360.
202. Wasserman, L. R., and Stats, D.: Clinical Observations on the effect of 3.3′-methyl-Enebis (4-Hydroxycoumarin), Am. J. M. Sc. **206**: 466-474, 1943.
203. Waterfield, R. L.: Biot's Respiration in Superior Vena Cava Obstruction, Guy's Hosp. Rep. **78**: 305, 1928.
204. Welch, C. E., and Faxon, H. H.: Thrombophlebitis and Pulmonary Embolism, J. A. M. A. **117**: 1502-1508, 1941.
205. Westman, S. K.: Thrombophlebitis in Obstetrics and Gynecology, Lancet **2**: 421-424, 1936.
206. White, P. D.: Pulmonary Embolism and Heart Disease: Review of Twenty Years of Personal Experience, Am. J. M. Sc. **200**: 577-581, 1940.
207. Wilson, L. B.: Fatal Postoperative Embolism, Ann. Surg. **56**: 809-817, 1912.
208. Wright, H. P.: Changes in Adhesiveness of Blood Platelets Following Parturition and Surgical Operations, J. Path. & Bact. **54**: 461-468, 1942.
209. Wright, H. P.: Adhesiveness of Blood Platelets in Normal Subjects With Varying Concentrations of Anticoagulants, J. Path. & Bact. **53**: 255-262, 1943.
210. Yahr, M. D.: The Treatment of Thrombophlebitis, Surg., Gynec. & Obst. **80**: 615, 1945.
211. Zambellini, F.: A Case of Obliteration of the Cava Superior (Extract), Lodi Tipolitograf C. Dell'avo, 1900.[153]
212. Zava, L.: Sui vantaggi del levar precoce degli operati, Policlinico (sez. prat.) **47**: 865-872, 1940. Cited by Ochsner.[146]
213. Ziak, cited by Aschoff, L.: Ueber Thrombose und Embolie, Wien. klin. Wchnschr. **51**: 1277, 1938.
214. Zucker, H. D.: Clinical Experiences With Dicoumarol: Report of Eighteen Cases, J. A. M. A. **124**: 217-220, 1944.

Review of Recent Meetings

FIFTY-NINTH ANNUAL SESSION OF THE SOUTHERN SURGICAL ASSOCIATION

HOLLYWOOD BEACH, FLA.

J. HARVEY JOHNSTON, JR., M.D., JACKSON, MISS.

Aneurysm Following Surgical Procedures, D. C. Elkin, Emory University, Ga.—Surgical trauma with resultant arterial injury occasionally produces arteriovenous fistulas. Such postoperative shunts are not infrequently found in amputation stumps or following hysterectomy, thyroidectomy, or thoracentesis, yet may follow any operation. Mass ligation of tissue containing multiple vessels should be avoided because it may be productive of arteriovenous aneurysms. Elkin presented six personal cases of aneurysm following surgical procedures: (1) Aneurysm of right brachial artery following venepuncture; (2) arteriovenous fistula of uterine vessels one year following hysterectomy for fibroids; (3) arteriovenous shunt of facial vessels subsequent to local anesthesia for tooth extraction; (4) aneurysm of external iliac artery due to trauma of inguinal hernioplasty; (5) arteriovenous aneurysm of left radial vessels at antecubital space following incision and drainage of abscess; and (6) renal vessel arteriovenous communication subsequent to nephrectomy. **Barney Brooks** reported three aneurysms following surgical trauma: two of the femoral artery following hernioplasty, and one following amputation. **J. M. T. Finney, Jr.,** cited a personal case in which the patient died of shock and collapse on the twelfth postoperative day following cholecystectomy for acute cholecystitis. Autopsy disclosed massive retroperitoneal hemorrhage due to rupture of a traumatic aneurysm of the right renal artery. This was unquestionably due to the force of a Deaver retractor traumatizing the vessel against the body of a lumbar vertebra. Finney warned against the use of such sharp-edged retractors. **Deryl Hart** told of a patient who had profuse gastrointestinal hemorrhages following a cholecystectomy in which deep sutures were taken in the liver bed to control bleeding. Operation revealed profuse bleeding from a false aneurysm, which had ruptured into the common duct. Bleeding was so brisk from an opening in the liver that control was difficult; it was, however, accomplished by packing the opening with muscle and suturing. Unfortunately, the patient left the hospital against advice and died at home of massive intraperitoneal hemorrhage. **J. E. J. King** cited a most interesting case depicting the danger of ligation of vessels with large suture such as umbilical tape. This patient presented a large arteriosclerotic aneurysm of the abdominal aorta. Bilateral lumbar sympathectomy caused the aneurysm to decrease to approximately one-half its original size. The sac was subsequently encased with cuffs of fascia lata and the aorta ligated proximally with umbilical tape. Death ensued at a later date from massive gastrointestinal hemorrhage. Post-mortem examination showed that the umbilical tape had eroded into the duodenum with resultant bleeding.

Arterial Aneurysm of the Left Common Iliac Artery Secondary to Arteriovenous Fistula of Left Popliteal Vessels, J. M. Donald, Birmingham.—A case report of a 61-year-old Negro man who had been shot through the left knee forty-three years previously was given. Large varicosities of the left lower extremity had been present for thirty-eight years. Examination revealed a pulsating mass with a continuous thrill over the left popliteal space; the left iliac artery was fusiformly dilated and presented as a pulsating mass with a systolic bruit. Treatment consisted of ligation and excision of the popliteal arteriovenous shunt. Six months later there had been a regression of the iliac aneurysm to approximately one-third its original size. In reviewing the literature, Donald was able to find nine similar cases in which an aneurysm of the proximal artery was associated with an arteriovenous fistula. In discussion, **Barney Brooks** pointed out the uncertainty of diagnosing a proximal aneurysm in such cases, as there is always tortuosity and dilatation of the artery in arteriovenous shunts.

Surgical Aspects in the Treatment of Aneurysms of the Aorta, Arthur H. Blakemore, New York.—An analysis of sixty-three cases of aneurysm of the aorta which had been treated surgically was given. There were twelve hospital deaths in this series, or a mortality of 19 per cent. Seventeen, or 27 per cent are now living; fifteen of these seventeen are carrying on normal activities. Treatment consisted of surgical exposure of the aneurysm with ''controlled'' stimulation of blood clotting by an electrothermic method, utilizing a 10 cm. segment of wire introduced into the aneurysm for ten seconds. Following production of the clot, impure polythene film was wrapped about the sac to produce chemical inflammation and fibrosis. A layer of pure, nonirritating polythene was used to overlay the first layer of polythene and limit the chemical inflammation. Blakemore found the electrothermic method of coagulation successful if the diameter of the orifice of the aneurysm was not greater than the diameter of the sac. The method has been sufficiently standardized so that there is little technical difficulty; most of the hospital deaths were due to the severity of the disease and not to the surgical treatment per se. This method should be more extensively studied as it holds promise of avoiding death from rupture of aneurysms and affords dramatic relief of pain with rehabilitation in some cases. **E. F. Parker** cited a personal case in which a ruptured aneurysm of the thoracic aorta was treated by proximal ligation. The patient survived two weeks without evidence of urinary suppression, but died of subsequent rupture with hemorrhage. **James Owings** has treated seven patients by the Blakemore method; there were excellent results in two. **A. O. Whipple** praised Blakemore for his untiring efforts in combating a heretofore hopelessly progressive disease.

Endometriosis, Joe V. Meigs, Boston.—The increased incidence of endometriosis seems directly related to late and infrequent childbearing. The disease is much less frequently seen in ward than in private cases. Meigs condemned the fact that our economic system is favoring late marriage and deferred pregnancy. Endometriosis is most commonly encountered in the age group from 30 to 50 years. The importance of acquired dysmenorrhea as a diagnostic point has been overemphasized, for in 32 per cent the pain was not dysmenorrheic. Infertility is important in the differential diagnosis of pelvic conditions, because it is so frequently associated with endometriosis. Meigs was emphatic in condemning oophorectomy as the treatment of choice. Although castration will cause regression and disappearance of endometrial implants, such patients are often more miserable as castrates than they were with the original disease. Oophorectomy should be reserved for those 45 years of age or older. Chocolate cysts of ovaries should be carefully shelled out. Bowel implants should be resected and not treated by castration. Testosterone has proved its value in selected cases.

In the discussion, all concerned heartily agreed in advocating conservatism in the treatment of endometriosis. Every attempt to salvage ovarian function must be made. **Curtis Tyrone** found endometriosis in 23 per cent of his private patients who had a pelvic laparotomy. **Walter Holmes** suggested observation when a diagnosis of endometriosis is made. Many of the associated symptoms will abate spontaneously. If surgery becomes necessary, hysterectomy with conservation of some ovarian tissue will frequently be the procedure of choice. Holmes agreed that bilateral oophorectomy was worse than the disease. **John Burch** stated that endometriosis is not such a progressive disease as is commonly believed. Observation has proved successful in most instances. The disease is characterized by a relatively low malignant potential. Burch contended that opening of endometrial cysts is all that is necessary in some cases. **Roger Doughty** rose to support further the conservative therapy in this disease.

Treatment of Acute Pancreatitis With Report of Cases, Mims Gage, New Orleans.—The etiologic factor in acute pancreatitis is reflux of bile into the pancreatic duct. This reflux is due to calculi in only 4 per cent of cases; spasm is much more likely to be the cause.

Rienhoff and Pickrell have shown a common ductal channel of the common and pancreatic ducts in 32 per cent of dissections. Gage showed a series of cholangiograms in which a reflux of lipiodal into the duct of Wirsung was evident. Severe acute pancreatitis may be associated with tetany; this is the result of hypocalcemia due to neutralization of the fatty acids in the areas of fat necrosis with calcium. The pain is of such severity that the diagnosis should be immediately considered. Confirmation with serum amylase studies is essential for diagnosis. Conservative treatment has proved to be the one of choice. In addition to the usual measures, such as transfusions, infusions, parenteral calcium, duodenal drainage, and sedation, Gage strongly advocated bilateral splanchnic block. This block not only dramatically relieves the excruciating pain, but seems to abort the pathologic process by overcoming the spasm of the blood vessels, common duct, and sphincter of Oddi. Six cases with no mortality in which the course of the disease was shortened and made less severe were cited. Approximately 65 per cent of the patients with acute pancreatitis have associated gall bladder disease and will require interval surgery.

Keith Grimson pointed out that splanchnic block interrupts visceral pathways to relieve pain, and warned against overlooking ruptured ulcer or acute cholecystitis. Certainty of diagnosis would be necessary before producing splanchnic anesthesia. **W. D. Gatch** stated that cessation of pain in acute pancreatitis is an ominous sign. **Alton Ochsner** stressed the importance of serum amylase determinations in the diagnosis. He is convinced that splanchnic block does much more than relieve pain; it halts the progress of the disease by overcoming the ductal and vascular spasm.

The Clinical Evaluation of Cholangiograms, Hart Hagan and **H. L. Townsend,** Louisville.—The need for more frequent cholangiography was stressed. Delayed cholangiograms should be routine procedure in all cases with T-tube or catheter drainage and fistulas. The value of immediate cholangiography has not been appreciated fully because its use has been restricted. That cholangiograms at the time of initial surgery are a valuable adjunct to the diagnosis of abnormalities of the biliary system, including stone, spasm, and strictures, is stressed. Employing immediate visualization will frequently broaden the scope of the primary operative procedure and thereby lessen the frequency of secondary operations. As there is no predicting when it will be needed most, it is urged that a casette and plate be properly placed as a routine procedure in biliary surgery. Excellent cholangiographic studies depicting the pathology frequently encountered were presented.

Acute Cholecystitis, J. W. Barksdale and J. Harvey Johnston, Jr., Jackson, Miss.—The importance of regarding acute obstructive cholecystitis as a surgical emergency was emphasized. Although a six- to eight-hour period of preoperative preparation is essential to restore electrolyte and fluid balance, surgery is then indicated. Most authorities agree that it is often impossible to determine the underlying pathology by laboratory-clinical methods; too often the disease advances to the stage of gangrene, empyema, and peritonitis with so-called conservative therapy. Barksdale and Johnston believe ''watchful waiting'' in reality to be ''wishful waiting.'' It is somewhat of a paradox that a policy of diligent observation is universally accepted as being an unsound one in acute appendicitis, but is all too frequently employed in acute cholecystitis. Instituting operative therapy before the period of complication (gangrene, empyema, and perforation) would obviously decrease the mortality and morbidity of the disease. Cholecystectomy is feasible in above 90 per cent of cases and is the procedure of choice in trained hands. Cholecystostomy should be reserved for those in whom the general condition is precarious or the local pathology so marked that identification of vital structures is not feasible. By questionnaire, it was determined that 67 per cent of the members of the Southern Surgical Association favored early operation in acute cholecystitis, 25 per cent preferred delayed surgical intervention, and 8 per cent utilized careful individualization to decide therapy.

W. H. Parsons regretted that so many of the patients he treated were first seen with advanced cholecystitis—usually ninety-six or more hours after onset of the disease. Any form of therapy at this time has its drawbacks, making meticulous individualization of cases essential. Stress was laid to the frequency of common duct stones in association with acute cholecystitis; **Parsons** has found a 50 per cent incidence of choledocholithiasis in his more recent acute cases. **J. Harvey Johnston** presented a series of 140 cases in which early operation (effected within the first seventy-two hours after the onset of symptoms) had proved to be much safer than conservative treatment. However, delayed intervention was the procedure of choice if at all possible in the period from four to eight days after the beginning of the illness.

Transverse Incisions in Lower Abdominal Surgery, John C. Burch, H. T. Lavely, Jr., and **Cloyce F. Bradley,** Nashville.—Transverse incisions of the Cherney type are especially useful in gynecologic and pelvic surgery. In the past few years, this approach has been used in over sixty cases with uniformly good results. Although the period of follow-up has been too brief, the authors have noted no wound weakness or hernias in their personal cases. Transverse incisions do require more operative time for execution; some difficulty in resuturing the rectus muscles to the pubis is not infrequently encountered. Burch believes these disadvantages are minor considerations when one considers the excellent exposure obtained for all pelvic surgery. He has found this incision to make Wertheim procedures technically much more feasible. **Joe V. Meigs** did not share this enthusiasm for transverse incisions. In a personal series of 150 cases he found the incidence of hernias to be too high. He favors a midline incision for radical pelvic surgery and questions better exposure with transverse incision.

Traumatic Wet Lung. An Experimental Study, Rollin A. Daniel, Jr., and **William R. Cate, Jr.,** Nashville.—The etiology of wet lung secondary to trauma and surgery was studied in dogs. A falling weight was used to produce controlled injury. This resulted in typical traumatic wet lung in the animals. As in human beings, fluid was found in parts of the lungs not subjected to trauma. The exact mechanism of this phenomenon is not known. These investigators found that simultaneous bleeding at the time of injury decreased the amount of fluid in the lungs. Animals, which had been subjected to previous cervical vagotomy, were given intravenous saline solution at the time of injury; nine of fifteen so studied developed a marked wet lung. However, if both a cervical sympathectomy and vagotomy had been done, controlled trauma and intravenous saline solution resulted in appreciable moisture in only one of seven. Daniel and Cate thus concluded that a reflex mechanism exists which plays a part in the pathogenesis of wet lung. In discussion, **J. M. Mason, III,** stressed the value of intercostal nerve block, bronchoscopy, and endotracheal catheter aspirations in the treatment of post-traumatic wet lung.

Paralysis of the Face Supported With Facial Grafts, Barrett Brown and **Frank McDowell,** St. Louis.—Demonstration by color movies showed the dramatic cosmetic results obtainable by support of paralyzed faces with fascial grafts. It was emphasized that this operative procedure was not to be considered as a competitor to the various nerve operations for the relief of facial paralysis. It is frequently a valuable adjunct to such procedures, but is especially indicated when they have failed or are not indicated. The technique of passing strips of fascia lata, obtained from the patient's thigh with a Masson fascia stripper, from the temporalis muscle and fascia to the upper and lower lips was well depicted in the movies. Only a small incision over the temporalis muscle is necessary to effect the procedure; the fascial strips are then passed subcutaneously to the upper and lower lips with long straight needles. The elevation of the face given by this fascial support overcomes much of the facial asymmetry and aids in closing the eyelids. A most important phase of the ultimate result is teaching the patient to use the facial muscles less. In discussion, **Louis T. Byars** stressed the importance of overcorrecting the deformity; he stated that he had never seen a patient in which the fascial strips had been too tight.

Preservation of Jaw Function Following Surgery, Trauma, and Infection, Louis T. Byars, St. Louis.—Many fundamentals of maxillofacial surgery aiding in attaining maximum jaw function were emphasized with case reports. More frequent use of subperiosteal resection with temporary wire splinting was urged for benign tumors. This uniformly gave excellent cosmetic and functional results, but is not applicable to malignant tumors. The importance of fixation of mandibular fragments following loss of substance to avoid contracture was stressed. This may be often accomplished with interdental wiring, but occasionally must be effected with internal bar fixation. In the operative treatment of temporomandibular ankylosis, adequate resection of bone to create a permanent false joint is necessary. **T. G. Blocker** presented several personal cases in which striking results had been obtained following extensive loss of mandible and overlying soft tissues as a result of gunshot injuries.

Prolapse of the Gastric Mucosa Through the Pylorus, Ira A. Ferguson, Atlanta.—Although prolapse of the gastric mucosa into the duodenum was formerly considered unusual, it is now found with increasing frequency as it is being looked for. In a series of 297 gastrointestinal series at the Henry Grady Hospital in Atlanta, 23 cases of herniation of the gastric mucosa through the pylorus were found, an incidence of 7.7 per cent. Six personal case histories, five of them of men, were reported. The symptomatology is not unlike that of peptic ulcer or any condition which produces pylorospasm. Diagnosis depends on careful x-ray interpretation; usually a characteristic mushroom deformity in the duodenal bulb with a "central streak" can be demonstrated. Occasionally the symptoms are so marked and refractory to conservative measures that surgery becomes necessary. Probably any procedure which resects the redundant mucosa and/or allows free passage to and from the duodenum would be successful. One of Ferguson's patients was treated surgically with resection of the mucosa and a Finney pyloroplasty; freedom of symptoms was obtained. The importance of considering this not infrequent entity in differential diagnosis of abdominal symptomatology was emphasized. One of the patients reported upon had had an appendectomy and subsequent cholecystectomy without relief before the diagnosis was established.

Mesenteric Vascular Occlusion With Special Reference to Venous Mesenteric Thrombosis Due to Causes Other Than Local Trauma and Infection, J. D. Rives, L. H. Strug, and **Irving Essrig,** New Orleans.—A series of nineteen cases of mesenteric vascular occlusion was presented. In thirteen, thrombosis was the cause of vascular occlusion; in six, embolism. The disease is a rapidly progressive one and passes through three stages: (1) period of intestinal cramps with associated hyperperistalsis, (2) period of intestinal obstruction, and (3) gangrene. The onset may be gradual, but is quite often sudden and dramatic. The symptomatology features pain, moderate distention, and shock after the development of massive gangrene. Jaundice, which has not been previously reported, was noted in four cases of this series. Although the results are poor, surgery with resection of involved bowel represents the only chance for cure. Of the eight patients in this series submitted to surgery, only one survived; this patient had twelve feet of bowel resected. Better results would be obtained if the diagnosis were established earlier and immediate surgery undertaken. The presence of copious peritoneal fluid is characteristic of these cases. The involved bowel is usually found in the pelvis; distention proximal and distal to the area of strangulation is equal.

Lymphangioma of the Mesentery, G. V. Brindley and **G. V. Brindley, Jr.,** Temple, Texas.—Mesenteric lymphangiomas are often denoted as "chyle cysts." Although there is usually a palpable abdominal mass with associated discomfort, the exact diagnosis is often not made until exploratory celiotomy is done. Excision has proved to be the treatment of choice when feasible; marsupialization is sometimes the necessary procedure, however. A case report was presented of a 4-year-old white male with the history of having an enlarged abdomen since birth, hospitalized because of abdominal pain. Palpation disclosed an abdominal mass. Roentgenologic studies including intravenous pyelograms were not diagnostic. At operation, a cystic mass ten inches in diameter filled the abdomen. As the jejunum was intimately incorporated into the mass, bowel resection with side-to-side anastomosis was done. Postoperative convalescence was entirely smooth and the child was well when seen six months later. This multilocular lymphangioma constituted one-seventh of the boy's total weight. **C. W. Mayo** commented on marsupialization of such cysts; this may be the only feasible surgical therapy. When done, it is imperative that all cystic compartments be ruptured. Infection should be anticipated and treated prophylactically with the various antibiotics. Sclerosing solutions are occasionally of value in aiding obliteration. The mistake of removing the drains too early is frequently made. In 175 cases of mesenteric cysts encountered at the Mayo Clinic only 7 were lymphangiomas. **D. B. Cobb** presented the case report of a 3-year-old child who, at operation for intestinal obstruction, was found to have a lymphangioma of the small bowel mesentery. It was possible to remove the cyst without resecting the bowel. At a subsequent operation, a second cystic mass was excised.

Enterogenous Cysts of the Duodenum With Report of a Case, Which Is Most Unusual, If Not Unique, W. L. Peple, Richmond, Va.—A most interesting cause of duodenal obstruction was found in the case of a 69-year-old white woman. In 1924, this patient was treated for gastric ulcer, but had freedom of symptoms until digestive disturbances reappeared in the spring of 1947. X-ray studies revealed an obstructing tumor of the duodenum. At operation, an enterogenous cyst was found. This was successfully resected through an incision in the pylorus of the stomach. Review of the literature revealed this to be the fifteenth reported case of enterogenous cyst of the duodenum. This case is most unusual from the age standpoint; most of the reported cases were in infants less than 4 months of age. **Deryl Hart** presented another case of enterogenous cyst of the duodenum. His 15-year-old patient presented a palpable mass in the right upper quadrant of the abdomen. At operation, a larger, noncompressible mass which seemed to be continuous with the stomach was found. As resection was not feasible, this cyst was anastomosed to the duodenum. Although the patient has been completely free of symptoms since operation, Hart believes a Roux or Y type of jejunal anastomosis would be a better operative procedure.

Diverticulitis of the Jejunum Complicated by Jejunocolic and Jejunojejunal Fistulas: Case Report, Carrington Williams and **L. H. Bosher, Jr.,** Richmond, Va.—In a study of 350 cases of jejunal diverticulosis, 60 patients developed surgical complications. A most unusual complication was manifest in the case reported of a colored woman hospitalized because of marked weight loss and the passage of undigested food by rectum. Barium enema disclosed a free communication between the transverse colon and jejunum; this opening was not demonstrable by gastrointestinal series. At operation, numerous mesenteric and antemesenteric jejunal fistulas were found. In addition to the jejunocolic fistula shown by barium enema, eight jejunojejunal fistulas were evident. These fistulas were disconnected and the openings in the bowel closed. Six months later the patient was much improved but barium enema disclosed another fistulous communication between the jejunum and the splenic flexure. **L. H. Landry** told of a personal case involving a large tympanitic mass in the epigastrium. Roentgenologic studies disclosed a huge jejunal diverticulum with a definite fluid level. **L. W. Grove** commented on a patient seen recently who had intestinal obstruction as a result of several large diverticuli of the ileum. **J. E. J. King** operated successfully upon a patient with a similar condition in which the intestinal obstruction was due to two large jejunal diverticula.

Rationale and Results of Retropubic Prostatectomy, Ousley Grant and **Robert Lich, Jr.,** Louisville.—Prostatectomy is usually effected by one of three standard methods: (1) suprapubic, which has the disadvantage of passing through the bladder to reach a gland lying outside of the bladder; (2) perineal, which is a true surgical procedure and has the great advantage of removing the prostate gland and its capsule (it has the decided disadvantages of creating temporary urinary fistulas and not infrequent loss of sex potency); (3) transurethral, which does not permit radical removal of carcinoma. Millan of London has recently revived interest in retropubic prostatectomy. Grant believes that the fears heretofore held about the space of Retzius are unjustified. By this approach, all the advantages of perineal prostatectomy are obtained without the complications of incontinence and impotence. A series of fifty retropubic prostatectomies without mortality, without fistulas, and with no impotence was presented. Grant believes this method is so far superior to the standard procedures that comparison is incredible. In the discussion **H. W. McKay** said he finds incontinence of one week to three months a usual sequela of perineal prostatectomy. **Guy Blackburn**, of London, has observed Millan perform this operation with great dispatch on any number of occasions. If retropubic prostatectomy follows a suprapubic cystostomy, a transverse incision has proved the one of choice in his hands. **Edgar Burns** expects to add the retropubic procedure to his therapeutic armamentarium, but believes each procedure has its individual merits. Grant concluded by stating that he and Lich have given up perineal prostatectomy. Hemorrhage has been minimal in the retropubic procedure; the operation can usually be completed in forty minutes.

Unusual Intracranial Lesions Producing Large Cranial Defects, J. E. J. King, New York.—A series of unusual intracranial lesions was depicted by x-ray pictures and lantern slides. Several large epidermoid cysts had been encountered. Diagnosis was established by the characteristic scalloped border with definite white line as found on roentgenologic examination. The defects resulting from excision of these large lesions were often closed, if the dura was intact, by cleaning and boiling the removed bone and replacing it as a bone graft. No untoward results were obtained from this practice. Another interesting case with a large extradural air pocket was reported. This was found to be due to a defect in the petrous portion of the temporal bone, which allowed the entrance of air.

Anatomical Observations on the Lumbar Sympathectics With Evaluation of Sympathectomies in Organic Peripheral Vascular Disease, G. H. Yeager and **R. A. Cowley,** Baltimore.—In a series of 162 patients with peripheral vascular disease who were subjected to sympathectomy, only 30 per cent were definitely improved. Feeling that nonfamiliarity with sympathetic anatomy may be partially responsible for the failures, careful anatomic studies were done on eighteen cases. Marked extremes of variation were found: no two cases were identically similar. No sex difference was noted. The most constant ganglion was that in relation to the second lumbar vertebra; it was usually found at the lower third, often extending on the intervertebral space. These anatomic studies showed only one of eighteen to have the four ganglia on one side, as is usually depicted in anatomy textbooks. **George Lilly** finds ''sympathetic failures'' are not infrequently due to not removing the sympathetic ganglia. In reoperating upon patients to effect an adequate lumbar sympathectomy, he finds it much easier to identify the chain if a posterior approach similar to the lower part of a Smithwick procedure is used instead of the usual anterolateral approach.

The Effects of Priscol (2-Benzyl-4, 5-Imidazoline HCl) on Vascular Diseases and Hypertension in Patients, Keith S. Grimson, F. A. Marzoni, M. J. Reardon, and **J. P. Hendrix,** Durham.—Priscol is more specific in its action than is tetraethylammonium chloride; it is able to block the action of adrenalin. Side reactions are not uncommon and include flushing, palpitation, nausea, ''goose flesh,'' and occasionally postural hypotension. These are rarely serious or distressing. When administered to seventeen hypertensive patients in dosage of 100 to 200 mg., eight showed a temporary drop of blood pressure to normal, four others had some reduction, and five presented no change. The cold pressor test was decreased or abolished in ten of the seventeen patients. Priscol proved to be of no value in determining which hypertensive cases would have significant lowering of blood pressure following sympathectomy. In peripheral vascular disease, it is felt that Priscol is able to equal the effects of sympathetic blocks and is thus of value in determining suitable candidates for surgery. Four of six patients with causalgia were aided by taking the drug. The most striking therapeutic response was in Raynaud's disease. Even those patients who had previously had a sympathectomy seemed to be aided. The drug increases the tolerance to ice water in vasospastic functional disease. Priscol, in dosage of 25 to 75 mg., is apparently a valuable adjunct to the treatment of peripheral vascular disease.

The Differentiation of Hyperthyroidism, George M. Curtis, Columbus, Ohio.—Since basal metabolism determinations are not wholly specific in determining thyroid activity, studies have been conducted to determine other tests to ascertain the degree of thyroid function.

After many thousands of determinations, it is evident that the protein-bound blood iodine is directly correlated with thyroid function. As is well known, there is a tendency in some cases of nontoxic goiter to develop toxicity. If these patients have suggestive symptoms, the protein-bound blood iodine is greater than 1.2 μg per cent, and the basal metabolic rate above plus 4, Curtis believes incipient hyperthyroidism to be developing and advises operation. It is possible to differentiate hyperthyroidism from hypermetabolism by determining the protein-bound blood iodine. Thus menopause, anxiety states, multiple myeloma, etc., can be excluded. Curtis concluded by stating the determination of the protein-bound blood iodine to be of distinct value in the diagnosis of hyperthyroidism—more so than basal metabolic rate alone. However, the best way to ascertain thyroid activity is to determine the level of the protein-bound iodine in the blood and the basal metabolic rate. **Frank Lahey** stated that the Lahey Clinic results fully confirmed the value of protein-bound iodine determinations in the diagnosis of thyroid disease. The main disadvantage is that the determination is a difficult and painstaking one. A direct relationship of storm to protein-bound blood iodine exists. The test is of especial value in the diagnosis of the occasional case of hyperthyroidism associated with a normal basal metabolic rate. The status of propylthiouracil has now been clarified; it provides an excellent method of preparing patients, but is not a substitute for surgery. No matter how long the drug is given, the percentage of recurrence of hyperthyroidism is the same. The incidence of complications is 1.25 per cent as contrasted to 9 per cent for thiouracil. It is certainly not a drug to be used indiscriminately, for deaths from agranulocytosis do occur. It has eliminated trial subtotal thyroidectomy, however, for propylthiouracil will demonstrate what can be accomplished by surgery. Dosage varies from 200 to 400 mg. daily. Children and pregnant women should be given full adult doses. Psychotic and cardiac patients should be allowed to get completely well for two to three months before operation is undertaken. Radioactive iodine should be reserved for experimental studies for the time being; otherwise, its use will be abused. It produces a marked degree of thyroiditis. Because of the danger of malignancy, it should not be given to patients with adenomatous goiter. **T. C. Davison** emphasized the occurrence of hyperthyroidism without an increased basal metabolic rate. In those patients with tachycardia, palpitation, and weight loss, the results of the ''tin-box'' should be disregarded and the patient given a thorough trial with propylthiouracil. Davison considers thiouracil so dangerous that it should be outlawed as a drug. **Rawley Penick, Jr.**, stated that basal metabolic rates of -17 and lower were so frequent in the Gulf Plain section that they are considered normal. Hence, a reading of plus 10 per cent would represent a real increase in these individuals.

Hyperthyroidism in Absence of Discernible Goiter, Harold L. Foss, Danville, Pa.—The frequency of thyrotoxicosis without enlargement of the thyroid gland is emphasized. Although these patients have classical hyperthyroidism, their physicians are often misled by the normal size of the thyroid gland. Foss found 8.4 per cent of all patients admitted for thyroid overactivity to have less than 30 Gm. of tissue removed at operation. While the milder cases may be cured with propylthiouracil, surgical resection is necessary in the majority. This entity is most frequently encountered in males. **Frank Lahey** stated that the size of the thyroid is in no way related to toxicity. In men, the thyroid gland is deeper and lower than in women; thus, an actual enlargement may be difficult to demonstrate clinically. **Donald Guthrie** is in favor of abandoning the term ''exophthalmic goiter.''

Further Study of Carcinoma of the Breast in the Negro, Isidore Cohn, Alfred Longacre, and **Robert Waters**, New Orleans.—The incidence of carcinoma of the breast in the colored race has remained the same. The disease seems to appear at an earlier age in the Negro. The average duration of symptoms at the time of first examination has diminished but is still one to two years. Obviously, further education is essential to have the patients present themselves for treatment earlier. When admitted to the hospital, 62 per cent of the colored and 42 per cent of the white patients had clinical evidence of axillary metastasis. A notable increase in the use of breast biopsy has occurred in the past decade.

Cancer of the Breast, W. P. Nicholson, Jr., and **Edgar D. Grady**, Atlanta.—A series of 905 charity patients with carcinoma of the breast was presented; 417 of the group were treated surgically. Since the series ended before 1942, no hormones were used. Two of the patients were under 25 years of age. Surprisingly, the rate of five-year survivals was as good in the 20 to 30 age group as in the 30 to 60. Pain alone was the presenting symptom in 5.3 per cent. Over 25 per cent of the malignancies had existed over one year. Less than 15 per cent had come in within one month of onset of symptomatology. The five-year survival rate was 18 per cent with positive axillary metastases; 54 per cent when the axillary lymph nodes were negative. Roentgen castration of patients in the premenopausal age group seems indicated. Although the series is small, a striking difference is noted: ten of eleven so treated survived five years. Simple mammectomy was done in patients over 60 years and in the poor operative risks. Following radical mastectomy, no swelling of the arm occurred in 56 per cent; 23 per cent had slight, 14 per cent moderate, and 7 per cent severe swelling. Eighty-six per cent of the malignancies were located at the upper half of the breast. Local recurrence occurred in 16 per cent. In discussion, **T. C. Davison** emphasized the striking difference in five-year survival rates in private and clinic patients: 55 per cent in the former and 28 per cent in the latter group. Testosterone in daily dosage of 50 mg. is helpful in those patients with osseous metastases.

Bacteriostatic Agents as Adjuvants to Anal Surgery, Curtice Rosser, Dallas.—Bacteriostatic agents are valuable adjuncts to the success of anal surgery: hemorrhoidectomy, fistulectomy, and sphincteroplasty. Reliance on constipating diets gives a false sense of security. Gelfoam or oxidized cellulose, when used as a covering to rectal wounds, seems to aid healing. Sulfone (NU-404) can be given without toxic effects and decreases the coliform bacterial count of the stool. It results in no change in the healing time of rectal wounds, but probably aids in increased function following fistulectomy. **A. R. Koontz** reminded the group that fibrin is converted into fibroblasts in the healing of wounds. Thus, frequent change of gauze dressings removes valuable fibrin and delays wound healing.

Current Trends in Surgery of the Distal Colon and Rectum for Cancer, A. S. Graham, Richmond, Va.—Fifty leading colon surgeons were contacted to determine their policies in the management of malignancies of the sigmoid, rectosigmoid, and rectum. A similar study in 1938 disclosed that most surgeons favored colostomy and stage resection of lesions of rectum and rectosigmoid. There is now a pronounced trend away from extraperitoneal procedures; primary anastomosis is increasingly favored. Routine proximal drainage is unpleasant and frequently unnecessary. Of the group consulted, 84 per cent use chemotherapeutic agents routinely; 36 per cent use one of these drugs locally at operation. The trend toward anterior resection for lesions of the upper rectum and rectosigmoid is apt to be short lived: 24 per cent never use the procedure, 58 per cent rarely, and only 18 per cent routinely. The classic abdominoperineal resection for rectal and rectosigmoidal lesions is used by 82 per cent; most prefer a one-stage procedure. In the discussion, **R. S. Daniel** of Los Angeles pointed out that the incidence of local recurrence following anterior resection was 15 per cent as compared to 3.4 per cent following abdominoperineal resection.

Familial Polyposis and Carcinoma of the Colon, W. L. Estes, Jr., Bethlehem, Pa.—Case reports of a remarkable family showing the marked familial tendency of diffuse polyposis of the colon with the strong probability of development of carcinoma were given. The mother died at the age of 41 years of cancer of the sigmoid. A 38-year-old daughter presents diffuse polyposis of the transverse and descending colon. A 29-year-old son presents similar lesions in the rectum and sigmoid. Both have refused surgery thus far. Another son, 25 years of age, has had an abdominoperineal resection for carcinoma of the rectum. He is alive and well five years postoperatively, but declines surgery for the numerous remaining colon polypi. A daughter died at the age of 24 years of carcinoma of the sigmoid superimposed on familial polyposis. Another member of the family died at the age of 29 years of cancer of the sigmoid; rectal polyposis had been detected eight years earlier. A 21-year-old daughter is alive with an ileosigmoidostomy following a colon resection for polyposis. There is no familial history of malignancy on the paternal side. Estes urged surgery in all cases of familial polyposis of the colon; he believes this to be a 100 per cent premalignant condition.

Complete colon resection with permanent ileostomy is usually the procedure of choice. Occasionally it will be possible to avoid an enterostomy by salvaging the rectum. **R. B. Cattell** reported a similar family group in which four children had multiple polyposis. The entity passes from generation to generation as a mendelian dominant. Total colectomy with ileostomy should be used in all cases because recurrence in the rectum is so likely. **C. W. Mayo** pointed out that 5 per cent of patients with colon polypi had polypi elsewhere, such as stomach, small intestine, etc.

Low Anterior Resection, With and Without Transverse Colostomy, C. W. Mayo, Rochester, Minn.—A comprehensive study of 200 unselected patients who had had low anterior resection for malignancy was carried out. All growths were from 5 to 15 cm. above the dentate margin. In 100 of the patients, complementary colostomy was done; in the other 100 no proximal decompressive or defunctionating procedure was carried out. The hospital mortality for the entire series of 200 was nine deaths, or 4.5 per cent. Only 3 per cent of those with colostomy died, while 6 per cent of those without colostomy died. However, four of the deaths in the latter groups were due to pulmonary embolism; thus, the corrected mortalities are not significantly different. The morbidity, as would be expected, was much higher in the colostomy group. While 82 per cent of those without colostomy were out of the hospital in one month, only 4 per cent of those with proximal enterostomy were. Mayo believes that low anterior resection has a definite place in the treatment of malignancies of the rectosigmoid and upper rectum, since retrograde lymphatic metastases are infrequent. He warns that careful case selection is essential, and urges that one get at least 2 cm. below the lesion to minimize recurrence. In discussion, **R. S. Daniel** reported forty-four personal cases of primary aseptic anastomosis following colon resection for malignancy. There were no deaths in the series. On the other hand, there were two deaths in a group of seven colon resections of the Mikulicz type. **R. G. Doughty** stressed the not infrequent occurrence of multiple primary malignancies in the colon. He cited a personal history in which the patient had multiple carcinoma of the sigmoid. **R. B. Cattell** and the surgical staff of the Lahey Clinic favor one-stage abdominoperineal resection for malignancies of the rectum and rectosigmoid. In a series of 383 abdominoperineal resections done from 1942 to 1945, only two two-stage procedures were done. Cattell questions one's ability to determine clinically ideal cases for anterior resection; he believes abdominoperineal resection should be employed routinely. Sulfathaladine is used preoperatively. Intraperitoneal antibiotics, that is, 200,000 units of penicillin, are used only when contamination occurs. Sulfa drugs are not used locally.

The Present Status of the Problem of Gastric Cancer, R. Lee Clark, Jr., Houston.—Review of the literature reveals an increasing resectability with a decreasing mortality for gastric cancer. In 1805, resection was done in only one in 200 patients; now one in three have gastric resection. The mortality has steadily declined from 75 to 5 per cent. Every effort to establish earlier diagnosis must be instituted, for here lies the great fallacy in present-day treatment. In spite of increasing resectability and lowering operative mortality, a patient with a gastric carcinoma has only a 5 per cent chance of five-year survival. Of the few fortunate enough to have gastric resection before lymph gland metastasis has occurred, 50 per cent survive five years. Every gastric ulcer should be regarded as a malignant one and treated surgically. In discussion, **Alton Ochsner** emphasized that treatment must be instituted before the diagnosis can be made by present-day standards. Every lesion must be treated as a carcinoma. Although roentgenograms are considered 90 per cent accurate in our present concept of gastric cancer, exploratory operation should be advised in those with weight loss and stomach complaints, even though roentgenologic studies are negative. **Frank Lahey** urges more total gastrectomies in the therapy of gastric malignancy. Since follow-up is so difficult, surgery should be advised for all gastric ulcers; one in ten are malignant. **Joe Meigs** cited two recent cases in which carcinoma in situ of the stomach was diagnosed by cytologic studies of the gastric juice. It is likely that extension of such studies will result in earlier diagnosis. **G. Blackburn** reported lowering of operating time in total gastrectomy by using two teams, one thoracic and the other abdominal.

The Surgical Treatment of Peptic Ulcer; A Comparison of the Results of Gastroenterostomy, Gastric Resection and Vagotomy at the Duke Hospital, C. E. Gardner, Jr., and **Deryl Hart,** Durham. An analysis of 265 surgically treated patients with peptic ulcer is given. Gastroenterostomy was done in 68 cases; it is the procedure of choice in older patients with cicatricial ulcer and pyloric obstruction. Hospital mortality was 7.3 per cent for the group; 88 per cent were relieved of symptoms. Malfunctioning stomas were present in 19 per cent; in 3 cases, secondary operation was necessary. Subtotal gastric resection was employed in 123 cases. Over-all hospital mortality was 8.9 per cent. If the patients with massive bleeding are excluded, the rate is lowered to 6.6 per cent. Five of the 8 deaths were due to injuries to structures about the duodenal stump: 2 duodenal leaks, 2 injuries to the common duct, and 1 damaged hepatic artery. Postoperative gastric retention occurred in 14 per cent of the patients; 84 per cent were relieved of symptoms; 5 per cent presented recurrences. Pyloric exclusion procedure was used in 27 per cent. Vagotomy was done in 77 patients and 80 per cent were improved; 36 per cent presented postoperative gastric retention; one-third of these (14 per cent of the total) required a secondary operation. Eight per cent complained of persistent intestinal cramps and diarrhea following vagotomy. The only death in the group resulted from rupture of a hugely distended stomach. As a result of their critical analysis, Gardner and Hart concluded: (1) none of the operations employed for the therapy of peptic ulcer give uniformly satisfactory results; (2) gastroenterostomy is applicable in only a few cases, but is the procedure of choice in elderly patients with cicatricial stenosis; (3) gastric resection remains the procedure of choice at this time; (4) vagotomy is contraindicated in the presence of hemorrhage, gastric ulcer, and pyloric obstruction. The status of vagotomy in association with gastroenterostomy or pyloroplasty is being determined. The greatest indication at present for vagotomy is marginal ulcer.

In discussion, **L. W. Grove** presented a personal series of 150 gastric resections with only one death, a mortality of 0.66 per cent. Three-fourths were of the Hofmeister antecolic type. **F. W. Bancroft** remarked that vagotomy is usually a first step operation for peptic ulcer. **Hart** emphasized that vagotomy can paralyze the stomach and thus it disturbs the stomach as much as resection. He believes vagotomy should be restricted to experimental projects until its indications and dangers are determined.

Surgical Treatment of Obstructive Lesions of the Esophagus, James M. Mason, III, Birmingham.—Brief case reports with illustrative roentgen studies of the usual obstructive lesions of the esophagus were given. Transabdominal esophagogastrostomy of the Finney type was favored for esophageal achalasia. The feasibility of resecting high esophageal lesions and effecting satisfactory intrathoracic esophagastrostomy was emphasized. An excellent result was obtained in a complete lye stricture of the cervical esophagus; a plastic procedure through an approach anterior to the sternomastoid was used to re-establish continuity.

Alton Ochsner opened the discussion by stressing the two bugbears of esophageal surgery which persist despite antibiotics: (1) contracted blood volumes, so frequently encountered in malignant disease and chronic infections, must be corrected if the patient is to withstand such massive surgical procedures; (2) anastomotic strictures remain a source of postoperative concern; these may be avoided if particular attention is paid to maximum enlargement of the severed end of the esophagus. The case report of a successfully resected carcinoma of the upper thoracic esophagus in a 77-year-old colored man was presented. **Dailey** emphasized three essentials of postoperative management: (1) avoidance of administering intravenous saline solution, thereby lessening anastomotic edema; (2) not passing the Levine tube through the site of anastomosis; and (3) allowing liquids as soon as the patient reacts, for they will cause no more harm than swallowed saliva. **Edgar Davis** prefers transthoracic esophagogastrostomy for achalasia.

Preliminary Report on the Use of Tantalum Mesh in the Repair of Ventral Hernias, Amos R. Koontz, Baltimore.—Realizing the need for improvement in the results of large ventral hernias, Koontz used tantalum mesh in experimental animals to determine its clinical value. In four dogs, the rectus muscles were resected. Repair was effected by interposing tantalum mesh between the peritoneum and subcutaneous tissue. In all four animals, a secure repair with no gross or microscopic tissue reaction was obtained. The experimental results were so gratifying that he used the method in five clinical cases—all patients with large or recurrent hernias. To date, each of the five repairs has been completely successful. In each case, the usual repair was re-enforced with a layer of tantalum mesh. Follow-up roentgenograms showed some fragmentation of the mesh, but no symptoms whatsoever were associated. All dead space should be carefully obliterated; it is essential to cover the mesh with skin that has attached subcutaneous tissue. Subsequent laparotomy is feasible, for the mesh can be cut with ordinary surgical scissors. **J. M. T. Finney, Jr.**, praised Koontz for his continued endeavors in overcoming the problem of large and recurrent hernias. **W. J. Prioleau** finds alloy steel wire to be the suture of choice in hernioplasty.

Spontaneous Perineal or Para-Rectal Hernia, Thomas Harrold, Macon, Ga.—The case report of a spontaneous levator or perineal hernia in a 36-year-old white man was presented. There had been no antecedent trauma. The patient complained of intermittent painful swelling to the left of the rectum. Examination revealed a 5 by 8 cm. mass in the left ischiorectal fossa. At operation, a fibromatous mass and hernial sac were excised; the opening in the levator muscle was closed with interrupted sutures. Pathologic study of the excised mass revealed it to be a fibrous hemangioma. In a review of the literature, five of the eight cases were associated with tumors, one of which was malignant. Thus, tumors seem to play a prominent part in the etiology of pararectal hernias.

Comparison of War and Civilian Experiences in Management of Perforating Abdominal Wounds, David H. Poer, Atlanta.—The recent war standardized the treatment of perforating abdominal injuries and lowered the mortality from 50 to 19 per cent. This was effected by better appreciation of the underlying pathology and the pathogenesis of shock, an increased knowledge of protein and electrolyte balance, and the routine use of chemotherapeutic and antibiotic agents. The importance of complete diversion of the fecal stream in wounds of the colon and rectum was emphasized. While the time factor is most important prognostically, multiplicity of wounds to intra-abdominal viscera is even more important. Oglivie has aptly classified deaths within the first two hours as due to hemorrhage, within the first two days as due to shock, and within the first two weeks as due to infection. **Pat R. Imes** emphasized the use of multiple transfusions in lowering mortality. He is not in full accord with the concept of fecal diversion in colon injuries. In a series of 168 such injuries in the Mediterranean theater treated by primary suture, there was a mortality of 12 per cent, which compares favorably with results obtained by exteriorization. **Ambrose H. Storck** urged the development of protective armor against atomic energy. **G. Blackburn** agreed with Imes in primary suture of colon injuries.

Construction of a Vagina With the Use of Skin Grafts and Vitallium Mold, Walter R. Holmes, Atlanta.—Excellent anatomic and functional results were obtained in three patients with congenital absence of the vagina. By careful sharp and blunt dissection a space between the vagina and rectum was developed. A split-thickness graft everted over a suitable vitallium mold was then inserted; care was taken to suture the edge of the graft to the vestibular mucosa. Approximation of the labia mucosa aids in immobilization of the mold and graft. Attention was called to the frequent association of urinary tract anomalies with congenital absence of the vagina. Each of these three cases had such congenital anomalies.

T. G. Blocker, Jr., presented a personal series of six patients treated by this method. He utilized an acrylic mold with an enlarged cephalic end; this remained in place well. **L. R. Wharton** stated that this method of construction of an artificial vagina was so simplified that it was the procedure of choice. Dissection of a wide space is essential to gain adequate depth; skin grafts should be used in every case. Making the mold of proper form is of more importance than is the material from which the mold is made. Postoperative care should feature daily dilatation; large Pyrex test tubes function as excellent dilators.

Announcement

Medical and Surgical Supplies Desperately Needed in War-Devastated Areas

Continued aid in the form of medical and surgical supplies from America is needed to prevent widespread suffering and death among the peoples of war-devastated areas throughout the world. It is earnestly requested that all members of our profession help us provide such aid through the Medical and Surgical Relief Committee, Inc.

During the past seven years, with little publicity and modest financial support, this committee has provided more than one million dollars worth of desperately needed medical, surgical, and dental supplies and applications to stricken areas overseas. These materials are sent to hospitals, physicians, and dispensaries giving free medical care to the needy.

Our colleagues in Europe and the East are still faced with an appalling lack of basic medical equipment. Some have not even seen a medical journal or textbook printed since 1939, and are woefully uninformed of many of the latest medical advances.

We are able to do a great deal to alleviate this situation through the Medical and Surgical Relief Committee which receives, sorts, reconditions, and ships material, ranging from physicians' samples to used instruments, in response to authenticated appeals from overseas.

The items most consistently requested and most vitally needed are:

Adhesive tape
Ampules—all types
Anesthetics (local, general)
Antiseptics
Aspirin
Aspirin combinations
Autoclaves
Baby supplies
  bottles
  cereals
  clothes
  canned food
  nipples
Cod-liver oil
Cotton—gauze, all forms
Dietary supplements
Germicides
Hospital ware
Hot-water bottles and syringes
Hypo needles and syringes
Liver and iron capsules
Microscopes
Penicillin
  (crystal, ointment, tablets)
Quinine—tablets, capsules
Rubber sheeting and tubing
Santonin and combinations
Scientific apparatus
Sedatives
Standard medication for various
  conditions
Sterilizers
Streptomycin
Sulfas—tablets, liquids
Surgeon's gloves
Surgeon's needles
Surgical instruments
Thermometers (fever, F. or C.)
Vitamins—all types and strengths
  for children and adults

—and the most pressing need of all is for recent medical, surgical, and dental textbooks and journals

Please forward any such supplies which you and your hospital can donate to this great need to:

The Medical and Surgical Relief Committee, Inc.
Room 328—420 Lexington Avenue
New York 17, N. Y.

Fleet Admiral Halsey is president and Edward R. Stettinius, Jr., is chairman of the board of directors and Dr. Allen Whipple, of New York, is chairman of the medical advisory council to the Medical and Surgical Relief Committee, Inc.

SURGERY

VOL. 23 MAY, 1948 No. 5

Original Communications

TREATMENT OF SHORT STRICTURE OF THE ESOPHAGUS BY PARTIAL ESOPHAGECTOMY AND END-TO-END ESOPHAGEAL RECONSTRUCTION

ROBERT E. GROSS, M.D., BOSTON, MASS.

(From the Surgical Service of the Children's Hospital and the Department of Surgery of the Harvard Medical School)

FOR several decades the standard form of therapy for congenital or for chemical burn strictures of the esophagus has consisted of repeated esophageal dilatations, combined in some instances with a gastrostomy for purposes of feeding or for retrograde bougienage. This form of treatment has usually been satisfactory; it has been practiced in this hospital for approximately thirty years in a large number of patients without fatality. While the method produces a good end result in the majority of cases, it has drawbacks in some instances because (1) the esophageal cicatrix may be unyielding, (2) repeated dilatations over a period of years may be necessary and (3) the economic factors may be formidable when many hospitalizations are required. These three considerations indicate that a more radical form of therapy might be advantageous (for a minority group of patients) since it would presumably offer a quicker, a less troublesome, and a much less expensive relief of the patients' swallowing difficulties.

A radical attack on the problem of impermeable stricture of the esophagus has been made previously by the establishment of some form of antethoracic esophagus. Such undertakings have had great impetus from the recent work of the Russian, Yudin,[4] who reported the surgical treatment of eighty patients by stage operations which consist of division of the jejunum, bringing up the distal loop of the jejunum in front of the thoracic cage for anastomosis with the esophagus in the neck above the stricture, and re-establishment of the continuity of the upper intestinal tract by anastomosing the proximal end of the divided jejunum to the lower jejunum or the upper ileum. Yudin's mortality rates have

Received for publication, Aug. 25, 1947.

been amazingly low and the end results have been satisfactory from the standpoint of function. Yudin's method has the disadvantage of completely sidetracking the stomach, duodenum, and upper jejunum; these are thrown out of function except for their activity in producing alimentary juices. It is important to point out that most of Yudin's subjects were adults. In our clinic, attempts at similar jejunal transplantation in children (for treatment of esophageal atresia) have been troublesome, or have failed, because of the shortness of the loop which can be brought up onto the chest or because of insufficient blood supply (and sloughing) of this limb. While the method of Yudin represented a tremendous advance in surgical thinking, I believe it is already relegated to a position of purely historical interest because of the more logical and the safer procedure developed by Sweet[2] and others, which consists of subtotal esophageal resection combined with a high intrathoracic esophagogastric anastomosis. This operation employs the stomach for replacement of that portion of the esophagus which has been removed. Most of the stomach is displaced upward into the thorax so that it can be joined at a high level to the proximal end of the esophagus. Sweet has accurately described this procedure and has recorded three cases in which it was successfully performed for treatment of extensive and impermeable esophageal stricture. While his method offers excellent relief if an esophageal stricture is extensive, I believe it would be unnecessarily radical in the treatment of a resistant stricture which is limited to a short segment of the esophagus. For this latter type of case, I would like to propose an excision of the narrowed portion of the esophagus and reconstruction of the esophageal tube by end-to-end suture of its remaining portions.

A decade ago an end-to-end suture of the esophagus would have been regarded as a technical impossibility; the risks attending such anastomoses were prohibitive. However, in recent years extraordinary advances have been made in the treatment of congenital atresia of the esophagus by end-to-end suture. Holt and associates[1] have reported twenty-six cases in which there has been survival following such reconstruction in newly born babies, and at the Children's Hospital of Boston thirty patients have been successfully treated by such primary anastomoses. This experience has convinced me that the esophagus can be widely raised from its bed with impunity, that large gaps in the esophageal tube can be overcome, and that end-to-end unions heal in a satisfactory way—provided one's technique is gentle, the esophagus is not traumatized unnecessarily, and the anastomosis is accurately and meticulously performed. The success which has attended the performance of such operations in small babies, combined with the recent experimental observations of Swenson and Clatworthy,[3] has led me to the conviction that it would be technically feasible to remove a stenosed segment of esophagus and then join the remaining ends of the esophageal tube by appropriate suture. Whenever this procedure is applicable for treatment of a short stenosis of the esophagus in a child, it would seem to be preferable to the method of Sweet wherein the stomach is displaced up into the chest because the former gives a more normal anatomic reconstruction of the alimentary pathway and because it does not in any way interfere with the functions of the stomach.

The practicality of excising portions of an esophagus and joining the remaining ends by direct suture is demonstrated by the case report which is made herewith. As far as I am aware, this is the first successful resection of an intrathoracic portion of the esophagus in a human being with reconstruction of the esophageal tube. Some technical considerations of such an operative procedure can be summarized as follows:

TECHNICAL CONSIDERATIONS OF OPERATION

1. *Avenue of Approach to the Esophagus.*—There is much to be said in favor of a retropleural approach to the esophagus, without traversing the pleural cavity. This has been preferred when making a direct anastomosis of the esophagus in babies with atresia of the esophagus. It maintains a reasonable degree of expansion of the lung during the operation, it eliminates contamination of the pleural cavity during operation, it gives maximum protection of the pleural cavity if there should be any postoperative leakage from the esophageal suture line, and it provides a direct route for external drainage if suppuration or esophageal leakage should occur. These considerations are all cogent reasons for using the retropleural approach in babies, where it is so important to maintain the integrity of the pulmonary system. In older subjects, such as those being explored for strictures of the esophagus, the more direct route to the esophagus by the transpleural approach seems to be preferable because it gives a wider exposure and because the mediastinal pleura will now be thick enough to permit its careful closure at the end of the operation for reconstruction of a partition between the mediastinum and pleural cavity.

2. *Side of Chest for Operative Approach.*—The esophagus can be approached satisfactorily by either the right or the left transpleural route, but mobilizing it from its bed (particularly beneath the aortic arch and at the thoracic apex) is accomplished much more easily from the right side. However, an exposure through the right side will not permit the stomach to be brought up into the chest if a longer segment of esophagus than anticipated has to be resected and the fundus of the stomach has to be employed for re-establishment of the alimentary tract continuity. If, before operation, it appears that the esophageal stenosis is short and an esophageal reconstruction can surely be effected (as in the case here reported), the operation is greatly facilitated by making the chest incision in the right side. But if before operation it is difficult to predict whether removal of an esophageal segment will allow esophageal reanastomosis—or whether a more formidable gastric mobilization and esophagogastric anastomosis will be required—then it is distinctly preferable to approach the esophagus via the left transpleural route.

3. *Chest Incision.*—A wide variety of chest incisions has been employed for gaining access to the esophagus, and indeed it is well to avoid rigid standardization, to allow for variation in the level of esophageal lesion which is being exposed. In the case herein reported a long intercostal incision running the entire length of the sixth interspace, with severance of the sixth and fifth costal cartilages, gave an entirely adequate view. In older subjects where the costal cage is less yielding, it might be necessary to divide several ribs posteriorly to provide a T-shaped wound. The severance of ribs posteriorly almost

certainly increases the patient's discomfort during the early postoperative period, but this should be accepted, when necessary, rather than hamper the proper performance of an operation by inadequate exposure.

4. *Entrance to the Mediastinum.*—Since the reconstruction of a protective bulkhead between the mediastinum and the pleural cavity at the end of operation is a highly important step, great emphasis should be placed upon the preservation of the parietal pleura, which covers the esophagus. The longitudinal opening of this layer should not be made directly over the bulge of the esophagus; it is preferably made in front of the esophagus so that a broad flap of pleura can be raised and turned backward in such a way that this tissue can be utilized later for covering over the esophagus.

5. *Raising the Esophagus From Its Bed.*—The esophagus must be widely freed and elevated from its bed, a point of great importance if its ends are to be brought together without too much tension after excision of a stenosed segment. The poor vascularity of the esophagus has been commented upon by many authors, but an increasing experience with esophageal surgery indicates that the esophagus can be mobilized from the diaphragm to the apex of the chest and still have sufficient blood supply to be viable. Of course, as much blood supply as possible should be saved, but there need be no hesitation about freeing the entire intrathoracic portion of the esophagus if this is essential for the resection and reconstruction which is being contemplated.

An esophagus is in some ways a very delicate structure and every effort should be made to avoid traumatizing it. Any part to be saved should not be grasped with forceps, hemostats, clamps, or other metallic instruments. By sharp and blunt dissection a tunnel can be made around the esophagus, and a linen tape can be drawn through this opening. Such traction tapes aid greatly in the further dissection of the esophagus from its bed.

Branches of the vagus nerve should be freed and protected, though this may be difficult if there are inflammatory changes in the periesophageal tissues. Posterior to the esophagus, the dissection should be kept as close as possible to the esophagus so that the thoracic duct can be left undisturbed.

6. *Identification of the Stenosed Portion of Esophagus.*—Inspection of the exterior of the esophagus may give little evidence of the exact site where the lumen is narrowed. To locate accurately the area of stenosis, a large, rather stiff catheter can be inserted through the mouth by the anesthetist and pushed down the esophagus until it meets the obstruction, at which point it can be palpated through the esophageal wall by the surgeon. Withdrawal of the catheter and severance of the esophagus will insure saving as much normal substance as possible. Probing of the lower segment under direct vision will locate the lower end of the stenotic portion and will indicate where the second transection of the esophagus should be made.

7. *Esophageal Anastomosis.*—The repair should be in two layers, interrupted stitches being used and fine, permanent, suture material, for which 00000 Deknatel silk serves admirably (in children). The outer layer includes muscularis and submucosa. The inner layer includes only the mucosa, the

stitches being so placed that the knots present in the lumen. A point of a great importance is the placement and tying of the sutures in the posterior surface of the muscularis. It is almost impossible to snug up and tie each stitch as it is placed, because this places great stress on each of the early stitches and they will tear out of the eophageal wall. Instead, it is better to place *all* of the posterior stitches and then draw them up simultaneously; this distributes the pull through all of the stitches, permits the ends of the esophagus to be drawn together, and then the individual sutures can be tied. Stitches in the outer and inner layers should be placed only 2 or 3 mm. apart.

While "closed" anastomoses would have some theoretical advantage, there is good reason to believe that "open" types of anastomoses in the esophagus are tolerated with a very low risk. It is hardly necessary to emphasize that serious contamination of the chest can be avoided by adequately packing off the small operative field from the remaining pleural cavity and by subsequently discarding these packs, any contaminated instruments, and the operator's gloves before proceeding with the chest closure.

After completion of the anastomosis, penicillin and streptomycin solutions can be flushed into the chest, but I rely more upon a careful operative technique which reduces soiling to a minimum than I do upon the indiscriminate dumping of chemotherapeutic agents into a chest.

While crushing of the phrenic nerve might reduce some of the tension or movement of the esophagus during the postoperative period, I have little faith in this procedure and do not believe that it is worth doing.

8. *Mediastinal Drainage.*—While it may be possible in some cases to close the mediastinum without drainage, it would seem far safer to provide some temporary opening for four or five days which allows for escape of serum or lymph. This can be accomplished by a stab wound through the back, just outside of the erector spinae muscles, leading through an intercostal space above (or below) the main chest incision and burrowing bluntly behind the parietal pleura to reach the mediastinum. A soft rubber drain can be pulled through the channel thus formed.

Of prime importance is the suture of the mediastinal pleura over the esophagus so that the mediastinal and pleural compartments will be sealed from one another. This gives the best assurance that the lung can be kept re-expanded and that the pleural cavity will probably be protected if infection or leakage should develop at the esophageal anastomosis during the postoperative period. Careful closure of the pleural sac will allow the pulmonary system to be returned immediately to its full function; at the same time provision can be made for any postoperative mediastinal suppuration by leading a mediastinal drain out through the back, as mentioned previously.

9. *Chest Closure.*—Before repair of the lateral chest wound, a rubber catheter is led out from the pleural cavity through the subjacent intercostal space. For four or five days following operation suction is constantly applied to this intrapleural catheter to keep the pleural space evacuated.

10. *Gastrostomy.*—Experience with anastomoses for atresia of the esophagus has shown that it is sometimes possible to feed in a few days through the reconstructed tube. As an alternative it is possible for an extended period of time to leave an inlying catheter which is threaded through the nose and esophagus and led into the stomach. However, it is becoming increasingly evident that it is far wiser to establish a gastrostomy routinely for feeding purposes so that the esophagus can be given the best chances for healing during the early postoperative period. Such a gastrostomy rarely needs to be kept open more than a few weeks. I believe the same general principles and precaution should be adopted for the postoperative care of patients who might be subjected to esophageal resection for esophageal stenosis. Indeed, it is almost inconceivable that patients in this latter category would be subjected to esophagectomy unless a gastrostomy had been previously established for purposes of improving the general nutrition.

CASE HISTORY

D. S., an 11-month-old boy, was admitted to the hospital Jan. 23, 1947, because of intermittent vomiting since birth. This had become much more severe in the past six weeks; during this interval the child could not retain any solid food and lost seven pounds. Immediately prior to hospital entry he had been studied in another institution for ten days where barium studies showed evidence of esophageal obstruction. For about ten days there had been a moist nonproductive cough.

On physical examination the child had some evidence of weight loss, but was fairly well hydrated. Weight was 19 pounds, 4 ounces. The respirations were rapid and auscultation disclosed numerous, moist, coarse râles throughout both lung fields.

A roentgenogram of the chest showed slight accentuation of the lung markings at the right base but no definite evidence of infiltration. Visualization with a barium swallow showed marked dilatation of the proximal half of the esophagus and an unusual congenital malformation with marked stenosis of the middle portion of the esophagus and a posterior, narrow communication between the dilated upper end of the esophagus and the smaller lower half of the esophagus (Fig. 1). There was considerable obstruction to the passage of thin barium through the esophagus.

Course.—Because of the progressive recent weight loss and inability to swallow a sufficient amount of milk to maintain adequate nourishment, a gastrostomy of a Stamm type was established on Feb. 3, 1947.

On Feb. 18, 1947, under general anesthesia an esophagoscope was passed from above to visualize the narrowed portion of the esophagus. On the posterior wall of the esophagus, just above its blind end, a tiny opening could be seen. Attempts were made to feed a ureteral catheter down through this opening in the hope that it could be threaded into the lower esophageal segment and fished out through the gastrostomy. It was our intention to pull a string through the narrowed area which would be employed as a guide for subsequent dilatations. The catheter would go through the tiny opening for only a short distance and then it constantly met some obstruction so that it could not be pushed downward. The gastrostomy tube was now removed and a small scope was introduced through this opening and led up into the lower end of the esophagus in an effort to pass a ureteral catheter (followed by a string) in a retrograde way through the tiny esophageal opening. A small opening, about 3 mm. in diameter could be viewed; the scope could not be passed through it, and a ureteral catheter could be pushed through it for only about 1 cm., at which point it constantly met some obstruction. It seemed unwise to continue the probing and efforts at placement of an inlying string. While it is possible that subsequent attempts might have been successful in placement of a string over which dilators could have been passed, the off-set alignment of the two esophageal segments was largely responsible for the decision to abandon conservative methods and to attempt resection of the involved portion of esophagus as soon as the general condition of the child could be built up to withstand such an undertaking. The child was discharged from the hospital on March 2, 1947, having gained to 22 pounds with the gastrostomy feedings.

On June 3, 1947, the patient was brought back to the hospital for surgical treatment of the esophageal defect. There was no evidence of respiratory infection. The general physical condition was excellent, there having been a striking gain in weight to 28 pounds, 3 ounces.

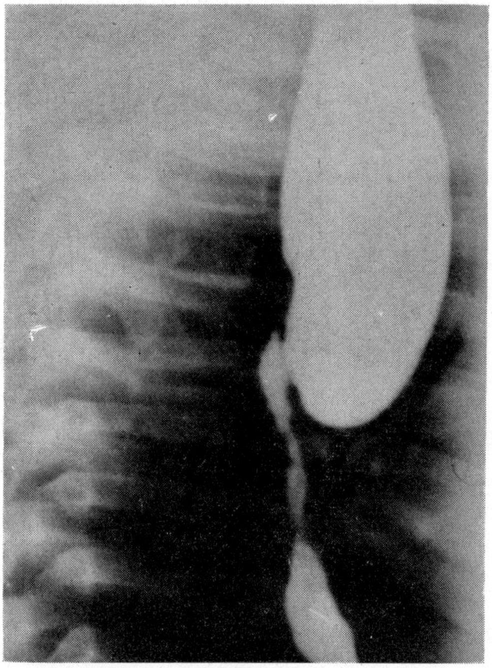

Fig. 1.—Preoperative roentgenogram of esophagus showing the stricture and the offset alignment of the upper and lower esophageal lumina.

Operation.—Exploration was undertaken June 6, 1947, under cyclopropane anesthesia, using a right transpleural approach, with a long incision in the sixth intercostal space, dividing the sixth and fifth costal cartilages. The mediastinal pleura was opened just behind the lung root, this incision being made from just above the diaphragm up to the apex of the chest, turning back a flap of pleura which had covered the esophagus. The azygos vein was doubly ligated and divided. The esophagus was exposed and was raised from its bed by sharp and blunt dissection from the second vertebral body to the diaphragm. The muscularis of the esophageal tube was a continuous layer, there being very little evidence externally of any internal derangement, in fact, it was impossible to determine accurately the level of the intrinsic obstruction. The anesthetist passed a stiff rubber catheter through the mouth and pushed it down into the esophagus to the point of obstruction, so that external palpation of the esophagus readily determined the point of blockage. A segment of esophagus 3 cm. in length was excised. The remaining ends of the esophagus were anastomosed by the technique indicated in Figs. 2 and 3. About twenty-four stitches were employed for the outer layer and a similar number for the inner layer of the anastomosis. The ends of the esophagus appeared to have an adequate blood supply. Mediastinal drainage was provided by a stab wound through the back; by blunt dissection a tract was made in behind the pleura to reach the mediastinum; through this tunnel a soft rubber wick was drawn into place. The pleural

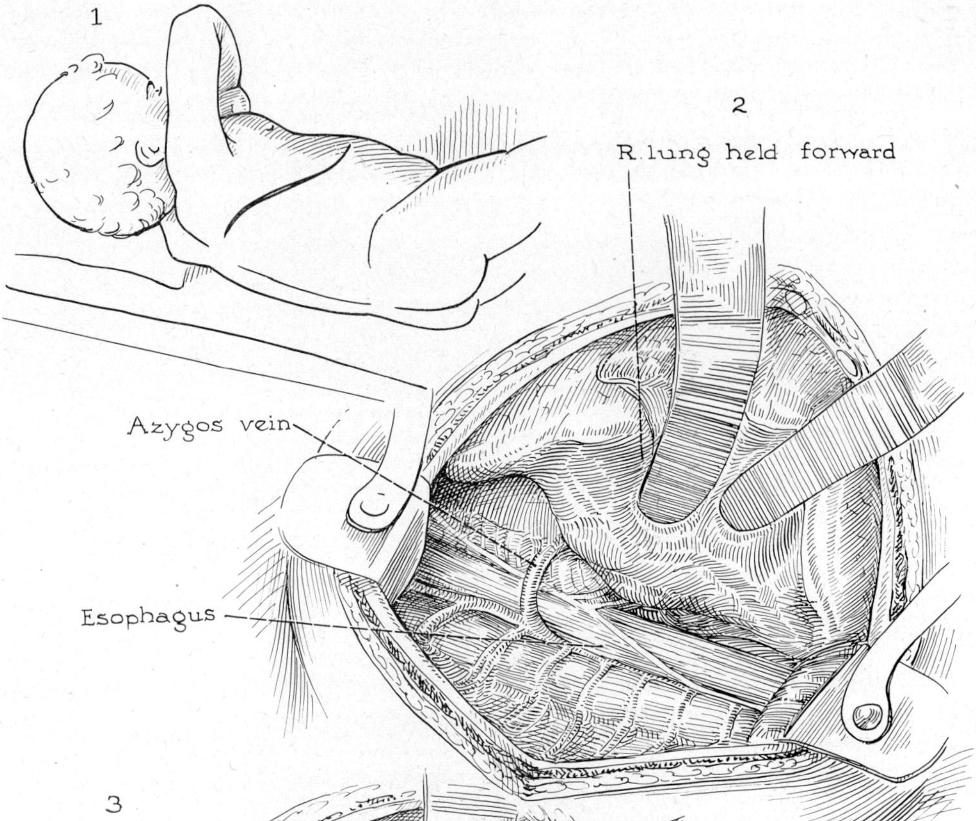

Fig. 2.—Operative procedure for partial esophagectomy. *1*, Position of thoracic wound; *2*, exposure through sixth interspace, and transpleural approach to the mediastinum; *3*, flap of mediastinal pleura reflected to expose the esophagus.

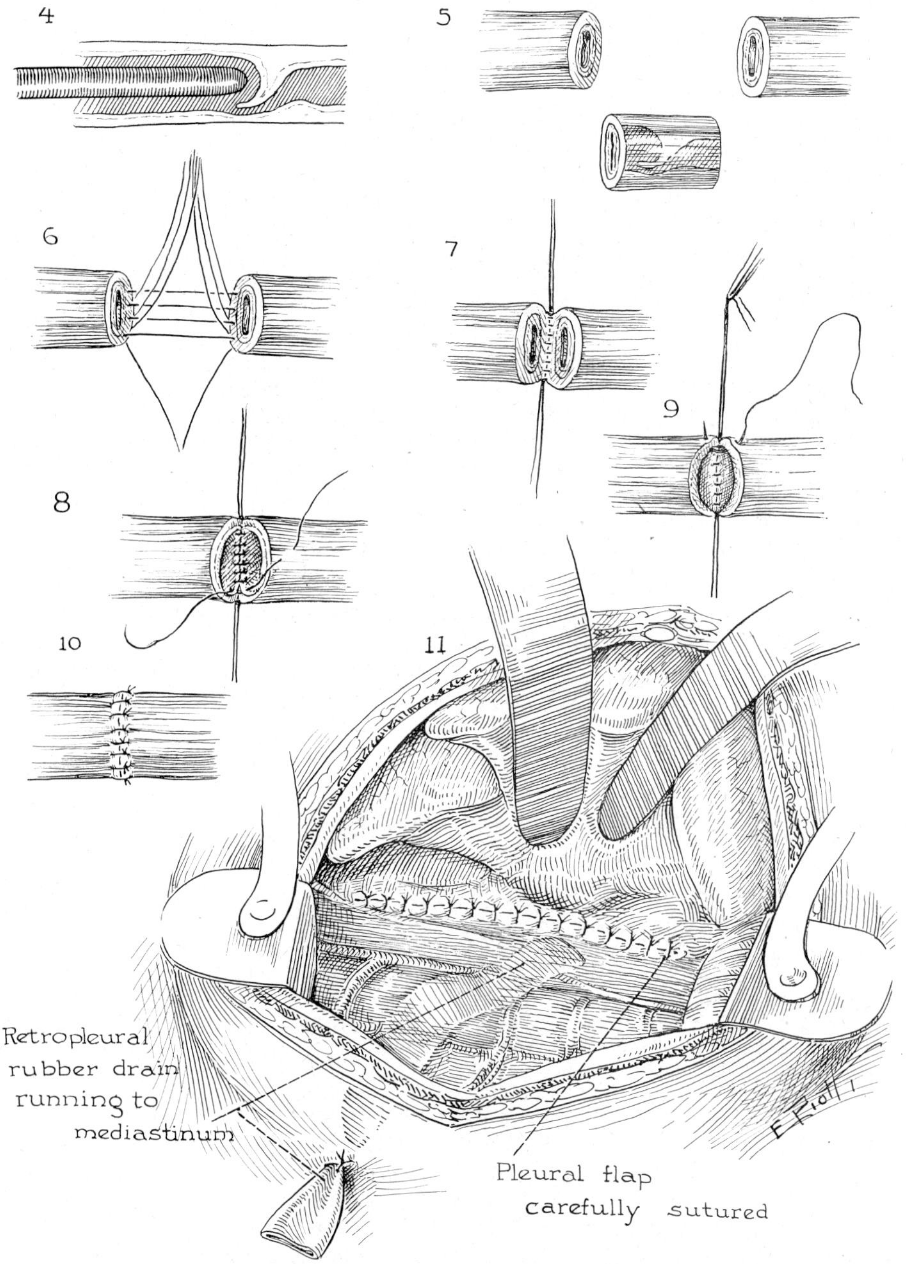

Fig. 3.—Operative procedure, continued. *4*, Large catheter passed down esophagus to identify point of obstruction; *5*, stenosed segment excised; *6*, placement of posterior row of interrupted silk sutures through muscularis and submucosa (actually, about a dozen sutures were used in this posterior row); *7*, posterior stitches drawn up and tied; *8*, mucosa being closed with interrupted fine silk sutures; *9*, mucosa entirely closed, external row of sutures being completed anteriorly in the muscularis-submucosal tissues; *10*, anastomosis completed; *11*, extrapleural drain led from back into mediastinum. Pleural covering of mediastinum closed tightly.

covering of the mediastinum was very carefully closed so that any accumulation of fluid within the mediastinum would be effectively barred from entrance into the pleural cavity. A catheter was led from the pleural cavity out through the lateral chest wall for subsequent aspiration of the pleural space.

Postoperative Course.—Suction was constantly applied to the intrapleural catheter for five days, at the end of which time the catheter was withdrawn. The posterior, soft rubber drain which led into the mediastinum by the retropleural route was withdrawn on the sixth day. There had been a slight discharge of thin serosanguineous fluid from this latter hole which ceased two days after removal of the rubber drain. The temperature reached a level of 102.4° F. on the first postoperative day and subsided to 100° F. by the fourth day. For the succeeding ten days there was a slight elevation of temperature but not above 100° F. at any time. The child had an extremely satisfactory postoperative course. Milk and other nourishing fluids were given through the gastrostomy tube during the early postoperative period. Penicillin was given by parenteral routes and sulfadiazine was given by gastrostomy for eleven days following operation. On the tenth postoperative day the child was allowed small amounts of water by mouth, which he took without the slightest hesitation. On the twelfth postoperative day sips of milk were offered and were swallowed without difficulty. On the fourteen day puréed vegetables were offered and were taken eagerly. On the sixteenth day all gastrostomy feedings were stopped and all milk was given by mouth. On this day soft solid foods were also offered and taken fairly well. The child was discharged home on the twentieth postoperative day; the gastrostomy tube was withdrawn and the opening allowed to close in six weeks. When last seen on Aug. 1, 1947, the weight was 30 pounds, deglutition was excellent, and the baby was swallowing a diet normal for his age without difficulty.

SUMMARY

Most strictures of the esophagus, whether of congenital origin or secondary to chemical burns, can be effectively treated by repeated dilatations. In certain instances intractable strictures which are extensive can be treated by the method of Sweet, wherein the diseased portion of esophagus is removed and the stomach is brought up to bridge the gap thus made. When a stenosis involves a short segment, and is not readily treated by the usual methods of dilatation, partial esophageal resection with end-to-end reconstruction is a feasible operation as is indicated by the case here reported.

REFERENCES

1. Holt, J. F., Haight, C., and Hodges, F. J.: Congenital Atresia of the Esophagus and Tracheo-Esophageal Fistula, Radiology **47:** 457, 1946.
2. Sweet, R. H.: Subtotal Esophagectomy With High Intrathoracic Esophagogastric Anastomosis in the Treatment of Extensive Cicatricial Obliteration of the Esophagus, Surg., Gynec. & Obst. **83:** 417, 1946.
3. Swenson, O. S., and Clatworthy, W.: Partial Esophagectomy With End-to-End Anastomosis in the Posterior Mediastinum. An Experimental Study. (To be published.)
4. Yudin, S. S.: The Surgical Construction of 80 Cases of Artificial Esophagus, Surg., Gynec. & Obst. **78:** 561, 1944.

LEIOMYOMA OF THE ESOPHAGUS AND CARDIA OF THE STOMACH

ROGER A. KENWORTHY, M.D., AND C. STUART WELCH, M.D., BOSTON, MASS.

(From the Department of Surgery, Tufts College Medical School, the Boston Dispensary and the Carney Hospital)

LEIOMYOMA involving both the esophagus and the cardia of the stomach is exceedingly uncommon. In a search of literature we were able to find only four cases of leiomyoma in this location. It is the purpose of this communication to report a fifth instance of leiomyoma in this location and to review the diagnosis, treatment, and reported data on these tumors. Particular attention will be given to the diagnosis of benign esophageal tumors, which, in the course of time, will undoubtedly be found and removed more frequently now that resection of the esophagus has found so sure a footing in the transthoracic resection with intrathoracic esophagogastric anastomosis.

Leiomyoma of the esophagus alone is likewise a rare disease. The clinical manifestations and symptoms of these tumors are mild or absent until great size has been attained. They are of particular interest to the surgeon because of the surgical procedures involved in their successful removal. More importantly, they are readily curable by operation and should be differentiated by clinical diagnosis from carcinoma of the esophagus and carcinoma of the stomach involving the esophagus. Leiomyomas may become leiomyosarcomas and, while the latter are usually found without metastasis, there are instances of more malignant types reported. In any event the questionable nature of some esophageal tumors may demand operative interference for diagnosis even if symptoms are minimal.

Leiomyoma of the stomach is generally considered to be a relatively rare lesion. However, Meissner,[1] in order to determine the incidence of leiomyoma of the stomach, carefully studied grossly and microscopically the organs obtained from fifty necropsies and found gastric leiomyomas in 46 per cent of these fifty individuals. The ages of the patients varied from 19 to 82 years, the majority being over 50 years. These studies indicate that leiomyoma of the stomach is a relatively common lesion. However, those tumors which give rise to symptoms remain relatively uncommon. The most alarming symptom of gastric leiomyoma is massive hemorrhage which results from ulceration of the overlying mucosa and erosion of the tumor. Gastric leiomyomas and benign gastric tumors are observed sufficiently often that preoperative diagnosis by roentgenologic examination is frequently made. The fact that operations on the stomach are a matter of almost daily occurrence in most hospitals has provided a great deal of information about gastric leiomyomas that has received careful correlation with clinical findings.

When leiomyomas involve both the stomach and the esophagus, diagnosis may be very difficult before operation. It is possible that erosion of the gastric portion of the tumor may result in massive gastric hemorrhage or chronic anemia; on the other hand the symptoms of esophageal obstruction may predominate.

Received for publication, June 27, 1947.

BENIGN ESOPHAGEAL TUMORS

The variety of benign tumors of the esophagus which are sufficiently large to produce clinical symptoms has provided little experience for clinicians and roentgenologists in diagnosis. There are, however, fairly good criteria for the diagnosis of benign esophageal tumors which can often make possible an accurate preoperative diagnosis.

Vinson[2] in 1926 stated that among approximately 4,000 patients complaining of dysphagia examined in the Mayo Clinic, benign tumor of the esophagus was found in only 3. In 1944 Moersch and Harrington[3] found 15 benign esophageal tumors among 11,000 patients complaining of dysphagia. These authors reported further that a review of 7,459 post-mortem examinations at the Mayo Clinic revealed 44 benign tumors of the esophagus. There were 32 leiomyomas among these 44 cases of incidentally found benign tumors in patients who had no esophageal difficulty in life. Shafer and Kittle[4] stated that in 6,001 post-mortem examinations at the University of Chicago Hospitals, 11 benign esophageal tumors were found. A great variety of benign tumors of the esophagus have been reported such as polyps, lipomas, papillomas, neurofibromas, adenomas, myxofibromas, hemangiomas, osteochondromas, and leiomyomas. Most authors have found that the common type of benign tumor of the esophagus is a polyp but the experience of Moersch and Harrington places leiomyomas first in frequency. In addition, Patterson[5] in a review of benign neoplasms of the esophagus found 61 cases between the years 1717 and 1932. There were 6 myomas among these reported cases. Bryant[6] in 1905 reviewed the literature on myomas of the esophagus and collected 9 cases and reported 2 more. All of these were found at autopsy and in only 2 were the symptoms referable to the esophagus. Fogge[7] in 1874 reported a case of myoma of the esophagus in the *Transactions of the Pathological Society of London.* The lesion was found at autopsy and was the first case of its sort reported before that society. The tumor measured 2 by 1.25 by 1 inch and projected into the esophageal lumen. In spite of this there was no history of dysphagia.

Miller[8] in 1912 reviewed the literature and collected five cases of leiomyoma of the esophagus between the years 1868 and 1897. One of these cases had been reported in 1872 by Coates[9] and dysphagia was a prominent symptom in that patient.

The most common sites for leiomyoma of the esophagus are the upper and lower thirds. The distribution between these two areas is generally considered to be equal although Rose[10] found the tumor most common in the lower third.

Benign tumors of the esophagus are divided into two main groups, extramucosal and mucosal. Leiomyomas arise from the smooth muscle of the esophagus and are classified as extramucosal or intramural. The growth of these tumors is usually slow and since they are extramucosal esophageal obstruction is rarely produced until they become unusually large. The association of a diverticula and myoma of the esophagus was reported by Stewart[11] in 1931.

Coates noted the relative absence of fibrous tissue in myoma of the esophagus as compared with uterine myoma but attributed this to the normal amount of fibrous tissue found in the uterus as compared with the muscular coat of the alimentary tract. The incidence of malignant change in these tumors is not known but probably bears the same relation to malignant transformation of smooth muscle tumors located elsewhere in the body. We were unable to find any case in which malignant change definitely occurred in a pre-existing benign myoma but it is difficult in many cases to be definitely sure that the tumor with which one is dealing does not have malignant characteristics. Howard[12] in 1902 reported the first case of myosarcoma of the esophagus. The histologic examination revealed a mixed-cell sarcoma apparently derived solely from the smooth muscle tissue of the esophagus. There was associated ulceration of the esophageal mucosa and metastasis to the stomach and regional lymph nodes. Pennes[13] in 1942 was able to find only five esophageal leiomyosarcomas in a study of the literature on the subject, to which he added one of his own.

LEIOMYOMA INVOLVING BOTH THE ESOPHAGUS AND STOMACH

A thorough search of the literature revealed only four cases of leiomyoma involving both the lower end of the esophagus and the upper portion of the stomach. Two of these were found incidentally at post-mortem examination, the first of which was reported by Milovanovic[14] in 1914. The patient was a 63-year-old man who at autopsy was found to have had a perforated peptic ulcer, bronchopneumonia, and malnutrition. At the junction of the esophagus and stomach was a bean-sized myoma and two other myomas the size of peas on either side of the larger one. The largest of the three tumors was located half in the esophagus and half in the cardia of the stomach. The microscopic report of the largest tumor confirmed its position. The very middle of the tumor corresponded with the transition between the mucous membrane of the esophagus and the mucosa of the stomach. The microscopic report of the tumor was typical of a leiomyoma.

The second case, reported by Miller, in which a large myoma involving the lower part of the esophagus and cardia of the stomach was found, occurred in a 20-year-old boy and was discovered at post-mortem examination. This tumor measured 6 by 2 by 5 inches but had produced no symptoms.

The third case was reported by Brock[15] in 1942. This was the first successful resection of the cardia and the lower end of the esophagus reported from the continent of Europe and, as far as the author knew, the first of its kind from Great Britian. This leiomyoma involving the lower end of the esophagus and cardia was removed through a combined thoracoabdominal approach with an intrathoracic esophagogastrostomy. The tumor presented the typical picture of a benign smooth muscle tumor with simple ulceration of the overlying mucosa on the gastric side.

The fourth case was reported by Harrington and Moersch[16] in 1944. The patient was a 56-year-old woman who, at operation, was found to have a large leiomyoma of the lower part of the esophagus and cardia extending through and enlarging the esophageal hiatus. The esophagus was partially obstructed at the cardia. The greater portion of the tumor was situated in the posterior mediastinum. The tumor was removed through an abdominal approach. An incision was made in the esophagus and stomach excising the tumor and the opening thus made was closed with interrupted silk sutures. These authors reported a second case of leiomyoma involving the lower five inches of the esophagus extending down to the cardia of the stomach but not involving it. This was removed through a transthoracic approach, and an intrathoracic esophagogastrostomy was performed. The patient died on the fourth postoperative day from bilateral bronchopneumonia.

DIAGNOSIS OF LEIOMYOMA OF THE ESOPHAGUS

The clinical manifestations and symptoms of all neoplasms of the esophagus are practically the same. The differential diagnosis cannot be made from carcinoma on the basis of symptoms alone but, as a rule, dysphagia is a more outstanding early manifestation of cancer of the esophagus and progresses more rapidly than in the case of benign tumors. Myomas of the esophagus may exist for years and attain huge size before symptoms become manifest. The most common symptom of these tumors is, of course, dysphagia. The first instance in which a leiomyoma produced symptoms referable to the esophagus was reported by Coates in 1871 and was found in the case of a 61-year-old man with symptoms of esophageal obstruction who died from inanition. At autopsy a large pedunculated tumor was found attached to the esophagus six and three-quarters inches below the glottis and extending to the cardiac orifice of the stomach. Microscopically the tumor was made up of spindle cells with a small amount of connective tissue.

A large leiomyoma of the esophagus and cardia of the stomach was reported by Miller. There were no symptoms referable to this esophageal tumor. Although these tumors are slow growing, they may produce obstruction resulting in marked dysphagia, nausea, and regurgitation of food. Symptoms are frequently intermittent because of the associated esophageal spasm. Pedunculated tumors may be regurgitated into the mouth as in the case reported by Moersch and Harrington or into the larynx causing hoarseness, paroxysmal cough, and intermittent obstruction of the larynx with dyspnea.

Tumors situated in the lower end of the esophagus give rise to epigastric discomfort. There may be an intermittent retrosternal sensation of dull pain or an aching sensation often aggravated by lying down. In those instances with tumors in which ulceration of the underlying mucous membrane has occurred, epigastric pain may be related to meals or there may be regurgitation of gastric fluid sometimes tinged with blood. Anorexia, nausea, weight loss, and occasional vomiting of rather large amounts of fluid due to dilatation of the esophagus similar to the situation found in achalasia are other symptoms which may be encountered.

Examination of the esophagus roentgenologically is necessary first in determining the presence and location of the growth. A definite histologic diagnosis can be established only by esophagoscopy and biopsy, although at times it may be difficult and inadvisable to obtain such specimens because of the necessity of penetrating the normal esophageal mucous membrane which overlies these tumors. Patterson stated that Sommer in 1923 reported the only case in which a diagnosis of benign tumor was made roentgenographically. In this case the tumor was lobulated and the diagnosis was based on the appearance of the barium as it passed in the clefts between the lobules. Pape and Spitznagel[17] in 1931 recognized that a diagnosis of myoma of the esophagus was possible by roentgenologic means. The smaller myomas differ from carcinoma by absence of infiltration of the wall and the smooth contour of the mucosa. Large polypoid myomas can be recognized by the fact that the contrast medium flows around them, the continuous band of the contrast shadow being split while it stays constant and continuous in the case of a substernal goiter which may displace it. In carcinoma of the esophagus usually only one fixed, narrow canal is observed. Harper and Tisceno[18] in 1945 reported a case of intrinsic extramucosal tumor (leiomyoma) of the esophagus verified by operation and described the roentgenologic characteristic features of these tumors in detail. The important diagnostic features in differentiating benign extramucosal tumors from carcinomatous deformities are few but careful observation may lead to the correct diagnosis. The presence of a bulky and mobile soft tissue mass attached to the deformed esophageal area and more or less bulging into the mediastinum is characteristic of benign tumor and quite unlike the elongated fusiform soft tissue density ensheathing a stenosing carcinomatous filling defect. Intrinsic extramucosal benign tumors additionally have the following characteristics: Dilatation of the walls or bulging of one wall at the level of and opposite the affected segment may be observed. Other findings include absence of undermining margins, smooth margins of the forklike appearance of the barium, variations of the shape and dimensions of the filling defect, absence of actual obstruction, the presence of a smooth variable mold effect, the absence of any erosion of the mucosal covering in the tumor, preservation of the normal folds in the immediate vicinity of the filling defect, and the observation of a barium ring or "ring sign." The probability of establishing a correct diagnosis of myoma of the esophagus by roentgenologic means is fairly good, nevertheless, the final diagnosis can be definitely established only by esophagoscopy and biopsy.

We have recently resected a leiomyoma involving the esophagus and cardiac end of the stomach by the transthoracic route and a detailed case report follows. In so far as we are able to determine, this is the fifth reported case in which a leiomyoma of the esophagus and cardia of the stomach has been found and the third resected. In the case of the patient reported by Brock, resection was performed through a combined thoracoabdominal approach. Moersch and Harrington's patient had the lesion successfully removed entirely by the transabdominal route. In the patient to be reported here, transthoracic esophagogastrectomy was performed.

CASE REPORT

A 56-year-old housewife was seen first at the Boston Dispensary and applied to the clinic because of abdominal pain of three days' duration. About five months before, anorexia and nausea accompanied by attacks of dizziness had been experienced. She had lost fifteen pounds in weight during this time. There was never any vomiting and at no time did she complain of dysphagia. Three days prior to admission the patient complained of generalized, persistent, mild abdominal pain. There was no radiation of this pain nor was it related to eating. Bowel movements had been regular and stools were normal color.

The past history revealed that twenty-five years previously she had suffered from ''indigestion'' for which gastric lavage and various powders had been prescribed. Twenty-two years before, a tumor had been removed from the uterus. Twenty years previously a cholecystectomy had been performed.

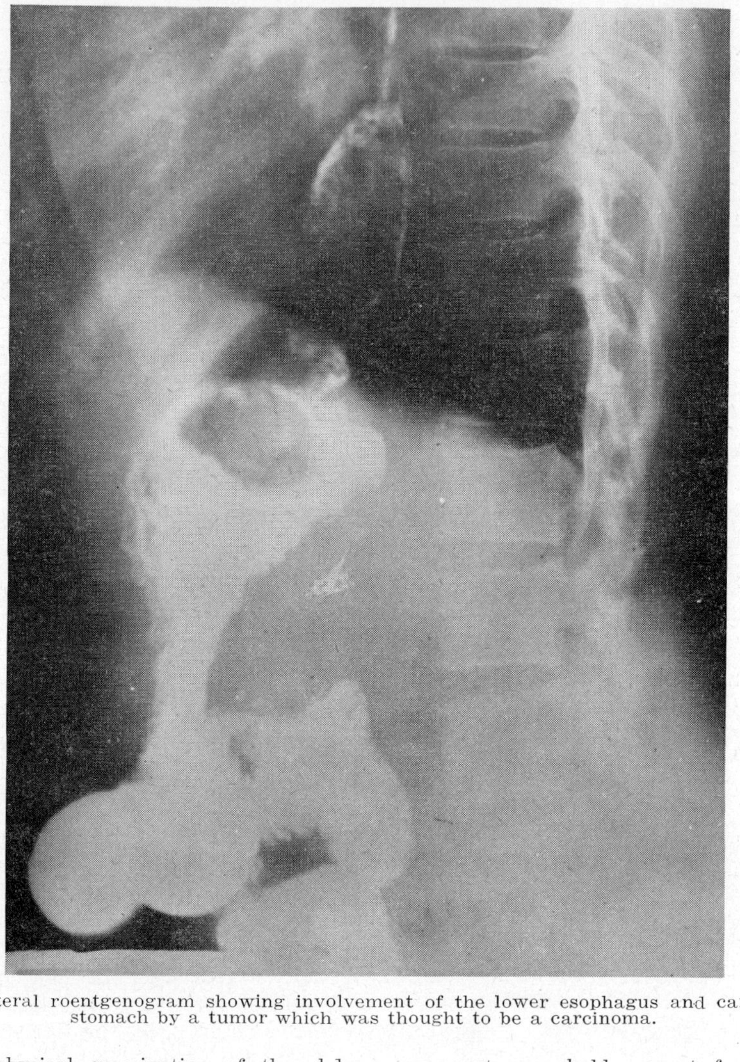

Fig. 1.—Lateral roentgenogram showing involvement of the lower esophagus and cardia of the stomach by a tumor which was thought to be a carcinoma.

The physical examination of the abdomen was not remarkable except for moderate tenderness on palpation of the midepigastric region. The red blood cell count was found to be 3.64 million per c.mm. of blood and the hemoglobin value 74 per cent.

Roentgenologic examination of the upper gastrointestinal tract revealed an irregularity of the lower end of the esophagus and, on several of the films, a suggestion of a filling defect within the lumen. The flow of barium was temporarily obstructed at the cardiac orifice and the lower end ballooned out with barium and air. The walls appeared distensible in this region. In the stomach a definite large mass was visualized in the cardia, which was polypoid in nature. There was some fixation and irregularity of the walls along the lesser curvature side. A re-examination two weeks later revealed a nodular mass in the fundus with multiple nodules extending to the lower end of the esophagus for a distance of 6 to 8 cm. A diagnosis of cancer of the cardiac end of the stomach involving the lower end of the esophagus was made.

The patient was prepared for operation with blood transfusions, gastric lavage, and general supportive therapy. Operation was performed using gas-oxygen-ether administered by endotracheal tube. The patient was operated upon in the prone position and postero-lateral thoracotomy performed with resection of the left eighth rib. In addition, the seventh and ninth ribs were divided. The phrenic nerve was crushed. A large smooth firm tumor was palpated within the two lower inches of the esophagus and was found to extend into the stomach. The diaphragm was opened and the stomach exposed. The lower portion of the

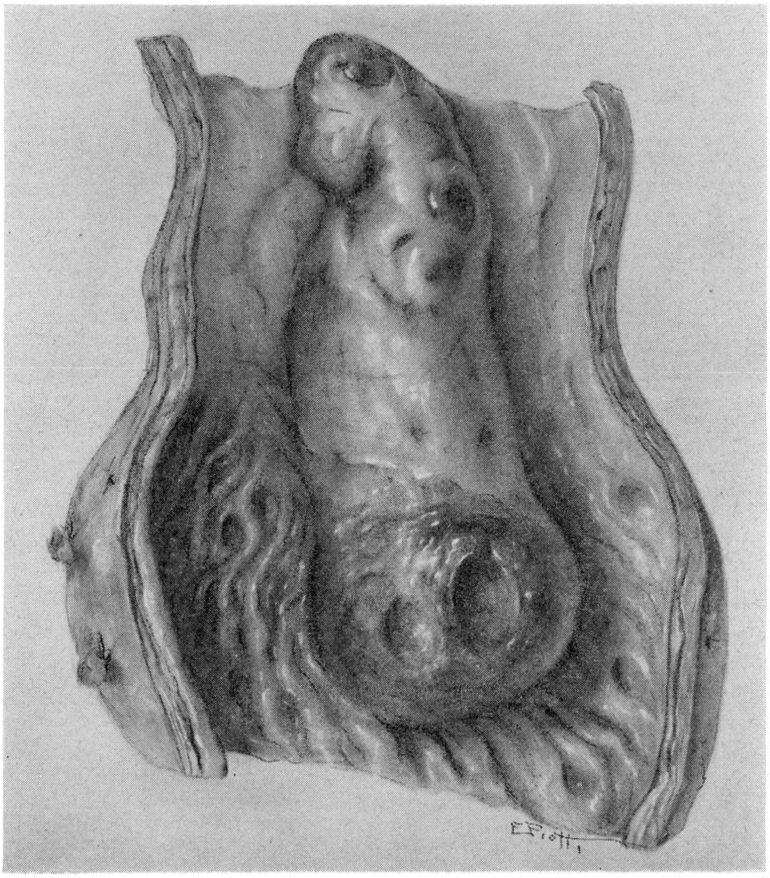

Fig. 2.—Artist's drawing of the resected esophagus and stomach showing the large leiomyoma involving both organs. Note the ulceration of the tumor on the gastric side.

esophagus and cardiac end of the stomach were then excised above and below the tumor mass in the usual manner. An incidental splenectomy was performed. The esophagogastric anastomosis was made on the posterior wall of the stomach, a more convenient placement when the patient is in the prone position. Catheter water-sealed drainage of the thoracic cavity was employed for forty-eight hours. The postoperative course of this patient was quite uneventful except for a moderate degree of discomfort along the line of incision. The patient ate without difficulty and was discharged on the thirty-eighth hospital day. A follow-up roentgenologic examination six months later revealed good function at the intrathoracic esophagogastrostomy.

The specimen was described as follows: Bulging into the lumen of the esophagus and the cardiac end of the stomach was a firm, rubbery, fusiform and grossly nodular tumor mass which appeared everywhere to be covered with mucosa except at its inferior end where there was an ulceration in the anterior surface measuring 1 cm. in diameter and .5 cm. in depth. At the proximal portion several small secondary nodules were attached to the main mass. Sections through the tumor mass revealed it to be well encapsulated and showed a rubbery, pale gray, finely trabeculated and finely whorled surface. The tumor mass measured 10 cm. in length and had an average diameter of 3.0 cm. The microscopic examination revealed a leiomyoma of the wall of the esophagus and stomach with ulceration of the gastric mucosa at two points.

In Fig. 1 the roentgenograms taken preoperatively showing the tumor involving both the stomach and the esophagus may be seen. In retrospect the diagnosis of benign tumor, possibly leiomyoma, could have been made if it were known that leiomyomas sometimes involve both of these structures at their junction and while carcinoma is by far the most common lesion in this area, the fact that benign tumors do exist here has been our reason for calling attention to this unusual lesion.

In Fig. 2 the artist's drawing of the resected specimen may be seen. The characteristic ulceration of the tumor through the gastric mucosa which so often results in massive hemorrhage from leiomyoma of the stomach, in the case of our patient resulted in some chronic blood loss with moderate anemia. The absence of dysphagia with so large a growth at this area can be easily understood since the tumor is intramuscular and does not constrict the esophageal mucosa.

REFERENCES

1. Meissner, W. A.: Leiomyoma of the Stomach, Arch. Path. **38**: 207-209, 1944.
2. Vinson, P. P., Moore, A. B., and Bowing, H. H.: Hemangioma of the Esophagus, Report of a Case, Am. J. M. Sc. **172**: 416, 1926.
3. Moersch, H. S., and Harrington, S. W.: Benign Tumor of the Esophagus, Ann. Otol., Rhin. & Laryng. **53**: 800-817, 1944.
4. Shafer, P. W., and Kittle, C. F.: Esophageal Leiomyoma, J. A. M. A. **133**: 1202-1205, 1947.
5. Patterson, Ellen J.: Benign Neoplasms of the Esophagus, Pennsylvania M. J. **36**: 244-246, 1933.
   Idem: Benign Neoplasms of the Esophagus, Report of a Case of Myxofibroma, Ann. Otol., Rhin. & Laryng. **41**: 942-950, 1932.
6. Bryant, John: Myoma of the Esophagus, J. A. M. A. **45**: 2008, 1905.
7. Fogge, Hilton: Myoma of the Oesophagus, Tr. Path. Soc., London **26**: 94-96, 1874.
8. Miller, James: Large Leiomyoma of the Esophagus, J. Path. & Bact. **17**: 278-281, 1912.
9. Coates, J.: Large Polypoid Myoma of the Oesophagus, Glasgow M. J. **4**: 201-206, 1872.
10. Rose, J. D.: Myomata of the Oesophagus, Brit. J. Surg. **24**: 297-308, 1936.
11. Stewart, J. D., Jr.: Myoma of the Esophagus With Associated Diverticula, Arch. Path. **12**: 77-84, 1931.
12. Howard, W. T., Jr.: Primary Sarcoma of the Esophagus and Stomach, J. A. M. A. **38**: 392-399, 1902.
13. Pennes, Alexander E.: Leiomyosarcoma of the Esophagus, Am. J. Roentgenol. **48**: 336-340, 1942.
14. Milovanovie, Milovan: Ueber Leiomyoma Des Oesophagus Und Der Kardia, Wein. klin. Wchnschr. **27**: 753-755, 1914.
15. Brock, R. C.: Cardio-Esophageal Resection for Tumor of the Cardia, Report of a Successful Case, Brit. J. Surg. **30**: 146-150, 1942.
16. Harrington, S. W., and Moersch, H. S.: Surgical Treatment and Clinical Manifestations of Benign Tumors of the Esophagus, J. Thoracic Surg. **13**: 394-414, 1944.
17. Pape, R., and Spitznagel: Myomas of the Esophagus, Radiology **17**: 571, 1931.
18. Harper, R. S. K., and Tisceno, E.: Benign Tumors of the Esophagus and Its Differential Diagnosis, Brit. J. Radiol. **18**: 99-107, 1945.

AN IN VIVO METHOD FOR EVALUATION OF DETERGENTS AND GERMICIDES

Charles A. Hufnagel, M.D.,* Carl W. Walter, M.D.,† and Rutledge W. Howard, M.D.,‡ Boston, Mass.

(From the Laboratory for Surgical Research, Harvard Medical School)

THERE have been many techniques for the evaluation of skin detergents and germicides. That of Price[1] has contributed greatly to the knowledge of the bacteriology of the skin and is an effective method for determining the relative efficiency of germicides. Because there are several major variables in this technique which are uncontrolled and because at least seven days must elapse between determinations for the numerical recovery of the bacterial flora on a subject's skin, experiments are necessarily protracted and strictly comparable determinations are impossible.

The technique to be described was intended to permit multiple determinations on contiguous areas of human skin so that various agents can be tested on the same skin on the same day.

An apparatus, Fig. 1, was designed and built to standardize the various mechanical factors involved in scrubbing techniques. This device isolates adequate areas of skin and scrubs it at a constant rate with a specially designed brush pressed against the skin by a constant force. The machine has three elements: a mechanical reciprocating scrubber, a stable brush, and a vacuum seal to isolate and hold the skin against the brush.

The reciprocating scrubber is driven by a gear reduction motor at 30 strokes per minute. Briefly, it consists of a rocker shaft mounted on a balanced arm. At the pivoted end of the balanced arm, the rocker shaft is actuated by a hinged rocker arm bearing a slide block which is driven by a crank mounted on the motor shaft. At the opposite end, the rocker shaft carries a rocker arm which supports a detachable brush. A small tray at this end of the balanced arm accommodates the weights used to load the brush.

The brush§ was designed to withstand repeated (300 times) sterilization by exposure to saturated steam at 121° C. for thirty minutes without a significant change in brushing characteristics. The nonwetting Nylon bristles are 0.25 mm. on centers. Two rows of tufts set in a heat-resistant plastic back were used.

The vacuum seal is created in a space around a square aperture, 4 by 4 cm., in the concave bottom of a stainless steel pan. The edges of the aperture are bent downward 0.5 mm. The radius of the concavity is of the same length as

This study was made under a grant from the Winthrop Chemical Company, Inc., New York, N. Y.

Received for publication, July 22, 1947.

*Arthur Tracy Cabot Fellow, 1944-1945.

†Director, Laboratory for Surgical Research.

‡Harvey Cushing Fellow, 1942-1943.

§No. 157, Prophylactic Brush Company, Florence, Mass.

the rocker arm and brush assembly so that the entire skin area is scrubbed uniformly and the bristles rub on the pan at either end of the stroke to divest themselves of organisms and detritus. The seal is made by mounting a second aperture, 4.2 cm. square, 1 mm. below the convex surface of the pan. Negative pressure applied to the space between the apertures effectively seals the skin to the pan. The entire pan can be detached for sterilization. Stainless steel was used because it has minimal oligodynamic action. An adjustable rest faced with sponge rubber is mounted beneath the aperture to support the hand. The rocker arm and brackets that support it are long enough to extend over the back of a prone subject.

TECHNIQUE

The pan and brush are sterilized in saturated steam at 121° C. for thirty minutes. The surface of the remainder of the apparatus is washed with 0.1

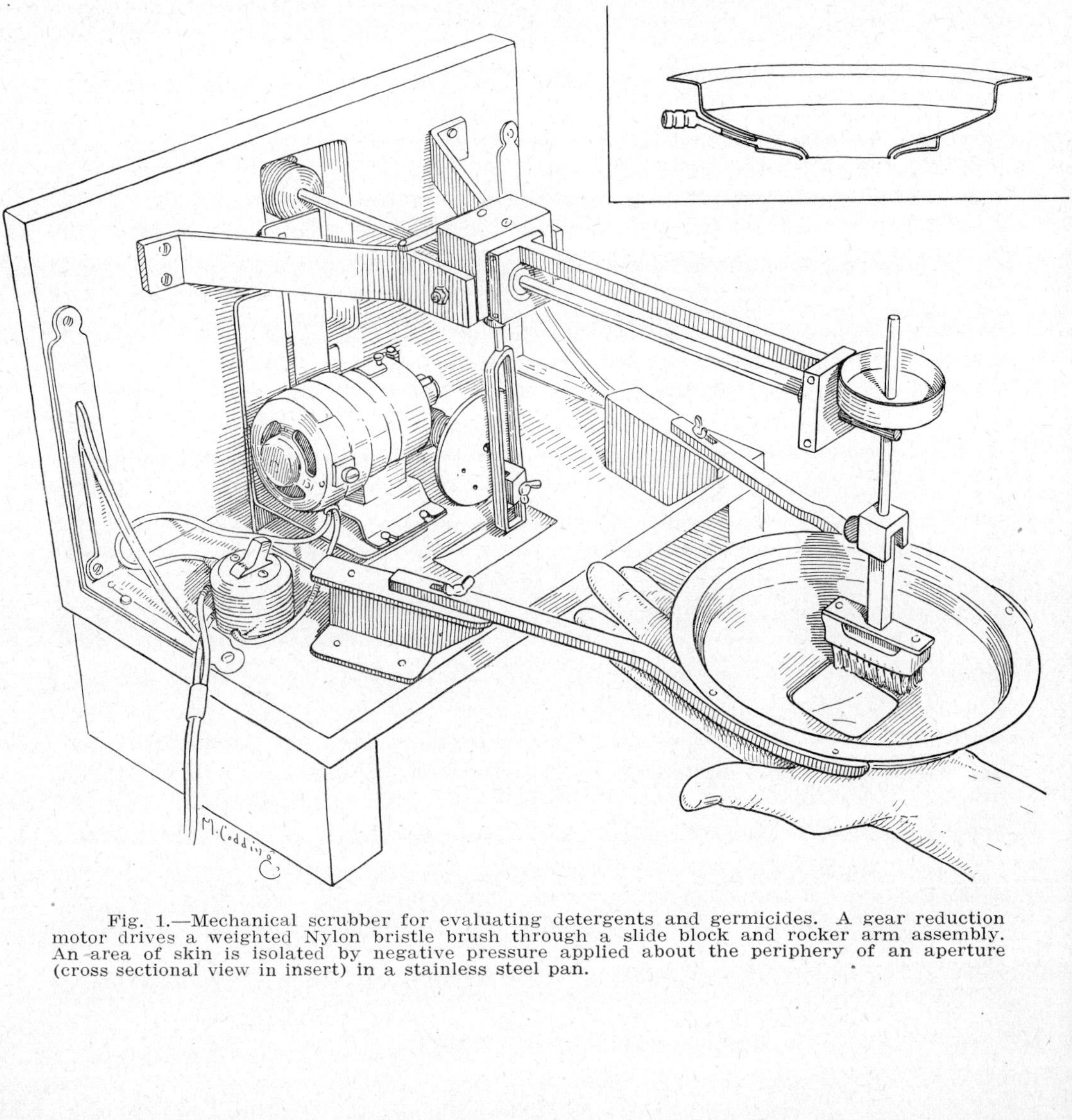

Fig. 1.—Mechanical scrubber for evaluating detergents and germicides. A gear reduction motor drives a weighted Nylon bristle brush through a slide block and rocker arm assembly. An area of skin is isolated by negative pressure applied about the periphery of an aperture (cross sectional view in insert) in a stainless steel pan.

per cent aqueous Zephiran and covered with a Pliofilm hood prior to each experiment to control air-borne contamination. The subjects are requested not to wash their hands for four hours before the test and are known not to have contacted germicidal solutions for four days. In this study the subjects were chosen at random from volunteers.

The hand is adjusted on the rest so that the flat mid-portion of the palm is in firm contact with the sealing chamber of the scrubbing pan and 250 mm. Hg negative pressure is applied to isolate the test area of skin. Five cubic centimeters of sterile distilled water are run on the test area of the skin. The brush is fixed in position and the skin is scrubbed with 110 Gm. pressure on the brush for ten complete reciprocating strokes. The water is aspirated with a sterile suction tip into a sterile test tube. Care is taken to remove as much water as possible. The same brush is used for subsequent test periods using similar amounts of distilled water and ten strokes. This process is repeated thirty times. On the thirty-first group of ten strokes, the pressure on the brush is made as hard as the subject can bear without discomfort. Thus, any remaining organisms which can be removed by increased pressure are detected. There were no cases in this study in which a variation beyond the predicted number was obtained, so that it appeared that at this point on the control curve there were few additional organisms available for removal. The complete series of scrubs was sufficiently traumatic to abrade soft skin such as that on either side of the midline of the back.

The technique for the evaluation of germicides is identical to that of the control curve except that the substance to be tested is introduced on the skin surface after the initial period of ten strokes with water, that is, at the second point of the curve. A new sterile brush is fixed and the hand scrubbed for ten strokes. The germicide then is aspirated, the brush removed from the pan, and, while the skin is rubbed with a cotton pledget, it is rinsed three times with 5 c.c. sterile water to remove the test substance. This simple washing with water and friction after an initial scrub with water removes an insignificant number of organisms. The original brush is then replaced and the scrub continued as in the control series, using 5 c.c. of water and ten strokes of the brush. The repeated scrubbing with fresh water further dilutes residual germicide beyond bacteriostatic levels and should break up any film the germicide may precipitate in the skin. Immediately following completion of the scrub, the contents of each tube are transferred to a sterile Petri dish and pour plates are made using Difco beef agar. Colony counts are made after twenty-four and forty-eight hours of incubation at 37.5° C. using a Quebec colony counter.

RESULTS

Control curves were obtained using sterile water. Colonies of "spreading" organisms on the plates caused a number of experiments to be discarded because it was impossible to count the colonies. Experiments yielding an initial count of below 500 colonies were likewise discarded because the paucity of organisms made these seem less reliable although, when plotted, the same general type of curve was obtained.

Nineteen experiments were finally accepted. These showed an average of 2,320 colonies on the initial ten strokes. When the curve of the average control experiment was plotted in conventional manner, number of bacteria removed against number of brush strokes, it corresponded to that of a rectangular hyperbola following the general formula of $y = f(x)^{-1}$ and closely approximated the calculated curve, Fig. 2. Thus, the second ten strokes should yield one-half, and the third ten strokes one-third the number removed by the first ten. It should be noted that this is not a simple dilution curve. Cumulative totals of organisms removed in successive intervals of scrubbing, a concept introduced by

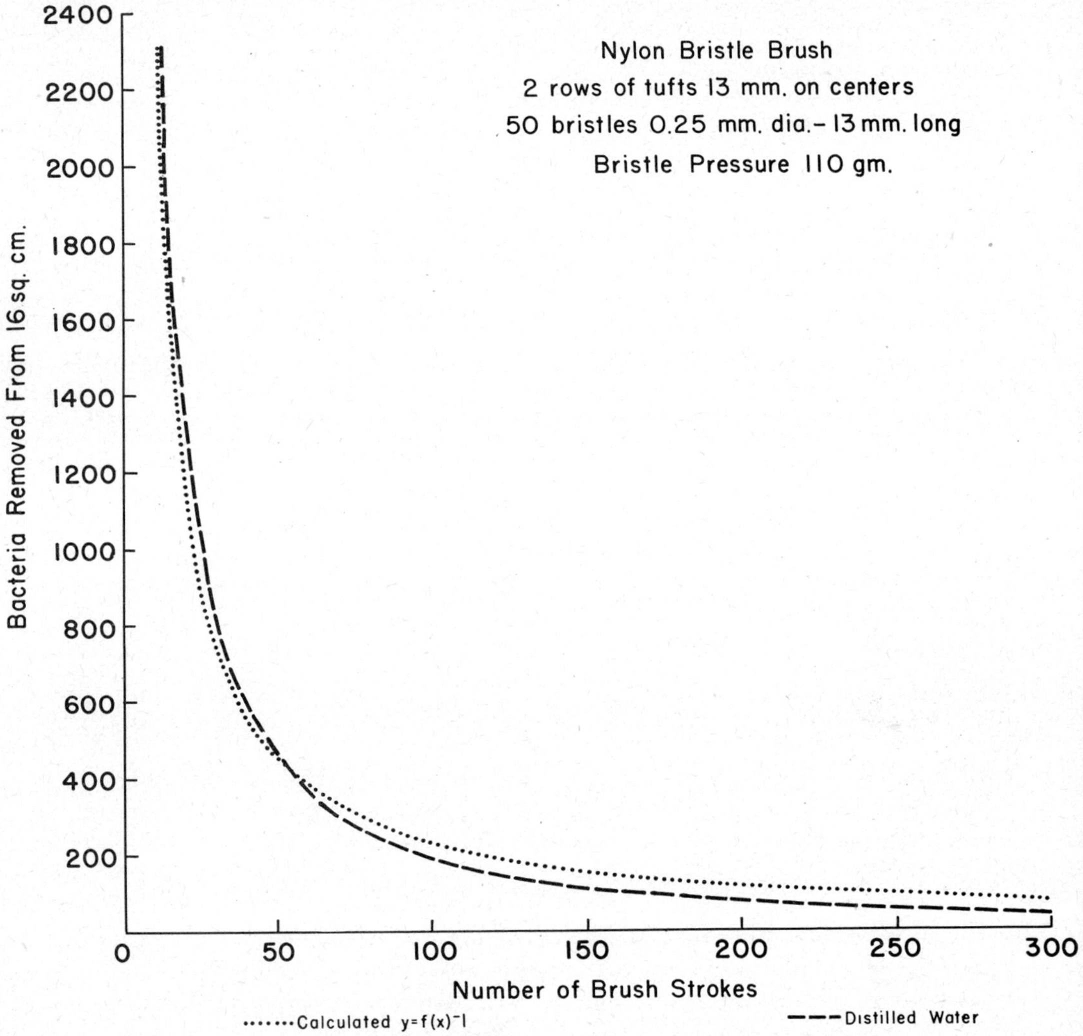

Fig. 2.—The effect of mechanical scrubbing. The distilled water, or control curve, demonstrates the effect of mechanical scrubbing alone. The curve expresses the average of nineteen experiments. It corresponds with that of the rectangular hyperbola $y = f(x)^{-1}$.

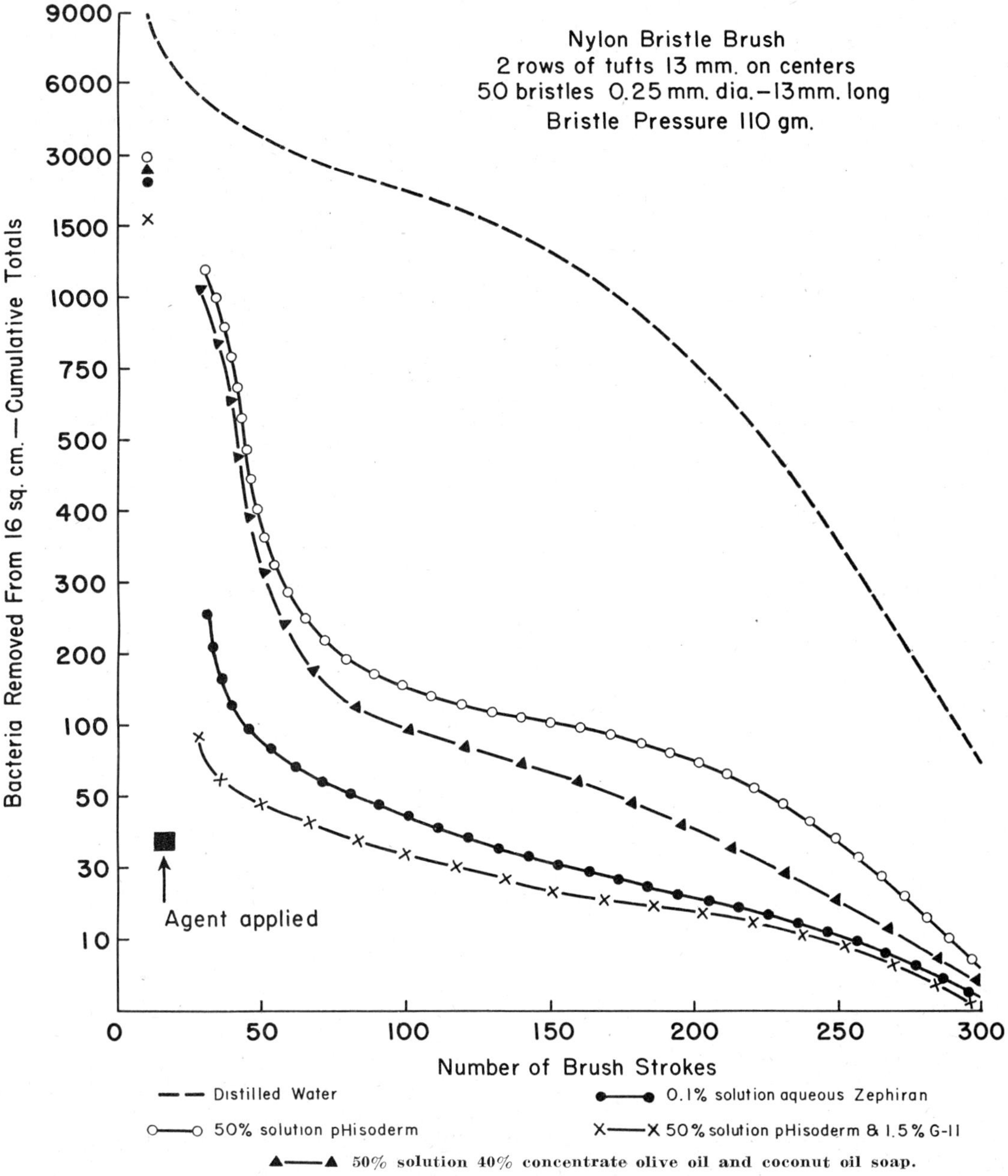

Fig. 3.—The comparative disinfecting effect of scrubbing, detergents, and germicides. The distilled water curve is made from the same data as Fig. 2, plotted cumulatively rather than in conventional fashion. The total counts for the other agents are given at ten brush strokes. The second period of ten strokes is that used to apply the agent. The third period, therefore, represents the total number of organisms removed following the application of the agent under study. The drop from the control curve portrays its relative effectiveness.

Price,[1] when plotted against the number of strokes applied, form a curve which portrays best the contrasts between experiments, Fig. 3.

Germicides or detergents were evaluated by applying them during the second interval of scrubbing. Ten strokes were thus used to apply them to the skin. The agent was then removed by suction and by dilution. Since only a film of fluid covering the skin was left each time, the triple rinsing with water reduced the concentration of each agent well below bacteriostatic levels. The effectiveness of the agent applied during the second interval of scrubbing was judged by comparing differences between the control curves and those obtained by plotting the counts of the subsequent periods of scrubbing with distilled water.

The agents tested were a 40 per cent concentrate of equal parts of coconut oil and olive oil soaps diluted equal parts with water; pHisoderm, diluted equal parts with water; 0.1 per cent aqueous Zephiran N.N.R.; pHisoderm containing 3 per cent G-11, diluted equal parts with water. G-11 is 2,2′-dihydroxy-3,5,6-3′,5′,6′ hexachlorodiphenylmethane, a promising new cutaneous germicidal agent.[2] A comparison of the result may be seen from Table I and Figs. 2 and 3.

The curves for ten scrubs each with coconut oil soap and pHisoderm are extremely similar. Both had average initial counts of close to 1700, and after

TABLE I

AGENT	CONTROL	COCONUT AND OLIVE OIL SOAP 20 PER CENT	PHISODERM #44 WATER āā	ZEPHIRAN 0.1 PER CENT AQUEOUS	PHISODERM AND 3 PER CENT G-11 WATER āā
NUMBER OF EXPERIMENTS	19	10	10	10	10
SCRUB PERIOD			AVERAGE COLONY COUNTS		
1	2320	1703	1665	2502	1568
2	1410	agent applied			
3	802	460	649	131	7
4	605	275	185	28	5
5	496	118	99	15	4
6	355	67	46	1	4
7	285	23	29	8	4
8	282	18	23	5	2
9	244	15	21	4	3
10	208	11	13	4	2
11	204	9	13	3	3
12	130	8	8	3	2
13	165	6	7	2	2
14	140	8	7	2	1
15	124	6	8	3	1
16	116	5	6	2	1
17	120	6	6	2	2
18	116	4	6	2	2
19	76	4	7	3	2
20	100	4	8	2	2
21	80	3	7	1	2
22	71	3	9	1	1
23	64	3	8	2	0.5
24	60	3	6	3	2
25	68	4	8	3	2
26	52	4	8	1	2
27	48	3	5	1	2
28	64	3	4	1	2
29	53	2	5	1	2
30	44	2	5	1	1

100 strokes, tube 9, had reached colony counts approaching ten in contrast to the control of 244.

Using Zephiran, however, the fall in the average number of organisms was much more rapid from an initial count of 2,500 to 130 organisms on the first ten strokes. Very few organisms could be removed after the ninth tube with an average of only two colonies per tube after that point and the majority of tubes were sterile. The total average number of organisms after the use of 0.1 per cent aqueous Zephiran for thirty seconds and ten strokes was 237 in contrast to 5,172 with water, 1,075 with coconut oil soap, and 1,207 with pHisoderm.

The results with pHisoderm and 3 per cent G-11 were even more striking. This agent was diluted with an equal amount of water before use. The initial count was 1,500 and the first tube after its use showed only seven colonies. Subsequent tubes showed further reduction and the total number of organisms removed by the water after its use averaged 65.

CONCLUSIONS

1. A technique is described which has been elaborated to permit multiple determinations of the bacterial flora of the human skin under standardized mechanical conditions.

2. The effectiveness of various agents is strikingly portrayed by the cumulative plotting of the data obtained.

3. The agents investigated are primarily detergents. The conventional practice is to use soap and pHisoderm for longer periods of time than employed in these experiments, yet comparable rates of removal of bacteria are detectable under the conditions employed. Zephiran exhibits marked germicidal properties on more prolonged exposure than the 60 seconds' maximal exposure possible in this technique.

4. Recent studies, to be elaborated in a subsequent report, indicate that pHisoderm fortified with G-11 displayed the most rapid disinfecting action. This combination appears to be more effective than any detergent commonly employed for the preoperative preparation of skin.

REFERENCES

1. Price, P. B.: The Bacteriology of Normal Skin; A New Quantitative Test Applied to a Study of the Bacterial Flora and the Disinfecting Action of Mechanical cleansing, J. Infect. Dis. **63**: 301-318, 1938.
2. Traub, E. F., Newhall, C. A., and Fuller, J. N.: New Cutaneous Bactericidal Agent Used in Soap, Arch. Dermat. & Syph. **52**: 385, 1945.

CHOLEDOCHOTOMY

Robert W. Buxton, M.D., and Lloyd B. Burk, Jr., M.D.*
Ann Arbor, Mich.

(From the Department of Surgery, University of Michigan)

CHOLEDOCHOTOMY is an important supplementary procedure of cholecystectomy, whether it be done at the time the gall bladder is removed or whether the later symptoms of the patient necessitate exploration of the common duct at a future date. At the time of every cholecystectomy the question arises before most surgeons as to whether or not the common bile duct should be opened and explored. To some, this question never arises—the common bile duct is explored in every instance. Certainly the criteria for choledochotomy are at variance with different surgeons, but most recognize certain factors which demand extrahepatic biliary exploration. In an attempt to understand better the dangers of this operative procedure, as well as to establish the criteria for choledochotomy more definitely, where this operation is not practiced routinely, we have reviewed 439 consecutive cases in which the common bile duct was opened and explored. This study encompasses a twelve-year period from July, 1934, to July, 1946. We have also enumerated the complications that seem peculiar to this operation. In each patient in whom the common bile duct was opened the duct was drained to the outside by means of a catheter or T tube. We have attempted to evaluate the length of time drainage should be employed, once it is instituted. This study has established certain beliefs which are worthy of note. We are impressed that choledochotomy is not the benign and uncomplicated procedure which it is sometimes believed to be.

In any discussion of choledochotomy, cholecystectomy cannot be excluded because of the close anatomic relations of the gall bladder and the common duct. The same dangers of cholecystectomy are ever present when the common duct is explored. Daseler and associates[2] have recently published their classic study of the anatomic variations of the hepatic pedicle. Accidents at operation, from sectioning the portal vein or hepatic artery, may result in a tragic ending to a "simple cholecystectomy." Or, injury to the extrahepatic ducts may result in death or a stricture of the duct, the result of which requires no emphasis. Certainly, too strong an emphasis cannot be placed upon a knowledge of the "anomalies" and the usual anatomy of the hepatic pedicle. Exact knowledge of the normal anatomy and its variations must be demanded of every surgeon before he operates upon the biliary system. Fig. 1 reflects well the improvements in technique and our greater knowledge of the preoperative and postoperative requirements of these patients. Because of the striking difference in mortality rate during this relatively short period, the factors which we have considered effective in reducing mortality should be mentioned.

Received for publication, July 29, 1947.

*Trainee of the National Cancer Institute.

Vitamin K.—It is well known that patients who are jaundiced or who have experienced repeated episodes of jaundice may have a prolonged prothrombin time. If the patient is not jaundiced, the possibility of prothrombin deficiency may be overlooked. It should be remembered that prothrombin deficiency may be due to any one of several factors—inadequate nutritional intake, absence of bile and hence inadequate absorption of vitamin K, or inadequate synthesis of prothrombin by a poorly functioning liver. It is well to emphasize that patients with an increased prothrombin time should have the operation deferred until the deficiency has been corrected. A prolonged preoperative period of preparation along with large doses of vitamin K parenterally are often necessary to correct this deficit.

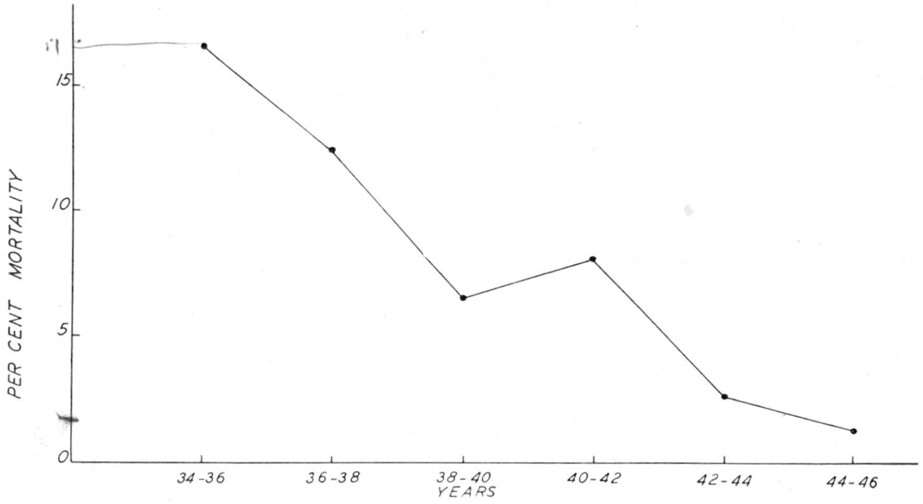

Fig. 1.—Mortality rates in choledochotomy (439 cases, 1934 to 1946).

Antibiotics.—Many times patients who have common duct obstruction have a concomitant cholangitis and hepatitis. It is only logical that the antibiotics would be beneficial.

Electrolyte and Fluid Balance.—An imbalance in either fluids or electrolytes may be overlooked in the preoperative period. This is a particularly important problem in the postoperative period when the patient has an external biliary fistula.

Nutrition.—Many of these patients have lost considerable amounts of weight because of inadequate food intake. Their admission of weight loss should be a reminder of a possible deficiency in proteins and vitamins. Certainly weight loss demands investigation with steps to correct the deficiencies that exist.

Blood.—The correction of a secondary anemia in the preoperative period, as well as the use of adequate amounts of whole blood at the time that it is lost at operation, has been shown to be of extreme importance.

With these therapeutic aids and the present low mortality rate it would seem that any discussion regarding criteria for opening the common bile duct is inconsequential. However, a statistically greater morbidity and mortality is associated with choledochotomy when this procedure is added to cholecystectomy. We have encountered certain complications which are directly related to the fact that the common duct was opened. And, although wound infection and subphrenic abscess are not unique following choledochotomy, we think the incidence is higher than it is in cholecystectomy alone. Choledochotomy certainly may be a factor in their occurrence. During the period of this study, from 1934 to 1946, the following complications (Table I) have occurred (excluding those cases in which death occurred).

Table I. Complications Following Choledochotomy in 439 Cases

Complications	Number
Retained calculi	26
Stricture	2
T tube broken in removal	2
Duodenal fistula	1
Subhepatic bile abscess	1
Subphrenic abscess	6
Wound infection	32
Total	70 (15.9%)

These seventy complications occurred in 439 patients so that the total morbidity from choledochotomy in this period was 15.9 per cent. If one contends that wound infection and subphrenic abscess are not uniquely related to common duct exploration, there still remain thirty-four cases (7.2 per cent) in which the complications seem definitely related to choledochotomy. These percentage figures lend support to the opinion that choledochotomy should not be performed routinely but should be carried out only when there is a definite indication for so doing.

The patients' historical background and the findings at operation, which formed the basis for our decision to open and explore the extrahepatic biliary system, are listed in Table II. The presence of any one of these criteria demands common duct exploration.

Table II. Criteria for Common Duct Exploration

1. Palpable stone in the hepatic or common bile ducts
2. Jaundice
   (a) Present on admission to the hospital
   (b) Recent (within 3 months)
3. Dilatation of the duct or thickening of the periductal structures
4. Clinical evidence of cholangitis
5. Multiple small stones in the gall bladder
6. Thickening or induration of the head of the pancreas
7. Biliary colic without stones in gall bladder

Certainly there is no disagreement regarding certain criteria for choledochotomy. The presence of a palpable stone is an obvious indication for duct exploration. The presence of jaundice at the time of operation or an unequivocal history of a recent episode of jaundice also demands duct exploration. The word "recent" is an ambiguous one. The arbitrary time is a difficult one to decide upon but it has seemed reasonable to set an interval of three or four months of freedom from jaundice as a minimum. In this series of cases two and one-half months was the longest interval without jaundice, in those cases in which the duct was opened for "recent" jaundice and in which stones were found within the duct. If the patient has had partial or recurring obstruction as the cause of the jaundice, changes in the duct will also be present.

A thickened or dilated duct suggests that obstruction may be present; common duct exploration is then indicated. Clinical evidence of cholangitis, in which the patient has had recurring chills and fever, with or without jaundice, is also a well-accepted reason for biliary exploration and drainage.

Small stones in the gall bladder have always been a debatable criterion for duct exploration. The size of the stones must be considered in relation to the size of the cystic duct. If the stones are extremely small it is always possible for one or more of these to have passed through even a small cystic duct. Such a small stone need not indicate its presence by jaundice; 37 per cent of the stones removed from the ducts of the patients in this series were not associated with jaundice. In only one case in this group of patients, in which the common duct was explored solely because of the presence of small stones in the gall bladder, was a stone found.

A small contracted gall bladder is sometimes referred to as an indication for common duct exploration. However, unless this finding has been associated with other more obvious indications for common duct exploration, none of the patients in this series had duct calculi upon duct exploration.

In this series of patients calculi were found in 190 instances. In only 92 cases (48 per cent) did the surgeon record his ability to palpate stones before opening the duct. In 38 instances the findings on palpation were not recorded. In 61 cases (32 per cent) the stone could not be palpated. This, of course, is excellent evidence that certain criteria for choledochotomy must be established so that stones, when not palpable, will not be missed. We have tabulated (Table III) the reasons for opening the common bile ducts in those patients in whom stones could not be palpated at the time of operation, but from whom stones were removed from the common duct.

TABLE III. INDICATIONS FOR CHOLEDOCHOTOMY IN NONPALPABLE CALCULI (61 CASES)

INDICATIONS	NUMBER
Jaundice	4
Jaundice, dilated duct	14
Jaundice, dilated, thickened duct	4
Jaundice, small stones in gall bladder	6
Jaundice, dilated duct, small stones in gall bladder	11
Dilated duct	3
Dilated, thickened duct	2
Dilated duct, small stones in gall bladder	4
Dilated, thickened duct, small stones in gall bladder	1
Thick duct, small stones in gall bladder, recent jaundice	1
Dilated duct, recent jaundice	4
Recent jaundice	1
Recent jaundice, small stones in gall bladder	1
Small stones in gall bladder	1
Indurated, thickened head of pancreas, dilated duct	1
Biliary colic without gall bladder stones	1
Choledochoduodenal fistula	1
No reason given	1
Total	61

The presence of a spontaneous choledochoduodenal fistula is an uncommon finding at operation and is seldom included in a listing of the more common indicators for duct exploration because of the rarity.

Whenever the common duct is opened and explored it has been drained routinely. If the duct is left completely patent at the conclusion of the operation, leakage may well not occur at the point of closure of the duct. However, it is entirely possible that a leak with the formation of a bile abscess or peritonitis may occur. This possibility is enhanced immeasurably if a residual calculus is present. It is often difficult to be certain that residual calculi do not remain, even after very careful exploration. Cholangiography at the time of operation does not always overcome this obstacle.[1]

During the twelve-year period under study, stones were found at the time of operation in 190 patients. In seventeen of these, subsequent cholangiograms showed the presence of a retained calculus. Eight calculi required removal at a second operation. At the same time 249 choledochotomies were performed in which stones were not found. Subsequent roentgen studies showed the presence of a common duct calculus in nine of these patients. Three of these patients required removal of the retained stone by operation. This is a total of 26 retained calculi in 439 choledochotomies (5.9 per cent).

This high incidence of retained calculi indicates the surgeon's difficulty in being certain that no stones are missed at the time of operation. The usual methods of common duct exploration were employed in all instances. Transduodenal removal of calculi was necessary in 18 of 190 cases of common duct stone. In only two of these cases did complications arise. In both instances only mild wound infections occurred.

The postoperative cholangiographic studies on five patients (Table IV) revealed one or more opaque shadows in the outline of the common duct, suggestive of residual calculi. In each instance the T tube was removed at the suggestion of the surgeon; the reason for this decision is no longer apparent. Recent information on each of these five patients indicates no residual symptoms of duct calculus. Only one patient had a single episode of jaundice following discharge from the hospital. No additional symptoms or recurrence of jaundice have occurred in this patient in a period of three and one-half years.

Several explanations can be offered for the excellent end results in these five patients. It is quite apparent that a single cholangiogram (two patients) offers no conclusive evidence of a residual calculus. In those patients upon whom repeated roentgenographic studies were carried out there seems good evidence of stone. We must presume that these have been discharged from the duct or

Table IV. Retained Calculi

1 cholang no good

CALCULI	NUMBER
Removed at reoperation	11
Gone after irrigations	8
Present last x-ray	5
Present last x-ray—death after leaving hospital	2
Total	26

∴ artefacts

are still present but have failed to produce symptoms of obstruction. The latter course seems unlikely since all of these patients were operated upon from three and one-half to eight years ago. While it is possible for a calculus within the common duct to remain silent for this length of time, it seems improbable that such a course would be followed in all of these patients.

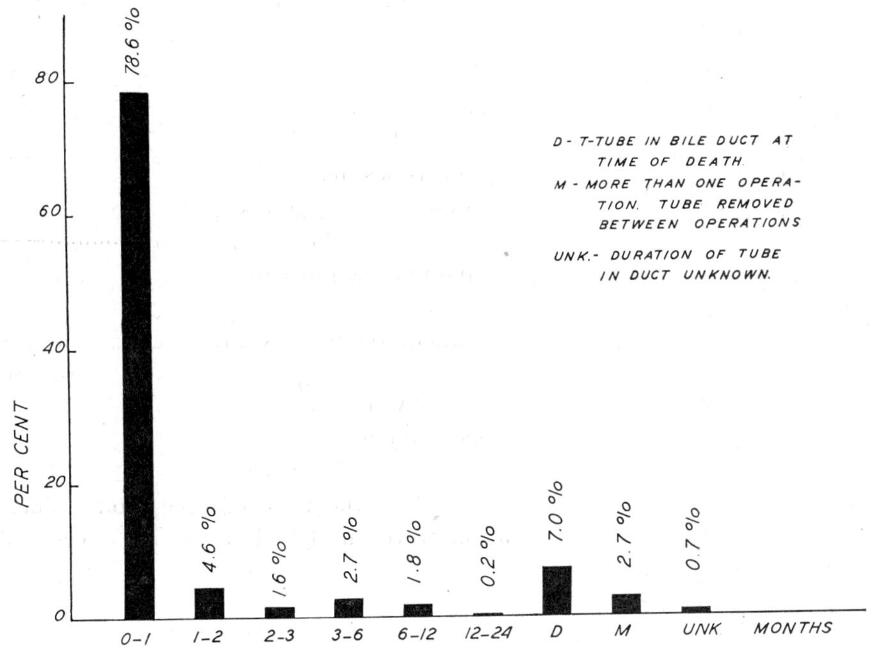

Fig. 2.—Duration of T tube or catheter in common bile duct.

With the high incidence of retained calculi some additional means of investigating the duct system at operation seems requisite. This need is answered in part by exploration of the biliary ducts by means of a cholangiogram at the time of operation and prior to closure of the abdominal wall. Such a procedure adds only a few extra minutes to the operation and may often insure a completely patent biliary system. The presence of a filling defect in the choledochogram is not unequivocal evidence of a retained calculus. Air bubbles, mucus, or debris may produce confusing defects and the diagnosis of a retained calculus is not entirely reliable from a single, and occasionally multiple, cholangiogram. In eight cases (Table IV) the roentgenographic evidence of obstruction disappeared postoperatively after irrigations of the duct system. Since a single cholangiogram is not complete evidence of a retained calculus, and if an obstructing defect is apparent, irrigations of the duct system are worthy of trial before resorting to a second operation.

Following exploration and drainage of the extrahepatic ducts, the surgeon must always decide the optimum time for withdrawal of this drainage tube (Fig. 2). After careful scrutiny of this group of patients, the following observations can be recorded:

1. When the duct is normal in appearance, slightly or moderately dilated or very slightly thickened, the catheter or T tube may be removed within eight to fourteen days following choledochotomy. Before withdrawal there must be cholangiographic evidence of freedom from obstruction, prompt spillage into the duodenum, and full visualization of the major hepatic radicles.

2. The presence of a catheter or T tube within the biliary ducts for as long as one to two years has not produced stricture or severe scarring.

3. In the presence of marked thickening and dilatation of the common bile ducts, it has been our policy to allow the catheter or T tube to remain in situ for two to six months, often longer. The patient is instructed to irrigate the tube with saline solution two to four times daily and is given an oral cholegogue which is to be taken as long as the tube remains within the duct.

With these observations in mind, it is proper to note that two patients developed a stricture, after exploration and drainage of the common bile duct, which necessitated reoperation. In one instance a tube, much too large for the duct, was inserted with some difficulty. It is obvious that necrosis of a portion of the duct wall may occur when it is stretched and distended by a large foreign body. In the other patient the common bile duct was accidentally transected at the time of cholecystectomy, anastomosed, and a T-tube splint left in place for two months. Subsequent obstruction by stricture necessitated reoperation. This instance has been instrumental in indicating to us that a transected duct, repaired over a T tube or catheter, should have that tube left in place for six to twelve months depending upon the amount of inflammatory reaction and scar present about the site of anastomosis and the preciseness with which the operator is able to approximate the severed duct ends.

We have concluded then, that following exploration and drainage of the common bile ducts, the T tube or catheter may be removed within the first two weeks provided the ductal lumen is adequate and unobstructed and that the walls of the duct are not markedly thickened. When there is evidence of marked choledochitis the drainage tube should be left in place, with frequent daily irrigations, for two to six months. If a stricture is present or anticipated, healing and contracture are expected and the tube splint should remain within the duct until these processes are complete. These simple observations have contributed greatly toward a satisfactory conclusion in the patients upon whom we have performed choledochostomy.

SUMMARY

Certain definite criteria should exist before the common bile duct is opened. These are:

1. Palpable stone in the hepatic or common bile ducts
2. Jaundice—on admission to the hospital or recent
3. Dilatation or thickening of the bile ducts
4. Clinical evidence of cholangitis
5. Small stones in the gall bladder
6. Thickening or induration of the head of the pancreas
7. Biliary colic without stones in gall bladder

The presence of any one of these criteria demands choledochotomy. A small contracted gall bladder is not considered as an indication for choledochotomy nor is a history of jaundice unless its occurrence has been recent.

The incidence of retained calculi in this group of patients is 5.9 per cent.

In all patients the common duct was drained through a T tube or catheter. The length of time the tube remained in situ depended upon the findings at operation. Conclusions, based upon the observations of the surgeon at operation, are made upon the length of time external drainage of the hepatic and common bile ducts should be carried out.

REFERENCES

1. Mixter, C. G., and Hermanson, L.: Am. J. Surg. **40**: 223-231, 1938.
2. Daseler, E. H., Anson, B. J., Hambley, W. C., and Reimann, A. F.: Surg., Gynec. & Obst. **85**: 47-63, 1947.

MYOTONIA ACQUISITA DUE TO CHRONIC CALCULOUS CHOLECYSTITIS AND CURED BY CHOLECYSTECTOMY

I. DARIN PUPPEL, M.D., AND EDITH KLINE, M.D., COLUMBUS, OHIO

(From the Department of Research Surgery of The Ohio State University)

MYOTONIA acquisita is a rare disease of muscle which presents the outstanding features of increased muscular irritability and contractility associated with diminution in the power of relaxation. It constitutes a syndrome which includes the *myotonic disorder of movement* with stiffness, tension, and spasm in the voluntary muscles when movements are initiated, the *myotonic reaction* with normal mechanical and electrical excitability of the motor nerves, but an increased mechanical and electrical excitability of the muscles, and *muscular hypertrophy*.

There have now been described to our knowledge thirty-six cases of myotonia acquisita.[1, 2] These have all occurred in men patients except one. The one case occurring in a woman was reported by Nosik and Shannon[3] in 1942.

The acquired form (myotonia acquisita or Talma's disease) has been usually differentiated from the congenital form (myotonia congenita or Thomsen's disease) although these may be different chronologic manifestations of the same underlying pathologic process. The underlying pathogenesis is as yet not fully understood even though we know Talma's disease is not congenital in origin but usually develops in adult life following or during an infection or following trauma or intoxication. In fact, myotonia acquisita frequently, if not always, is secondary to some other disease entity. It has already been described to have occurred following trauma, dysentery, gastroenteritis, alcoholism, lead poisoning, tuberculosis, and typhoid fever. The disease tends to improve spontaneously or go on to complete recovery. Frequently, however, it is important to search for an underlying primary cause in the secondary form since removal of this factor may decrease the severity and length of morbidity of the myotonia such as is demonstrated in our case. Myotonia apparently followed chronic calculous cholecystitis with an associated chronic hepatitis and was cured after cholecystectomy, choledochostomy, and adequate follow-up treatment of the hepatitis in the case we are about to report.

CASE REPORT

The data up to 1942 on this patient are fully described in the report of Nosik and Shannon.[3] While at the Cleveland Clinic in 1942 she complained of cramping muscles and swelling of joints. She became aware for the first time of cramping pain in the right calf with radiation down to the foot in 1936, three months following a panhysterectomy for menorrhagia. The pain often awakened the patient during the night and was not related to exercise. Marked inversion and plantar flexion of the right foot frequently were associated with the severe pain. The other calf and both arms were similarly involved in pain. Fibrillary twitching of the muscles accompanied the pain in 1937. Painful swelling of various joints of the body and particularly those of the hands, shoulders, and ankles was noted in 1941. This was accompanied by a weight gain of twenty pounds. She then complained of practically a con-

Received for publication, July 30, 1947.
Aided by a grant from the Comly Fund for Research of The Ohio State University.

stant "spasm" of the right calf of four years' duration, whereas in the beginning the spasms were intermittent in character, each lasting about thirty minutes. A cramping sensation in the left arm and shoulder girdle, and in the muscles of the back then developed. The right arm and shoulder girdle were similarly involved and during 1941 retardation of movements of this side and severe headaches occurred. The patient had always been of a nervous temperament. There had been an exaggeration of this symptom following the surgical menopause in 1936. She stated she had a "nervous breakdown" in 1937 which required sanatorium care. Neurologic examination in 1942 revealed negative findings. The right calf was in a continuous state of contraction. Reflexes were all brisk and nonpathologic. Faradic and galvanic stimulation of the motor nerves was normal but there was a hyperirritability of the right calf muscles. A piece of the right gastrocnemius muscle was taken for biopsy. Sections of it showed normal striated muscle with areas of degeneration and hyalinization of muscle fibers. Some fibrosis of the intermuscular septa was present without a sign of active inflammatory reaction, parasites, or neoplasm. Pain was then the outstanding symptom. No hypertrophy of the muscles was found although the myotonic syndrome was present. The patient was unable to relax the affected muscles or to initiate a rapid movement. The myotonic reaction to mechanical and electrical stimuli was observed.

After leaving the Cleveland Clinic the patient continued to have almost constant severely painful spasms of the right calf muscles. Cramps often occurred at night but were worse on walking. Because of stiffness of these muscles, difficulty in arising from the sitting position and in beginning to walk was associated. The patient was exhausted after walking a short distance. There later occurred a constant increase in the size of the calf which was present even when there was no spasm. Frequently this area felt stone hard. Mental and emotional upsets did not seem to agitate the condition. Climbing stairs aggravated the pain. It finally became necessary for her to hire help to do the housework. She visited several physicians for treatment of this disease but without permanent improvement. Local application of heat gave only temporary and partial relief of pain. Liniments and pills produced similar temporary results. The sciatic nerve was injected at one time with novocain which, the patient believed, accentuated the pain. She became much depressed because of this continued disability and was discouraged by the many unsuccessful attempts to remedy the disease.

The patient entered University Hospital on Jan. 14, 1945, complaining of this condition but principally of episodes of epigastric distress which began approximately seven years prior to admission. These were characterized by gaseous eructations and abdominal distention. They occurred frequently after eating fatty foods. The patient had four to six attacks a year of vertigo, nausea, and vomiting of bile-stained fluid, each of which lasted for from twenty-four to forty-eight hours. The accompanying pain was sharp and intermittent in type. It frequently radiated to the tip of the right scapula and was aggravated by body movement. Often epigastric and upper right quadrant tenderness remained following the pain. Fever was associated during the attacks, but there were no chills. Jaundice of the scleras and the skin with marked pruritus was present intermittently for several years. During these attacks of jaundice the stools were clay-colored. Cholecystography revealed the presence of many gallstones in the gall bladder.

Physical examination showed the patient to be well developed and rather obese. Her stated age was 49 years. She did not appear acutely ill. The temperature was 98.4° F., with the pulse 70, respirations 20, and the blood pressure 126 systolic and 80 diastolic. The skin was warm, dry, and showed no evidence of jaundice. The pupils were regular, round, and reacted well to light and accommodation. The scleras were normal in color. The conjunctivae appeared normal. Nasal examination revealed no abnormalities. She wore a complete upper artificial denture. The lower teeth were in good repair. Examination of the oropharynx gave negative findings. There were no abnormalities of the neck, and no gross abnormalities of the chest. The breasts were obese and pendulous but otherwise normal. The lungs were clear to percussion and auscultation. The heart was normal in size to percussion; its sounds were of normal quality and no murmurs were present. There was marked tenderness on moderate pressure of the upper right quadrant of the abdomen. The point of maximum tenderness was at the Mayo-Robson area. The liver extended 1½ fingerbreadths below the right costal margin on deep inspiration. It was tender and definitely enlarged on percussion. There was present a well-healed hysterectomy scar. Otherwise results of the remainder of the abdominal examination were negative. The right leg, even when relaxed, was definitely larger than its mate on inspection and measured 2.5 cm. greater in circumference

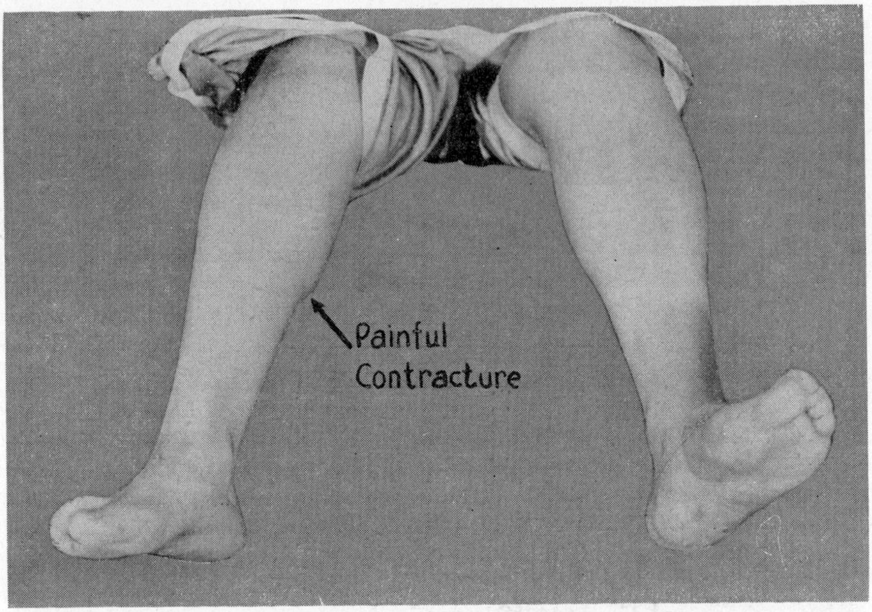

A.

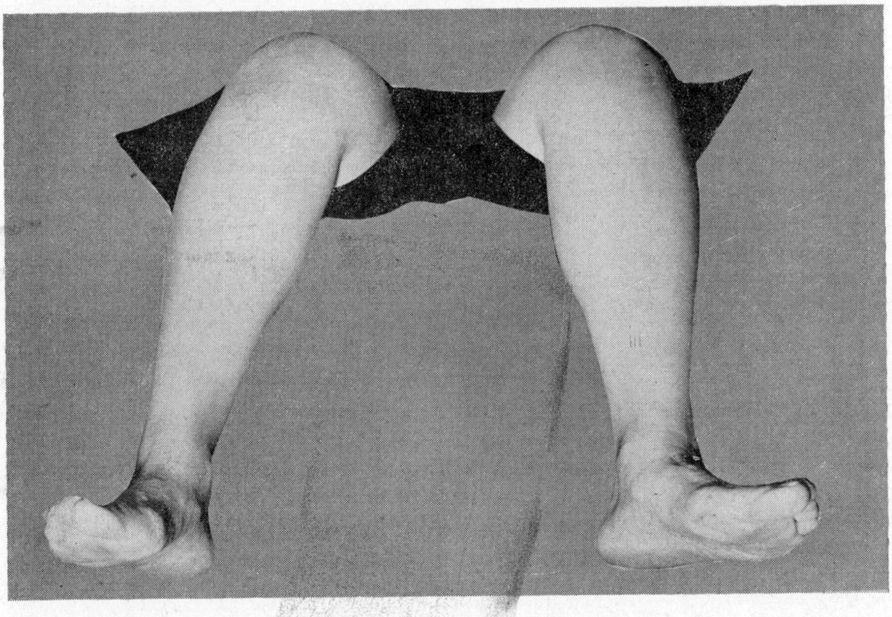

B.

Fig. 1.—*A*, The calf muscles of the right leg were outstanding, hard as wood, and very tender to palpation on Jan. 16, 1945, two days prior to cholecystectomy and choledochostomy. *B*, The right calf muscles returned to normal contour, size, and consistency and were nontender by April 12, 1947.

than the left at the mid-calf area. The calf muscles of the right leg when contracted were outstanding, hard as wood, and very tender to palpation (Fig. 1, *A*). There were no evidences of atrophy (Fig. 1, *A*). Gait was slow and labored and she walked the stairs with considerable difficulty. The reflexes were physiologic throughout.

On admission the red blood count was 4,800,000 with hemoglobin 13.2 Gm. per cent. The white blood cells were 13,500 with neutrophiles 69 per cent, lymphocytes 27 per cent, monocytes 2 per cent, eosinophiles 1 per cent, and basophiles 1 per cent. The segmenters were 64 per cent and the non-segmenters 5 per cent. The blood Kahn and Mazzini tests for syphilis gave negative results. The bleeding time using the Duke method was 1 minute 20 seconds and the clotting time using the Lee and White method was 4 minutes 40 seconds, which are normal. The icterus index was 5.0; the direct van den Bergh, negative; and the indirect less than 0.2 mg. per cent, which are normal. The blood urea nitrogen was 25.0 and the blood sugar 101.0 mg. per cent. The blood cholesterol was 190 mg. per cent, which is normal. The hippuric acid test for liver function yielded 2.90 Gm., which is also normal. The blood prothrombin was 60 per cent of normal, which is slightly decreased.

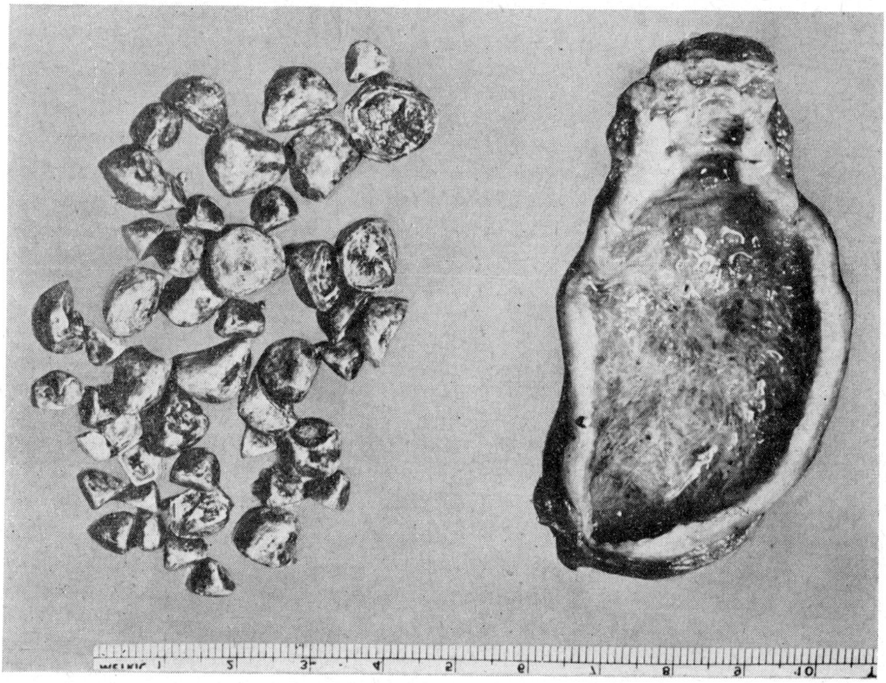

Fig. 2.—Chronic cholecystitis with cholelithiasis.

Preoperatively the patient received a high carbohydrate, high protein, low fat, and high vitamin diet. Glucose-reinforced fruit juices were given between meals and 1 ampule of synkayvite (vitamin K) was given on each of two days before operation. On Jan. 18 1945, exploratory celiotomy revealed the gall bladder to be greatly distended with many stones (Fig. 2). Its wall was edematous, thick, and showed evidence of chronic inflammation (Fig. 2). Dense pericholecystic adhesions were present which bound the gall bladder down to the common bile duct. The latter structure was easily uncovered and definitely dilated. The common bile duct was therefore explored just below the juncture of the cystic duct through an incision about 1 cm. in length. Stones could not be discovered and the duct seemed to be patent throughout. A small Kehr tube was therefore trimmed and placed in the common bile duct. The wound of the duct was then closed by interrupted sutures of black silk to prevent leakage of bile around the tube. The cystic duct as well as a cystic artery was then uncovered and individually ligated with double sutures of medium black silk. The gall bladder was excised in the usual fashion and the uncovered area of the liver was reperitonealized with interrupted sutures of fine black silk. A medium-sized cigarette drain was placed in the pouch of Morison. Both the long end of the Kehr tube and the cigarette drain were brought through the abdominal incision. Five grams of microform sulfathiazole were then dusted lightly about the intra-abdominal operative area. The abdominal incision was closed in a routine manner using interrupted sutures of black silk in layers throughout.

The postoperative course remained uneventful. Adequate amounts of 10 per cent glucose in distilled water as well as normal saline solution were given during the first two days postoperatively. The cigarette drain was completely removed on the fourth day. Postoperatively the diet was increased rapidly as tolerated to the preoperative type of intake. Early ambulation was carried out. Synkayvite in adequate amounts was administered. The bile appeared dark green and cloudy so that two tablets of ketochol were given three times daily beginning on January 22. Twenty-four hours later definite increase in the amount of bile drainage was noted and this became more golden yellow in color by Jan. 25, 1945. The skin sutures were removed on the seventh day. Cholangiography was done on January 30, the twelfth postoperative day, using lipiodol, which visualized the left and right hepatic ducts, the common hepatic duct, and the common bile duct to be normal in appearance without evidence of stones or of obstruction. The lipiodol passed freely into the duodenum. The Kehr tube was therefore clamped. The patient remained symptom-free and this tube was removed on the fourteenth postoperative day. The patient was discharged on Feb. 3, 1945, to return to our office.

By Sept. 25, 1945, the spasms referable to the right lower extremity, which had been present for eight years prior to surgery, had practically subsided. She had been treated by various physicians throughout these years without relief. However, after cholecystectomy with choledochostomy the pain referable to the right calf muscles rapidly disappeared. Thereafter, the contracture of these muscles also disappeared gradually. At this examination she complained only of an occasional slight stiffness but no contractions of the muscles. Frequent follow-up examinations since September, 1945, showed the muscular hypertrophy to remain for a long time after the myotonic symptoms had disappeared. However, this limb gradually returned to a normal size so that on April 12, 1947, measurements of the lower extremities revealed them to be equal in circumference (Fig. 1, *B*) at 45.0 cm. above (7.5 cm.) the knees, 34.0 cm. below (7.5 cm.) the knees, 35.5 cm. at mid-calf (12.5 cm. below the knees), and 20.5 cm. at the ankles. Mental depression had disappeared since cholecystectomy so that she felt that life was now worth living. The headaches had completely disappeared. The symptoms referable to other parts of the body had disappeared to a great extent. Gait was normal and she was able to carry out all normal activities including housework.

SUMMARY

Apparently the etiologic factor which explained the myotonia and muscular hypertrophy in this case was a chronic calculous cholecystitis with an accompanying chronic hepatitis of several years' duration. After removal of the gall bladder and adequate treatment of the hepatitis the whole syndrome completely subsided. This case was also of unusual interest since it appeared to be the first of its kind reported to have occurred in a woman.

REFERENCES

1. Krabbe, Knud H.: The Myotonia Acquisita in Relation to the Postneuritic Muscular Hypertrophy, Brain **57**: 184, 1934.
2. Moore, M. T.: Myotonia Acquisita. A Case Showing Myotonia in Both Lower Limbs Following Injury, Am. J. Syph. & Neurol. **19**: 409, 1935.
3. Nosik, William A., and Shannon, E. W.: Myotonia Acquisita (Talma's Disease), Cleveland Clin. Quart. **9**: 185, 1942.

HERPES ZOSTER AND THE SURGICAL ABDOMEN

LEWIS H. BOSHER, JR., M.D., AND CARRINGTON WILLIAMS, JR., M.D.
RICHMOND, VA.

(From the Department of Surgery, Medical College of Virginia)

AMONG the many causes of abdominal pain which must be differentiated in the diagnosis of the surgical abdomen, herpes zoster may offer a difficult challenge to the examiner. That this syndrome may mimic intra-abdominal pathology has been pointed out by various investigators in the past, but the close simulation of conditions requiring surgical intervention is not clearly or readily appreciated. Two patients with abdominal pain as the primary symptom have recently been seen in whom the clinical picture of intra-abdominal disease was so closely simulated by herpes zoster as to cause difficulty in correct diagnosis.

In brief, the major clinical manifestations of herpes zoster are as follows: the disease is frequently preceded by an upper respiratory infection which antedates the onset of symptoms from the zoster infection by several days. The chief complaint is usually that of rather severe and steady, sometimes stabbing pain distributed in a radiating course along the extent of one or more peripheral nerves, usually in the trunk region. The skin eruption which is characterized by groups of vesicles on an erythematous base ordinarily comes on several days after the onset of the pain and is distributed also along the course of the sensory nerve. The disease usually attacks the dorsal root ganglia of the thoracic segments but commonly involves also the areas supplied by the trigeminal and first lumbar nerves. It is in the preherpetic stage of herpes zoster that confusion with visceral disease usually occurs.

The possibility of confusing herpes zoster with visceral disease has been previously noted by several authors. In 1902 Curtin[9] reported one case of "catarrhal appendicitis" which subsided and then was followed by herpes zoster. He also described mimicry of intrathoracic and renal pathology by the syndrome. In his *Differential Diagnosis* Cabot[4] listed herpes zoster as the cause of lumbar pain as often as all renal diseases combined. Litchfield[12] in 1913 wrote on acute posterior ganglionitis simulating surgical conditions in the abdomen. He cited cases where ureteral colic and cholecystic disease were ruled out by the appearance of herpetic rashes and quoted Marinacci's description of a case thought to be generalized peritonitis but later proved to be herpes. Barney,[1] Blanton,[2] and Young[14] have described cases of herpes zoster simulating renal disease. Boland[3] remarked on the lack of comment in dermatology books concerning the possibility of confusing herpes with acute abdominal disease. He then cited a case erroneously diagnosed as acute appendicitis, in which operation was fortunately delayed until the appearance of the herpetic eruption. Among other authors who have listed herpes zoster with diseases to be considered in the differential diagnosis of the acute abdomen are Paullin[13] and Comroe.[8]

Received for publication, Aug. 8, 1947.

In an extensive review of 137 hospitalized cases of herpes zoster, Gais and Abrahamson[11] found that pain was the chief complaint in 118 patients. Of 34 cases in which abdominal or lumbar pain was the primary symptom, erroneous diagnoses were made in 26 cases. Failure to diagnose herpes zoster led to surgery in 2 instances. The erroneous diagnoses covered a wide range of abdominal diseases. Since this is the only large series of such cases yet presented in the literature, certain statistics supplied by Gais and Abrahamson are of interest. Most frequently the pain involved the right upper quadrant but all regions of the abdomen were included. Tenderness, rigidity, anorexia, nausea, and vomiting were present in many. The difficulty in diagnosis led to x-ray studies in 10 patients. Of the 6 patients with lumbar pain, all had costovertebral angle tenderness, 4 had dysuria, 3 frequency, 2 hematuria; and 1 nausea and vomiting. Retrograde pyelography was carried out in 5 of the 6 cases.

Intercostal neuralgia or posterior radiculoganglionitis is a syndrome described by Carnett[5, 6] and by Davis,[10] and this is said to account for many otherwise unexplained cases of abdominal pain. Carnett referred to intercostal neuralgia as the cause of pain in "pseudo-appendicitis," a designation for those cases of "appendicitis" which the pathologist is unable to confirm. Whereas skin hyperesthesia is usually explained on the basis of the viscerosensory reflex, Carnett attributed it to an intercostal neuralgia. In a report of over 250 school children suffering from pain in the area of distribution of the lower thoracic nerves, Davis concluded that the pains were due to a radiculoganglionitis (segmental neuralgia) caused by a neurotropic virus associated with the common cold. He suggested that vesiculation may be unusual in zoster and that subherpetic manifestations may be the rule. In only 2 of his 250 cases did herpes develop. The characteristic features of this syndrome are segmental pain and skin hyperesthesia. Davis pointed out the similarity of this condition to appendicitis, renal colic, cholelithiasis, pleurisy, colitis, etc. Fever is usually not present but vomiting may be associated. However, in constrast to the unilateral nature of herpes zoster, 40 per cent of the cases reported by Davis showed bilateral symptoms. In the cases referred to by Carnett the symptoms were frequently bilateral.

We have recently seen a patient admitted to the hospital with a presumptive diagnosis of perinephric abscess in which the diagnosis of segmental neuralgia seemed justified. A brief report follows.

CASE REPORT

A 15-year-old colored boy was admitted to St. Philip Hospital complaining of left lower quadrant and left flank pain of two weeks' duration. Three weeks prior to admission, the patient had been discharged following treatment for diabetic acidosis and mild bronchopneumonia. The pain was described as originating in the back and radiating anteriorly into the left lower quadrant. Anorexia was present but no nausea, vomiting, bowel disturbances, or urinary symptoms. The pains had increased in severity during the three days before admission. On admission the temperature was 99.6° F., pulse 70, respirations 22. With the exception of a mild conjunctivitis, the positive findings were limited to the trunk and abdomen. Examination revealed a soft abdomen without spasm. There was apparent tenderness in the left lower quadrant, flank, and costovertebral angle. The tenderness did not appear to be increased by deep palpation. It was still present on examination with the abdominal muscles tensed, thus indicating that most of the pain at least was parietal (positive Carnett's sign). There was a definite band of hyperesthesia extending from the midline of the back in the approximate distribution of the eleventh thoracic nerve and stopping sharply at the midline anteriorly. The white count and urine were normal. A spinal fluid examination showed only 3 lymphocytes and a protein of 50.

Following an intercostal nerve block with 1 per cent novocain in the region of the tenth and eleventh thoracic nerves posteriorly, the pain and hyperesthesia completely disappeared and palpation no longer elicited tenderness. This relief was permanent with the exception of some persisting hyperesthesia in the distribution of the posterior ramus of the tenth thoracic nerve. During a period of observation lasting over ten days, herpetic lesions did not develop.

The following two cases simulating surgical disease presented definite evidence of herpes zoster.

CASE 1.—A colored man, aged 30 years, was admited to St. Philip Hospital on Oct. 11, 1946, complaining of abdominal pain and vomiting of one day's duration. Approximately twenty-four hours before admission he had become nauseated and vomited. Shortly thereafter he noted the onset of crampy pain in the right lower quadrant which soon involved the entire abdomen and later localized again in the right lower quadrant. He continued to vomit intermittently until admission. No history of urinary symptoms or other gastrointestinal disturbances could be elicited. For four days prior to admission he had noted some tenderness in the right flank and right lower abdomen.

Temperature on admission was 100.4° F., but this shortly afterward was recorded as 99° F., per rectum. Pulse was 77, respirations 28. Abdominal examination revealed tenderness with rebound in the right lower quadrant near McBurney's point, with associated skin hyperesthesia. One observer thought that muscle spasm was present in the right lower quadrant. There was some tenderness high on the right by rectal examination. Inspection of the skin revealed small groups of vesicles on an elevated base extending in a linear fashion from the midline of the back into the right lower quadrant in the approximate distribution of the eleventh intercostal nerve. There was a small group in the region of McBurney's point, approximately 3 cm. in diameter.

Laboratory examination revealed a red blood cell count of 2,900,000, with 60 per cent hemoglobin, white count of 6,900, 72 per cent polymorphonuclears, and 28 per cent lymphocytes. Urinalysis was negative except for 1 plus albumin. Despite the obvious presence of herpetic lesions it was felt that the symptoms and signs were sufficiently suggestive of acute appendicitis to warrant an exploratory laparotomy.

The abdomen was opened through a McBurney incision. The appendix appeared grossly normal; there were a few small mesenteric nodes which did not appear to be inflamed. Pathologic report on the appendix was chronic healed appendicitis with fibrous obliteration of the lumen. There was some round-cell infiltration but no evidence of acute inflammation. The patient's abdominal pain was not relieved by operation and at the time of discharge five days later the rash was still present.

CASE 2.—A white man, aged 70 years, was admitted to the Medical College Hospital on Nov. 5, 1946, complaining of abdominal pain of six days' duration. Six days before admission the patient had noted the sudden onset of severe pain in the right lower quadrant, radiating at times into the right flank. The pain became dull and aching, was severe enough to interfere with sleeping, and persisted until admission. There were no crampy or colicky pains. Anorexia had been present, but no nausea or vomiting. A vague history of recent nocturia and dysuria was obtained. The past history was not directly contributory. Six weeks before admission the patient had suffered a short period of constipation. For forty years he had passed bright red blood per rectum intermittently. There was no history of weight loss and the appetite had been good until the presenting illness.

On admission the temperature, pulse, and respirations were normal. Physical examination revealed a soft, scaphoid abdomen with diffuse tenderness in the right lower quadrant extending into the flank and with some costovertebral angle tenderness. No hyperesthesia of the skin was noted. Rebound tenderness was not present. No organs or masses were palpable. Peristalsis was somewhat hyperactive and continuous. Rectal examination was negative with the exception of tender external hemorrhoids and an enlarged prostate.

Laboratory examination revealed a white blood cell count of 6,800, with 63 per cent polymorphonuclears, 30 per cent lymphocytes, 2 per cent eosinophiles, and 5 per cent monocytes. The hemoglobin was 96 per cent, with a red blood cell count of 4,650,000. Initial urine examination showed a specific gravity of 1.012 and was otherwise normal. A definite diagnosis could not be made on admission, but a carcinoma of the right side of the colon or some kidney lesion was considered most likely. Blood chemistry revealed a sugar of 93, nonprotein nitrogenof 30, total proteins 6.6, with albumin 4.0. Flocculation was negative. Total phenolsulfonphthalein excretion was 43 per cent and Mosenthal concentration 1.020. Stools were negative for blood. A proctoscopic examination showed only internal and external hemorrhoids. Intravenous pyelogram and barium enema were likewise normal.

On the fourth day after admission, ten days after the onset of pain, herpetic lesions consisting of vesicles arranged in small groups surrounded by areas of erythema appeared on the trunk. The groups were separated by areas of normal skin. The lesions extended from the right side of the spine almost around to the umbilicus in the distribution of the tenth intercostal nerve. By the time of the appearance of these lesions the patient's abdominal soreness and tenderness had practically subsided. At the time of discharge on the eighth hospital day the lesions were beginning to fade.

DISCUSSION

In the first case of herpes zoster presented, in which the additional diagnosis of appendicitis was made, a posterior intercostal nerve block would have permitted more accurate evaluation of the apparent deep tenderness. The application of Carnett's test, that is, palpation with the abdominal musculature tense, would probably have suggested that the pain and tenderness were predominantly parietal. Under such conditions, one would expect that the tenderness would remain unchanged or be only slightly diminished, in contrast to disappearance of tenderness in intra-abdominal disease. The absence of severe systemic symptoms and the normal white count were consistent with the diagnosis of herpes. Rarely does the temperature rise above 100° F. in herpes. In the large series of cases presented by Gais and Abrahamson the leucocyte count ranged between 5000 and 7000, and in none was it reported above 10,000.

In the second case, the long interval of ten days between the onset of symptoms and the appearance of the rash postponed the correct diagnosis and permitted an unnecessary number of expensive laboratory procedures to be carried out. This interval, though longer than the average reported, is certainly not unusual. An examination of the spinal fluid may or may not be of value. Though a lymphocytosis of the spinal fluid is usually stated to be present in herpes zoster, Gais and Abrahamson found it in only 50 per cent of the eleven patients so examined. Davis stated that in the cases of so-called intercostal neuralgia mentioned previously, the spinal fluid was almost always negative.

A recognition of the radicular nature of the pain, of the presence of hyperesthesia, the degree of which may vary considerably, and a careful examination to demonstrate the segmental distribution with limitation at the midline anteriorly will aid materially in the differential diagnosis of herpes zoster and the surgical abdomen. Gais and Abrahamson point out that careful examination of the back sometimes will reveal a single vesicle indicating the correct diagnosis.

SUMMARY

1. Herpes zoster may offer a difficult challenge to the examiner in differentiating causes for abdominal pain.

2. The characteristic pain in herpes zoster is one radiating from the back to the midline anteriorly in the distribution of one or more spinal nerves, usually in the lower thoracic segments.

3. The syndrome usually follows an upper respiratory infection by several days and may be manifested as an intercostal neuralgia without the herpetic eruption.

4. Carnett's test, to suggest whether the pain and tenderness arise in the abdominal wall or in the viscera, is a useful adjuvant in the examination of a patient with abdominal pain.

5. Careful plotting out of the area of skin hyperesthesia and novocain block of the nerves supplying this area may aid in establishing the origin of the patient's presenting complaint.

6. Two cases of herpes zoster and one case resembling intercostal neuralgia are reported to show the close simulation of the acute surgical abdomen by these conditions.

REFERENCES

1. Barney, J. D.: A Case of Herpes Zoster Mistaken for Renal Disease, New England J. Med. **203**: 1012, 1930.
2. Blanton, W. B.: Herpes Zoster Simulating Nephrolithiasis, J. A. M. A. **85**: 1811, 1925.
3. Boland, F. K.: The Interpretation of Abdominal Pain, South. M. J. **28**: 133, 1935.
4. Cabot, R. C.: Differential Diagnosis, Philadelphia, 1911, W. B. Saunders Company.
5. Carnett, J. B.: Acute and Recurrent Pseudoappendicitis Due to Intercostal Neuralgia, Am. J. M. Sc. **174**: 833, 1927.
6. Carnett, J. B.: Chronic Pseudoappendicitis Due to Intercostal Neuralgia, Am. J. M. Sc. **174**: 579, 1927.
7. Carnett, J. B.: Pain and Tenderness of the Abdominal Wall, J. A. M. A. **102**: 345, 1934.
8. Comroe, B. I.: Non-Surgical Causes of Abdominal Pain, Ann. Surg. **101**: 438, 1935.
9. Curtin, R. B.: Herpes Zoster and Its Relation to Internal Inflammations and Diseases, Especially of the Serous Membranes, Am. J. M. Sc. **123**: 264, 1902.
10. Davis, J. H.: Segmental Neuralgia in Childhood Simulating Visceral Disease, J. A. M. A. **107**: 1620, 1936.
11. Gais, R. S., and Abrahamson, R. H.: Herpes Zoster and Its Visceral Manifestations, Am. J. M. Sc. **197**: 817, 1939.
12. Litchfield, L.: Acute Posterior Ganglionitis Simulating Surgical Conditions in the Abdomen, J. A. M. A. **60**: 1691, 1913.
13. Paullin, J. E.: Symptoms and Signs Referred to the Abdomen the Result of Disorders Elsewhere, South. M. J. **27**: 331, 1934.
14. Young, E. L.: Herpes Zoster, as a Differential Diagnosis in Surgical Conditions of the Abdomen and Kidneys, Am. J. Surg. **22**: 335, 1933.

MESENTERIC THROMBOSIS

J. E. McClenahan, M.D., and Bernard Fisher, M.D., Pittsburgh, Pa.

(From Department of Surgery, Mercy Hospital, and University of Pittsburgh, Medical School)

The purpose of this paper is to review briefly the subject of mesenteric thrombosis from the standpoint of current literature and to present a series of forty cases encountered at the Mercy Hospital during the last twenty years. Of more importance, it will stress two ideas which are deserving more emphasis than they have previously received. One is that mesenteric thrombosis occurs more commonly in a milder form than is often appreciated, accounting for many vague abdominal symptoms in older people without there necessarily being a massive abdominal accident. The picture may be compared to "angina" caused by coronary insufficiency, "cerebral spasm" which results from cerebral circulation insufficiency, or "intermittent claudication" due to insufficiency of the circulation of the extremities. A similar syndrome may occur in the abdomen where intestinal circulation is impaired in a gradual manner as by arteriosclerosis. We believe that it is possible to predict or anticipate a massive abdominal occlusion in some of these people, just as severe coronary occlusion may be predicted in people with angina, and gangrene of extremities in people with intermittent claudication. As is pointed out by Dunphy,[1] this condition has been described for years, but a lack of post-mortem evidence has prevented its acceptance as a clinical fact. As early as 1905, Pal[2] of Austria stressed this idea when writing about vascular crises.

Second, it will be emphasized that in spite of what one's thoughts may be in regard to surgery in general, there is no place for conservatism in the treatment of this condition when it presents itself as an acute abdominal emergency. Radical surgery is the only hope in saving life.

INCIDENCE

Ficarra,[3] in November, 1944, brought the medical literature up to date. He reported at that time 569 cases with 35 successful resections. Since then, no large series has been presented. A review of the literature since his article adds 7 more cases with 3 successful resections. To these we now add 40 cases with 5 successful resections; thus bringing the totals to 616 cases with 43, or 7 per cent, successful resections. Since there was an average of 10,000 admissions per year in the Mercy Hospital over this period of time, we find that the incidence in this institution was one case in 5,000, or .002 per cent.

Of our 40 patients, 23 were men, 17 women. All 40 occurred in white people; no Negro receiving the diagnosis in spite of the fact that many are admitted to this institution. In comparing the incidence with other places, we find that the Michael Reese Hospital in Chicago had 44 cases in ten years, or .105

Received for publication, Aug. 8, 1947.

per cent of all *surgical* admissions. The Kings County Hospital in New York had 35 cases in eight years. Warren and Eberhard[4] found that only .041 per cent of the admissions in their institution received this diagnosis.

Although the incidence of mesenteric thrombosis is greatest between the third and sixth decades, it may occur at any age. In our series the youngest patient was 27 years old, the oldest 82. Of our cases, 57 per cent occurred between the ages of 40 and 60 years. Laufman and Scheinberg[5] reported cases where infants 10 days, 11 days, and 5 years of age were operated on for this condition. These are the exceptions and for the most part the condition occurs at the age where degenerative diseases begin to appear.

In this series of 40 cases, the diagnosis was definitely proved in 27, or 67 per cent, by either operation or autopsy. Of these 27 cases, 11 came to autopsy, 16 were operated upon, and 3 came to autopsy after operation. The remaining 13, or one-third of the total, were diagnosed clinically and, of course, it is quite impossible to prove the diagnosis in this group.

Proven Dg

MORTALITY

The group which was not proved by operation or autopsy, that is, the 13 cases, may be dismissed by saying that of this number 12 patients died, for a mortality of 92 per cent. Of these 13 cases, 8 were the results of a primary heart disease, 3 followed previous surgery, and 2 were primary in nature. Operation was not attempted in any of these cases because of the generally universal feeling by the surgeon that the patient could not tolerate surgery. Perhaps it is wishful thinking that at least one of these patients might have benefited by surgery.

In the proved group of 27 cases, 19 patients were operated upon and 5 lived, for a mortality rate of 73 per cent. Of this group of 19, there were 6 patients in whom nothing but the diagnosis was established by opening and closing the abdomen. One cannot consider these individuals as having been operated upon in the ordinary conception of surgery. All 6 died. Of the remaining 13, where some operative procedure was done, 5, or 39 per cent lived. So, of all cases where some operative procedure, other than just opening and closing the abdomen was performed, the mortality rate was 61 per cent. In the group in which nothing was done, the mortality rate was 95 per cent. Thus, it would seem that surgery gives the patient about one chance in three to survive, while watchful waiting has little to offer but death.

Our operative mortality figures compare favorably with those of other clinics. Michael Reese has a rate of 67 per cent; Kings County, 71 per cent; a review of 104 cases from the literature by Brown[6] in the American Journal of Surgery, 68.2 per cent; and Whittaker and Pemberton[7] reported from Mayo Clinic a mortality of 84 per cent following surgical intervention.

ANATOMY AND PATHOLOGIC PHYSIOLOGY

The blood supply to the small bowel is derived from the superior mesenteric artery which also supplies the large bowel as far as the middle of the transverse colon. Large bowel distal to this is nourished by the inferior mesenteric artery.

The superior mesenteric artery gives off from ten to sixteen intestinal branches which are divisible into two groups, jejunal and ileal, passing between the layers of the mesentery toward the small intestine. Each of these divides into two branches which anastomose with those of adjacent arteries to form a series of arcades from which secondary branches are given off. With the lower ileal arteries this may happen four or five times so that there may be four or five tiers or arcades. In the jejunum there may be only two arcades present. From the terminal arcades, straight vessels pass to supply the intestinal wall. These so-called "vasa recta" do not anastomose. Of prime importance in knowledge of circulation of the abdomen is the fact that the inferior pancreaticoduodenalis, another branch of the superior mesenteric artery, anastomoses with the superior pancreaticoduodenalis which comes from the coeliac axis. This forms an obvious channel for the development of collateral circulation in cases of occlusion of the superior mesenteric artery. The greatest benefit derived from this collateral circulation is in cases of gradual occlusion rather than in those of a sudden nature. This collateral circulation no doubt plays an important role in those occasional patients with mesenteric thrombosis who get well even though no surgery is done.

The superior mesenteric artery arises from the aorta at such an angle immediately below the celiac axis that its main stem parallels to some extent the abdominal aorta. Thus, it has almost a direct connection with the heart and for this reason is particularly vulnerable to emboli from it. As a matter of fact, of any 100 cases of arterial occlusion of the abdomen, 96 per cent occur in the superior mesenteric artery, while the remaining 4 per cent are distributed in the inferior mesenteric artery and the celiac axis.

In contrast to the arterial distribution, all blood collected into the veins of the abdominal part of the digestive tract passes into the portal vein by which it is filtered into the liver and then through the hepatic veins to the vena cava. A thrombus arising in the lumen of a vein may do one of two things: (1) give off an embolus into the cephalic channels, or (2) block off venous channel so that a descending thrombosis extending toward the bowel might occur.

The pathologic picture which results from vascular occlusion is infarction and hemorrhage throughout all layers of the bowel with accumulation of blood in the lumen. It seems strange that this should occur in an organ where the collateral circulation is so abundant. The reason was proposed by Litten in 1889 when he showed that the superior mesenteric artery acts as an end artery. Sudden occlusion of a branch may set up a severe spasm of the musculature of the intestines, sometimes as far as from the ligament of Treitz to the middle of the transverse colon. This spasm is due to the sudden anemia which results from the cessation of arterial blood flow. At this stage the bowel appears as a firm, white, rippled structure; then, in a matter of three or four hours, as the musculature fatigues, it relaxes, some parts more rapidly than others. The result is a splotching of the bowel with bluish-red areas of discoloration. In forty-eight hours the musculature is completely relaxed and the entire bowel has a dark blue, blood-soaked appearance. These facts lead to the emphasis of the idea that wide radical resection is absolutely necessary. Although the surgeon may feel that he is wide of the gangrenous bowel in the resection, if he is not sufficiently far away, he may be making the anastomosis in a part of bowel which has not yet relaxed, but within a few hours will become engorged and gangrenous. The exact mechanism of hemorrhagic infarction has always been controversial. Experimental work has shown that, as the musculature of the intestine relaxes, the negative pressure created in both arterial occlusion and venous occlusion is sufficient to draw blood into the walls of the bowel, causing it to become markedly engorged, thus having the characteristics of other infarcted tissue. Whenever venous obstruction occurs it is quite easy to see why the damming back and congestion of blood should occur. Pathologically, then, the picture of mesenteric thrombosis shows microscopically an involved segment of bowel which is thickened, edematous, dark red in color, and rapidly becoming gangrenous. The lumen contains blood and the peritoneal cavity contains bloody fluid. Microscopically the lumen of the bowel is filled with a large amount of hemorrhagic edema fluid. The mucosal lining shows all stages of degeneration ranging from edema to necrosis. Edema is seen in the submucosa. The muscular layer and serosa show a hemorrhagic reaction. Frequently the vessels are seen to be dilated and filled with erythrocytes. The mesentery itself is usually markedly thickened, containing large patches of hemorrhage, and the mesenteric glands may be swollen and hemorrhagic.

ETIOLOGY

Many authors have written at length on the etiologic factors of mesenteric vascular occlusion. It may suffice to present a simple outline of the numerous predisposing conditions.

Arterial embolus of the mesentery is seen most frequently in patients with heart disease and the embolus usually arises in the left side of the heart, either from vegetations on the valves or a thrombus in the auricle.

Venous emboli are practically nonexistent.

Arterial thrombosis of the mesenteric artery may be most frequently traced to atheromatous degeneration of the vessel wall, or arteriosclerosis.

Venous thrombosis on the other hand is most frequently associated with infections in organs or viscera that are tributaries to the portal vein. Thus, appendicitis, pelvic disease, or ulcerating carcinoma of the colon may lead to venous thrombosis. Also, surgery of the stomach, appendix, strangulated hernia, and pelvis are predisposing factors.

Primary venous thrombosis, unlike arterial thrombosis, is quite rare. When it occurs it is due to endophlebitis or phlebosclerosis.

Other conditions which have led to thrombosis of the mesenteric artery or vein have been (1) blood dyscrasias, such as polycythemia vera and splenic anemia; (2) trauma to the mesenteric vessels; (3) mechanical causes, as portal stasis, pressure from tumors, adhesions and bands; (4) following ablation of the lumbar sympathetic chain (mentioned in the literature recently[5] (the mode of action here is unknown); and (5) a small group of cases in which no primary cause of thrombosis can be demonstrated.

Of our series of cases we have found the etiologic factors to be as follows:

(1) 8 of 11 autopsies showed primary intimal arteriosclerosis with thrombosis of the superior mesenteric arteries
11 other cases were probably primary arteriosclerosis with thrombosis; we say, "probably," because no other factors as heart disease, trauma, infection, etc., were present

(2)	Heart disease	14 cases (2 proved by autopsy)
	Arteriosclerotic H.D.	4 cases
	Rheumatic H.D.	3 cases
	Coronary H.D.	3 cases
	Unclassified H.D.	4 cases
(3)	Following surgery (probably venous thrombosis)	5 cases (none autopsied)
	Strangulated hernia	2 cases
	Gynecologic operation	1 case
	Appendectomy	1 case
	Gastroenterostomy	1 case
(4)	Following delivery	1 case
(5)	Primary portal vein thrombosis	1 case (autopsied)
(6)	Undetermined etiology	2 cases

Thus, in this series, 7 were venous thrombosis and 19 were arterial thrombosis; 14 were arterial emboli and 2 were undetermined. This does not conform with findings in the literature. Moore[8] blamed venous obstruction for 75 per cent of the cases. Shively and Renshaw,[9] from the Cleveland Clinic, reported that 70 per cent of all cases are venous in origin; Boyd,[17] that the venous type is more common. Whittaker and Pemberton in 60 cases found 19 to be arterial and 27 to be venous. However, both Larson[10] and Trotter[11] concurred with our findings that arterial thrombosis occurs more frequently than venous thrombosis.

CLINICAL PICTURE

Two cases on our service in the last year summarized the clinical picture. These are cases which will help prove (1) that radical surgery is necessary to save life, and (2) that oftentimes this condition may cause unexplained abdominal symptoms due to the mildness and gradual onset of the pathologic process. Both of these patients recovered.

CASE 1.—F. S., a white man, 69 years of age, was admitted to the emergency room on May 26, 1945. Five days previously he had suddenly complained of pain in the stomach with mild indigestion. The next night he had a sudden severe pain in the lower abdomen which radiated from the midline to both sides. The following day, three days after onset, the pain continued and he vomited. It was necessary to give morphine to obtain relief. Since the onset of the symptoms he had had no normal bowel movement. Stools were loose and on three occasions contained blood. Pain grew worse until the time of admission on May 26, 1945. Physical examination on admission showed a man slightly cyanotic, obviously in pain, with a distended abdomen and generalized abdominal tenderness. There was an occasional peristaltic tinkle and a fair amount of diffuse rigidity. Temperature was 102° F., pulse 96, respirations 20, white blood cells, 15,700. He was immediately taken to the operating room and when the abdomen was opened, pink, blood-stained fluid occupied the peritoneal cavity. About 14 cm. of blue-black gangrenous bowel were present. The bowel was resected very wide of the gangrene on either side so that it was felt that we were well beyond the involved area of bowel. A wedge-shaped piece was removed from the mesentery and an end-to-end anastomosis was performed. Aside from some mild atelectasis and breakdown of the wound, he left the hospital July 29, 1945, sixty-two days after admission, apparently well. During his stay in the hospital, a cardiovascular survey showed no cardiac disease. This man was well and doing his normal work when last seen in April, 1948.

CASE 2.—W. H., a white man, aged 49 years, was admitted to the emergency room on our service April 5, 1946. His history revealed that four days before admission he was seized with severe abdominal pain, sharp and generalized, over the entire abdomen. He took several enemas, with no effect. At no time was there any blood in the stool. Nausea and vomiting began the day of admission. Examination on admission revealed a rather heavy-set pale, clammy individual with a greatly distended abdomen. There was diffuse tenderness and peristalsis was absent. A roentgenogram of the abdomen failed to reveal air or obstruction. Electrocardiogram was normal. He was given plasma and taken to the operating room immediately. Upon opening the abdomen, pink, hemorrhagic fluid filled the peritoneal cavity. About two-thirds of the small bowel was gangrenous. This bowel was resected well beyond the gangrenous areas on both sides and it measured 56 inches in length. A wedge of the mesentery was likewise removed. The laboratory found extensive mesenteric artery thrombosis. An enteroanastomosis was performed. The patient made a rather uneventful postoperative recovery and was discharged May 4, 1946, twenty-nine days after operation, apparently well. A most interesting fact was concerning his past medical history. Approximately three and one-half years before, in October, 1942, he had been operated upon by one of us for a very similar complaint. At that time nothing was found in the abdomen to account for the symptoms. Between the two operations, for a period of two years, he had some vague abdominal distress. The following is a follow-up note written in the records Jan. 15, 1943, which is very impressive: "Patient was in the office today for a follow-up examination. He now has the same type of complaints that he had preoperatively, namely, distention, swelling, and some cramplike pains in the upper abdomen; also tenderness in the same area in which he was tender preoperatively. I am still at a loss to explain this patient's symptoms."

In review of the literature, one is amazed at the lack of unanimity as to the symptoms and physical findings in this condition. Some authors state that continuous pain is a feature, others that pain is intermittent; some show much concern about vomiting, others about the lack of it. We feel that very frequently the diagnosis of mesenteric thrombosis is one which is made by exclusion. In our cases, no definite picture is universally present. Bloody stools about which so much is written occurred in only two cases. Furthermore, it is felt that to differentiate mesenteric artery thrombosis from mesenteric venous thrombosis is clinically practically an impossibility. In the differentiatial diagnosis, one should bear in mind such conditions as (1) acute hemorrhagic pancreatitis, (2) acute cholecystitis, (3) ruptured peptic ulcer, (4) ruptured abdominal viscus, (5) diverticulitis, and (6) atypical heart disease. While the actual diagnosis may be difficult, the condition almost always presents itself as an "acute surgical belly."

COMMENTS

Both cases confirm the fact that when actual gangrene of bowel is present, radical surgery is the only treatment. Resection and anastomosis are advocated as the most desirable surgical procedures. Resection must be sufficiently wide to remove edematous bowel adjacent to the gangrenous area. It is generally agreed by all that exteriorization of the bowel, enterostomy, and cecostomy are futile. Every patient in our series, six in number, in whom these procedures were done, died. Such men as Brown,[6] Beigler,[12] Thomas Moore[8] of London, and Renshaw[9] of Cleveland Clinic, in their writings on the subject, all confirmed this idea.

Of the five patients who lived following surgery in our series, only the two cases reported in detail in this paper were cases of extensive gangrene of bowel. Of the other three, two had only small areas of gangrene and one had a small area of terminal ileum involved. Thus, actually only two patients with extensive gangrene of the bowel have recovered by surgery and in both of these cases, both on our service within the last year, very wide resection with anastomosis was performed. Thus, it would seem, although the number of cases admittedly is relatively few, that for extensive gangrene no other procedure is acceptable.

The second case emphasizes the fact that mesenteric thrombosis may occur in a mild form and cause vague abdominal symptoms. Several others in our series and many more reported in the literature[13] confirm the idea that if the history of people who have primary mesenteric thrombosis due to atheromatous change in the vessels of the mesentery is gone into, one will find that over a period of months or years these individuals have had some abdominal distress, perhaps after a heavy meal, after severe exertion, or other times when blood supply to the gut may be impaired. Therefore, when the surgeon opens the abdomen of an elderly individual and finds nothing, he may presume that this condition is a possibility.

TREATMENT

The treatment of this condition is primarily surgical, the aspects of which have already been mentioned. Regarding the use of dicumarol and heparin, one thing is certain—they will never act as a cure. Dicumarol will be tried in our next case. However, our appraisal of it will be conservative. It would have been very easy to have given these drugs credit, if they had been used, for the success in the two reported cases. The value of these drugs in reducing operative mortality by preventing propagation of the parts of the thrombus which may remain following surgery is questionable. Moses,[14] of the University of Pittsburgh, showed experimentally that heparin and dicumarol in adequate dosage did not prevent the development of experimental intravascular thrombosis in the presence of stasis of the venous circulation. On the other hand,[15] they are reported to be of great usefulness particularly in arterial occlusion. Here they prevent extension of the thrombosis. However, it must be emphasized that in venous thrombosis especially, it may be extremely dangerous to use these drugs preoperatively. Death may be hastened because of continued bleeding into a bowel which is already hemorrhagic.

Other treatment of this condition is purely supportive and symptomatic. Plasma and saline solution for combating shock and fluid loss, opiates for the relief of pain, oxygen and circulatory stimulants, Levine tube for the relief of distention—all are to be used when indicated.

SUMMARY AND CONCLUSIONS

1. Radical surgery, that is, wide resection and anastomosis, is the only tenable treatment in those cases where there is extensive gangrene of bowel.

2. The condition may often present itself in a mild form, not always as the massive accident as is so commonly thought.

3. Mortality rate of the patients in the Mercy Hospital was, for those operated upon, 61 per cent, and for those not, 96 per cent. The total mortality rate was 85 per cent for 40 cases.

4. Of 40 cases, 57 per cent of the patients were between the ages of 40 and 60 years, with the youngest 27 and the oldest 82.

5. A brief discussion of the anatomy and pathologic physiology was presented with emphasis on collateral circulation.

6. An outline of etiologic factors was presented and arterial thrombosis of arteriosclerotic origin was the most common cause in our series. This is not the case in the literature.

7. Presentation of two cases on our service demonstrated the clinical picture of this condition. The signs and symptoms are not consistent.

8. We believe that the use of heparin and dicumarol must be considered. They may possibly be of great value postoperatively.

REFERENCES

1. Dunphy, J. E.: Abdominal Pain of Vascular Origin, Am. J. M. Sc. **192**: 109-113, 1936.
2. Pal: Gefaskrisen, Leipzig, 1905.
3. Ficarra, B. J.: Occlusion; Presentation of 15 Cases, Am. J. Surg. **66**: 168-177, 1944.
4. Warren, S., and Eberhard, T. P.: Mesenteric Venous Thrombosis, Surg., Gynec. & Obst. **61**: 102, 1935.
5. Laufman, H., and Scheinberg, Shayel: Arterial and Venous Occlusion; Analysis of 44 Cases, Am. J. Surg. **58**: 84-92, 1942.
6. Brown, M. J.: Venous Occlusion; Clinical Entity, Am. J. Surg. **49**: 242-249, 1940.
7. Whittaker, L. D., and Pemberton, J. deJ.: Mesenteric Vascular Occlusion, J. A. M. A. **111**: 21-24, 1938.
8. Moore, T.: Vascular Occlusion, Brit. J. Surg. **28**: 347-356, 1941.
9. Shively, F. L., Jr., and Renshaw, R. J. F.: Mesenteric Thrombosis; Report of Case, Cleveland Clin. Quart. **10**: 133-137, 1943.
10. Larson, G. M.: Mesenteric Vascular Occlusion, Surg., Gynec. & Obst. **53**: 45, 1931.
11. Trotter, G.: Embolism and Thrombosis of Mesenteric Vessels, London, 1913, Cambridge University Press.
12. Beigler, S. K.: Occlusion of Vessels; Case, Harper Hosp. Bull. **3**: 76-78, 1945.
13. Conner, L. A.: Discussion of Role of Arterial Thrombosis in Visceral Diseases of Middle Life. Based Upon Analogies Drawn From Coronary Thrombosis, Am. J. M. Sc. **185**: 13, 1933.
14. Moses, C.: Effect of Heparin and Dicoumarol on Thrombosis Induced in the Presence of Venous Stasis, Proc. Soc. Exper. Biol. & Med. **59**: 25-27, 1945.
15. Luke, J. C.: Venous Thrombosis; Treatment With Heparin, Lancet **1**: 552-553, 1943.
16. d'Abreu, F.: Mesenteric Venous Thrombosis, Recovery After Resection With Heparin, Lancet **1**: 534-536, 1946.
17. Boyd, Wm.: Text Book of Pathology, 1939, p. 567.

OBSERVATIONS ON AN ABSORBABLE POWDER TO REPLACE TALC

E. L. MacQuiddy, M.D., and J. P. Tollman, M.D., Omaha, Neb.

(From the College of Medicine, University of Nebraska)

THE use of talc as a lubricant on gloves in surgery has been questioned for the past ten years. Several authors have called attention to the dangers of talc as a factor in the production of adhesions and of talc granulomas. Difficulty has been encountered in finding an acceptable substitute for talc. We present a review of the present literature on this subject and offer a specially processed starch as a substitute for talc.

The study of talc and its effect on the human body begins with Thorel[1] in 1896. He found talc or soapstone remaining in the incinerated lung of a woman supposedly dying from tuberculosis, who had worked for some years in the handling of products made from soapstone. In 1913, Harrison[2] suggested cultures of living tissue as a means for the study of the response of cells to directive stimuli. Lambert,[3] the year previous to this, had employed the same method and reported the formation of foreign body giant cells in vitro by the addition of foreign objects such as Lycopodium spores and cotton spores to cultures of chick embryo spleen. Sayers,[4] in 1924, began studies at the Pittsburgh Station of the United States Bureau of Mines to determine the action of various dusts when injected into the peritoneal cavity of guinea pigs. The conclusion he reached was that live animal tissue in all parts of the body tended to react in essentially the same manner to foreign bodies. This work was further reported by Miller and Sayers[5, 6] in 1934 and 1935. In the 1935 article Miller described the effect of soapstone and the formation of giant cells.

Lanza[7] in 1938 described the physiologic effects of different forms of talc. Talc produced a less active response than some of the other materials tested, but of a similar character.

Gardner,[8] in 1938, also described the irritative effect of talc, in his article on pneumoconiosis. When talc was injected directly into the testes of guinea pigs, it was found that a very active cellular proliferation was produced within six months.

Since 1919 there have appeared various articles describing a condition, found particularly in the peritoneum, resembling tuberculosis, but which was recognized as not being a true tuberculous lesion. Hertzler[9] in 1919 described it as a pseudotuberculosis. In 1933, Haythorn[10] described nodular lesions of the peritoneum, among these a pseudotuberculosis and foreign body granulomas. In 1933 also, Antopol[11] in reporting on granulomas caused by lycopodium, reported the case of a man 34 years of age who had had a laparotomy. Granulomas were found and within the giant cells refractile bodies were discovered, morphologically identified as crystals of talc. In his conclusions he stated

This study was supported by a grant from the Ethicon Suture Laboratories, Division of Johnson & Johnson, New Brunswick, N. J.

Received for publication, August 18, 1947.

definitely that granulomatous lesions may be caused by talc. Erb,[12] in 1935, described Lycopodium granuloma and urged against the use of Lycopodium as a dusting powder in operating rooms.

Owen,[13] in 1936, described a patient in whom granulomas were found due to talc. This prompted her to study the effect of talc intraperitoneally in 120 rabbits. Autopsies were done on these animals at 35, 45, 60, 90, 120, 180, 210, and 300 days after the dusting operation. Eighty-eight of these animals were autopsied. In each instance a varying number of small, slightly elevated, grayish-pink nodules were found on the peritoneal surface of the intestine. She suggested that talc be removed from the surface of the gloves before operating.

In 1937, Fienberg[14] reported on two cases of granuloma caused by talc, and was able to produce a similar lesion in the peritoneum of the mouse. He stated that indiscriminate use of talc in the operating room may produce granulomatous lesions. He suggested also the use of polarized light in recognition of the crystals in these lesions. In 1940, Ramsey and Douglass[15] called attention to the production of granulomas by talc and reported three such cases. They warned against the indiscriminate use of this powder in abdominal or other surgery, and in the use of rectal or vaginal suppositories containing talc.

Byron and Welch,[16] in 1941, discussed complications from the use of glove powder and suggested that, in addition to the formation of granulomas, sinus tracts might be formed. They stressed the necessity of washing off as much of the powder as possible before surgery. Ramsey,[17] in 1942, described four more cases of talc granulomas, and stated that the use of polarized light was of great help in making the diagnosis. He further stated that more attention should be given to possible sources of irritation in the operating room itself, from surgical dressings, rubber gloves, and drains. He urged that no excess be left in the finger tips of the gloves. A tear while working in the peritoneum or any other body cavity could heavily contaminate the area. Weed and Groves,[18] in 1942, published a most interesting article regarding surgical gloves and wound infections. They called attention to the fact that in 4,549 operations, 35,763 gloves were used, and that of this number 8,103, or 22.6 per cent, showed perforations which had occurred during the surgery. Not only would this allow infections to travel from the hand to the surgical field, but would allow powder as well to escape.

German,[19] in 1943, described dusting powder granulomas following surgery and stated that talc, while chemically inert, promptly induces a marked tissue reaction in the form of granulomas. The formation of the granulomas is a protective mechanism which might interfere with the normal healing process depending on the site and the abundance of the granulomas which are present. German felt that adhesions do not develop without some form of traumatization of the peritoneum sufficient to produce exudation of fibrin. It was his opinion that in the presence of peritoneal trauma with exudation of fibrin, talc plays a secondary role in that it is caught up in the fibrin and is incorporated in the adhesions. Seelig, Verda, and Kidd,[20, 21] in 1943, called attention to the disadvantages of talc in surgery, and suggested potassium bitartrate as a substitute.

Seelig,[22] and Seelig and Verda,[23] in 1944, stated that talc can produce pathologic changes that may deceptively resemble cancer or tuberculosis. He urged the abandonment of the use of talc in surgery and suggested the use of potassium bitartrate. Seelig,[24] again in 1945, called attention to the danger of the use of talc on gloves in surgical ampitheatres, and urged strongly a substitute powder for talc; he proposed the use of a formaldehyde-treated starch, and stated that after using it for four months he found it completely safe. In 1945, Seelig and Verda[25] redescribed the dangers of talc, and showed photographs of the effect, intraperitoneally, of talc in rats.

Talc may exert deleterious influences in industrial applications as well as surgery. Its use is ubiquitous according to Lichtman and associates.[33] It may be employed for many purposes such as a cleaning agent for barley, beans, and coffee, as a packing and conserving agent for fruits and vegetables, as a filler in toothpaste, and is found in some chewing gums, candies, and suppositories—to mention but a few of the many fields where it is employed. It is a question whether in these industrial uses as well, its dangers, though perhaps less recognized, may be as real as in surgery.

In a study of plants engaged in the crushing and milling of talc, Dreessen,[26] in 1933, reported that silicate dust of tremolite talc and slate induces a fine, diffuse, bilateral fibrosis of the lungs which is definitely demonstrated in the x-ray view. In 1935 the same author[27] investigated two talc mills in Northern Georgia in an effort to determine whether there was a connection between the talc dust exposure and the high tuberculosis mortality rate reported in the county in which the industry was located. Physical examinations and radiographs were made on sixty-six men and women who were exposed or had been exposed to talc dust. Of thirty-three men exposed to heavy concentrations of dust, eight were found to have pneumoconiosis grade 1, and eight to have pneumoconiosis grade 2 or 3. He could not attribute the high tuberculosis mortality rate in the county to the talc industry.

Kronenberg,[28] in 1937, called attention to the danger to nurses using talc to prepare gloves for surgery, and urged proper care so that the nurses need not breathe injurious quantities of this powder. In his report he stated that he found dangerous concentrations of the powder from air samples taken near the breathing zone of the nurses.

In 1942, Porro, Patton, and Hobbs[29] called attention to the danger of pneumoconiosis in the talc industry, and reported fifteen cases in talc workers. These included five autopsies. He stated that the pneumoconiosis causes disability, but that death did not result directly from this cause in talc workers. The tissue changes were due to talc itself.

Schulz and Williams,[30] in discussing commercial talc, found that lesions were present only in the organs where talc had been deposited. Progressive fibrosis, such as produced by crystalline-free silica, was not observed. The fibrosis which does occur is only to hold and limit the space for storing of foreign material.

In 1935, Bethune[31] suggested the use of talc as a means of artificially creating adhesions around the lung so that it would remain in position during resection. He was able satisfactorily to produce adhesions using an iodized talc blown in with a special blower. Ten months after the first clinical patient was operated upon, he observed no ill effects from the presence of this insoluble powder between two pleural surfaces.

In 1940, Thompson[32] suggested talc to produce pericardial adhesions. He said: "From our experiments with animals, it was found that placing talcum powder in the pericardial sac would produce an adhesive pericarditis, which, in turn, would furnish collateral circulation adequate to overcome a deficiency of blood supply to the heart following ligation and diversion of a main branch of the coronary artery. On the basis of this experiment, ten patients with coronary artery disease have been operated upon. Although two have died, and one patient has been operated upon too recently to evaluate the recovery, seven have received very marked benefits."

In 1946, Lichtman and co-workers,[33] working at Rochester, Minn., presented evidence to show that extensive tissue damage may be caused by talc. Granulomatous lesions of the peritoneum, draining sinuses, scar nodules, and malfunctioning intestinal stomas were found at secondary operations. Talc implanted intentionally around fistulas in dogs caused persistence of the fistulas. They observed that in human beings the tissue reacts by forming pseudotubercles and they believe that, as Lycopodium powder has been removed from use in the operating room, talc likewise must go. It was their impression that talc granulomas would be recognized more frequently if there were greater use of polarized light microscopy.

Lee and Lehman,[34] in 1947, contrasted the physiologic effect of talc with that of a powder similar to the one used in this investigation. Their work substantiated the previous reports that have been published emphasizing the irritative lesions caused by talc. They found that this new nonirritating powder (starch powder No. 108)* was completely absorbed by the peritoneum without inflammatory reaction and without the formation of adhesions.

The absorbable starch powder (No. 108) with which we have been working for approximately one year, and with respect to which our findings are presented in this paper, is the same material used by Lee and Lehman[34] and Lindenmuth.[35] It consists of a mixture of amylose and amylopectins, derived from cornstarch, which has been treated by physical and chemical means to improve its lubricating value and to prevent gelatinization when autoclaved.

The first portion of our investigation was an allergenic study to determine whether human beings could have become previously sensitized to this or similar starches. We also attempted, by means of parenteral injections, to sensitize animals.

The second section of the study consisted of injecting powder No. 108 intraperitoneally and subcutaneously in rabbits and guinea pigs, and intraperitoneally alone in dogs, to observe its effect. These particular experiments

*For the sake of convenience, starch powder No. 108 has been given the trade name of Bio-sorb.

were also contrasted with similar experiments on animals, using talc. The talc experiments were carried out to confirm previously reported work on the use of this powder.

The third portion of our work consisted of inhalation experiments in which rabbits were exposed to atmospheres of talc and of powder No. 108 under the same conditions.

Studies were made to determine existence of a previously acquired sensitivity to this starch. Patch tests were made on fifty adult males. The tests were applied and left in place for seventy-two hours with readings recorded at the end of twenty-four, forty-eight, and seventy-two hours. No positive reactions were obtained.

An extract was made of this starch in the manner used to prepare allergens for use in the allergy department. Eighty-one patients with allergenic backgrounds in the allergy clinic at the University of Nebraska were tested both by scratch and by intracutaneous tests. No reactions were found in this group. In so far as our results go we could not find that a previous sensitivity to this starch existed.

In the rabbits in which parenteral inoculations of the starch had been done, ophthalmic tests were made from time to time, and at no time was a positive reaction obtained. Ten virgin female guinea pigs were given injections of 0.5 Gm. of the starch. At the end of fourteen days strips of uterine muscle were removed and tested by the approved methods for sensitivity. Testing with extracts of the starch, no contractions were elicited. Histamine and Pituitrin used on the same muscle proved its contractibility. We were not able to sensitize rabbits and guinea pigs with powder No. 108.

As a matter of interest in further confirming the excellent work of Lee and Lehman,[34] a laparotomy was performed on a medium-sized dog under strict surgical technique and 1.0 Gm. of the absorbable powder was dusted over the intestines and omentum. The dog was allowed to survive for three weeks and the abdomen again opened. No adhesions were found, and we were not able to detect any of the starch.

A similar operation was performed on another dog but, instead of using the absorbable powder, 1.0 Gm. of talcum powder was dusted over the intestines and the omentum and the wound was closed. This dog was sacrificed at the end of three weeks. Almost the entire peritoneal cavity was covered with adhesions. Sections taken from these adhesions also showed talc.

Under general anesthesia, the peritoneal cavities of two rabbits were opened and 0.5 Gm. of powder No. 108 was placed within. At the end of twenty-four days the rabbits were sacrificed; no adhesions were found, and we were not able to detect any of the powder. Under similar conditions two rabbits were operated upon but 0.5 Gm. of talc was used in place of the absorbable powder. At the end of twenty-four days these rabbits were sacrificed and the peritoneal cavities were found to contain massive adhesions. The general picture was the same as that in the dog (Figs. 1, 2, 3 and 4).

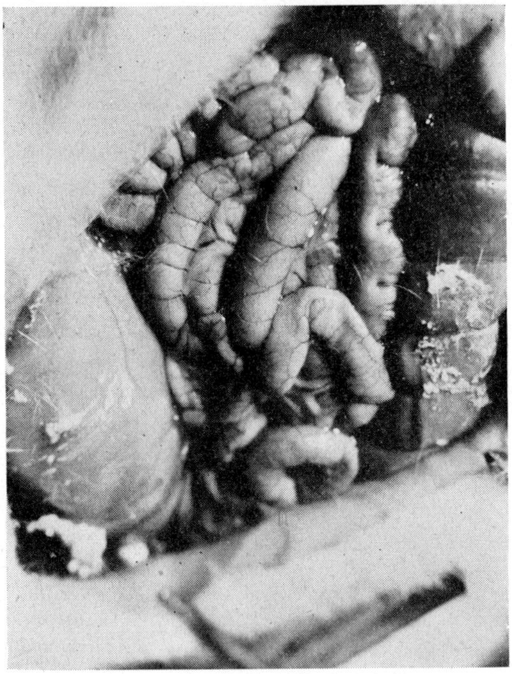

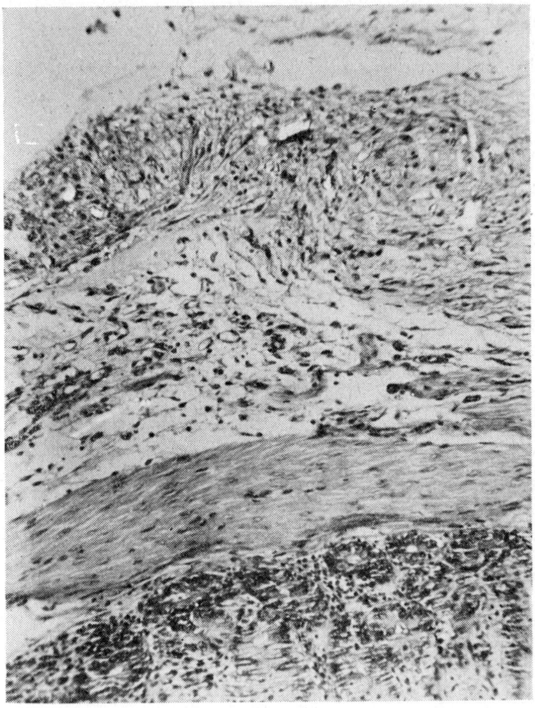

Fig. 1.—Peritoneum of rabbit, three weeks after introduction of talc; many collections of talc may be seen, and several adhesions are evident.

Fig. 2.—Wall of bowel (×120) after use of talc, under polarized light, partial extinction. The subserosa has been greatly thickened by fibrosis and granuloma formation. White spots are talc granules.

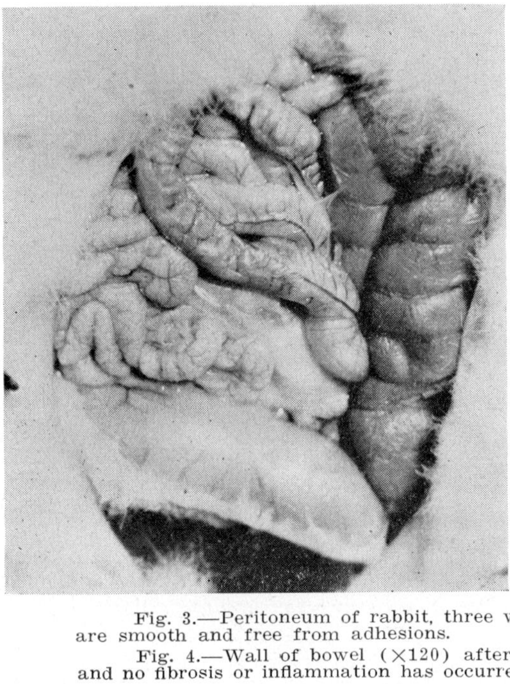

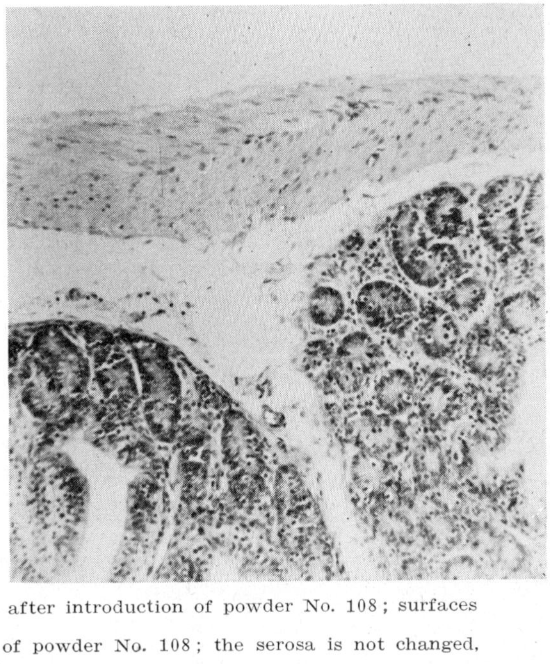

Fig. 3.—Peritoneum of rabbit, three weeks after introduction of powder No. 108; surfaces are smooth and free from adhesions.

Fig. 4.—Wall of bowel (×120) after use of powder No. 108; the serosa is not changed, and no fibrosis or inflammation has occurred.

The absorbable starch powder under investigation was made into pellets weighing 200.0 mg. These pellets were placed subcutaneously in the interscapular region of twenty-five rabbits. The pellets were allowed to remain in ten rabbits for fourteen days, in ten rabbits for twenty-eight days, and in five rabbits for fifty-six days. The impression from these studies is of a persistent activity, but not intense reaction to the presence of the material, and very little, if any, of the material was to be found at the end of fifty-six days. It should be pointed out that this is a very severe test since absorption of a fairly hard pellet of material from the subcutaneous tissue would be expected to proceed slowly.

In line with the studies of Lindenmuth,[35] 500 mg. of powder No. 108 were injected intraperitoneally into the abdomen of each of ten guinea pigs. These guinea pigs were allowed to survive for fourteen days and then were autopsied; no adhesions or other evidences of irritation were found.

Since the inhalation of mineral dusts is potentially dangerous, and to obtain information with respect to the reactivity of the experimental powder in lung tissue, six rabbits were subjected to an inhalation experiment in which they were placed in an enclosure approximately four feet in diameter and two feet high, and a heavy concentration of powder No. 108 was kept in atmospheric suspension by means of a circulating fan. These animals were exposed forty minutes a day for fifty days. At the end of this time the animals were sacrificed; no lung pathology could be demonstrated.

A similar experiment was carried out with two rabbits, using talc instead of the absorbable powder. The lungs of these rabbits showed scattered silicate particles with some giant-cell formation.

CONCLUSIONS

1. We were unable to find any sensitivity to this starch in the group of human beings tested.

2. We were unable to prove that the animals became sensitive when injected parenterally with this absorbable powder.

3. No peritoneal adhesions occurred in any of our animals in which powder No. 108 was used.

4. Our work shows that a chemically modified starch powder (No. 108), when placed in the tissue of animals, is nonirritating and is readily absorbed from the peritoneal cavity.

5. Our work confirms that of previous authors that talc is irritating when placed in the peritoneal cavity of dogs and rabbits, and in the lungs of rabbits.

6. The evidence indicates that powder No. 108 is a safe replacement for talc for surgical and other purposes for which this commodity is widely used.

REFERENCES

1. Thorel, C.: Die Specksteinlunge, Betr. z. path. Anat. **20**:84-101, 1896.
2. Harrison, R. G.: The Life of Tissues Outside the Organism From the Embryological Standpoint, Tr. Cong. Am. Phys. & Surg. **9**:63-76, 1913.
3. Lambert, R. A.: The Production of Foreign Body Giant Cells in Vitro, J. Exper. Med. **15**:510-515, 1912.

4. Sayers, R. R.: Health Hazards in the Mining Industry, U. S. Bureau of Mines Report of Investigation, No. 2660, December, 1924.
5. Miller, John W., and Sayers, R. R.: The Physiological Response of the Peritoneal Tissue to Dusts Introduced as Foreign Bodies, Pub. Health Rep. **49**:80-89, 1934.
6. Miller, J. W., and Sayers, R. R.: Microscopic Appearance of Experimentally Produced Dust Nodules in the Peritoneum, Pub. Health Rep. **50**:1619-1628, 1935.
7. Lanza, A. J. (Gardner, Leroy U.): Silicosis and Asbestosis, New York, 1938, Oxford University Press, p. 257.
8. Gardner, Leroy U.: Etiology of Pneumoconiosis, J.A.M.A. **111**:1925-1936, 1938.
9. Hertzler, Arthur E.: The Peritoneum, vol. 2, St. Louis, 1919, The C. V. Mosby Company, p. 713.
10. Haythorn, Samuel R.: Nodular Lesions of the Peritoneum, Am. J. Path. **9**:725-737, 1933.
11. Antopol, Wm.: Lycopodium Granuloma, Arch. Path. **16**:326-331, 1933.
12. Erb, I. H.: Lycopodium Granuloma, Surg., Gynec. & Obst. **60**:40-44, 1935.
13. Owen, May: Peritoneal Response to Glove Powder, Texas State J. Med. **32**:482-485, 1936.
14. Fienberg, Robert: Talcum Powder Granuloma, Arch. Path. **24**:36-42, 1937.
15. Ramsey, T. L., and Douglass, F. M.: Granulomatous Inflammation Produced by Foreign Body Irritants, J. Internat. Coll. Surgeons **3**:3-10, 1940.
16. Byron, F. X., and Welch, G. Stuart: A Complication From the Use of Glove Powder, SURGERY **10**:766-769, 1941.
17. Ramsey, Thos. L.: Magnesium Silicate Granuloma, Am. J. Clin Path. **12**:553-558, 1942.
18. Weed, L. A., and Groves, J. L.: Surgical Gloves and Wound Infections, Surg., Gynec. & Obst. **75**:661-664, 1942.
19. German, W. M.: Dusting Powder Granulomas Following Surgery, Surg., Gynec. & Obst. **76**:501-507, 1943.
20. Seelig, M. G., Verda, D. J., and Kidd, F. H., Jr.: The Talcum Powder Problem in Surgery and Its Solution J. A. M. A. **123**:950-954, 1943.
21. Seelig, M. G., Verda, D. J., and Kidd, F. H., Jr.: The Talcum Problem in Surgery and Its Solution, Proc. Interst. Postgrad. M. A. North America (1943) pp. 205-208, 1944.
22. Seelig, M. G.: Abdominal Silicosis (Due to Talcum Powder) and Cancer, S. Clin. North America **24**:1162-1171, 1944.
23. Seelig, M. G., and Verda, D. J.: Talcum Used as a Surgical Dusting Powder is Hazardous, Hospitals **18**:32-34, 1944.
24. Seelig, M. G.: Talcum as an Operating Room Hazard, South. M. J. **38**:470-472, 1945.
25. Seelig, M. G., and Verda, D. J.: The Talcum Powder, J. Mt. Sinai Hosp. **12**:655-666, 1945.
26. Dreessen, W. C.: Effects of Certain Silicate Dusts on The Lungs, J. Indust. Hyg. & Toxicol. **15**:66-78, 1933.
27. Dreessen, W. C.: The Effects of Exposure to Dust in Two Georgia Talc Mills and Mines, Pub. Health Rep. **50**:131-143, 1935.
28. Kronenberg, M. H.: Dust Dangers Exposed, Mod. Hosp. **49**:84, 1937.
29. Porro, F. W., Patton, J. R., and Hobbs, A. A.: Pneumoconiosis in the Talc Industry, Am. J. Roentgenol. **47**:507-524, 1942.
30. Schulz, R. Z., and Williams, C. R.: Commercial Talc, Animal and Mineralogic Studies, J. Indust. Hyg. & Toxicol. **24**:75-79, 1942.
31. Bethune, N.: Pleural Poudrage, J. Thoracic Surg. **4**:251-261, 1935.
32. Thompson, S. A.: An Operation for the Relief of Coronary Artery Disease, Quart. Bull., Sea View Hosp. **5**:175-182, 1940.
33. Lichtman, A. L., McDonald, J. R., Dixon, C. F., and Mann, F. C.: Talc Granuloma, Surg. Gynec. & Obst. **83**:531-546, 1946.
34. Lee, C. M. Jr., and Lehman, E. P.: Experiments with Non-Irritating Glove Powder, Surg., Gynec. & Obst. **84**:689-695, 1947.
35. Lindenmuth, W. W.: Personal Communication. (To be published.)

THE MAGNUSON-STACK PROCEDURE FOR RECURRENT DISLOCATIONS OF THE SHOULDER

N. J. GIANNESTRAS, M.D., CINCINNATI, OHIO

THE multiplicity of procedures described for repair of recurrent traumatic subcoracoid and subglenoid dislocations of the shoulder is ample evidence that no procedure has yet proved completely successful. During the last few years two procedures have held out more hope for permanent reduction; one is the Bankart[1] operation of repair of the capsule, and the other the Magnuson-Stack[2] procedure of transportation of the tendon of the subscapularis from the lesser to the greater tuberosity of the humerus. The author is concerned with the latter procedure, and wishes to report a follow-up study of thirty-one such operations which vary in follow-up from three years to one and one-half years. It is conceded that the length of time elapsed is insufficient for a complete and final analysis, but it is hoped that this report will serve as an added impetus for more bone and joint surgeons to use this procedure. It appears to be quite promising, and only by reviewing a large series of cases, at least five years after surgery, can any definite conclusions be reached.

The incentive for the use of the Magnuson-Stack procedure in preference to other operative techniques has been based on the following observations. It was noticed that the Nicola[3] procedure and its various modifications, even when performed by men in the armed services who were capable and qualified, still permitted recurrences to develop in approximately 20 to 25 per cent of the instances. The use of the Henderson[4] suspension was not particularly appealing because the recovery of the average enlisted man and his return to duty diminished in proportion to the number of skin incisions, particularly where elective surgery was concerned. Certainly there are multiple such incisions in the Henderson procedure. Use of the bone peg procedure or of the various fascial and muscle plasties was not particularly advocated in the armed services, due to the long healing time required and the difficulty in mobilizing such shoulders after a prolonged period of immobilization. As for the Bankart procedure, I attempted it on three occasions, and it is admitted that decisions based on three attempts are inconclusive. However, the consensus of opinion of a number of other men who had also attempted the same procedure was that, (1) it was extensive surgery, and with this statement even the exponents of the Bankart procedure must agree, (2) the reattachment of the capsule to the lip of the glenoid process was not the reason for the success of the procedure for the capsule could again be avulsed with sufficient trauma, but rather the amount of scar and adhesions which developed following such extensive dissection, which was unphysiologic, and, (3) the drilling of the holes just posterior to the rim of the glenoid process was not the easiest procedure to perform. Furthermore,

Received for publication, Aug. 8, 1947.

Magnuson and Stack's[2] reasoning as to the causes of recurrent subglenoid and subcoracoid dislocations of the shoulder and the corrective surgery for this condition sounded more reasonable and convincing.

CAUSES OF RECURRENCE

The exact cause of recurrent dislocations has not been adequately explained. Certainly not all shoulder dislocations recur, and furthermore dislocations have recurred in many patients who have received adequate immobilization after the initial episode. Originally it was thought to be due to a poorly healed tear of the capsule. Another theory propounded was that it was due to the shallowness of the glenoid fossa. Bankart attributed it to a tearing of the capsule at the anterior inferior lip of the glenoid with an avulsion of the capsule with subsequent lack of healing and gapping at the point of tearing. Magnuson has brought forth another line of thought as to the cause of recurrent dislocations, which is, that it is due to "a lack of balance, traction, and leverage of muscles which ordinarily resists the downward and forward displacement of the head." Magnusons's idea is well worth considering. In reasoning out this thought he stated:[5]

> I do not feel that the glenoid, which is very slightly cup-shaped, has much supporting function for the head of the humerus in contradistinction to the acetabulum, which is much deeper and serves as a weight-bearing structure. There are no such ligaments in the shoulder capsule as are in the hip, where the Y-ligament acts as a strong reinforcing band to resistance of hyperextension of the hip. The shoulder muscles are the only structures which maintain the head of the humerus in contact with the glenoid and in proper position. This is plainly evident, for if these muscles are paralysed, the head of the humerus will drop away from the glenoid and may lie clear below it. That is not true of the hip; even if the muscles between the pelvis and the femur are completely paralysed, the hip will not easily dislocate and certainly will not drop as a result of the drag on the leg. Patients who have had infantile paralysis and have a subsequent fracture of the leg must have traction applied. Never have I seen a hip pulled out of the acetabulum, but I have seen the head of the humerus pulled away from the glenoid as a result of improperly applied traction to the humerus. When the shoulder muscles are relaxed, it takes very little pull to separate the head of the humerus from the glenoid, and if traction is left on for a few hours, it is not difficult to create as much as a half inch separation between the faces of the joints.

Certainly such reasoning cannot be cast aside as simply another theory even by the most ardent exponents of the Bankart procedure, who claim that the reason for recurrence was the avulsion of the capsule from the glenoid labrum. Furthermore, tear of the capsule was not found to be present in all of the shoulders which were exposed in this series. If, as Bankart contends, the cause of the recurrent dislocation is the shallow glenoid and the tear of the capsule, then what is to prevent a future recurrence of the tear of this capsule if sufficient trauma should be applied?

THE OPERATION

The operation was designed to meet and counteract certain conditions which Magnuson and Stack believe exist in recurrent shoulder dislocations.

Ordinarily the subscapularis tendon is broad and strong and blends with the capsule of the shoulder, thus reinforcing the capsule in this region and tending to counteract the pull of the strong adductors, namely, the pectoralis major, the teres major, and the latissimus dorsi (Fig. 1). If, on the other hand, the tendon of the subscapularis is thin and narrow or if it does not blend fully with

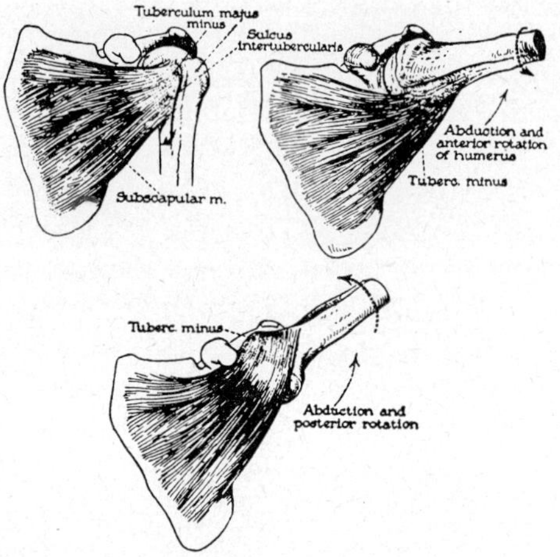

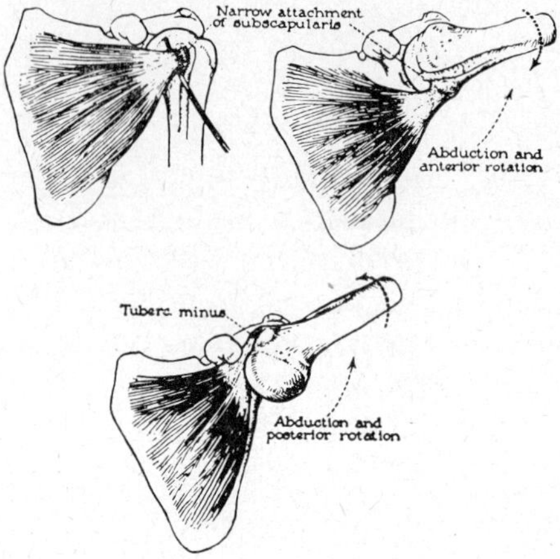

Fig. 1.—Attachment of subscapularis to lesser tuberosity of humerus. (Figs. 1 to 5 from Magnuson and Stack, J. A. M. A. December, 1943.[2])

Fig. 2.—Tendon slipping between head of humerus and coracoid when arm is placed in abduction and extension.

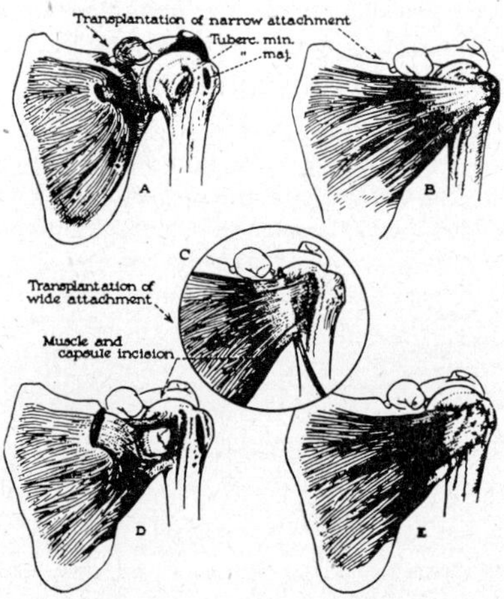

Fig. 3.—Medial reflection of tendinous attachment and exposure of head of humerus.

the capsule, then the space between the subscapularis tendon, which latter attaches to the lesser tuberosity, and the supraspinatus, infraspinatus, and teres minor muscles, which attach to the greater tuberosity, is so increased as to permit the head to dislocate downward and forward between these two groups of muscles (Fig. 2). The abnormality of a loose tendon, and therefore slipping of this structure in between the head and the coracoid was not seen in any of the series of cases reported here. The tendon was found to be quite thin and narrow in a number of instances.

The operation, therefore, was designed to overcome this weak point in the musculotendinous cuff by transplanting the subscapularis from the lesser to the greater tuberosity (Fig. 3), thus forming a musculotendinous cup around the anterior surface of the head of the humerus which is controlled by the subscapularis, which reinforces the capsule in the region of the insertion of the supraspinatus, infraspinatus and teres minor, and which overcomes the spread which exists ordinarily (Fig. 5).

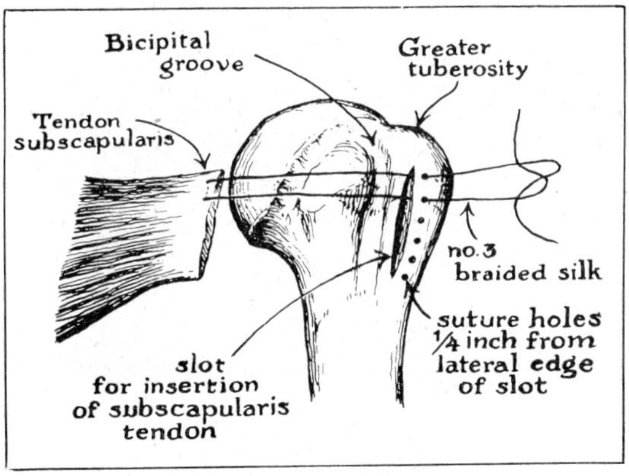

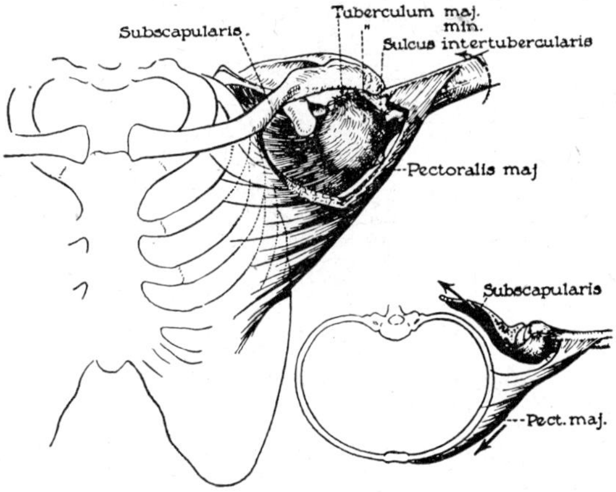

Fig. 4.—Method of application of braided silk No. 3 suture to draw tendon into slot.
Fig. 5.—Tendon and muscle of subscapularis winds firmly around head of humerus.

OPERATIVE PROCEDURE

A four to five inch incision is made on the anterior aspect of the shoulder beginning just below the acromioclavicular joint and extending distally parallel to the fibers of the deltoid. The muscle fibers are split at the region of the anterior and middle thirds exposing the capsule. Bleeding is controlled by the use of the coagulating current, which latter is quite an efficient and certainly a time-saving device. The extremity is externally rotated thus bringing into view the tendon and the musculotendinous junction of the subscapularis. A blunt dissector is then slipped under the musculotendinous junction just lateral to the area where the tendon blends in with the capsule, the dissector being inserted at the lower border and coming out at the upper border. This portion of the structure is easily identified and requires very little sharp dissection. Traction is then applied by lifting up on the blunt dissector, thus bringing into relief the insertion of the muscle into the capsule and also the upper and lower borders of the tendon where they blend to the capsule (Fig. 3). The incision is made along the upper and lower borders of the tendon through the capsule, the scalpel is then slipped under the tendon and the tendon and capsule are then incised, thus freeing these structures to the area of their insertion into the lesser tuberosity.

During the first three or four operations an attempt was made to free the tendon from the capsule, but it was found to be almost impossible, and furthermore the tendon itself was much thinner and thus a weaker structure. Magnuson and Stack in their procedure then recommended removing a wedge-shaped piece of bone at the insertion of the tendon, for transposition into the greater tuberosity. This step has not been followed. Instead, the tendon is detached from the lesser tuberosity, a suture is passed through it so that it can be brought into the field whenever necessary, and the extremity is then internally rotated to bring the bicipital groove and the greater tuberosity into view. The joint can be inspected at this time and any tear of the capsule noted. After the arm has been internally rotated, the tendon is pulled across the bicipital groove to the greater tuberosity to determine the new location of the tendon. During this time the arm should be externally rotated to observe how much external rotation is permitted with the tendon in its new position. The amount of external rotation should never be less than 50 per cent of the normal amount and not more than 75 per cent of the normal amount. Two thin-bladed chisels, one-half inch wide, should then be driven into the greater tuberosity next to one another and parallel to the outer edge of the bicipital groove, thus forming a slot approximately one inch in length. The two chisels should then be rocked back and forth in opposite directions to widen this slot. A heavy, small tenaculum or a towel clip should be used to make six holes approximately one-quarter of an inch lateral to the lateral edge of the slot. Three No. 3 braided silk mattress sutures are used to immobilize the tendon (Fig. 4). They are inserted through the most proximal hole out through the slot, through the tendon from the dorsal to the ventral surface, up through from the ventral surface to the dorsal surface through the slot, and out through the second hole. After all three sutures have been placed, they are drawn tightly, thus pulling the tendon into the slot, and are tied securely. The upper and lower borders of the tendon are then sutured to the surrounding capsular structure with interrupted No. 40 white cotton sutures so that there will be no tendency of the tendon to slip up toward the coracoid process when the arm is held in a position of abduction. This part of the procedure is very important, for it is felt that the two failures which occurred in this series are due to the fact that this step was not carried out in either instance. The arm should again be externally rotated and if the operation has been properly performed, there should be no more than a 50 per cent limitation of external rotation. The deltoid fibers are allowed to fall back into place, and the soft tissues are closed in the usual anatomic manner. The upper extremity is then immobilized against the chest using a Velpeau bandage.

The period of absolute immobilization is three weeks. At the end of this period of immobilization active and passive exercises are instituted in the form of pendulum exercises actively, three times daily for ten minutes, and gentle external rotation passively once daily by the physiotherapist. Active external rotation and abduction were not instituted until the end of six weeks, at which time these motions are included in the daily exercise routine. At the end of eight weeks the average patient has almost complete range of all motions, except for external rotation which is usually limited to about 110 degrees of the normal, the normal being between 130 to 140 degrees.

ANALYSIS

Thirty-one shoulders were operated upon in thirty patients. All had had a minimum of at least three, and usually five, dislocations, and quite a number of them had lost count of the number of dislocations. In one patient the shoulder dislocated whenever it was abducted beyond 90 degrees. Twelve months after the operation he passed a West Point physical examination. Another patient stated that his main concern was that the shoulder dislocated in his sleep as frequently as twice a night. The maximum follow-up has been three years, and the minimum one and one-half years.

Avulsion.—In nineteen shoulders, or 60.6 per cent, there was definite evidence found of avulsion of the capsule from the anteroinferior glenoid rim. This was determined by inspecting the shoulder joint when a small section of the capsule was removed along with the tendon of the subscapularis. A blunt dissector was then inserted into the joint, the glenoid rim palpated, the tear located, and, when present, inspected. No attempt was made to repair it. In the other twelve shoulders no tear could be found. It was possible to dislocate these shoulders quite easily at the operating table, but no definite pathology could be found other than a general relaxation of the capsule.

Recurrences.—There were only two recurrences to date, or 6.4 per cent. Both of these shoulders dislocated approximately six to eight months after surgery. It is felt, however, that the fault does not lie with the procedure, but rather with the operator. In each of these instances the upper and lower borders of the transposed tendon were not sutured to the surrounding capsular structures, and, therefore, probable slipping of the tendon occurred because of it. It would be interesting to re-explore these shoulders, but to date the patients concerned have been unwilling to submit to further surgery.

Motion.—The primary motion concerned in each instance is, of course, external rotation. As previously mentioned, at the end of eight weeks postsurgery, there was limitation of external rotation in almost all of the patients. At the present writing, however, only eight or 27.6 per cent, had any definite limitation of external rotation. One had a 30 degree limitation of motion. Of the rest, one had 20 degrees loss, and the general average was approximately 10 degrees. However, none of the patients, except the one with the 30 degrees limitation of external rotation, were particularly incapacitated because of this loss, nor did they complain about it. The remaining twenty-one shoulders, or 72.4 per cent, had a trace or no limitation of external rotation, and it was less than 10 degrees in comparison to the opposite shoulder. Abduction through the scapulohumeral joint, which is the next important factor to consider, was limited in five patients. The maximum loss was 45 degrees in one patient, 25 degrees in another, and 15 degrees in three patients. Two patients showed a loss of forward extension—15 degrees in one, and 10 degrees in the other.

Pain.—Regarding pain upon use of the operated extremity, eight patients reported its presence. One patient who had a recurrence stated that the shoulder ached constantly. The other seven noticed pain or stiffness only after strenuous use or upon changes in weather. Thus, 77.5 per cent had asymptomatic shoulders.

It is important to remember that this operative procedure was performed on military personnel and that the strenuous use of these shoulders in the armed services is usually far and above the amount required in civilian life. These patients were able to return to limited duty at the end of eight weeks, and at the end of three months all were able to return to full duty, except for three patients who had continued symptomatology of the operated shoulder, and in two of these the shoulders subsequently dislocated. In the follow-up study from the reports solicited from the patients and their physicians, the majority of these men had been able to carry on a full day's work without any difficulty whatever. Some are able to ski and perform other strenuous physical activities without any difficulty. One patient proudly wrote that he was able to chin himself fourteen times on a chinning bar in spite of the operated shoulder.

CONCLUSIONS

1. The Magnuson-Stack Procedure has been successful in 91.6 per cent of the present series of cases, with a minimum follow-up of one and one-half years.
2. In 72.4 per cent there was a trace or no limitation of external rotation.
3. In 77.5 per cent of the patients, the shoulder operated upon was entirely asymptomatic, and the patient concerned was able to perform a gainful occupation.
4. The two postoperative recurrences were not due to failure of the operative procedure, but were due to errors in technique on the part of the operator.
5. The Magnuson-Stack procedure is a well-planned operation, and this report is presented at this time in the hope that others will use this procedure, and thus amass a large enough series of cases within the next five to ten years so that definite conclusions can be reached as to the final value of the operation.

The author wishes to take this opportunity to thank Dr. Edmond Uhry and Dr. Charles A. Hulse, whose able assistance and suggestions have been of great value in performing this work.

REFERENCES

1. Bankart, A. S. B.: The Pathology and Treatment of the Recurrent Dislocation of the Shoulder Joint, Brit. J. Surg. **26**:23-29, 1938.
2. Magnuson, Paul B., and Stack, James K.: Recurrent Dislocation of the Shoulder, J. A. M. A. **123**:889-892, 1943.
3. Nicola, Toufick: Recurrent Anterior Dislocation of the Shoulder, J. Bone & Joint Surg. **2**: 128-132, 1929.
4. Henderson, M. S.: Habitual Dislocation of the Shoulder, J. A. M. A. **95**: 1653, 1930.
5. Magnuson, Paul B.: Treatment of Recurrent Dislocation of the Shoulder, S. Clin. North America **25**:14-20, 1945.

A PLASTER TRACTION SPLINT FOR COMPOUND COMMINUTED FRACTURES OF THE TIBIA AND FIBULA

MARSHALL R. URIST, M.D.,* BOSTON, MASS., LINCOLN RIES, M.D.,† YAKIMA, WASH., AND THOMAS B. QUIGLEY, M.D.,‡ BOSTON, MASS.

(From the Department of Orthopedic Surgery, Massachusetts General Hospital, the Department of Surgery, Peter Bent Brigham Hospital, and Harvard Medical School)

THE efficiency of the plaster traction splint described in this communication was evaluated under military circumstances in the 22nd United States Army General Hospital at Blandford, England, and the 97th General Hospital at Frankfurt, Germany, between May, 1944, and December, 1945. During this period we personally used it in sixty-five battle-incurred fractures of the tibia and fibula in sixty-three patients and in eleven simple and compound comminuted accidental fractures of the same bones. During the early months of the same period an approximately equal number of similar fractures, which served, in effect, as a control series, were treated in the Böhler-Braun splint or in the Thomas splint with Pearson attachment. As the advantages of the combination splint, which at first was used only tentatively, became clarified, standard splints were used less and less frequently.

From the standpoint of providing skeletal traction and securing immobilization of the fractures in plaster, the combination splint was found to compare very favorably with the classical traction splints. It was also found to possess several additional advantages. It furnishes better protection for the reduced fractures. It makes movement less painful during the early days of healing. It eliminates the uncomfortable counterpressure of the ischial ring of the Thomas splint and the painful play at the fracture site permitted by the Böhler-Braun frame. It does not require the time-consuming, continuous, expert attention necessary when the Thomas splint with Pearson attachment is used, which made it of particular value during the war when heavy casualties were received. Finally, it proved of great usefulness in patients received more than eight to twelve hours after injury, when internal fixation was contraindicated by the risk of infection or when extensively comminuted fractures of the shaft of the tibia would have required undesirable dissection of the whole leg for the safe application of plates and screws.

The plaster traction splint would seem to be as applicable to compound fractures of the tibia and fibula in civilian practice as it was in military surgery, and it is presented with this thought in view.

The traction splint, which is made of materials in standard supply in all fracture clinics, is constructed and applied as follows (Figs. 1 to 3): A plaster

Received for publication, July 8, 1947.

*Formerly Major, Medical Corps, Army of the United States.

†Formerly Captain, Medical Corps, Army of the United States.

‡Formerly Lieutenant Colonel, Medical Corps, Army of the United States.

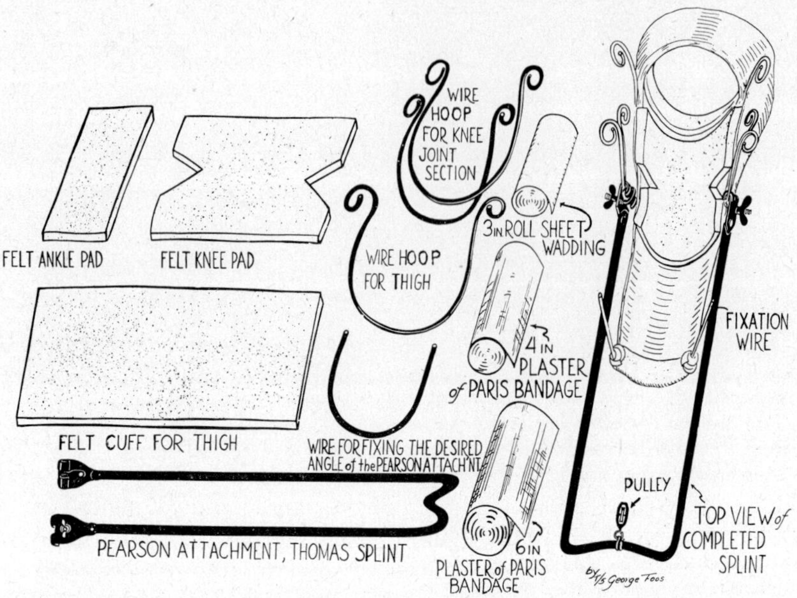

Fig. 1.—Materials used in construction of plaster traction splint for compound fractures of the tibia and fibula, with interior view, from above, of assembled splint.

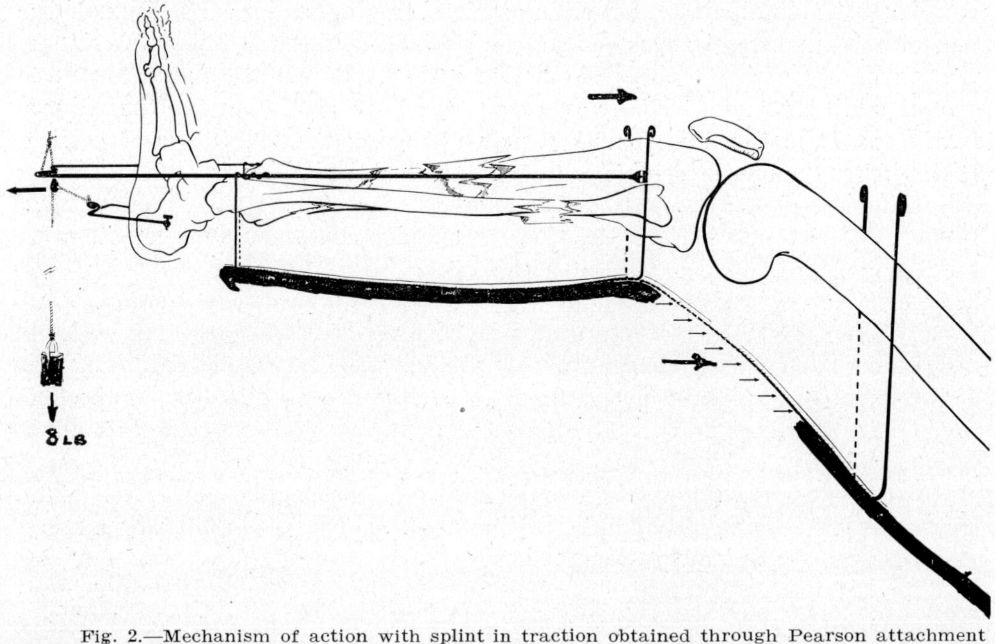

Fig. 2.—Mechanism of action with splint in traction obtained through Pearson attachment incorporated in long leg plaster cast. The countertraction is mainly from a hoop to which the Pearson attachment is clamped at right angles, and also, but slightly, from the ventral aspect of the cast around the thigh.

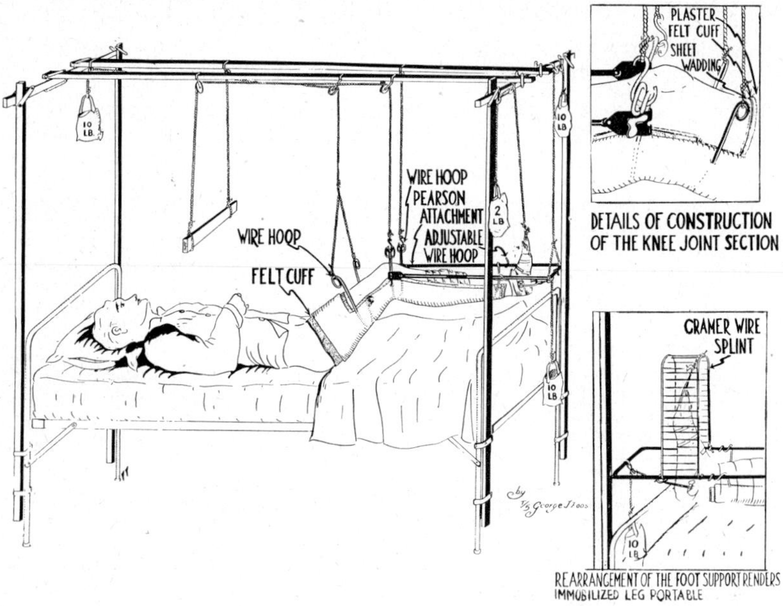

Fig. 3.—Diagrammatic showing of method of suspension of splint and use of trapeze by which patient can lift himself off bed and aid in his own nursing care. Details of construction of the knee joint section are shown in upper right insert. Method of mobilizing splint and adding foot support is shown in lower right insert.

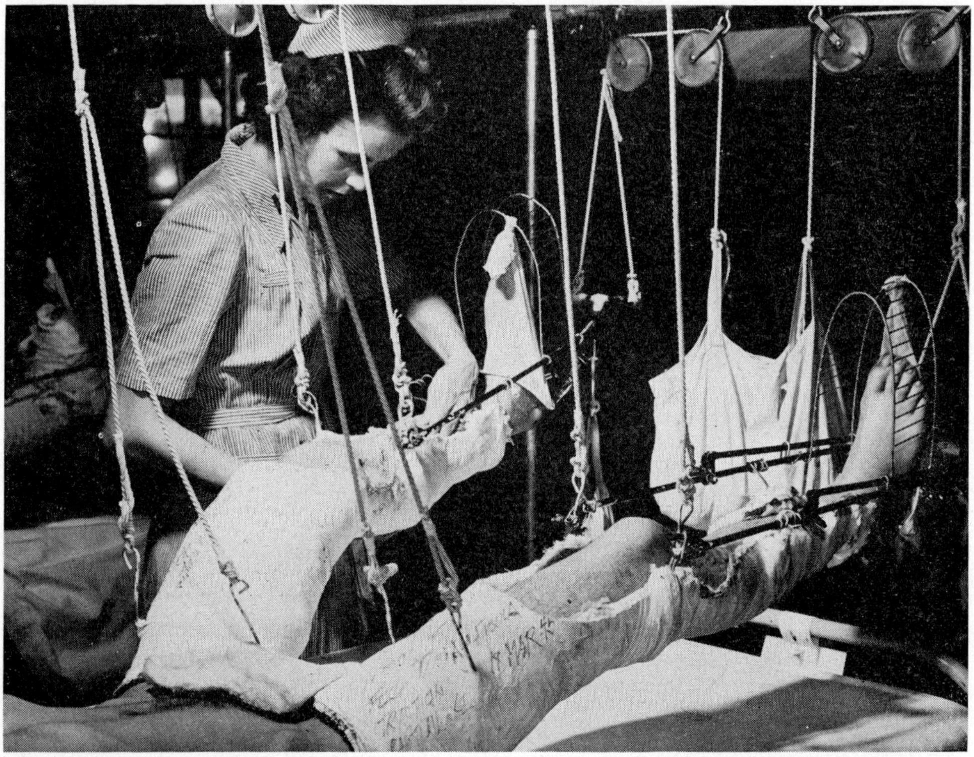

Fig. 4.—Traction splints applied for bilateral compound fractures of tibia and fibula. The wounds were closed by delayed suture seven days after the splints had been applied. The physiotherapist is supervising early muscle-setting exercises during third week of healing.

cylinder, padded with felt in the upper thigh and the popliteal and malleolar regions, is applied from the groin to the ankle while the knee and hip are flexed 45 degrees. U-shaped wire hoops, fashioned from No. 12 iron wire, or any other available metal rod, are incorporated in the plaster at the midthigh and the malleolus, so that the closed portion circles the lateral and posterior aspects of the leg. Two similar wire hoops (or a single heavier metal hoop) are similarly incorporated in the plaster at the knee. A Pearson attachment, with a pulley fastened to the crossbar, is placed over the leg in the sagittal plane and clamped in place to the hoops at the knee (Fig. 1). The ends of the wire at the malleolar level are wound about the Pearson attachment. The anterior portion of the cast between the open ends of the hoop is cut away from the superior pole of the patella to the ankle, and windows are cut, if necessary, on the posterior and lateral aspects to give access to soft tissue wounds.

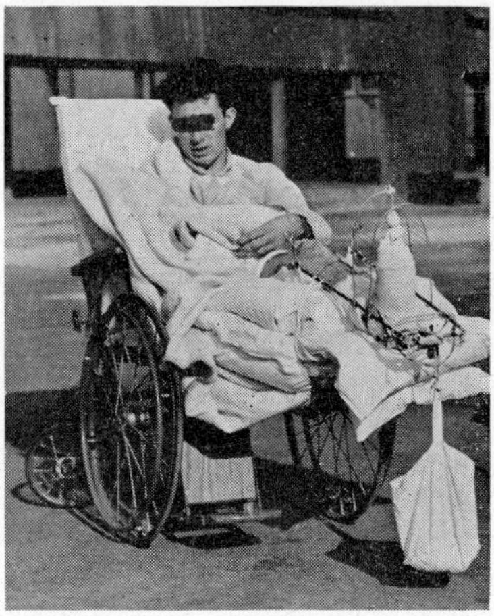

Fig. 5.—Patient in traction splint after overhead suspension has been discontinued.

A suitable weight is attached and traction is applied with the leg suspended in a Balkan frame (Figs. 3 and 4). The foot is supported by a stockinet or moleskin sling fastened to a loop of Cramer wire attached to the long bars of the Pearson attachment. When minor corrections in alignment become necessary, the distal fragment can be moved up to 10 degrees in the sagittal or coronal planes by shifting the pulley from side to side and elevating or lowering the end of the Pearson attachment.

Overhead suspension is continued during the first two weeks of healing, when the nursing ritual, including the bath and the use of the bedpan, are painful undertakings. As healing progresses, overhead suspension is discontinued and the patient is allowed more freedom in bed. At the end of three to five weeks, when movement is practically painless, he can be placed in a wheel chair (Fig. 5). At the end of six weeks, when callus formation is usually adequate or the fracture site is sufficiently stable, traction can be discontinued and the extremity transferred to a long leg cast, after which ambulation on crutches is instituted as rapidly as possible.

The treatment followed in fractures on which this apparatus was used in World War II is applicable to similar civilian injuries. Thorough débridement was done and the wound was closed by primary suture if the patient was received within eight hours of injury and if damage to the soft parts had not been too extensive. If he was received after this period, the wound was left open at the initial operation and, in the absence of gross infection, was closed by delayed suture within five days or, later, by grafting.

At the first operation in a general hospital skeletal traction was instituted by the application of a Kirschner wire. In fractures of the upper third of the tibia the wire was inserted about one-half inch above the distal epiphyseal line of the tibia. In fractures of the middle and lower thirds it was inserted through the tuberosity of the os calcis, in line with the posterior margin of the fibula. A small Steinmann pin was used in some cases, with complete satisfaction. It was soon found that it was essential to insert the wire or the pin at an exact right angle to the weight-bearing line, without tension on the soft tissues, and with the limb in the position it was to occupy in the completed splint. If these criteria were not met when the wire was applied, it was withdrawn and reapplied. Lack of care in these respects was responsible for several instances of pin seepage and sepsis.

The fractures were reduced by traction and manipulation and held on a fracture table, with the hip and the knee each at 135 degrees. The tautening bow of the Kirschner wire served as a useful handle on the distal fragment for manipulation purposes and was fixed to the footpiece of the table after the reduction had been secured. With this arrangement the position of the reduced fracture was secure while the plaster bandage was being applied and traction was being established.

SUMMARY

1. A combination plaster traction splint is described which was used for simple and compound comminuted fractures of the tibia and fibula during World War II. It proved as effective as classical traction splints in providing skeletal traction and securing immobilization, and it was found to possess several additional advantages which other splints lack.

2. It is believed that this splint is as applicable to simple and compound comminuted fractures of the tibia and fibula in civilian practice as it was to battle-incurred fractures.

SUBCUTANEOUS RUPTURE OF THE BRACHIORADIALIS MUSCLE

ALFRED T. HAMILTON, M.D., RALEIGH, N. C.

AFTER an exhaustive review of the literature, it is evident that subcutaneous rupture of the brachioradialis is probably hitherto unreported. Other muscle rupture is, of course, very common. It may result from excessive tension or from direct trauma, especially if the muscle involved in under voluntary tension at the time. The most common point of rupture is at the musclotendinous juncture, but the rupture may occur at the muscle's origin, at its insertion, or across its belly. Common predisposing factors are: (1) diseases, such as the acute generalized infections, local tumor, local trauma, trichinosis, and local infections; (2) previous wear and tear; and (3) age, with attendant muscle brittleness, inelasticity, and associated arthritis. Certain occupations provide the second factor of wear and tear. Hence, in plasterers, one sees rupture of the long head of the biceps; in drummers, rupture of the extensor pollicis longus; in climbers, rupture of the Achilles tendon; in loaders, rupture of the muscles of the neck; and in horsemen, rupture of the adductors of the thigh. Other ruptures not infrequently encountered are that of the extensor tendon of the finger at its distal insertion, the so-called "mallet finger," those of the supraspinatus tendon, of the rectus abdominis muscle, the gastrocnemius, and the quadriceps. All these muscles have in common one characteristic, the constant liability of great strain while in a state of voluntary contraction.

This characteristic is not possessed to a great degree by the brachioradialis and this fact probably explains its relative immunity of this injury. The muscle is the most superficial on the radial side of the forearm; it arises from the upper two-thirds of the lateral supracondylar ridge of the humerus, from the lateral intermuscular septum, and from the lateral humeral epicondyle. Fibers from the large muscle belly end above the mid-forearm in a flat tendon which is inserted into the lateral side of the base of the styloid process of the radius. It is apparent that supination, while undoubtedly induced to some degree by the muscle, is not its major function, and that the name "supinator longus" is, for this reason, misleading. Actually, the muscle's primary function is flexion of the radius on the humerus and is most efficiently undertaken with the forearm in the neutral position between supination and pronation, that is, with the radial side of the forearm faced directly upward.

CASE REPORT

R. B., on Jan. 29, 1947, caught the right hand and forearm and elbow between a rotary conveyor belt and the drive wheel of a machine he was operating. He sustained a mild abrasion of the forearm, but rapidly developed a tremendous hematoma of the entire arm. There was no evidence of nerve injury, and x-ray examination showed no fracture. The patient was kept in the hospital for three days, the arm being wrapped in grease dressings and kept constantly elevated. He was then allowed to go home, heat, a sling, and medication

Received for publication, July 8, 1947.

for the relief of pain being prescribed. He remained away from work for about two weeks, at the end of which time the arm was very much improved in appearance, and entirely asymptomatic. The patient returned to light work and after about two more weeks the swelling had subsided sufficiently for there to be apparent a gap in the brachioradialis at approximately the point where it normally joins its tendon. The patient complained of weakness in the whole forearm, but particularly weakness of flexion. On March 2, 1947, the forearm was explored under pentothal anesthesia. An Esmarch tourniquet was applied and a vertical incision made over the body of the brachioradialis. The deep fascia was incised, revealing a serum-filled cavity between the rounded, retracted, annealed belly of the brachioradialis and the scarred adherent tendon. The rounded belly was freed from the interosseous membrane and adjacent structures, care being taken to preserve the radial artery running along its medial border. The muscle belly was unfortunately nearly devoid of fascia. The

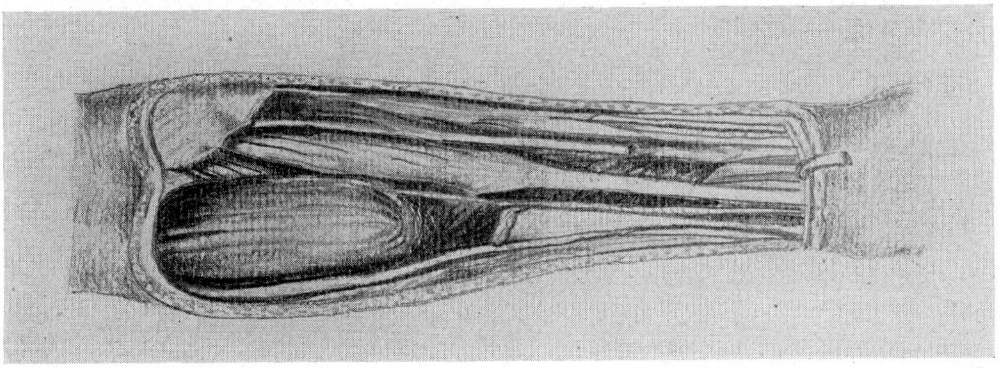

Fig. 1.

tendon was dissected up, its proximal scarred tip was excised, and the tendon itself divided vertically in the midline. With deep chromic catgut sutures the muscle belly was sutured into the tendinous V thus formed. The fascia, subcutaneous tissue, and skin were closed with fine catgut, a petrolatum gauze dressing overlain with sheet cotton applied, and the arm encased from axilla to wrist in plaster, the elbow at right angles, the forearm in supination. The case remained on for four weeks, at the end of which time the wound was well healed. The patient began active motion upon being released from plaster, and at the end of twelve weeks had normal motion and apparently normal strength in the involved arm.

In review, two possible mechanisms by which this muscle was ruptured are apparent. Either the original trauma, with the voluntary effort on the part of the patient to release himself, ruptured the muscle directly, or, following trauma, muscular hemorrhage, and partial recovery, the patient, on resuming light work, subjected the weakened muscle to sufficient strain to bring about its rupture.

FOUR METACHRONOUS MALIGNANT LESIONS OF THE COLON

An Unusual Case

Monte Edwards, M.D., M.R.C.S. (Eng.), Baltimore, Md.

SIMULTANEOUS involvement of the large intestine by two or more malignancies, usually on the basis of polyposis, has been given its full share of publicity, with the consequence that concomitant lesions are usually recognized and dealt with at the one appropriate time.[1-3] Metachronous lesions may be viewed more leisurely in that each provides a new train of symptoms with no incident between. Interest in the case to be reported lies in the absence of polyposis, the survival of the patient for nineteen years between the first and the fourth lesions, and his resumption of professional activities, limited only by his age, following the most recent resection.

A somewhat similar case, in which four resections were performed within a period of five years, presents features which suggest overlap of consecutive lesions.[4]

CASE REPORT

The patient was a practicing physician, 79 years old at the time of this communication. Subjective evidence of gastrointestinal disturbance first manifested itself in 1926.

First Lesion.—The patient was admitted to Maryland General Hospital on May 3, 1927. He gave a history of general abdominal distress with much flatulence and increasing difficulty with the bowels for one year. For six weeks before admission there had been a dragging sensation in the abdomen and cramps in the left lower quadrant, most noticeable during defecation. Small amounts of blood were occasionally seen in the stool. Abdominal palpation revealed a mass in the left lower quadrant. There was no distention. X-ray studies made prior to admission showed a deformity at the upper end of the pelvic colon. Except for an untransmitted systolic bruit at the apex, the rest of the physical examination was essentially negative.

At operation on May 5, 1927, performed under ether anesthesia, a low left pararectus incision was made and approximately 15 cm. of sigmoid colon, containing a tumor, were removed. The severed ends of the bowel were exteriorized through the original incision. At the time of discharge, on May 25, 1927, the bowel ends were said to be in good condition, draining freely.

Pathologic report (No. 7625, Maryland General Hospital) showed adenocarcinoma. There was no recognizable malignancy in mesocolic lymph glands.

Closure of the colostomy was effected on Oct. 12, 1927, at a subsequent admission, and healing was complete before the end of the year.

Second Lesion.—Because of an attack of nausea and vomiting lasting several hours, followed by persistent constipation relieved only by enemas, a barium study of the colon was performed on June 10, 1935. In the right third of the transverse colon there was a definite obstruction to the progress of the opaque medium, and a tentative diagnosis of neoplasm was made. The patient was admitted to University Hospital on June 18, 1935. At operation, performed two days later, a constricting lesion was freed and exteriorized through an upper right pararectus incision. Complementary cecostomy was performed through a stab wound in the right loin. On June 28, 1935, the tumor mass was removed and a clamp applied to the spur.

The patient was discharged Sept. 4, 1935, with cecostomy and transverse colostomy draining freely. The cecostomy closed spontaneously, and the colostomy yielded some months

Received for publication, July 10, 1947.

later to the unusual maneuver of insertion of a purse-string suture in the parietes around the stoma.

Pathologic report (No. 25487, University Hospital) revealed adenocarcinoma of colon. The patient came under my observation for the first time on July 14, 1941.

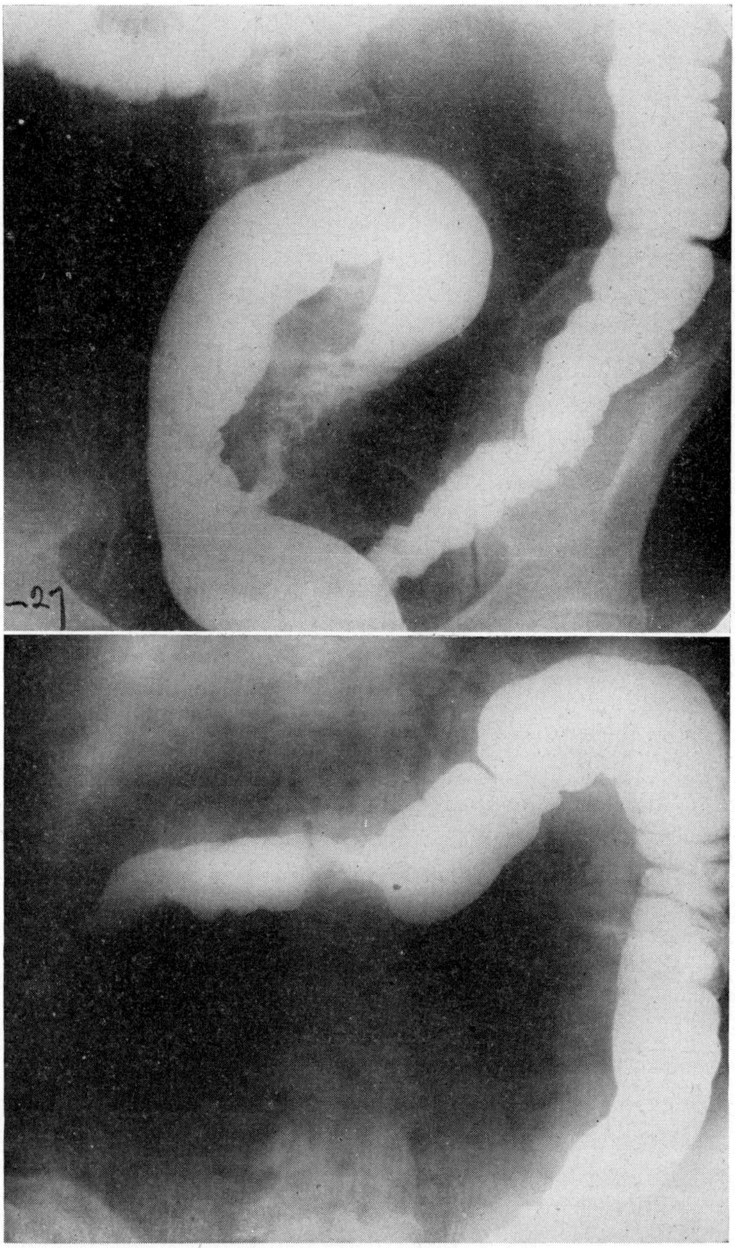

Fig. 1.—Roentgenograms showing filling defects in sigmoid colon of first lesion and in transverse colon of fourth lesion. Other films had been destroyed. (Courtesy of Dr. John Evans, who made all x-ray studies.)

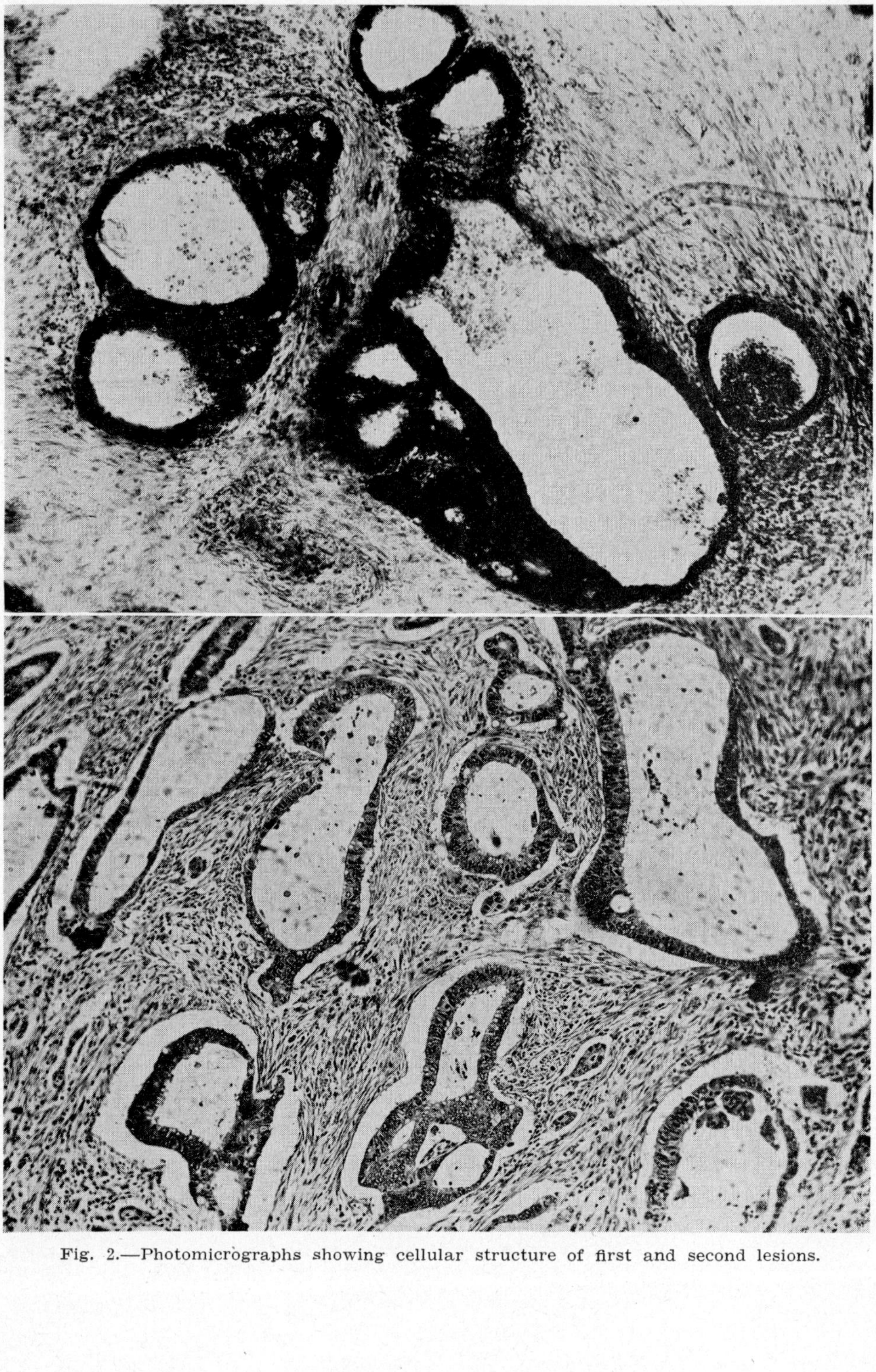

Fig. 2.—Photomicrographs showing cellular structure of first and second lesions.

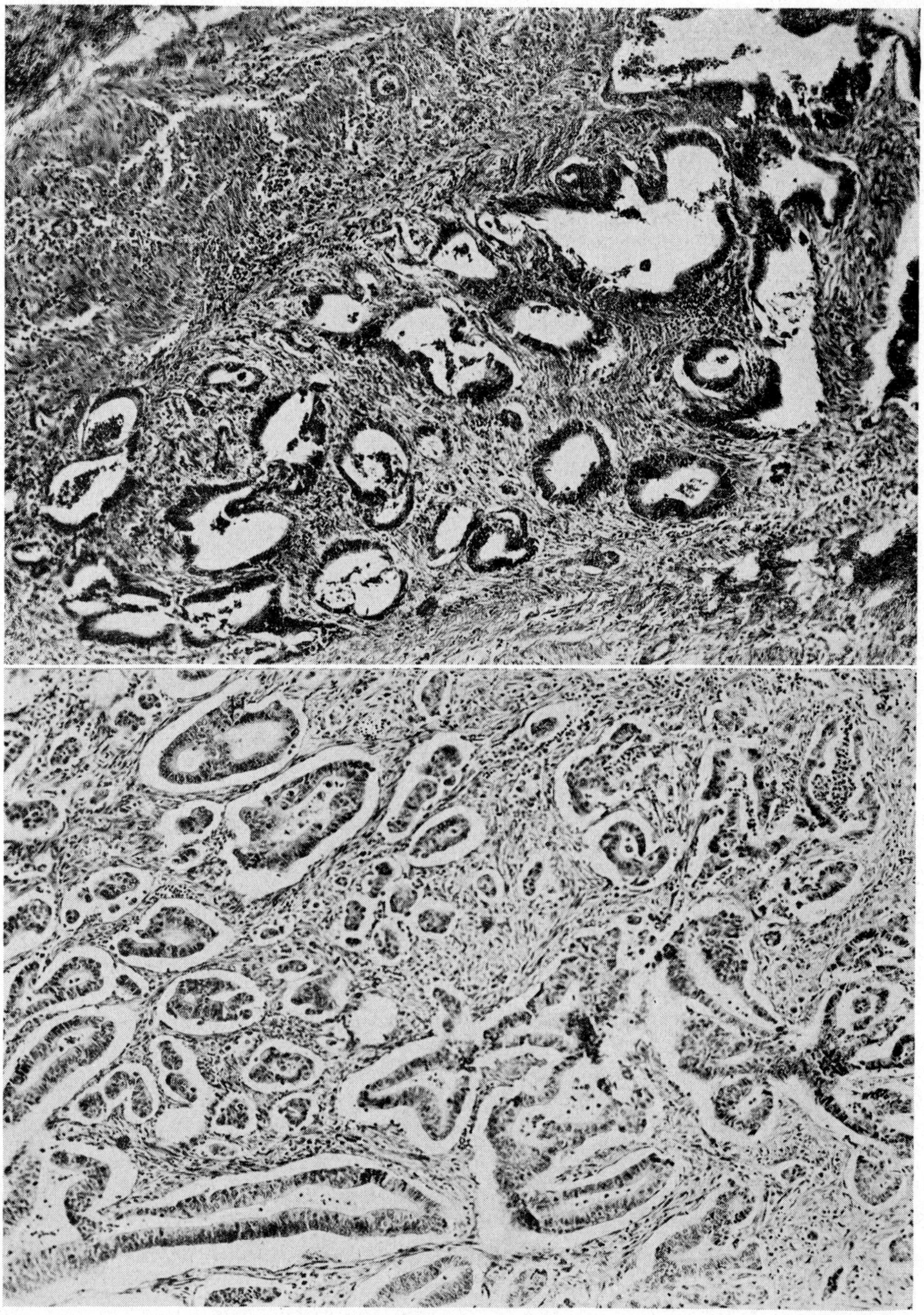

Fig. 3.—Photomicrographs showing cellular structure of third and fourth lesions.

Third Lesion.—For two months prior to admission to University Hospital on July 28, 1941, the patient's suspicions were aroused by a gradual postponement of morning defecation for several hours later than was customary for him. The stools were normal, containing neither gross blood nor mucus. A barium enema performed on July, 10, 1941, showed some delay in the advance of the barium column in the sigmoid, attributable, perhaps, to constriction at the site of the first operation. However, at proctoscopy on July 14, 1941, a well-defined vegetative lesion was seen at 18 cm. from the anus.

On Aug. 5, 1941, following an eight-day sulfaguanidine preparation, laparotomy was performed through a low left paramedian incision. A small, firm mass with slight dimpling on its serosal surface was found 8 cm. above the pelvic peritoneal reflection. Many organized adhesions between omentum, viscera, and parietal peritoneum prevented any attempt at manual exploration. In spite of a previous resection, there remained sufficient sigmoid colon to permit adequate resection and open end-to-end anastomosis.

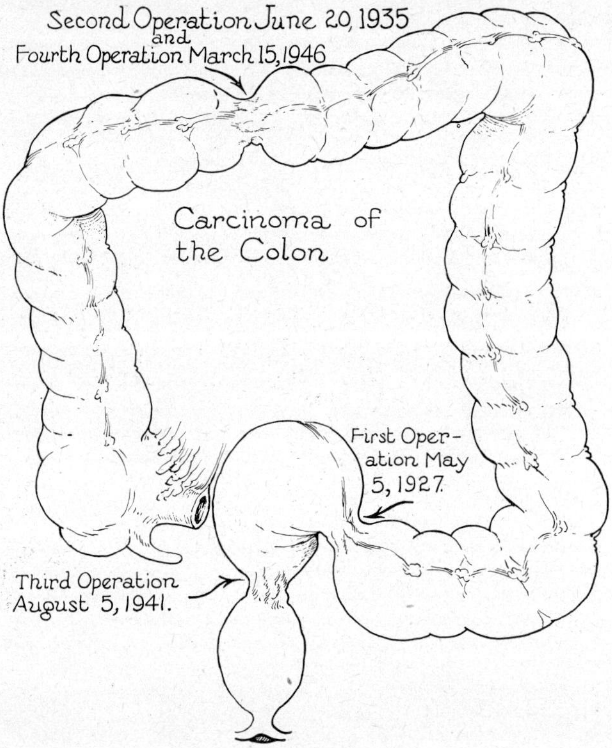

Fig. 4.—Schematic drawing showing approximate location of all four lesions. That removed at third operation was at a slightly higher level than indicated.

Convalescene was without incident and the patient was discharged from the hospital on Aug. 23, 1941. Proctoscopy on Sept. 24, 1941, revealed no narrowing at the level of the anastomosis.

Pathologic report (S.P. 41665, University Hospital) showed adenocarcinoma of sigmoid, grade II, with mucinous change.

Fourth Lesion.—During August, 1945, the patient became conscious of tenderness and an increasing firmness in the scar of the second operation in the right upper quadrant. He described a gurgling sensation, as of gas passing through a narrowed section of bowel beneath the scar. Barium enema confirmed this observation. Proctoscopy performed to 20 cm. was negative. A sulfasuxidine preparation, begun prior to admission to University Hospital on

March 13, 1946, was continued until operation two days later. A lens-shaped piece of scar and skin were included in the initial incisions, which were carried down to the peritoneal cavity wide of indurated tissue. Dense adhesions were severed in an attempt, with but somewhat limited success, to mobilize the transverse colon toward right and left flexures. It was possible to resect all involved tissue with two inches of gut to spare on each side of the lesion. End-to-end open anastomosis was effected with slight tension. Approximation of the parietes and skin was aided by contralateral incisions and Tiffany wire tension sutures. Slight separation of the skin margins at the middle of the wound with escape of watery material on the fifth postoperative day persisted for three weeks but did not interfere seriously with the convalescence, which had advanced sufficiently to permit discharge from the hospital on April 11, 1946.

Healing was complete two weeks later, by which time the patient had resumed his practice. Examination on Feb. 1, 1947, revealed the abdomen to be free from palpable recurrence. The patient's weight was 205 pounds, and he was very active for his age.

Pathologic report (S.P. 53931, University Hospital) revealed adenocarcinoma of transverse colon, with involvement of skin and parietes.

COMMENT

Of the four lesions removed, the first three were undoubtedly primary. The fourth may represent a recurrence of the second lesion. At least the scaffolding may have survived the ten intervening years. The pathologic findings are very similar in each of the four tumors.

The limitations for further interference in this case would appear to be either from lack of years or lack of available colon. Parenthetically, the patient has outlived two of his surgeons.

REFERENCES

1. Bargen, J. A., and Rankin, F. W.: Multiple Carcinomata of the Large Intestine, Ann. Surg. **91**: 583-593, 1930.
2. Stalker, L. K., Phillips, R. B., and Pemberton, J.: Multiple Primary Malignant Lesions, Surg., Gynec. & Obst. **68**: 595-602, 1939.
3. Schweiger, L. R., and Bargen, J. A.: Multiple Primary Malignant Lesions of the Large Bowel, Arch. Int. Med. **66**: 1331-1340, 1940.
4. Mayo, C. W.: Multiple Primary Malignant Lesions of the Colon With Resection. Report of an Unusual Case, Proc. Staff. Meet., Mayo Clin. **15**: 479-480, 1940.

BENIGN LYMPHOMA OF THE RECTUM

IRENE Y. LI, M.D., NEW YORK, N. Y.

(From the Laboratory of Surgical Pathology, College of Physicians and Surgeons, Columbia University)

AMONG the polypoid tumors of the rectum, clinically suspected of being adenoma or some other benign or even malignant tumor, some of them when examined microscopically prove to be composed of lymphoid tissue. This may occasion doubt as to whether one is dealing with a benign process, either hyperplastic or neoplastic, or a lymphosarcoma. Therefore, an analysis of the clinical and morphologic data obtained both from the literature and from the material of the Laboratory of Surgical Pathology of Columbia University may help one to know more about the nature of this growth.

Table I summarizes forty-nine cases of which those numbered 1 to 23 have been previously reported from other clinics, while the remainder were collected in this laboratory during a period of twenty-seven years, from 1920 to 1946.

Case 1 reported in 1890 by Ball[1] was clinically diagnosed as adenoma. The author presumed that the growth originated in the solitary lymphatic follicles of the rectum. He also mentioned that tumors like this unassociated with obvious lymphoid tissue disease in other parts of the body were previously not observed.

Case 2 reported in 1908-1909 by Greig[2] was termed "lymphoma" by this author, who agreed with Ball as to the origin and rarity of this growth at that time.

Cases 3 and 4, reported in 1925 by Lehmann,[3] were described as submucosal, nodular tumors with no tendency to bleed. He attributed the bleeding in one of his cases to the complicating hemorrhoids.

Case 5 reported in 1927 by Knoflach[4] was complicated by stomach cancer.

Case 6 was reported in 1931 by Konjetzny.[5]

Case 7 reported in 1931 by Siemens[6] was polypoid and considered benign by the author.

Cases 8 to 13 reported in 1932 by Dick[7] under the term of lymphadenoid rectal polyp were among seventy cases of polypoid rectal tumors of various natures. He concurred in the opinions of various investigators that this condition of growth is invariably considered to be hyperplasia of previous existing lymphoid tissue of the rectum and has never been proved to be a true tumor or granulaton tissue.

Case 14 reported in 1933 by Epstein[8] was described microscopically as a lobulated, submucosal nodule breaking the muscularis mucosae and penetrating into mucosa, and composed of large cells of a lymphocytic variety forming germinal centers. He described this growth as differing from the structure of a normal lymph node by the absence of a definite capsule, marginal sinuses, and medullary cords. He illustrated a number of cases reported, such as those of Gripp, Felizet, Branca, Broca, and Malgat. He also quoted Schwab's case of multiple polypi which was named diffuse lymphadenoma.

Cases 15 to 17 were reported in 1934 by Dukes.[9] Two of them were pedunculated tumors and the other was a submucosal induration. Histologically the three cases were identical with each other. He emphasized that the case with submucosal induration deserved to be mentioned because it resembled lymphosarcoma, which needs an entirely different treatment.

Case 18 reported in 1940 by Hayes and his associates[10] showed symptoms bearing no direct relation with the rectum except constipation. He agreed with others that the lesion he described is a benign lymphoid tumor or lymphomatosis.

Received for publication, July 25, 1947.

Cases 19 and 20 reported in 1942 by Gruenwald[11] were called by him, "Accumulations of lymph follicles in the digestive tract."

Cases 21 to 23 were reported in 1943 by Smith[12] under the name of primary lymphoid tumors of the rectum. The first of his cases was diagnosed lymphosarcoma but may well be considered as growth allied with the present group as illustrated in Table I.

From these tabulated data there are some general features which can be considered characteristic for this growth:

1. All these cases are free from associated generalized lymphoid disease.
2. The chief associated lesions are hemorrhoids and prolapse.
3. The chief symptoms are rectal bleeding, pain, and constipation.
4. The common pattern of the growth is a small, usually polypoid and commonly solitary nodule.
5. The nature of this growth is believed to be benign since in 33 out of the 49 cases in which follow-up has been carried out for different lengths of time there was no evidence of recurrence.

The general histopathologic study of our material and the review of some of the other authors' observations can be summarized as follows:

It is a noncapsulated yet well-circumscribed and often lobulated nodular growth which is composed exclusively of lymphoid tissue. This in turn is framed or supported by reticular tissue. The submucosal nodule often extends through the muscularis mucosae and involves the mucosa. Invasion of the underlying muscular coat has never been observed. The nodule is made of units of lymph follicles which contain all the cellular elements normally found in the lymphoid follicles of the intestine. Mitotic figures, regardless of their number, remain well within the limit of the germinal center and have not been found elsewhere. The number of mitoses varies among different follicles from the same case as well as from one case to another. A diffuse infiltration of different forms of wandering cells in varying intensity is many times encountered. The overlying mucosa suffers from compression of the underlying nodular growth, becomes therefore thin and straightened, and is thus exposed to mechanical injury.

So often and so closely does this growth resemble an adenomatous polyp of the rectum that it is difficult to differentiate one growth from the other. From the descriptions of the reported cases and the ones studied in this laboratory it would seem that the lymphoma, though often polypoid, is invariably broad based, feels firm and nodular, and is covered by comparatively normal looking mucosa. The adenomatous polyp is usually redder because of the congested capillaries near its surface. Since the lymphoma originates in the submucosa and only secondarily extends into the mucosa, it has a more solid base and is less often pedunculated than is the one with the adenomatous polyp in which the submucosa is unaffected.

Also, our observation inclines to separate this growth from lymphosarcoma by means of the histologic and cytologic study of the present material. In short, this growth is made of units of follicles with mitotic figures strictly limited to the germinal center, while lymphosarcomas are made of one type of cells such as small lymphoblasts in the case of the lymphocytic cell lymphosarcoma or of

TABLE I

CASES	SEX	AGE (YR.)	CHIEF SYMPTOMS*	DURATION	ASSOCIATED LESION†	NUMBER‡	SITE (DISTANCE ABOVE ANUS IN CM.)§	TREATMENT‖	FOLLOW-UP¶
1	M	6	0	?	P	M	Prolapse	Ex	0
2	F	30	a	?	P	S	Ant. wall	Ex	For some time
3	F	45	b	?	P	S	Post. wall, 5 cm.	Ex	0
4	M	35	a, b	2 yr.	0	M	7 cm.	Ex	0
5	F	59	b, d	?	Stomach cancer	M	?	Ex	0
6	F	40	b, c	Several mo.	0	M	Post. wall, 5 cm.	Ex	6 mo.
7	F	43	a, b	?	0	S	Post. wall, 5 cm.	Ex	0
8	M	44	b	?	0	S	Above sphincter	Ex	6 yr.
9	F	57	Tenesmus	Several mo.	0	S	5 cm.	Ex	2 yr.
10	F	56	b	Several mo.	0	S	?	Ex	1 yr.
11	M	26	a, b	?	0	M	?	Ex	6 mo.
12	F	39	(Foreign body feeling for several months and acute appendical symptoms)			M	Ampulla	Ex	3 mo.
13	F	50	a	Several mo.	Epithelioma of anus	M	?	Resection	0
14	?	46	a	15 yr.	H	S	Ant. wall, 5 cm.	Amputation	0
15	M	38	a	4 yr.	P	S	?	Ex	5 yr.
16	M	32	a	2 yr.	P	S	Ampulla	Ex	3 yr.
17	F	59	0	?	0	S	Lat. wall	Ex	0
18	F	31	c	?	Ant. fissure	M	8 cm.	Ex, x-ray	2 yr.
19	F	48	0	?	H, polyp of colon	S	?	Ex	0
20	F	60	0	?	0	S	?	Ex	0
21	F	42	0	?	H	S	?	X-ray	18 mo.
22	F	36	a, c	?	H	S	?	Ex	1 yr.
23	F	21	a	?	H, P	S	?	Ex	1 yr.

24	M	43	a, c	3 weeks	0	M	Ant. wall, 2 cm.	Ex	1½ yr.
25	F	34	a, b, c	1 week	H, P	S	Post. wall, 8 cm.	Ex	3 mo.
26	M	24	a, b	2 weeks	H, P, venereal dis.	M	Ampulla	Ex	3½ yr.
27	F	50	0	?	0	S	Ant. wall, 2 cm.	Ex	0
28	F	43	a, b, c, d	1 mo.	Ulcerative colitis	S	Lat. wall, 8 cm.	Ex	1 yr.
29	M	42	a, c	2 yr.	Gonorrhea	M	Left & rt. ant. wall	Ex	4 mo.
30	M	45	a, c	1 yr.	0	S	Ant. wall, 6 cm.	Amputation	28 mo.
31	F	71	c, d	9 yr.	0	S	5 cm.	Ex, x-ray	6 mo.
32	F	31	a	13 yr.	P	S	Post. levator	Ex	4 mo.
33	M	17	a	6-7 mo.	H, P	M	Ant. wall	Ex	3 yr.
34	M	45	a	?	H	S	Among hemorrhoids	Ex	11 mo.
35	M	40	a, c	5 yr.	H, P, fistula	M	Among hemorrhoids	Ex	4 mo.
36	F	27	b	3 days	0	S	Anal orifice	Ex, biopsy	0
37	M	22	d	29 hr.	0	M	Post. wall	Ex, biopsy	0
38	M	39	0	?	H	S	Ant. wall	Ex	0
39	M	56	c	?	H	S	Ant. wall	Ex	5 mo.
40	M	25	a, c	Many yr.	P	M	?	Ex	2 yr.
41	F	29	a	9 yr.	0	S	?	Ex biopsy	0
42	M	17	a	2 mo.	Fistula	S	Lat. wall, 4 cm.	Ex	3 yr.
43	F	49	a, b	3 mo.	P, ca. of rectum	S	Distal part	Resection	0
44	M	56	a	8 mo.	H	S	Ant. wall, 5 cm.	Ex	3 mo.
45	M	19	a, c	?	0	S	Lat. wall, 3 cm.	Ex	7½ yr.
46	F	7	a	2 weeks	P	S	Post. wall, 4 cm.	Ex	1 yr.
47	M	27	b, c	1 yr.	H, pruritus	M	Above anus	Ex	13 mo.
48	M	50	c	?	0	S	Ant. wall, a few mm.	Ex	8 yr.
49	M	44	0	?	Pruritus	S	Lat. wall, 2 cm.	Ex	6½ yr.

*a, Bleeding.
b, Pain.
c, Constipation.
d, Diarrhea.
0, None.

†P, Prolapse.
H, Hemorrhoid.
‡M, Multiple.
S, Single.

§The size of the tumor is small.
‖Ex, Excision.
¶There were no recurrences.

large cells in the case of reticulum cell lymphosarcoma. The difficult differentiation occurs in the tumors with giant follicles. If these growths are restricted to the mucosa and submucosa as occurred in a number of the cases here reported, the growth gives no clinical evidences of malignancy. If, on the

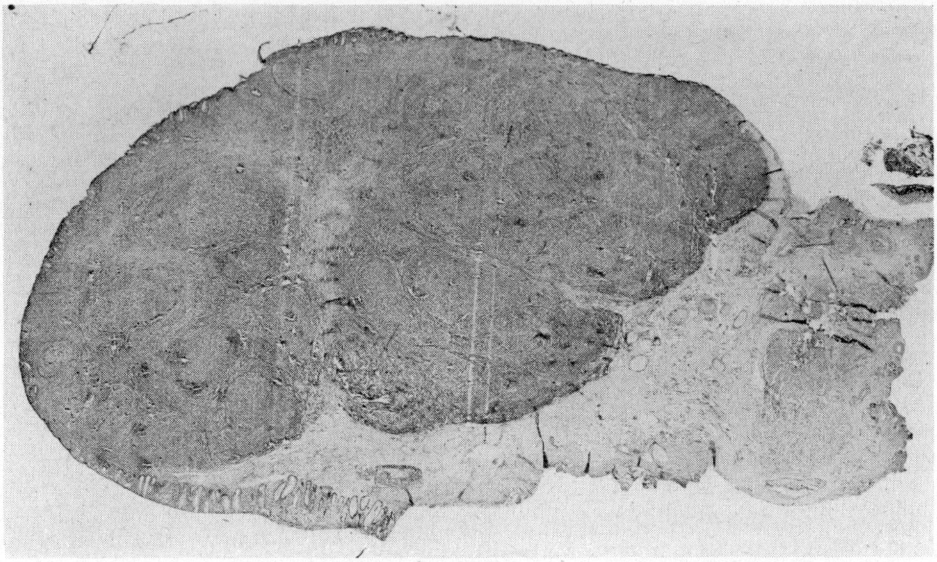

Fig. 1 (Case 33).—A wide-based polypoid growth of rectum showing a submucosal nodule of lymphoid tissue and the atrophied-covering mucosa.

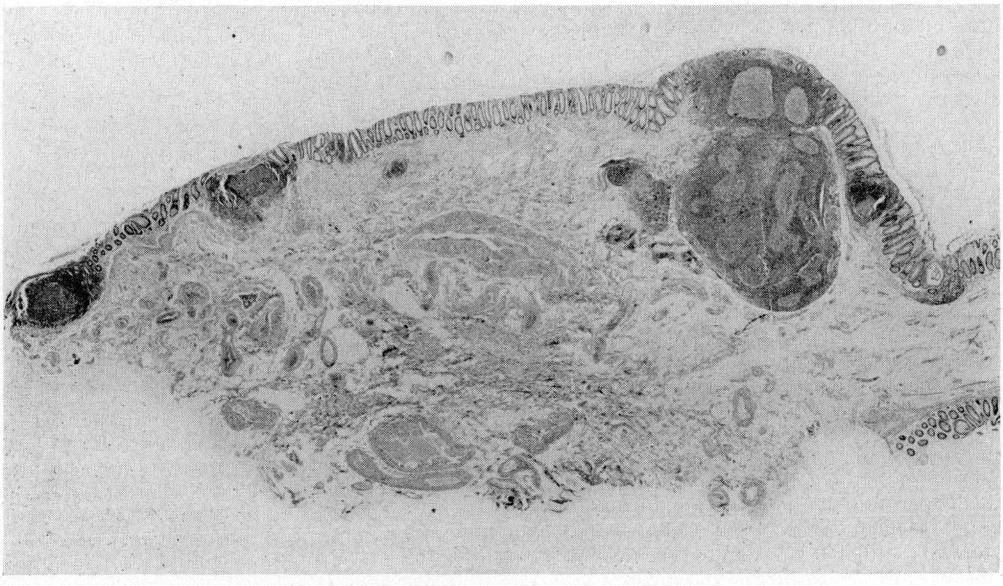

Fig. 2 (Case 43).—A small lymphoid growth of rectum in comparison with the coexisting normal solitary lymph follicles in the wall.

other hand, there is infiltration into or through the muscular coat, the growth may be considered a lymphosarcoma.

It does not seem possible to decide from the data at hand whether this lesion should be considered a simple localized hyperplasia, as was originally suggested by Stout[13] in reporting Cases 46 and 49 of this series, or a true neoplasm. There does not even exist any proof that a lymphosarcoma can develop from one of these nodules. It is abundantly clear that these are benign growths. Since they are tumorlike it seems more reasonable to call them lymphoma, which is the

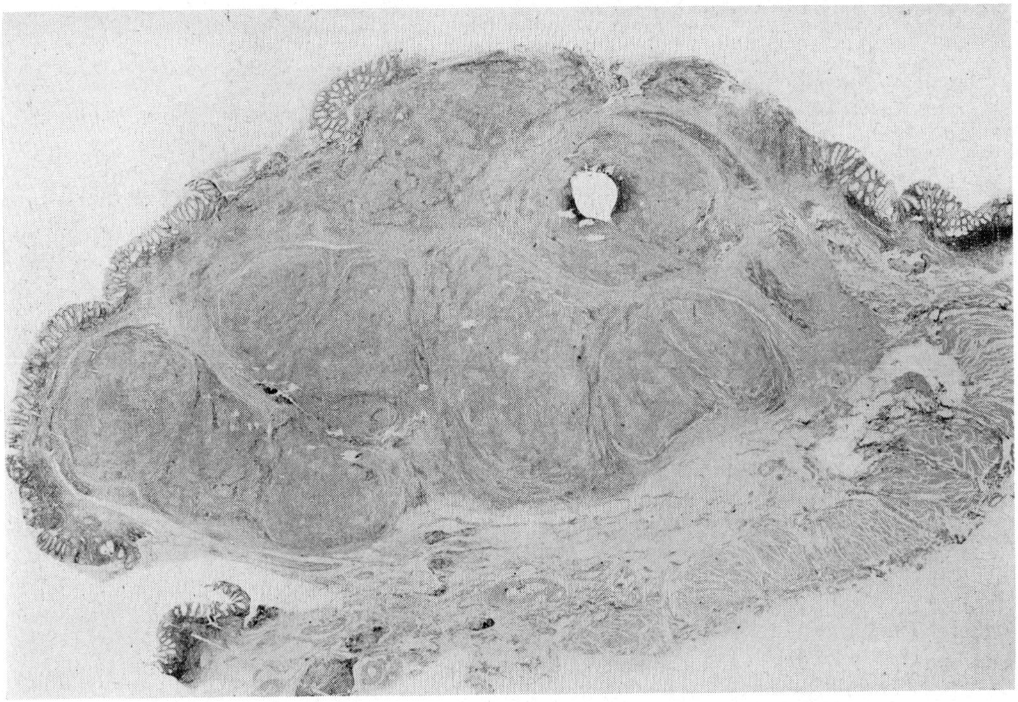

Fig. 3 (Case 48).—A very broad-based lymphoid growth of the rectum showing extension to mucosa through the muscularis mucosae and no invasion of the muscular coat of the rectum.

proper term to apply to a benign tumor of lymphoid tissue. Because this word "lymphoma" has been used by many clinicians as a loose term to cover all of the malignant lymphoid neoplasms it seems necessary to use the qualifying adjective "benign" with it in order to remove all doubt as to its nature.

SUMMARY

Forty-nine cases of benign lymphoma of the rectum are reported including twenty-six previously unreported ones. It is established that the growth involves the submucosa and mucosa, is often polypoid, resembles the adenomatous polyp, and is always benign.

The author expresses great appreciation to Dr. Arthur Purdy Stout for his kind supervision in the preparation and completion of this paper.

REFERENCES

1. Ball, C. B.: The Benign Neoplasms of the Rectum, Brit. M. J. **2**: 1353-1355, 1890.
2. Greig, D. M.: Lymphoma of the Rectum, J. Path. & Bact. **13**: 49-50, 1909.
3. Lehmann, H.: Unter dem Bilde der ''Polyposis'' in Erscheinung tretende, umschriebene Hyperplasie des lymphatischen Gewebes im Dickdarm, Deutsche Ztschr. f. Chir. **190**: 391-396, 1925.
4. Knoflach, J. G.: Ein Beitrag zur Pathologie und Chirurgie der Mastdarmpolypen, Wien. klin. Wchnschr. **40**: 876-877, 1927.
5. Konjetzny, G. E.: Lymphadenoide Polypen des Rektum; Bemerkung zu dem Aufsatz von Siemens, Zentralbl. f. Chir. **58**: 3154, 1931.
6. Siemens, W.: Lymphadenoider Polyp des Rektums, Zentralbl. f. Chir. **58**: 2070-2072, 1931.
7. Dick, W.: Lymphadenoide Rektumpolypen, Beitr. z. klin. Chir. **156**: 263-274, 1932.
8. Epstein, A. A.: Ueber Lymphadenome des Rectum, Arch. f. klin. Chir. **175**: 351-356, 1933.
9. Dukes, C.: Lymphoma of the Rectum: With Report of Three Cases, Proc. Roy. Soc. Med. **27**: 926-927, 1934.
10. Hayes, H. T., Burr, H. B., and Pruit, L. T.: Lymphoid Tumors of the Colon and Rectum, Surgery **7**: 540-545, 1940.
11. Gruenwald, P.: Abnormal Accumulations of Lymph Follicles in the Digestive Tract, Am. J. M. Sc. **203**: 823-829, 1942.
12. Smith, T. E.: Primary Lymphoid Tumors of the Rectum Resembling Internal Hemorrhoids; Report of Three Cases, J. A. M. A. **121**: 495-498, 1943.
13. Stout, A. P.: Isolated Lymphoid Hyperplasia in the Cecum and Appendix of Children, Am. J. Dis. Child. **34**: 797-806, 1927.

GASTROSTOMY

A Statiscal Review of One Hundred Ninety-nine Cases

Donald R. Cooper, M.D., and Robert W. Buxton, M.D., Ann Arbor, Mich.

(From the Department of Surgery, University of Michigan)

GASTROSTOMY, as a measure for the control or betterment of the nutrition of ill patients, long has been a standard surgical procedure to be carried out upon selected cases. A recent editorial, however, by Meyer and Kozoll* indicated that the life expectancy of the majority of patients upon whom this procedure is carried out is little, or possibly adversely, affected by this operation. A review of the literature failed to reveal any recent significant statistical studies on a large group of patients. It was thus decided to review all the instances for which gastrostomy was performed at the University Hospital from 1934 to 1946 in an effort to evaluate further the procedure as palliative or therapeutic.

One hundred ninety-nine patients upon whom gastrostomy was performed form the basis of this study. Five of these are considered separately in the latter portion of this review and are not included in the discussion or statistical tables. It has been possible to obtain a recent follow-up report in all instances. Table I lists the primary diagnoses for which these operations were carried out. The vast majority were patients with neoplasms of the esophagus who comprise 109 (55 per cent) of the total. Other patients with neoplasms included 22 with carcinoma of the gastric cardia, 11 with carcinoma of the larynx, and 2 with bronchiogenic carcinoma. Thus, in all there were 144 patients (72 per cent) with malignant neoplasms. The patients with nonmalignant disease included 20 infants with congenital atresia of the esophagus, 10 patients with esophageal stricture as a result of caustic burns, 5 patients with cardiospasm, 1 patient with congenital stricture of the esophagus, and 14 patients with less common lesions (Table I).

Fig. 1 graphs the age incidence of these patients by decades. The majority of these patients were, of course, those with malignant neoplasm. Of the 25 infants and children in the first decade, 20 were operated upon because of congenital atresia of the esophagus.

There were 134 patients with inoperable neoplasms, so determined at the time of abdominal or thoracic exploration or because of evident widespread or distant metastases. Six additional patients were classified as inoperable. In this group were 4 patients with congenital atresia of the esophagus operated upon before it became apparent that primary anastomosis of the esophageal segments was feasible. One patient had widespread gastrointestinal tubercu-

This study was aided by grants from the John Harper Seeley Fund and from the Elsa U. Pardee Foundation Cancer Research Fund.

Received for publication, July 14, 1947.

*Meyer, K. A., and Kozoll, D. D.: Editorial, Surg., Gynec. & Obst. **81**: 221, 1945.

TABLE I. DIAGNOSES FOR WHICH GASTROSTOMY WAS CARRIED OUT

DIAGNOSIS	NUMBER
Esophageal carcinoma	109
Carcinoma of gastric cardia	22
Congenital esophageal atresia	20
Esophageal stricture (caustic)	10
Laryngeal carcinoma	11
Cardiospasm	5
Esophagobronchial fistula	4
Bronchiogenic carcinoma invading esophagus	2
Congenital esophageal stricture	1
Tuberculous esophageal ulcer	1
Postgastrectomy stomal stricture	1
Bulbar palsy, traumatic	1
Esophageal stricture of other etiology	5
Histoplasmosis	1
Thyroid carcinoma with esophageal invasion	1

losis and another histoplasmosis. In both instances, gastrostomy was performed in an attempt to control severe malnutrition. Thus, 140 (72 per cent) of the patients were considered inoperable; another 13 patients were estimated to have operable carcinomas. Only 41 patients (21 per cent) were in the nonmalignant group in which the primary lesion was either correctable or upon whom operation was unnecessary (Table II).

TABLE II. OPERABILITY OF PRIMARY LESION

LESION	NUMBER
Inoperable, neoplasm	134
Operable, neoplasm	13
Operable, nonneoplastic	38
Inoperable, nonneoplastic	6
No further operation required	3

The performance of gastrostomy is one of the earliest of surgical procedures. Because of some of the technical difficulties encountered in carrying out this simple operation, or because of the subsequent unsatisfactory functioning of the gastrostomy, many methods and variations have been advocated by various surgeons. At the present time the fashioning of a gastrostomy is varied by each surgeon to meet the needs of a particular situation and little importance is attached to the use of difficult or elaborate techniques. Since many gastrostomies are considered temporary expedients and not permanent fistulas the simpler procedures are felt to be most suitable. In many instances, because of the poor general condition of patients, the simplest procedure carried out under local anesthesia is obligatory. In Table III are listed the types of gastrostomy performed upon the patients under consideration in this study. Interpretation

TABLE III. TYPES OF GASTROSTOMY

TYPE	NUMBER
Stamm (Kader, Fontan)	96
Witzel	86
Janeway	8
Beck-Jianu	2
Transthoracic	1
Simple gastric cone	1

of the technique used was given wide latitude since the surgeon seldom utilized the exact technique described by the author to which the operation is ascribed.

In attempting to correlate the surgical complications and the difficulties entailed in the postoperative feeding regimes, a detailed examination of each complication in relation to the surgical technique used was made. The percentage of complications encountered in each instance was, with one exception, without significant difference; a significantly greater number of patients experienced stomal malfunction after the Stamm type of gastrostomy.

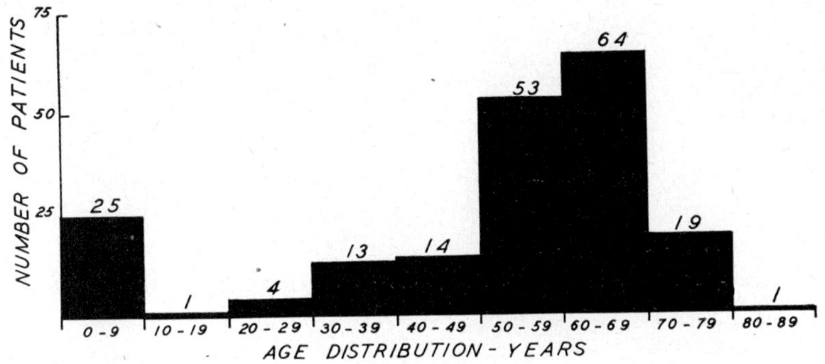

Fig. 1.

Again, the type of anesthetic agent has been implicated in the production of increased morbidity and mortality rates. In each case the anesthetic agent in this series of patients was chosen to meet the qualifications of the patient and the requirements of the surgeon. In this group of 194 patients, gastrostomy was carried out 109 times with local procaine infiltration anesthesia, 79 times under general inhalation anesthesia and 6 times with spinal anesthesia. No clear-cut correlation with postoperative complications or cause of death, definitely attributable to the incorrect choice of anesthetic agent, was noted.

There were 82 patients (42 per cent) of the 194 upon whom gastrostomy was performed in whom no postoperative complications occurred. In the remaining 112 patients there occurred a total of 147 complications. These complications are listed, in the order of their frequency of occurrence, in Table IV.

It will be noted that pneumonitis was the most frequent complication. There appeared to be close correlation between the severity of malnutrition and the incidence of pneumonitis in these patients, in that 41 of the 47 patients gave evidence of extreme weight loss, anemia, and hypoproteinemia. Twelve of these 47 patients had congenital esophageal atresia with tracheoesophageal fistulas. This primary lesion may well have contributed importantly to the incidence of pneumonitis.

The discrepancy between the incidence of phlebothrombosis or thrombophlebitis and pulmonary embolism can be explained only by the failure of the attending physician to look for or find evidence of venous thrombosis in the lower extremities. Three of these five patients were operated upon before this entity and its relationship to pulmonary embolism was fully recognized. In one of the other two patients the peripheral venous thrombosis was either not

Tarle IV. Postoperative Complications

Complication	Number
Pneumonitis	47
Wound infection	29
Unsatisfactory stoma (leakage outside)	23
Peritonitis	6
Mediastinitis	5
Pulmonary embolism	5
Wound dehiscence	4
Urinary tract infection	2
Thrombophlebitis or phlebothrombosis	1
Others (see text)	25
82 gastrostomies	No complications
112 gastrostomies	147 complications

present or not recognized. Two of the patients who died from pulmonary embolism did so after subsequent thoracotomy.

A most distressing postoperative complication, occurring in 23 patients, was persistent leakage of formula and gastric secretion from about the gastrostomy tube. These patients complained bitterly of constant leakage excoriation of the parastomal skin, and a constantly wet, ill-smelling wound dressing. In 17 of the 23 patients encountered with this complication, the Stamm type of gastrostomy had been performed. Of the remaining 6 patients, 4 had a gastrostomy of the Witzel type and on 2 patients a Janeway procedure had been carried out. Thus, it appears that, in our hands, a high incidence of unsatisfactory stomal function is to be expected from the utilization of the Stamm technique of gastrostomy.

Despite this large number of patients with malfunctioning gastrostomy stomas serious wound infections occurred in only 4 of these patients.

Twenty-five patients developed postoperative complications often seemingly unrelated to the performance of gastrostomy. In many instances these complications were more directly related to the age of the patient (cerebrovascular accident) or to the sequelae of the underlying disease (chylothorax, empyema, esophagopleural fistulas, lung abscess). In a few patients a totally unrelated complication occurred such as acute gangrenous appendicitis, otitis media, and strangulating femoral hernia.

It is evident that an over-all view of the survival time of the entire group of 194 patients (Table V) is of no value in deciding the degree of palliation

Table V. Survival

Time interval of gastrostomy and last follow-up or death	Alive	Dead	Cumulative dead (per cent)
Less than 1 mo.		83	43
1 to 3 mo.		39	63
3 to 6 mo.		22	74
6 to 12 mo.	1	21	84
1 to 2 yr.	3	6	87
2 to 3 yr.	4	3	89
3 to 4 yr.	4	2	90
4 to 5 yr.	2		90
Over 5 yr.	4		90
Total	18	176	90

TABLE VI. SURVIVAL BY DIAGNOSIS

DIAGNOSIS	TOTAL PA-TIENTS	LESS THAN 1 MO.	PATIENTS LIVING AFTER INDICATED TIME INTERVAL FOLLOWING GASTROSTOMY 1-3 MO.	3-6 MO.	6-12 MO.	1-2 YR.	2-3 YR.	3-4 YR.	4-5 YR.	LIVING OVER 5 YR.	TOTAL DEAD	PER CENT MOR-TAL-ITY
Esophageal carcinoma	109	63	34	18	7	2	1	1	1	1	108	99.1
Esophageal stricture, caustic	10	10	9	9	8	8	8	7	7	7	3	30.0
Cardiospasm	5	4	3	2	2	2	2	2	2	2	3	60.0
Congenital atresia of esophagus	20	5	5	5	4	4	4	4	4	4	16	80.0
Bronchiogenic carcinoma involving esophagus	2	1	1	0	0	0	0	0	0	0	2	100.0
Carcinoma of gastric cardia	22	14	8	6	1	1	0	0	0	0	22	100.0
Esophago-broncho fistula	4	4	3	2	2	2	2	1	1	1	3	75.0
Laryngeal carcinoma	11	5	4	3	0	0	0	0	0	0	11	100.0
Congenital esophageal stricture	1	1	1	1	1	1	1	1	1	1	0	00
Other rare feeding problems*	10	5	4	3	2	2	2	2	2	2	8	80.0

*See Table I.

offered by gastrostomy where palliation alone is desirable, nor is it evident to what degree nutrition is facilitated or improved where this feature is of utmost importance. An examination of survival time in relation to diagnosis (Table VI) is more illuminating but cumbersome for such a study.

Therefore, in an effort to determine further whether or not true palliation was achieved by the performance of gastrostomy in patients with hopelessly unresectable neoplasms, these patients were considered in a single group in Table VII, *A* and their survival time was determined to five years. Eighty-three per cent of these patients were dead within six months, the majority dying within less than one month. It then appears that the 18 patients who have survived longer than this period were possibly greatly aided by this operation.

It will be noted that 3 of these 18 patients lived longer than one year. A close scrutiny of these indicates that they were still capable of ingesting food orally and that the gastrostomy was done primarily for future need. In 2 of these patients the gastrostomy tube was removed shortly after it had been placed and the third patient received gastrostomy feedings only the last two or three months of his existence. One patient in this group had excellent palliation from x-ray therapy given to the esophageal lesion.

The remaining 15 patients living longer than six months showed a somewhat lesser degree of malnutrition as well as neoplastic lesions which progressed more slowly. Four of these patients had carcinomas of the larynx, 6 had neoplasms of the gastric cardia, and 5 had carcinomas of the esophagus. We have concluded from observations on this group of patients that life expectancy, from the time the diagnosis was verified, was directly related to the degree of starva-

TABLE VII. SURVIVAL BY PREOPERATIVE INDICATION

PREOPERATIVE INDICATION	TOTAL PATIENTS	0-1 MO.	1-3 MO.	3-6 MO.	6-12 MO.	1-2 YR.	2-3 YR.	3-4 YR.	4-5 YR.	OVER 5 YR.	TOTAL DEAD	TOTAL LIVING
A. Palliation, hopeless carcinoma	109	50	29	12	15	2	1	0	0	0	109	0
B. Control nutrition operable carcinoma	18	4	4	3	2	4					17	1
C. Palliation; hopeless not neoplasm	6	6									6	0
D. Therapeutic (1)	33	12	2	3	2			2			21	12
Total patients, 41 (2)	8	1	1		1						3	5
E. Neoplasm, hopeless; radium application	20	9	4	5	2						20	0
Total	194										176	18

tion present and that nutrition was not aided materially by the performance of a gastrostomy. Therefore, when a hopelessly irremovable neoplasm of the larynx, esophagus, or gastric cardia is present, the performance of a gastrostomy did not appear, in the patients studied, as an important means of improving nutrition and thus prolonging life.

Gastrostomy was performed on 18 patients (Table VII, *B*), with lesions of the esophagus and gastric cardia as a preliminary procedure to surgical resection of the primary lesion. In 5 of these patients resection was later abandoned because of the wide extent of the lesion. All 5 of these patients died within six months and their course apparently was not modified by the gastrostomy.

The remaining 13 patients, with one exception, died within two years of the time of resection of the neoplasms. Four patients in this group should be considered operative mortalities since they failed to survive longer than several days postoperatively. The remaining patients died from progression or recurrence of the original neoplasms.

One patient of this group survived to date and is now living, seven years after esophagectomy, with a cervical esophagostomy. The entire nutrition is well maintained through the gastrostomy.

Six patients (Table VII, *C*) were considered to have incurable, nonmalignant disease. Four of these were patients with congenital esophageal atresia. At the time these patients were seen, esophageal anastomosis for restoration of the esophageal continuity was not considered feasible. One patient with widespread miliary tuberculosis and a second patient with histoplasmosis were operated upon in an attempt to improve nutrition. All of these patients died within less than one month following operation and none were benefited by the operation.

Forty-one patients (Table VII, *D*) had non-neoplastic operable lesions for which gastrostomy was performed. These patients were further divided into two subgroups; the first includes those patients for whom the gastrostomy was done in order to combat starvation and in whom treatment of the causative lesion must of necessity depend upon nutritional control. The second group is comprised of patients for whom the gastrostomy was done primarily to facilitate the treatment of the causative esophageal lesion. In this latter group nutrition was, in general, good—the gastrostomy functioned not as a palliative measure and minimally, if at all, as an adjunct to nutrition.

In the first subgroup of Table VII, *D* (1) are a total of 33 patients, 12 of whom are living. The lesions for which the gastrostomy was performed in these 12 living individuals were as follows: cardiospasm, 2 patients; bronchoesophageal fistula, 1 patient; congenital atresia of the esophagus, 4 patients; caustic stricture of esophagus, 3 patients; traumatic bulbar palsy, 1 patient; operative stricture of hypopharynx, 1 patient.

At the time of this writing, the gastrostomy is still functioning in only 2 of these patients; it has been present for five years in 1. Retrograde esophageal dilatations are still being carried out through one gastrostomy stoma, and the second patient has refused surgical correction of the bronchoesophageal fistula and thus depends greatly upon the gastrostomy intake.

In all 10 of the patients in whom the gastrostomy was closed, it was possible to supplement, early, the gastrostomy feeding with an increasing oral intake. In some instances the gastrostomy was maintained long after its utilization for feeding was required in order to facilitate treatment of esophageal obstruction.

In this small group of 12 patients, now living, gastrostomy was performed primarily for feeding but soon became only a supplementary means of increasing the oral intake. As such, it has probably contributed materially in the maintenance of good nutrition in these individuals.

Twenty-one patients in this first subgroup died. Twelve of these were infants with tracheoesophagal fistulas, 10 of whom died of aspiration pneumonitis, 1 of hemorrhage, and 1 of tuberculous meningitis. Of the remaining patients, 3 were operative deaths, the deaths resulting from operations carried out subsequent to gastrostomy in order to correct the primary diseases. One patient with a bronchoesophageal fistula died of a suppurative pneumonitis, 1 patient committed suicide, and 1 died of a drug reaction. One severely psychotic patient presumably died of inanition, and in 1 patient the cause of death was unknown. One patient with a postoperative esophagopleurocutaneous fistula failed to improve following gastrostomy, because of regurgitation of the gastrostomy feedings through the fistula, and also failed to improve after jejunostomy.

In the group of patients now dead, 7 survived longer than three months from the time at which gastrostomy was performed. These patients undoubtedly derived some benefit from gastrostomy. In 2 patients with bronchoesophageal communications, benefit may well have been derived simply from defunction of the esophagus as a food passage, thus delaying the onset of aspiration pneumonitis. In the remainder, satisfactory supplementation of a diminished oral intake must be ascribed to the gastrostomy.

Eight patients are considered in the second subgroup of Table VII, *D* (2). In each instance gastrostomy was performed in order to facilitate esophageal dilatation. Three patients in this class died. One of these died of a cerebral thrombosis, another from a mediastinitis following instrumental esophageal rupture, and a third from an unknown cause. All patients now living have the gastrostomies closed.

In this group of 41 patients with non-neoplastic, curable lesions, gastrostomy finds its most important use as a means of aiding the surgical treatment of the obstructing lesion. Feeding, as a means of prolongation of life, has been aided only by supplementation of oral intake.

Between 1934, the date from which this study was begun, until 1939, 20 patients with carcinoma of the esophagus were treated by gastrostomy and retrograde implantation of radium (Table VII, *E*). Eight of the patients so treated failed to tolerate this procedure and died within fifteen days of operation. The great majority of the patients who lived longer than one month was able to ingest a soft or general diet for a variable period of time after operation due to the dilatations attendant upon the treatment. In two instances the gastrostomy tube was removed. The life expectancy after this form of treatment was less than one year in all instances and depended primarily upon the rate of neoplastic extension and the occurrence of aspiration pneumonia. In no instance did the life expectancy or improvement in nutrition appear to be aided materially by the performance of gastrostomy.

Thus, of 194 patients upon whom gastrostomy has been performed over a period extending from 1934 to 1946, 18 patients (9 per cent) are still living at the time of this communication. Seventeen of these surviving patients are those with non-neoplastic, presumably curable disease. In this group alone does gastrostomy appear as a most useful and worth-while surgical operation.

Five patients, not included in the foregoing discussion, were somewhat unique in that each was subjected to gastrostomy upon two occasions. Two of these patients had far-advanced carcinomas of the esophagus. In one, radium implantation was done, a short period of symptomatic improvement occurred, and the gastrostomy was permitted to close. Early recurrence of symptoms required re-gastrostomy and the patient's subsequent course was no different than that of the other patients discussed in the preceding portion of this study. In the second patient, gastrostomy was performed as a preliminary to esophagectomy. Esophagectomy was later abandoned and the gastrostomy was allowed to close for lack of use. Eventual total obstruction necessitated reopening of the gastrostomy. This individual survived less than one month postoperatively.

Three patients with esophageal strictures also required gastrostomy on two occasions. In each instance, following satisfactory response to dilatation, the gastrostomy was permitted to close. Subsequent recurrence of obstruction necessitated reoperation. Two of these patients were alive and well more than five years following the original gastrostomies. One patient died of an aspiration pneumonitis.

These patients offer no different problems or conclusions than those referred to in our previous discussion.

DISCUSSION

The value of the palliative gastrostomy in patients with inoperable malignant neoplasms or other hopelessly incurable lesions is certainly brought to question by the data herein presented. It seems certain that no significant extension of life has been gained for these patients. The question then resolves itself into one of the degree of physical or mental comfort afforded these patients by this operation.

The difficulties encountered in the utilization of the artificial stoma for feeding are noted in Table VIII. In 57 per cent of the patients no adverse feeding complications occurred. In these, both physical and mental comfort may have been afforded by the operation. Thirty per cent of the patients, however, experienced one or more complications associated with feeding through the gastric stoma. The majority of these were associated with actual discomfort. Those patients listed as "uncooperative" apparently experienced minimal palliation as they repeatedly and willfully removed the gastrostomy tubes against the physicians' orders.

TABLE VIII. FEEDING COMPLICATIONS

COMPLICATIONS	NUMBER OF PATIENTS
No complications encountered	110
No feeding attempted	26
65 complications occurred in	58
Leakage, outside	23
Diarrhea	17
Vomiting	10
Leakage, intraperitoneal	6
Uncooperative patient	4
Regurgitation into leaking esophageal anastomosis	4
Abdominal pain (severe)	1

Thus, the value of a contemplated "palliative" gastrostomy must be judged for each individual patient and the basis for this judgment must lie on an estimate of the patient's ability to cope with the problems of this manner of feeding, and upon his physical and mental reaction to the degree of starvation already present.

Gastrostomy is obligatory for those patients from whom the entire esophagus has been removed. It apparently functions satisfactorily either as a means of direct feeding or as a site of junction for an antethoracic esophagus. Today total extirpation of the esophagus for neoplasm by the method of Torek has been abandoned in this hospital. Under such circumstances the gastrostomy in patients with esophageal neoplasms falls again entirely within the realm of palliation, and as such seems of little aid.

However, in those patients for whom esophagectomy has been performed the gastrostomy has been of obvious value. Its use in such patients is necessary and therefore justifiable. It should be noted here that this group of patients offers the best test example of the adequacy of the present-day methods of tube feeding. It has been our experience that gastrostomy-fed patients seldom attain the nutritional improvement and sense of well-being that is usually expected from a carefully selected, suitably calculated diet.

While the outstanding place for the use of a gastrostomy lies in those individuals upon whom total esophageal resection has been done, this is the least gratifying group of patients. The life expectancy is frequently not great and many of these elderly individuals find much difficulty in mastering the simple technique of tube feeding. Fortunately, the frequency of this indication for gastrostomy is small.

For the more hopeful non-neoplastic lesions, gastrostomy would seem ideal. This is our experience where the gastrostomy is necessary primarily to facilitate surgical correction in the esophagus or hypopharynx. In the group of patients in this study the gastrostomy has been of much aid in facilitating subsequent dilatations of the esophagus. It has been somewhat less satisfactory in this same group of individuals where its need has been dictated by starvation. Here again we have been impressed by our inability to gain the desired nutritional control over patients when the customarily diversified oral diet is replaced by an unvaried scientifically calculated one. However, when it has been possible to augment the gastrostomy formula early by an oral diet, such gastrostomy-fed patients have shown good nutritional response.

The fact that a large number of individuals in this group are now dead does not necessarily reflect discredit upon the procedure of gastrostomy. The causes of death in these patients seem directly attributable to their primary diseases or to complications resulting from the treatment thereof. In no instance was the patient's course adversely affected by the performance of the gastrostomy. However, the degree of positive nutritional support offered by the gastrostomy, although difficult to estimate, is certainly less than was desired or hoped for. It is even possible that the high mortality associated with the treatment of the primary diseases in this group of patients may reflect to some degree the inadequacy of the nutritional regimen afforded by the gastrostomy feedings.

In evaluation of the operation of gastrostomy it must be remembered that frequently, as in other palliative operations, brilliant results are seldom expected or observed. These operations are often carried out in the desperation of the surgeon and the patient's family. Such operations are probably justified, since they frequently add to the comfort of the patient and help to maintain the aggressive attitude of the surgeon in attacks upon lesions that are far advanced and frequently hopeless.

CONCLUSIONS

1. A palliative gastrostomy in patients with inoperable malignant neoplasms or other hopelessly incurable lesions produces no significant extension of life and no demonstrable nutritional improvement.

Since neither life expectancy nor outstanding nutritional improvement is to be gained by "palliative" gastrostomy, the use of this procedure for hopeiessly incurable lesions must depend upon the surgeon's judgment of each individual patient as to the degree of physical and mental satisfaction which will be afforded by such an operation.

2. Gastrostomy in patients with non-neoplastic curable lesions of the hypopharynx, esophagus, and esophagogastric junction serves admirably as a means of furthering the local treatment of these areas. When the nutritional need is great in these patients, the nutritional response is maximum only when the gastrostomy feeding is supplemented by an oral diet.

3. A satisfactory state of nutrition is best maintained in esophagectomized patients when they are able to ingest a diversified diet through either an artifical or a surgically reconstructed esophagus.

AN IMPROVED DRAIN FOR PERITONEAL LAVAGE

STEPHAN S. ROSENAK, M.D., AND GORDON D. OPPENHEIMER, M.D.
NEW YORK, N. Y.

(From The Mount Sinai Hospital)

INTEREST has again been revived in the use of peritoneal lavage for the relief of certain types of azotemia.

In the early work with this method[1, 2] glass cannulas with multiple perforations were utilized; however, considerable difficulty was encountered because of the plugging of the perforations by omentum and there was evidence of irritation of the intestinal wall. Recent authors[3] successfully used a sump drain as described by Babcock,[4] for removal of irrigation fluid. However, the disadvantages of this type of drain are:

(1) Rigidity of the tube with resulting pressure to intestines
(2) Constant suction of contaminated air into the peritoneal cavity
(3) Occasional plugging of the small openings
(4) Leakage of lavage fluid into the dressing, which is a potential source of infection and which makes exact determination of nitrogen output difficult
(5) Difficulties of proper aseptic fixation of the tube on the abdominal wall.

To obviate these drawbacks in our setup for peritoneal lavage a new drain was devised.* Figs. 1 and 2 are photographic representations of the assembled and disassembled drains, respectively. The average drain consists of an upper rigid tube 3⅛ inches long and 5⁄16 inches inside diameter (*A*), with an interchangeable lower, spiral, flexible, stainless steel coil extension of 3 or 4 inches in length (*B*).

A straight inner tube (*C*), 3½ inches long, extends from beyond the outlet of the right angle tube (*D*), down into the upper half inch of the flexible tube. This inner tube is fitted with a rubber tube connection for suction aspiration.

There is an air space between the inner and the outer tube which connects with a right angle air inlet tube (*D*). This tube is connected to a rubber tubing to which is attached a suitable air filter.

We used a glass funnel covered with several layers of sterile gauze. It is obvious that when suction is applied to the outer tube, and there is no fluid available, filtered air will enter into the drain.

Since no negative pressure of significance can develop in the drain, omentum will not be drawn into the interstices of the spring coil.

At the outer portion of the steel tube there is an adjustable tie plate (*E*) for fixation by means of adhesive plaster.

Using a Stedman pump on a five gallon bottle attached to the drainage tube, a maximum flow of 240 c.c. per minute of fluid can be obtained, while during peritoneal lavage a maximum outflow of only 30 to 60 c.c. of fluid is required.

To test the possibility of development of a negative pressure, measurements taken on the bottom of the rigid tubing by attaching it directly to a manometer

Received for publication, Aug. 25, 1947

*Manufactured by Speedo Manufacturing Company, New York, N. Y.; patent pending.

at maximum rate of suction showed a negative pressure of less than minus 2 mm. of water.

We have used the drainage tube described here for peritoneal lavage in dogs and have found it satisfactory without the drawbacks previously mentioned. It will be used for clinical purposes.

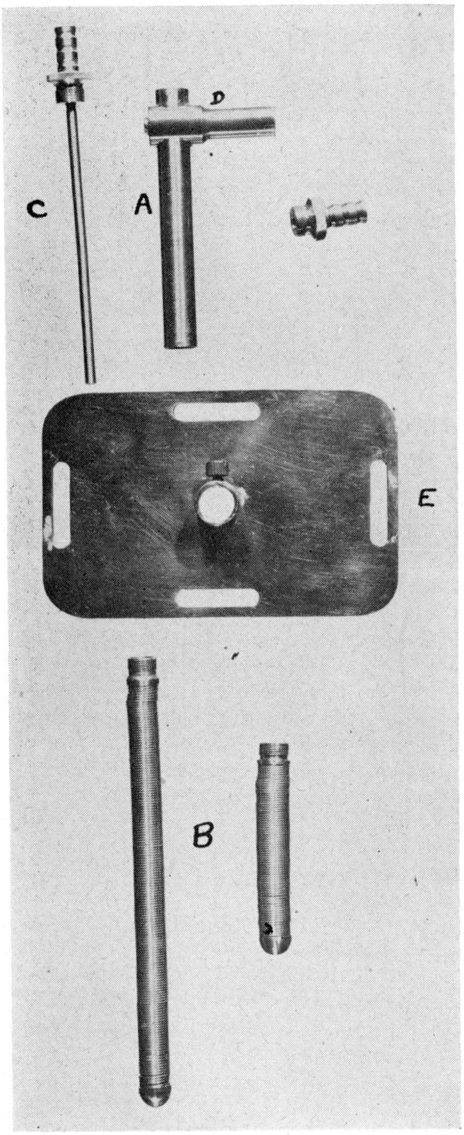

Fig. 1.

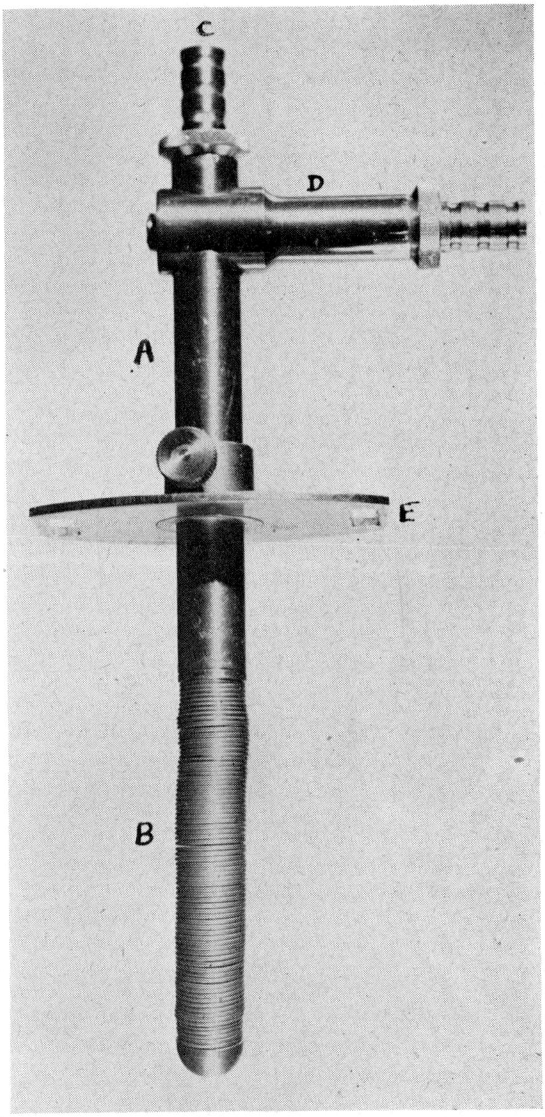

Fig. 2.

REFERENCES

1. Rosenak, S., and Siwon, P.: Experimentelle Untersuchungen über die Peritoneale Ausscheidung Harnpflichtiger Substanzen aus dem Blute, Mitt. a. d. Grenzgeb. d. Med. u. Chir. **39**: 391-408, 1926.
2. Balázs, J., and Rosenak, S.: Zur Behandlung der Sublimatanurie durch Peritoneale Dialyse, Wien. klin. Wchnschr. **47**: 851-854, 1934.
3. Fine, J., Frank, H. A., and Seligman, A. M.: The Treatment of Acute Renal Failure by Peritoneal Irrigation, Ann. Surg. **124**: 857-878, 1946.
4. Babcock, W. W.: Abdominal Drainage, Arch. Surg. **54**: 365-373, 1947.

Recent Advances in Surgery

CONDUCTED BY ALFRED BLALOCK, M.D.

PROGRESS IN SURGERY OF THE AUTONOMIC NERVOUS SYSTEM, 1943-1946

JAMES C. WHITE, M.D., BOSTON, MASS.

(From the Neurosurgical Service of the Massachusetts General Hospital and the Department of Surgery, Harvard Medical School)

IN THE four-year period since the last review of progress in surgery of the autonomic nervous system[1] many papers of interest have been published. These concern particularly wartime studies of the role of the sympathetic innervation in painful post-traumatic states and the value of sympathectomy for increasing blood flow in cases of injury to major arteries; also the continued and increasing experience with the surgical treatment of essential hypertension. Even while the war was still in progress laboratory investigators in this country and England continued to turn out much profitable work. This was brought up to date in the recently published Spanish monograph of Pi-Suñer[2] and in an article on visceral functions of the nervous system by Hare in the *Annual Review of Physiology.*[3]

This review is intended for neurologic and general surgeons. It is from this point of view that I have undertaken to summarize physiologic investigations of direct clinical bearing which have been conducted in the laboratory, as well as procedures established in the clinic and operating theatre in attempts to correct abnormal visceral function or to relieve pain connected therewith. Nothing of the sort has been attempted in the works just mentioned. The subject of surgical intervention for relief of essential hypertension was, however, well reviewed by Smithwick[4] from just this angle and has therefore been omitted from this article.

ANATOMY

Investigations carried out by means of careful anatomic dissection and by stimulation of the efferent sympathetic fibers in the course of spinal operations have given us a much clearer understanding of the distribution of the peripheral sympathetic impulses and how to interrupt them effectively. Pick and Sheehan[5] studied the connections of the sympathetic chains in twenty-five human dissections. The thoracolumbar outflow in man was found to leave the spinal cord between its first thoracic and second lumbar segments, with occasional apparent contributions from the eighth cervical root. While the uppermost origin of the major splanchnic trunk was usually from the sixth, occasional variations in this level were found as high as the fourth and as low as the eighth thoracic roots.

In view of the fact that many textbooks illustrate the white ramus as leaving the spinal nerve proximal to the gray, it is of interest to note that in this careful study exactly the opposite arrangement was found, at least in the thoracic region. Double, occasionally triple, sympathetic chains were found at times, but as these never extended over a greater extent than the space between two neighboring ganglia, this is of no surgical concern. The same is true of transverse connections between the two sympathetic trunks, which were never encountered above the fifth lumbar level. The possibility of any bilateral innervation of the limbs via such transverse connections can be almost certainly excluded. Variations in the position and number of the paravertebral ganglia are of interest, especially in the lumbar region, where it was rarely possible to define the separate ganglia with any certainty.

Determination of the spinal origin of the pupillary dilator and vasoconstrictor fibers was carried out in the human being for the first time by Ray, Hinsey, and Geohegan.[6] Pupillary dilation was obtained by electrical stimulation of anterior roots and was found to travel over one or more roots between the eighth cervical and fourth thoracic, most commonly in the first and second thoracic. In sixteen patients in whom the level of preganglionic innervation to the hand was investigated it was found that the usual source of the sympathetic outflow arose from the second to ninth thoracic, although in one case stimulation of the first thoracic root, and in two others of the tenth thoracic, gave rise to a definite change in the electrical resistance of the skin. It is also of interest that if a single one of these roots was left intact the degree of sympathectomy was far from complete and resulted in very partial clinical improvement.

From the more fundamental viewpoint, Hillarp's[7] microscopic studies of the peripheral endings of the autonomic neurones are of considerable interest. Previous microanatomists, Stohr and Boeke (referred to by Hillarp), had claimed that the connections at the ganglionic synapses and between the terminal nerve endings and the effector cells were formed by a nervous syncitium. This Swedish microscopist by more refined staining of the terminal fibers found that the construction of the ganglionic pericellular apparatus is incompatible with the existence of a terminal reticulum. The peripheral nerve network consists of "a terminal Schwann plasmodium, within which terminal axon ramifications are running. . . . Within the ground plexus each axon has a certain extension, and innervates in its course a certain number of cells. . . the neuro-effector unit. . . . A neuro-effector unit is not innervated by one neurone alone, however, but several neurones converge towards it. . . . By the overlap thus present . . . the response of the autonomic effector system on indirect stimulation may be modified both by temporal and by spatial summation effects." The objections raised by Stohr and Boeke against the neurone doctrine were evidently based on unreliable neurohistologic methods.

The importance of sensory fibers in the visceral nerves was emphasized by Langworthy,[8] who pointed out that many terminate in smooth muscle and glandular structures. Their cells of origin are in the sensory ganglia of the spinal and cranial nerves. No sensory cells have been demonstrated in the autonomic ganglia, so no reflex arc can be mediated through the peripheral autonomic structures. Smooth muscle reacts to stretch stimuli, and the tone of hollow viscera (for example, bowel and bladder) is maintained by afferent stimuli from the muscle itself. While proprioceptive impulses from the viscera rarely reach the level of consciousness, the splanchnic and other visceral nerve trunks contain large numbers of sensory fibers whose role in the appreciation of pain in many chronic diseases is of particular importance to the surgeon. The role of sympathectomy in these conditions will be discussed.

PHYSIOLOGY

To the modern medical man brought up on the concept that the parasympathetic and sympathetic divisions of the autonomic nervous system are of exactly equal importance in the nicely balanced control of homeostasis, Langworthy's[8] discussion of the general principles of autonomic innervation will be most provocative reading. Basing his arguments against the universally accepted theory that the craniosacral and lumbar divisions are functionally antagonistic, Langworthy pointed out that in such dually innervated organs as the iris and the bladder the parasympathetic is of paramount importance in the innervation of smooth muscle, while the sympathetic exerts its influence solely through the medium of the circulation.

In the case of the urinary bladder the sympathetic fibers have been referred to as the nerves of bladder filling and the sacral parasympathetics as the nerves controlling bladder emptying. This is obviously an oversimplification, as resection of the superior hypogastric plexus (presacral neurectomy) has no effect on micturition, while section of the second to fourth sacral roots or the inferior hypogastric plexus produces complete paralysis. In so far as the bladder is concerned there is no doubt that many of the phenomena ascribed to sympathetic nerve-muscle action can be explained by changes in the caliber of the blood vessels or by contraction of the smooth muscle in their walls.

In the case of the iris it must be realized that the constricted pupil seen in the Claude-Bernard-Horner syndrome is still capable of undergoing reflex widening as well as narrowing through the unopposed action of the oculomotor nerve. The role of the sympathetic in pupillary dilatation is ascribed by Langworthy[8] to constriction of the blood vessels and reduction of the spongy vascular tissue of the iris, while he believes that all adjustments in the actual muscle fibers are controlled solely by the parasympathetic outflow over the third nerve. Ophthalmologists agree that engorgement of the spongy iris tissue may make the pupil smaller; such is the condition seen in iritis; but the impressively thick wall of the iris vessels is made up uniquely of hyaline material, and not of smooth muscle fibers as Langworthy assumed.

The work and writings of the late Walter B. Cannon have made such a clear-cut case for the antagonistic action of the two divisions of the autonomic nervous system on smooth muscle in general that any exception of this sort in such an important structure as the iris deserves most careful scrutiny. In going back through the literature the classical investigations of Langley and

Anderson[9] published in 1892 seem to refute Langworthy's criticism in an unequivocal fashion. These British physiologists made radial cuts through the iris to eliminate the action of the circular sphincter muscle. In dogs and cats there was definite retraction of this free wedge-shaped strip of iris each time the cervical sympathetic trunk was stimulated. They furthermore proved that this movement could be explained only by the presence of an active dilator muscle, and not through any action of its radially arranged blood vessels. Not only does the radial muscle contract before its blood vessels constrict, but it contracts so forcibly that they become angulated and tortuous, indicating a purely passive shortening on their part. Langley and Anderson also cited earlier experiments by Budge and François-Franck showing that pupillary dilatation on sympathetic stimulation continued even after the animal was bled to death. In addition it is important to recall Bean and Bohr's[10] observation that even in vitro the smooth muscle of the radial muscle contracts directly under the influence of adrenaline, proving that there must be a direct sympathetically mediated pupillodilator response.* The work of Cannon showed that the craniosacral outflow is of prime importance in the control of adjustments of single organs, while the sympathetic acts on the body as a whole under emergencies such as fear, exertion, and exposure. Langworthy's conclusion that there is no real antagonism between the two systems appears to be true in the case of the bladder, but he does not produce convincing proof against the dual control of the iris, nor any evidence whatever against the dual control of other important organs such as the heart.

Another fundamental principle discussed by Langworthy is the comparative differentiation of the various types of motor nerves. The skeletal motor fibers are of the highest differentiation and are most dependent on control through the central nervous system. The sympathetic fibers show the least differentiation, are least dependent on control through the central nervous system, and are least responsive to voluntary control. The parasympathetic fibers hold an intermediate position. The sympathetic fibers reach all portions of the body in their role of vasoconstrictors, whereas the parasympathetic have both a more limited distribution and a more specific action. While total removal of the sympathetic ganglionated chains can be tolerated with only limited inconvenience by the cat, dog, and man, deprivation of the craniosacral outflow would lead to far more serious consequences.

Our understanding of the central control of homeostasis has been forwarded by the experimental studies of Beaton and his co-workers.[11-13] Three distinct mechanisms serve to maintain a constant body temperature, namely, heat loss, heat conservation, and heat production. Local heating of the preoptic hypothalamic nuclei with the high frequency current causes sweating, vasodilatation, and increase in respiratory rate. Conversely, an inability to eliminate excess heat and a consequent rise in body temperature follows bilateral lesions placed in the anterior hypothalamus. Sweating is inhibited, the cutaneous blood vessels

*I am indebted for these pertinent earlier references to Dr. Francis H. Adler, Professor of Ophthalmology, University of Pennsylvania; Dr. David G. Cogan, Director of the Howe Laboratory of Ophthalmology, Harvard Medical School; and Dr. Arturo Rosenblueth, Instituto Nacional de Cardiologia, Mexico City.

are constricted, and there is intermittent piloerection and shivering. Intravenous administration of soluble pentobarbital suppresses this mechanism for heat conservation and heat production, and reduces body temperature in the experimental animal to the normal level. These investigators suggested that the administration of intravenous barbiturate should be effective in cases of human hyperthermia following surgical or other injuries to the hypothalamus. (This has since been tried on numerous occasions and has unfortunately failed.) In contrast to excessive heat conservation produced by anterior hypothalamic lesions, Stoll[14] has found that bilateral electrolytic lesions placed more caudally in the central hypothalamus cause a complete loss of heat regulation with poikilothermia.

Interesting human cases of disturbed temperature regulation have been observed in the presence of tumors invading or compressing the hypothalamic nuclei. Davison and Friedman[15] have described a newborn infant with hydrocephalus whose body temperature fluctuated from 93° to 103° F. throughout the four weeks' course of its life. At post-mortem, in addition to generalized dilatation of the ventricles, most of the hypothalamic nuclei were found to be destroyed by an infiltrating neuroblastoma. A second patient, 31 years old, with mild diabetes insipidus, adiposogenital dystrophy, hypersomnia, and prolonged subnormal temperature, was studied by Davison and Selby.[16] For the last three months of his life the temperature had ranged from below 90° to 96.6° F. In this instance an angioma situated in the floor of the third ventricle had partially destroyed the rostral portions of the supraoptic and paraventricular nuclei, together with the right mammillary body. Disturbances in the sleeping-waking mechanisms also arise from lesions in the hypothalamus and neighboring structures (Davison and Demuth[17]).

While Heinbecker, White, and Rolf[18] produced obesity in dogs after removal of the pars distalis of the pituitary, it is probable that this was caused by concomitant injury to the inferior hypothalamus. Hetherington,[19] who reinvestigated this problem, concluded that the hypothalamic disorder is the sole factor involved. Brobeck, Tepperman, and Long[20] found that rats with injuries to the hypothalamus get fat because of their increased appetite. Cox[21] reported a case of voracious appetite with rapid gain in weight and increased somnolence in an 8-year-old boy after recovery from a severe head injury. He died from attacks suggestive of autonomic epilepsy, and post-mortem examination showed areas of gliosis just posterior to the hypothalamus and surrounding the aqueduct.

In his Balfour lecture of 1932, Cushing[22] first presented evidence that acute ulceration of the upper gastrointestinal tract may follow various cerebral lesions and operations which injure the parasympathetic centers in the hypothalamus. Strassmann[23] who made a post-mortem study of acute pathologic changes in the gastrointestinal tract, reported that gross lesions of the brain were absent in only two out of thirty cases of perforation of the esophagus or stomach. These patients had been in coma for hours or days before death and evidence of specific lesions to the hypothalamic centers is lacking. The type of cerebral pathology ranged over a wide variety of acute and chronic conditions, including intracranial injury, vascular accidents, tumor, inflammatory lesions, and barbiturate poisoning.

Kennard[24] has shown that the highest centers of autonomic control are situated in the cortex of the frontal lobes and that the orbital surface is the control area for vagal representation. While she has observed the phenomenon of "sham rage" in cats following bilateral removal limited to the frontal lobes, in monkeys there were only temporary signs of increased sympathetic activity. Very little effect is seen in man. The reason for the different result in these three species must depend on the process of encephalization and upon the integration of emotion with the complex associative functions known to be represented in the frontal lobes. "In the simpler cortex of the cat these are more immediately related to segmental autonomic reactions than they are in man in whom all of the autonomic manifestations of the mechanisms of fight and flight have become minimized."

The fundamental problem of sensitization of denervated smooth muscle to adrenaline has been found to have less clinical importance in man than was at first suggested by animal experiments. Doupe,[25] however, confirmed the observation that denervated blood vessels are rendered abnormally sensitive to circulating adrenaline and pointed out that the reactions after peripheral nerve lesions are similar to those following sympathetic ganglionectomy. These observations bring the results of denervation in human beings into agreement with those in other mammals. He has also found a difference between the reactions of digital vessels following preganglionic and postganglionic sympathectomy. Fingers after complete degeneration of the peripheral nerves remain abnormally cold, due to the fact that there is both a lowered threshold and a more prolonged response to the action of adrenaline, whereas the vessels of preganglionectomized digits show only a lowered threshold. This chemical mediation of denervated blood vessels explains in part the peculiar early and late effects of peripheral nerve injury. Immediately following nerve transection the paralyzed extremity becomes hot and dry through interruption of the sympathetic components in the nerve trunk. However, as the severed fibers degenerate, the skin in the paralyzed area loses its initial vascular dilatation and becomes cool, although it remains dry. Doupe concluded that the diminished circulation of paralyzed fingers is due in large part to local sensitization of arteriolar smooth muscle to moderate cold. This sensitization to cold which takes place with degeneration of sympathetic innervation is made more manifest by the increased action of adrenaline and by disuse with secondary diminution in the formation of acid muscle metabolites.

Using the denervated finger as an indicator, Doupe[25] was able to make some interesting observations of the rate of adrenal secretion. Adrenaline was found to be liberated in response to psychogenic stimuli, whereas the need for heat conservation did not consistently evoke its secretion. It was found that adrenaline could be liberated in the body in amounts comparable to the rapid intravenous injection of 2 μg and for longer periods at the rate of 6 μg per minute. Under other circumstances much larger amounts might be liberated and would suffice to initiate a persistent vasoconstriction of a denervated digit.

Richards,[26] who also studied the control of circulation in the hand after injuries to the peripheral nerves, reached exactly similar conclusions, except that he believed that the loss of axone reflexes contributes to the maintenance of the chronic cold phase.

While the secretion of sweat has long been ascribed to the action of hypothalamic stimulation of the sympathetic fibers, Bucy and Pribram[27] found its highest representation within the precentral area of the cerebral cortex in man. Reflex sweating, caused by a variety of stimuli, may be produced by spinal reflex arcs below the level of a complete transection of the spinal cord (List and Pimenta[28]). In several cases perspiration in paralyzed areas was so profuse that sympathetic ganglionectomy had to be performed for its relief. Doupe and Sharp[29] showed that sebaceous secretion, unlike sweating, continues unaltered after sympathectomy. By analogy with the growth of hairs and of the epidermis, it was concluded that sebaceous secretion is the result of a continuous growth of the cells in the sebaceous glands.

de Takats,[30] who tested the clotting mechanism by the response to heparin, found that it is under the influence of the autonomic innervation. Adrenergic stimuli arising under the influence of fear, nervous strain, and hemorrhage increase the tendency to thrombosis, whereas this is reduced by the cholinergic action of prostigmine.

Both overactivity and paralysis of the sympathetic thoracolumbar fibers have been mentioned as factors in the production of shock. The theory advanced by Cannon[31] and Freeman[32] assumes that the emergency function of the sympathetic nervous system, called into action by hemorrhage, fright, or pain, is at once a protecting and a damaging response—protecting in that it maintains the circulating blood volume of the vital centers, and damaging in that it causes peripheral capillary damage with loss of blood plasma from increased permeability. In recent animal experiments prolonged and intense vasoconstriction produced by Schafer[33] by resection of the aortic depressor and carotid sinus nerves failed to produce shock. These dogs tolerated hemorrhage in approximately the same manner as normal animals. Schafer stated that the experience at the University of Chicago fails to support the theory that sympathoadrenal hyperactivity may act as a cause of shock during injury or operation except in patients with a pheochromocytoma.

One of the oldest theories of traumatic shock is that excessive afferent stimulation may exhaust the vasomotor center and thereby produce a fall in blood pressure of such magnitude that the circulation becomes inadequate. Phemister and co-workers[34] tested this hypothesis in rabbits by inducing prolonged periods of hypotension at a shock level by stimulation of the aortic depressor nerve. Judging by the relative harmlessness of long periods of low blood pressure, by the inability to produce more than a brief slight lowering of blood pressure by direct stimulation of somatic nerves, and by the comparatively short duration of reflex lowering of blood pressure during syncope and abdominal manipulations, it is extremely improbable that "primary shock" is ever produced in man by the action of afferent depressor nerve impulses.

Another physiologic finding of fundamental interest in connection with hemorrhagic shock, the crush syndrome, and transfusion reactions is the neurogenic alteration in renal blood flow described by Trueta and his co-workers[35] at Oxford. Experiments on animals, both with the abdomen unopened and with the kidneys exposed, have demonstrated the development of cortical ischemia through a neurogenic mechanism. Arteriograms taken at the time of stimulation of the nerves in the renal pedicle show complete shut down of circulation in the cortical glomerular zone. The simultaneous appearance of pulsating red arterial blood in the renal vein indicates a short-circuiting of the blood in the medullary subcortical vessels while the circulation through cortical glomeruli is entirely cut off. Under these circumstances the secretion of urine decreases or may be entirely suppressed. If this mechanism is confirmed, further work along these lines may demonstrate that certain varieties of postoperative, traumatic, and toxic uremia may be amenable to splanchnic block, and also that this mechanism may be concerned in the etiology of essential hypertension.

TESTS

Therapeutic sympathectomy cannot be utilized intelligently without preliminary evaluation of the degree of vasoconstrictor tone. In cases of peripheral vascular disease there is often both a functional element of vasospasm and an organic element of vascular obliteration. It is therefore important to find out the degree to which neurogenic constriction predominates. This has been done in the past by blocking the sympathetic vasoconstrictor outflow in the peripheral nerves, paravertebral rami, or anterior spinal roots by injecting procaine hydrochloride.

Differential spinal block, a refinement of spinal anesthesia, has been developed by Sarnoff and Arrowood.[36] By gradual injection of 0.2 per cent solution of procaine into the lumbar subarchnoid space it is possible to block the spinal root fibers carrying vasoconstrictor impulses and also those concerned with pain and temperature sense without materially affecting fibers concerned with touch, proprioception, vibratory sense, or motor power. This differential blocking of the anterior root fibers probably depends on the size of the fibers and their degree of myelinization, the fine, poorly myelinated axones, which carry sympathetic, thermal, and pain-conducting impulses, being the first to be impregnated by the drug. The fall in blood pressure is not the result of muscular flaccidity or diminished thoracic excursions, but a specific result of the interruption of sympathetic vasoconstrictor fibers. By gradually raising the level it is possible to produce a vasomotor and sudomotor block of the entire body. This technique has proved to be a safe and simple method of determining the degree of vasospasm. Southworth and Russek[37] have advocated the caudal or epidural injection of procaine to block the lower portion of the thoracolumbar vasoconstrictor outflow, but this is both more difficult from a technical and less specific from a physiologic viewpoint. (Preliminary observations at the

Massachusetts General Hospital have not confirmed the hope that these methods would be helpful in the preoperative testing of hypertensive patients.)

An entirely new method of testing the effect of sympathectomy by blocking synapses between the pre- and postganglionic autonomic neurones (both sympathetic and parasympathetic synaptic transmission is blocked) has been developed as a result of the study of Acheson and Moe[38] on the pharmacologic action of tetraethylammonium chloride and bromide at Harvard Medical School. Clinical evaluation of the drug, administered by intravenous or muscular injection, was carried out by Berry and his co-workers[39] at the University of Michigan. This demonstrated the efficiency and safety of the drug in producing a blockade of the autonomic ganglia to a degree comparable with that obtained following the usually accepted methods of sympathetic block. These investigators reported useful diagnostic and even therapeutic results by single or repeated injections in 500 patients with peripheral vascular disease, posttraumatic painful syndromes in the extremities, and hypertension. (Preliminary studies at the Massachusetts General Hospital, however, have shown a far greater tendency for the blood pressure to fall after administration of the drug than after radical resections of the thoracolumbar chains and splanchnic trunks.)

Despite the accurate evaluation of the degree of acute dilatation which is gained by all of these methods, it is still desirable to find a method of more prolonged diagnostic block of the vasoconstrictor fibers. Only in this way can the surgeon who deals with peripheral occlusive vascular disease gain an idea of the long-term improvement in collateral circulation which often develops gradually after sympathectomy. Promising efforts toward developing temporary but longer lasting paravertebral sympathetic block of the vasoconstrictor fibers for use in preoperative testing of patients with thromboangiitis obliterans and arteriosclerosis have been reported. Lee, Macht, and Pierpont[40] used 4 per cent monobromhydroxybenzyl alcohol in peanut oil and Rasmussen and Alessi[41] 5 per cent benzyl alcohol and propylamine-benzoate in procaine. The resultant vasoconstrictor block has lasted from several days up to a maximum of several months.

In cases of traumatic injuries of the larger arteries, wartime experience has shown that increased vasomotor tone hinders the development of adequate collateral circulation. As Rector[42] has stated, "The majority of patients who presented clinical evidence of high vasomotor tone as shown by cyanosis, sweating, and constricted veins developed symptoms of vascular insufficiency unless they were subjected to sympathectomy. By comparison, those with a low or normal vasomotor tone appeared to develop collateral circulation spontaneously." A simple method of separating individuals into these categories was suggested by Naide and Sayen.[43] This consists of observing the cutaneous temperature response of the finger tips under standard cooling conditions. Individuals are classified as having "a high grade of vascular tone if the hands are cool (below 25° C.) 15 minutes after the patient has been in a constant temperature room at 20° C., unclothed except for a light gown. . . . If, on the contrary, the hands remain warm (25° C. or above) after this same exposure, the patient is in a low vascular tone group." The majority of individuals with a high grade of vascular tone do not develop an adequate collateral circulation after occlusion of major arteries. These constitute the group of individuals who respond well to sympathectomy, whereas those with a low vascular tone are not strikingly benefited.

The application of skin resistance measurements has greatly simplified previous methods of mapping the extent of interruption of the sympathetic fibers to the skin. The resistance offered to the passage of a minute, imperceptible, direct current through the body is localized almost entirely in the skin. Cutaneous resistance is controlled largely by the activity of the sudomotor impulses and therefore depends on the sympathetic components of the peripheral nerves. Simple portable "dermometers" have been described by Richter[44] and Jasper.[45] Denervated skin (after either paravertebral sympathectomy or injury to the peripheral nerves) shows a marked increase in electrical resistance which remains at a relatively high level unless neurotization takes place. The method, which was studied intensively by Richter and associates,[46-48] is an objective, practical, and precise test for mapping out the sympathetic dermatomes or the area of peripheral nerve degeneration, and also gives evidence of subsequent regeneration.

Previous methods of mapping areas of sweating have consisted of the color reactions of cobalt chloride, quinizarin, and the starch iodine reaction. An improvement in bringing out the details of the sweating pattern, which makes it possible to visualize the orifices of the individual glands, was devised by Silverman and Powell.[49] This is extremely simple and consists of painting the skin with tincture of ferric chloride. On dusting tannic acid powder onto the skin or pressing the sweating surface against paper impregnated with tannic acid, the smallest droplets of sweat turn black as the iron and tannic acid unite to form ink. Photographs may be taken if permanent records are desired.

SYMPATHECTOMY IN PERIPHERAL VASCULAR DISEASE

The value of sympathectomy in many forms of peripheral vascular disease is still a highly controversial subject. If interruption of the peripheral sympathetic fibers dilates only the cutaneous vessels and fails to release the much more important arterial tree in the muscles, sympathectomy would not be justified, either for the treatment of threatened peripheral gangrene or intermittent claudication. Under such circumstances the pooling of blood in the relatively unimportant cutaneous bed would actually starve the muscles and favor the onset of a Volkmann lesion (Cohen,[50] Siddons[51]). Through ingenious human experiments, Barcroft and Edholm[52] proved that this is fortunately not the case. By measuring the circulation through the human forearm with the plethysmographic technique, these investigators have reached the conclusion that blood flow in acutely denervated mucles is more than doubled. After sympathectomy, however, there is a gradual return of vasoconstrictor tone in about a week. Vasodilatation, which normally takes place in the muscles of the forearm after fainting, does not occur in sympathectomized extremities. During syncope there is active vasodilatation in the normally innervated extremity, as the blood flow increases to a greater extent than in the acutely denervated arm. It is also noteworthy that release of sympathetic tone cannot explain the increase in circulation during exercise.[53] Release of vasoconstrictor tone in muscles would probably increase blood flow by about 1.5:1, whereas in strenuous exercise the increase is nearer 20:1. It is therefore evident that sympathectomy should be of value in preventing acute gangrene after injury to the major arteries of an extremity. It should likewise help in the treatment of threatened gangrene in peripheral vascular disease, even though it may not improve the walking capacity in intermittent claudication. Such theoretical conclusions fit well with clinical observations.

Direct measurements of capillary blood pressure have been made by Eichna[54] before and after preganglionic sympathectomy in cases of Raynaud's disease and scleroderma. He found a striking rise of pressure in the arteriolar limb (9.3 mm. of mercury) and the establishment of a more favorable pressure gradient, which is generally low in the abnormally dilated capillary loops in the presence of chronic digital ischemia. The abnormal capillaries with slowly flowing, bluish-red blood became smaller and narrower, with rapidly flowing, better oxygenated blood. This change was attributed not to the removal of sympathetic innervation per se but to the improvement in digital circulation which followed the abolition of periods of circulatory arrest.

Grimson[55] made a careful review of the causes that impair the results of sympathectomy in the upper extremity. In the first place, man with his upright posture has a lesser degree of vasoconstrictor tone in the arm than in the leg. Hence upper thoracic sympathectomy is not followed by such a striking increase in blood flow as follows resection of the lumbar ganglia. Several other factors are involved in the inferior late results. The inherent ability of smooth muscle of blood vessels to maintain an independent tone probably limits the general effectiveness of sympathectomy more than any other single factor. The sympathetic nerve supply largely modulates, but only partially maintains vascular tone. Following total or near-total sympathectomy or high transections of the spinal cord, there is a striking acute fall in blood pressure and a severe degree of postural hypotension. These effects do not last long. It is therefore difficult to avoid the conclusion that the regain of tone results from an intrinsic property of smooth muscle, although why residual tone should be so much greater in the hand than the foot is not explained on this basis.

Another factor which militates against the prolonged effectivenes of upper extremity sympathectomy is nerve regeneration. Severed preganglionic sympathetic fibers have an extraordinary ability to re-establish connections with other remaining ganglia, even over a considerable gap. When a 5 cm. length of lumbar chain is removed regeneration is rare, but after the less extensive gap which is achieved after the usual operation for the upper extremity, recovery is not uncommon. Kirgis and Ohler,[56] who investigated this problem in cats, were able to find regenerating fibers bridging the operative gap within a period of four months. These findings emphasize the necessity of taking special measures to obviate re-establishment of functional connections by preganglionic fibers with upper thoracic ganglia when the latter are not extirpated. They also demonstrate the futility of removing such a limited area as the second thoracic ganglion, as recommended by Goetz and Marr.[57] (At the Massachusetts General Hospital some fifteen years ago removal of the second and third thoracic ganglia was carried out in three patients with Raynaud's disease of the upper extremity. Although the early results were all that could be desired, all had recurrences within one year.) Grimson,[55] who reviewed the relative value of pre- versus postganglionic sympathectomy for increasing circulation in the upper extremity, reached the conclusion that the "adrenaline sensitization" phenomenon, upon which the preganglionic type of sympathectomy is based, is not sufficiently important clinically to warrant the risk of regeneration. He employed the preganglionic operation only in cases of poor circulation in a single arm in order to avoid the disfiguring effect of a unilateral Horner's sign. Illustrating the frequency of relapses following preganglionic sympathectomy in Raynaud's disease of the upper extremity, Telford[58] admitted that only sixteen out of thirty-seven patients maintained their original improvement in circulation some years afterward. While he was not convinced that these late recurrences are necessarily due to regeneration, Simmons (cited by Telford), who made a careful study of the problem in his clinic, reached this conclusion.

Recent evaluations of sympathectomy in cases of peripheral vascular disease have brought out the following points:

Shumacker[59] stated that in his hands sympathectomy gives excellent results in the treatment of Raynaud's disease and other purely vasospastic states. In a small proportion of cases there were no further attacks from emotional stimuli, but the extremities continued to cool abnormally on exposure to cold. Late cases with subcutaneous fibrosis and digital ulceration responded less well than those with early uncomplicated Raynaud's phenomenon. However, he believed that improvement will take place in most instances of scleroderma, although in the more advanced cases progress of the disease will only be stopped or definitely slowed. In general the good effects of sympathectomy can, as pointed out previously, be fairly well assayed by careful preoperative tests. The fact that severe scleroderma may become a generalized disease with visceral as well as cutaneous involvement has been disclosed by reports of clinical and post-mortem examinations published by Goetz[60] and Pugh and associates.[61]

Other conditions with a primary underlying element of vasospasm in which impressive results have been recorded in recent reports include acrocyanosis, pernio,[58] and the vasomotor disturbances which often follow poliomyelitis (Telford,[58] Collins and co-workers[62]). Telford[58] claimed that even in erythromelalgia he was able to obtain good results, although the reason for this is far from clear.

Further confirmation has been given by Shumacker[59] and others (Trimble and associates,[63] Gautier,[64] Telford and Simmons,[65] de Takats and co-workers[66]) that selected cases of thromboangiitis obliterans and other varieties of obliterative arterial deficiency may be justifiably submitted to sympathectomy by surgeons experienced in this field. Shumacker also drew the interesting conclusion that any patient with obliterative arterial disease who has significant superimposed vasospasm can be treated more effectively and with a shorter period of hospitalization by sympathectomy than by more prolonged daily treatment with the pavex boot, intermittent venous occlusion, various sorts of intravenous injections, and other varieties of so-called conservative measures. Time and money-saving are most important considerations to patients, many of whom come for help only after they have been impoverished by prolonged medical treatment and inability to work.

Past reports have led to considerable confusion in regard to the increase in walking tolerance which results from sympathectomy in patients with Buerger's disease and arteriosclerosis. A number of encouraging experiences have been published in the last four years (Trimble and associates,[63] Telford and Simmons,[65] de Takats and associates[66]). The results, as might be expected, are not as good in arteriosclerosis as in thromboangiitis obliterans (Barringer[67]). It may be concluded that lumbar sympathetic ganglionectomy is well worth a trial if there is concomitant evidence of increased vasomotor or sudomotor activity, or if exercise tolerance increases as a result of diagnostic paravertebral block. While only a certain number of patients are entirely relieved of their pain, many are benefited, and even the failures usually show other worth-while evidence of improvement such as warmer feet, elimination of sweating, etc.

Traumatic Arterial Injury.—The tendency of long segments of arteries to go into spasm following local thrombosis or trauma has long been stressed by Leriche.[68] Spasm of this sort may be so intense that collateral circulation fails and the limb is threatened with gangrene. Learmonth[69] gave an interesting discussion of this subject, showing that neither complete interruption of sympathetic vasoconstrictor impulses nor the reflex mechanism of heating the remainder of the body can be counted on to release the spasm. Similar observations were made by Siddons.[51] Learmonth stated that "it is undoubtedly possible . . . for a thrombosed segment of artery to impose spasm on its collateral circulation when the limb is denervated." He described a number of instances in which resection of the injured portion of the artery restored an adequate circulation through the collateral bed.

Once the source of traumatic vasospasm has been removed by adequate local surgery in penetrating battle wounds, the recent wartime experience of American Army surgeons has favored repeated postoperative injections of the sympathetic ganglia with procaine. Rose, Hess, and Welch[70] advocated a first injection at the close of the operation followed by repeated blocks at six- to twelve-hour intervals until the fate of the extremity is established. They also suggested injection with 5 c.c. of 95 per cent alcohol when the procaine block was effective. DeBakey and Simeone,[71] who reviewed the statistics of arterial injuries in the recent war, stated that from their analysis there is "no substantial evidence that this method [chemical block] was of any value. The incidence of amputation in the group in which sympathetic block was performed is only slightly less than the incidence for the group as a whole, while the incidence in the cases in which ganglionectomy was done is greater than for the entire series." They explained, however, that familiarity with the material permits a different, more accurate interpretation. Sympathectomy, as a rule, was used only as a last resort, while sympathetic block was instituted more frequently as part of the immediate postoperative routine. They therefore concluded that there is considerable evidence in favor of both sympathectomy and sympathetic block in these arterial injuries and that the experience of most American surgeons is to the effect that both methods were "useful and beneficial procedures, regardless of inconclusive statistical evidence to prove the point."

The results of sympathectomy in the prevention of late arterial deficiency as manifested by coldness, ulceration, and intermittent claudication which so often follows ligation of the major arteries in the upper leg have been definitely encouraging (Kirtley,[72] Crutcher[73]). Recent experience has also shown that preliminary sympathectomy is of unquestionable value for the safe surgical resection of aneurysms and arteriovenous fistulas (Kirtley,[72] Richards and Learmonth,[74] Linton and White,[75] Harbison[76]).

A final type of war lesion in which the value of sympathectomy remains of debatable value is the so-called trench and immersion foot. After prolonged exposure to mild freezing and thawing, as occurred so frequently during the campaigns in Attu, northern Italy, and Europe, or in the course of prolonged immersion after torpedoings in the North Atlantic, the preliminary reaction of the injured feet was an intense hyperemia. In the late phase, however, the feet developed deep tissue fibrosis with persistent ulceration, and they were often sweaty, painful, and excessively sensitive to cold. Hyperhidrosis often led to maceration of the skin and chronic secondary infection. Resection of the lumbar ganglia has a limited value in the late phase, as it stops the excessive sweating, tends to reduce the sensitivity to cold, but is unlikely to diminish pain (Shumacker and Abramson,[77] Kirtley,[78] White and Scoville[79]).

Treatment of Thrombophlebitis by Sympathetic Block.—Treatment of phlegmasia alba dolens in the acute stage by chemical block of the sympathetic outflow to the lower extremities was first proposed by Leriche in 1927 and popularized in this country by Ochsner and DeBakey. In a recent discussion of venous thrombosis, Ochsner[80] gave a clear description of the two varieties of this condition. In phlebothrombosis, where the thrombi are loosely attached to the walls of the veins and there is no superimposed arteriolar spasm or block of the lymphatics, symptoms are minimal, but the danger of death by pulmonary embolism is great. In deep thrombophlebitis, on the other hand, there is often prolonged incapacity and much discomfort from fever, vasospasm, edema, and pain. This results in the classical picture of phlegmasia alba dolens. Ochsner explained the paradox of a white, cold extremity in the presence of pyrexia and elevation of surface temperature in the other uninvolved extremities on the basis of arteriolar spasm. Because the symptoms and signs are due to spasm of the arterioles with secondary ischemia and increase in capillary permeability, vasodilatation by chemical interruption of the regional sympathetic ganglia with procaine is rational. By daily repetition of the block until the fever subsides, the symptoms and signs are quickly alleviated and the postphlebitic sequelae of prolonged pain, edema, and ulceration eliminated. The painful ischemia is relieved at once. Sixty-two per cent of Ochsner's patients were able to leave the hospital within eight days and only 10 per cent remained on the wards after twelve days.

De Sousa Pereira[81] and also Papper and Imler[82] have attempted to show that there is also active reflex constriction of the veins in thrombophlebitis. The importance of sympathetic innervation of the veins is still uncertain. While numerous nerve fibers are present in their walls, it is not known how active a role they play in regulating their caliber. Definite dilatation of the veins of patients with thrombophlebitis is clearly shown in contrasting venograms taken before and after procaine block which are reproduced in these two papers. This clear demonstration of increased venous flow, although most convincing evidence of the therapeutic value of procaine block, does not prove that the increased diameter of the veins is due to release of spasm in their walls. Exactly the same result would follow increased arterial inflow and secondary distention. De Sousa Pereira, however, illustrated an increase in caliber of the internal saphenous vein in phlebograms taken before and after the intravenous injection of 15 c.c. of procaine in a single patient. This should not have increased arterial inflow and therefore constitutes fairly convincing evidence that a certain degree of active neurogenic venous constriction may be present.

Treatment of Polycythemia Vera by Total Sympathectomy.—The intriguing possibility that polycythemia may be treated surgically by radical sympathectomy has been suggested recently. In an experimental study, Schafer[83] found that dogs, following denervation of the carotid sinus and section of the cardio-aortic depressor nerves, became not only hypertensive but also developed polycythemia. After extensive resections of the paravertebral sympathetic chains these animals had a significant decrease in the red cell mass and total blood volume, as well as a reduction in hypertension. Support is given to the theory that the formation of red blood cells by the bone marrow is under the control of the sympathetic nervous system and that some cases of polycythemia in man are due to contraction of the perisinusoidal blood vessels in the bone marrow. The case of a 27-year-old man with intractable polycythemia rubra vera is presented and the striking effect of bilateral removal of the paravertebral ganglionated chains from the first thoracic to second lumbar inclusive and the splanchnic nerves is recorded. Immediately following surgery the total blood volume, red cell mass, hemoglobin, and hematocrit fell abruptly, and then gradually increased in a space of two years to approximately their preoperative values. This recurrence took place with the regeneration of nerves to the sweat glands and is presumably due to a partial recovery of bone marrow innervation. It is of interest that despite the return of objective evidence of the disease the patient remained symptom-free and able to work strenuously as a hospital orderly for fourteen hours a day for a period of three years.

VISCEROMOTOR DENERVATION

Carotid Sinus Syndrome.—Reflex adjustments of blood pressure and cardiac rate are largely effected by an autonomic proprioceptive mechanism mediated by the pressoreceptor innervation of the carotid sinus. Current knowledge of this subject has been well reviewed in an editorial of the *Journal of the American Medical Association.*[84] Attacks due to a hyperactive carotid sinus reflex may result in syncope or convulsions due to cardiac asystole or primary reflex depression of the blood pressure.

The syndrome is most common in males, increases with advancing age, and is often related to coronary disease. In Nathanson's[85] study of 115 patients with a hyperactive carotid sinus reflex, only twenty-three had clinical symptoms and only four had attacks of sufficient severity to cause actual incapacity. Nathanson believed that it is not the afferent arc (glossopharyngeal) that is hypersensitive, but the vagus center in the medulla. This localization of the site of sensitivity is of more than theoretical significance, as a certain number of failures of sinus denervation may be explained by an hyperactive response of the vagus to stimuli from other proprioceptive-depressor areas, such as the aortic arch.

Value of Vagus Resection in the Treatment of Peptic Ulcer.—Experimental work performed by Dragstedt and Owens[86] suggested that among other factors the corrosive action of gastric juice is responsible for peptic ulcer. Some ulcer patients display an excessive secretion of gastric juice in response to stimulation by food, histamine, and alcohol. A considerable number secrete large amounts when there is no obvious stimulant, such as between meals or at night. In addition to hyperacidity one occasionally finds increased motility. Both these abnormal factors are probably neurogenic in origin and may be reduced by total interruption of the vagi. Many physicians have called attention to the high incidence of ulcer in individuals whose occupations subject them to continuous mental strain and anxiety, and to the tendency for exacerbations to occur during periods of emotional stress. These observations suggest the possibility that ulcer is a psychosomatic disorder (Dragstedt[87]). The earlier observations of Cushing showed that acute ulceration and perforation of the stomach could take place with lesions in the region of the hypothalamus, the higher center of visceral control. Increased activity in the hypothalamic parasympathetic centers induced by psychic disturbances in the frontal lobes therefore is probably one etiologic factor in this disease.

In a study of secretion in various forms of gastric pouches in dogs, Weinstein and associates[88] found that only in the Heidenhain type of pouch, in which all the vagal fibers are divided, is neurogenic secretion totally abolished. The fact that copious secretion is maintained in partially denervated pouches is evidence of an important principle in surgery of the autonomic nervous system, namely, that any denervation to be effective must be complete (White and Smithwick[89]). Smithwick,[4] who has reviewed this subject, pointed out that early attempts at partial vagectomy in the treatment of peptic ulcers failed for this reason.

The anatomic arrangement of the vagal trunks along the lower esophagus and their distribution to the stomach was well described by Bradley and his colleagues at the Mayo Clinic.[90] Dragstedt[91] outlined the technical procedures for complete division of all the vagal rami to the stomach. This can be performed by either a transthoracic or an upper abdominal approach. While a greater length of the vagal trunks can be removed by the former route, the latter is of advantage when it is desirable to explore and resect a questionably malignant gastric ulcer, and also when it is necessary to perform a gastroenterostomy or resection for relief of pyloric obstruction.

After the supradiaphragmatic transthoracic resection of the vagi along the lower esophagus, as proposed by Dragstedt and his co-workers,[91, 92] the following alterations in gastric physiology have been observed: the operation has no effect on the secretory response of the stomach to histamine or food, but abolishes the stimulating effect of insulin hypoglycemia or a sham meal. The abnormally copious continuous secretion of gastric juice at night in the empty vulnerable stomach is reduced from 50 to 60 per cent. There is also a great reduction in free and combined gastric acidity, and the excessive tonus and hunger contractions are decreased.

By the end of 1946, ninety vagotomies had been reported by Dragstedt,[87] eighteen by Grimson,[93] and fifteen by Moore and co-workers.[94] The latter have given particularly clear and impressive evidence of the postoperative changes which lead to healing of the ulcer. The first twelve of Dragstedt's patients, followed for three years, remained well, took no medication, and were under no dietary restrictions. The nocturnal secretion of gastric juice was still within the normal range and tests of gastric secretion by the sham meal and insulin hypoglycemia showed that regeneration of the secretory fibers in the vagi had not yet occurred.

Moore and associates[94] discussed the indications and contraindications for vagotomy. The most favorable group of individuals for this operation is made up of young or middle-aged men with a long history of peptic ulceration, possibly with previous perforation or hemorrhage, unobstructed and not bleeding acutely, who have been refractory to careful medical therapy, and who have severe ulcer pain in times of stress, which can be relieved temporarily by the usual antacid, milk, or food. Gastric ulceration proximal to the pylorus should be approached with the greatest caution because of the difficulty of distinguishing ulcer from cancer. Resection should therefore usually be employed in such cases. Patients who have had previous surgery, such as pyloroplasty, posterior gastroenterostomy, or gastric resection, and who present themselves with renewed ulceration, are the most suitable subjects for this procedure. The operation is contraindicated in acute perforation, massive hemorrhage, or advanced cicatricial obstruction. Its mortality rate has been remarkably low.

Before any final evaluation can be made of the ultimate value of vagotomy, many more cases must be studied and more time must pass for nerve regeneration and recurrent ulceration from other causes to become manifest. Papers published in 1947 already give evidence of unsatisfactory features about the operation which were not stressed in earlier publications. From his own experience up to this date at the Massachusetts General Hospital and from correspondence with others, Moore found that vagotomies have now been performed in nearly 1,000 patients. In two recent papers[95, 96] he reached certain opinions which, even though out of place in a review of this four-year period, must be included here in order to present a judicial evaluation of this new and important subject. These recent observations bring out a 10 to 15 per cent incidence of annoying postoperative symptoms, especially diarrhea and sensation of "fullness" with odoriferous eructation. There is already a known incidence of recurrent ulceration in 5 per cent of patients. Though both disagreeable side-effects and recurrences have been observed in all surgical and medical therapies for ulcer, the final usefulness of vagotomy must depend on the relative frequency of its ill effects. These, as Moore pointed out, are just coming to the surface.

The role of the sympathetic innervation of the stomach is of far less importance than the vagus, as the splanchnic nerves carry mainly vasoconstrictor and sensory fibers. To a certain limited extent they exert an antagonistic effect on the vagi, and excessive activity on their part might lead to spasm of the cardia and pylorus with atony of the stomach. No changes in gastric secretion would be expected, but generalized or local vasoconstriction and stasis might result (Dragstedt[87]). The idea that peptic ulceration is due to local ischemia of the gastric mucosa has been proposed and in recent years an attempt has been made in France (Froelich[97]) to treat duodenal ulcer by sympathectomy. While this operation is known to relieve gastric distress, the release of unopposed vagal activity carries with it the risk of acute perforation. This complication has led to a fatal result reported by Weeks, Ryan, and Van Hoy.[98]

Neurogenic Dysfunction of the Gastrointestinal Tract.—Evidence is lacking to prove that the sympathetic fibers play an important antagonistic role to counteract the peristalsis-promoting, sphincter-controlling action of the vagi and sacral parasympathetic nerves. Nevertheless, the similarity of esophageal dilatation secondary to cardiospasm and megacolon, which is occasionally accompanied by great dilatation of the ureters as well, suggests that the idiopathic enlargements of the hollow viscera are of neurogenic origin. Furthermore, degenerative changes have been found in the plexus of Auerbach in megacolon (Penick[99]).

The value of sympathectomy, however, remains extremely questionable in these conditions. In cardiospasm, Eggers[100] concluded that it is not justifiable to advocate extensive neurosurgical procedures, as evidence is lacking that sympathetic denervation can benefit patients with advanced degrees of a disease in which mechanical factors are so prominent.

The same viewpoint may also apply to the treatment of megacolon, as Scott and Serenati[101] pointed out. In this condition they believe that there are two clinical groups. In one the interference in emptying of the bowel is primarily neurogenic in origin, whereas in the other it is due to mechanical obstruction from the kinking of an abnormally long colon. Evidence that certain cases are primarily of neurogenic origin is their response to parasympathetic stimulating drugs and the evacuation of the dilated lower bowel by spinal anesthesia. These writers advised sympathectomy in the small group of patients who respond dramatically to spinal anesthesia, but fail to gain sufficient relief from this and other forms of conservative treatment. When an extreme redundancy of the colon with kinking exists and conservative methods are ineffective, they recommend resection of the redundant colon combined with left lumbar sympathectomy. They have not yet proved whether this combination offers more than resection alone.

If sympathectomy is to be undertaken, surgeons are not in agreement as to the best type of denervation. This is brought out in Midon's[102] extensive review of the literature, in which the results of a half-dozen different operations are recorded. These include resection of one or both lumbar chains with or without the added removal of the splanchnic nerves, as well as several varieties of presacral neurectomy and resection of the inferior mesenteric plexus. The most interesting and convincing discussion of sympathetic denervation was given in a paper by Penick.[99] He summarized the results in eleven patients from the department of surgery at Tulane treated by left lumbar sympathectomy, in seven of whom highly satisfactory results were obtained. Three others were greatly improved, although occasional cathartics or enemas were still required. The remaining very advanced case was a complete failure. Essentially the same figures were obtained from 178 cases he abstracted from the literature. Penick therefore favored a trial of left lumbar sympathectomy in children who have reached the age of 3 without improvement on a medical regime and in whom spinal anesthesia produces a copious bowel movement. Should this fail, one has to decide whether the right lumbar chain or the splanchnic trunks are to be resected as well. In the discussion of this paper Bargen commented on the fact that extensive bilateral operations may cause sterility in males, and that unfortunately in this condition males predominate over females in the ratio of 5:1. When all these factors are kept in mind the operation is bound to have a limited application, as the results of resection are uniformly good and permanent, although at the risk of a distinctly higher mortality rate.

A recent French publication by Luzuy[103] contained the interesting suggestion that pylorospasm in infants is of neurogenic origin and can be treated by repeated splanchic block with procaine.

VISCEROSENSORY DENERVATION

Although the pioneer work of Bernard, Gaskell, Langley, and Cannon has defined the function of the autonomic nervous system as purely a motor mechanism for the control of homeostasis, all its visceral rami nevertheless carry large numbers of sensory fibers. These differ structurally from the visceromotor fibers because they are more heavily myelinated, leave the spinal cord in the posterior roots, and run to their sensory end organs without any ganglionic synapse. Posterior root section, paravertebral ganglionectomy, or interruption of the peripheral trunks and plexuses are all capable of relieving pain in otherwise intractable visceral disease.

Angina Pectoris.—Now that interest in Beck's attempts to increase coronary circulation by muscle grafts has waned on account of its excessively high rate of mortality (37.8 per cent according to Feil[104]), and since total thyroidectomy has also fallen into disfavor, the neurosurgical control of cardiac pain appears to be the most effective method of treating the rare sufferer from angina pectoris who cannot be controlled on a medical regime and cannot be freed from the nervous and physical exhaustion caused by continued pain and loss of sleep.

In their large series of cases White and Smithwick[89] showed that ipsilateral precordial and arm pain are constantly relieved after excision of the upper three thoracic sympathetic ganglia or effective interruption of their cardiac rami by chemical block with alcohol. Statistics from other neurosurgical clinics in this country also show that laminectomy and section of the upper four thoracic posterior roots will give equally effective results. A complete analysis of these cases will soon be published by White and Bland. In brief, surgical interruption of the sensory fibers to the heart is highly effective, although it carries a greater mortality risk (10 per cent) than the injection with alcohol. On account of the technical difficulty in obtaining perfect accuracy of injection, the latter gives results comparable with operation in only two-thirds of the cases. As it may also produce a temporary but disagreeable intercostal neuralgia, it should be reserved for those patients who present too serious an operative risk.

Less extensive cardiac denervations, such as removal of only the stellate ganglion, result in a considerable proportion of failures because they leave intact accessory pain fibers in the thoracic cardiac nerves. Gallavardin and Froment,[105] in summarizing their series of thirty cases of limited stellectomy, reported excellent lasting relief of pain in one-third, moderate improvement in a second third, and failure in the remaining third. Wertheimer,[106] who used the more extensive anterior exposure to the stellate ganglion recommended by Gask and Ross[107] and thereby was able to remove the second and possibly third thoracic ganglia as well, had correspondingly better results—twenty-eight cases with seventeen good results, four failures, and four deaths, with three others with inadequate follow-up.

Another type of cardiac denervation was recently proposed by Fauteux,[108] who utilized a direct exposure of the heart with pericoronary neurectomy and additional ligation of the coronary vein. In sixteen reported cases there was the high proportion of three deaths "during or rapidly after operation" and one soon after from progressive cardiac failure. Although the results in the survivors seem to have been satisfactory, one is led to wonder whether there will not be rapid regeneration of the pericoronary rami and whether the mortality rate of an operation comparable in extent with Beck's will not be prohibitively high. Only if ligation of the coronary vein leads to a significant increase in myocardial circulation can this transthoracic operation on the heart be superior to the far more innocuous and simpler interruption of its nerves in the posterior paravertebral space. (From experience with vein ligation in other forms of obliterative vascular disease and from recent, as yet unpublished, measurements made on experimental animals and man at this hospital by F. A. Simeone and W. H. Sweet, this seems most unlikely.)

The explanation as to why sympathectomy and posterior rhizotomy have relieved angina pectoris probably lies in the de-afferentiation of the heart. In the past the question has often been raised as to whether the clinical improvement could not be explained better on the basis that cardiac sympathetomy also results in coronary dilatation. This would imply that the coronary vasoconstrictor fibers run in the sympathetic and is based on past uncertainty concerning the pathway of vasomotor nerves to the heart. Gregg,[109] who reviewed this subject, concluded that constrictor fibers predominate in the vagi and that coronary flow increases with sympathetic stimulation, although this effect can be accounted for, in part at least, by the increased work of the heart with the consequent increase in local production of metabolites. Since the heart can also increase its activity and coronary blood flow by the direct action of adrenaline, as well as by vagal inhibition, sympathectomy does not have any deleterious effect. In all the cases that have been submitted to this operation there has been no evidence of subsequent impairment of cardiac function.

Pain From the Abdominal Viscera.—A new field of surgery for the relief of intractable gastrointestinal pain has been opened in the last few years, and credit for most of the pioneer work is due to Leriche and his school in France. The monographs of Servelle[110] and Luzuy[103] give an interesting description of the conditions in which the sensory conduction of the splanchnic and other thoracic sympathetic trunks has been tested and the great value of temporary chemical block with procaine in the experimental study of human pain. Of particular importance are the studies of Mallet-Guy and Guillet[111] on the innervation of the biliary tree and pancreas. These surgeons in Lyons have studied the contractions of the gall bladder by direct observation in dogs and by cholecystography in man. It is evident that the splanchnic trunks inhibit contractility of the biliary tree which, together with relaxation of the sphincter of Oddi, is increased by vagal stimulation. These findings have been corroborated in this country by Johnson and Boyden[112] in experiments on cats. A series of twenty-three patients with biliary stasis treated by injection or resection of the right splanchnic nerve showed definite improvement in gall bladder emptying and relief of pain. Similar relief of otherwise intractable pain due to distention of the liver capsule by carcinoma and postoperative constriction of the biliary ducts have been reported by White and Smithwick.[89]

Chronic pancreatitis with fibrosis and calculi blocking the ducts is another cause for severe bouts of epigastric pain. Although this condition is amenable to cure by pancreatectomy, the extent of the disease or poor condition of the patient may make such a radical procedure extremely dangerous, if not impossible. Mallet-Guy and associates[113] have treated ten such cases with splanchnicectomy, with nine successful results and a single recurrence after five months. At the Massachusetts General Hospital four further cases of pancreaticolithiasis have been treated in similar fashion with equally striking results. One of these patients had residual pain on the side which was not operated upon nearly one year after a unilateral denervation. We have felt it wise to employ more extensive thoracolumbar resections of the ganglia and splanchnic trunks than is possible through the infradiaphragmatic operation used by Mallet-Guy, and feel that nerve regeneration is the probable explanation for his single failure.

Although pain from the stomach and intestines can usually be treated effectively by direct surgical attack on the lesion itself, experimental observations made in dogs have shown that afferent impulses from the stomach (Balchum and Weaver[114]) and the upper small intestine (Herrin and Meek[115]) are transmitted over the greater splanchnic nerves.

Chronic intractable attacks of renal colic in which there is no pathologic explanation for the pain, which can be simulated by retrograde distention of the renal pelvis, can also be relieved by regional sympathetic denervation. Bauer[116] reported an impressive series of eleven patients with intermittent attacks of severe renal colic. On urologic examination nothing abnormal was found with the exception of low-grade hydronephrosis and delayed emptying of the opaque medium from the pelvis or from a single calyx. All of these individuals developed their typical pain when tested by the ureteral distention test, and were relieved by careful dissections of all the nerve bundles that run along the renal pedicle and upper ureter. In a second paper[117] a five-year follow-up examination was reported as showing lasting good results with no evidence of functional impairment in the denervated kidneys.

The sympathetic fibers do not play an important role in micturition or conduction of bladder pain. Their action is primarily concerned with vasomotor control, while filling and emptying as well as vesical pain are mediated by the parasympathetic fibers in the second, third, and fourth sacral nerves. Workers at the Mayo Clinic have long been interested in the possible value of presacral neurectomy. Jacobson, Braasch, and Love[118] reviewed their extensive series of sixty-two cases and concluded that "the operation has been found wanting," although temporary or partial relief of vesical pain has often been observed. They found some cystoscopic evidence of relaxation of the muscular tissues in the region of the trigone and vesical neck, but concluded that other operative procedures such as transurethral resection "have proved to be of greater effectiveness in providing the desired relief."

Pain in Causalgia and Other Posttraumatic States.—The effectiveness of sympathectomy and increasing blood flow in the treatment of chronic painful states found after certain traumatic lesions of the extremities has been recognized since Leriche first described its value during World War I. Literature on this subject published prior to 1941 has been reviewed by White and Smithwick.[89] No animal experimentation has advanced knowledge as much as clinical experience in this field. Experiences in World War II have been particularly valuable in providing large numbers of cases for study with consequent better evaluation of the specific indications, the value, and the limitations of sympathetic interruption.

Unfortunately the mechanism which causes pain in such conditions as causalgia, postraumatic dystrophy (Südeck's atrophy), amputation neuralgia, etc. are still not known. Pain often develops in the presence of vasomotor and sudomotor dysfunction, and relief following sympathetic denervation is most likely to occur when these evidences of abnormal sympathetic activity are present. There is no valid evidence that sensory fibers run in the peripheral, as distinguished from the visceral, nerve trunks, and the fact that Berry and associates[39] reported relief following intravenous injection of tetraethylammonium salts indicates that the site of interruption is on the side of the sympathetic motor outflow. Sensory axones, which run in continuity to the posterior root ganglion cells without a synapse in the paravertebral ganglia, are not interrupted by this drug. Therefore, as Mandl[119] aptly stated, "although we are successfully treating 'reflex dystrophy,' we are unable to explain the mechanism of the therapeutic effect."

In the preoperative evaluation of all these conditions the preliminary test by paravertebral injection with procaine is a most valuable method. Not only does temporary interruption of pain give a favorable prognosis for permanent relief by sympathectomy, but the action of chemical block is often prolonged. During this period active physiotherapy and mobilization of painful joints may be begun. Mahorner,[120] as well as many others, advocated a trial of repeated injection of procaine, and many patients have thereby regained use of the painful extremities without the need of surgical denervation.

In typical major causalgia, as described by Weir Mitchell during the Civil War, the relief of pain rarely lasts more than a brief period following diagnostic procaine block, but is nearly always permanent following sympathectomy. The impressive series of cases which has been reported to date following this method is shown in Table I.

Table I. Sympathectomy in Major Causalgia

Authors	No. of Cases	Satisfactory Result	Failure	Comment
Doupe, Cullen, and Chance[121]	5	5	0	1 incomplete sympathectomy failed to relieve pain until denervation was completed by secondary operation; 1 failure following periarterial sympathectomy
Speigel and Milowsky[122]	9	0	0	1 patient treated by paravertebral injection of alcohol
Mayfield and Devine[123]	12	12	0	
Allbritten and Maltby[124]	30	27	3	In 2 failures following lumbar ganglionectomy the level of sympathetic denervation did not reach the point of nerve injury
Rasmussen and Freedman[125]	40	29	11	Many patients listed as failures had only slight degree of residual pain
Ulmer and Mayfield[126]	58	58	0	
Total	154	131	14	

Successful results in causalgia depend on selection of typical cases of Weir Mitchell's syndrome. These generally follow a penetrating wound which has caused only partial injury of a peripheral nerve. They are characterized by burning pain and hyperesthesia of the hand or foot, with vasomotor, sudomotor, and trophic changes. All these patients have profound aggravation of the symptoms with excitement or emotion, and improvement when in a quiet environment, asleep, or after medication which reduces the activity of the sympathetic discharge from the hypothalamus. Failure may result from incomplete sympathectomy or, in cases in the lower extremity, when the level of denervation has not been brought up to the level at which the nerve is injured. This means that in cases of injury to the upper portion of the sciatic nerve the sympathectomy may have to be carried upward as high as the eleventh thoracic ganglion (Ulmer and Mayfield[126]). The reason for this may depend on Doupe, Cullen, and Chance's[121] theory that causalgic pain is due to a short-circuiting at the point of nerve injury of the sympathetic motor discharge across to the somatic sensory fibers.

So-called reflex or postraumatic dystrophy of an extremity, which leads to spotty atrophy of bone as described in 1900 by Südeck, usually follows comparatively mild injury of the tissues without any definite lesion to a nerve. With the onset of spreading neuralgia and immobilization of the extremity, vasodilatation is generally present at first, although in the late stage the extremity is often cold and discolored. Miller and de Takats[127] and also Evans[128] published carefully conducted studies of their cases. In the first series treated by sympathectomy all patients did extremely well, with the exception of a single recurrence at the end of one year. Seven treated by repeated chemical blocks did nearly as well. Of three others, treated by periarterial sympathectomy, one had an excellent and two mediocre results. It is of interest that only in this condition have a number of American writers reported favorable results from arterial stripping.

Evans published the results on fifty-seven patients treated at the Lahey Clinic during the last five years. Of twenty-nine submitted to sympathectomy, twenty-two obtained satisfactory to complete relief of pain. Eleven others obtained adequate relief following one or more sympathetic nerve blocks with procaine, sometimes reinforced by local injection of "trigger areas."

Neuralgia in peripheral amputation stumps, related to excessive coldness and moisture, can often be relieved by sympathetic surgery (White[129]), but few successful cases have been reported after amputations above the wrist or ankle. Major amputation-stump neuralgia of this sort usually requires a cordotomy for relief, but if there is a superimposed element of phantom pain this may not be effective. Woodhall,[130] who performed a sympathectomy for a combined phantom hand with burning sensation in the lower forearm stump, was able to secure complete relief of the latter without any alteration in the phantom.

In concluding this review of the painful posttraumatic syndromes it is well to stress the importance of early effective treatment. Watchful waiting, in the hope that severe pain will disappear spontaneously, is not advisable for more than a very limited period. The surgeon should consider active intervention as soon as he is convinced that conservative orthopedic, physiotherapeutic, and psychiatric measures are unavailing.[129] He should bear in mind that repeated resection of neuromas, neurolyses, neurotomy, and posterior root section have all failed consistently. Each useless surgical intervention will make ultimate cure more difficult by adding further psychic trauma and further reduction in the patient's morale. As de Takats[131] has written, "in cases of the late severe form, the spreading neuralgia may involve the shoulder, the thoracic wall and the opposite limb. The patient has a severe psychoneurosis, either because of his original make-up or because of continued, unrelieved pain." Add to this a compensation complex or narcotic addiction and the problem may become insoluble. In these situations, section of the spinothalamic tract has often failed. The most hopeful method of rehabilitating such individuals is by bilateral frontal leucotomy.

REFERENCES

1. White, J. C.: Progress in Surgery of the Autonomic Nervous System, 1940-1942, SURGERY **15**: 491-517, 1944.
2. Pi-Suñer, A.: Sistema Neurovegetativo, Mexico, 1947, Unión Tipografica Editorial Hispano-Americana, pp. 817.
3. Hare, K.: The Visceral Functions of the Nervous System, Ann. Rev. Physiol. **8**: 375-420, 1946.
4. Smithwick, R. H.: Surgery of the Autonomic Nervous System, New England J. Med. **236**: 662-669, 1947.
5. Pick, J., and Sheehan, D.: Sympathetic Rami in Man, J. Anat. **80**: 12-20, 1946.
6. Ray, B. S., Hinsey, J. C., and Geohegan, W. A.: Observations on the Distribution of the Sympathetic Nerves to the Pupil and Upper Extremity as Determined by Stimulation of the Anterior Roots in Man, Ann. Surg. **118**: 647-655, 1943.
7. Hillarp, N. A.: Structure of the Synapse and the Peripheral Innervation Apparatus of the Autonomic Nervous System, Acta anat. (Suppl. IV, Lund, 1946, Håkan Ohlssons Boktryckeri) p. 153, 1946.
8. Langworthy, O. R.: General Principles of Autonomic Innervation, Arch. Neurol. & Psychiat. **50**: 590-602, 1943.
9. Langley, J. N., and Anderson, H. K.: On the Mechanism of the Movements of the Iris, J. Physiol. **13**: 554-597, 1892.
10. Bean, J. W., and Bohr, D. F.: Effects of Adrenalin and Acetylcholine on Isolated Iris Muscle, in Relation to Pupillary Regulation, Am. J. Physiol. **133**: 106-111, 1941.
11. Beaton, L. E., Leininger, C., McKinley, W. A., Magoun, H. W., and Ranson, S. W.: Neurogenic Hyperthermia and Its Treatment With Soluble Pentobarbital in the Monkey, Arch. Neurol. & Psychiat. **49**: 518-536, 1943.
12. Beaton, L. E., Leininger, C. R., and McKinley, W. A.: Thermoregulatory Pathways in the Cat Brain Stem, J. Neurophysiol. **6**: 29-36, 1943.
13. Beaton, L. E., McKinley, W. A., Berry, C. M., and Ranson, S. W.: Localization of Cerebral Cortex Activating Heat-Loss Mechanisms in Monkeys, J. Neurophysiol. **4**: 478-485, 1941.
14. Stoll, W. A.: Beziehungen des Hypothalamus zur Temperaturregulierung, Helvet. physiol. et pharmacol. acta **1**: 329-357, 1943.
15. Davison, C., and Friedman, E. D.: Poikilothermia With Hypothalamic Lesions. A Clinicopathologic Study, Arch. Neurol. & Psychiat. **38**: 1271-1281, 1937.
16. Davison, C., and Selby, N. E.: Hypothermia in Cases of Hypothalamic Lesions, Arch. Neurol. & Psychiat. **33**: 570-591, 1935.
17. Davison, C., and Demuth, E. L.: Disturbances in Sleep Mechanism: A Clinicopathologic Study. II. Lesions at the Corticodiencephalic Level, Arch. Neurol. & Psychiat. **54**: 241-255, 1945.
18. Heinbecker, P., White, H. L., and Rolf, D.: Experimental Obesity in the Dog, Am. J. Physiol. **141**: 549-565, 1944.
19. Hetherington, A. W.: The Production of Hypothalamic Obesity in Rats Already Displaying Chronic Hypopituitarism, Am. J. Physiol. **140**: 89-92, 1943.
20. Brobeck, J. R., Tepperman, J., and Long, C. N. H.: Experimental Hypothalamic Hyperphagia in Albino Rat. Yale J. Biol. & Med. **15**: 831-853, 1943.
21. Cox, L. B.: A Hypothalamic Syndrome and Periventricular Epilepsy as a Late Sequel of Brain Injury. Report of a Case With Autopsy, SURGERY **19**: 669-683, 1946.
22. Cushing, H.: Peptic Ulcers and the Interbrain, Surg., Gynec. & Obst. **55**: 1-34, 1932.
23. Strassmann, G. S.: Relation of Acute Mucosal Hemorrhages and Ulcers of Gastrointestinal Tract to Intracranial Lesions, Arch. Neurol. & Psychiat. **57**: 145-160, 1947.
24. Kennard, M. A.: Focal Autonomic Representation in the Cortex and its Relation to Sham Rage, J. Neuropath. & Exper. Neurol. **4**: 295-304, 1945.
25. Doupe, J.: Studies in Denervation. B. The Circulation in Denervated Digits, J. Neurol. & Psychiat. **6**: 97-111, 1943.

Idem: E. Observations Concerning Adrenaline, J. Neurol. & Psychiat. **6**: 121-128, 1943.

26. Richards, R. L.: Vasomotor Disturbances in the Hand After Injuries of Peripheral Nerves, Edinburgh M. J. **50**: 449-468, 1943.
27. Bucy, P. C., and Pribram, K. H.: Localized Sweating as Part of a Localized Convulsive Seizure, Arch. Neurol. & Psychiat. **50**: 456-461, 1943.
28. List, C. F., and Pimenta, A. DeM.: Sweat Secretion in Man. VI. Spinal Reflex Sweating, Arch. Neurol. & Psychiat. **51**: 501-507, 1944.
29. Doupe, J., and Sharp, M. E.: Studies in Denervation. G. Sebaceous Secretion, J. Neurol. & Psychiat. **6**: 133-135, 1943.
30. de Takats, G.: Nervous Regulation of Clotting Mechanism, Arch. Surg. **48**: 105-108, 1944.
31. Cannon, W. B.: A Consideration of Possible Toxic and Nervous Factors in the Production of Traumatic Shock, Ann. Surg. **100**: 704-713, 1934.
32. Freeman, N. E.: Decrease in Blood Volume After Prolonged Hyperactivity of the Sympathetic Nervous System, Am. J. Physiol. **103**: 185-202, 1933.
33. Schafer, P. W.: Hyperactivity of Vasoconstrictor Nerves in Relation to Shock: An Experimental and Clinical Study, Surg., Gynec. & Obst. **79**: 163-174, 1944.
34. Phemister, D. B., Laestar, C. H., Eichelberger, L., and Schachter, R. J.: Afferent Vasodepressor Nerve Impulses as a Cause of Shock: Tested Experimentally by Aorticdepressor Nerve Stimulation, Ann. Surg. **119**: 26-63, 1944.
35. Trueta, J., Daniel, P., Barclay, A. E., Franklin, K. J., and Prichard, M. M. L.: Renal Pathology in the Light of Recent Neurovascular Studies. Preliminary communication, Lancet **251**: 237-238, 1946.
36. Sarnoff, S. J., and Arrowood, J. G.: Differential Spinal Block, SURGERY **20**: 150-159, 1946; Differential Spinal Block. II. The Reaction of Sudomotor and Vasomotor Fibers, J. Clin. Investigation **26**: 203-216, 1947.
37. Southworth, J. L., and Russek, H. I.: A Technic for Testing Hypertensive Patients Preoperatively, Ann. Surg. **125**: 119-125, 1947.
38. Acheson, G. H., and Moe, G. K.: The Action of Tetra-ethyl-ammonium Ion on the Mammalian Circulation, J. Pharmacol. & Exper. Therap. **87**: 220-236, 1946.
39. Berry, R. L., Campbell, K. N., Lyons, R. H., Moe, G. K., and Sutler, M. R.: The Use of Tetraethylammonium in Peripheral Vascular Disease and Causalgic States. A New Method for Producing Blockade of the Autonomic Ganglia, SURGERY **20**: 525-535, 1946.
40. Lee, F. C., Macht, D. I., and Pierpont, R. Z.: A Preliminary Report on a Method for Lengthening the Effect of a Sympathetic Nerve Block, Bull. Johns Hopkins Hosp. **74**: 119-120, 1944.
Idem: The Use of Bromsalizol in Lengthening the Effect of a Sympathetic Nerve Block, Am. J. M. Sc. **209**: 314-324, 1945.
41. Rasmussen, T. B., and Alessi, A. A.: A Method for the Chemical Production of a Prolonged Sympathetic Paralysis: Report of Its Use in Two Patients With Causalgia, SURGERY **20**: 360-363, 1946.
42. Rector, E. W.: Evaluation of the Basal Vascular Tone Test as an Indication for Sympathectomy in the Treatment of Surgical Lesions of the Major Arteries, SURGERY **21**: 630-635, 1947.
43. Naide, M., and Sayen, A.: The Primary Influence of Basal Vascular Tone on the Development of Postocclusive Collateral Circulation and in Selecting Patients for Sympathectomy, Am. J. M. Sc. **209**: 478-483, 1945.
44. Richter, C. P.: Instructions for Using the Cutaneous Resistance Recorder, or ''Dermometer,'' on Peripheral Nerve Injuries, Sympathectomies, and Paravertebral Blocks, J. Neurosurg. **3**: 181-191, 1946.
45. Jasper, H.: An Improved Clinical Dermohmmeter, J. Neurosurg. **2**: 257-260, 1945.
46. Richter, C. P., Woodruff, B. G., and Eaton, B. C.: Hand and Foot Patterns of Low Electrical Skin Resistance: Their Anatomical and Neurological Significance, J. Neurophysiol. **6**: 417-424, 1943.
47. Richter, C. P., and Katz, D. T.: Peripheral Nerve Injuries Determined by the Electrical Skin Resistance Method, J. A. M. A. **122**: 648-651, 1943.
48. Richter, C. P., and Woodruff, B. G.: Lumbar Sympathetic Dermatomes in Man Determined by the Electrical Skin Resistance Method, J. Neurophysiol. **8**: 323-338, 1945.
49. Silverman, J. J., and Powell, V. E.: A Simple Technic for Outlining the Sweat Pattern, War Med. **7**: 178-180, 1945.
50. Cohen, S. M.: Traumatic Arterial Spasm, Brit. M. Bull. **2**: 1-6, 1944.
51. Siddons, A. H. M.: Sympathetic Block in Vascular Injuries, Lancet **249**: 77, 1945.
52. Barcroft, H., and Endholm, O. G.: Sympathetic Control of Blood-Vessels of Human Skeletal Muscle, Lancet **151**: 513-515, 1946.
53. Barcroft, H., Bonnar, W. McK., Edholm, O. G., and Effron, A. S.: On Sympathetic Vasoconstrictor Tone in Human Skeletal Muscle, J. Physiol. **102**: 21-31, 1943.

54. Eichna, L. W.: Capillary Blood Pressure in Man. Direct Measurements in the Digits of Patients With Raynaud's Disease and Scleroderma Before and After Sympathectomy, Am. Heart J. **25**: 812-825, 1943.
55. Grimson, K. S.: Sympathectomy and the Circulation: Anatomic and Physiologic Considerations and Early and Late Limitations, SURGERY **19**: 277-298, 1946.
56. Kirgis, H. D., and Ohler, E. A.: Regeneration of Pre- and Postganglionic Fibers Following Sympathectomy of the Upper Extremity: An Experimental Study, Ann. Surg. **119**: 201-210, 1944.
57. Goetz, R. H., and Marr, J. A. S.: The Importance of the Second Thoracic Ganglion for the Sympathetic Supply of the Upper Extremities, With a Description of Two New Approaches for Its Removal in Cases of Vascular Disease: A Preliminary Report, Clin. Proc. **3**: 102-114, 1944.
58. Telford, E. D.: The Results of Sympathectomy in Chronic Vascular Diseases, Proc. Roy. Soc. Med. **37**: 621-624, 1944.
59. Shumacker, H. B., Jr.: Sympathectomy in the Treatment of Peripheral Vascular Disease, SURGERY **13**: 1-26, 1943.
60. Goetz, R. H.: The Pathology of Progressive Systemic Sclerosis (Generalised Scleroderma) With Special Reference to Changes in the Viscera, Clin. Proc. **4**: 337-392, 1945.
61. Pugh, D. G., Kvale, W. F., and Margulies, H.: Scleroderma With Involvement of the Viscera: Report of Case, Proc. Staff Meet., Mayo Clin. **20**: 410-414, 1945.
62. Collins, V. J., Foster, W. L., and West, W. J.: Vasomotor Disturbances in Poliomyelitis, With Special Reference to Treatment With Paravertebral Sympathetic Block, New England J. Med. **236**: 694-697, 1947.
63. Trimble, I. R., Cheney, W. S., and Moses, W. R.: The Operative Attack on Organic Peripheral Vascular Disease, SURGERY **15**: 655-678, 1944.
64. Gautier, R.: Les résultats éloignés de la thérapeutique chirurgicale dans les artérites oblitérantes des membres (d'après 274 observations), Lyon, 1946, Imprimerie des Beaux-Arts, pp. 128.
65. Telford, E. D., and Simmons, H. T.: Sympathectomy in Peripheral Arteriosclerosis, Brit. M. J. **1**: 386, 1946.
66. de Takats, G., Fowler, E. F., Jordan, P., and Risley, T. C.: Sympathectomy in the Treatment of Peripheral Vascular Sclerosis, J. A. M. A. **131**: 495-499, 1946.
67. Barringer, F. S.: The Results of Lumbar Sympathectomy for Arteriosclerosis of the Lower Limbs, Queen's M. Mag. **39**: 34-35, 1946.
68. Leriche, R.: Physiologie Pathologique et traitement chirurgical des maladies artérielles de la vaso-motricité, Paris, 1945, Masson & Cie, pp. 304.
69. Learmonth, J. R.: Reflex Vasodilatation in Surgery, Edinburgh M. J. **50**: 140-154, 1943.
70. Rose, C. A., Hess, O. W., and Welch, C. S.: Vascular Injuries of the Extremities in Battle Casualties, Ann. Surg. **123**: 161-179, 1946.
71. DeBakey, M. E., and Simeone, F. A.: Battle Injuries of the Arteries in World War II: An Analysis of 2,471 Cases, Ann. Surg. **123**: 534-579, 1946.
72. Kirtley, J. A.: Arterial Injuries in a Theater of Operations, Ann. Surg. **122**: 233-234, 1945.
73. Crutcher, R. R.: Sympathectomy for Ischemia Following Femoral Artery Ligation, Ann. Surg. **123**: 304-310, 1946.
74. Richards, R. L., and Learmonth, J. R.: Lumbar Sympathectomy in Treatment of Popliteal Aneurysm, Lancet **242**: 383-384, 1942.
75. Linton, R. R., and White, P. D.: Arteriovenous Fistula Between the Right Common Iliac Artery and the Inferior Vena Cava: Report of a Case of Its Occurrence Following an Operation for a Ruptured Intervertebral Disk With Cure by Operation, Arch. Surg. **50**: 6-13, 1945.
76. Harbison, S. P.: Experiences With Aneurysms in an Overseas General Hospital, Surg., Gynec. & Obst. **81**: 128-137, 1945.
77. Shumacker, H. B., Jr., and Abramson, D. I.: Sympathectomy in Trench Foot, Ann. Surg. **125**: 203-215, 1947.
78. Kirtley, J. A., Jr.: Experiences With Sympathectomy in Peripheral Lesions, Ann. Surg. **122**: 29-38, 1945.
79. White, J. C., and Scoville, W. B.: Trench Foot and Immersion Foot, New England J. Med. **232**: 415-422, 1945.
80. Ochsner, A.: Venous Thrombosis, J. A. M. A. **132**: 827-833, 1946.
81. de Sousa Pereira, A.: The Innervation of the Veins: Its Role in Pain, Venospasm, and Collateral Circulation, SURGERY **19**: 731-742, 1946.
82. Papper, E. M., and Imler, A. E.: The Use of Phlebography and Lumbar Sympathetic Block in the Diagnosis of Venospasm of the Lower Extremities: A Preliminary Report, SURGERY **15**: 402-412, 1944.

83. Schafer, P. W.: The Etiology and Treatment of Polycythemia Rubra Vera: Observations Based Upon Studies of Body Fluid Changes in Dogs Subjected to Proprioceptor Depressor Neurotomy and Extensive Sympathectomy, Including the Case Report of a Man With Polycythemia Rubra Vera Treated by Extensive Paravertebral Sympathectomy, Ann. Surg. **122**: 1098-1124, 1945.
84. Editorial: Carotid Sinus Syndrome, J. A. M. A. **132**: 24-25, 1946.
85. Nathanson, M. H.: Hyperactive Cardioinhibitory Carotid Sinus Reflex, Arch. Int. Med. **77**: 491-503, 1946.
86. Dragstedt, L. R., and Owens, F. M., Jr.: Supra-diaphragmatic Section of the Vagus Nerves in Treatment of Duodenal Ulcer, Proc. Soc. Exper. Biol. & Med. **53**: 152-154, 1943.
87. Dragstedt, L. R.: Section of the Vagus Nerves to the Stomach in the Treatment of Peptic Ulcer, Surg., Gynec. & Obst. **83**: 547-549, 1946.
88. Weinstein, V. A., Colp, R., Hollander, F., and Jemerin, E. E.: Vagotomy in the Therapy of Peptic Ulcer, Surg., Gynec. & Obst. **79**: 297-305, 1944.
89. White, J. C., and Smithwick, R. H.: The Autonomic Nervous System: Anatomy, Physiology, and Surgical Application, ed. 2, New York, 1941, The Macmillan Company, pp. 469.
90. Bradley, W. F., Small, J. T., Wilson, J. W., and Walters, W.: Anatomic Considerations of Gastric Neurectomy, J. A. M. A. **133**: 459-461, 1947.
91. Dragstedt, L. R.: Vagotomy for Gastroduodenal Ulcer, Ann. Surg. **122**: 973-989, 1945.
92. Thornton, T. F., Jr., Storer, E. H., and Dragstedt, L. R.: Supradiaphragmatic Section of the Vagus Nerves: Effect on Gastric Secretion and Motility in Patients With Peptic Ulcer, J. A. M. A. **130**: 764-771, 1946.
93. Grimson, K. S.: See Discussion in Thornton and others,[92] pp. 769-770.
94. Moore, F. D., Chapman, W. P., Schulz, M. D., and Jones, C. M.: Transdiaphragmatic Resection of the Vagus Nerves for Peptic Ulcer, New England J. Med. **234**: 241-251, 1946.
95. Moore, F. D.: Vagus Resection for Ulcer: An Interim Evaluation. I. Operative Techniques and Hospital Management, Arch. Surg. **55**: 164-174, 1947.
96. Moore, F. D.: Vagus Resection for Ulcer: An Interim Evaluation. II. Clinical Results, Ann. Surg. **126**: 664-678, 1947.
97. Froehlich, F.: À propos de 25 cas d'ulcères gastro-duodénaux traités par la splanchnicectomie et l'ablation du premier ganglion lombaire, Presse méd. **49**: 336, 1946.
98. Weeks, C., Ryan, B. J., and Van Hoy, J. M.: Two Deaths Associated With Supradiaphragmatic Vagotomy, J. A. M. A. **132**: 988-990, 1946.
99. Penick, R. M., Jr.: Problems in the Surgical Treatment of Congenital Megacolon, J. A. M. A. **128**: 423-426, 1945.
100. Eggers, C.: Cardiospasm, Ann. Surg. **115**: 215-227, 1942.
101. Scott, W. J. M., and Serenati, Q. J.: Megacolon, Mechanisms and Choice of Treatment, SURGERY **20**: 603-618, 1946.
102. Midon, J.: Le méga-dolichocolon: Pathogénie, traitement, Nancy, 1944, Imprimerie Nancéienne, pp. 197.
103. Luzuy, M.: Les infiltrations du sympathique: Physiologie, indications, techniques, Paris, 1946, Masson & Cie, pp. 200.
104. Feil, H.: Clinical Appraisal of the Beck Operation, Ann. Surg. **118**: 807-815, 1943.
105. Gallavardin, L., and Froment, R.: Sur trente cas d'angine de poitrine traités par la stellectomie, J. de méd. de Lyon **27**: 785-801, 1946.
106. Wertheimer, P.: Faut-il opérer l'angine de poitrine? Presse méd. **53**: 325-326, 1945.
107. Gask, G. E., and Ross, J. P.: The Surgery of the Sympathetic Nervous System, ed. 2, Baltimore, 1937, William Wood & Company, pp. 191.
108. Fauteux, M.: Surgical Treatment of Angina Pectoris: Experiences With Ligation of the Great Cardiac Vein and Pericoronary Neurectomy, Ann. Surg. **124**: 1041-1046, 1946.
109. Gregg, G. E.: The Coronary Circulation, Physiol. Rev. **26**: 28-46, 1946.
110. Servelle, M.: La chirurgie du splanchnique, Paris, 1942, Ed. Maloine, pp. 374.
111. Mallet-Guy, P., and Guillet, R.: Innervation des voies biliaires et chirurgie, Lyon chir. **38**: 436-452, 1943.
Idem: Documents expérimentaux et cliniques sur l'innervation des voies biliaires, Rev. d. Mal. du Foie, No. 1, Jan., 1944.
112. Johnson, F. E., and Boyden, E. A.: The Effect of Sectioning Various Autonomic Nerves Upon the Rate of Emptying of the Biliary Tract in the Cat, Surg., Gynec. & Obst. **76**: 395-410, 1943.
113. Mallet-Guy, P., Jeanjean, R., and Servettaz, P.: Résultats éloignés de la splanchnicectomie unilatérale dans le traitement des pancréatites chroniques, Lyon chir. **40**: 293-314, 1945.
114. Balchum, O. J., and Weaver, H. M.: Pathways for Pain From the Stomach of the Dog, Arch. Neurol. & Psychiat. **49**: 739-753, 1943.

115. Herrin, R. C., and Meek, W. J.: Afferent Nerves Excited by Intestinal Distention, Am. J. Physiol. **144**: 720-724, 1945.
116. Bauer, G.: Treatment of Hydronephrosis and Renal Pain by Denervation of the Kidney, Acta chir. Scandinav. **83**: 160-184, 1939.
117. Bauer, G.: Late Results of Denervation of the Kidney for Renal Pain, Acta chir. Scandinav. **90**: 460-468, 1944.
118. Jacobson, C. E., Braasch, W. F., and Love, J. G.: Presacral Neurectomy for Intractable Vesical Pain and Neurogenic Vesical Dysfunction, Surg., Gynec. & Obst. **79**: 21-26, 1944.
119. Mandl, F.: Reflex Dystrophy of Extremities. A Clinical Report, Acta med. orient. **3**: 169-182, 1944.
120. Mahorner, H.: Control of Pain in Posttraumatic and Other Vascular Disturbances: The Rôle of the Sympathetic Nervous System in the Treatment of Peripheral Vascular Diseases, Ann. Surg. **119**: 432-444, 1944.
121. Doupe, J., Cullen, C. H., and Chance, G. Q.: Post-traumatic Pain and the Causalgic Syndrome, J. Neurol., Neurosurg. & Psychiat. **7**: 33-48, 1944.
122. Speigel, I. J., and Milowsky, J. L.: Causalgia: A Preliminary Report of Nine Cases Successfully Treated by Surgical and Chemical Interruption of the Sympathetic Pathways, J. A. M. A. **127**: 9-15, 1945.
123. Mayfield, F. H., and Devine, J. W.: Causalgia, Surg., Gynec. & Obst. **80**: 631-635, 1945.
124. Allbritten, F. F., Jr., and Maltby, G. L.: Causalgia Secondary to Injury of the Major Peripheral Nerves: Treatment by Sympathectomy, SURGERY **19**: 407-414, 1946.
125. Rasmussen, T. E., and Freedman, H.: Treatment of Causalgia. An Analysis of 100 Cases, J. Neurosurg. **3**: 165-173, 1946.
126. Ulmer, J. L., and Mayfield, F. H.: Causalgia: A Study of 75 Cases, Surg., Gynec. & Obst. **83**: 789-796, 1946.
127. Miller, D. S., and de Takats, G.: Posttraumatic Dystrophy of the Extremities: Sudeck's Atrophy, Surg., Gynec. & Obst. **75**: 558-582, 1942.
128. Evans, J. A.: Sympathectomy for Reflex Sympathetic Dystrophy: Report of Twenty-nine Cases, J. A. M. A. **132**: 620-623, 1946.
129. White, J. C.: Painful Injuries of Nerves and Their Surgical Treatment, Am. J. Surg. **72**: 468-488, 1946.
130. Woodhall, Barnes: Personal communication.
131. de Takats, G.: Nature of Painful Vasodilatation in Causalgic States, Arch. Neurol. & Psychiat. **50**: 318-326, 1943.

In Memoriam

ELLIOTT CARR CUTLER
1888-1947

IN THE premature death on Aug. 16, 1947, of Elliott Carr Cutler at 59 years of age—recipient of the Bigelow Medal of the Boston Surgical Society in 1947—medicine and surgery throughout the world have lost a virile figure and beloved teacher; his community has lost a loyal, generous friend; and his country a soldier who gave his life for her as surely as if a bullet had snuffed it out during his long years of battlefront service. Taken ill while still on active duty, his true disability unrecognized despite his own sure knowledge that he was a sick man, his devotion to his work made him as expendable as any soldier of the line.

Not until his job was complete and he had returned home was the true nature of his malady recognized. Very few men could, or would, have faced the next two years with the courage, cheerfulness, optimism, and refusal to quit which he showed. A great soldier is gone.

Elliott Cutler was born in Bangor, Maine, July 30, 1888, of sturdy colonial heritage, stemming from our earliest history. As a young man he gave prompt indication of the driving energy, lofty ambition, and love of a good fight so characteristic of his whole life. Both public and private schools in Brookline, Mass., set his feet in the educational pathway. He entered Harvard in 1905 where his scholastic record was one of distinction, and where he found time as well to captain a victorious Harvard crew. He graduated from Harvard Medical School *cum laude* in 1913, doing special work in pathology during his fourth year under Dr. F. B. Mallory at the Boston City Hospital.

The following summer was spent at postgraduate work in Heidelberg under Professor Krehl. He returned to become the ardent pupil of Dr. Harvey Cushing at the Peter Bent Brigham Hospital as a surgical house officer. In 1915 and 1916 he was resident surgeon at the Massachusetts General Hospital, and followed this with one year's work under Dr. Simon Flexner at the Rockefeller Institute. His first war experience came immediately after; a period of willing and distinguished service for which he seemed especially adapted, and which gave him his first award of the Distinguished Service Medal and a personal citation from General Pershing.

He returned to the Brigham Hospital as chief resident surgeon in 1919, serving for two years in this post. His climb up the academic ladder from that time was rapid and sure. He became professor of surgery at Western Reserve University School of Medicine in Cleveland in 1924, and director of the surgical service at the Lakeside Hospital. On the retirement of his teacher, Dr. Cushing, he came back to Boston as Moseley Professor of Surgery at Harvard, and as

Surgeon-in-Chief at the Peter Bent Brigham Hospital. His great and oft-expressed ambition was to teach Harvard medical students, and knowing how much he admired and even subconsciously copied many of Dr. Cushing's characteristics, it is understandable that this post seemed to him the crowning touch of his academic career.

He was one of the first to recognize the inevitability of our participation in World War II. In addition to his hospital and medical school work in the days preceding universal recognition and the actual step of war declaration, he worked long hours in the organization of civilian safety here at home. He was largely responsible for imbuing many of his pupils and colleagues with the need to organize themselves early into a new base hospital ready for their country's

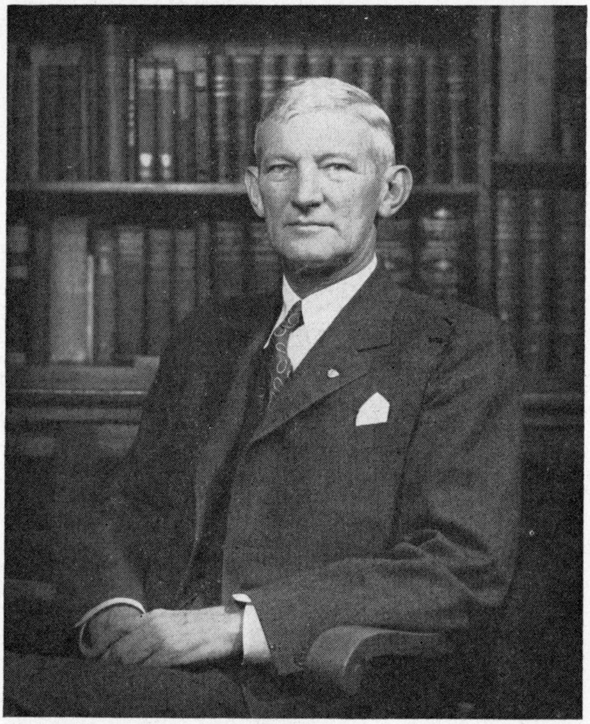

Elliott Carr Cutler
1888-1947

call. It is understandable that he could not leave them to face such service alone. In July, 1942, with the approval of the University and the Hospital, he became active again in the Army of the United States as a colonel in the Medical Corps. He became Chief Surgical Consultant in the European Theatre of Operations from August, 1942, to February, 1945, and Chief of the Professional Service Division from February, 1945, to August, 1945, with the rank of Brigadier-General.

Major-General Paul R. Hawley, Surgeon-in-Chief of the European Theatre, has spoken of him in the following terms: ''His wisdom and his wide experience made him invaluable. His inexhaustible energy became proverbial among his fellow officers. He organized, he planned, he criticized, he praised. He was here, he was there, and he invariably subordinated his personal comfort and the prerogatives of his position to the task at hand. To him, more than to any other man, is due the credit for the fine medical care given the wounded in the European Theatre.''

As a surgeon he was not spectacular. His technique was a direct heritage from Halsted, through Cushing. His pupils have all often heard his admonition —''These tissues are mostly water; we must never forget this!''—a typical exaggeration for the sake of emphasis. Careful hemostasis, gentleness, and a sacrifice of speed to obtain other more vital things as exposure and avoidance of trauma made his operations frequently lessons in anatomy for his assistants. He believed wholeheartedly in the importance of preoperative and postoperative care, more often than not doing the dressings himself and always seeing his patients daily. His best known work is remembered as his insistence on the embolic theory of postoperative pulmonary complications as opposed to the widely accepted belief that inhalation played the major role; his pioneer work in cardiac surgery; and his work in the relief of congestive heart failure through the medium of total thyroidectomy. He will be remembered as the surgeon who performed the first pericardiectomy in this country and who successfully carried out the first direct operative attack on the stenosed postrheumatic mitral valve. It was his pioneer work in this field which laid the foundation for the present-day spectacular enlargement of this field which we all know so well in the work of Beck, Elkin, Gross, Blalock, and others.

As a teacher he maintained that the fundamentals of good surgery should be presented to the students by senior teachers, and acted on this preachment. His own long training in pathology and laboratory study was all that was needed to emphasize his insistence on such preparation among his pupils. A large number of his published writings dealt with the education of the surgeon, a subject upon which he was always ready to speak; in fact, this was the subject of his Bigelow Medal Address, his last published work. In spite of many problems of personal interest which his restless, even somewhat feverish mind, urged him to pursue personally, he was always ready with helpful, pertinent suggestions in connection with the work of his younger colleagues. The weekly ''Surgical Teas'' over which he presided in his beloved surgical laboratory, where over a cup of tea and a biscuit all the younger staff listened to one of their fellows present his work for general discussion, were stimulating beyond measure for these young men. It was here more than anywhere that his breadth of interest and wide familiarity with almost every phase of modern surgery showed itself to its best advantage. A nearly continuous stream of distinguished visitors—his personal friends—were regularly taken to these exercises and brought into the friendly, informal discussions. The Laboratory to Dr. Cutler was the proving ground for any new or difficult clinical problem.

He was a prolific writer (his publications numbered well over 260) and an exceptionally able administrator. The duties incident to conducting a busy department of surgery, so often the greatest hindrance to scientific productivity, never bothered him. Budgetary limitations meant nothing to him. If the need arose, one or another of his host of friends seemed always ready to listen to his persuasive tongue and supply the necessary funds.

It is not possible here to enumerate all the honors which were his. He belonged to forty medical societies in many of which he held important offices. Even as the end came he was busily planning, as President of the American Surgical Association, for its meeting in 1948. Seven medical journals listed his name on their editorial boards. Honorary university degrees were his, and among his ten military decorations are three from the governments of England, France, and Norway. Few families can boast the proud story of patriotic service of the Cutlers during the last war. Twenty members of his family served in the armed forces, among them one commodore and two generals. Topping this remarkable record stands General Cutler's own, for his was a service of help and rehabilitation to the wounded. He alone in our military history stands out as the only medical officer to have received two Distinguished Service Medal awards.

But those who knew him best will not so much remember him as a great surgeon, a stimulating teacher, a person of many talents and unbounded energy, a charming host and wonderful companion, but as a man who faced with supreme courage, in a manner few may duplicate, those darkest hours of his last two years—a man to whom the laying down of arms was unknown.

His career and achievements furnish inspiration for all, and afford an example any young man might hope to emulate—never was it more inspiring than during the last long months. He found his own reward in his consciousness of service, in the approval and recognition of his fellows, and in seeing his own great desire to improve the medical care given to our sons and daughters who served in the armed forces become a reality.

—*Francis C. Newton*

SURGERY

Vol. 23 | June, 1948 | No. 6

Original Communications

Symposium on Cancer of the Esophagus and Gastric Cardia

INTRODUCTION TO SYMPOSIUM ON CANCER OF THE ESOPHAGUS AND GASTRIC CARDIA

George T. Pack, M.D., New York, N.Y.

THE recent upsurge of interest and improvement in surgical treatment of cancers of the esophagus and gastric cardia has occurred chiefly since the year 1940. The census figures covering deaths from cancer of the esophagogastrointestinal tract in the United States for 1940 list 2,805 esophageal cancers (3.9 per cent) and 26,133 gastric cancers (35.9 per cent). In our personal experience at the Memorial Hospital, 17 per cent of patients with carcinomas of the stomach have the tumor originating in or involving the cardiac segment. Seventeen per cent of 26,133 gastric cancers would be 4,443 occurring in the region of the cardia and accounting for 6 per cent of all deaths from cancer of the esophagogastrointestinal tract. In short, approximately 10 per cent of all malignant tumors of the esophagogastrointestinal tract, that is, those of the esophagus and cardia, are now suitable for the increasingly popular operation of transthoracic esophagogastrectomy and intrathoracic esophagogastric or esophagojejunal anastomosis.

The classical esophagectomy of Torek with anterior thoracic esophagostomy was done in 1913 and a similar operation by Zaaiger with axillary esophagostomy was successfully accomplished in the same year. Von Mikulicz (1904) and Sauerbruch (1906) and others had suggested and attempted with failure the transthoracic resection of the gastric cardia until Brun in 1916 reported for the first time an operative survival following a transpleural gastric cardiectomy. It seems incredible that with proof existent of the feasibility of surgical removal of cancers of the esophagus and gastric cardia, a quarter of a century must elapse before these operations became improved and standardized so as to be routinely employed. The rare operation of a decade ago has now become a commonplace procedure, practiced not only in the major surgical centers but in the smaller general hospitals as well. This great host of people comprising 10 per cent of all patients who have cancer of the gastrointestinal tract now, for the first time, enjoy a reasonable prospect of cure. It is another

Received for publication, March 30, 1948.

epochal milestone in the surgical conquest of cancer; the credit for it belongs not only to the large number of surgeons who have perfected the technical details of the operation but importantly to the improvements in anesthesia and the contributions of physiologists who have solved so many of the attendant problems dealing with the cardiovascular and pulmonary systems. It does seem appropriate at this time, therefore, to publish this symposium embodying as it does the efforts, results, and opinions from a considerable number of the surgical clinics where these operations are done with some frequency.

It is high time that attention is focused on esophageal tumors. Cancer of the esophagus is of more frequent occurrence than all malignant tumors of bone and is even more common than cancers of the lip, tongue, larynx, or kidney. Carcinoma of the esophagus resembles the intraoral group of cancers more than it does the gastrointestinal cancers of glandular origin; the resemblance is evident in three ways: (1) the epidermoid carcinoma is the common histologic type; (2) the age and sex distribution are strikingly similar; (3) there is a common etiologic relationship to chronic irritants, and because of the increasing knowledge of these factors, carcinoma of the esophagus may become one of the preventable cancers.

The medical profession as a whole has had a justifiable pessimism concerning the treatment of esophageal cancer, for the end results have been discouraging. The explanation of this point of view may be found in the following:

1. The obscurity of symptoms renders the diagnosis usually late.

2. The esophagoscope is used infrequently. Only a small minority of patients with symptoms referable to the gullet or cardiac end of the stomach are subjected to early endoscopic examination of the esophagus. There are relatively few physicians trained and equipped for esophagoscopy, certainly not one for every community which can support a hospital. Part of the blame for this unhappy situation has been the attitude of the early specialists who made the procedure so ritualistic and its study so specialized as to discourage general surgeons from using peroral endoscopy as one of their routine diagnostic measures. For the past fifteen years every interne, assistant resident, and Fellow of the Memorial Hospital has become proficient in esophagoscopy, bronchoscopy, and gastroscopy; in fact the technique is only slightly more complicated than sigmoidoscopy. The esophagoscopies and bronchoscopies are done on ambulatory outpatients under local anesthesia and the manipulation can be done by a single operator, unassisted.

3. The esophageal wall is perforated by the carcinoma not infrequently at an early stage in its development, although suppurative mediastinitis and fistulous communication with other viscera may not occur until much later. The esophagus does not have the serosal coat which serves as such an efficient barrier to perforation in the organs of the lower gastrointestinal system.

4. Esophageal carcinoma is usually highly malignant, a statement that is contrary to many recorded opinions. Metastases often occur early and widely, to a far greater extent than would be expected from epidermoid cancers of their histologic grade of malignancy. It extends intramurally up and down the esophagus for surprising lengths, sometimes far beyond the palpable margins

of the tumor; the operator is sometimes profoundly shocked to learn that the pathologist has discovered cancer cells at the very level of transsection. Esophageal cancers tend early to invade contiguous organs within the chest. During the performance of the transthoracic resection with anastomosis, the surgeon frequently discovers that the epidermoid carcinomas of the esophagus have extended greatly below the diaphragm to involve the stomach, the juxtacardiac lymph nodes, and even the liver. A review of necropsy findings following death from cancers of the esophagus will impress one with the widespread extent of the metastases even to distant sites.

5. The tumor is often inoperable at the time the diagnosis is established due to the degree of local invasion, the presence of regional and distant metastases, and the poor general condition of the patient.

6. The patient with esophageal cancer is not always a fit subject for radical treatment, surgical or otherwise. He is often elderly, with the senile changes concomitant with aging. Malnutrition is another important factor inasmuch as the esophagus is an essential organ of the gastrointestinal tract and its functional incapacity leads to early inanition. Coexistent pulmonary complications, such as emphysema, bronchitis, tracheal or bronchial fistula, bronchiectasis, tend to handicap surgical intervention.

7. The technique of transthoracic esophagocardiectomy with intrathoracic anastomosis involves grave physiologic and anatomic problems as well as requiring skill, judgment, resourcefulness, special equipment, and well-trained assistance. The contents of this symposium clearly indicate that these conditions are being constantly improved and the operation will undoubtedly be more generally employed in the future.

8. Radiation therapy of esophageal cancers has given only palliative end results as it has been employed in the United States. Intracavitary radium therapy using heavily filtered tubes of radium, arranged in tandem formation, has been successful in disengaging the esophageal lumen with improvement in deglutition, but has not completely sterilized these cancers. The radium tandem has been inserted as an intubating applicator, often under fluoroscopic and esophagoscopic guidance, with or without a supplementary gastrostomy. Even when it is perfectly applied and the dose administered with meticulous exactitude, the results are beneficial, but not curative. There are three common reasons for this failure of radium therapy, namely, (1) impossible adequate distribution of dosage throughout the tumor from such a source, (2) necrosis and sloughing of the infected tumor because of its solution by radium therapy and the consequent occurrence of suppurative mediastinitis, and (3) failure of a linear local source of radiation to reach the distant sites of extension of the cancer. Gold radon seeds used interstitially are also palliative, but fail of cure for the same previously mentioned reasons, to which should be added the extra hazard of their caustic action.

X-ray therapy of esophageal cancers has been used sporadically in the United States with confirmatory evidence of palliative relief. Sufficient regression of the cancers has occurred, avoiding the necessity for gastrostomy in many instances; swallowing is improved, weight is gained, symptoms disappear, and postradiation x-ray studies have often shown complete or nearly complete disappearance of the tumor. The direct esophagoscopic view corroborates the clinical and radiographic evidence of regression of the cancer following x-ray therapy. The million volt x-ray apparatus has been the most satisfactory modality, using a target-skin distance of 70 cm., a half-value layer of 3.8 cm. of lead, four rectangular ports (two parasternal and two paravertebral), treatment to one port daily of 300 r, and alternating on successive days until a total skin dose of 3000 r × 4 has been administered. The cause of ultimate failure in these patients has occasionally been not local recurrence but distant metastases, which is the same explanation for many surgical failures.

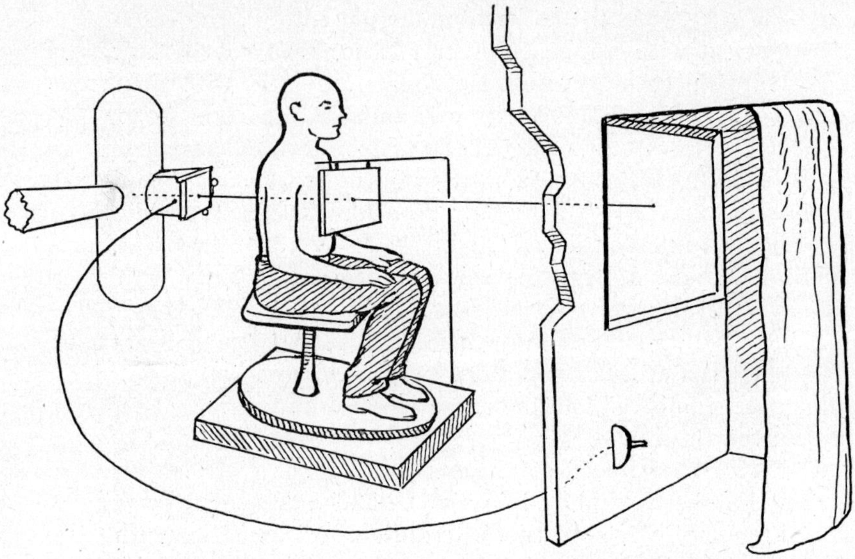

Fig. 1.—Arrangement for rotatory irradiation with the patient seated and screening control (Nielsen).

ROTATION ROENTGEN THERAPY OF ESOPHAGEAL CANCER

Although the present symposium is devoted to the consideration of surgical treatment of esophageal cancers, it would seem appropriate to consider in summary what recent accomplishments in radiation therapy have paralleled these advancements. To this end we must turn to the Scandinavian school of radiologists, and in particular to Dr. Jens Nielsen, Chief of the Radium Center in Copenhagen, Denmark, who by the application of original and scientific methods has made the most important contributions to this field. We have installed a preliminary crude motor-driven rotation table at the Lendrim Tumor Clinic in the Paterson General Hospital, but it is too early to comment on our personal experience with this apparatus. The following principles, therefore, are direct expressions of the work of Nielsen. Although the idea of rotatory irradiation is comparatively old, being mentioned by Kohl in 1906 and suggested by Pohl in 1913, it has been only during the recent postwar years that it has been developed on a scientific basis. The principle of rotation radiation therapy is to rotate the patient about an axis through the tumor at right angles to the x-ray beam, or vice versa, to rotate the x-ray tube around the stationary patient. It is Nielsen's contention that cancers of the esophagus are especially suitable for rotation x-ray therapy, because the esophagus is situated in an almost central location in the longitudinal axis of the thorax and these cancers, both by direct extension and lymphatic dissemination, spread in the same axial direction.

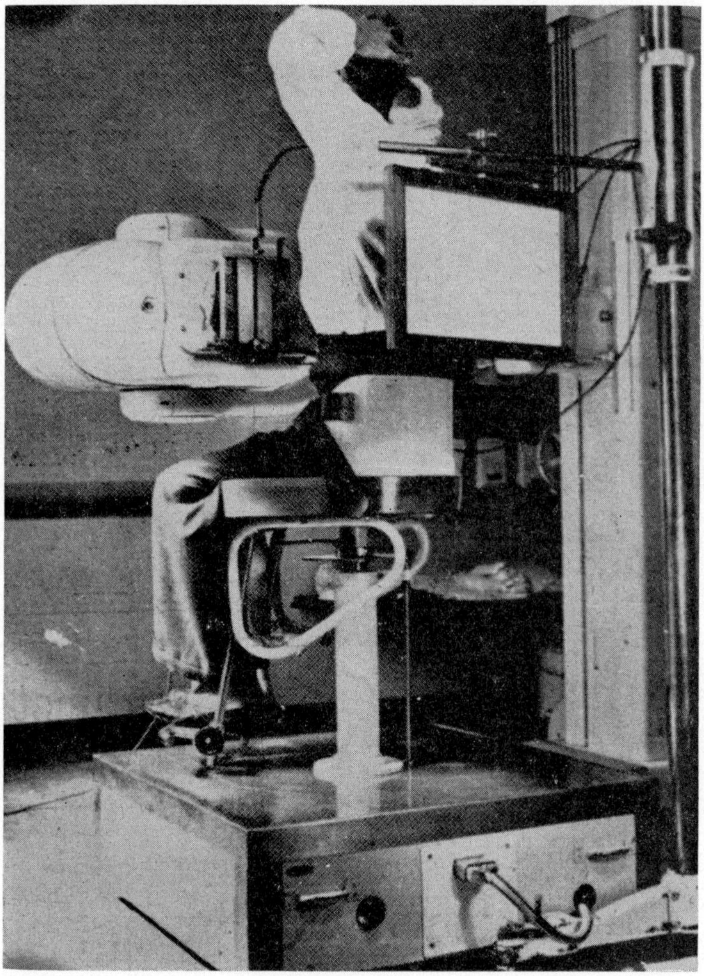

Fig. 2.—Clinical photograph of patient in position for treatment (Nielsen).

The patient is placed on a motor-driven rotating stool, which is turned at a uniform rate, that is, one complete turn in ten to thirty minutes depending on the plan of the therapist. The distance from the x-ray taret to the focusing diaphragm is 20 cm., and the distance from the focus to the axis of rotation, that is, the esophageal cancer, is an additional 50 cm. or a total of 70 cm. target-tumor distance. The size of the skin portals are from 4 by 6 to 6 by 10 cm., averaging 30 to 35 sq. cm. A current of 6 ma. and a potential of 180 kv. are commonly used. The filtration varies from a half-value layer (H.V.L.) of 0.32 mm. cu. (118 cases), to an H.V.L. of 0.9 mm. cu. (56 cases). The stool on which the patient sits is so located that the esophagus lies in the axis of the stool's rotation, which positioning is secured and maintained by fluoroscopic control. The patient is given a mouthful of a thick barium mixture to swallow and the centering of the x-ray beam is done on this opaque objective, which of course localizes the esophageal cancer. During the entire exposure to treatment, that is, while the patient is being rotated, the observer, who is outside the treatment room, watches this shadow on the fluoroscopic screen interposed between the patient and the lead glass window for the therapist. If the esophageal cancer should fall without the direct beam of radiation, the operator can recenter it by moving the diaphragm of the x-ray machine from one side to the other by means of remote control via a Bowden cable.

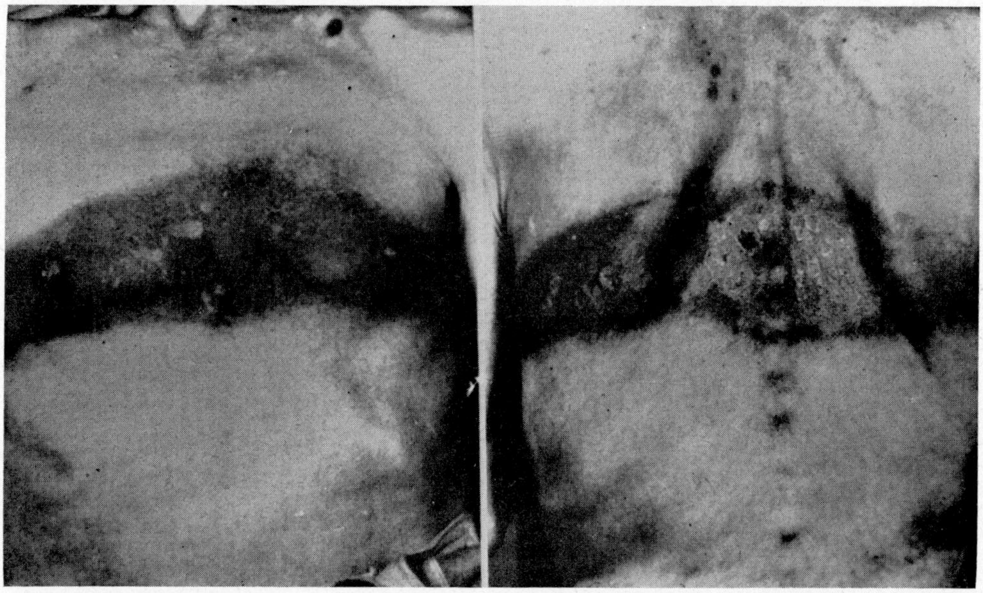

Fig. 3.—Cutaneous reaction at the end of rotatory irradiation treatment of cancer of the esophagus. Tumor dose, about 5,000 r (fifty-four sittings in the course of thirty-seven days). (Nielsen.)

By this rotation method a circular band of skin around the chest is irradiated and tanned. Nielsen considered this method as similar to the employment of many small fields, "which are irradiated in succession, each with a fraction (from a fifteenth to a twentieth) of the full dose." The result of this method of x-ray therapy is that the skin and normal thoracic organs receive a relatively small amount of radiation, while, conversely, the esophageal cancer receives an enormous dose because of the constant centering of the beam where it should be. This method takes full advantage of the differential sensitivities of normal and cancerous tissues to radiation therapy and fulfills as far as possible the primary tenet of successful irradiation, namely, to spare the normal tissues, while destroying the cancer.

Nielsen found the most suitable daily dosage to be a tumor dose of 100 to 200 r (usually 150 r) given in two daily sittings. The total dose approaching 500 r into the substance of the tumor is consummated in the course of five to six weeks. The bodily effect of these treatments is only a mild degree of radiation sickness characterized by slight nausea, anorexia, leucopenia, fatigue, lowered blood pressure, and loss of weight.

SUMMARY OF NIELSEN'S RESULTS WITH ROTATION ROENTGEN THERAPY

In only eight patients was it deemed unwise to administer this treatment. In thirty-four patients the treatment was solely for palliative purposes inasmuch as the tumor dose was consistently less than 3000 r. In 140 patients an attempt at curative x-ray therapy was made using the rotation method; 96 of these patients received more than 4000 r into the substance of these esophageal cancers. In four-fifths of Nielsen's patients who received the full dose, complete or nearly complete immediate freedom from symptoms was obtained. The patients could swallow and there was radiographic evidence of improvement. Death was due to metastases and cachexia, but the majority of patients were able to swallow until the fatal day. The survival curve for months and years revealed that with rotation x-ray therapy, 25 per cent of the patients as against a former 10 per cent were alive at the end of one year and 15 per cent as against a former 4 per cent were alive at the end of two years.

EPICRISIS

The technique of radiation therapy of esophageal cancers, epitomized here, and the end results given represent the best that can be accomplished in the world today by methods other than surgical removal. Nielsen and other Scandinavian radiologists are frankly skeptical that esophagectomy can compete with radiation therapy as a means of affording the greatest relief to the largest number of patients and for the longest time. To quote Nielsen, "To us, there is no doubt that the difficult task of trying to treat esophageal cancer both radically and symptomatically will to a very great extent continue to be the domain of radiotherapy. All imaginable advances of thoracic surgery notwithstanding only a small percentage of carcinomas in the esophagus will be amenable to surgical treatment, and the number of these in which a complete cure will be obtained will be smaller still." The answer to Nielsen's challenge may or may not be given in this symposium, but it is my opinion that a review of the accomplishments of our radiologic colleagues toward the common goal of the control or cure of esophageal cancer should be presented in this surgical forum.

REFERENCES

1. Pack, G. T., and Livingston, E. M.: Introduction: Treatment of Cancer of the Esophagus, Vol. II, Chap. 53, In Treatment of Cancer and Allied Diseases, New York, 1940, Paul B. Hoeber Inc., Pp. 923-927.
2. Nielsen, Jens, and Jensen, Sv. Hoeffer: Some Experimental and Clinical Lights on the Rotation Therapy, Its Basis and Possibilities, Acta radiol. 23: 51-66, 1942.
3. Jensen, Sv. Hoeffer, Nielsen, Jens, and Thayssen, V.: Evaluation of Different Factors in Rotation Therapy, Acta radiol. 25: 95-104, 1944.
4. Nielsen, Jens: Clinical Results With Rotation Therapy in Cancer of the Esophagus, Acta radiol. 26: 361-391, 1945.

THE ROENTGEN DIAGNOSIS OF CANCER OF THE CARDIAC REGION OF THE STOMACH

ROBERT S. SHERMAN, M.D., NEW YORK, N. Y.

(From the Department of Diagnostic Roentgenology, Memorial Hospital)

GENERAL PRINCIPLES IN ROENTGEN DIAGNOSIS OF STOMACH CANCER

ROENTGEN examination in the hands of the competent is the most important method for the detection and subsequent diagnosis of gastric neoplasm. In contrast to other means of direct study of the stomach, this procedure is relatively harmless. Not only are there no significant contraindications, but the number of unsatisfactory examinations is few. As far as the patient is concerned, x-ray examination is comparatively simple and readily available. Thorough training, precise technique, modern equipment, and a special interest in the subject are as necessary for dependable results as these factors are deemed to be in gastric surgery.

Present-day roentgenology places emphasis on the fluoroscopic study with mucosal and pressure technique on the filming fluoroscope. The practice of multiple film taking in a routine manner deserves little attention. There are many instances where film examination of conventional type might be dispensed with altogether. The term gastrointestinal, or G. I. series, might well be abandoned since six, twenty-four, and forty-eight hour films are no longer taken routinely.

Since gross pathology is the foundation for reliable x-ray diagnosis in gastric cancer, a classification based upon morphology is used. Three types of carcinoma, polypoid, infiltrating, and ulcerating, are recognized. While most carcinomas contain more than one of these features, one usually predominates, permitting classification. The fundamental units upon which the roentgenologist must rely for diagnosis are mass, either seen or felt, infiltrate and ulcer. These elements occur in various degrees and in manifold guises, making their recognition simple or difficult as the case may be. The same situation holds regarding interpretation, for only when these findings are present in certain patterns do they justify cancer as the correct roentgen diagnosis. The functional changes which have been described in detail in the past play little role in the diagnosis of tumors of the stomach.

Most gastric cancers when first seen by the roentgenologist can be diagnosed with assurance on x-ray findings alone. Symptomatology and information from the laboratory are not held to be of basic importance, and in practice rarely influence roentgen diagnosis significantly in this field.

The greatest contribution of gastric roentgenology lies in the ability to *detect* organic abnormality. Potentially any lesion of macroscopic size which does not exhibit a physiologic feature as its sole characteristic can be uncovered. Experience demonstrates that this ideal is attainable. It follows that x-ray is of equal importance in excluding organic gastric change as a possible cause of a patient's complaints. Kirklin[1] has expressed these beliefs by emphasizing that errors in detection should no longer be charged to roentgenology, but should be blamed upon the examiner himself.

Received for publication, Aug. 13, 1947.

In the *diagnosis* of an organic lesion roentgenology is generally less reliable than in its detection. Nevertheless, the method is the most accurate available for the diagnosis of gastric cancer. Because of the morphologic similarity of certain stomach lesions, the roentgenologist is occasionally unable to make a differentiation with full assurance, especially upon the initial examination. His difficulty concerns some of the ulcerating processes and some of the localized and clinically significant cases of gastritis. He is unable to discern the histologic varieties of stomach cancer, and he cannot always tell whether a tumor is benign or malignant.

Since surgery is the proper management for most of the cases falling into these categories, and since histologic diagnosis can thereby be gained with little or no added risk, the inability of the roentgenologist to differentiate in all instances does not necessarily constitute a serious deficiency. The rarity of the simulants of malignant tumors tends to lessen further the problem of differential diagnosis. Finally, the treatment test for selected ulcerating lesions of the stomach, when critically applied and carefully carried out, is another instance where proper management of the patient may provide a diagnosis. In essence, the crux of the problem of differential diagnosis is the ability to tell with assurance whether a process is surgical or medical.

Statistical and comparative studies which have failed to integrate these principles cannot provide a reliable evaluation of roentgenology in cancer of the stomach. Their value is further lessened when there has been indiscriminate grouping of novice and competent work, a neglect to judge the technical methods employed, and a massing of old and new material.

While the roentgenologist's statement concerning resectability may be correct more often than otherwise, sufficient discrepancy has been shown to discredit the practice. An accurate statement as to tumor type, extent, location, and complications is of more practical value than an x-ray appraisal of resectability. Since the patient's only chance for cure is in resection, it is fitting that the surgeon determine resectability in the operating room.

Fluoroscopy has been used as a screening procedure for symptomless persons in an effort to find resectable cancer of the stomach.[2] Sufficient material has now been accumulated to demonstrate the reliability of this step, but it remains to be proved that such studies are feasible from other standpoints.*

FUNDAMENTALS IN ROENTGEN DIAGNOSIS OF CANCER OF THE CARDIAC REGION

Anatomy.—Roentgen anatomy is fundamentally different from cadaver and surgical anatomy, and this is especially true in the upper part of the stomach. There is a wide range of developmental variation with which the roentgenologist must become familiar. The effects of respiration, change of body position, results of stomach distention, and alterations due to varying degrees of intra-abdominal pressure must be integrated and evaluated in each instance. These varying, complex, and manifold details, a full knowledge of which is so vital to dependable interpretation in diseases of this area, can be gained only by experience.

*The writer is carrying out such a survey in conjunction with the Strang Cancer Prevention Clinic at Memorial Hospital.

The mucosal anatomy of the cardiac region is subject to variations within normal limits equal in degree to those listed for the grosser aspects of roentgen anatomy. There seems to be a fairly constant, basic mucosal pattern upon which may be superimposed the changes related to respiration, increase and decrease in intra-abdominal tension, extrinsic pressure, gastric distention, type of media used, and functional alterations.

In the roentgen terminology that we employ, the cardia is considered to be an area about one inch square surrounding the esophageal orifice. A line drawn horizontally from its upper margin when the patient is upright separates the fundus above from the body below. In the erect sagittal position the lesser curvature forms the medial and the greater curvature the lateral border of the stomach. The greater curvature is continued over the fundus to end at the esophageal orifice. It is evident that the radiographic curvatures may not correspond exactly to the anatomic ones, although generally speaking the association is sufficiently close for practical purposes. In many instances there is a notchlike recess superiorly where the abdominal esophagus enters the stomach. This is called the cardiac angularis. The intra-abdominal part of the esophagus varies considerably, not only from person to person, but with the position of the diaphragm and of the patient as well. In the high transverse type of stomach there is a tendency for the abdominal part of the esophagus to be short or absent. The uppermost portion of the fundus follows the curve of the left side of the diaphragm and normally contains some air, the amount being subject to extreme variation.

Developmental Variations.—The cascade stomach is a developmental form, not necessarily significant in itself, that may complicate interpretation at times. A bizarre appearance in the sagittal view caused by cascading is often easily resolved when the study is continued into the oblique and the lateral positions. Cascade stomach may occur in various degrees from slight posterior pouching to an essentially bilocular stomach. Once the condition is recognized, the detection of disease in this form of stomach may be carried out with assurance.

A false appearance of cascading may be brought about when intra-abdominal pressure is high due to failure to relax on the part of the patient. We have found that the best way to bring about abdominal wall relaxation is to instruct the patient to "push the stomach out in front." A false cascade appearance may also be encountered in certain upper body, posterior wall lesions, particularly ulcerations with fixation. Oblique and lateral studies should help to resolve such instances.

The various degrees of stomach rotation or torsion occasionally found might also act as a deterrent to a satisfactory examination unless their nature were recognized at the onset. Once the condition is evaluated there should be no particular difficulty in telling whether there is also a tumor present. The same holds regarding gastric herniation through the diaphragm.

Technical Aspects.—There are certain procedural handicaps in the x-ray examination of the upper part of the stomach. The most important of these is that the area is usually inaccessible to palpation. Spot film studies employing pressure techniques are likewise generally excluded. However unlikely it might appear that the cardiac portion of the stomach can be felt, one should always attempt to do so. By deep pressure coupled with forced inspiration on the part of the patient, the examining fingers will occasionally contact the cardia. A mass may be uncovered for the first time by this maneuver.

Peristalsis which may be of considerable aid in evaluating the finer degrees of wall stiffening and mucosal motion in the distal stomach cannot be utilized in the upper third because of the weakness or absence of the wave.

Among the advantages of a technical nature that the radiologist enjoys in the examination of the upper stomach is the absence of local functional changes. The different varieties of spasm, hypersecretion, altered peristalsis, gastric dilatation, tone changes, and abnormal emptying rates which may plague the examiner studying the distal part of the stomach do not occur in a significant degree in the upper third.

Another advantage in roentgen study of this region is the wide lumen which is air containing. This permits a dependable barium and air visualization to be carried out. We have not seen the need for the introduction of air into the stomach by means of a tube, and the use of effervescent powders for the same purpose is advised against. Judicious positioning of the patient and increasing the air content by rapid, small swallows are the means favored for satisfactory double contrast studies.

The close association of the fundic region with the left side of the diaphragm makes the effect of respiration a valuable source of information at fluoroscopy. With forced inspiration the contour of the upper stomach changes, position is altered, the mucosa moves, and the barium-coated walls show a characteristic undulating motion. Occasionally cardiac and aortic pulsations may be used to shed further light upon wall mobility.

Changes in the lower esophagus are so frequently related to cancer of the cardiac region that careful esophageal study may provide essential information. Obstruction, narrowing, wall stiffening and irregularity, mucosal derangement or destruction, ulceration and mass formation are among the types of lower esophageal involvement that may be due to extension of tumors of gastric origin.

There are features in the fluoroscopic part of the examination of the upper stomach which deserve special mention. Before the opaque material is swallowed, careful attention is given to the air bubble, particularly as it is seen in the erect sagittal view. Tumors of the cardiac area can often be seen as a mass of water density protruding into the air sac usually from the lesser curvature side.

The first swallow of the barium and water mixture is of the consistency of thick batter. As this slides down the esophagus, it leaves traces which demonstrate the mucosa. This canalizing bolus, as it traverses the lower esophagus and the upper part of the stomach, warrants particular attention. Repeated deep inspiration is used to help the bolus along, to demonstrate diaphragmatic pinchcock action, and to bring out the normal undulating motion of the lower esophagus and the upper stomach. Deep palpation with forced inspiration is carried out. Both oblique and lateral positions as well as the sagittal are employed at this stage.

The patient is then placed horizontally and the procedures described are repeated. When the erect position is reassumed, barium should be found coating the mucosa, giving a double relief pattern. Either "spot" or conventional films may be used advantageously at this point.

Finally, the patient is given barium of cream consistency and told to swallow several mouthfuls rapidly. In this way the lower esophagus is distended providing additional test of wall flexibility. With the thinner barium, a splashing or divided stream appearance may rarely be uncovered. This is due to the presence of the tumor in the barium pathway. With the stomach moderately distended with the thinner mixture, the fluoroscopic examination is concluded by directing attention to contour changes.

A careful film technique is of fundamental importance for visualization of the upper third of the stomach. The movable grid is regularly employed with exposures of one-tenth of a second at thirty-inch distance. The appropriate cone and the smallest focal spot permissible are utilized. The patient is rotated in the recumbent position before the films are exposed and all are secured with a small amount of barium in the lower esophagus.

No film routine is followed. An attempt is made to get information indicated by the fluoroscopic study from as few films as possible. The general principle of obtaining two views, one at right angles to the other, is sound. We now tend to rely considerably upon erect sagittal and lateral views. Occasionally a small tumor, readily visible in the erect position, has been hidden with the patient recumbent. We do not recall having seen the opposite occur.

GENERAL PRINCIPLES IN DIFFERENTIAL DIAGNOSIS OF CANCER OF THE CARDIAC REGION

Even though peptic ulcer occurs relatively less often in the upper third of the stomach, it represents one of the common sources of difficulty in differential diagnosis. For the most part peptic ulcer can be diagnosed with as much assurance as when it is seen in the distal parts of the stomach, particularly when it is possible to obtain both full face and profile views. The inability to use mucosal studies with graded pressure, however, means that the finer changes occasionally important for differentiation are seen fortuitously if at all. It appears to us that most peptic ulcers seen in the upper stomach have fallen into a surgical category from the onset. In any case the principles of diagnosis and management of the ulcerating lesions of the stomach hold with equal force irrespective of the cardiac location.

It is occasionally a problem to tell whether a malignant tumor is of lower esophageal or upper stomach origin. Mere identification of the bulk of the cancer above the diaphragm does not assure that it is esophageal since intrathoracic gastric cancer is not uncommon. The basis for accurate differential diagnosis is a mucosal one, although in certain instances it is impossible to tell site of origin with full assurance. In our experience most cancers involving the lower esophagus are found to be of stomach origin. Most lesions in this group would be available for biopsy diagnosis through the esophagoscope and would have the same type of surgical treatment.

The various forms and degrees of herniation of stomach through the diaphragm may provide a stumbling block to the diagnosis of cancer of the cardiac region. One must exclude the possibility of intrathoracic gastric cancer in all hernia cases. If the condition is kept in mind and the technique employed is satisfactory, the diagnosis is not necessarily difficult.

In the obstructive lesions occurring at the lower esophageal orifice it is important to get enough barium into the stomach to be able to rule out gastric cancer. To accomplish this the period of the examination may have to be considerably extended. If an air bubble is present, a careful study of its contour may provide essential information. It is well to remember that cancer and cardiospasm may occur together. The general x-ray principle that both ends of an obstructive lesion must be seen to determine its nature should be borne in mind.

The localized forms of gastritis and the simulants of cancer of specific etiology are almost nonexistent in the cardia area alone.

Polypi and myomas are usually seen in the distal portions of the stomach. It should be pointed out that in spite of their "benign" appearance their treatment is surgical removal after which the true nature can be accurately determined by the pathologist. Aberrant pancreas, a rare condition in itself, infrequently occurs in the upper part of the stomach. An example of how complicated diagnosis may be at times is seen in an unusual case mentioned by Templeton,[3] in which a sarcomatous nodule of the spleen adjacent to the fundus gave the appearance of gastric tumor.

Varices may protrude into the lumen of the lower esophagus and the adjacent stomach as polypoid serpentine masses resembling cancer. The absence of wall stiffening or narrowing, the preservation of organ mobility and peristaltic contraction, the smoothness of outline and the slight inconstancy of pattern are among differential points from the roentgen standpoint.

Other conditions concerned in the problem of differential diagnosis are peptic esophagitis, gastric diverticulum, benign stenoses, and extrinsic involvement from near-by tumor. The stellate configuration is of little importance as a simulant of cancer. The manifold types of extrinsic pressure from aorta, spleen, liver, colon, tail of pancreas, left adrenal, left kidney, as well as certain developmental variations, may at times enter into differential diagnosis. The distinguishing features of these conditions cannot be discussed here.

EVALUATION OF ROENTGEN FINDINGS IN CARCINOMA OF THE CARDIAC REGION

In a group of 205 resected carcinomas of the stomach at Memorial Hospital it was found that 22 per cent were located in the cardiac region. For the purposes of this discussion the cardiac region or upper stomach is considered to be the superior one inch of the body, the entire fundus and the cardia. Twenty-five of the more recent cardiac cases were selected on the basis of adequacy of x-ray coverage, presence of a satisfactory description of the resected specimen, and completeness of the histologic survey. Cases in which operation had been done were studied because the earliest and most significant carcinomas would be included. All patients were seen in the past five years and were examined radiographically either by the resident, fellow, or staff member of the x-ray department. In several instances repeat examinations within a short time interval were required before a final diagnosis was advanced. In each case the lesion was detected and the correct diagnosis of cancer of the cardiac region was made.

Under the following headings points are presented which are considered to be most significant in the detection and diagnosis of cancer of the upper stomach as revealed in a film study of the twenty-five resected cases. While the features noted are primarily based upon films, their integration with fluoroscopy should provide no difficulty.

Mucosal Alteration.—Mucosal alteration was a constant finding in the stomach. This was of the same type as encountered in the esophagus when it was involved. The mucosal changes were due to the basic features of infiltration causing fold stiffening, thinning, and destruction; of ulceration with fine irregularities; and of mass formation showing fold erasure and change in course of the rugae.

Infiltrate.—There was evidence of wall infiltration of some degree in each case. In addition to that mentioned for the mucosa, there was always a more severe induration extending into the musculature and producing wall rigidity, fixation, and frequently local contour change.

Mass.—There were sixteen of the twenty-five cases where a mass was seen as a shadow of water density in the air bubble. In four more cases a mass was suspected, while in the remainder none could be determined in the gas bubble area. While mass in this form was less often seen than some of the other diagnostic features, it was occasionally the most definite and provided valuable supporting information. A mass was usually seen in this way more easily on the erect sagittal view, but in a few instances the oblique or lateral position provided the best visualization. No mass was palpated in this series.

Ulcer.—Generally speaking ulceration played a minor role as a diagnostic aid. In nine cases there was evidence of ulcer, but in most it was thought to be superficial and of secondary significance. In three instances the area of tissue loss seemed to be sufficiently prominent for it to be considered as the outstanding roentgen feature. The ulcerations were shallow, elliptical in configuration, and were always accompanied by infiltration and usually mass formation. These associated changes emphasized the malignant character of the ulceration.

Esophageal Involvement.—Cancer extension into the lower esophagus was diagnosed radiographically in nineteen of the twenty-five cases. It was suspected in an additional two and was absent in the remaining four. The smallest segment of involvement was 1.5 cm. and the longest was 6 cm. In diagnosing esophageal invasion special attention was paid to the abdominal part of the esophagus as revealed in the erect position.

Miscellaneous Findings.—There are roentgen findings commonly mentioned as being of diagnostic importance in cancer of the cardiac region of the stomach which ultimately depend upon varying degrees of infiltration, mass formation, or ulceration for their presence. Obstruction, gross contour changes, general widening between the fundus and the dome of the diaphragm, lateral displacement of the stomach at the cardia, and diaphragmatic alteration are among the findings.

In one patient there was sufficient obstruction in the lower esophagus to warrant its being noted as an outstanding x-ray finding. There were two other cases where there was mild obstruction. Mucosal alteration continuous with a similar change in the adjacent part of the stomach and infiltration of the wall with mass formation were actually the basic findings in these cases which indicated cancer extension.

In the group there was no example of generalized contour change. In twenty-one cases there were local contour alterations at the tumor site in the upper portion of the body and adjacent cardia. There were eighteen instances where a local contour alteration was encountered at the tumor site in the fundic portion adjacent to the cardia. Local contour change of this order seems to be a less critical way of pointing out the presence of mass, infiltrate, or ulcer as the case might be.

In this series no instance of general widening between the diaphragm and the gastric fundus was encountered. This is a late sign and probably one of little practical importance, particularly since there may be other causes for its occurrence. We observed no dependable evidence of lateral displacement of the stomach at the cardiac area. This is thought to be a quite unreliable sign, because not only is it a late one, but it is dependent upon unrelated and uncontrollable influences. There were no cases showing diaphragmatic changes that could be related to the presence of the tumor itself. The appearance of diaphragmatic alteration must be a late sign.

There were two instances where a cascade type of stomach was present. It is thought that there might have been more examples but the absence of a lateral view on many of the cases prohibited confirmation. There were two examples of intrathoracic cancer. Although the surgeon made no mention of herniation in either instance, the clearness of the x-ray demonstration established the condition as being present. In three instances it was possible to see the tumor on a chest film by studying the appearance of the gas bubble. It might be well to note this area on photoroentgen surveys of the chest.

There were sixteen cases where the cancer was classified morphologically by the department of pathology. Eleven were called polypoid, three ulcerating, and two infiltrating. In eight of the sixteen there was close correlation between the x-ray and the pathologic classification, in four more there was slight correlation, and in four the radiographic opinion as to type was completely erroneous.

The smallest tumor measured 2.5 by 1.5 cm. while the largest was 18 by 8 cm. The average size seemed to be 7 by 5 by 2 cm. The judgment of the roentgenologist as to tumor size was about 50 per cent dependable. This deficiency seemed to be related to the difficulty in typing these tumors. It may be that the more frequent use of lateral views would help the roentgenologist in evaluating these two aspects by providing a three dimensional concept.

As for location, it was found that all cancers involved the cardia to some extent, and most had the cardia as the principal site. All were located at the lesser curvature side of the stomach. While it is true that cancer may appear in any area, fundic and greater curvature carcinomas of the upper third are relatively uncommon.

There were fifteen cases where the department of pathology recorded the presence or absence of esophageal involvement. There was invasion by cancer in eleven and none in four. The roentgenologist's appraisal of the lower esophagus was correct in thirteen. One case thought to show involvement was found to have tumor protruding into the lumen of the lower esophagus. Five of the fifteen cases were evaluated correctly at operation and no remark was made in four more. In six judgment was erroneous. Tumor was found histologically in five instances extending to the upper line of resection.

ROENTGEN DIAGNOSIS OF INFREQUENT CANCERS OF THE CARDIAC REGION

Lymphosarcoma of the stomach occurs either in the primary form or as a manifestation of the generalized disease. In either case the appearance is similar. Lymphosarcoma of the stomach cannot be differentiated from carcinoma with assurance on roentgen findings alone. Even the presence of a generalized lymphoblastoma does not prove conclusively that the stomach lesion is of the same etiology, although in lymphosarcoma it may be considered as very strong presumptive evidence. The features suggesting that a cancer may be lymphosarcoma are the younger age (one carcinoma of the cardia at Memorial Hospital was in a patient 31 years of age), a better physical state than a carcinoma of the same size would seem to permit, a pattern suggesting considerable fold enlargement, a bulky tumor that cannot be palpated, a tumor that feels "soft," and tendency for the tumor to cross stomach orifices. From a number of primary lymphosarcomas at Memorial Hospital there is one that involves principally the cardiac region of the stomach.

Stomach origin for the other lymphoblastomas is distinctly less common than for lymphosarcoma. There are only a few established cases of isolated Hodgkin's disease of the stomach. Leucemia, especially the lymphatic form, is said to have involved the stomach rarely. There is at least one case of myelogenous leucemia at Memorial Hospital where the stomach cancer was found at autopsy to be a carcinoma.

In a single case of resected sarcoid of the stomach studied in this department several small ulcerations in the distal segment were found.

Myosarcoma is usually seen as a rounded mass with smooth mucosal surface protruding into the stomach lumen from a relatively broad base. An area of ulceration on the surface or the presence of a sinus tract is the feature pointing to the muscular origin of the tumor. When occurring in a polyp form these cancers cannot be differentiated from epithelial tumors at times. In this connection it is well to note again that the roentgen criteria for a tumor's benign character are relatively unreliable. Myosarcoma may be located anywhere in the stomach; one of the few seen at Memorial Hospital was in the cardiac region.

There were two patients with cancer metastases to the stomach wall examined radiographically. In neither of these was there involvement of the cardiac region.

ROENTGEN FINDINGS FOLLOWING GASTRIC CARDIECTOMY

Resection of the gastric cardiac area with esophagogastric anastomosis was the operation performed in these cases. In operations of this type the stomach and duodenum are mobilized, drawn upward and to the left, and the involved portion is removed. In most of these patients the transthoracic approach was used. The anastomosis was usually done within the thorax. As a result the stomach is smaller than normal to a degree attendant upon the amount of tissue removed. The stomach axis is often vertical in both sagittal and lateral planes. Varying portions of the stomach are found within the chest. The duodenal bulb is usually found on the left side of the abdomen and inferior in position to the pyloric canal. The pyloric canal is vertical in direction. The vagus innervation of the stomach is interfered with and some of the sympathetic connections may also be lost by this operation.

There were but ten of the twenty-five cases of resected cancer of the upper part of the stomach where there were sufficiently complete postoperative x-ray views to make study worth while. In these ten cases the first examination was usually made in three to six weeks after the resection. There were a few patients where the follow-up period was continued from one to four years. In all but one of these cases the transthoracic approach was used.

In a general way an estimation was made of the degree of stomach and duodenal mobilization from the roentgenograms. It was found that in nine instances there was significant gastric and duodenal displacement. In about one-half of the cases the stomach was vertical. An estimation was also made of the amount of stomach removed. This varied from about one-tenth to as much as five-sixths, the average being about one-fourth of the stomach area.

Functionally these postoperative stomachs appeared relatively quiet with little effective peristalsis. Barium fell through the stomach as though by gravity and came to rest abruptly against the closed pyloris. There was no significant alteration noted in the gastric tone. The stomach could not be distended and it appeared that barium left the stomach after a certain point in filling. Emptying seemed to be largely through simple opening of the pyloris unaccompanied by any effective peristaltic wave. In two cases a mild dilatation of the second portion of the duodenum was seen initially. This disappeared after several months. We wish to emphasize that we pretend no controlled or detailed survey of stomach function in these cases at this time.

In all but one of the ten cases the anastomosis was made above the diaphragm level. There were three patients who developed fistulas both clinically and radiographically. There were three in whom blind pouches formed. One patient having blind pouching showed this unchanged after four years. One developed a stenosis at the esophagogastric junction. The appearance was specific for cancer recurrence of the infiltrating type. In another there was evidence of recurrence within the intrathoracic portion of the stomach. This showed mucosal destruction and wall fixation.

REFERENCES

1. Kirklin, B. R.: Am. J. Roentgenol. **49**: 259, 1943.
2. St. John, F. B., Swenson, P. C., and Harvey, H. D.: Ann. Surg. **119**: 225-231, 1944.
3. Templeton, Frederic E.: X-ray Examination of the Stomach, Chicago, 1944, University of Chicago Press, p. 378.

PREOPERATIVE, OPERATIVE, AND POSTOPERATIVE CARE IN ESOPHAGEAL RESECTIONS

HERBERT C. MAIER, M.D., NEW YORK, N. Y.

DURING the past few years radical resection of the esophagus for carcinoma has been attended by a considerable decrease in morbidity and mortality. More satisfactory surgical procedures which permit re-establishment of the continuity of the alimentary tract have been developed. These advances have been due to better preoperative preparation of the patient, improvements in anesthesiology, chemotherapy, a better understanding of the physiologic alterations during and following operation, improved surgical technique, and better postoperative care.

Preoperative Preparation of the Patient.—Carcinoma of the esophagus is associated with varying degrees of obstruction. The stagnation of food and secretions above the tumor may cause an esophagitis. Ulceration of the carcinoma may lead to secondary infection. Therefore, the preoperative preparation of the patient for esophageal resection includes cleansing of the esophagus above the tumor. All retained material and secretion should be aspirated and daily lavage of the esophagus instituted. Care should be taken that no aspiration into the lungs occurs due to an overflow from the obstructed esophagus. Preoperative lavage is not necessary in those patients with no esophageal retention. The importance of good mouth hygiene at the time of esophageal surgery has been appreciated for many years. Infection of the gums increases the hazard of pulmonary complications and is usually associated with an unfavorable bacterial flora in the esophagus. The extent of dental work to be done prior to operation is a matter of judgment.

Almost all patients undergoing surgery for carcinoma of the esophagus have lost weight and may have nutritional deficiencies. These disturbances may be due to inadequate food intake or be caused by secondary chemical changes associated with the presence of the malignant tumor. It is preferable to correct these deficiencies if possible through feeding by mouth, together with supplementary parenteral injections, rather than to perform a preliminary jejunostomy. The latter operative procedure is reserved for those cases in which the obstruction is so marked that adequate intake by mouth is impossible. Preliminary gastrostomy is to be avoided in any case in which the stomach requires mobilization at the time of the esophageal resection. Hypoproteinemia is a common finding in esophageal cancer. The protein depletion may be more marked than the plasma protein determination would seem to indicate. In interpreting the report on the plasma protein level the state of hydration of the patient must be borne in mind. The correction of the hypoproteinemia as well as the other nutritional deficiencies may require a week or two of preoperative preparation. A fluid diet or, if feasible, a soft diet high in proteins, carbohydrates, and vitamins is given. In some cases preoperative blood or plasma transfusions and amigen are indicated. Many patients with carcinoma of the esophagus have a

Received for publication, Aug. 13, 1947.

deficiency in vitamin C which should be corrected by a daily dose of 200 to 1,000 mg. of ascorbic acid parenterally. Both hypoproteinemia and deficiency in vitamin C are important factors in poor wound healing and especially in late leakage at the site of anastamosis. These deficiencies also tend to cause edema of the tissues and consequently tend to increase the fluid content of the lung. The incidence of postoperative pulmonary complications can be reduced by avoiding the tendency to edema of the lung associated with hypoproteinemia and ascorbic acid deficiency.

The hematocrit and the plasma specific gravity should be determined in order to obtain a better index of the degree of anemia present. Red blood cell and hemoglobin determinations alone may give an erroneous impression because of hemoconcentration due to dehydration. Transfusions are given if the hemoglobin is less than 80 per cent after dehydration is corrected. Preoperative infusion of saline solutions is occasionally indicated, but due to the infrequency of vomiting in carcinoma of the esophagus, sodium chloride deficiency may not be prominent as it frequently is in carcinoma of the stomach.

The preoperative work-up should also include an evaluation of the cardiac and renal status. In some cases preoperative digitalization may be indicated. Any clinical or laboratory evidence suggesting coronary sclerosis requires constant effort to avoid anoxia at all times during and following operation. The prevention of any circulatory depression during operation is most essential in such cases because diminution in blood flow to the heart and kidneys impairs their function. Pulmonary emphysema is a common finding in the age group in which carcinoma of the esophagus is most prevalent. The importance of emphysema of the lung in postoperative morbidity and mortality has not been fully appreciated. An emphysematous lung has a greatly diminished resistance to infection, hence, the greater risk of pulmonary complications. Slight changes in pulmonary expansion in the emphysematous individual may lead to respiratory insufficiency with resultant anoxia, which may in turn bring about cardiac complications.

The induction of a pneumothorax in preparation for esophageal surgery was employed more widely a decade ago than it is at the present time. Preoperative pneumothorax used to be recommended because it was thought that there would be less physiologic disturbance at the time the thorax was opened and the lung collapsed. It must be borne in mind that the degree of diminution in function of a lung is not equivalent to the percentage of collapse. A 50 per cent collapse of the lung does not connote a similar percentage reduction in function. Therefore, in order to obtain a marked reduction in the blood flow and function of one lung, a fairly complete pneumothorax would be necessary. Moreover, during an operation upon the esophagus the lung does not need to be completely collapsed. If pulmonary emphysema is present, little collapse of the lung can be obtained by pneumothorax. An attempt to collapse the lung preoperatively may result, therefore, in more physiologic disturbance in pulmonary function than would ordinarily occur during operation, provided the surgeon has the cooperation of an experienced anesthetist. With recent advances in anesthesiology, preoperative pneumothorax does not seem advisable for esophageal surgery.

Preoperative penicillin therapy is indicated. It is usually satisfactory to start the penicillin twenty-four to forty-eight hours prior to operation, unless there are signs of secondary infection in or around the tumor which indicate more prolonged preoperative treatment. Before operation a Levine tube is introduced through the nose and placed in the esophagus so that the end of the tube is just above the site of obstruction. The upper esophagus can thus be kept empty during operation by aspiration through the indwelling tube.

Care of the Patient During Operation.—The fundamental principles of successful esophageal surgery include (1) the avoidance of obstruction of the airway and adequate oxygenation throughout the operation; (2) adequate blood and fluid replacement throughout operation; (3) minimizing reflex disturbances in the operative field by the avoidance of unnecessary trauma; (4) minimizing contamination of the operative field; (5) maintaining an excellent blood supply and avoidance of tension at the site of anastomosis; (6) periodic inflation of the lung during the intrapleural part of the operation, and (7) complete reexpansion of the lung as the pleural cavity is closed.

It is not the object of this paper to discuss the technique of esophageal resection. Only those factors relating to the development of postoperative complications will be considered. The postoperative morbidity and mortality are often influenced by apparently minor violations of such basic principles.

The choice of anesthesia and the technique of its administration are very important factors in this type of surgery. An anesthetic agent which permits normal oxygenation of the blood at all times, even during the physiologic disturbances associated with the operation, should be chosen. Ether and oxygen are most satisfactory. An anesthetic technique which permits good ventilation of the lungs at all times is mandatory. Some type of intratracheal tube is desirable. The anesthetist should be allowed sufficient time for a slow, smooth induction of the anesthesia and intubation of the patient. Breathing should be quiet at the time the pleura is to be opened, so that there will be a gradual collapse of the lung on that side unassociated with marked mediastinal motion. If abnormal respiratory effort and mediastinal motion occur due to an improper plane of anesthesia or obstruction of the airway, the anesthetist should be permitted to correct the situation before the difficulty is aggravated by further stimulation on the part of the surgeon. It is desirable that the lung be completely reexpanded at fifteen-minute intervals, even though this may necessitate a brief interruption in the operative manipulations.

The use of clamps across the esophagus or stomach at the time the anastamosis is being performed is theoretically undesirable. Such clamps render the tissue temporarily anoxic, which results in edema in these tissues following relief of the constriction. This may lead to disturbances in healing. Traction sutures can be employed if necessary in order to maintain adequate control of the gastric and esophageal segments. Before the esophagus is transected it should be thoroughly emptied by aspiration through the Levine tube in the upper esophagus. One must make sure that the tube is not coiled up in the esophagus so its tip is much above the level at which the esophagus is opened. Coiling of the tube within the esophagus is more likely to occur if that organ is dilated. Drainage from the stomach can be controlled by adequate and repeated suction after it has been opened. In the performance of the anastomosis the surgeon must be certain that the blood supply of the part is in no way compromised and that there is no tension on the suture line, either due to insufficient mobilization of the parts or due to traction from other causes. Anchoring sutures are often important, but these also should not be associated with tension. Stricture formation is likely to occur at the anastomotic line between esophagus and stomach if continuous sutures are utilized and if care is not taken to obtain accurate approximation of the mucosa. The external aspect of the anastomotic line should be covered by other tissues such as the omentum or mediastinal pleura. Careful repair of the defect in the diaphragm is necessary to avoid postoperative herniation. Some surgeons prefer to leave the indwelling Levine tube above the site of the anastomosis, whereas others pass it through the anastomosis into the stomach.

During the freeing of the esophagus, the mediastinal pleura of the opposite pleural cavity may have been traversed or inadvertantly torn. Sometimes it is difficult to tell whether an opening has been made in the opposite pleura. Air trapped in the mediastinal tissues may make a noise similar to that heard through an opening in the contralateral pleura. It is erroneous to assume that a small opening in the pleura is necessarily less serious than a large one. A small opening may cause air to enter the pleural space during inspiration and may permit only a part of this air to escape during expiration. Thus air may be trapped in the opposite pleural cavity in spite of the fact that the anesthetist is maintaining a positive intrabronchial pressure. If the mediastinal pleura of the opposite side has been torn, and there is an unexplained difficulty with breathing or deterioration of the patient's condition, it is best to enlarge the opening into the opposite pleura so that any trapped air can escape. The anesthetist can then maintain expansion of both lungs by controlling the intratracheal pressure. In any case in which there is even a suspicion that the opposite pleural cavity may have been entered, a roentgenogram of the chest is taken in the operating room at the conclusion of the operation and inspected at once. If this shows any appreciable degree of pneumothorax on the opposite side, aspiration of the air by a syringe fitted with a three-way stopcock and connected to a monometer is indicated. It has been our practice to institute closed drainage on the side of operation. A fairly large-sized rubber tube is introduced through an intercostal space and connected to a waterseal bottle. It is highly desirable that this tube be connected to the bottle while the chest wall is being closed. The practice of clamping off the tube and connecting it later in the patient's room is to be condemned because the best time for immediate expansion of the lung has been lost, and an extensive pneumothorax may have been allowed to remain for some time. It must be emphasized that maintaining a positive intratracheal pressure during closure of the chest wall does not necessarily exclude the possibility of extensive collapse of the lung or even of a tension pneumothorax because the thoracic wall wound may act like a sucking wound during part of the time that it is being closed. If a Torek type of procedure is being performed, the anesthetist must maintain positive intratracheal pressure until the cervical wound is airtight, because air could enter the pleural space through the cervical wound after the thoracotomy wound has been closed.

In any operative procedure of the magnitude of an esophageal resection, a considerable reduction in blood volume may occur during operation. The amount of blood lost is often larger than the surgeon estimates. Blood transfusions should be started at the beginning of the operative procedure and blood should be replaced as it is lost. It is unwise to give large quantities of saline solution intravenously during the earlier part of the operation. Whole blood and plasma, particularly the former, are the most effective means of maintaining an adequate blood volume without increasing the hazard of pulmonary edema.

Postoperative Care.—During the postoperative period, conditions which promote healing should be maintained at an optimum level. This may be difficult unless feeding is started early. It is a rather frequent practice to withhold food by mouth for as long as four to seven days after operation. This results in a marked tendency toward depletion of the protein reserve. In my experience, hypoproteinemia has occurred following esophageal resection in spite of plasma transfusions, blood transfusions, amigen, or other protein derivatives administered parenterally. Perhaps the hypoproteinemia resulting from delayed feeding entails more risk of leakage from the suture line than would occur due to feeding started early by mouth. Experimental studies have shown that sutured wounds are often weakest between the fourth and seventh days, just when feeding is customarily started. Early feeding following esophageal surgery has been employed in several clinics, and there has been no definite evidence so far that this practice is dangerous. It would seem advisable, therefore, to start using a high protein and high carbohydrate fluid diet by mouth within one or two days of operation, rather than run the risk of a marked drop in the plasma protein about one week after operation. The combination of careful placing of the sutures at the time of operation, plus maintenance of optimum conditions for healing in the postoperative period, would seem to be the wisest course. Plasma or blood transfusion and amigen should be employed. Liberal doses of vitamin C should be given. Numerous studies in the last few years have amply demonstrated the importance of the maintenance of an adequate level of vitamin C in body tissues. Not only is this vitamin an important factor in obtaining satisfactory wound healing, but it has also been shown to be related to the distribution of fluid in tissues. Recent reports show that when vitamin C deficiencies are corrected the incidence of postoperative pulmonary complications is decreased. Other vitamins should also be administered.

A quantitative point of view with respect to replacement therapy in the postoperative period is essential to intelligent management of the patient. Too often, in an attempt to avoid dehydration, a large amount of fluid is administered in the form of isotonic sodium chloride. Patients with carcinoma of the esophagus do not tend to have the sodium and chloride depletion associated with frequent vomiting which is found in carcinoma of the stomach. The regurgitation which occurs in carcinoma of the esophagus leads to a different type of chemical loss than that seen with true vomiting associated with gastric neoplasm. The aim should be to replace minerals and salts as they are lost, quantity for quantity. Determinations of plasma proteins and minerals in the blood without correction for variations in the total blood volume are of limited value. Carcinoma of the esophagus is often associated with a diminution in blood volume due to reduction in the fluid and food intake. In the postoperative period sharp fluctuations may occur in the blood volume and hence seriously alter serum protein levels. When postoperative complications develop which tend to produce a further reduction in the total blood volume, the total circulating plasma protein may be much lower than an analysis of the grams of protein per 100 c.c. of plasma would lead one to suspect. I believe, therefore, that the determination of total plasma volume is essential for the best management of the patient following resection for carcinoma of the esophagus. Improvements made in this direction would not only lower the incidence of complications due to poor healing at the site of the anastomosis, but would also reduce the frequency of postoperative pulmonary complications. Protein depletion produces changes in the fluid content of pulmonary tissue and may cause the abnormal passage of fluid into the alveoli which is an important initiating factor in many postoperative pulmonary complications.

Following intrathoracic surgical intervention, early and complete pulmonary expansion is an important factor in reducing pulmonary or pleural complications, in lessening the risk of anoxia which may have secondary cardio-circulatory effects, and in obtaining optimum restoration of pulmonary function. Closed drainage of the pleural space allows air and fluid to escape from the pleural cavity in the first few hours following operation, and permits contact of the visceral with the parietal pleura. This lessens the incidence of pleural fluid accumulation later.

It should always be borne in mind that pulmonary emphysema is a common occurrence in the age group undergoing surgery for carcinoma of the esophagus. Whenever a needle is inserted into the pleural space for the aspiration of fluid or air, the technique employed should minimize the risk of laceration of pulmonary tissue. The breath sounds are often hard to hear on auscultation in an emphysematous patient. It is therefore often difficult to ascertain on the basis of physical examination alone whether a pneumothorax is present. If the presence of a pneumothorax, especially on the contralateral side, is suspected in the postoperative period, a bedside roentgenogram should be made before a needle is introduced into the pleural space, unless the clinical findings are very obvious and the signs of tension pneumothorax are such as to necessitate immediate action. The position of the trachea as determined by palpation in the neck is an unreliable index to mediastinal shift. Serious displacement of the lower portion of the mediastinum may occur without obvious deviation of the cervical portion of the trachea.

The length of time that the drainage tube is left in situ depends upon (a) the completeness of pulmonary expansion, (b) the thoroughness of evacuation of air and fluid from the pleural space, (c) whether the tube is still functioning or has been sealed off inside the thorax, and (d) whether the tube in situ would be a factor of safety should complications develop in the region of the anastomosis. It is obvious that the drainage system must be kept airtight at least during the first week after operation if drainage has to be maintained for such a period of time. It is equally important that when the drainage tube is removed within the first few days following operation, no air be permitted to enter the drainage tract and thus result in secondary collapse of the lung. If at the time of operation a mattress suture of heavy silk is inserted in the skin and subcutaneous tissues at the margins of the stab wound through which the drainage tube has been introduced, this suture can be tied by an assistant as the tube is rapidly withdrawn. If a drainage tube with several fenestrations is withdrawn slowly, air may enter some of the fenestrations and gain access to the pleural space. This hazard is increased by the fact that the patient often takes a sudden deep breath as the tube is being withdrawn. For this reason the importance of rapid withdrawal of the tube and immediate tying of the previously placed suture, to close the opening, is stressed.

Cardiovascular complications play an important role in postoperative morbidity and mortality following esophageal resection for carcinoma. Much can be done to diminish the incidence of these complications if certain fundamental principles are constantly borne in mind. Although many patients with carcinoma of the esophagus have some impairment of the coronary blood flow due to arteriosclerosis, and there is often weakening of the myocardium due to degenerative changes, the main cause of postoperative heart failure and death is a reduction in the amount of oxygen delivered to the cardiac muscle. One must avoid (1) reduction of the arterial oxygen saturation, (2) reduction of cardiac output which would affect the coronary blood flow, and (3) factors which reduce effective blood flow, such as vasospasm or an increased tendency to coagulation of the blood. The tendency to regard a sudden death from coronary thrombosis a few days after operation as an unfortunate and more or less unavoidable accident is unwarranted. It is well known that any undue strain, such as occurs with strenuous exercise, is detrimental to a damaged heart. Labored breathing during operation, even a brief period of cyanosis, or any other factor which reduces the oxygen supply to the myocardium, can initiate a chain of events which may result in a cardiac death in the postoperative period. The principles which must be observed to reduce postoperative cardiac complications are (1) avoidance of anoxia at all times; (2) the avoidance of any interference with pulmonary ventilation, because pulmonary circulation and cardiac function are closely interrelated; (3) the avoidance of any appreciable drop in blood pressure which would reduce the effective blood flow and hence the ability to deliver sufficient oxygen to the tissues; (4) reduction of vasospastic factors as far as possible, and (5) the avoidance of an increased tendency to intravascular clotting due to changes in the blood constituents and blood flow. Such considerations are far more important in reducing cardiac complications than routine preoperative digitalization as some have advocated. Naturally, digitalis has an important place in the therapy of postoperative auricular fibrillation and cardiac failure, but more emphasis should be placed upon prevention of these complications by the means indicated. Cardiac arrhythmias are not very unusual following esophagogastrectomy. In addition to auricular fibrillation, auricular flutter occasionally occurs. There may be a relationship between auricular flutter and the intrathoracic position of the stomach. A dilated intrathoracic stomach may increase the likelihood of reflex changes in the cardiac rhythm. The treatment of arrhythmia after esophageal resection is similar to that employed in other cardiac cases.

The chief factors initiating pulmonary complications in the postoperative period are depressed respirations and retained bronchial secretions. The importance of a clear airway throughout operation and its influence on the incidence of postoperative pulmonary lesions has already been discussed. Equally important is the avoidance of any retained secretion in the first few hours and days following operation. The early removal of secretion by cough or suction may eliminate the further tendency to formation of secretion which is produced by the partial bronchial obstruction caused by the original secretion. The principles to observe in avoiding retention of bronchial secretion are (1) proper nursing assistance with manual support of the area of incision during coughing, so as to diminish pain and increase expulsive effect of cough; (2) proper use of sedation with avoidance of undue pain so that the patient will not be unwilling to take a deep breath or give an effective cough (small doses of narcotics given more frequently rather than large doses at longer intervals), and (3) the early use of intratracheal suction if voluntary cough is impossible or ineffective. If these measures are employed, postoperative atelectasis and bronchopneumonia will occur much less frequently, and bronchoscopy, which is also an important therapeutic measure, will be necessary only occasionally. When indicated, however, there should be no hesitation in employing early therapeutic bronchoscopic aspiration. Frequent changing of a patient's position, encouraging deep breathing, and placing the patient so that he can effectively raise the secretions are all measures that have their place. The great value of antibiotics as a prophylactic measure against pulmonary complications should not lead one to neglect the mechanical factors necessary for the maintenance of a clear tracheobronchial tree. Bedside roentgenograms should be taken frequently in the postoperative period if it is felt that they might give information of value in the diagnosis and management of postoperative complications. It has been our practice to make x-ray examination of the chest routinely within the first twenty-four hours following operation to ascertain the status of the lungs with respect to infiltration and re-expansion. Subsequent roentgenograms are taken as indicated.

Whether or not it is advisable to introduce a Levine tube past the gastroesophageal anastomosis into the intrathoracic portion of the stomach at the time of operation is a moot point. Some have advocated leaving the tube in the upper esophagus above the anastomotic site so that swallowed saliva may be removed. Others have advanced the tube into the stomach to keep it deflated as well as to permit the administration of a fluid diet through the tube. That such an indwelling tube resting on the suture line may predispose to ulceration and interference with healing cannot be denied. It still remains to be seen whether the disadvantages are outweighed by the advantages. Some surgeons recommend jejunostomy so that alimentary feedings can be begun promptly after operation. Further experience will be necessary to assess the value of these various measures.

Complications occasionally arise due to gastric dilatation. Since the operation of esophagogastrectomy involves division of the vagus nerves, disturbances associated with vagotomy may occur. Reflex pylorospasm may be present. Whether certain measures which have been found useful in vagotomy performed for peptic ulcer will also be beneficial following esophagogastrectomy for carcinoma of the esophagus and stomach remains to be seen. Such drugs as urecholine deserve a trial. When there is retention in the intrathoracic stomach, care must be taken to avoid pulmonary complications due to a spillover of the gastric contents through the larynx into the lung. Occasionally a temporary edema at the site of the gastroesophageal anastomosis may result in aspiration into the lung. Therefore, these patients should be instructed to swallow fluids very slowly until it has been definitely ascertained that regurgitation does not occur. Strictures at the site of the anastomosis between esophagus and stomach are still encountered, although not as frequently as formerly. Later dilatation of the strictured area may be indicated.

Since some patients in the older age group with carcinoma of the esophagus have disturbances in the peripheral blood flow, thromboembolic phenomena have been a common postoperative complication. Opinions are divided concerning the indications for vein ligation as compared to the use of anitcoagulants in both the prophylaxis and management of thrombophlebitis and phlebothrombosis. Anticoagulants such as dicumarol and heparin would seem to have a logical place in the prevention and treatment of intravascular clotting. In some cases the combination of ligation and anticoagulants might be the best procedure.

Oxygen therapy, either by tent, nasal catheter, or mask, should be given to every patient. Almost all patients who have had a major thoracotomy have a reduction in the arterial oxygen saturation for a few days because of various factors interfering with a proper correlation between pulmonary ventilation and pulmonary circulation. Since considerable anoxia can be present without cyanosis, the absence of this clinical sign should not be considered as indicating adequate oxygenation. It is far wiser to employ oxygen prophylactically than to permit the persistence of subclinical anoxia. Early ambulation should be encouraged as much as possible in patients undergoing esophageal resection. Because of the use of oxygen therapy and the presence of a closed drainage system, it may be impractical to get the patient out of bed on the first postoperative day. Leg exercises can be performed, however, before the patient is out of bed.

CONCLUSIONS

Attention to details in the care of the patient before, during, and after operations on the esophagus will aid greatly in reducing the morbidity and mortality. Preoperative preparation aims to correct deficiency states. During operation cardiocirculatory and respiratory conditions should be maintained as near normal as possible. An operative technique which provides optimum conditions for healing is most desirable. Proper postoperative care will lower the relatively high incidence of cardiovascular and respiratory complications which have been encountered in the past. Improvements in the present-day methods of meeting nutritional requirements in the first week after operation should result in a further reduction in morbidity and mortality.

CANCER OF THE CERVICAL ESOPHAGUS

A Discussion of Treatment

William L. Watson, M.D., and John L. Pool, M.D., New York, N. Y.
(From the Thoracic Surgical Service, Memorial Hospital)

A BRIEF historical review of the surgical progress evolved in dealing with cancer of the cervical esophagus will show that the ultimate aim of the individual operator has always been to devise a safe and adequate operation for the cure of this otherwise fatal neoplastic condition. In general, it may be said that the multitude of procedures devised and recommended together with the paucity of reported cures by any form of treatment would indicate a decided need for a more satisfactory method of handling malignant disease in the first portion of the gullet.

The cervical esophagus was not considered a suitable province for surgical endeavour until 1877 when Czerny[3] extirpated the first human cervical esophagus for cancer in that organ. He made an incision along the left anterior border of the sternocleidomastoid muscle, mobilized and excised a segment of cervical esophagus 6 cm. in length, sutured the distal opening into the lower angle of the wound and used it for feeding purposes. His patient made a satisfactory postoperative recovery, but died of recurrent cancer fifteen months after this pioneer operation had opened the cervical esophagus to surgical attack.

The second, major, surgical advance in this work was by Mikulicz.[6] In 1884 he resected the cervical esophagus of a patient with cancer and fashioned a plastic flap repair of the fistula which was technically successful and permitted his patient to enjoy eating solid food ten days after operation. Recurrent cancer caused the death of this patient sixteen months later.

Up to 1908, twenty-five cervical esophagectomies had been reported with an operative mortality rate of 48 per cent. The longest postoperative survival in this group was sixteen months. At this time von Hacker[13] reported the first successful resection of the cervical esophagus together with complete extirpation of the larynx. His patient lived more than sixteen months, but the final result was not recorded.

Arthur Evans,[5] in 1934, reported a twenty-three-year survival after surgical excision of a cervical esophageal cancer, and in 1937 Sir Wilfred Trotter[11] reported a ten-year surgical cure. The four surgical resections reported by Wookey[17] in 1942 showed freedom from disease in two cases at two years, three months and at seven months, and death from recurrence at two years and at one year, nine months in the other two.

W. L. Watson[14] in 1942 reported three controlled cases of cancer of the cervical esophagus. Two of the patients had been treated by a combination of surgical and radiation measures and were alive and free of disease, respectively, five and one-half and five years after treatment. Both of these patients are still alive and free of disease, one for ten and one-half years and the other just

Received for publication, Sept. 8, 1947.

ten years after treatment (Table III). The cervical esophagus of the third patient was surgically excised in the spring of 1940, and plastic reconstruction of the gullet subsequently carried out. This patient is now alive and free of disease more than seven years later.

MATERIAL

The clinical material for this report consists of a consecutive series of seventy-seven patients with cancer of the cervical esophagus admitted to Memorial Hospital in the seven-year period from 1940 to 1947. During the war period, 1942 through 1945, both authors were in the Armed Services and interest in the problem lessened; twenty-six patients were admitted during this period and one was operated upon.

INCIDENCE

In metropolitan New York, cancer of the esophagus accounts for nearly 4 per cent of all deaths due to malignant disease; cancer of the cervical esophagus alone is responsible for about 18 per cent of all the esophageal deaths,[16] and it is therefore an important disease from the standpoint of incidence alone. About 3.8 per cent of all patients admitted to Memorial Hospital have cancer of the esophagus.

MICROPATHOLOGY

Compared with cancer of the esophagus in general, it is noted (Table I) that a higher percentage of squamous-cell lesions falling into the grade 3 classification is encountered, and also that adenocarcinoma is rarely found at the cervical level. Biopsies from cancers of the cervical esophagus are difficult to classify accurately into rigid groups, in part due to the small size of the specimens. One case showed only intraepithelial carcinoma.

TABLE I. PATHOLOGY

CERVICAL ESOPHAGEAL CANCER	NO. OF CASES	PER CENT	ESOPHAGEAL CANCER	PER CENT
Squamous carcinoma			Squamous carcinoma	
Grade I	3	4	Grade I	7
Grade II	37	48	Grade II	65
Grade III	18	23	Grade III	17
Grade IV	2	3		
Ungraded carcinoma	12	16		
Adenocarcinoma	1	1	Adenocarcinoma	8
No pathology	4	5	Epidermoid carcinoma	3
Total	77			

ETIOLOGY

It is not possible to give exact etiologic data, although it is now quite generally believed that there are certain definite factors which predispose the esophagus to new growth activity. If the oral cavity presents broken, irregular, or sharply worn teeth, ill-fitting dentures, leucoplakia, and intraoral sepsis, one may be certain that the esophagus as well as the oral cavity has been subjected to chronic irritation. One of us (W. L. W.)[15] has reported sixteen cases of cancer of the esophagus in which each patient had a second and independent primary cancer, and in 87.5 per cent of these cases the other primary cancer was in the intraoral region, indicating the likelihood of a common causative agent. Excessive pipe smoking, incomplete or hasty mastication of food, together with thermal irritation as a result of drinking large quantities of hot liquids, and even syphilis may all play a role in preparing the groundwork for the inception of cancer in the cervical esophagus.

AGE AND SEX

Of the patients in this series, twenty-three per cent were women, whereas in a series of well over 1,000 cases of cancer of the entire esophagus the percentage of women patients was only 15.7 per cent.[16] No explanation for the relative frequency of cancer of the esophagus in men has been offered, and this study does not elicit any reason why women should have cancer of the esophagus so frequently in the cervical portion of the organ. Women also tend to develop this disease at an earlier age than men. In this series the average age of women was 55 years, and men 63 years.

Videback[12] reported comparable figures. In 296 cases of esophageal cancer, 67, or 23 per cent, occurred in women. There were 48 lesions (15 per cent) in the cervical esophagus and 36 per cent of them were in women patients.

SYMPTOMATOLOGY

The results of treatment for cancer of the cervical esophagus have been discouraging up to the present time for a variety of reasons. In the first place, the symptomatology of cancer in this site is vague and not alarming to the patient in the early stages of the disease. Dysphagia, the most prominent symptom of esophageal cancer at any level, is usually a late symptom, because it does not manifest itself until there is fixation of a large enough portion of the pliable esophageal wall to cause sufficient blockage of the gullet to interfere with the passage of food. As the esophagus does not contain pain fibers, symptoms are necessarily due to pressure on adjacent organs and structures. Early in the disease, a feeling of roughness in the throat, halitosis, or slight vague and ill-localized discomfort on swallowing occurs. The patient is likely to shrug off these premonitory symptoms, or, if a doctor is consulted for such symptoms, tonsillitis, postnasal drip, carious teeth, or excessive smoking may be indicted as the causitive agent. Also, when diagnosed, the treatment of esophageal cancer in the neck may be dropped between the nose and throat specialist, the general surgeon, and the x-ray therapist, unless the patient falls, or is steered, into the hands of a physician particularly interested in this disease and capable of treating it.

DIAGNOSIS

For the purpose of this report, the lesion under discussion is considered to occur in the upper 10 cm. of the esophagus, thus including a portion of the gullet which extends into the thoracic inlet. Early diagnosis can be established only if consulting physicians will bear in mind the possibility of the existence of this disease in any patient complaining of difficulty in swallowing. Globus hystericus and thyroid disease are the two most frequent diagnostic errors encountered in our series. The esophagus should be studied carefully under the fluoroscope, not only with a thick barium suspension in order to outline the gullet, but also to assess the mucosal pattern after the bolus has passed. Esophagoscopy should be carried out in every suitable case as the next diagnostic measure. Proper evaluation of persons who complain of a "scraping throat" or who have minimal swallowing difficulties is arduous, and this may even be true of people with prominent swallowing difficulty. When leucoplakia is present in the mouth, an investigation of the esophagus is not amiss, as there is a definite association of precancerous leucoplakia in the whole of the upper digestive tract.

The early diagnosis may be confused with foreign bodies retained immediately beneath the cricopharyngeal constriction or with traumatic ulceration in this area of narrowing. One of the major symptoms of the Plummer-Vinson syndrome is dysphagia and, when not accompanied by other findings such as glossitis, anemia, achlorhydria, cracked fingernails, etc., may be difficult to differentiate from carcinoma. Furthermore, the two diseases may coexist. For instance, Akerlund and Welin[2] surveying twenty-nine microscopically proved cases of early cancer at the esophageal mouth found twenty-four in women, and seventeen of these women had, in addition, signs and symptoms of Plummer-Vinson disease. In our series of eighteen women, three had sufficient evidence to warrant the diagnosis of a Plummer-Vinson syndrome.

Prominent osteoarthritic spurs of the lower cervical vertebrae can cause dysphagia in the elderly. Other extrinsic factors which can produce disorder of the swallowing mechanism in the neck include retropharyngeal abscess, tuberculosis of the cervical vertebrae, recurrent laryngeal nerve paralysis, and thyroid or lymph node enlargements.

TREATMENT METHODS

If a patient with carcinoma of the cervical esophagus is put on a high caloric, supportive, liquid diet, the life expectancy is approximately five months from onset of symptoms (Table II). A satisfactory gastrostomy increases life expectancy slightly. In two-thirds of the cases, x-ray therapy directed toward the esophagus brings about some degree of amelioration of the symptoms and temporarily reduces the size of the growth, thus at least allowing saliva to be swallowed and by this mechanism does much to prevent aspiration pneumonia. The life expectancy of such a patient after x-ray therapy and gastrostomy is more than one year, and an occasional patient may have complete arrest of the cancer. This desirable result has occurred in two cases in our experience.

TABLE II. AVERAGE DURATION OF LIFE FROM ONSET OF DISEASE*
(In Fifty-two Cases of Failure to Arrest Disease)

	DURATION (MO.)	NO. CASES
No treatment	5	2
Gastrostomy	5½	8
X-ray therapy	15	23
Gastrostomy and x-ray therapy	14½	18
Resection	24	1

*Compiled from records of fifty-two patients who died while follow-up was being carried out.

Metastasis to cervical lymph nodes is an early event, and these secondary deposits may be bilateral. The node groups most frequently involved are the supraclavicular, the deep jugular, and the prevertebral. This last group has proved to be the most difficult to control. On admission to Memorial Hospital, 22 per cent of our patients had lymph node metastases. A fatal termination of this disease is usually hastened by a superimposed aspiration pneumonia due to complete blockage of the esophagus and spillage into the trachea. Hemorrhage may cause sudden death, or the end may come slowly due to generalized carcinomatosis.

There are three established methods of surgical attack on this problem of cancer of the cervical esophagus: First, the Torek[10] procedure is indicated in high intrathoracic lesions, or those at the thoracic inlet, where, on fluoroscopy, the esophagus is found to be movable. Mobilization and transection of the intrathoracic esophagus distal to the lesion can be accomplished through either the right or the left transpleural approach. In those lesions whose upper limit is within the neck, more dissection will be required through the cervical approach than is described in the original Torek procedure. The incision may still be along the anterior border of the left sternomastoid muscle, but the sternal head of this muscle should be divided to provide added exposure and the esophagus approached between the carotid sheath and the thyroid gland. The cervical esophagus is then brought out through the neck wound, the tumor excised, and the margin of the proximal esophagus sutured to the skin at a suitable level. A skin-lined anterior chest wall esophagus can be constructed later, as described by Stevenson.[8]

Second, Trotter,[11] Eggers,[4] and Wookey[17] have described a radical operation for cancer of the cervical esophagus which invades the postcricoid region, the arytenoids, the thyroid gland, or the trachea itself. This operation consists in resection of the larynx and esophagus and adjacent jugular lymph nodes en bloc. A preliminary gastrostomy is made and a low tracheostomy is provided under local anesthesia to furnish an airway and an opportunity to introduce oxygen. Sodium pentothal has proved to be a satisfactory anesthetic agent. Bilateral rectangular skin flaps including platysma are elevated, the prelaryngeal muscles resected, and the sternal origins of both sternocleidomastoid muscles divided. The thyroid isthmus is severed and the lobes of this gland reflected laterally. Lymph nodes along the jugular veins are mobilized and reflected medially, and, if necessary, one internal jugular vein may be resected. The middle thyroid veins on one side are divided and the lateral wall of the esophagus is visualized to determine the lower limit of the disease.

The trachea is next transected at the level of the second or third tracheal ring, somewhat higher posteriorly than anteriorly. The superior laryngeal nerves and arteries are divided at the level of the greater cornu of the thyroid cartilage. The hypopharynx is then entered through the thyrohyoid membrane, and the mucous membrane overlying the epiglottis is carefully preserved, but the epiglottis itself is removed with the larynx. When the superior limit of the tumor is identified, the mucosa of the hypopharynx is incised 2 cm. cephalad and stay sutures are applied to maintain control of it. The esophagus is then mobilized from the prevertebral fascia. Considerable mobilization distal to the tumor can be secured by this maneuver.

The esophagus is then divided 2 cm. distal to the lower margin of palpable and visualized disease. Again support of mucous membrane margin is secured with stay sutures. The trachea is sutured to the margin of the replaced skin flaps in the midline with interrupted silk sutures, not more than 3 mm. apart. In a similar way, the inferior esophageal stoma is sutured in one of the lateral incisions at least 2 cm. from the permanent tracheostomy, and the pharyngeal opening is also sutured superiorly. A Levine tube is introduced through the nose and into the stomach.

At a later stage, the cervical esophagus is reconstructed. Each stoma should readily admit a No. 40 French bougie, but, if it is tight, it may be enlarged by an incision through skin and mucosal membrane with resuturing of skin to mucosa along this vertical line. Reconstruction of the gullet is effected by a skin-lined tube turned in upon itself and sutured with interrupted triple chromic catgut sutures of the inverting type. Adequate patency can be secured, as advocated by Stevenson,[8] if an envelope-like flap is used at each end of the skin-lined tube. Finally, the lateral skin flaps are mobilized to cover the reconstructed esophagus, or a Padgett graft may be used.

Third, segmental resection, a less radical resection of the cervical esophagus, is feasible when cancer has not extended completely through the muscular coat. This holds true even for those lesions at the cricopharyngeal pinchcock where the tumor is partially on the anterior wall. In such cases resectability without sacrifice of the larynx cannot be determined until exploration of the postcricoid space is undertaken. Lesions as low as the sternal notch can be resected in this manner.

Preliminary gastrostomy may be indicated and tracheostomy is essential to allow the use of sodium pentothal anesthesia and provide protection against postoperative laryngeal edema or bilateral abductor cord paralysis due to recurrent laryngeal nerve injury.

In this operation, a single rectangular flap with its base laterally is elevated on the side of the greater tumor prominence (Fig. 1, *A*). Again the sternal and clavicular heads of the sternocleidomastoid muscle are mobilized and the lateral surface of the esophagus is identified after dividing the middle thyroid veins and inferior thyroid artery. Exposure is greatly improved and the plastic tube reconstruction is facilitated by thyroid lobectomy at this stage. The esophagus is then mobilized from the prevertebral fascia by blunt dissection. Next, the tracheoesophageal groove is developed below the tumor by blunt dissection (Fig. 1, *B*). The esophagus is completely mobilized at this level, and the recurrent laryngeal nerve identified and dissected out from caudad of the disease until it dips behind the thyroid cartilage. The esophagus should be separated from the posterior wall of the larynx for at least 4 cm. above the palpable tumor. In almost all cases, the opposite inferior thyroid artery can be secured without separate dissection through the other side of the neck (Fig. 2).

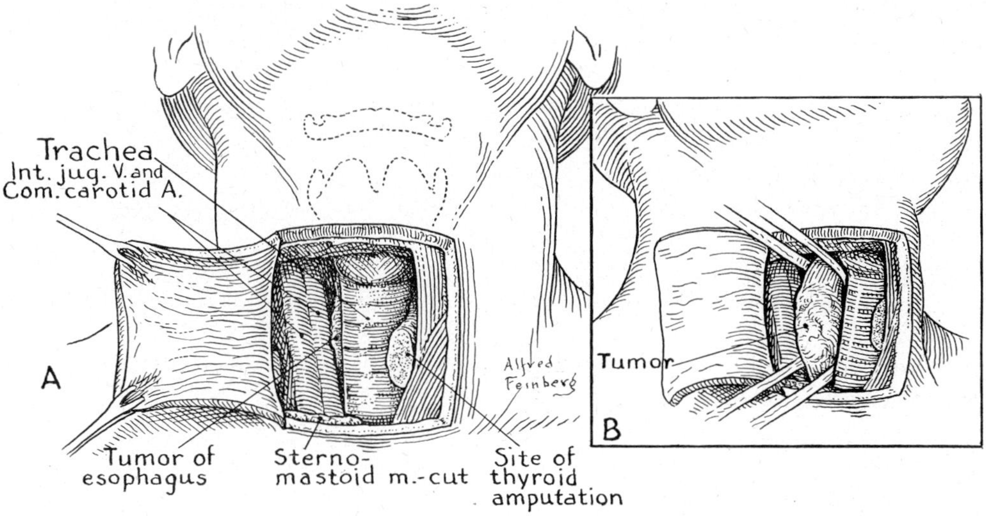

Fig. 1.—*A*, The trap-door incision has been made, the sternocleidomastoid and pretracheal muscles and right lobe of thyroid excised, and the cancer of cervical esophagus exposed. *B*, Cervical esophagus and tumor mobilized.

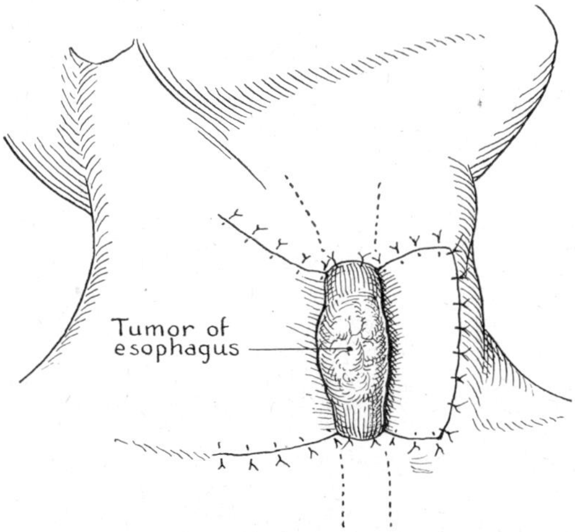

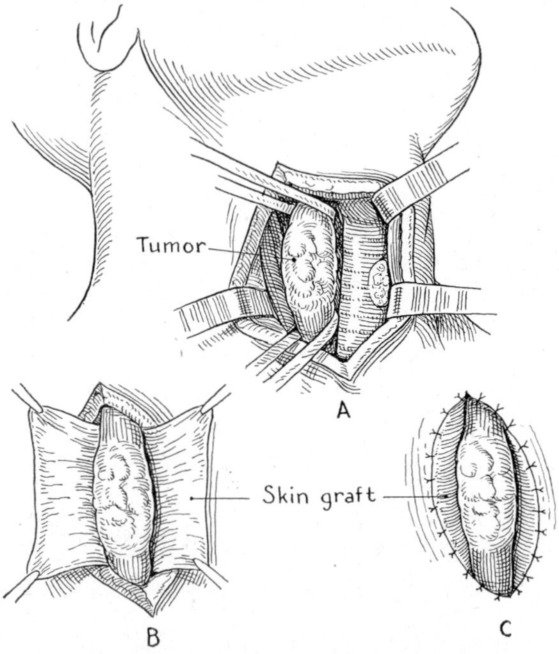

Fig. 2.—Trap door of skin and platysma has been placed beneath the esophagus as a cradle and wound edges closed.

Fig. 3.—*A*, Incision has been made along the anterior border of sternocleidomastoid muscle, and the tumor exposed as in Fig. 1. *B*, Padgett skin graft 22/1000 inch in thickness is placed beneath the esophagus and sutured to skin edges. *C*, Skin graft, raw surface down, has been sutured in place.

Two methods are available for completing the operation. If the lesion is particularly ulcerated and infected, the esophagus may be exteriorized by suturing a Padgett graft behind it, covering the carotid sheath, the prevertebral fascia, and the lateral aspect of larynx and trachea (Fig. 3). Four to seven days later, the involved segment of the esophagus is resected. It is well to leave in place black silk sutures on the esophagus at the desired levels of resection at the first procedure, as later palpation of the esophageal wall is not accurate due to edema and granulation tissue. This method leaves some stenosis of each stoma, requiring later plastic mobilization prior to final reconstruction of a skin-lined esophageal tube.

It is more satisfactory to resect the esophagus at this stage and suture the superior and inferior stoma to the replaced skin flap margins. A graft is often needed over the prelaryngeal muscles, and later tubular reconstruction is as previously described (Fig. 4).

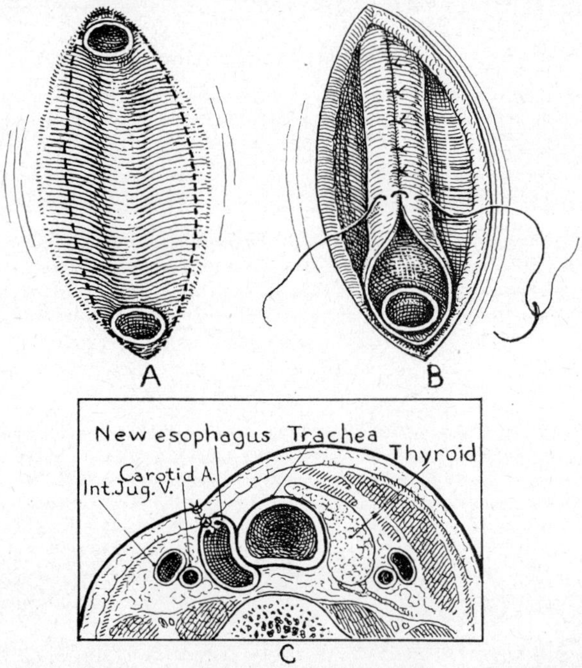

Fig. 4.—*A*, Local condition satisfactory for reconstruction of esophagus. Stomata are adequate and skin graft viable. *B*, Method of reconstruction of new plastic tube esophagus. *C*, Cross section showing relationship of new esophagus to neck structures.

In the present series of seventy-seven cases, there have been eleven operations on the cervical esophagus, an operability rate of 14 per cent. In seven cases (64 per cent), the tumor was resectable. Of the seven patients whose cervical esophagus was resected, one died on the second postoperative day of pulmonary edema and myocardial infarction. The immediate convalescence of the other six patients was uncomplicated. Four patients were alive and without evidence of disease seven years, one year, nine months, and six months after resection. Two were alive with recurrence three years, and three months following surgery (Table III).

TABLE III. RESULTS OF TREATMENT, 1940 TO 1947

TREATMENT	NO. OF CASES	DEATH AFTER TREATMENT 3 MO.	6 MO.	12 MO.	LONGER	ALIVE (MO.)	NO FOLLOW-UP
No treatment	5	2	0	0	0	None	3
Gastrostomy	9	8	0	0	0	None	1
X-ray therapy*	28	5	7	4	7	10, 13, 17, & 56	1
Gastrostomy and x-ray therapy	27	4	5	8	1	4, 6, 9, 13, 15, & 19	3
Gastrostomy, tracheostomy, and resection of cervical esophagus	7	1	0	0	0	4, 6, 9, 12, 36, & 84	0
Torek	1	0	1	0	0	None	0

*Not included in this group are two patients treated by radiation measures alive and well more than ten years after treatment.

CASE REPORTS

CASE 1.—S. I. was 49 years of age when admitted to Memorial Hospital in the spring of 1940. She had complained of dysphagia for seven years, and esophagoscopy and biopsy had established a diagnosis of squamous carcinoma, grade 2, of the first portion of the cervical esophagus. A preliminary Janeway type gastrostomy was done for feeding purposes.

Treatment was entirely by surgical measures and the procedure required five major stages and extended over a period of more than twelve months. The first stage was carried out under intratracheal cyclopropane anesthesia. A wide rectangular incision was made across the lower part of the neck with its base on the left side. The lower half of the right sternocleidomastoid muscle was excised revealing a hard, adherent, right lobe of thyroid gland, which was also removed. (Histologically, this proved to be a Hashimoto struma and not cancer infiltration.) The esophagus was mobilized, the prepared skin flap placed behind it, and the wound closed. During the subsequent ten days, tension and interference with blood supply caused necrosis of the exteriorized portion of the esophagus, and at the second operation the necrotic portion was removed by cautery and the upper and lower apertures sutured to the skin.

During the next eight months various unsatisfactory measures were employed in an attempt to maintain a communication between the pharynx and esophagus. When the stricture finally closed and obstruction became complete, the first step in the plastic reconstruction was carried out under local anesthesia by opening the right side of neck, excising old scar, mobilizing trachea and larynx, and placing in the defect a large Padgett skin graft. This graft was obtained from a comparatively hairless portion of the right lower abdomen, and it healed in place by primary union.

After an interval of three months, the patient was readmitted, a retrograde esophagoscopy was undertaken, and a small olive-tipped bougie was passed upward to the point of obstruction in the lower neck. A small incision was made in the graft at the point where the bougie could be palpated. A black silk thread was then tied to the bougie and brought out through the gastrostomy stoma. The optimum point for incising into the pharynx was located in the same fashion, and the same black silk thread was then brought out the patient's mouth and anchored to the skin of the cheek.

After a short interval, the apertures were greatly enlarged and an accurate approximation of skin and mucous membrane was obtained.

The final operative step was carried out June 3, 1941. The anterior wall of esophagus was formed by infolding the lateral portions of the graft so as to form a continuous tube from pharynx to esophagus. Five grams of sulfathiazole powder were then placed in the wound, and the skin edges closed without tension over the tube. A full liquid diet was taken on the seventeenth postoperative day; the patient was soon allowed to take a normal diet and the gastrostomy was closed.

Comment.—This patient had a very early cancer of the cervical esophagus developing in an area of leucoplakia, probably the result of chronic partial obstruction of thyroid origin. She was well more than seven years after excision of the esophagus. One can only hope that disease will not recur in the future or an overgrowth of hair cause esophageal obstruction.

CASE 2.—M. H.,* a woman aged 50 years, was admitted to Memorial Hospital, April 25, 1944. She complained of difficulty in swallowing of six weeks' duration, and pain in the back of the throat which gradually extended down into the chest. X-ray studies revealed a defect in the cervical esophagus, and esophagoscopy and biopsy established a diagnosis of papillary epidermoid carcinoma, grade 2.

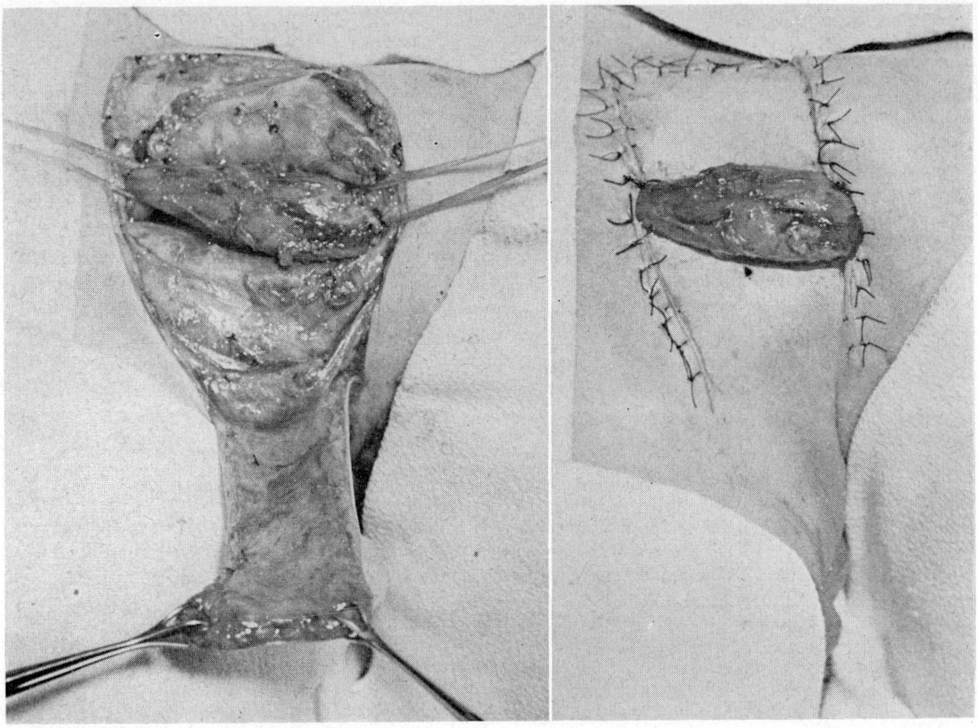

A. B.

Fig. 5 (Case 2, M. H.).—*A*, The cervical esophagus including the cancer has been mobilized between larynx and carotid sheath. *B*, The tumor-bearing portion of the esophagus is exteriorized on top of the trap-door flap. The patient's head is to the right.

A Janeway type gastrostomy was established under local anesthesia April 28, 1944, and exteriorization of the cervical esophagus was carried out May 10, 1944. A rectangular skin flap was raised on the left side of the neck and portions of the left sternocleidomastoid, sternohyoid, and sternothyroid muscles, and the left lobe of thyroid were resected. The cervical esophagus was mobilized and exteriorized (Fig. 5). The patient could then swallow liquids without difficulty, these liquids passing through the intact esophagus over the skin flap. As soon as healing had taken place at the upper and lower margins of skin and esophageal musculature, cautery excision of the exteriorized esophagus was carried out (May 22, 1944). The superior and inferior stomas were dilated with bougies and skin-lined esophagus was reconstructed from mobilized skin of the neck. Swallowing was satisfactory.

*A patient of Dr. G. T. Pack.

A. 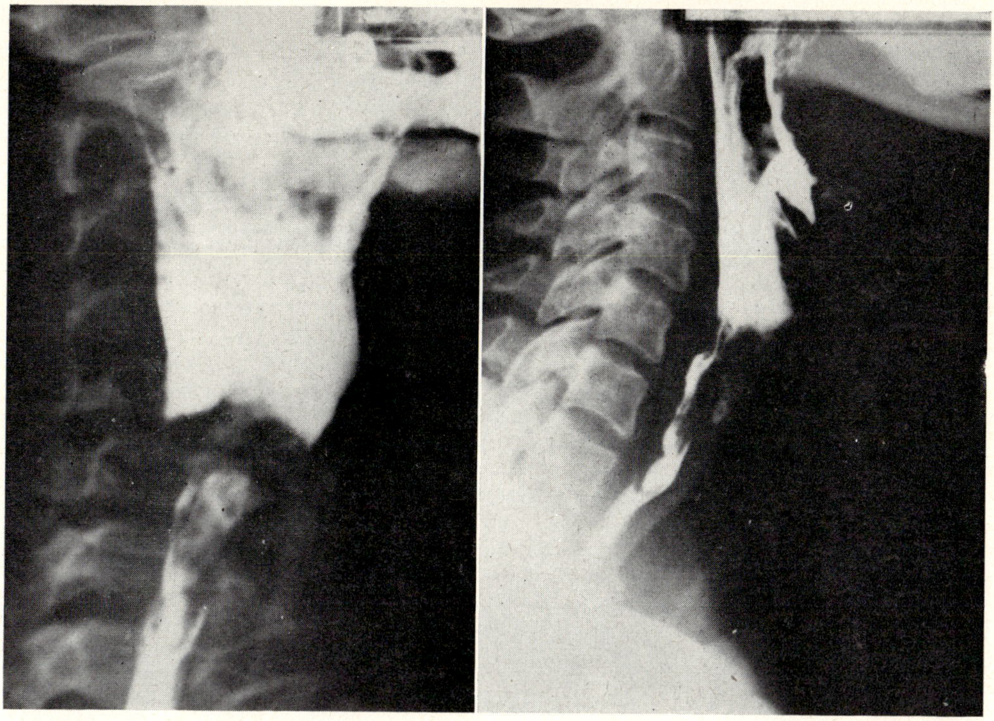 B.

Fig. 6.—*A* and *B*, Esophagram shows normal filling of the pyriform fossae and a mottled irregularity in the first portion of the cervical esophagus, the lower limit of which is well defined. There is increased distance between vertebral bodies and air column over the length of the tumor.

A. 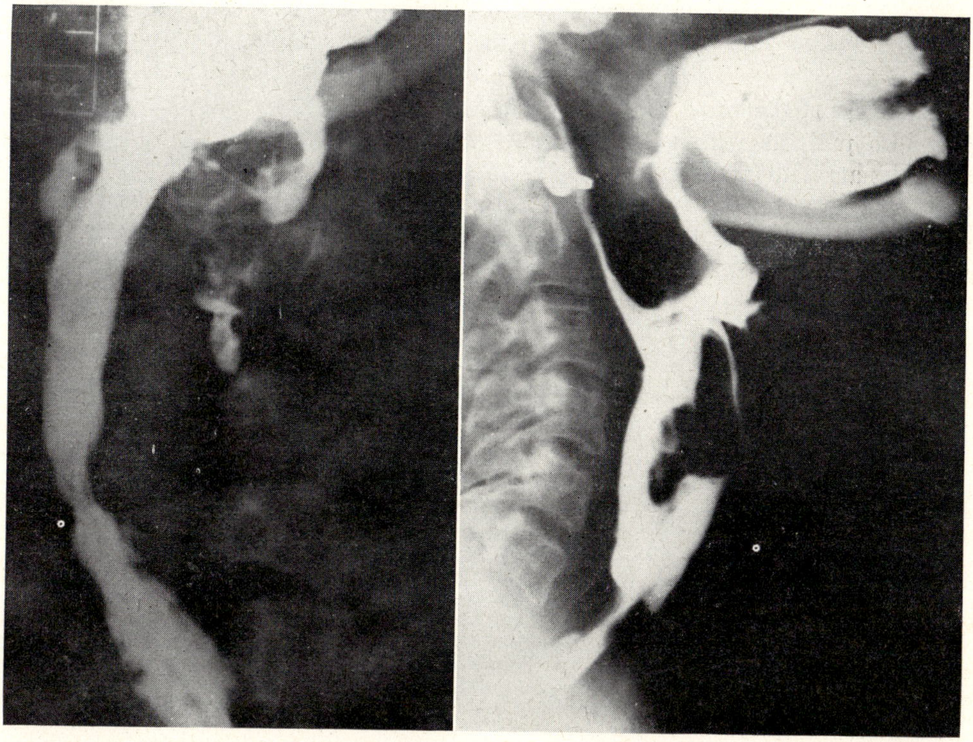 B.

Fig. 7.—*A* and *B*, The reconstructed skin-lined esophagus is in the right side of the neck. Some stricture persists at junction with esophagus. Barium spills into larynx because of right recurrent laryngeal nerve paralysis.

Metastatic disease appeared in the neck in March, 1947, and a surgical resection was done followed by high voltage x-ray therapy. The patient was alive, with evidence of recurrent disease, three years, four months after operation.

CASE 3.—T. K., a woman aged 52 years, was admitted to Memorial Hospital Feb. 20, 1947. The patient had complained of difficulty in swallowing solid food over a period of fifteen years. The dysphagia became severe about eight months before admission to the hospital, and she was finally unable to swallow anything but liquids. X-ray studies revealed an irregular stenosis of the lower portion of the pharynx and the upper portion of the esophagus (Fig. 6), which caused marked difficulty in the passage of the barium. There was also an anterior displacement of the larynx by a soft tissue mass in that region. Esophagoscopy and biopsy established a diagnosis of squamous carcinoma, grade 3, of the cervical esophagus.

A preliminary gastrostomy for feeding purposes was done Feb. 26, 1947. The cervical esophagus and lower hypopharynx, along with adjacent paravertebral nodes and the right recurrent laryngeal nerve, which was adherent to a lymph node, were resected on March 6, 1947. The stomas, superior and inferior, were carefully sutured to adjacent skin and a split graft was placed over the exposed larynx. Healing was satisfactory, except that one-half of the graft on the lateral laryngeal surface did not take. The removed nodes did not contain metastatic cancer. Plastic reconstruction of the esophagus was carried out May 15, 1947, and the patient was later able to take a soft diet (Fig. 7).

There was no evidence of local recurrence nor palpably enlarged cervical lymph nodes six months after excision of the cervical esophagus.

SUMMARY

Cancer of the cervical esophagus differs somewhat from cancer occurring in the lower portions of the gullet in that it occurs at an earlier age and is noted with relatively greater frequency in women.

A higher percentage of grade 3 squamous-cell cancers occur in this portion of the esophagus, and a much smaller number of adenocarcinomas is encountered.

Of seventy-seven patients, 22 per cent had cervical lymph node metastases from cancer of the esophagus at the time of admission to the hospital.

Two patients with advanced cancer of the cervical esophagus, treated by a combination of radiation and surgery, were alive and well ten and ten and one-half years, respectively. One patient had a surgical extirpation of the cancer of the cervical esophagus and a surgical, skin-lined, tubular, reconstruction seven years previously, and is alive and free of disease at the time of this communication.

Cancer of the cervical esophagus, if discovered reasonably early in its course, can be cured surgically, and even when the disease is advanced and cervical metastases are present a control of growth may be obtained by aggressive surgery plus substantial irradiation.

In some detail three methods of surgically dealing with this disease have been discussed.

REFERENCES

1. Adams, W. E.: The Pathological Considerations Relating to the Early Diagnosis and Curative Surgical Treatment of Carcinoma of the Esophagus, Internat. Abstr. Surg. **72**: 105-110, 1941.
2. Akerlund, A., and Welin, S.: Roentgen Diagnosis of Malignant Tumors Within the Boundary Region Between the Pharynx and Esophagus, Acta radiol. **25**: 883-909, 1944.
3. Czerny: Neue Operationen, Zentralbl. f. Chir. **4**: 433-434, 1877.
4. Eggers, C.: Carcinoma of the Upper Esophagus and Pharynx, Ann. Surg. **81**: 695, 1925.

5. Evans, Arthur, quoted by Turner: Recent Advances in the Treatment of Carcinoma of the Esophagus From the Surgical and Radiological Aspects, Proc. Roy. Soc. Med. (Sect. Laryngol.) **27:** 7-17, 1934.
6. Mikulicz, J.: Ein Fall von Resection des carcinomatosen Esophagus mit plastischem Ersatz des excidirten Stuckes, Prag. med. Wchnschr. **11:** 93, 1886.
7. Nielson, Jans: Clinical Results With Rotation Therapy in Cancer of the Esophagus, Acta radiol **26:** 361-393, 1945.
8. Stevenson, T. W.: Reconstruction of the Esophagus by a Skin-lined Tube, Surg., Gynec. & Obst. **84:** 197-202, 1947.
9. Tomlinson, W. J., and Wilson, L. A., Jr.: Esophageal Carcinoma in British West Indies and Panamanian Negroes, Arch. Path. **39:** 79-80, 1945.
10. Torek, F.: Carcinoma of the Larynx, Trachea, and Esophagus, Ann. Surg. **84:** 889, 1926.
11. Trotter, quoted by Pilcher, R.: Carcinoma of the Cervical Oesophagus, Lancet **1:** 73-76, 1937.
12. Videback, A.: Solitary and Multiple Carcinomas of the Upper Alimentary Tract, Acta radiol **25:** 339-350, 1944.
13. Von Hacker, V.: Ueber Resection und Plastik am Halsabschnitt der Speiserohre insbesondere beim Carcinoma, Verhandl. d. deutsch. Gesellsch. f. Chir., Berl. **37:** 359-425, 1908.
14. Watson, W. L.: Cancer of the Cervical Esophagus, Ann. Surg. **116:** 86-96, 1942.
15. Watson, W. L.: Cancer of the Esophagus; Some Etiological Considerations, Am. J. Roentgenol. **41:** 420-424, 1939.
16. Watson, W. L.: Cancer of the Esophagus, Surg., Gynec. & Obst. **56:** 884-897, 1933.
17. Wookey, Harold: The Surgical Treatment of Carcinoma of the Pharynx and Upper Esophagus, Surg., Gynec. & Obst. **75:** 499-506, 1942.

PROGRESS IN THE SURGICAL TREATMENT OF CARCINOMA OF THE ESOPHAGUS AND UPPER STOMACH

JOHN H. GARLOCK, M.D., NEW YORK, N. Y.

(From the Surgical Service of the Mount Sinai Hospital)

THE present symposium on the problem of cancer of the esophagus and cardia is indicative of the increasing importance that is being accorded this subject throughout the world. In comparison with the surgery of cancer of other parts of the gastrointestinal tract, it is true that esophageal surgery is still a young child. However, progress in this field of surgery has been so rapid in the last few years that it remains to accumulate a large mass of data, especially with respect to long-term follow-up studies, in order to appraise properly the efficacy of surgery as a curative measure. These facts are being gathered with surprising speed, because surgery of esophageal cancer has been taken up as a group study in most of the major clinics of this country and in many clinics in other lands. I might cite the excellent clinic for diseases of the esophagus established in Argentina by Finochietto and conducted by Resano.

In this article I would like to indicate in a general way observations based on an operative experience with approximately 250 cases, emphasizing particularly the progressive steps that have been taken in the development of this branch of surgery and the changes that have occurred in the preoperative, operative, and postoperative management. Progress in any field can take place only by a process of trial and error and this is particularly applicable to the subject under discussion. It must be emphasized that the tremendous progress in esophageal surgery during the past ten years can in large measure be attributed to the great development of American surgery during the past twenty-five years, the understanding of the altered physiologic relationships attending open thoracic procedures, the rapid studies in the field of anesthesiology, and the recent discovery of the newer antibiotics.

It has been repeatedly demonstrated that early diagnosis constitutes one of the most important phases of the therapy of this disease. Early ulceration of the esophageal wall or minimal diminution in the caliber of the lumen will produce symptoms more quickly than will similar aberrations in any other part of the gastrointestinal tract. It, therefore, becomes important to view with concern any sudden change in the function of deglutition and to adopt measures to establish a positive diagnosis. It is unnecessary to stress the importance of a thorough radiographic examination of the esophagus, cardia, and the so-called silent area of the stomach along the beginning of the greater curvature. In my opinion, esophagoscopy should be done in every patient with radiographic

Received for publication, Aug. 13, 1947.

Part of address delivered before Congrès Francais de Chirurgie, Paris, Oct. 10, 1947, and The Royal College of Surgeons, London, Oct. 16, 1947.

evidence suspicious of carcinoma. It is sometimes extremely difficult to differentiate a benign from a malignant lesion on the radiographic evidence alone. I have seen smooth conical obstructions at or near the cardia which indicated probable benign cardiospasm. Yet the biopsy specimen obtained at esophagoscopy disclosed the presence of a neoplasm. On the other hand, it is not uncommon to encounter instances where the x-ray evidence strongly suggests a neoplasm but the esophagoscopic examination discloses a benign stricture, a peptic esophagitis, or a chronic inflammatory reaction as seen in syphilis. These are some of the important reasons for routine esophagoscopy and biopsy in establishing a diagnosis of carcinoma.

The pathologist's report of squamous-cell cancer from the biopsy specimen indicates that the tumor has originated in esophageal mucosa. When the finding is one of adenocarcinoma, the indication is clear that the tumor has had its origin at the cardia or upper stomach. We have encountered many examples of extensive upward growth along the esophageal wall of tumors arising at the cardia. This extension may be entirely submucosal and may not be evident to the esophagoscopist. Growth of squamous-cell carcinomas in the opposite direction apparently does not occur. Such tumors will grow as far as the esophagogastric junction and will not proceed beyond this point. This has been a curious pathologic differentiation between these two types of cancers.

Increasing operative experience during the past ten years in the treatment of this disease has disclosed certain pathologic information concerning lymph node spread which was not known heretofore. Until recent years, all our knowledge concerning the pathology of this disease was based on autopsy material and represented the terminal stages. It is now known that some of the tumors of the thoracic esophagus may grow in a peripheral direction and quickly become inoperable by reason of fixation to the aorta, hilus of the lung, left main bronchus, or vertebral column. On the basis of this operative experience in the various stages of the disease, it has also become clear that spread to the lymph nodes may be not only to the immediate vicinity of the tumor but also to nodes far removed from the growth. That is to say, tumors of the middle third of the esophagus may spread to the paracardial or peripancreatic nodes below the diaphragm as well as to the regional nodes in the mediastinum or hilus of the lung or proximally to the lower cervical region (node of Virchow). Adenocarcinoma arising at the cardia or upper stomach may show no extension below the diaphragm, yet exploration may disclose extensive dissemination to the structures in the chest, namely, mediastinal nodes, pleura, or pericardium. Squamous-cell tumors rarely, if ever, metastasize to the liver. However, hepatic involvement via the portal system is frequently seen with adenocarcinoma of the cardia.

Increasing experience with the surgical treatment of this disease has demonstrated very clearly that it is desirable to consider it as a group co-operative problem to include the combined efforts of roentgenologist, esophagoscopist, internist, anesthetist, surgeon, operating room staff, and nurses for postoperative care. This experience has also emphasized the value of careful preoperative preparation, frequently prolonged for two or three weeks. A study of the postoperative complications and causes of mortality has shown the great preponderance of cardiovascular accidents over all other complicating factors. Postoperative cardiac difficulties or cerebral accidents are in the main in the imponderable group and cannot usually be predicted preoperatively or even guarded against. However, the internist becomes an important member of the team in his appraisal of the cardiovascular capacity of the patient to withstand an extensive operative procedure. The incidence of postoperative pulmonary complications has been materially decreased since we began to utilize preoperative nebulization of penicillin of the bronchial tree. This has been a real advance in the preoperative preparation. The low incidence of chest and wound sepsis in our series is indicative of the great importance that we attach to scrupulous wound protection, nontraumatic operative technique, thorough hemostasis, and meticulous suture anastomoses. This extra effort at the operating table will pay dividends in the form of a low wound and chest morbidity.

It seems superfluous to stress the importance of meeting the patient's protein, carbohydrate, fluid, electrolyte, and vitamin requirements during the period of preoperative preparation. Deficiencies, as indicated by blood studies and clinical appraisal, are made up by intravenous injections of proteins, plasma, whole blood transfusions, parenteral vitamins, etc. Checking of the patient's weight by daily measurements aids the surgeon materially in determining the degree of nutritional improvement. Repetition of the original blood studies in the latter part of the preoperative period is also desirable for comparative purposes.

The progressive improvement in the operative management of cancer of the esophagus and cardia may perhaps best be emphasized in the form of a step-by-step tabulation.

1. There seems to be fairly general agreement now that the question of anesthesia is of paramount importance. I am convinced that, unless the anesthetist is thoroughly competent, the surgeon should not undertake this operation. In talking to many surgeons who have attempted esophageal resections in appreciable numbers, I have been impressed with the fact that many of them have been severely handicapped by serious problems on anesthesia. This has been particularly noticeable with the foreign surgeons, who are now visiting America in increasing numbers. The anesthesia of choice today, on the basis of an extensive experience with various modalities, is intratracheal gas-oxygen-ether.

2. For cancers of the middle third of the esophagus it is no longer necessary to utilize the Torek operation. It is now possible to restore normal gastrointestinal continuity by the operation of supra-aortic esophagogastrostomy, originally described in January, 1944. By an accurate ligation of the blood supply of the stomach, one can mobilize the organ to such an extent that it can be brought to the apex of the chest without jeopardizing its vitality and anastomosed to the stump of the esophagus. Recently, in a patient with a carcinoma just above the arch of the aorta, I was able to bring the stomach through the apical aperture of the chest and anastomose its cardiac end to the esophagus in the lower part of the neck without impairment of its blood supply. The utilization of the stomach in effecting these high anastomoses has made unnecessary the various complicated plastic procedures which employed tubes of stomach

wall and loops of jejunum in an attempt to restore esophagogastric continuity. The operation of supra-aortic esophagogastrostomy is a recent development in esophageal surgery.

3. Since Phemister's first successful esophagogastric anastomosis in 1938 for cancer of the distal part of the esophagus, most surgeons have adopted this procedure as a routine measure for tumors of the lower esophagus and upper stomach. Until recently, this was accomplished by a transthoracic transdiaphragmatic route. Frequently, after the patient had been subjected to a formidable transthoracic exploration, an inoperable tumor was disclosed by reason of extensive metastases below the diaphragm. It is for this reason that I suggested some years ago the great desirability of demonstrating a resectable tumor by the simpler expedient of an abdominal exploration alone. If the growth was found operable, the abdominal wound was closed and a transthoracic resection was then done. A recent development of this thought has been the perfection of a combined abdominothoracic incision with simultaneous exposure of both the upper abdomen and the left thoracic cavity. This incision has simplified in no small measure the whole problem of the surgical treatment of cancer of the lower esophagus and upper stomach. Because the incision is a large one, the approach is more direct and all operative maneuvers can be carried out under direct vision with minimal trauma. This has been clearly discernible in the much smoother postoperative course, the lower mortality, and decreased incidence of postoperative complications. The combined abdominothoracic approach has a wide field of applicability and should be the exposure of choice for total gastrectomy.

4. Increasing experience during the past five years has effected some changes in the technical details of these operations. The important ones may be mentioned briefly.

(a) The left leaf of the diaphragm should be put at rest by pinching the phrenic nerve above the diaphragm.

(b) It is not necessary to apply clamps to either the esophagus or stomach in order to minimize contamination. The esophagus may be kept empty by an indwelling Levine tube during the operation. The stomach can be emptied by suction.

(c) In the performance of the anastomosis, it has been clearly demonstrated that interrupted silk sutures should be used if one is to avoid a stricture. I am inclined to agree with Sweet that the excision of a button of gastric wall the approximate size of the esophageal lumen also aids in the prevention of stricture.

(d) Slight telescoping of the suture line by drawing the stomach over it and anchoring of the stomach to both edges of the mediastinal pleura will prevent drag on the suture line.

(e) It is important to anchor the diaphragm around the transplanted stomach in such a way as to prevent herniation of abdominal contents into the chest.

(f) We have never found it necessary to use an indwelling Levine tube during the postoperative period. In fact, there may be some danger from pressure necrosis on the suture line.

(g) There seems to be general agreement that underwater drainage of the chest for at least a few days postoperatively is desirable.

(h) Before closure of the operative wound, 50,000 to 100,000 units of penicillin should be injected into the pleural and abdominal cavities. It probably has some local beneficial effect.

The postoperative care of these patients is concerned mainly with the early detection of chest complications and the immediate application of the necessary therapy. Collections of trapped air should be aspirated as quickly as possible. Serious respiratory and cardiac difficulties may ensue if this is not done. Oxygen therapy should be utilized for the first day or two. Swallowing is interdicted until the fourth day, when sips of water are permitted. The fluid intake is increased rapidly thereafter. Soft food is usually given on the seventh or eighth day. In the last two years we have given penicillin parenterally during the early postoperative period. The latter has probably been a large factor in the reduction of pulmonary complications.

The problem of palliative surgery in cancer of the esophagus and upper stomach is one open to considerable discussion. The question resolves itself into whether or not a surgeon is justified in subjecting a patient to an extensive resection in the presence of nonresectable local and distant metastases which would preclude any possibility of a cure. Some surgeons feel that palliative surgery of this sort is justifiable solely for the purpose of restoring the act of swallowing, if only for a few months. The majority of surgeons, I believe, feel that the risk is too great and that the results do not justify the effort. I bring up this much debated question because it is important for surgeons, when they report a series of cases, to indicate most clearly which resections are palliative and which are otherwise. If all surgeons adopted a similar plan of reporting their operations for cancer, a great mass of valuable material could be collected and a clearer picture could be obtained of the value of surgical therapy as opposed to other methods. It is suggested, that, in reporting results of resections for cancer of the esophagus and upper stomach, the following tabulation be utilized:

CANCER OF ESOPHAGUS

Resectable group

Middle Third
1. No local extension or node involvement
2. Local node involvement
3. Distal node involvement
4. Local extension beyond esophagus

Lower Third
1. No local extension or node involvement
2. Local extension
3. Local node involvement
4. Distal node involvement

Palliative group

Middle Third—extent of metastases
Distal Third—extent of metastases

CANCER OF CARDIA

Resectable group

1. No extension
2. Local node involvement with removal of same

Palliative group

1. Liver involvement
2. Extensive nonresectable node involvement
3. Peritoneal metastases
4. Thoracic metastases

The operative mortality should be calculated separately for the resectable group and the palliative group and also for the supra-aortic anastomosis and the low anastomosis. The over-all mortality of all groups can also be reported if the surgeon so desires. The period of follow-up should be clearly indicated in each group. Only by some such method can a clear picture be obtained of the whole problem of the surgical therapy of this disease.

Progress in this field of surgery has been so rapid in the past ten years that it can be safely predicted that the next decade holds great promise of a steadily decreasing operative mortality and a rapidly increasing number of long-term survivors.

REFERENCES

Adams, W. E., Escudero, L., Aronsohn, H. G., and Shaw, M. M.: Resection of the Thoracic Esophagus: A Clinical and Experimental Study, J. Thoracic Surg. **7**: 605-620, 1938.

Adams, W. E., and Phemister, D. B.: Carcinoma of the Lower Thoracic Esophagus; Report of a Successful Resection and Esophagogastrostomy, J. Thoracic Surg. **7**: 621-632, 1938.

Garlock, John H.: The Surgical Treatment of Carcinoma of the Thoracic Esophagus; With a Report of Three Successful Cases, Surg., Gynec. & Obst. **66**: 534-548, 1938.

Garlock, John H.: The Surgical Treatment of Carcinoma of the Thoracic Esophagus, Internat. Clin. **1**: 28-45, 1939.

Garlock, John H.: The Surgical Treatment of Carcinoma of the Thoracic Esophagus, Surg., Gynec. & Obst. **70**: 556-569, 1940.

Garlock, John H.: Surgical Treatment of Carcinoma of the Esophagus, Arch. Surg. **41**: 1184-1214, 1940.

Garlock, John H.: Surgical Treatment of Diseases of the Esophagus. Bancroft's Operative Surgery, New York, 1941, D. Appleton-Century Company, Inc.

Garlock, John H.: The Problem of Cancer of the Esophagus, J. Mt. Sinai Hosp. **7**: 349-352, 1941.

Garlock, John H.: The Problem of Carcinoma of the Cardiac End of the Stomach, Surg., Gynec. & Obst. **73**: 244-256, 1941.

Garlock, John H.: The Present Status of the Surgical Treatment of Carcinoma of the Thoracic Esophagus, Am. J. Surg. **54**: 262-272, 1941.

Garlock, John H.: Radical Surgical Treatment for Carcinoma of the Cardiac End of the Stomach, Surg., Gynec. & Obst. **74**: 555-560, 1942.

Garlock, John H.: The Re-establishment of Esophagogastric Continuity Following Resection of the Esophagus for Carcinoma of the Middle Third, Surg., Gynec. & Obst. **78**: 23-28, 1944.

Garlock, John H.: Causes of Mortality Following Radical Resection of the Esophagus for Carcinoma, J. Thoracic Surg. **13**: 415-423, 1944.

Garlock, John H.: Technical Problems in Surgical Treatment of Carcinoma of the Esophagus and Upper Stomach, J. Thoracic Surg. **21**: 215-224, 1947.

TRANSTHORACIC GASTRIC RESECTION FOR LESIONS OF CARDIA OF STOMACH AND LOWER PART OF ESOPHAGUS

Review of Cases

John H. Payne, M.D.,* and O. Theron Clagett, M.D.,† Rochester, Minn.

During recent years the transthoracic approach for the surgical removal of lesions of the mid- and lower portions of the esophagus and lesions of the cardia and fundus of the stomach has been used with a gratifying measure of success.[1-8] The exposure obtained by this approach makes it suitable for resection of, and complete removal of, malignant lesions in the lower and mid-portions of the esophagus and for malignant lesions arising in the cardia, the fundus, and the upper portion of the lesser curvature of the stomach. Benign lesions of the esophagus and stomach, such as leiomyomas, can be handled in the same manner as the malignant lesions.

The majority of malignant lesions of the esophagus are squamous cell carcinomas although adenocarcinomas do occur infrequently. These latter come from either aberrant gastric mucosa, which Rector and Connerly[9] have shown might occur anywhere in the esophagus, or from gastric mucosa extending up from the stomach into the lower part of the esophagus.

The malignant lesions of the fundus, cardia, and lesser curvature are adenocarcinomas and generally are of grade 3 or grade 4 (Broders' method). The leiomyomas may arise in the lower part of the esophagus, the fundus, or the cardia. They are quite vascular, bleed easily, and may grow to a moderate-sized lesion.

Malignant lesions of both the lower part of the esophagus and the stomach can spread by direct extension to adjacent structures and by lymphatic invasion. The mid-esophageal lesions may spread and invade the left main bronchus, the left recurrent laryngeal nerve, the left inferior pulmonary vein, and the aorta. The lower esophageal lesions may invade the adjacent diaphragm, pericardium, and aorta.

The esophageal lesions may spread through the lymphatics to the regional lymph nodes at an early period. Usually the spread is downward from the original lesion. Those nodes around the hilus of the lung, around the lower part of the esophagus, above the diaphragm, and the subdiaphragmatic nodes are the ones most frequently involved. Esophageal malignant lesions often spread in the submucosa and muscular layers of the esophagus so that in resecting the esophagus one must go well above the lesion to be sure of having removed it in its entirety.

The malignant lesions of the stomach and abdominal portion of the esophagus may invade by direct extension the spleen, the tail of the pancreas, the left

Received for publication, Aug. 13, 1946.
*Fellow in Surgery, Mayo Foundation.
†Division of Surgery, Mayo Clinic.

leaf of the diaphragm, and the left lobe of the liver. These lesions may spread through the lymphatics to involve the nodes in the subphrenic region and those around the left gastric artery. They can also spread into the periaortic nodes and into the nodes of the gastrolienal and gastrocolic ligaments.

The diagnosis of the esophageal lesions can be readily established. There is a history of progressive dysphagia, often an associated feeling of fullness in the retrosternal region, and loss of weight in proportion to the dysphagia. Esophagoscopy can, of course, establish an exact diagnosis, substantiated by specimens taken at the time of examination. It cannot, however, tell the extent of the lesion or whether adjacent structures have been invaded by it. Roentgenoscopic and roentgenographic examinations can, of course, tell the extent of the lesion and its anatomic location.

These malignant lesions of the stomach usually are associated with a history of atypical epigastric discomfort and pain for varying periods. Occasionally these patients have hematemesis and melena but this is not the usual finding. They may have achlorhydria and usually they have lost a moderate amount of strength and weight. Roentgenoscopic and roentgenographic examination of these patients is of the greatest value because the lesions are readily identified. Occasionally lesions near the cardia may be difficult to visualize and in these few cases gastroscopic examination may aid one in establishing the true nature of the lesion.

In all cases in which these lesions are present one should perform a careful physical examination to exclude the possibility of distant metastasis. Routine roentgenograms of the thorax should be taken to be certain that there are no metastatic lesions in the lungs. Patients who have back pain should be carefully examined and should have complete roentgenograms of the spinal column and pelvis, together with a determination of alkaline phosphatase to exclude the possibility of spinal metastasis.

PREOPERATIVE PREPARATION

As Churchill and Sweet[10] have stressed, the preoperative preparation of these patients is important. In all instances these patients should receive a high carbohydrate, high protein diet in either a soft or a liquid form. Should they be completely obstructed and unable to swallow, preliminary jejunostomy should be done, and the patients fed in this manner. The portion of the jejunum used should be 2 feet (61 cm.) from the ligament of Treitz and every precaution should be taken to avoid formation of adhesions from abdominal exploration.

These patients should also be given large amounts of vitamins B, C, and K in their daily diet or by the intravenous route. If there is any anemia or hypoproteinemia, transfusions of whole blood should be given until a normal value is obtained. Every effort must be made to have these patients in the best possible general condition.

We usually give penicillin (160,000 units daily) intramuscularly to these patients for three or four days before operation. On the morning of operation we aspirate the stomach whenever it is possible to do so and remove all the gastric contents.

ANESTHESIA

For these cases we use nitrous oxide, ether, and oxygen anesthesia, using an intratracheal tube in all cases. Administration of fluids is started routinely in one of the veins in the foot in all of these cases.

OPERATION

After the patient has been anesthetized and intravenous administration of fluids has been started he is turned on the right side with both arms drawn forward and the right arm fastened securely on an arm board. An oblique incision is then made over the left ninth rib. A long segment of the ninth rib is then resected, the edges of the incised area are covered with large gauze pads, and the Tudor Edwards chest retractor is put in and spread open. Any adhesions of the left lung are then freed up with sharp dissection and the lung is retracted out of the way with a gauze pad and an overlying Harrington retractor. Exploration of the thorax is then carried out, feeling carefully for any involvement of the lungs and lymph nodes around the esophagus, the diaphragm, and the hilus of the left lung. If the growth seems to be resectable, a few cubic centimeters of procaine hydrochloride (1 per cent) are injected into the phrenic nerve and an incision is made in the central tendinous portion of the diaphragm. The cut edges are then grasped with long tenacula and held open. Exploration of the abdomen is then carried out to determine the final operability of the lesion. The stomach, spleen, gastrocolic and gastrolienal ligaments, the retroperitoneal nodes, the liver and pelvis are all carefully palpated. If resection is feasible, the incision in the diaphragm is enlarged with division of the crura and ligation of the left inferior phrenic vessels.

In cases of lesions of the lower part of the esophagus and lesions of the fundus and cardia of the stomach, to which the scope of this paper is limited, partial gastrectomy and esophagectomy with esophagogastric anastomosis is the procedure of choice. After incision of the pulmonary ligament, mobilization of the esophagus is undertaken by blunt dissection. Care must be exercised in this step since tiny esophageal arteries arise directly from the aorta. The vagus nerves and any vessels accompanying them are then ligated and sectioned.

The upper portion of the stomach is mobilized by division and ligation of the vasa brevia and the gastrolienal ligament. The left gastroepiploic vessels are identified and carefully ligated. The lesser omental sac can then be explored easily. Should the tail of the pancreas or the spleen be invaded it can be removed along with the other organs. The stomach is gently pulled upward and to the left and the left gastric vessels are visualized and doubly ligated with No. 1 chromic catgut. These vessels are ligated close to their origin from the celiac axis, and all surrounding node-bearing tissue is removed at this time. The gastrohepatic ligament is divided and any bleeding points are ligated, dissection being continued down toward the antrum of the stomach and care being exercised to preserve the right gastric artery and vein. Dissection along the greater curvature is then continued down past the gastrolienal ligament and into the gastrocolic ligament with ligation and division of all vessels lying in the gastrocolic ligament. Care is taken to preserve the right gastroepiploic vessels since these and the right gastric vessels constitute the blood supply to the entire stomach.

When the stomach has been adequately freed so that enough of it can be brought up into the thorax to enable one to perform a satisfactory anastomosis, two large stomach clamps are placed on the stomach well below the lesion and division of the stomach is done with a knife. A gauze pad is carefully fastened over the proximal cut end and it is pulled up out of the incision. The lower cut surface of the stomach is then closed with a double row of continuous chromic catgut (No. 00) and one row of interrupted silk sutures.

With the stomach well pulled up into the thorax and a gauze pad carefully placed to prevent contamination, a circular incision about 2.5 to 3 cm. in diameter is made in the anterior wall of the stomach near the greater curvature. All bleeding points of the serous and muscular layers of the stomach are controlled and a sucker is introduced into the stomach to aspirate all gastric contents. The lower segment of the stomach is then covered carefully with a gauze pad and the esophagus is divided at a suitable point above the lesion. We have been dividing the esophagus between a proximally placed Smith-Thomas bowel clamp and a distal straight clamp. It is our feeling that the esophageal tissue is not damaged when the Smith-Thomas bowel clamp is put on carefully, and the proximal esophageal segment can be drawn down to the stomach more easily than if the clamp is not used. Gauze pads are carefully placed to prevent any soiling of the adjacent thoracic structures and the anastomosis.

The esophagogastric anastomosis is then begun. Interrupted mattress sutures of No. 000 braided silk are placed between the seromuscular layer of the posterior wall of the stomach and the muscularis layer of the esophagus. The proximal Smith-Thomas clamp is removed and a second layer of interrupted silk sutures (No. 000) is placed between the mucosa of the stomach and the mucosa of the esophagus. The posterior layer is put in first, then a similar anterior layer is put in and an anterior layer of interrupted silk mattress sutures is placed between the muscularis of the esophagus and the seromuscular layer of the stomach. If any omentum is available it is carefully tacked around the esophagus. At this point in the operation, a Levine tube is inserted through the patient's nose and is pushed down through the anastomosis into the stomach. All sutures are placed close together in making the anastomosis and all are carefully tied to prevent undue tension and cutting through of the sutures. All tension on the anastomosis is prevented by fixing the stomach to the mediastinal pleura with sutures.

The cut edges of the diaphragm are then sutured to the stomach below the level of the anastomosis and the rest of the diaphragmatic incision is closed. The phrenic nerve is crushed for temporary paralysis. The operative site is irrigated with aqueous solution of Zephiran (1:10,000) and saline. A stab wound is put in the tenth interspace. A mushroom catheter is inserted and negative pressure instituted at once. The lung is carefully and fully re-expanded and the incision is closed in layers.

Bronchoscopy is performed while the patient is in the operating room. The bronchial tree is carefully inspected and all secretions are removed.

POSTOPERATIVE CARE

The patient is placed in an oxygen tent as soon as he returns to his room. Nasal suction is started on the inlying nasal catheter and suction of from –10 to –15 cm. of water is maintained on the thoracic drainage catheter. Administration of penicillin is started at once and usually is continued for five to seven days. Glucose, blood, and isotonic saline solution are given parenterally as needed for the first three or four days.

The oxygen tent is discontinued after twenty-four to forty-eight hours, nasal suction is discontinued after forty-eight hours, and 1 fluidounce (30 c.c.) of water is injected hourly into the nasal tube. If this is tolerated well, the volume of the fluid is increased. Usually about the fifth day after operation administration of liquids by mouth is begun. If this is well tolerated, we remove the nasal tube, gradually adding soft foods to the diet such as cereals, eggs, puréed vegetables, ground meat and fish, and custards.

Roentgenograms of the thorax are made daily for the first three or four days by means of a portable x-ray apparatus and the thoracic catheter is checked frequently to insure its patency. When the lung has been well expanded for forty-eight hours, we usually remove the thoracic catheter, using an airtight dressing over the incision. Generally we remove the thoracic catheter about seventy-two hours after operation. Supplementary vitamins and fluids (such as blood, glucose, and so forth) are given in the postoperative period as needed by the individual patient. We allow these patients up about the fifth day after operation.

REVIEW OF CASES IN WHICH OPERATION WAS PERFORMED AT THE MAYO CLINIC

Until Jan. 1, 1946, one of us (O. T. C.) had performed transthoracic exploration in seventy cases. In thirty-one (44 per cent) of these there was an inoperable malignant lesion of the esophagus, cardia, or fundus of the stomach. In all of these thirty-one cases of inoperable malignant lesions there were no postoperative deaths and the immediate postoperative course was uneventful.

In three cases (4 per cent) there were benign gastric ulcers high in the cardia or the lesser curvature. Transthoracic resection was carried out in these cases without difficulty; all of the patients recovered uneventfully and have remained well since operation. In two cases (3 per cent) there were leiomyomas of the stomach. In one case a segmental resection of the cardia was done without disturbing the esophagus, and in the other case a simple enucleation of the leiomyoma was done. Both patients withstood the procedure well and have been entirely well since operation. In one case (1 per cent) transthoracic resection was performed because of severe cardiospasm which could not be handled conservatively and the patient was having a progressive downhill course. She tolerated the operation well and has been in good health without any dysphagia ever since.

In thirty-three cases (47 per cent), transthoracic resection was performed for a malignant lesion of the esophagus or stomach. Of these cases three patients had a squamous-cell carcinoma arising in the lower third of the esophagus, while thirty patients had an adenocarcinoma arising in either the fundus or cardia of the stomach. Many of the latter lesions extended up to the esophagogastric junction. In these thirty-three cases, eight of the patients were women, twenty-five were men. Our youngest patient was 21 years old, our oldest patient was 68 years old, and each had a malignant lesion, grade 4, arising in the cardia of the stomach. Table I shows the age distribution of these patients.

TABLE I. AGE DISTRIBUTION OF PATIENTS HAVING TRANSTHORACIC RESECTION FOR MALIGNANT LESION

AGE (YR.)	PATIENTS	
	NUMBER	PER CENT
20 to 29	2	6.1
30 to 39	2	6.1
40 to 49	9	27.2
50 to 59	16	48.5
60 to 69	4	12.1
Total	33	100
Mean	50.5 yr.	
Youngest	21 yr.	
Oldest	68 yr.	

There is a fairly wide variation in the nature and severity of the symptoms manifested by these patients. Dysphagia was the most frequent symptom that these patients complained of, and the severity of this varied a good deal. Twenty-seven of the patients (69 per cent) on whom resection was performed had dysphagia of varying degrees. Five of these twenty-seven patients had complete dysphagia and were unable to take either liquids or soft foods. The duration of the dysphagia in the individual cases was an interesting feature. The shortest time was three weeks and the longest time was one year; the average time of all these cases was two and one-half to three months.

Epigastric pain and abdominal discomfort were the next most frequent symptoms that these patients had. There was considerable variation of these two symptoms, as in many cases the pain resembled that of a gastric ulcer, while in other cases the pain was quite atypical and did not have any periodicity about it. Many of these patients complained of abdominal discomfort and a feeling of epigastric fullness. Twenty-six patients (67 per cent) complained of epigastric pain or discomfort. The shortest duration of these symptoms was one month; the longest was two years. In the three cases of benign gastric ulcer in which transthoracic resection was performed pain had been a prominent symptom. It had been present for six months, four years, and eight years, respectively. In each instance the nature of the pain was changing and it was increasing in its intensity. In all three of these cases of benign ulcer the patients had lost weight recently; twenty pounds (9.1 kilograms), twenty-three pounds (10.4 kilograms) and twenty-seven pounds (12.2 kilograms), respectively. In view of the changing symptoms and loss of weight manifested by these three ulcer patients, transthoracic resection was undertaken because of the possibility of malignant degeneration in a benign ulcer.

In three cases of malignant lesions hematemesis was a symptom but in none of them was there severe bleeding. In these same cases melena developed. In one of our cases of leiomyoma there was hematemesis, while in the other case of leiomyoma there was melena. In each instance these were the only symptoms the patients manifested.

Anemia was a variable finding in these cases. Only twelve patients (31 per cent) had a concentration of hemoglobin less than 12.9 Gm. per 100 c.c. of blood. The lowest concentration of hemoglobin was 8.0 Gm. per 100 c.c. of blood; erythrocytes numbered 2,730,000 per cubic millimeter of blood.

Loss of weight was present in twenty-two cases (56 per cent). The smallest loss of weight was seven pounds (3.2 kilograms) and the largest loss was fifty pounds (22.7 kilograms).

Regurgitation of food occurred in only five cases.

The establishment of an accurate diagnosis was made in thirteen cases (33 per cent) by esophagoscopic examination and removal of tissue for pathologic diagnosis. In thirty cases (77 per cent) roentgenoscopic and roentgenographic diagnosis was possible. The roentgenologic diagnosis agreed with the pathologic diagnosis.

Of the thirty-nine cases in which some type of operative procedure was undertaken in this series, five patients died postoperatively, giving a hospital operative mortality rate of 13 per cent. The cases and times of death are given in Table II.

TABLE II. HOSPITAL DEATHS IN CASES OF RESECTION

CASE	DEATH (DAYS AFTER OPERATION)	CAUSE OF DEATH
1	3	Bilateral pleural effusion, marked on left side with collapse of left lung
2	4	Bilateral bronchopneumonia
3	6	Atelectasis and pneumonia of left lung
4	10	Fibrinous pericarditis with effusion
5	45	Brain abscess which followed the development of empyema (left side of thorax)

There were surprisingly few complications in these cases. In four cases (10 per cent) a mild wound infection developed, which was of minor importance, and cleared up with conservative measures. In three cases (8 per cent) empyema developed. In one of these cases the patient died from an associated brain abscess on the forty-fifth postoperative day. The other two patients recovered uneventfully following adequate surgical drainage. In seven cases (18 per cent) slight dysphagia developed after operation. In several of these dilatation was performed and the patients recovered completely; in the other cases dilatation was not performed and the patients improved gradually. In only one case was there a recurrence of the malignant lesion at the anastomosis; this occurred four months after operation and the lumen was dilated successfully. The patient died six months after operation from generalized carcinomatosis.

In sixteen cases (41 per cent) it was necessary to remove the spleen in addition to doing transthoracic resection. This was done because of either extension of the malignant growth into the gastrolienal ligament or invasion of the spleen.

Seventy per cent of the lesions were grade 3 or grade 4; also the regional lymph nodes were involved in 70 per cent of the cases. Of the thirty-three malignant lesions that were resected, Table III shows the grade of malignancy of the lesion and the presence or absence of nodal involvement at the time of operation.

TABLE III. GRADE OF MALIGNANCY (BRODERS' METHOD)

GRADE	TOTAL CASES	NO NODES INVOLVED	NODES INVOLVED
1	1	1	–
2	9	3	6
3	11	3	8
4	12	3	9
Total	33	10	23

In only two of our cases was preliminary jejunostomy necessary. Both of the patients responded well and resection was performed at a later date. In one case it was necessary to perform pyloroplasty because of persistent postoperative vomiting. After this pyloroplasty the patient did well and did not have further vomiting.

The prognosis for all of these malignant lesions should be guarded, for in spite of adequate and presumably radical surgical removal of the lesion and the node-bearing regions, many of our patients who had undergone resection still died of the malignant lesions. We have divided the malignant lesions that were resected into two main groups, including in one group all patients who survived operation but who subsequently had died of the malignant lesions, and in the second group all patients who were alive and well following the operations (Table IV). These follow-ups were made as of April 1, 1946. We were unable to trace two patients.

TABLE IV. TRANSTHORACIC RESECTION FOR MALIGNANT LESION; CONDITION AT LAST REPORT

INTERVAL,* FROM TIME OF OPERATION (YR.)	LAST REPORT	
	LIVING	DEAD
0 to ½	7	5
½ to 1	3	2
1 to 2	5	6
2 to 3	1	1
3 to 4	2	0
4 to 5	1	0
Total	19	14

*Inquiry as of April 1, 1946.

In some of our cases regurgitation and belching have occurred following resection. These are handled satisfactorily by feeding small quantities of food five or six times a day, resting after eating, and elevating the head of the bed on retiring. A few patients have complained of epigastric fullness following eating and some few complained of vague abdominal gas pains.

SUMMARY

1. Transthoracic gastric resection offers the best method of surgical management of malignant lesions of the lower part of the esophagus and the cardia and upper part of the fundus of the stomach.

2. Simple transthoracic exploration has not resulted in any deaths in our hands. Our immediate postoperative mortality rate for the cases in which resection was performed was 13 per cent.

3. Although the numbers are small, calculation by the actuarial method as described by Berkson[11] indicates the following survival rates: 71 per cent lived for one year, 40 per cent lived for two years, and 31 per cent lived for three years.

REFERENCES

1. Adams, W. E., Escudero, L., Aronsohn, H. G., and Shaw, M. M.: Resection of the Thoracic Esophagus; a Clinical and Experimental Study, J. Thoracic Surg. **7**: 605-620, 1938.
2. Garlock, J. H.: The Re-establishment of Esophagogastric Continuity Following Resection of Esophagus for Carcinoma of Middle Third, Surg., Gynec. & Obst. **78**: 23-28, 1944.
3. Graham, R. R.: A Technique for Total Gastrectomy, SURGERY **8**: 257-264, 1940.
4. Sweet, R. H.: The Surgical Management of Carcinoma of the Mid-thoracic Esophagus, Tr. Am. Acad. Ophth. pp. 75-88, 1942.
5. Sweet, R. H.: Total Gastrectomy by the Transthoracic Approach; Report of Seven Cases, Ann. Surg. **118**: 816-837, 1943.
6. Sweet, R. H.: Transthoracic Gastrectomy and Esophagectomy for Carcinoma of Stomach and Esophagus, Clinics **3**: 1288-1315, 1945.
7. Torek, Franz: The First Successful Resection of the Thoracic Portion of the Esophagus for Carcinoma; Preliminary Report, J. A. M. A. **60**: 1533, 1913.
8. Yudin, S. S.: The Surgical Construction of 80 cases of Artificial Esophagus, Surg., Gynec. & Obst. **78**: 561-583, 1944.
9. Rector, L. E., and Connerly, M. L.: Aberrant Mucosa in the Esophagus in Infants and in Children, Arch. Path. **31**: 285-294, 1941.
10. Churchill, E. D., and Sweet, R. H.: Transthoracic Resection of Tumors of the Stomach and Esophagus, Ann. Surg. **115**: 897-917, 1942.
11. Berkson, Joseph: Quoted by Walters, Waltman, Gray, H. K., and Priestley, J. T.: Carcinoma and Other Malignant Lesions of the Stomach, chap. 23, Philadelphia, 1942, W. B. Saunders Company, pp. 487-507.

CARDIOESOPHAGEAL CANCERS TREATED VIA THE TRANSTHORACIC AND TRANSDIAPHRAGMATIC ROUTE

Felix de Amesti, M.D., and Eliseo Otaiza, M.D., Santiago, Chile
(From the School of Surgery, University of Chile, Salvador Hospital)

IN THE three-year period extending from September, 1943, when we first performed a resection of a cancer located in this region, until September, 1946, 39 patients with cancers in the cardioesophageal region have been treated in Section B of Surgery of the Salvador Hospital. Of this number, 1 patient refused intervention; in 2, the tumor was considered inoperable; and in the remaining 36 patients intervention was carried out.

Resection was performed in 14 of the 36, or 38.88 per cent, and a simple exploration by the transthoracic and transdiaphragmatic route because of the nonresectability of the lesion was performed in 21, or 58.33 per cent. In 1 patient a jejunostomy was performed prior to exploration because of undernourishment caused by the obstruction, but it was not possible to carry out the planned radical operation as the patient died in the first days of the postoperative period.

Age and Sex.—The average age and relation between the two sexes is practically the same as it is with the rest of the gastric cancers; as with the latter, the greater frequency occurred in the fifth decade of life (Table I).

Symptomatology.—In our patients, the initial symptoms which were manifested were either dysphagia (in 27, or 69.23 per cent) or dyspepsia (in 10, or 30.76 per cent). We consider "dyspepsia" as discomfort after meals, indefinite epigastric pain, acidosis, anorexia, flatulence, etc. If we relate the initial symptom of the illness with the resectability of the lesion, we can show that those patients initially complaining of "dyspepsia" have cancers that are more likely to be resectable (Table II).

The duration of the illness from the appearance of the first symptoms until the time of consultation at the hospital varied in our patients from one to twenty-four months. If we compare this with the resectability or inoperability of the neoplasm, we can show that in those with clinical symptoms of less than three months' duration the inoperability is more frequent than in those with symptoms of six to twelve months. This same phenomenon we have observed in general with all gastric cancers, regardless of their location (Table III).

In our group of 39 patients with gastroesophageal cancers, we did not encounter any family history of cancer.

Two outstanding signs in our patients because of their consistency were anemia of varied intensity and loss of weight.

X-ray Examination.—The radiographic examination was carried out on the 39 patients. Only on two occasions was the first examination negative, but upon a second examination, the diagnosis of the suspected neoplasm was confirmed.

Received for publication, Aug. 26, 1947.

TABLE I. AGE AND SEX

AGE	TOTAL	MALE	FEMALE
31 to 40 yr.	2	1	1
41 to 50 yr.	7	6	1
51 to 60 yr.	17	16	1
61 to 70 yr.	13	10	3
Total	39	33	6
Percentage of total		84.61	15.38

TABLE II. TYPE OF SYMPTOMS

SYMPTOMS	TOTAL	RESECTABLE		NONRESECTABLE	
		NUMBER	PER CENT	NUMBER	PER CENT
Dysphagia	25	8	32.0	17	68.0
Dyspepsia	14	6	42.85	8	57.14
Total	39	14		25	

TABLE III. DURATION OF SYMPTOMS

DURATION	TOTAL	RESECTABLE		NONRESECTABLE	
		NUMBER	PER CENT	NUMBER	PER CENT
1 to 3 mo.	13	5	38.46	8	61.58
3 to 6 mo.	10	3	30.0	7	70.0
6 to 12 mo.	14	6	42.85	8	57.14
More than 1 yr.	2			2	100.0
Total	39	14	35.89	25	64.10

TABLE IV. LOCATION BY RADIOGRAPHY

LOCATION	NUMBER
Carcinoma of cardia	3
Carcinoma of cardia and esophagus	21
Carcinoma of lower third of esophagus	15
Total	39

In the remaining, the diagnosis was specified as in Table IV. In order to evaluate the exactness of the x-ray examination, we have compared the radiologic location (or location as determined by radiography) with a study of the resected operative specimen, being able to prove that of 14 stomachs resected, in 8 the diagnosis of the cardioesophageal cancer coincided exactly with that which was pointed out by the anatomicopathologic study of the resected specimen; in 6, the radiologic study showed it as cancer of the lower third of the esophagus without showing the involvement of the stomach.

Esophagoscopy.—Esophagoscopy was carried out in 23 patients; the operator indicated the location of the neoplasm by measuring the distance from the dental arch to the site of the neoplasm or to the hiatus or the cardia, in those

TABLE V. LOCATION BY ESOPHAGOSCOPY

LOCATION	NUMBER	PER CENT
From 29 to 44 cm. from the dental arch	15	65.22
Hiatus	2	8.69
Cardia	6	26.08
Total	23	

TABLE VI. PATHOLOGIC FINDINGS BY ESOPHAGOSCOPY

PATHOLOGIC ANATOMY	NUMBER OF PATIENTS	NUMBER OF RESECTIONS
Squamous-cell carcinoma	7	3
Adenocarcinoma	7	4
Carcinoma solidum	1	1
Mixed	2	2
Lymphosarcoma	1	
Negative for carcinoma	5	
Total	23	10

cases in which he could reach these different zones (Table V). In general, the location by esophagoscopy is possible to perform only in the upper limit of the tumor without being able to determine gastric invasion.

In the 23 patients submitted to esophagoscopy, biopsy was taken with the results shown in Table VI. There is not always a relationship between the level of the esophagoscopic location (centimeters from the dental arch) and the histologic type of tumor, since at 34 cm. from the arch, the diagnosis is adenocarcinoma, which could correspond to a tumor of gastric origin or simply to one developing in the superficial esophageal glands, which are identical with those found in the first centimeters of the cardia. The result of the negative biopsy for neoplastic cells in 5 of the patients only indicates the insufficiency of the biopsy and the necessity of another esophagoscopy.

TABLE VII. OPERABILITY AND RESECTABILITY IN THIRTY-NINE CASES

CASES	NUMBER	MORTALITY (PER CENT)	TOTAL
Total	39		
Inoperable	2		
Operation refused	1		
Operations	36		36
Jejunostomy	1		
Thoracotomies	35		35
Transthoracic explorations	21	28.80	
Resections	14	57.14	14
Total gastrectomies	2		
Partial esophagogastrectomies	12		

Treatment and Results.—Of the 39 patients under treatment with gastroesophageal cancer, 36 were operated upon. In 1, jejunostomy was performed, and in the remaining 35, exploration through the thorax and the diaphragm was carried out. Of the latter, resection was performed in 14, or 38.88 per cent, and simple exploration of the tumor, considered nonresectable, in 21, or 58.33 per cent. Of the 14 radical operations, 2 were total gastrectomies with esophagojejunostomy, and 12 were partial esophagogastrectomies with esophagogastrostomy (Table VIII).

All the cancers of the distal third of the esophagus or cardioesophagus were explored through the thorax (resection of the ninth rib) and the diaphragm. In the cancers of the cardia without invasion of the esophagus (proved by esophagoscopy) we consider, at present, that the most favorable route for intervention is the abdominal. As absolute contraindication to the surgical exploration, we consider the following, which we found in two of our patients: Distant

TABLE VIII. END RESULTS

TYPE OF OPERATION	NUMBER OF PATIENTS	THORACIC INCISION	LOCATION OF CANCER	OPERATIVE MORTALITY NO.	OPERATIVE MORTALITY PER CENT	SURVIVAL
1. Gastroesophageal resection, esophagogastric anastomosis	6	Left 9th rib	Cardia infiltrating esophagus	4	75.00	1 patient survived 3 yr. and 4 mo. in perfect health 1 patient survived 2 yr., now recurrence in the anastomotic stoma
2. Gastroesophageal resection, removal of the tail of the pancreas; esophagogastric anastomosis	1	Over the left 9th rib	Distal third of esophagus with invasion of stomach and tail of pancreas	1	100.00	
3. Gastroesophageal resection, splenectomy; esophagogastric anastomosis	2	Over the left 9th rib	Lesser curvature of the stomach and cardia, with invasion of esophagus	1	50.00	1 patient well 3 mo.
4. Gastroesophageal resection, splenectomy; esophagojejunal anastomosis (very little of the stomach remained)	2	Over the left 9th rib	Cardia with invasion of stomach and esophagus	1	50.00	1 patient died at 6 mo. with cachexia
5. Resection of the entire stomach and distal segment of the esophagus; esophagojejunal anastomosis	2	Over the left 9th rib	Cancer involving entire stomach with invasion up to cardia	1	50.00	1 patient died at 6 mo. with recurrence
6. Gastroesophageal resection, splenectomy, removal of the tail of the pancreas; esophagogastric anastomosis	1	Over the left 9th rib	Cardio-esophageal cancer			1 patient living at 3 mo. with cachexia
Total	14			8	57.14	

metastatic invasion which is manifested by a palpable nodular liver, supraclavicular lymph nodes (proved by biopsy), periumbilical tumor masses, implants in the pouch of Douglas, etc.

We consider nonresectable: (1) Those tumors which at exploration of the thorax are accompanied by hemorrhage freely collected in the pleural cavity, neoplastic nodules disseminated in the pleura (histopathologic study by frozen section), adhesions en bloc with the diaphragm determining an immovable tumor and very extensive infiltration, extensive invasion of neighboring organs, as the aorta, the bronchus, spinal column, etc.; (2) those which, after incision of the diaphragm, are shown to be accompanied by liver metastases, implants in the adjacent peritoneum or the pouch of Douglas (not revealed by clinical examination), extensive infiltration of the adjacent epiploon (omentum) and the pancreas, etc.

We performed 14 radical operations of various types according to the different location and the degree of cancerous invasion. In Table VII are grouped the different procedures.

As can be seen, the transthoracic resections of cardioesophageal cancers on our service resulted in a mortality of 57 per cent, the patients dying within thirty days postoperatively.

In a little longer period on this same service, we have performed 24 total gastrectomies for gastric cancer employing the abdominal route with a mortality of 33.33 per cent. In two of these, the cancer was located in the cardia and both patients survived the intervention. Another patient, who presented cancer of the cardia and very limited esophageal invasion, was operated upon by the abdominal route, effecting the resection of the lower portion of the esophagus and the upper middle portion of the stomach with esophagogastric anastomosis; the patient died two months later from an intestinal fistula (produced by rubber tube drainage). These latter two patients are not included in the statistics which are presented since they were treated by the abdominal route. If these are added to the statistics, we have a total of 17 gastroesophageal resections (3 by the abdominal route, 14 by the thoracic) with a mortality of 52 per cent.

The mortality of the simple transthoracic exploration was, in 21 cases, 23.8 per cent (5 deaths considered also within the first thirty days postoperatively).

Anesthesia.—The anesthesia used was always the same, cyclopropane mixed with ether and administered by tracheal intubation.

Complications.—Of the 6 patients who survived the radical intervention, 2 presented as a complication "left purulent cystic pleurisy" of late appearance, more than one month after the operation, which was treated by drainage, and the third, simple hemorrhage one month later for which the treatment was a simple thoracentesis. In the simple explorations, in none of which drainage of the pleural cavity was established, there were complications, the majority of them with serosanguineous effusion of medium amounts, which was treated by thoracentesis.

Cause of Death.—

Resections: The cause of death in patients who underwent resection and died during the first thirty days postoperatively was acute pleuropulmonary infection in 6. In all, autopsy revealed partial separation of the sutures of the anastomatic stoma. One patient died as the result of operative shock and the other (total gastrectomy) of generalized peritonitis (also due to separation of sutures).

Simple transthoracic explorations: Three of the patients who had simple transthoracic explorations died from acute pleuropulmonary infection; one died during the operation from anesthesia syncope, and the other as the result of hematemesis and melena.

Pathologic Anatomy.—In 28 of the 39 patients with cardioesophageal cancer, histologic examination was made either from the resected specimen or from a specimen obtained by biopsy (esophagoscopy). The results obtained were as shown in Table IX.

TABLE IX. PATHOLOGIC FINDINGS

PATHOLOGIC ANATOMY	NUMBER	PER CENT
Adenocarcinoma	14	50.0
Carcinoma solidum	3	10.72
Mixed	3	10.72
Squamous-cell carcinoma	7	25.0
Lymphosarcoma	1	3.55
Total	28	

In a total of 14 cases of resections, the histopathologic examinations revealed neoplastic invasion of regional lymph nodes, that is, the cancer had extended from outside the limits of the organ (advanced cases). The invasion of the regional lymph nodes was as shown in Table X.

TABLE X. INVOLVEMENT OF LYMPH NODES

LYMPH NODES INVOLVED	NUMBER
Lesser curvature	6
Greater and lesser curvatures	1
Cardia	5
Cardia and greater curvature	2
Total	14

The proof of these are of great importance as it shows that in the great majority of cases, and in all of ours, the lymphatic routes effected by the cardioesophageal tumors are on the abdominal side.

The histopathologic examination, carried out on the 14 resected specimens with the purpose of studying specifically the limits of the tumor in relation to the section of the esophagus and stomach, revealed the following: In 5 cases, the surgical section of both organs was performed on healthy tissue. In 8 cases, the tumor invaded up to the same limit of the esophagus (esophageal section). In 1 case, the tumor invaded the site of both sections, esophageal and gastric. The opinion of the pathologist regarding the point of origin of the neoplasia drawn from the studied specimens was as shown in Table XI.

TABLE XI. LOCATION OF THE RESECTED CARCINOMA

ANATOMICPATHOLOGIC LOCATION	HISTOLOGIC TYPE	NUMBER
Cardia infiltrating esophagus	Adenocarcinoma	9
Esophagus infiltrating stomach	Squamous-cell carcinoma	2
Esophagus infiltrating stomach	Carcinoma solidum	1
Stomach infiltrating esophagus	Mixed	2
Invasion of regional lymph nodes		14

Survival After Resection.—By survival after resection we mean those individuals who did not die in the immediate postoperative period, that is to say, in the course of the first thirty days after the intervention.

Of the 14 patients undergoing resection, 6 survived. Of these, 1 (Case 1) survived three years and four months (follow-up in January, 1947), enjoyed perfect health, and is working and living an active life. The esophagoscopic examination on that visit revealed a healthy and well-healed, functioning anastomatic stoma proved by its good functioning, and also with the radioscopic and radiographic examinations (see Fig. 1).

Another patient (Case 3) survived two years, but at present a neoplastic invasion of the anastomatic stoma has been proved by biopsy. Two died six months postoperatively with cachexia (Cases 2 and 4). One was living at the time of this communication, three months after operation, in poor health with liver metastases (Case 6). One has survived three months and is in a splendid state of health (Case 5). (See Table XII.)

TABLE XII. SURVIVAL AFTER RESECTION

SURVIVAL	WELL	CACHEXIA	DIED
More than 3 yr.	1		
More than 2 yr.		1	
More than 6 mo.			2
More than 3 mo.	1	1	

In Conclusion.—Of 39 patients who had cardioesophageal cancer treated by us between September, 1943, and September, 1946, in 14, or 35.89 per cent, it was possible to perform a radical operation. Six, or 42.85 per cent, of those undergoing resection were discharged, in other words, 15.38 per cent of the total, the average survival having been 13 months.

CASE REPORTS

CASE 1 (43-8677).—M. P. P., a 54-year-old railroad laborer, was admitted to the hospital Aug. 21, 1943, and discharged Sept. 28, 1943.

Clinical History.—Symptoms began ten months before hospitalization with belching, eructations, gastric pyrosis, and sensation of fullness in the stomach, at times with alimentary vomiting. These attacks were periodic and alternated with weeks of well-being and perfect health. There was asthenia and also loss of weight. The dysphagia increased, resulting in an obstruction causing vomiting.

The blood count indicated a definite anemia.

Radiography.—Radiography showed a filling defect with narrowing of the cardioesophageal region with irregular contours, also involving the proximal segment of the stomach. There was difficulty in emptying esophagus and an increase of diameter was noticed (see Fig. 1).

Conclusion.—It was decided that there was a gastroesophageal carcinoma.

Operation.—Preoperative preparation was made Sept. 3, 1943, with transfusions, hypoproteinemia regime, gastroesophageal lavages, etc. Cardioesophagectomy via the transpleural and transdiaphragmatic route was performed under general anesthesia, nitrous oxide with intratracheal intubation.

Anatomicopathologic Examination.—Examination revealed ulcerated gastroesophageal carcinoma, Borrmann III type.

Histopathologic Type.—For the most part, the type of carcinoma was *undifferentiated;* in a small part, adenocarcinoma; metastasis to regional lymph nodes.

Postoperative Course.—In the postoperative period, a left cystic pleurisy developed which was treated by evacuation of 400 c.c. of pus.

Follow-up.—After three years and four months the patient was in a perfect state of health, actively at work. There were no manifestations of recurrence, as shown by radiography and esophagoscopy.

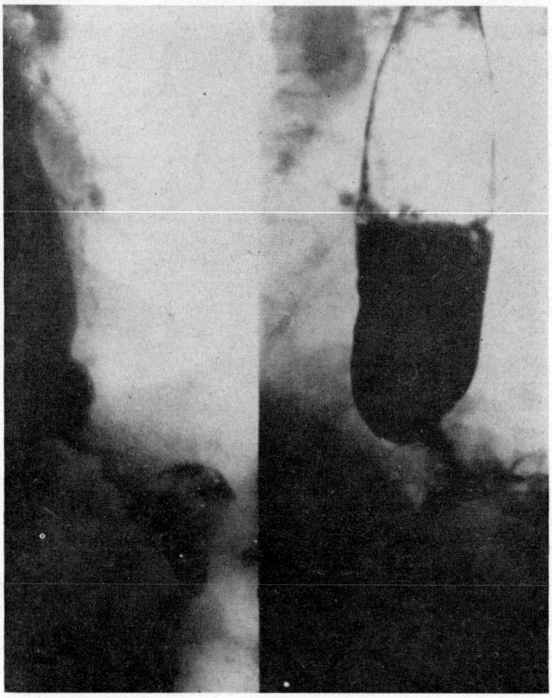

Fig. 1 (Case 1, M. P. P.).—Preoperative x-ray views of gastroesophageal cancer.

Comment.—This was a patient of 54 years with ulcerated gastroesophageal carcinoma (solidum and adenocarcinoma); cardioesophagectomy was performed by the transthoracic route. The survival of three years and four months is due to a probable total removal of the neoplasm since the tumorous elements nearest the superior operative section remained at *2 mm. from it* and at *8 mm. from the distal portion.* Nodes containing cancer were located around the cardia. At the time of this communication, the patient lives an active life of employment without presenting symptoms and is in perfect health.

CASE 2 (43-8498).—R. C. L., a 50-year-old miner, was admitted to the hospital Aug. 28, 1943, and discharged Feb. 24, 1944.

Clinical History.—For one year there had been postprandial meteorism and, at times, vomiting. Three months later, dysphagia for solids continued to increase, as did anorexia, alimentary vomiting, dysphagia for liquids, constipation, and weight loss of 9 kilograms in a year.

X-ray Examination.—Examination of the esophagus and stomach showed a filling defect of the gastroesophageal region with retention of the barium in the esophagus. The rest of the stomach and the duodenum were normal (see Fig. 2, *A*).

Conclusion.—Gastroesophageal carcinoma was indicated.

Operation.—Esophagogastrectomy (subtotal gastrectomy) and splenectomy via the transpleural and transdiaphragmatic route were carried out Sept. 10, 1943. Esophagojejunostomy and jejunostomy were done. Anesthesia used was cyclopropane and ether with tracheal intubation.

Anatomicopathologic Examination.—Examination revealed adenocarcinoma of the cardia constituting for the most part an annular carcinoma, Borrmann type III, with multiple lymph node metastases. There was chronic gastritis (see Fig. 2, *B*).

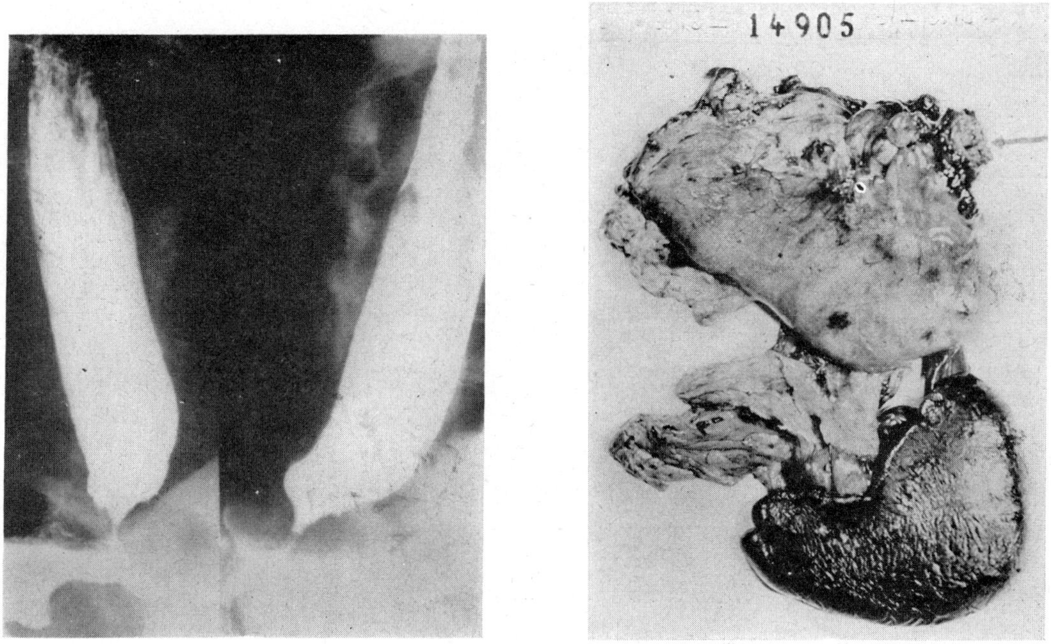

A. *B.*

Fig. 2 (Case 2, R. C. L.).—*A*, Preoperative x-ray views of gastroesophageal cancer. *B*, Macrophotograph anterior to resected specimen following esophagogastrectomy and splenectomy.

Postoperative Course.—The patient had pain, buccal aphthae, left pleural hemorrhage, suppuration through the operative wound, and later suppuration through the pleural cavity. He was treated by repeated transfusions, sulfonamide, stimulants, etc. In the third postoperative month, the patient was very well. There occurred soon afterward an encysted pleural abscess, which was opened through the operative wound, leaving an opening which drained purulent secretion and later serous fluid. This presented a medium amount of ascites. The patient did not improve after operation and died at home six months later of cachexia.

Comment.—This was a patient of 50 years on whom an esophagogastrectomy (subtotal gastrectomy) and splenectomy were performed through the transthoracic route for adenocarcinoma of the cardia.

The survival was only of six months' duration due to a very advanced tumor which had deeply invaded the gastric serosa with extension up to the proximal limit of the section and in the serosa to the distal limit of the section. The metastasis to the lymph nodes included the lymph nodes of the lesser curvature and the hilum of the spleen. The resection was incomplete considering the extension of the tumor, as a result of which the survival was short.

CASE 3 (43-11676).—L. A. G., a 44-year-old chauffeur, was admitted to the hospital Jan. 4, 1945, and discharged March 29, 1945.

Clinical History.—Two months before admission the illness commenced with dysphagia for solids and later for liquids; weight loss began at that time. Red and white blood counts and differential were normal. Proteinemia was 65.5 Gm. per cent.

X-ray Examination.—Examination showed carcinoma of the distal third of the esophagus (see Fig. 3).

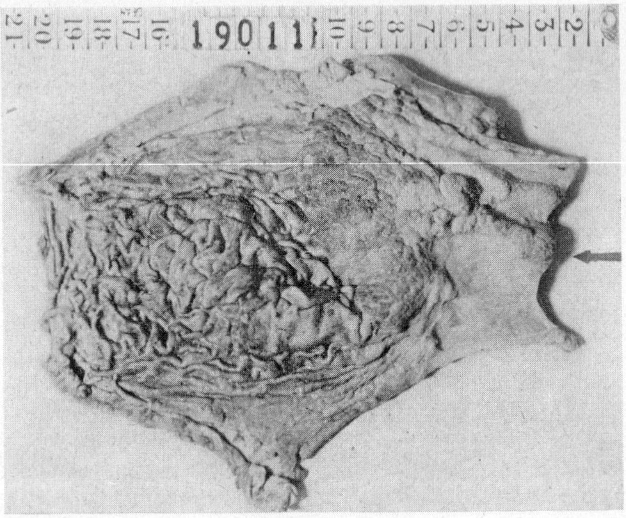

Fig. 3 (Case 3, L. A. G.).—Macrophotograph of cardiac region of the stomach and distal portion of the esophagus.

Esophagoscopy.—At the level of the cardia, the surface was found to be irregular with infiltration of the wall.

Biopsy.—Biopsy revealed adenocarcinoma.

Operation.—On Jan. 26, 1945, after previous preparation, general anesthesia (cyclopropane and ether) was given with tracheal intubation and cardioesophagectomy was performed by the left transpleural and transdiaphragmatic route. An esophagogastric anastomosis was made.

Anatomicopathologic Examination.—Cardioesophageal cancer was found at examination, with invasion of part of the body of the stomach and with lymph node metastasis.

Macroscopic Form.—Diffuse infiltrating carcinoma was found.

Histologic Type.—Histologic type for the most part was adenocarcinoma and several sections were carcinoma solidum.

Postoperative Course.—There were left pleuropulmonary complications. The patient was discharged on the sixty-third day in good condition.

He returned four days later because of gastroesophageal stenosis which was treated by dilatation, continuing with dilatations periodically for a year and nine months, during which period recurrence in the anastomosis occurred, proved by biopsy (adenocarcinoma). *At the end of two years, the patient was living, with cachexia.*

Comment.—This was a patient of 44 years who underwent a cardioesophagectomy via the transthoracic route for adenocarcinoma with sections of carcinoma solidum. The neoplasm did not invade the serosa; *the limit of the esophageal section was performed through infiltrated tissue* causing the recurrence which appeared in the twenty-first postoperative month, as proved by the biopsy. In the resected specimen, *metastatic cancer in lymph nodes was present in the region of the cardia.*

CASE 4 (45-14852).—A. L. L., a 58-year-old guard (watchman), was admitted to the hospital Nov. 29, 1945, and discharged Feb. 5, 1946.

Clinical History.—The illness actually began eleven months before admission with progressive dysphagia and pain in the upper part of the epigastrium which radiated to the left hemithorax. The patient had anorexia and a distaste for meat. There was a weight loss of 20 kilograms in eight months.

X-ray Examination.—Findings in the radiologic examination performed in the ninth month of symptoms were negative for cancer. On gastroscopy, there was encountered a firm obstruction at the level of the cardia which impeded the passing of the instrument. One month later, a new radiologic study revealed *probable gastroesophageal cancer* and a perforated lesion located in the region near the cardia.

Esophagoscopy.—In the region of the cardia, in the anterior left segment, the mucosa was seen to be somewhat inflamed and with a smooth surface and normal folds of cardia, permitting the passage of a medium sound. Biopsy showed carcinoma solidum.

Operation.—The anesthesia used, Dec. 14, 1945, was ether by intubation. Transthoracic gastrectomy was done, with a terminolateral esophagojejunostomy, Braun's enteroanastomosis, and splenectomy.

Anatomicopathologic Examination.—Gelatinous gastric cancer was found with cardioesophageal invasion and regional node metastasis.

Postoperative Course.—The postoperative course was satisfactory. There was a left pleural hemorrhage one month after operation which was controlled without recurrence. Six months later, there was recurrence in the anastomotic stoma, proved by biopsy, and liver metastasis. The patient died of cachexia and jaundice.

Comment.—This was a patient of 58 years on whom a transthoracic total gastrectomy and splenectomy were performed for gelatinous carcinoma with metastasis to the lymph nodes of the lesser and greater curvatures. The invasion of the tumor extended in depth down to the serosa and to the esophageal line of section. In six months, there was recurrence in the esophagojejunal anastomosis due to incomplete resection.

CASE 5 (46-11021).—Q. D. A., a 61-year-old merchant, was admitted to the hospital Sept. 14, 1946, and discharged Nov. 5, 1946.

Clinical History.—Illness actually began four months before hospitalization with dysphagia for solids located in the distal third of the sternum. Two months later, the dysphagia which had become acute and was painful was accompanied by anorexia. There was a weight loss of 19 kilograms.

X-ray Examination.—The opaque media was delayed at the level of the distal third of the esophagus, forming a peculiar cone with irregular edges and with small filling defects underneath this site.

The slow, small amount of opaque substance evacuated into the stomach did not permit its study.

Conclusion.—Carcinoma of the distal third of the esophagus was found.

Operation.—Anesthesia (cyclopropane and ether by intubation) was given Sept. 30, 1946. Partial resection of the esophagus and stomach was done, and gastroesophageal anastomosis and splenectomy.

Anatomicopathologic Examination.—Examination showed cardioesophageal carcinoma with lymph node metastasis.

Histologic Type.—Squamous-cell carcinoma was the type found.

Postoperative Course.—The postoperative course was satisfactory.

Follow-Up.—Three months later the patient was in excellent health, with an increase of 3 kilograms in weight.

Comment.—This was a patient of 61 years, with squamous-cell cardioesophageal carcinoma for which an esophagogastrectomy and splenectomy were performed. The tumor was ulcerated and circumscribed, reaching the upper limit *to 2 cm. of the esophageal edge* and the lower *to 4 cm. of the edge of the gastric section.* There were metastases to the pericardial lymph nodes and those of the greater and lesser curvatures.

At the time of this communication, the patient is living, three months after operation, with increase in weight and in an excellent state of health. The probabilities of survival are greater because of radical operation beyond the line of section and removal of the regional lymph nodes.

CASE 6 (46-11222).—M. M. D., a 55-year-old housewife, was admitted to the hospital Aug. 24, 1946, and discharged Nov. 1, 1946.

Clinical History.—For one year, there was progressive asthenia and sialorrhea after meals; nine months later there was dysphagia with solid foods which increased to include liquids. The dysphagia, which was painful, was localized in the lower third of the sternum irradiating to the right interscapular region. This caused vomiting for fifteen days for relief. There was weight loss of 5 kilograms in two months.

The hematologic examination indicated slight anemia.

Esophagoscopy.—The esophagus was dilated in its entire extent. No suspicious signs of a neoplasm were encountered.

X-ray Examination.—The esophagus was normal. The proximal third of the stomach including the fundus extending 7 cm. on the lesser curvature was transformed into a rigid narrow tube.

The distance which separated the fundus from the left diaphragmatic sac was unusually large. The rest of the stomach was normal, as was the duodenum.

Operation.—On Oct. 9, 1946, cardioesophagectomy, splenectomy, and partial pancreatectomy (tail of pancreas) were done. Transpleural esophagogastric anastomosis was made. Anesthesia used was cyclopropane and ether.

Anatomicopathologic Examination.—Cardioesophageal carcinoma with metastasis to regional lymph nodes was found and carcinomatous peritonitis and carcinomatous peripancreatitis.

Histologic Type.—The carcinoma was for the most part solidum with a few areas of scirrhous glands.

Postoperative Course.—In spite of the severity of the intervention, the postoperative period was uneventful; the patient was discharged in good condition on the twenty-second day.

Follow-Up.—Three months later cachexia with liver metastasis was present.

Comment.—This was a patient of 55 years with a cardioesophageal carcinoma for which there was performed a cardioesophagectomy, splenectomy, and partial pancreatectomy (tail of the pancreas) by the transthoracic route.

Examination of the resected specimen revealed that it was a very advanced carcinoma which infiltrated the neighboring organs, producing a *carcinomatous peripancreatitis and carcinomatous peritonitis with lymph node metastasis located around the cardia and lesser curvature of the stomach.* The upper limit of the tumor extended to 1.5 cm. from the esophageal edge of the specimen. The lower limit was 2 cm. from the line of the lower edge of the specimen.

This was an unfavorable case for a radical operation which was proved by the presence of liver metastasis and cachexia three months after operation.

COMMENTS

The critical analysis of the statistics which we have presented permits us to arrive at certain conclusions which we consider of interest, since they enable us to adopt different attitudes in the future, as compared with the present, in relation with certain aspects of cancers of the cardia and distal portion of the esophagus.

1. There is evidence in our studies, in the first place, of the advanced stage of these cancers in all the patients at the time of consultation, as revealed by the *low percentage of resectability obtained,* just about 25 per cent. In addition, the resected specimens show that in *100 per cent of them, the regional lymph nodes show invasion* by the cancer, that is to say, that the cancer has spread beyond the region of origin in all cases. In our entire experience with *gastric cancer, at different locations,* regional node metastasis reaches a total of 75 per cent.

The remedy for this situation is for the most part educational, not only of the public, but especially of the medical profession in whom the idea is predominant that cancers in this location are for that very reason incurable. In reality, it is not the patients who ignore the initial symptoms without attention to them, for the nature of them, especially the dysphagia, causes them to consult a doctor for their relief. It is then, in general, the medical practitioner who is responsible in the most part for the lost time.

2. A point of extraordinary importance, which should be stressed, is that which refers to the primary route of the first exploration of these cancers, once the diagnosis is determined, and the exact location of them *(fluoroscopy* and *radiography, esophagoscopy* and *biopsy).*

Up to the present time, and agreeing with the opinion of the majority of surgeons who know the subject, we have carried out the first exploration by thoracotomy, usually by resection of the ninth rib from the base itself to its cubit, adding, in some cases, the section of the eighth and tenth ribs at the level of the spinal muscles. The thoracic abdominal region of exploration, once the diaphragm is sectioned, has been sufficient; the operation is not possible in cases of advanced gastric cancer. The simple transthoracic diaphragmatic exploration was followed by immediate death (up to thirty days postoperatively) in 23.8 per cent. On the other hand, the mortality from exploratory laparotomy, in general, in cases of gastric cancer has been in our experience only 7.3 per cent.

In addition, the anatomicopathologic study of the specimens removed has led us to believe that in 100 per cent of the patients, the lymph nodes containing metastatic cancer were limited to the perigastric group (see Table X).

We found in cases of resection that the greatest difficulty was encountered on the gastric side.

These considerations make us believe, exactly as Garlock, that the cardioesophageal cancers should be explored first through the abdomen, for the purpose of determining their operability. In case it is judged resectable, the procedure should be continued through the laparotomy incision toward the thorax (eight or nine degrees), actually practicing a phrenothoracic laparotomy. In agreement with that author, the facility for completing the radical operation is greater with this route than through the thorax and the sectioned diaphragm.

3. The invasion of the esophageal tumor takes place in a peculiar manner, the macroscopic delimitation process being difficult. In some of our specimens,

we could prove that the neoplasia penetrated into the mucosa and submucosa in irregular *vertical prolongations.* The difficulty in palpating the limit of the tumor is shown in our statistics, as in 9 of 14 resections, the *cancer invaded up to the limit of the esophageal section,* and from there, from what we have observed, there was frequency of recurrence in the anastomotic stoma.

One, therefore, has to be extraordinarily cautious in order to determine the exact level for surgical section of the esophagus and, furthermore, we believe that before starting the anastomosis, the surgeon should wait for the pathologic report of a frozen section for the study of the esophageal and gastric sections.

4. The high mortality rate in our resections is due in greater part to *dehiscence of the sutures at the level of the gastroesophageal or jejunoesophageal anastomosis.*

The reason for this we can find in the aforementioned: The anastomosis has been made directly on the neoplasia in several of the operative cases, and it is assumed that the healing under such circumstances is defective or impossible.

The technique used by us in joining the stomach and the esophagus is the following:

(a) Fine silk Halsted sutures in the posterior part joining the gastric seromuscular layers with the esophageal muscularis layer

(b) Continuous catgut chromic 00 sutures, with atraumatic needle, which will include all of the gastric and esophageal layers in the posterior part

(c) The same method in the anterior circumference of the anastomosis

(d) Fine silk Lembert sutures, for reinforcement, in all the circumference of the anastomosis

(e) Fixation of the suspended stomach in the thorax at the edge of the diaphragm

(f) Levine tube for five or six days, passed above the anastomosis

(g) Underwater drainage of the left thoracic cavity

We have tried not to submit the anastomosis to any sort of tension. It is possible that what Carter and his associates* say is correct, that the important point of the anastomosis is the fixation of the stomach and the esophagus by means of the separate fine silk sutures which fix these organs in the diaphragm and the spinal column (intervertebral adjacent discs) with the purpose of eliminating the tension on the suture lines.

We do not wish to stress in particular, in this review, the importance of the operative preparation, the postoperative care, the means to avoid operative shock (plasma therapy, blood transfusion), the avoidance of infection (sulfa drugs and penicillin given in sufficient doses before and after the operation), and anesthesia, especially by tracheal intubation.

It is these and other well-known points which have been insisted upon and are insisted upon every day in such a way that, in relation to them, precise standards have been obtained by those who dedicate themselves to this type of surgery.

---

*Carter, Stevenson, and Abbott: SURGERY 8: 587, 1940.

SUBTOTAL ESOPHAGECTOMY AND ESOPHAGOGASTROSTOMY FOR HIGH INTRATHORACIC ESOPHAGEAL LESIONS

Michael E. DeBakey, M.D., and Alton Ochsner, M.D., New Orleans, La.

(From the Departments of Surgery, Tulane University School of Medicine and the Ochnsner Clinic, and Charity Hospital of Louisiana)

LITTLE more than ten years has elapsed since Churchill, in a presentation of his own experience with surgery of the esophagus, pointed out how limited and unsuccessful were even the boldest pioneering efforts which had been made in this field of surgical endeavor up to that time. Since then, however, truly gratifying progress has been made in this area of surgery, particularly in the surgical management of malignant lesions of the esophagus.

By 1941, when this subject was reviewed by us, a satisfactory method of dealing with lesions of the lower third of the esophagus and cardia had become well developed. The procedure consisted essentially of extirpation of the involved area, with restoration of the continuity of the alimentary tract by intrathoracic esophagogastrostomy. Since then Garlock and Sweet have demonstrated that the stomach can be adequately mobilized to permit the application of this procedure to lesions higher in the esophagus. This important development now obviates the need for employing the unsatisfactory Torek operation and the tedious and usually disappointing multi-staged antethoracic esophagoplasties. Thus, it is now possible to employ a safe and satisfactory surgical procedure with immediate restoration of function for lesions involving almost all levels of the intrathoracic esophagus.

This report is concerned with our personal experiences with this procedure as it is applied to lesions of the upper portions of the intrathoracic esophagus and with certain technical aspects of the operation.

REPORT OF CASES

Case 1.—R. R. B., a 32-year-old white man, was admitted to the Foundation Hospital, New Orleans, La., on Feb. 25, 1947, because of difficulty in swallowing, which began at the age of 2 years, following the ingestion of a solution of lye. A gastrostomy had been performed for feeding purposes on two occasions; first, immediately after the accident and again at the age of 12 years. He has always had to eat soft foods and well-ground meat. Esophagoscopies and dilatations had to be done periodically since the accident (107 times) because food would become lodged in the esophagus, but in recent years the dilatations became progressively less effective.

Physical examination revealed a white man of slight build but in moderately good general condition. The temperature and pulse rate were normal; the blood pressure was 120 mm. Hg systolic and 70 mm. Hg diastolic. There were no significant findings except for the presence of an upper abdominal scar in the midline, a mastoid scar on the right side, and an uncomplicated pilonidal sinus. Laboratory studies of the urine, blood, and feces showed no abnormalities.

Roentgenographic examination of the esophagus following ingestion of barium revealed the presence of a smooth narrowing of the esophagus over about 8 cm. of its length extending from the superior end of the sternum to the seventh thoracic vertebra (Fig. 1). Most pronounced narrowing was just above the level of the superior margin of the aortic arch. The diameter of the lumen measured about 5 mm.

Received for publication, Aug. 12, 1947.

Esophagoscopy revealed a tendency of some scarring of the pharynx with a glazed smooth appearance of the mucous membrane; there was a good opening and normal movement of the pharyngeal musculature. At the level of the suprasternal notch a stricture was encountered which could be expanded to about 4 to 5 mm. in diameter. This was due to a dense, fibrous tissue scar which could not be safely dilated.

On March 6, 1947, a subtotal esophagectomy with esophagogastrostomy was performed. Under intratracheal ether-oxygen anesthesia and with the patient in the right lateral position an incision was made over the seventh rib on the left side from the paravertebral line posteriorly to the parasternal line anteriorly and extended upward posteriorly and paravertebrally to the fifth rib. The incision was carried down through the skin, subcutaneous tissue, and musculature to the seventh rib, which was then resected subperiosteally. The fifth and sixth ribs were sectioned subperiosteally and paravertebrally. The chest was entered through the bed of the seventh rib. The lung was mobilized

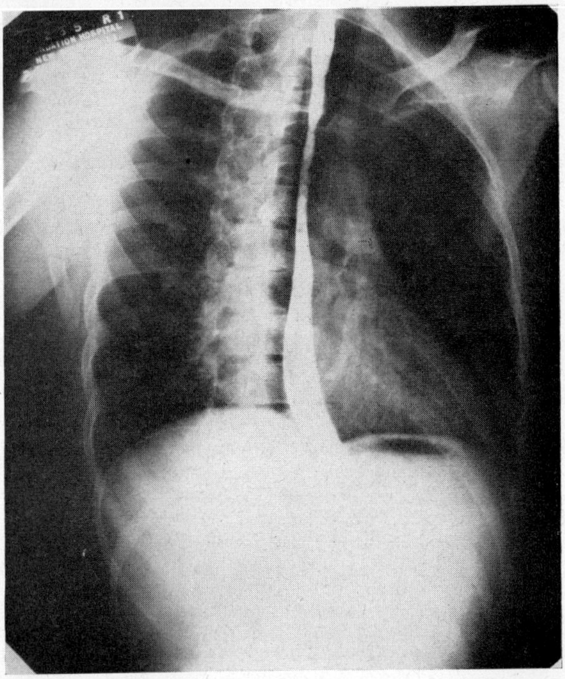

Fig. 1 (Case 1).—Preoperative roentgenogram of esophagus following ingestion of barium showing stricture of esophagus extending just above jugular notch to seventh thoracic vertebra.

forward and the mediastinal pleura was opened below the aortic arch and then above this structure behind the subclavian artery to expose the esophagus. Both in the region just above and in the region just behind the aortic arch the esophagus was surrounded by much dense fibrous tissue which made its mobilization extremely difficult. The stricture was high up in the esophagus above the aortic arch but it was believed that there was sufficient normal esophagus above the stricture to permit anastomosis to the stomach. This actually consisted of about 4 cm. of the esophagus after it entered the thoracic cavity. The remaining portion of the esophagus in the chest was completely mobilized from its bed after the vagus nerve and thoracic duct had been carefully drawn out of the way to prevent injury. Several esophageal arterial branches of the aorta were isolated and ligated. After the phrenic nerve had been crushed, the diaphragm was opened by a radial incision from the hiatus to its peripheral margins and the peritoneal cavity entered. In the effort to mobilize the stomach it was found that its anterior wall near the pylorus was intimately attached to the abdominal wall. In order to permit visual dissection of this region better exposure was required and for this reason the thoracic incision was converted into a thoracicoabdominal approach by extending the anterior end of the incision in the thoracic wall obliquely across the sixth costal cartilage into the abdomen and downward paramedially almost to the umbilicus. The stomach was completely mobilized by dividing the vasa brevia, the left gastric and left gastroepiploic vessels, and the gastrolienal, gastrocolic, and gastrohepatic ligaments; the right gastric and right gastroepiploic arteries were carefully protected from injury. Adhesions between the anterior wall of the stomach and the abdominal wall, as a result of the former gastrostomy, were carefully freed without injury to the gastric wall. The pylorus was further mobilized in order to permit almost complete mobilization of the stomach into the chest. Small Payr clamps were then placed across the esophagus at the cardiac level and the esophagus was severed between them. The gastric stump was closed by two layers of atraumatic chromic catgut sutures. The proximal end of the esophagus was then drawn out from behind the aortic arch and the stomach pulled up into the chest. The fundus of the stomach was tacked to the pleura at the apex of the chest with several interrupted sutures.

The esophagus was then anastomosed to the anterior wall of the stomach near the cardia with two rows of interrupted quilting cotton sutures, mattress sutures being used for the outer seromuscular layer and simple interrupted sutures for the inner mucosal layer. Although the esophagus was severed just above the stricture, the opening in the proximal end appeared still somewhat narrowed. It was believed, however, that the esophagus could not be severed at a higher level and still permit performance of the anastomosis, but a larger stoma was considered desirable and this was achieved by incising the esophagus upward on one side, as shown in Fig. 11.

The stomach was then fixed along its greater curvature to the pleura of the posterior thoracic wall by a row of interrupted quilting cotton sutures. After completion of the esophagogastrostomy, the nasal tube connected to suction, which had been previously passed down the esophagus to the point of obstruction, was passed through the anastomotic opening into the stomach. The incision in the thoracic wall and abdomen was then closed in layers with interrupted cotton sutures throughout. Before the thoracic wall was closed, a thoracotomy tube was inserted through the eighth intercostal space.

The patient was under the anesthetic for approximately six hours, but during the entire time the blood pressure remained well stabilized at a normal level, the systolic ranging between 120 and 130 mm. Hg and the diastolic between 70 and 80 mm. Hg; the pulse rate varied from 120 at the beginning of the operation to 80 at the end. During the operation he received 2,500 c.c. of whole blood.

Pathologic examination of the specimen showed chronic inflammation and fibrous stricture of the esophagus involving a distance of about 5.5 cm., which was densely sclerotic and scarred. The diameter of the lumen in the stricture at its most narrowed point was about 4 mm.

The postoperative course was uneventful except for the development of partial atelectasis of the right lung on the second day. This was adequately treated early and by the fifth postoperative day the temperature became normal and remained normal thereafter. The patient began taking liquids on the second day, a soft diet on the fourth, and a full diet on the sixth postoperative day. Penicillin therapy, which was started on the day before operation, was discontinued on the sixth postoperative day. On the eighth postoperative day the sutures were removed, the wound had completely healed, and the patient was feeling well and was up and about. He was permitted to leave the hospital on March 18, 1947, the twelfth postoperative day.

Fluoroscopic examination of the esophagus and stomach following ingestion of barium showed a well-functioning stoma with no obstruction to the passage of barium (Fig. 2).

On March 28, 1947, esophagoscopy was performed* in Phoenix, Ariz. After the piriform sinus had been anesthetized with 2 per cent pontocaine, the esophagoscope was

*By Dr. Thomas H. Bates, who was kind enough to send us the description of his examination.

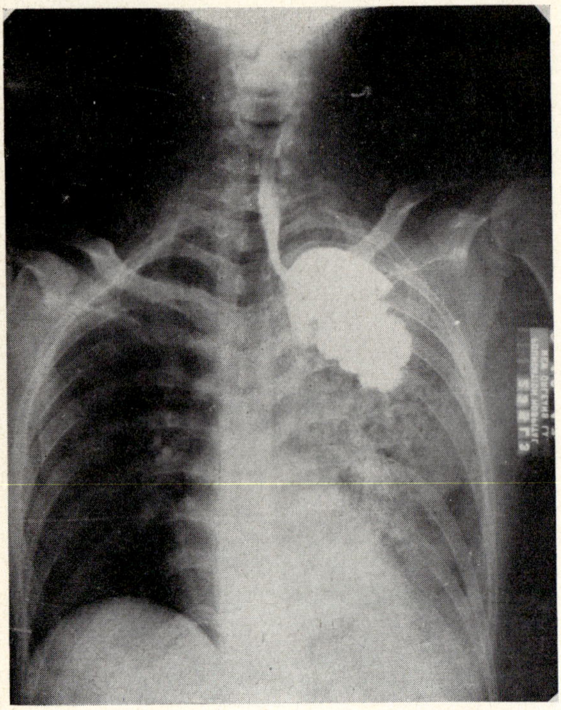

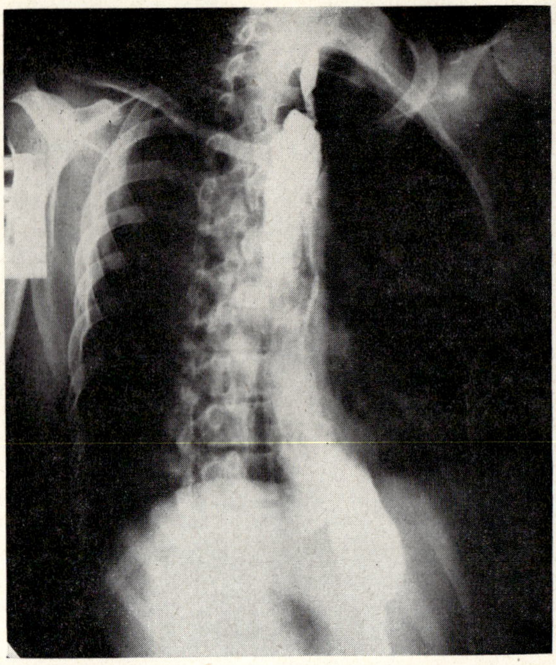

Fig. 2 (Case 1).—Postoperative roentgenogram after ingestion of barium showing esophagus and stomach with anastomosis a few centimeters above the jugular notch.

Fig. 3 (Case 1).—Roentgenogram following ingestion of barium taken almost four months after operation showing esophagus, stomach, and duodenum in almost vertical position. The flow of barium observed fluoroscopically revealed well-functioning anastomosis with no obstruction to inlet or outlet of stomach.

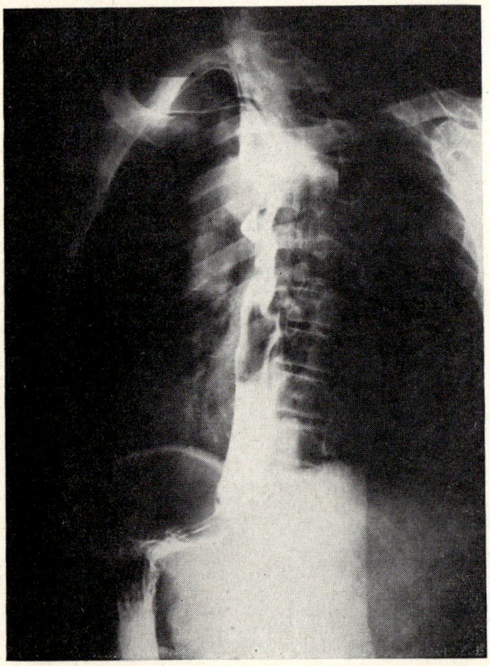

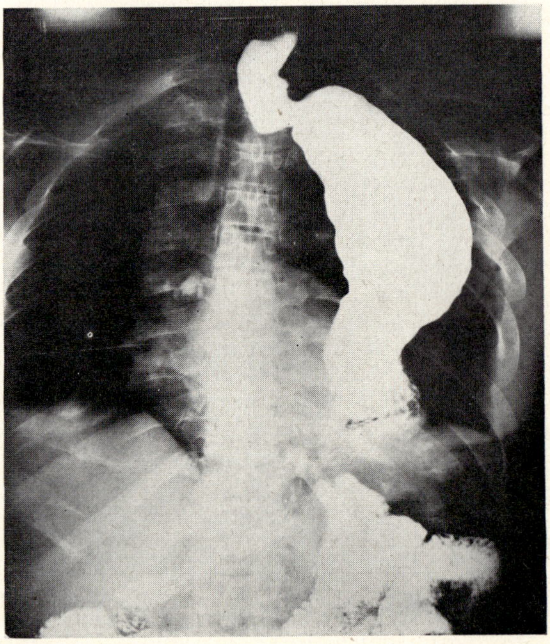

Fig. 4 (Case 2).—Preoperative roentgenogram of esophagus following ingestion of barium showing irregular constriction in middle third of esophagus.

Fig. 5 (Case 2).—Roentgenogram of esophagus and stomach following ingestion of barium, taken on eleventh postoperative day, showing well-functioning stoma about the level of the jugular notch.

thrust through the right sinus. Considerable spasm of the cricopharyngeus muscle was encountered. About 16 cm. from the alveolar ridge the line of anastomosis was encountered. There was no edema at this point. The lumen accepted the scope with ease. The upper portion of the stomach appeared normal. The stoma between the esophagus and the cardiac end of the stomach lying at the level of the lower cervical portion of the esophagus appeared to be well functioning.

On May 13, 1947, the patient was doing very well. The only complaint he had was that when he swallowed "it splashes." After the patient arrived in Phoenix, he had some dysphagia but this relieved itself in about one week's time. He used some belladonna.

The patient returned to the hospital on June 23, 1947, almost four months after the operation, complaining of some digestive disturbances and occasional vomiting, but no difficulty in swallowing. Fluoroscopic examination of the esophagus and stomach following ingestion of barium was reported as follows: The esophagogastric anastomosis was a little above the level of the suprasternal notch and functioned very satisfactorily. There was no obstruction at the outlet of the stomach and the duodenum filled immediately (Fig. 3).

It was evident that the vague digestive disturbances and occasional vomiting were not caused by mechanical obstruction to the passage of food either into or out of the stomach, at least in the vertical position. Closer questioning of the patient revealed the fact that the essential disturbance was regurgitation of gastric contents upon lying down. This disurbance was considerably relieved by remaining in the vertical position for some time after eating or lying down with the head elevated.

Similar disturbances in digestive function and gastrointestinal motility were observed by Churchill and Sweet in some of their patients upon whom esophagogastric anastomosis had been performed. They found evidence of diminished or absent gastric motility and hypertonicity of the pylorus, confirming their belief that this was due to an imbalance of the neurogenic influences as a consequence of division of the vagus nerves.

CASE 2.—J. G., a 77-year-old Negro man, was admitted to Charity Hospital in New Orleans on March 14, 1947, complaining of substernal pain and progressive dysphagia of four months' duration. The patient had lost a considerable amount of weight but was unable to say how much. He also complained of transient diplopia and scotomas and some dyspnea and dizziness for the previous three or four years during which he had been treated for hypertension by a local physician. Past history, social history, and family history were not significant.

Physical examination revealed an elderly Negro man, somewhat undernourished but otherwise in fairly good general condition and with no observable gross abnormalities. Temperature was normal, pulse rate 88, respiratory rate 24, blood pressure 210 mm. Hg systolic and 110 mm. Hg diastolic. Laboratory findings were as follows: Klein reaction negative; red blood cell count 4,600,000; hemoglobin 10.6 Gm.; hematocrit 36 per cent; white blood cell count 6,840, with 67 per cent polymorphonuclear cells; urinalysis, no abnormalities; blood urea nitrogen 26.1 mg. per cent; blood chloride 654 meq. per liter.

Roentgenographic studies showed an irregular constriction of the middle third of the esophagus extending from about the fifth to the ninth thoracic vertebra (Fig. 4). Esophagoscopy showed a friable granular mass projecting into the lumen of the esophagus beginning about 25.5 cm. from the upper incisor teeth; it appeared annular, bled easily on manipulation, and had the gross appearance of a malignant lesion. The biopsy specimen taken at this examination was reported as epidermoid carcinoma, grade II.

On April 19, 1947, after the patient was considered adequately prepared, operation was performed. Under intratracheal ether-oxygen anesthesia and with the patient lying in the right lateral position, an incision was made over the left sixth rib posteriorly where it was extended upward to the level of the fourth rib. The sixth rib was resected subperiosteally and the fifth rib divided posteriorly. The pleural cavity was entered through the bed of the sixth rib. The lung was gently retracted forward and the mediastinal pleura opened to expose the esophagus. By careful sharp and blunt dissection the esophagus was mobilized from its bed in the mediastinum below the aortic arch. As was indicated by the roentgenogram, the tumor was found to involve the middle third of the esophagus from about the junction of the eighth and ninth thoracic vertebrae below to the upper surface of the aortic arch above. The entire esophagus including several adjacent firm lymph nodes at this level was freed from its attachments and the esophageal

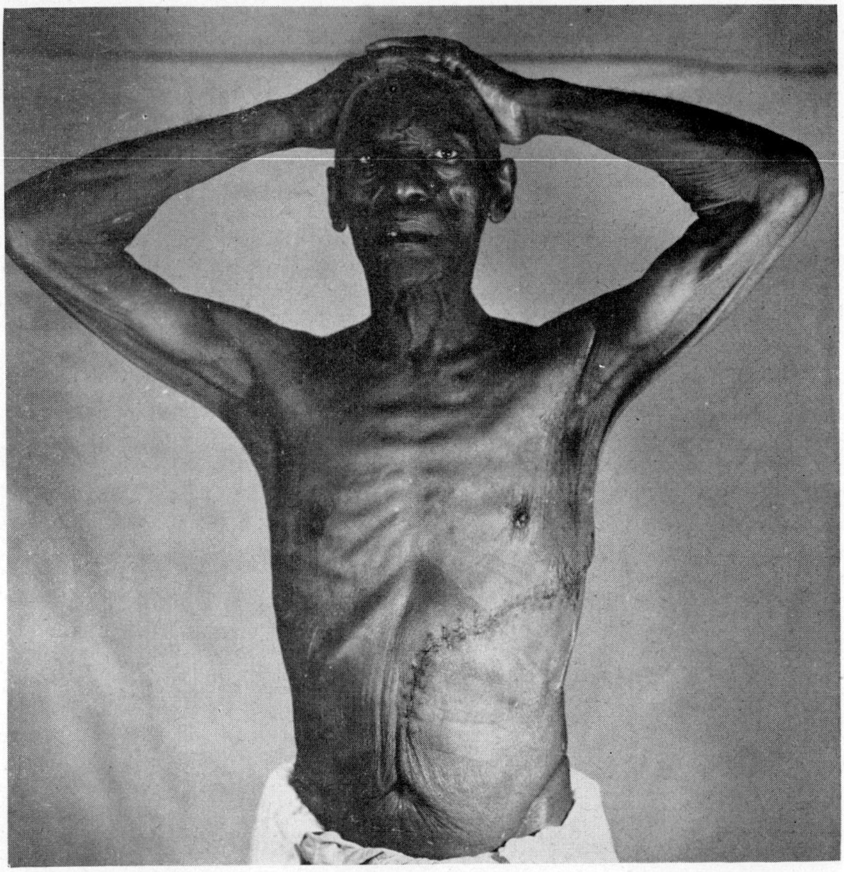

Fig. 6 (Case 2).—Photograph of patient taken approximately ten days postoperatively.

vessels were ligated and sectioned. Further mobilization of the esophagus above the level was then carried out after the mediastinal pleura had been opened above the aortic arch behind the left subclavian artery. After the phrenic nerve had been crushed, a radial incision was made in the diaphragm and the peritoneal cavity entered. The stomach was mobilized by division of its vascular and ligamentous attachments as described in Case 1, care being taken to preserve the right gastric and right gastroepiploic arteries. In order to provide better exposure for thorough mobilization of the stomach it was considered desirable to extend the anterior end of the incision in the thoracic wall across the costal cartilage and through the rectus sheath paramedially into the peritoneal cavity. The esophagus was divided between clamps at the cardioesophageal junction and the distal stump closed with two layers of interrupted sutures.

The proximal end of the severed esophagus was then covered with a rubber tampon and tied securely; the esophagus was brought out from under the aortic arch, through the opening in the mediastinal pleura above the aorta, and behind the left subclavian artery. The stomach was then brought up into the chest and the fundus attached to the pleura at the dome with several interrupted sutures. The esophagogastric anastomosis was then performed, as described in Case 1 and shown in Fig. 11. This type of anastomosis provided an L-shaped opening between the esophagus and the stomach and thus increased the size of the stoma. The stomach was then attached along its greater curvature to the pleura of the posterior thoracic wall with a row of interrupted sutures. The diaphragm was closed around the stomach just above the pylorus. The incisions in the thoracic wall and peritoneal cavity were closed in layers with interrupted cotton sutures after a catheter had been placed in the pleural cavity through the ninth interspace in the posterior axillary line.

The operation, which required about five hours, was well tolerated by the patient. He received 1,500 c.c. of whole blood during the course of the operation. Except for slight dyspnea, which disappeared by the sixth postoperative day, the postoperative course was uneventful. Penicillin, which was started the day before operation, was continued until the fifth postoperative day. The thoracotomy tube was removed on the fourth day.

On the fifth postoperative day the patient was eating a full diet. The sutures were removed on the eighth postoperative day; the wound had completely healed and the patient was up and about in the ward (Fig. 6). The subsequent course continued satisfactorily and he was discharged from the hospital on May 14, 1947. At the last follow-up examination in February, 1948, approximately ten months after operation, the patient was found to be in good condition with no complaints and no evidence of recurrence.

On April 30, 1947, the eleventh postoperative day, fluoroscopic examination of the esophagus and stomach following ingestion of barium showed a normally functioning stoma with no evidence of obstruction to the passage of barium (Fig. 5).

The pathologic report of the specimen removed was epidermoid carcinoma grade II, with extension into the muscularis, but no invasion of the outer layers.

TECHNICAL CONSIDERATIONS

It has now been established that lesions involving the upper portions of the intrathoracic esophagus and producing permanent functional disturbances can be successfully attacked surgically with restoration of normal function. This is achieved by resection of all but a sufficient segment of normal esophagus above the lesion to permit primary anastomosis to the mobilized stomach. The feasibility of this procedure, which was first demonstrated by Garlock and Sweet, permitting anastomosis at the highest level in the chest, is illustrated by the two cases reported in this paper, in one of which the lesion was benign and in the other malignant. The procedure, however, is not simple as presently performed and there are certain technical considerations of the operation that deserve comment.

Perhaps the most difficult feature of the operation is the performance of esophagogastric anastomosis at such a high level in the chest. If the incision in the thoracic wall is made sufficiently high to facilitate this procedure, difficulty will be encountered in adequately mobilizing the stomach, whereas if the incision is made low enough in the chest to facilitate the latter procedure, the former becomes difficult. For these reasons a proper surgical approach to the problem is important. To solve this problem, Garlock opened the chest through the sixth or seventh interspace and then divided the fourth to the eighth or fifth to the ninth ribs posteriorly to form a T-shaped incision in the thoracic wall.[7, 9] Clark used a somewhat similar approach in his case but entered through the bed of the subperiosteally resected seventh rib and Sweet achieved this purpose by entering the chest through the bed of the eighth rib and then dividing the seventh, sixth, fifth, and fourth ribs paravertebrally. An essentially similar approach was used by Adams in his case.

These approaches appeared rather extensive to us and we therefore attacked the problem somewhat differently. In the first case the chest was entered through the bed of the left seventh rib and the sixth and fifth ribs were divided paravertebrally. In the second case the chest was entered through the bed of the left sixth rib and the fifth rib was divided paravertebrally. Neither of these approaches proved completely satisfactory for in both in order to provide adequate exposure for mobilization of the stomach it was found desirable to extend the incision across the costal arch anteriorly into the abdomen. Extension of the thoracic incision across the costal arch into the abdomen to produce a combined thoracicoabdominal approach affords excellent exposure to the lower segment of the esophagus and to the stomach. Like others[2, 3, 8, 10, 11, 14, 21] we have often found it useful for lesions in this area, and Carter recently, in a comprehensive historical and technical consideration of this approach, also proposed it for splenectomy. Although it was well tolerated in both of our reported cases, it obviously increases the time and magnitude of the operation. For this reason and because it is probably unnecessary in most cases of high esophageal lesions, we believe that it should be avoided unless there are special reasons for its use. It was found necessary in the first case because of the adhesions from the low placement, near the pylorus, of the old gastrostomy and in the second because of the more highly placed incision in the thoracic wall. Although this latter factor made the esophagogastric anastomosis easier to perform in the second patient than in the first, it was still done with difficulty.

Ideally, the incision should permit adequate exposure low in the chest in order to facilitate mobilization of the stomach and high in the chest to provide ready access to the esophagogastric anastomosis but with a minimum of operative trauma. It is possible that these desiderata may be better met by an incision in the left thoracic wall which begins paravertebrally over the fourth rib, extends caudad to the seventh rib, and then curves anteriorly to follow the seventh rib to its costochondral junction. The pleural cavity could then be entered through the bed of the subperiosteally resected seventh or eighth ribs. After it had been determined that the lesion was resectable, especially in malignant cases, and the esophagus freed from its bed, the stomach could be mobilized through the diaphragm, brought up into the chest, and the diaphragm closed around it. The remainder of the operation, that is, the esophagogastric anastomosis, could then be done through a higher level by mobilization of the upper flap of the incision in the thoracic wall and entrance into the pleural cavity through the bed of the subperiosteally resected fourth rib. In this way only one incision is made in the soft parts of the thoracic wall with provision for two levels of exposure. It thus meets the requirements for adequate exposure for two essential features of the procedure, mobilization of the stomach and esophagus and performance of the high esophagogastric anastomosis, while at the same time avoiding extensive operative trauma. For these reasons we believe that this proposed approach has much to recommend it and are looking forward to trying it at the next opportunity.

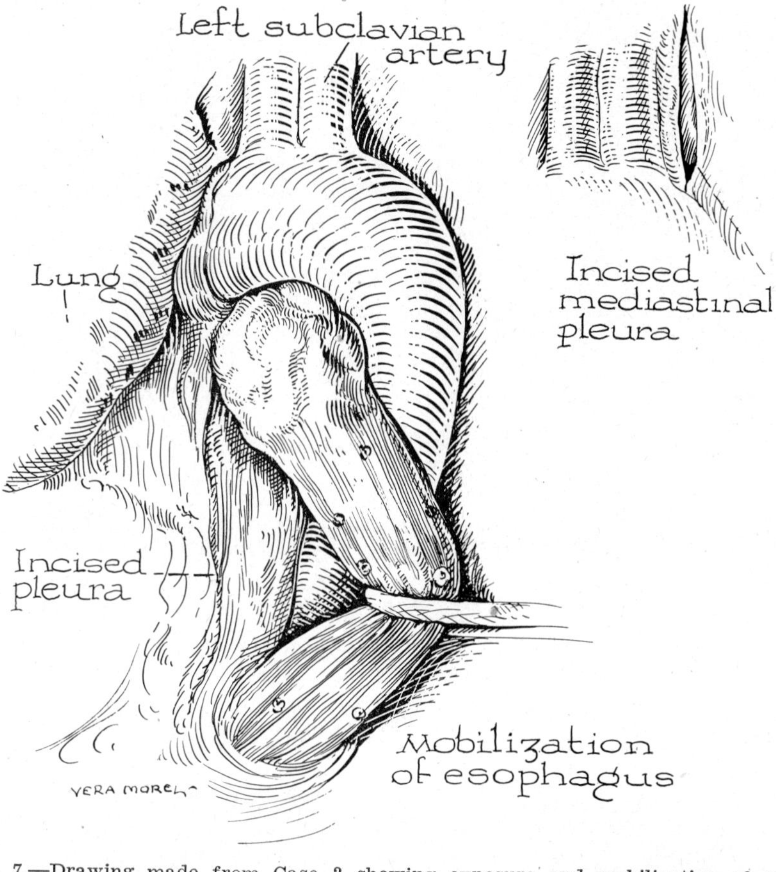

Fig. 7.—Drawing made from Case 2 showing exposure and mobilization of esophagus. The mediastinal pleura has been opened from the aortic arch to the hiatus. The esophagus has been mobilized from its bed by careful sharp and blunt dissection and the esophageal vessels have been divided between ligatures. The lower portion of the tumor beneath the aortic arch has been exposed and freed. The mediastinal pleura is then opened above the aortic arch and behind the left subclavian artery (inset) and the remaining portion of the esophagus including the tumor is mobilized by working from above and below the arch.

After the pleural cavity has been entered, the next step is exposure and mobilization of the esophagus. This is done by gentle retraction of the lung forward and opening of the mediastinal pleura from the aortic arch to the hiatus. By careful blunt and sharp dissection the esophagus is mobilized from its bed in the mediastinum at this level (Fig. 7). The esophageal vessels from the aorta and bronchial arteries are carefully ligated and divided. Considerable care must be exercised in freeing that portion of the esophagus behind the aortic arch for in both benign (Case 1) and malignant (Case 2) lesions, the esophagus tends to be closely adhered to its surrounding structures. In fact the dissection is usually easier in the latter if the lesion is resectable because a cleavage plane is more readily identified, whereas in the former the esophagus is usually surrounded by much dense scar tissue. The esophagus above the aortic arch is exposed through an opening in the mediastinal pleura behind the left subclavian artery (Fig. 7). This permits dissection of the esophagus behind the aortic arch to be carried out from above and below. Care should be exercised to avoid injury to the thoracic duct in this region.

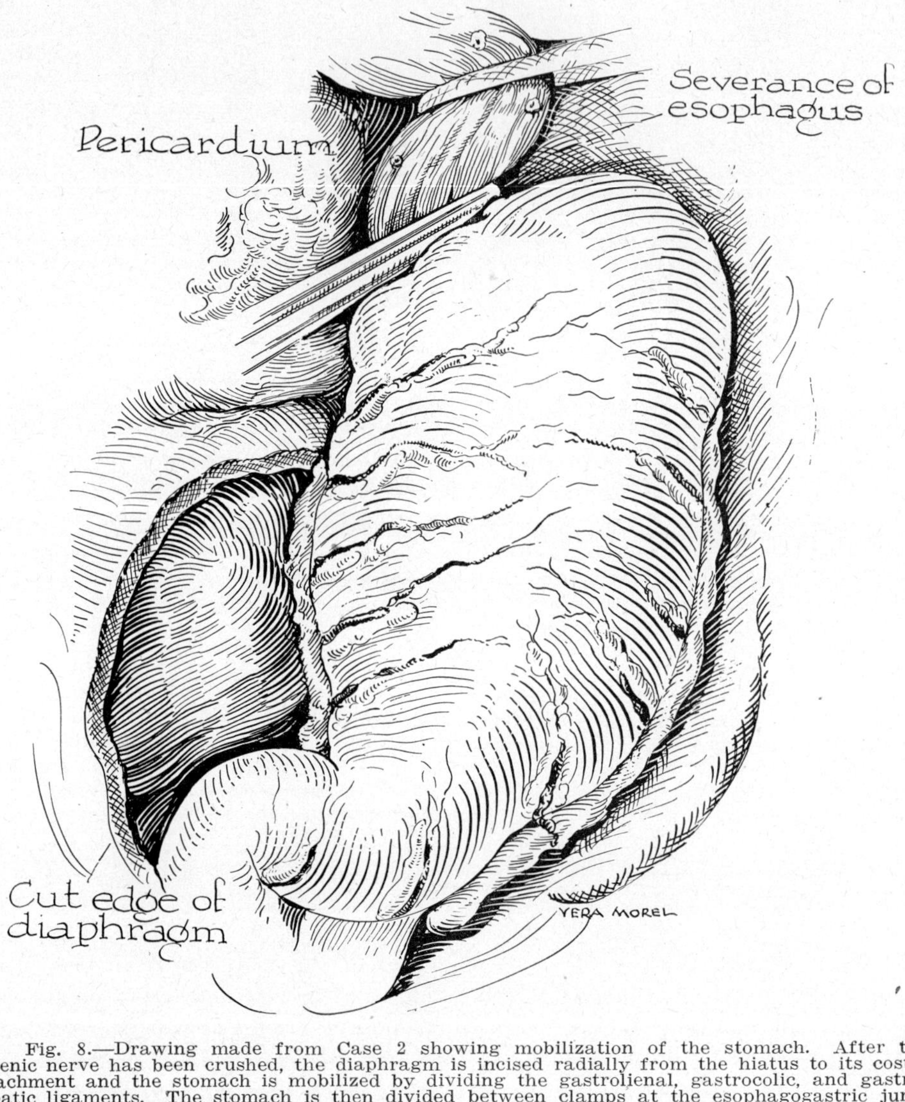

Fig. 8.—Drawing made from Case 2 showing mobilization of the stomach. After the phrenic nerve has been crushed, the diaphragm is incised radially from the hiatus to its costal attachment and the stomach is mobilized by dividing the gastrolienal, gastrocolic, and gastrohepatic ligaments. The stomach is then divided between clamps at the esophagogastric junction and the gastric stump closed by two layers of fine atraumatic catgut sutures and an inverting layer of interrupted quilting cotton sutures.

After the esophagus has been completely freed from its bed, the next step in the procedure is mobilization of the stomach (Figs. 8 and 9). After the phrenic nerve has been crushed to provide immobility of the diaphragm, the peritoneal cavity is entered through a radial incision in the diaphragm from the hiatus to its costal attachment. The stomach is mobilized by section of the gastrolienal, gastrocolic, and gastrohepatic ligaments and the vessels contained in them, care being taken to preserve the vascular arches along the greater and lesser curvatures. Division of the left gastric artery close to its origin, as recommended by Sweet, is preferred to division of its branches as proposed by Garlock. The remaining blood supply to the stomach arises from the right gastric and right gastroepiploic arteries and had proved adequate (Fig. 9).

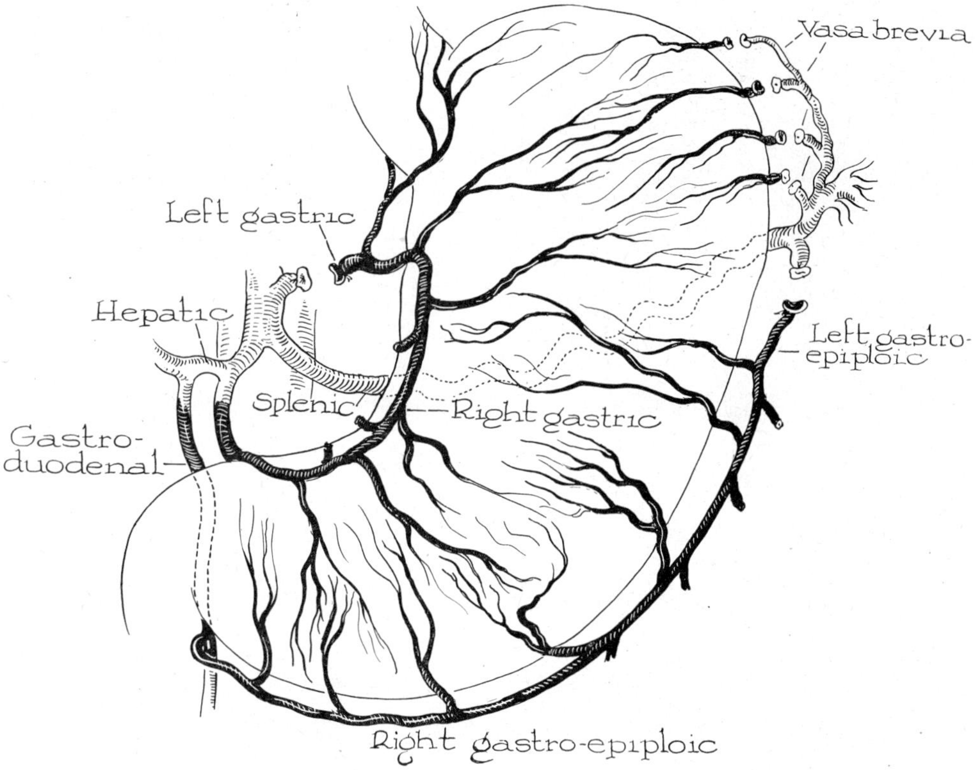

Fig. 9.—Diagrammatic drawing of blood supply of stomach showing vessels that must be ligated in mobilization of the stomach. The only remaining blood supply of the stomach arises from the right gastric and right gastroepiploic arteries (shown in black).

Obviously, this step in the operation, mobilization of the stomach, should be done gently and with a minimum of manipulative trauma in order to avoid injury or compromise of the intramural vascular integrity of the stomach. This is particularly important in freeing an adherent stomach to the abdominal wall as a result of a pre-existing gastrostomy (Case 1).

The stomach is then divided between clamps at the esophagogastric junction and the distal stump closed by two layers of fine atraumatic chromic catgut sutures and inverted by a layer of interrupted quilting cotton mattress sutures. The proximal end of the severed esophagus is covered with a rubber tampon and tied securely. The esophagus is brought out from under the aortic arch and to the left and above the aorta through the opening in the mediastinal pleura behind the left subclavian artery (Fig. 10). The stomach is brought up into the pleural cavity and attached to the pleura at the dome and along the paravertebral gutter with interrupted quilting cotton sutures. In one of our cases (Case 1), in order to permit the cardia of the stomach to be brought up to the apex of the chest without tension, it was found desirable to mobilize the pylorus and first portion of the duodenum by incision of the peritoneal covering along their lateral margins as suggested by Phemister.

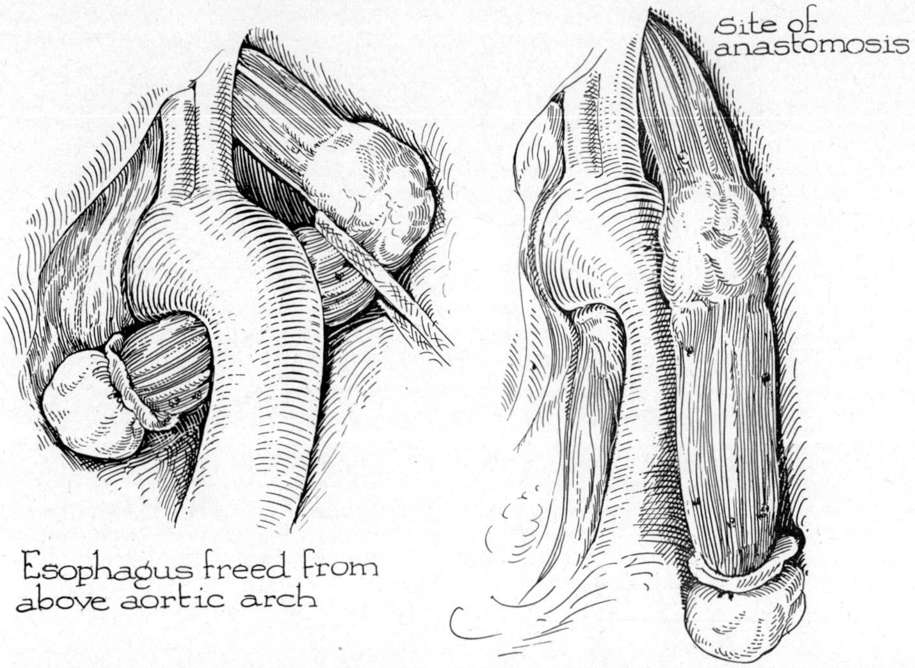

Fig. 10.—Drawing made from Case 2 showing the completely free esophagus being drawn out from under the aortic arch and to the left of the aorta through the opening in the mediastinal pleura behind the left subclavian artery. The stomach is then brought up into the pleural cavity for performance of the esophagogastric anastomosis.

The next step in the operation is performance of the esophagogastric anastomosis. This is accomplished by a two-layer row of interrupted cotton sutures, the outer layer being of a mattress type, as shown in Fig. 11. This method of anastomosis differs somewhat from those previously described and we believe has certain advantages, especially in some cases. For example, in our Case 1 the highest level at which the esophagus could be divided and at the same time provide sufficient proximal length to permit the technical performance of the anastomosis was immediately above the stricture. At this level, however, the esophagus was still somewhat narrowed and had the anastomosis been done with only the cross-sectional diameter of the esophagus the stoma would have been undesirably small. The problem was readily solved by incision of the esophagus longitudinally along its left lateral margin and performance of the anastomosis as shown in Fig. 11. This maneuver provided a much larger stoma. It is believed also to be preferable to beveling the esophageal opening for this purpose

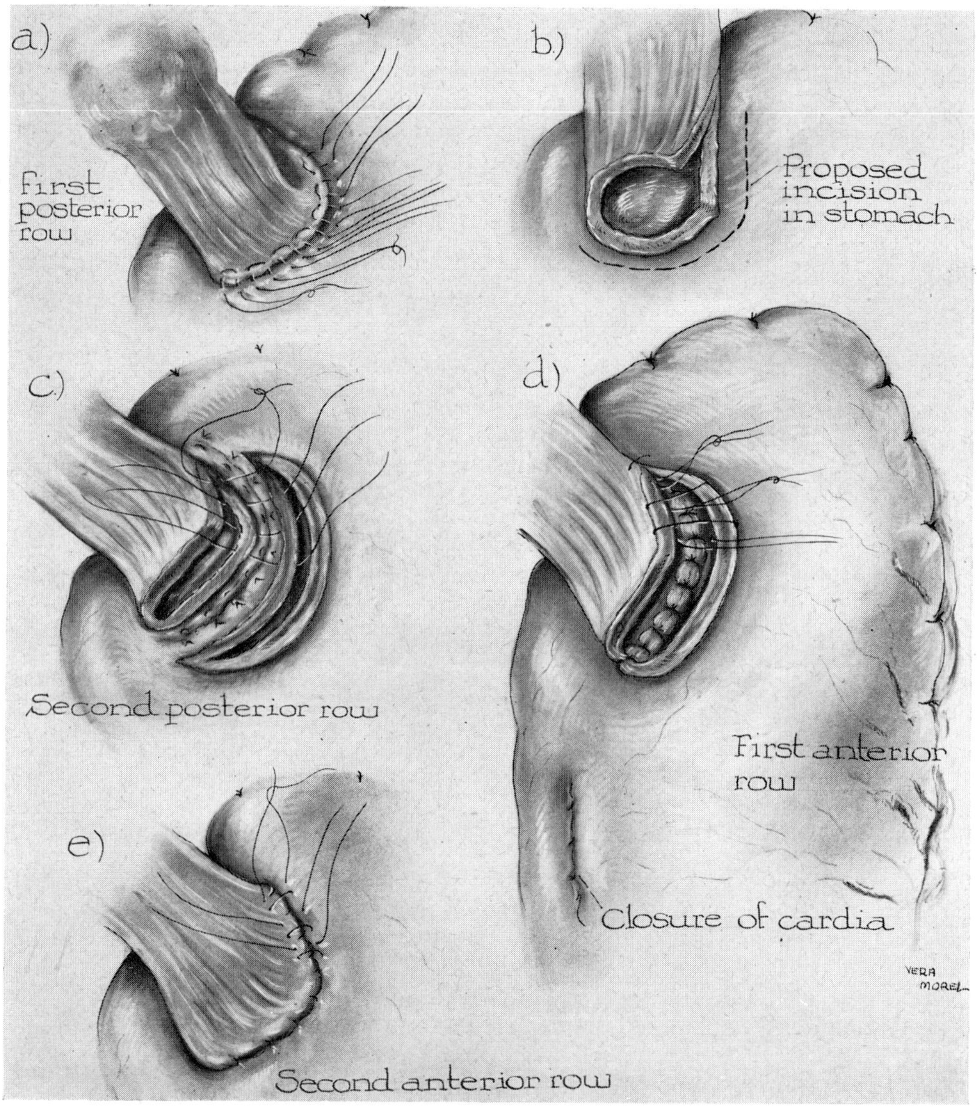

Fig. 11.—Drawing showing technique of esophagogastrostomy performed in the cases reported. (*a*) The first posterior layer of interrupted mattress sutures of quilting cotton is placed between the posterior wall of the esophagus and the anterior wall of the stomach. This layer of sutures is carried upward for a short distance along the left lateral margin of the esophagus. (*b*) The esophagus is divided just distal to the first posterior row of sutures and at right angles to its longitudinal axis and then incised longitudinally upward for a short distance along its left lateral margin paralleling the first posterior row of sutures. A comparable L-shaped opening in the stomach is then made as shown by the dotted line. (*c*) Placement of second posterior row of simple interrupted sutures of quilting cotton for careful approximation of the mucosal edges. (*d*) First anterior row of interrupted sutures to close opening, care being taken to place sutures so that knots are within the lumen as suggested by Churchill and Sweet. (*e*) Final anterior row of interrupted mattress sutures of quilting cotton. This type of anastomosis provides an L-shaped opening between the esophagus and stomach and thus increases the size of the stoma.

because it is less likely to compromise the intramural vascularity than the latter procedure. We have employed this method of anastomosis in all our cases during the past year, believing that by this means, that is, the provision of a relatively large stoma, the prevention of subsequent stricture formation can be better assured. This does not minimize the importance, however, of the gentle handling of the edges of the esophagus and stomach or the careful placement of the sutures, as emphasized by Churchill and Sweet, particularly with regard to the mucosal layers.

After the completion of the esophagogastric anastomosis the stomach is attached to the parietal pleura posteriorly with interrupted sutures (Fig. 12).

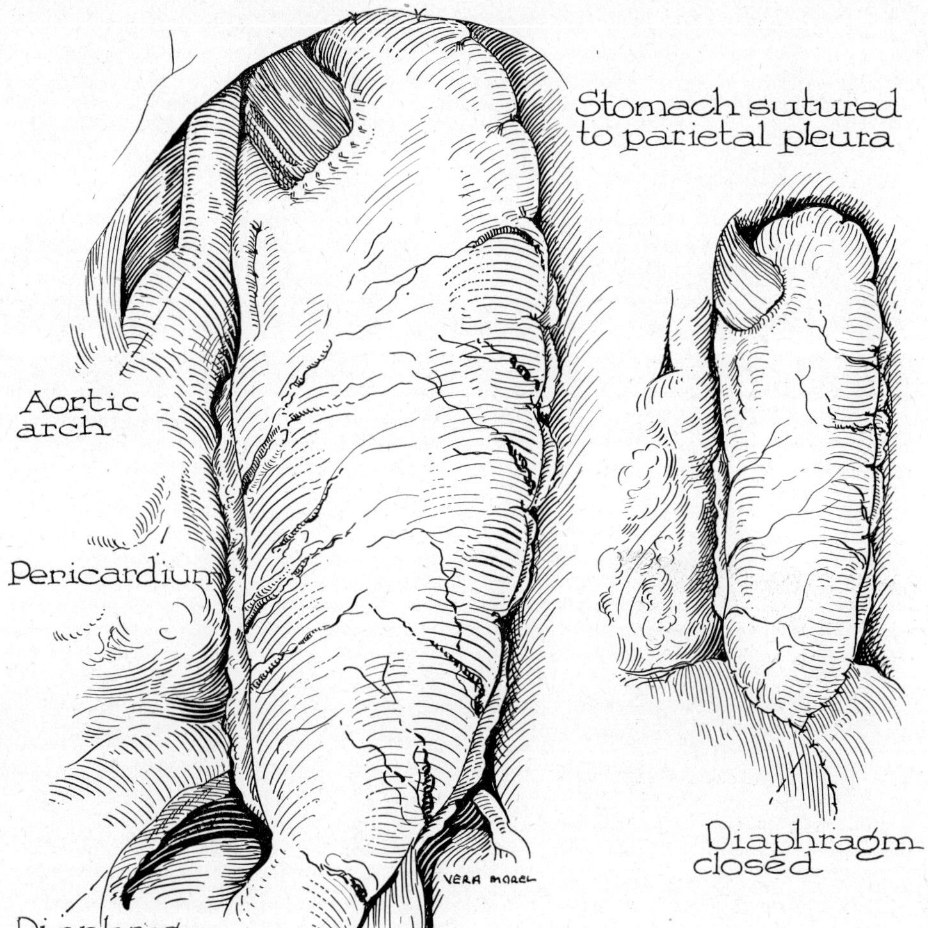

Fig. 12.—Drawing made from Case 2 showing relation of structures following completion of esophagogastric anastomosis. The stomach has been attached to the parietal pleura at the apex and along the paravertebral gutter. The diaphragm is closed by attachment of its edges around the stomach just above the pylorus and approximation of the remaining edges with interrupted cotton sutures.

The opening in the diaphragm is then closed first by attachment of its edges around the stomach just above the pylorus and then by approximation of the remaining edges anteriorly with interrupted cotton sutures. After a catheter has been inserted in the pleural cavity through one of the lower interspaces, the lung is expanded and the thoracic wall closed in layers with interrupted cotton sutures.

PREOPERATIVE AND POSTOPERATIVE MANAGEMENT

The preoperative preparation of these patients and their postoperative care require careful attention.[16] Half starved by their inability to swallow, these patients characteristically manifest obvious evidence of nutritional depletion with pronounced loss in weight, muscular weakness, vitamin deficiency, oral sepsis, and secondary anemia. Moreover, in malignant cases they are often elderly individuals with diminished cardiovascular reserve. For these reasons and because of the formidable nature of the surgical procedure, the preoperative preparation of these patients becomes particularly important. Since much emphasis has been placed upon these matters in the recent literature, their detailed discussion is considered unnecessary here.

Except in patients with complete obstruction, the restorative program can be carried out adequately by the oral administration of a properly planned liquid diet having a high caloric and vitamin content. Depending upon the indications, this can be supplemented by the parenteral administration of fluids, electrolytes, vitamins, and whole blood. Even in the presence of complete obstruction, unless the patient is in an extremely depleted state, we prefer to rely upon parenteral therapy and to avoid the use of preliminary gastrostomy or jejunostomy for feeding purposes. Increasing experience in the management of these cases has strengthened our conviction that by these measures and particularly with the ample use of blood transfusions[12] both before and during the operation, most of these patients can be safely carried through the procedure. For these reasons and because of certain disadvantages associated with the procedure, we have become increasingly reluctant to employ preliminary gastrostomy or jejunostomy.

During the course of the operation, blood is administered in amounts sufficient to compensate for blood loss and to maintain proper hemodynamic function. This will vary depending upon the patient's general condition, extent of operative trauma and manipulation, blood loss, and other factors. Thus, the amount of blood administered during the operation was 2,500 c.c. in Case 1 and 1,500 c.c. in Case 2, although the patient was younger and in better general condition in the former case than in the latter. In both cases, however, the blood pressure and the pulse rate remained well stabilized during the entire operation, which lasted six hours in the first and five in the second case.

In order to empty the esophagus and stomach and minimize soiling, an intranasal gastric tube connected to a suction apparatus should be inserted prior to the operation, preferably into the stomach but, if this is not possible, to the level of the obstruction. It should be allowed to remain in place during the procedure, maintaining continuous suction; just before the stomach is severed from the esophagus, if the tube has been passed into the stomach, it should be drawn up until its lowest end is at the level of the site of anastomosis. After the anastomosis has been completed, the tube is passed through the stoma and into the stomach for use during the early postoperative period.

Chemotherapy is administered systemically to control infection, penicillin being the preferred agent. This is begun one or two days before the operation and continued postoperatively for four or five days until the temperature remains normal for forty-eight hours.

It appears desirable to administer oxygen during the first twenty-four hours after the operation. Parenteral fluids and blood are administered postoperatively as required. The patient is allowed to drink fluids early. He can usually take a soft diet by the third and a full diet by the fifth postoperative day. During this early period frequent small feedings have been found preferable to the usual dietary regimen. Both the character and schedule of the diet during this period should be adjusted to the individual patient's tolerance. Early ambulation is considered desirable and most of these patients can be out of bed by the fifth postoperative day, unless there is some definite contraindication.

SUMMARY

The two cases of subtotal esophagectomy and esophagogastrostomy for high intrathoracic lesions described in this communication illustrate the feasibility of the performance of esophagogastric anastomosis as the highest level in the chest and demonstrate its applicability in both benign and malignant esophageal lesions. The superiority of this procedure over others which have been employed for such lesions lies in the fact that it provides immediate restoration of function.

Certain technical aspects of the operation are discussed. It is suggested that further improvement in the operative approach is desirable in order to minimize trauma and facilitate the two essential features of the operation, mobilization of the stomach and performance of the esophagogastric anastomosis. An approach directed toward this objective is proposed. A method of anastomosis is described which is believed to have some advantages over those previously employed, especially under certain conditions. Its purpose is to permit the formation of a larger stoma than that obtained by ordinary methods and thus provide greater assurance against the development of subsequent stricture.

REFERENCES

1. Adams, W. E.: Surgery of the Mediastinum, S. Clin. North America **26:** 130-142, 1946.
2. Brock, R. C.: Cardio-oesophageal Resection for Tumour of the Cardia. Report of a Successful Case, Brit. J. Surg. **30:** 146-150, 1942.
3. Carter, B. N.: The Combined Thoracicoabdominal Approach With Particular Reference to Its Employment in Splenectomy, Surg., Gynec. & Obst. **84:** 1019, 1947.
4. Churchill, E. D.: Oesophageal Surgery, Surg., Gynec. & Obst. **60:** 417-423, 1935.
5. Churchill, E. D., and Sweet, R. H.: Transthoracic Resection of Tumors of the Stomach and Esophagus, Ann. Surg. **115:** 897-920, 1942.
6. Clark, D. E.: Transthoracic Esophagogastrostomy for Carcinoma of the Middle Third of the Esophagus. Report of a Successful Resection, Ann. Surg. **121:** 65-73, 1945.
7. Garlock, J. H.: The Re-establishment of Esophagogastric Continuity Following Resection of Esophagus for Carcinoma of Middle Third, Surg., Gynec. & Obst. **78:** 23-28, 1944.
8. Garlock, J. H.: Combined Abdominothoracic Approach for Carcinoma of Cardia and Lower Esophagus, Surg., Gynec. & Obst. **83:** 737-741, 1946.

9. Garlock, J. H.: Technical Problems in the Surgical Treatment of Carcinoma of the Esophagus and Upper Stomach, J. Thoracic Surg. **16:** 215, 1947.
10. Harper, F. R.: Thoracicoabdominal Approach to the Upper Abdomen, Surg., Gynec. & Obst. **84:** 331-332, 1947.
11. Humphreys, G. H.: An Approach to Resections of the Esophagus and Gastric Cardia, Ann. Surg. **124:** 288-299, 1946.
12. Lyons, C., and Mayerson, H. S.: The Surgical Significance of Hemoglobin Deficiency in Protein Depletion, J. A. M. A. **135:** 9-11, 1947.
13. Ochsner, A., and DeBakey, M.: Surgical Aspects of Carcinoma of the Esophagus, J. Thoracic Surg. **10:** 401-445, 1941.
14. Ohsawa, T.: The Surgery of the Esophagus, Arch. f. jap. Chir. **10:** 605, 1933.
15. Phemister, D. B.: Transthoracic Resection for Cancer of the Cardiac End of the Stomach, Arch. Surg. **46:** 915-929, 1943.
16. Sweet, R. H.: Transthoracic Resection of Esophagus and Stomach for Carcinoma Analysis of the Postoperative Complications, Causes of Death, and Late Results of Operation, Ann. Surg. **121:** 272-284, 1945.
17. Sweet, R. H.: Surgical Management of Carcinoma of the Midthoracic Esophagus. Preliminary Report, New England J. Med. **223:** 1-7, 1945.
18. Sweet, R. H.: Subtotal Esophagectomy With High Intrathoracic Esophagogastric Anastomosis in the Treatment of Extensive Cicatricial Obliteration of the Esophagus, Surg., Gynec. & Obst. **83:** 417-427, 1946.
19. Sweet, R. H.: Carcinoma of the Midthoracic Esophagus; Its Treatment by Radical Resection and High Intrathoracic Esophagogastric Anastomosis, Ann. Surg. **124:** 653-666, 1946.
20. Torek, F.: First Successful Resection of Thoracic Portion of Esophagus, J. A. M. A. **60:** 1533, 1913.
21. Wu, Y. K., and Loucks, H. H.: Surgical Treatment of Carcinoma of the Esophagus, Chinese M. J. **60:** 1-33, 1941.

THE TREATMENT OF CARCINOMA OF THE ESOPHAGUS AND CARDIAC END OF THE STOMACH BY SURGICAL EXTIRPATION

Two Hundred Three Cases of Resection

Richard H. Sweet, M.D., Boston, Mass.

(From the Surgical Services of the Massachusetts General Hospital and Palmer Memorial Hospital)

WITH the exception of certain attempts to remove by local excision small lesions in the cervical segment and a few successful results following the use of the Torek operation in the thoracic portion, carcinoma of the esophagus has remained until recent years a relatively inaccessible disease. The first successful resection and esophagogastric anastomosis to be performed in this country was reported by Adams and Phemister in 1938.[1] During the ensuing decade this operation has been modified and its utilization extended so that now it can be applied in the treatment of carcinoma of the esophagus at all levels with the exception of the cervical segment, where an entirely different technique is required. Furthermore, the incidence of postoperative complications has fallen appreciably and the postoperative mortality rate has reached an acceptable level.

Success in this field of surgery depends upon the application of a detailed knowledge of anatomy and an understanding of the principles of physiology as they apply to the organs within the thoracic cavity. The esophagus traverses three important anatomic regions, the *neck,* the *thorax,* and the *abdomen.* In the neck and chest it lies in close contact with various important, even vital, structures such as the vagus nerves with their recurrent laryngeal branches, the great vessels of the carotid sheath, the aortic arch and descending aorta, the trachea, the left pulmonary artery, the left main bronchus the pericardium, the inferior pulmonary veins, the thoracic duct, and the azygos vein. Injuries to any of these structures during the operation are likely to be followed by serious inconvenience or troublesome physiologic disturbances if not by immediate or ultimate death. The esophagus furthermore must be handled with much greater care and gentleness than any other portion of the gastrointestinal tract. It lacks a serous coat. Its musculature is largely longitudinal and does not hold sutures well. The long-established principle of avoiding tension on the suture line is therefore of pre-eminent importance in any anastomosis involving this organ. Its strictly segmental blood supply must be considered in every resection in order to avoid necrosis at the suture line. It is wise never to perform an anastomosis more than 2 or 3 cm. below the next highest vessel and in every case where the dissection has been carried to a level above the arch of the aorta,

Received for publication, Feb. 18, 1948.

the anastomosis must be made at or above the level of the arch because of the fact that the only remaining arterial supply is from the inferior thyroid arteries in the neck. Fig. 1 illustrates the blood supply of the esophagus.

To these important observations must be added the fact that at least in some portions it is difficult if not impossible to carry out a wide removal of the growth and surrounding tissues. It is axiomatic in the surgery of carcinoma of any organ that in addition to the removal of a large portion of uninvolved tissue in all directions beyond the growth, it is necessary to excise en masse

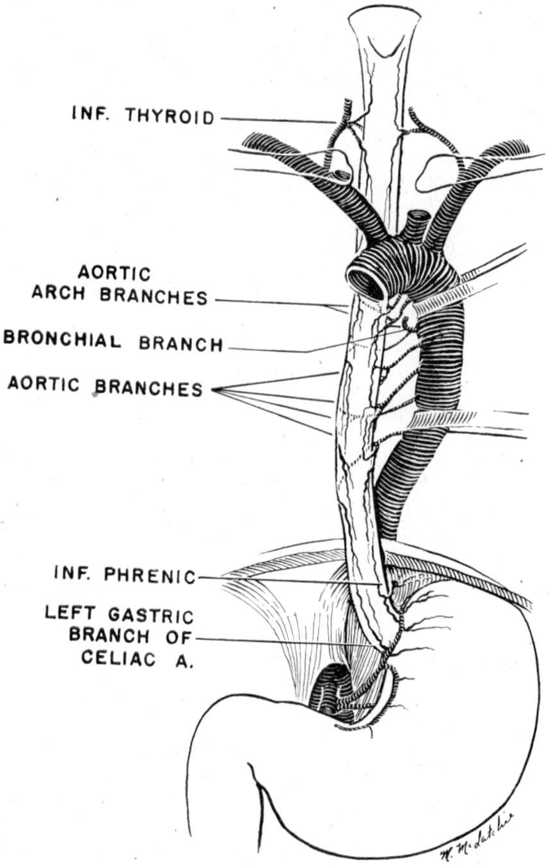

Fig. 1.—Drawing showing the segmental origin and distribution of the principal arterial blood supply to the esophagus. Several smaller vessels such as the branches from the pericardiophrenic and superior suprarenal arteries are not shown. Note: The segment between the base of the neck and the superior surface of the aortic arch depends upon branches from the inferior thyroid arteries.

with the growth-containing area as many as possible of the regional lymph nodes to which metastases may be expected to go. In this respect the esophagus presents a peculiar and varied problem. The close proximity of the organ to important anatomic structures in the neck and superior mediastinum and in the region of the aortic arch and hilum of the lung makes it difficult if not impossible to remove an adequate amount of periesophageal tissues and regional lymph nodes when the growth arises in any of these regions. From the level of the hilum of the lung down to the cardia, however, it becomes increasingly possible to perform a satisfactory cancer operation with the removal of larger numbers of the regional nodes. These facts inevitably have a definite bearing upon the end results obtained after surgical extirpation. Reference to Fig. 2 serves to illustrate the most important lymph node groups which are frequently invaded by metastases from carcinoma of the esophagus.

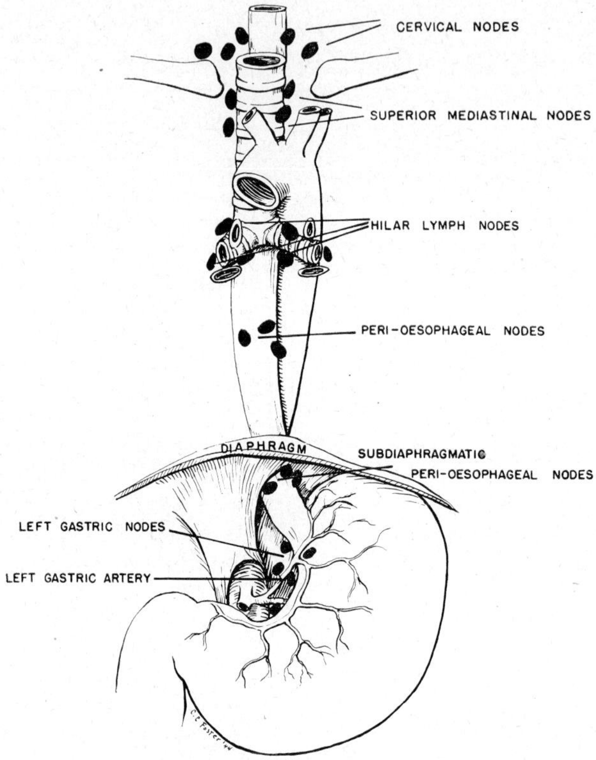

Fig. 2.—Marks show the most frequent sites of lymph node metastases from carcinoma of the esophagus.

THE APPLICATION OF SURGERY IN THE TREATMENT OF CARCINOMA OF VARIOUS SEGMENTS OF THE ESOPHAGUS

The technical problem presented by a carcinoma of the esophagus varies according to the region where the tumor lies. It is necessary, therefore, to give separate consideration to the various levels (Fig. 3). In the cervical segment the restoration of continuity after resection depends upon the substitution of a turned-in portion of skin for the excised portion of esophagus. This is accomplished by the method described by Wookey.[2] In the thoracic segment, three different modifications of the operation of partial esophagectomy with primary esophagogastric anastomosis must be used, depending upon the location of the growth. If the tumor lies in the upper fourth (or superior mediastinal segment), a very difficult obstacle to be overcome is the passage of the mobilized stomach through the apex of the chest into the neck. A technique to accomplish this has been developed very recently.[3] This involves performing an intracervical esophagogastric anastomosis. When the growth involves the middle half of the thoracic segment of the esophagus, a high intrathoracic esophagogastric anastomosis must be made. Two modifications of this procedure are required, depending upon the relation of the tumor to the aortic arch. In some cases because of the high location of the growth the anastomosis must be made above the arch. In others where the growth lies in the lower portion of the middle half, it is possible to make it just below the aortic arch. In the lower fourth of the thoracic segment and in the abdominal segment, a low intrathoracic anastomosis is performed.

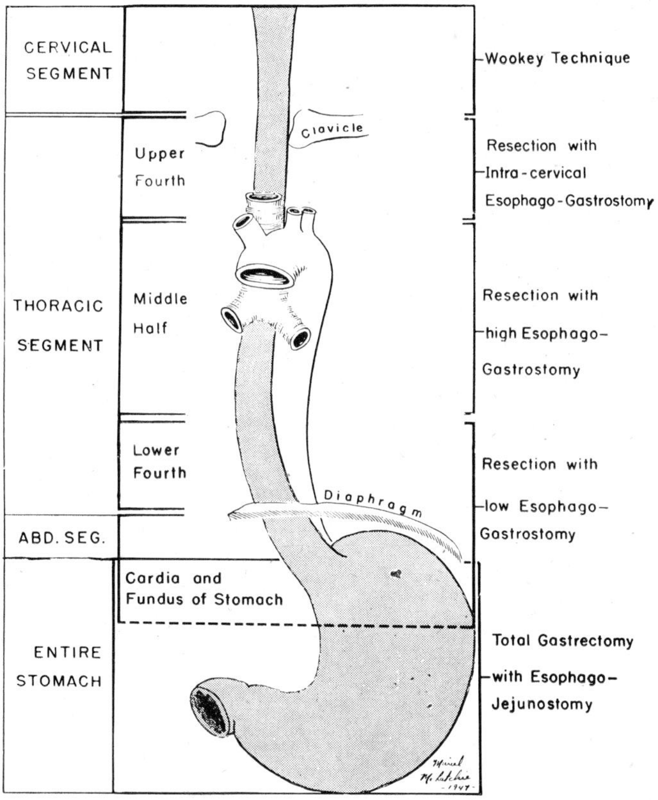

Fig. 3.—Anatomic regions of the esophagus and cardiac end of the stomach illustrated to facilitate the understanding of the technical problems involved in the surgical management of carcinoma arising at various levels.

Carcinoma of the Cervical Segment of the Esophagus.—The cervical segment of the esophagus is short, extending from the hypopharynx to the level of the suprasternal notch. It lies directly behind the larynx and trachea. It is bounded laterally by the carotid sheath and its contents and the lobe of the thyroid gland on each side of the neck. It is crossed by the recurrent laryngeal nerves and the superior and inferior thyroid arteries. A large group of lymph nodes lies in close apposition to it on each side. This group of nodes communicates with other cervical nodes and with the nodes in the superior mediastinum. It is a frequent occurrence to find a large number of these nodes involved in metastases from a carcinoma arising in this region. Thus a large portion of the carcinomas of the cervical segment are inoperable or at least incurable when seen for the first time by the surgeon. In the earlier more favorable

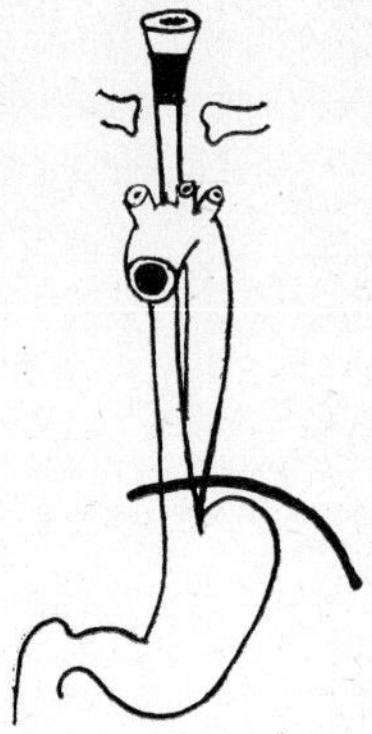

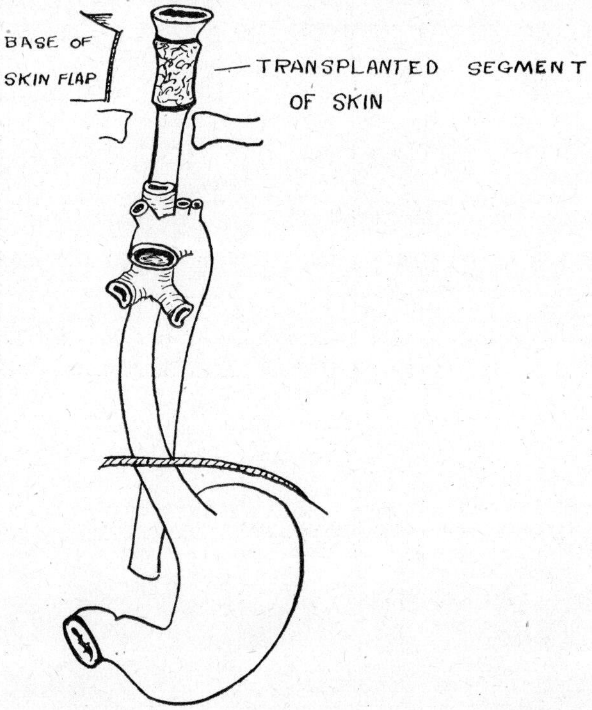

Fig. 4.—Drawing showing the principle of the Wookey operation for resection of the cervical segment of the esophagus with the substitution of a flap of skin from the neck to restore continuity. The base of the skin flap and the transplanted segment are shown diagrammatically. Insert gives in black the region in the esophagus where this operation should be applied.

cases the growth can be resected and the resulting defect bridged with a skin tube constructed from the skin of the neck. The operation described by Wookey[2] which makes this performance possible is brilliantly conceived. It is performed in two stages. The first consists in the resection of the cervical segment of the esophagus and the turning-in of a rectangular flap consisting of skin, subcutaneous fat, and platysma muscle. This flap is sutured to the hypopharynx above and to the distal esophagus below, leaving a temporary lateral groove. At the second stage of the operation, which is performed several weeks later, the lateral groove is closed so as to restore completely the continuity of the esophagus (Fig. 4). The immediate results of this operation are highly successful (Fig. 5). The patient is able to swallow without any functional difficulties and with no discomfort. It is a serious fault of the procedure, however, that it cannot be made to include a wide regional dissection with the removal of the neighboring lymph nodes. The result of this drawback is that although from the standpoint of restoration of function it is

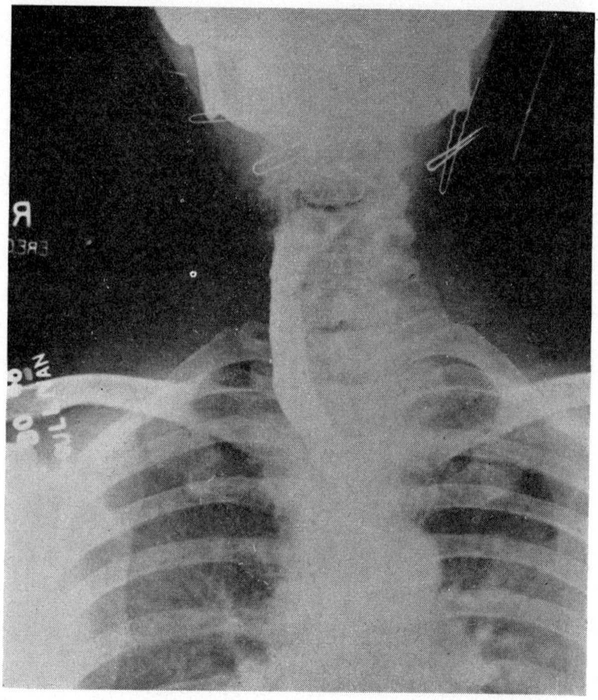

Fig. 5 (Case M. O'S.).—Roentgenogram showing ingested barium passing through the tube constructed from the skin of the neck by the Wookey technique. Film obtained a few weeks after completion of the second stage.

nearly perfect, the operation is in the great majority of cases a failure as a method of cure. I have used it in seven cases with excellent immediate results. In each case, however, sometime from six months to a year after the operation a local recurrence or, more often, evidence of cervical lymph node metastases has been observed. With the exception of one patient who is still alive with extensive metastatic disease in the cervical lymph nodes, all have died (Fig. 6, *A* and *B*). This result, although not surprising, is a great disappointment, but in view of the anatomic and technical aspects of the problem, it is difficult to conceive how a more favorable outcome could be insured. The usefulness of the Wookey operation would seem, therefore, to be confined to the rare early case of carcinoma of the cervical segment with a low-grade malignancy.

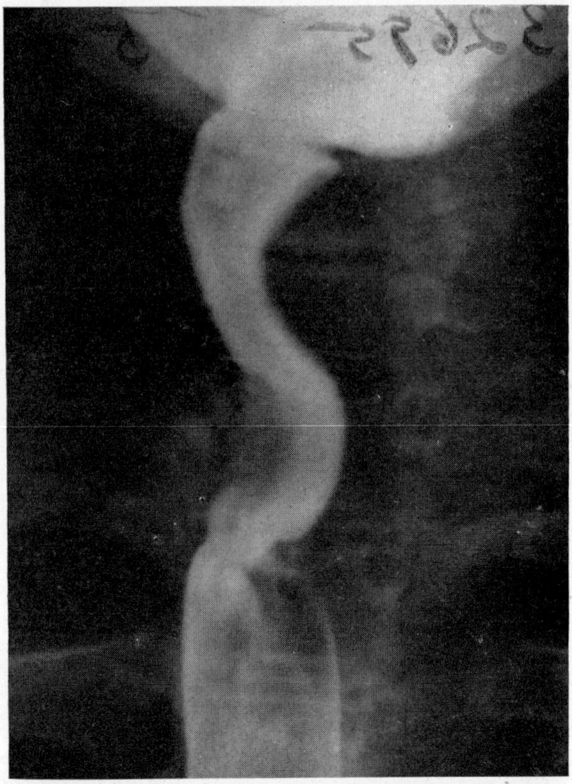

A.

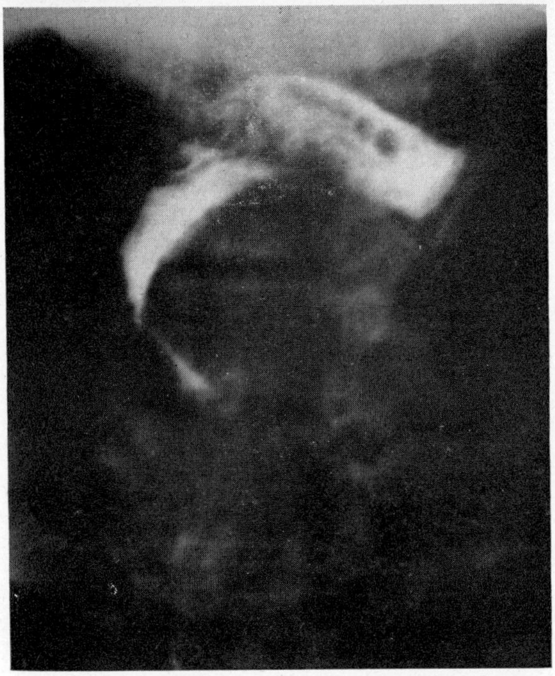

B.

Fig. 6 (Case L. R.).—*A*, Roentgenogram obtained ten months after successful completion of Wookey operation, showing first evidence of filling defect produced by recurrent or metastatic carcinoma in the adjacent region of the neck. *B*, Fifteen months after original operation, illustrating the complete obstruction which developed as a result of the recurrent disease.

Carcinoma of the Thoracic Segment.—

Upper fourth—resection with primary intracervical esophagogastrostomy (Fig. 7): A carcinoma located in the upper fourth of the thoracic segment of the esophagus has until recently presented an insurmountable difficulty. It lies obviously too low for the use of the Wookey operation and too high for the performance of an intrathoracic esophagogastric anastmosis. Recently a new

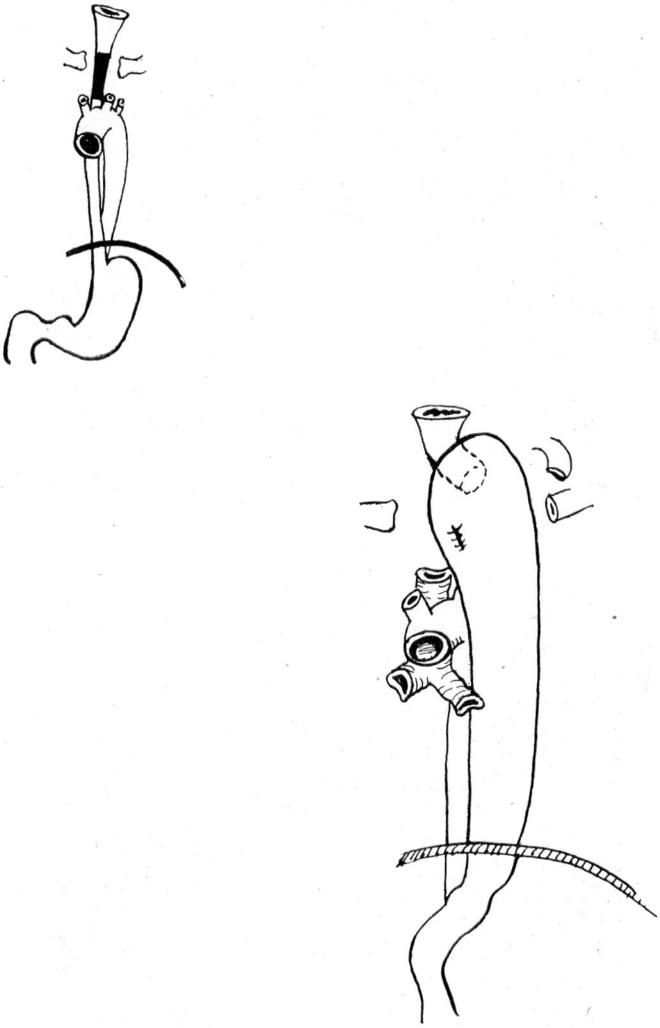

Fig. 7.—Drawing showing the arrangement of the viscera after completion of the resection of carcinoma of the superior mediastinal segment with an intracervical esophagogastric anastomosis. Insert shows the region in the esophagus which requires the use of this procedure. Note: The anastomosis shown in dotted line is on the posterior surface of the fundus. The cut ends of the left clavicle and first rib are shown.

procedure has been applied successfully in the resection of a carcinoma in this region. This operation, which is performed in one stage, involves the making of two incisions. The first is the usual left thoracotomy incision through which the entire esophagus from the base of the neck to the cardia is dissected free

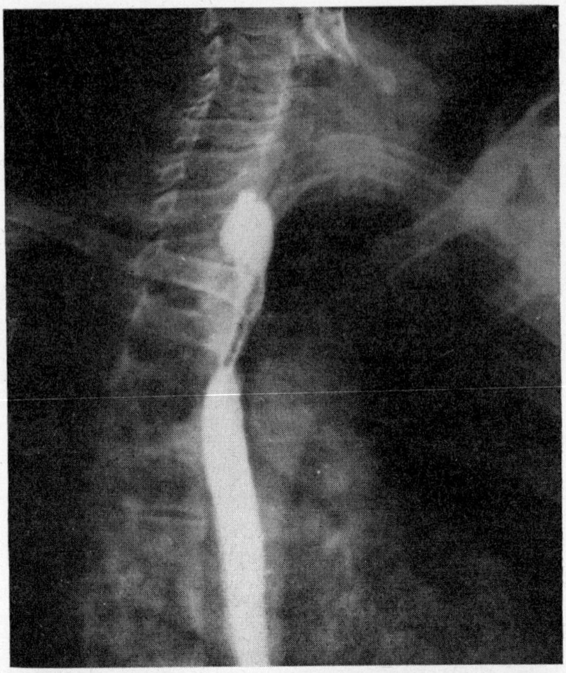

A.

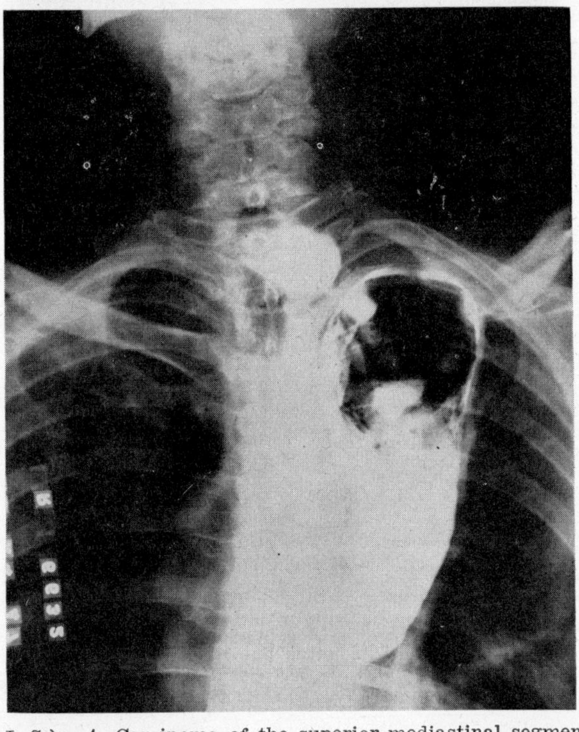

B.

Fig. 8 (Case J. S.).—*A*, Carcinoma of the superior mediastinal segment of the esophagus. Preoperative roentgenogram showing the filling defect outlined by ingested barium. *B*, Postoperative roentgenogram showing the new location of the stomach with its fundus in the neck, the short proximal portion of the esophagus, and the anastomosis several centimeters above the level of the suprasternal notch.

and the stomach completely mobilized. The stomach is pulled up high in the chest and the thoracic incision is closed. The second part of the operation is performed through an anterior incision over the lower cervical and upper sternal regions. Through this incision the inner half of the left clavicle and a corresponding segment of the left first rib are resected. The pleural cavity is then entered, the fundus of the stomach is drawn up, and an esophagogastric anastomosis is performed within the neck above the level of the clavicle. A detailed description of the procedure is reported elsewhere.[3]

The operation has been used in one case so far. It is subject to the limitation that it is not possible to perform a wide regional dissection in the region of the growth, but it offers promise of being the most effective method of palliation in the treatment of the relatively few patients whose misfortune it is to have a carcinoma in this region (Fig. 8, *A* and *B*).

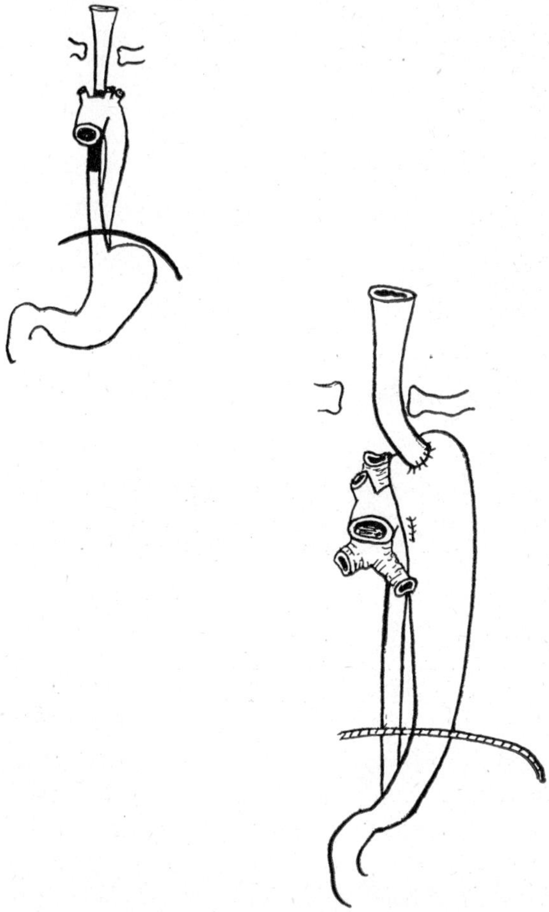

Fig. 9.—Drawing showing arrangement of the viscera after resection of a carcinoma of the upper portion of the middle half of the thoracic segment of the esophagus with a supra-aortic arch anastomosis. The stomach lies anterior to and to the left of the aortic arch. The anastomosis is made at the apex of the fundus of the stomach. The closed-over cardia is shown. Insert shows the level of growth where this procedure is required.

Middle half—resection with primary high intrathoracic esophagogastrostomy: The middle half of the esophagus comprises two regions, each with a different relation to the aortic arch. The first extends from the level of the superior margin of the aortic arch to a point several centimeters below its inferior margin. A growth in this portion of the esophagus lies at least in part behind the aortic arch and in such a case it is necessary to carry the dissection above the level of the arch to make it possible to pull the esophagus up over the arch for the performance of a supra-aortic esophagogastric anastomosis high in the chest. Fig. 9 illustrates the anatomic relations in such a case and Fig. 10, *A* and *B* shows the preoperative and postoperative roentgen-ray appearance in a patient who was operated upon for a carcinoma in this region.

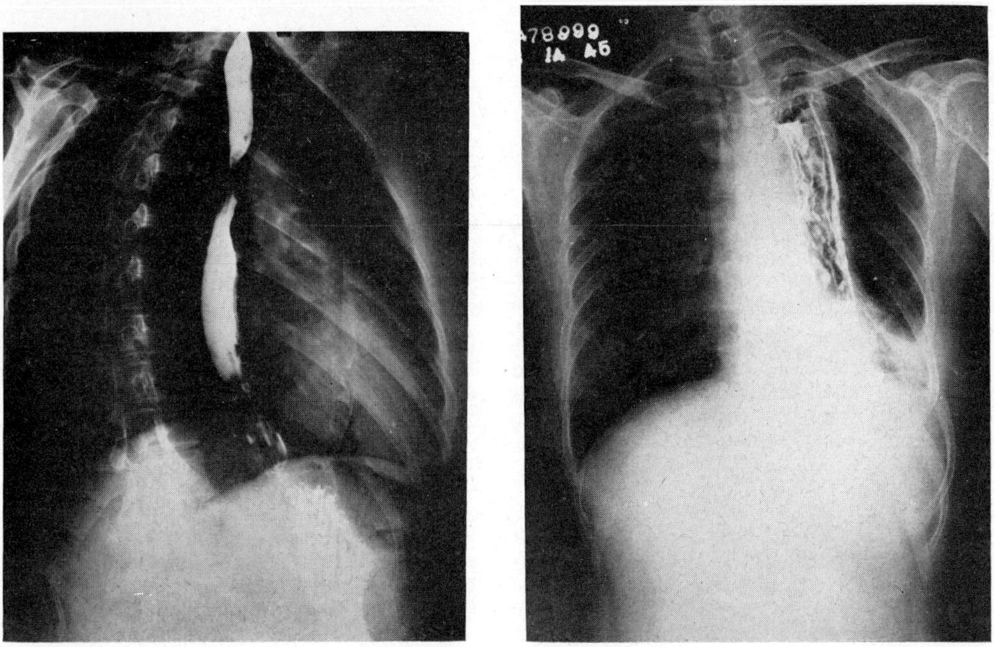

A. *B.*

Fig. 10 (Case P. T.).—*A*, Carcinoma of the midthoracic segment of the esophagus extending behind the aortic arch. Preoperative roentgenogram showing the appearance caused by the growth after ingestion of barium. *B*, Postoperative roentgenogram showing the stomach lying in the left hemithorax with the apex of the fundus in the dome of the pleural cavity above the level of the clavicle. The anastomosis lies at the level of the sternoclavicular articulation.

The second region in the middle half of the thoracic segment of the esophagus extends from several centimeters below the inferior margin of the aortic arch to the level of the inferior pulmonary vein. In such a case, although a high esophagogastric anastomosis is required, there is enough normal esophagus below the aortic arch to make it possible to perform the anastomosis just below the arch (Fig. 11). If it is at all possible, it is wise to make the anastomosis at this level instead of above the arch because of the lower postoperative mortality (19 per cent as compared to 24 per cent[6] and the lower incidence of postoperative complications. It is not to be assumed, however, that an anastomosis at the infraaortic arch level is easier to perform. It is actually often more difficult than the average supra-aortic anastomosis because of the limited space, bounded by the aortic arch above the hilum of the lung anteriorly, and the descending aorta posteriorly, in which the anastomosis must be made.

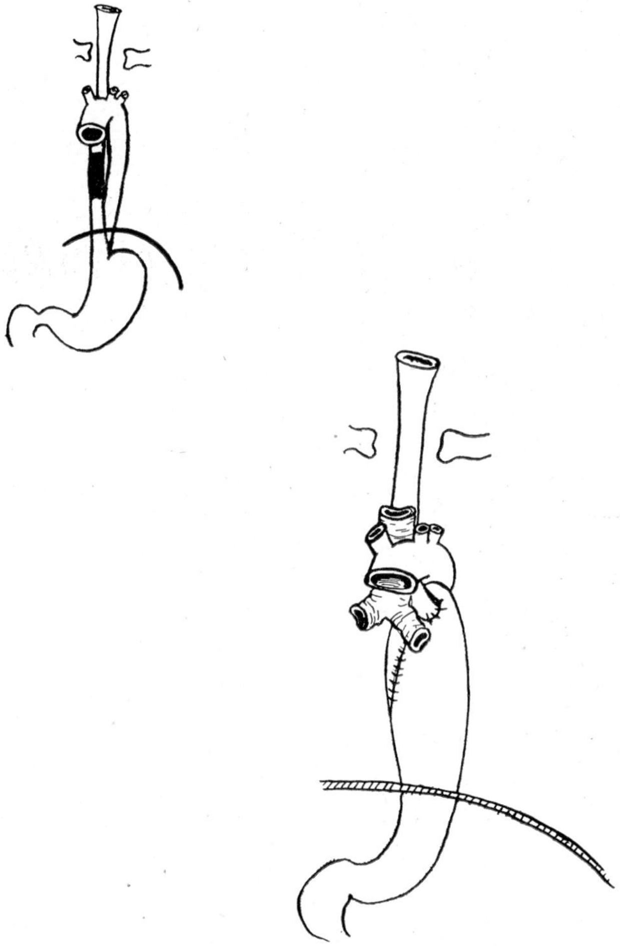

Fig. 11.—Drawing showing relations of the viscera after resection of a carcinoma of the lower portion of the midthoracic segment of the esophagus. In such a case a portion of the fundus is removed along with the cardia and the upper portion of the lesser curvature which must be removed to excise the lymph nodes which lie in relation to the left gastric vessels. The anastomosis lies just below the aortic arch. Insert shows the location of a growth after removal of which the anastomosis can be made at this level.

Fig. 12, *A* and *B* represents the preoperative and postoperative roentgenograms of a patient in whom the growth lay in the lower portion of the middle half of the thoracic segment.

Lower fourth of the thoracic segment and the abdominal segment—resection with primary low intrathoracic esophagogastrostomy (Fig. 13): A carcinoma in the lower fourth of the thoracic segment of the esophagus or in the relatively short abdominal segment lends itself to resection by the technique used for carcinoma of the cardiac end of the stomach. In fact in a large proportion of the cases of carcinoma located in the lower end of the esophagus, the growth actually invades the cardia as well. Of all cases of carcinoma at the cardia approximately 20 per cent are of this type, arising in the lower esophagus and invading the cardia. These tumors are of the squamous-cell variety. The remaining 80 per cent of cases of carcinoma of the cardia invade the esophagus as well in the

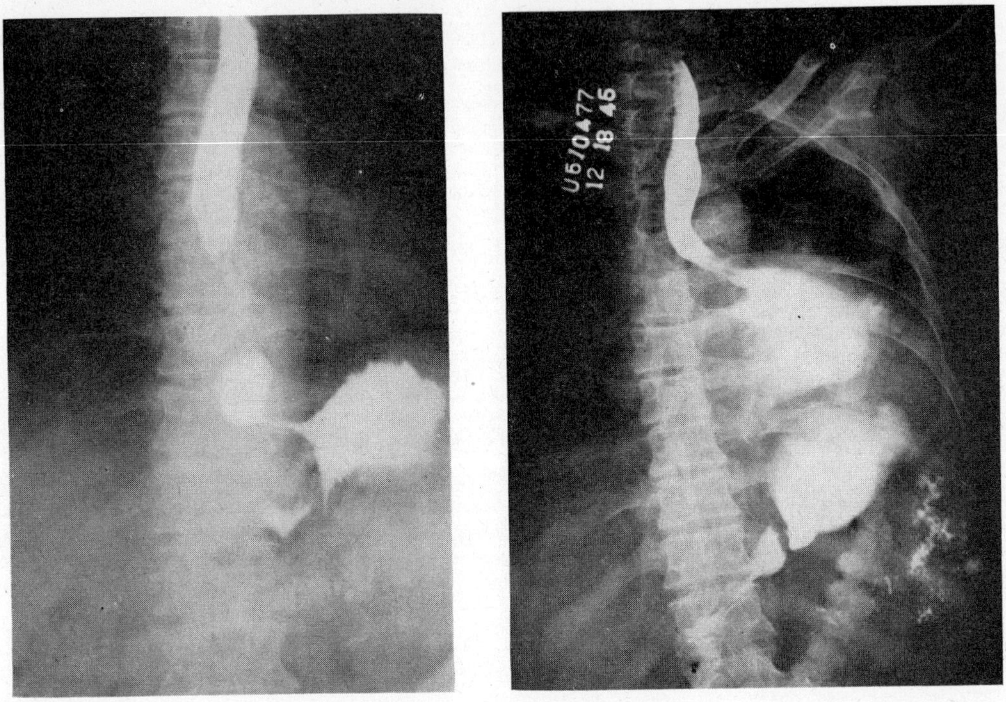

A. *B.*

Fig. 12 (Case H. S.).—*A*, Carcinoma involving the lower portion of the middle half and a portion of the lower fourth of the thoracic segment of the esophagus. Preoperative roentgenogram after ingestion of barium; large filling defect shown. *B*, Postoperative roentgenogram after the ingestion of barium, showing anastomosis just beneath the aortic arch.

great majority of instances, although they are all primarily gastric in origin and adenocarcinomas histologically. From the standpoint of the operative technique it is unimportant to distinguish between these types of cases on the basis of the exact origin of the tumor. In all cases a transthoracic partial gastrectomy and esophagectomy followed by a low intrathoracic esophagogastric anastomosis are performed. (Fig. 13.)

It has been suggested that the epidermoid lesions of purely esophageal origin ought to present a better prognosis when it comes to ultimate survival than the adenocarcinomatous lesions of gastric origin. A careful study of end results of two such groups failed to show any significant difference between the three-year survival rates of both groups. Subsequent investigations based upon larger groups of cases will be made, but there is little to suggest at the present time that any difference is to be anticipated.

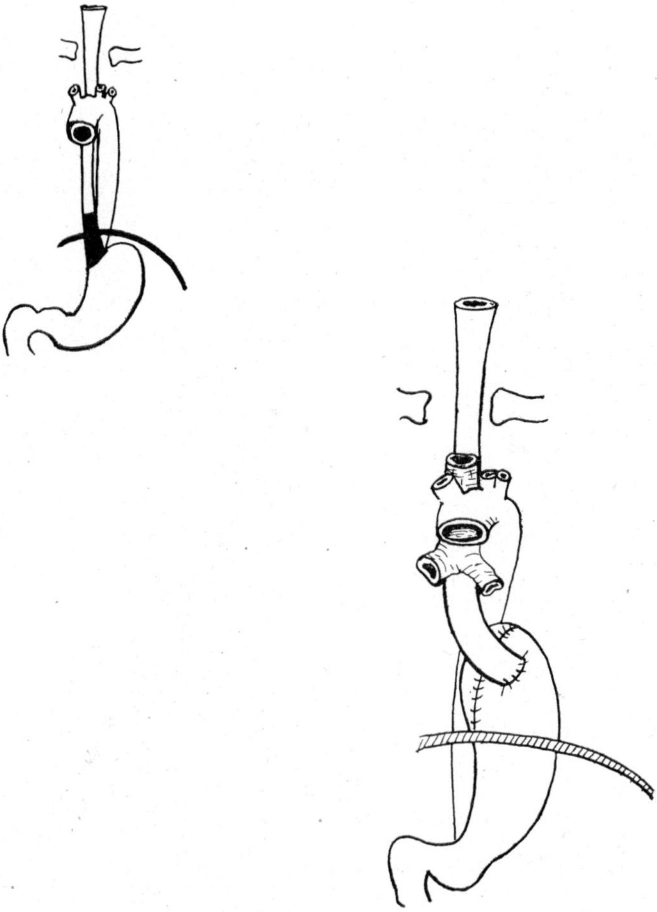

Fig. 13.—Drawing showing relations of the viscera after resection of a carcinoma of the lower fourth of the thoracic segment and the abdominal segment of the esophagus. The proximal esophagus is relatively long and a large segment of the stomach including the lesser curvature, cardia, and fundus has been resected. The anastomosis lies in the lower portion of the mediastinum at or just below the level of the inferior pulmonary veins. Insert shows the location of the tumor in such a case.

Fig. 14, *A* and *B* represents preoperative and postoperative roentgenograms in the case of a patient with carcinoma of the lower esophagus treated by resection and low intrathoracic esophagogastric anastomosis.

TECHNIQUE OF THE OPERATION

The technical details which must be observed in the surgical management of carcinoma of the esophagus have been described elsewhere[2-5] and need not be repeated here. No important changes have been made excepting the modification of the operation of resection with primary esophagogastric anastomosis which has been applied to the difficult problem of carcinoma in the upper fourth of the thoracic segment.[3]

POSTOPERATIVE COMPLICATIONS AND MORTALITY

Since the advent of the antibiotics, the postoperative occurrence of infection which was formerly the most frequent complication has been practically eliminated. Furthermore, by exerting special precautions against the development of cardiac arrhythmias and the occurrence of congestive failure, considerable progress has been made recently in reducing the incidence of cardiac complications which had become the most frequent after the elimination of the element of infection. A detailed report dealing with the incidence of postoperative complications and the causes of death during the immediate postoperative period has been made elsewhere.[6]

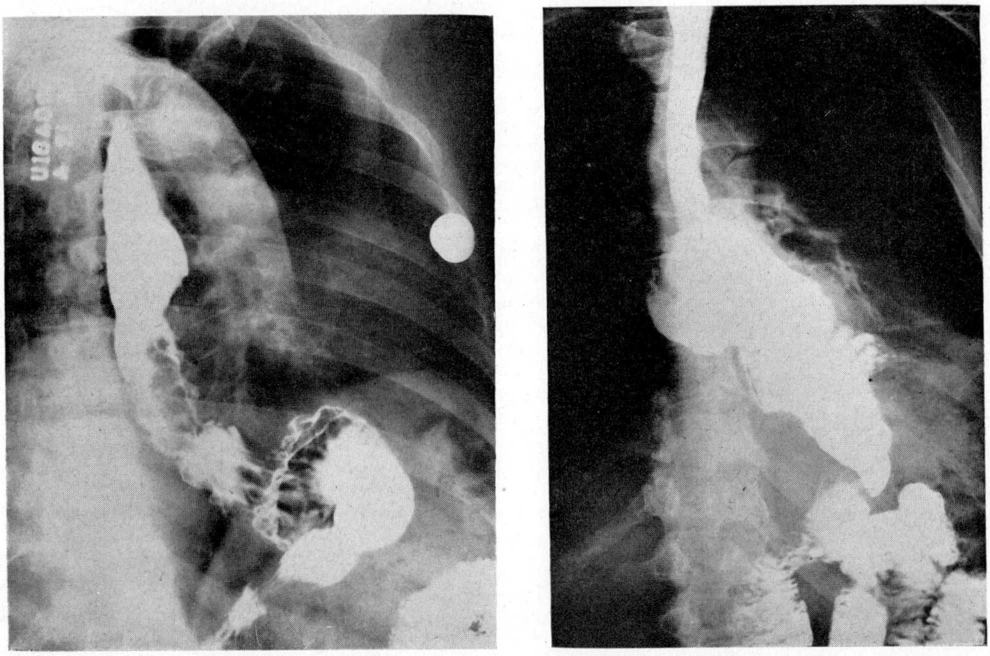

A. *B.*

Fig. 14 (Case J. W.).—*A*, Carcinoma involving the lower fourth of the thoracic segment and the abdominal segment of the esophagus. Preoperative roentgenogram showing the outline of the growth produced by the ingestion of barium. An unusually large polypoid tumor, histologically adenocarcinoma, arising in gastric mucosa within the lower esophagus. *B*, Postoperative roentgenogram after ingestion of barium, showing the esophagus and the distal portion of the stomach. The anastomosis is well demonstrated.

MANAGEMENT OF THE CONVALESCENT PERIOD

During the three years which have elapsed since the last detailed discussion of the postoperative care after esophagectomy was presented,[7] certain changes have been made which make it worth while to outline the present-day routine.

Early Postoperative Period.—

Administration of antibiotics: After the completion of the anastomosis, 60 c.c. of a solution containing 100,000 units of penicillin and 1 Gm. of streptomycin are instilled, one-half in the upper abdomen and the other half in the mediastinum and thoracic cavity. The administration of these agents is then continued by intramuscular injection during the first five days after operation or until any suspicion of infection has subsided. The dosage used at present is 0.5 Gm. of streptomycin and 100,000 units of penicillin administered intramuscularly every eight hours.

The results of the adoption of this medication have been very striking. Whereas the occurrence of sepsis was at first the principal source of postoperative complications even when the sulfonamides were used, after the administration of penicillin alone was begun the occurrence of infection was reduced to a very occasional loculated small empyema, in every instance confined to the high anastomosis cases. Since the addition of streptomycin as a part of the routine antibiotic administration, there have been no cases of infection of any kind in over one year. This involves fifty-two consecutive cases of carcinoma at all levels.

Use of sulfonamides: The administration of sulfonamides has been abandoned since the adoption of the use of penicillin and streptomycin. This is because in the first place they are not as effective as the antibiotics, and in the second place their use may be dangerous, especially in the group of elderly patients which comprises the largest number of cases of carcinoma of the esophagus.

Use of oxygen: During the past three years the method of administering oxygen postoperatively has been changed from the use of an oxygen tent to the intranasal insufflation method through an inlying nasal catheter. This method is not only more efficient but is better tolerated by the majority of patients and eases the nursing problem considerably. The administration of oxygen after esophagectomy need not be continued more than twenty-four hours in the average case. In the high-lying tumor cases, however, where the anastomosis must be made above the aortic arch, the large incision required and the extensive dissection within the mediastinum as well as the presence of almost the entire stomach within the left thoracic cavity make the readjustment of the respiratory and circulatory functions more difficult. In such cases the inhalation of oxygen may have to be continued at least intermittently for four to five days.

Aspiration of the esophagus and stomach: Continuous suction on an inlying Levine tube inserted with its tip just above the level of the growth is used during the course of the operation. The tube is removed, however, as soon as the patient regains consciousness. It is rarely necessary to reinsert a Levine tube although in the high supra-aortic anastomosis cases aspiration of an overdistended stomach may occasionally be required to overcome respiratory embarrassment. The tube should not be left lying through the anastomotic stoma for any long period of time because of the danger of its interference with the prompt healing of the anastomosis.

Aspiration of the thoracic cavity: Just before the closure of the thoracic incision is begun, a catheter of large caliber (No. 26F) is led out through one of the lower interspaces. A Foley catheter with an inflatable rubber bag near the tip is very convenient for this purpose. A few hours after the completion of the operation, continuous suction of not over 8 to 10 cm. of water is applied to the end of the catheter. The maximum effusion of serosanguineous fluid occurs during the first twenty-four hours. During the second twenty-four hours there is relatively little drainage, and in the majority of cases the catheter can be removed after the expiration of forty-eight hours from the time of the operation. Subsequent removal of fluid by thoracentesis is rarely necessary since the routine use of antibiotics has overcome the element of infection, the onset of which was always heralded by the reaccumulation of a large amount of fluid after the first effusion was over.

Cardiac regimen and medication: A low sodium dietary regimen which is begun one week before the operation is continued after operation to diminish the tendency of the tissues to retain too much fluid which might otherwise lead to the development of pulmonary edema. All patients are seen in consultation by a cardiologist, and pre- and postoperative administration of digitalis if indicated and quinidine in all cases is supervised by him. Since these measures have been adopted, there has been a striking reduction in the incidence of alarming cardiac arrhythmias on the operating table and during the early postoperative period and of congestive failure during the first few days after operation. In spite of these measures the administration of fluids intravenously must be carried out with special care to avoid giving excessive amounts and too rapid flow.

Maintenance of nutrition and oral feeding: During the first few days the patient's requirements of food and fluid are maintained almost entirely by intravenous alimentation. By this means glucose, amino acids, vitamins, and whole blood if indicated are administered taking care always to avoid embarrassment of the circulatory system as mentioned previously.

Oral administration of fluids is begun after twenty-four hours with 30 c.c. of water given each hour. The second day after operation 60 c.c. of clear fluids, not including fruit juices, may be given hourly. It is unwise to increase this amount, however, on the third day or even in some cases on the fourth. By the fifth postoperative day liquids made with milk may be added and slightly larger amounts administered at a time. From that day on the amount and character of the feedings can be adjusted to suit the abilities of the patient to take them. The patient should not be urged to eat, however, until he feels the inclination to do so or at least until after the expiration of ten to twelve days when the danger of overloading the stomach is not great. The majority of patients, however, are able to eat a six-meal soft solid diet by the twelfth postoperative day.

Early ambulation: The majority of patients who have had an esophagectomy are well enough to get up from bed on the second postoperative day. Many of them are allowed to begin ambulation on the first day after operation. A few patients, however, must be kept in bed four or five days before the readjustment of the respiratory and circulatory functions is sufficiently well established to allow greater activity. This rule applies almost exclusively to the patients with a growth which necessitates the performance of a high supra-aortic arch anastomosis.

The Late Recovery Period.—The majority of patients on whom an esophagectomy has been performed (excluding the cervical segment cases) are able to return home within two to three weeks after operation, depending upon the distance to be traveled and the possibilities of care at home. Then there is a period of readjustment which may present difficulties and lead to anxieties from which the surgeon should seek to protect the patient by explanation and advice.

Functional disturbances of the gastrointestinal tract: In common with patients who have been subjected to a total gastrectomy, patients who have had operations of the sort described frequently complain that they do not regain a normal appetite. This may correct itself after weeks or months have elapsed, but in many cases the return of appetite is incomplete at best. This occurrence is associated with and possibly explained in part by the fact that many patients experience a functional delay in the emptying time of the stomach. The interruption of the vagus nerves is a contributing factor because of the resulting diminution in the amplitude of the gastric peristaltic activity and because of the hypertonicity of the pyloric sphincter. The result is that the stomach remains partially filled much of the time. It is a common observation among these patients that they are able to eat a large breakfast, but that they have little appetite for their noonday meal and are able to accommodate hardly any of their supper. This functional difficulty is most pronounced in the cases with carcinoma of the cardia which require excision of large segments of the stomach leaving only a small distal portion which accomodates a limited volume of food. It has been observed, however, that pronounced examples of the inability of the stomach to empty after the performance of a partial gastrectomy and esophagectomy have become much less frequent than formerly and that the difficulty arises least often in patients who have had a high esophagectomy. A possible explanation for this is that the division of the gastrocolic and gastrohepatic ligaments is now carried all the way to the level of the pylorus in every case, thus probably interrupting many of the sympathetic nerve fibers which would otherwise be overactive because of the absence of the vagus inhibition.

In evaluating the postoperative digestive function of these patients it should be kept in mind also that except in the case of lesions high in the esophagus where the whole stomach is preserved, it is necessary to resect portions of the fundus of the stomach. In some cases this causes a very large reduction in gastric volume which further limits the capacity of the patient to take food.

The inability of patients to handle large quantities of food during the first few months of their convalescence is sometimes so great that there is a progressive loss of weight. Such patients should be advised to take nothing but the most nourishing types of food and to avoid wasting valuable space on materials, either liquid or solid, which have a low caloric content. As time goes on, however, in the majority of cases the patient's capacity for food increases as the gastric remnant enlarges and the emptying time of the stomach approximates a normal rate. In spite of this it is unusual for the patient to regain his customary weight. More often he will gain a few pounds, or in many cases he will be able merely to hold his weight at a reduced level without further loss.

It is interesting to note that although it is frequently necessary to ligate the thoracic duct, particularly in the cases where the position of the growth requires a supra-aortic arch anastomosis, no disturbance of nutrition which can be attributed to this procedure has been observed. The nutritional status of such patients does not vary in any respect from that of those whose thoracic duct remains undisturbed.

A troublesome occurrence frequently observed is the tendency to regurgitation from the stomach if a recumbent posture is assumed soon after eating. All patients who have had the operation should be advised not to lie down during the first two hours after meals.

Occasionally a patient may develop diarrhea which lasts sometimes a few days, sometimes several weeks before it subsides. This is probably caused by the disturbance of function resulting from bilateral vagus section. But this phenomenon is observed in these cases much less frequently than among patients who have had a vagotomy performed in the treatment of duodenal ulcer. Relief is obtained by means of the usual symptomatic treatment.

Recurrences of dysphagia are exceedingly unusual after esophagectomy with esophagogastric anastomosis. Cicatricial stenosis of the anastomosis has been observed in only one of a series of resections for carcinoma of the esophagus amounting now to 189 cases. This stricture responded to treatment by bougienage and the patient has remained well four years after resection. Recurrence of carcinoma at the anastomosis occurs occasionally, but the majority of the patients who succumb to the disease die from the effects of distant metastases or local recurrences within the mediastinum and retain their ability to swallow normally as long as they live.

Incisional pain: Incisional pain lasting more than a few weeks is unusual. It is a frequent observation that after the period of immediate postoperative pain is over, there is very little discomfort. If any uncomfortable sensations are experienced, they are described as a slight pain, an aching or sore feeling, or in some cases as a numbness beneath and medial to the anterior end of the incision in the abdominal and lower thoracic distribution of the terminal branches of the corresponding intercostal nerves. In many cases a transitory sensation of numbness or anesthesia in this area gives way to a period of hyperesthesia when the slightest touch gives rise to discomfort. This in turn subsides in a few weeks and the patient remains comfortable. Long lasting incisional pain or discomfort of any kind is extremely unusual.

Dyspnea: Although a large portion of the left thoracic cavity may be occupied by the transplaced stomach, patients on whom an esophagectomy has been performed almost never experience any sensations which might make them aware of the presence of the stomach within the thorax. Gastric peristaltic sounds are occasionally heard, but they are more often noticed by other people than by the patient himself. Furthermore, after the immediate postoperative period of readjustment has gone by, there is rarely any striking dyspnea or evidence of circulatory disturbances.

Rehabilitation: The return of strength and the ability of the patient to resume an active life depend, of course upon the age, general condition, and mental outlook of the individual patient. Because the majority of the patients with carcinoma of the esophagus are elderly,[4] the return to a normal degree of strength may be very gradual and often never complete. It is not unusual, on the other hand, for patients to return to their customary daily routines and often to their usual occupations. The majority of them are so happy to be able to swallow normally again after a more or less prolonged period of dysphagia and chronic starvation that they usually maintain a cheerful outlook and are eager to become useful citizens once again.

TOTAL EXPERIENCE WITH 203 CASES OF CARCINOMA OF THE ESOPHAGUS AND CARDIAC END OF THE STOMACH*

From 1939 to Jan. 1948, 189 patients with carcinoma of the esophagus and cardiac end of the stomach have been treated by radical resection followed by restoration of continuity of the alimentary canal by primary esophagogastric anastomosis or by the use of the Wookey operation in a few cases of carcinoma of the cervical segment. Before the Torek operation was finally abandoned in 1944 in favor of resection and high intrathoracic esophagogastrostomy, 14 patients with carcinoma of the midthoracic region of the esophagus were operated upon by that method. If these are included, the total series consists of 203 cases. The results in the 14 Torek cases have been reported previously and the reasons for discarding this procedure have been set forth elsewhere.[4, 8] Because the Torek operation is inadequate and because the technique employed is so entirely different from resection and anastomosis it seems best to exclude these cases and confine the discussion to the 189 cases of resection and anastomosis. Table I enumerates the types of cases and the immediate result of the operative procedure used in each group.

TABLE I. IMMEDIATE RESULTS OF RESECTION IN CASES OF CARCINOMA OF THE ESOPHAGUS AND CARDIA (PRIMARY ANASTOMOSIS GROUP)

LOCATION	NO. CASES	COMPLICATIONS WITH RECOVERY	DEATHS	MORTALITY PER CENT
Cervical esophagus, Wookey technique	7	2	0	0
Superior mediastinal segment	1	0	0	0
Midthoracic segment	72	12	17	23.6
Lower thoracic and abdominal segments	23	7	3	13
Gastric carcinoma invading the cardia and lower esophagus	86	16	10	11.6
Total	189	37	30	15.9

*The entire series comprises a large number of personal cases and in addition a few performed by Dr. E. D. Churchill, by my associates, Dr. C. C. Miller and Dr. Lamar Soutter, and by such members of the resident surgical staff of the Massachusetts General Hospital as have shown themselves to be qualified to perform these difficult technical precedures. The techniques employed and the principles observed in the management of the cases have been uniform throughout.

Selection of Cases for Operation.—Because of the hopeless prognosis of the disease and the pitiable plight of these patients who are unable to swallow because of the obstruction produced by the growth, it is justifiable to make an effort to remove the growth in every case. As with carcinoma elsewhere in the gastrointestinal tract the ultimate decision regarding the resectability of the growth depends upon the findings at exploration. No patient has been refused the benefits of an exploratory operation in the hope that a resection of the tumor might be performed, unless there was some obvious contraindication. The most frequent contraindications are the occurrence of metastases to the neck, spine, or lungs, serious cardiac or renal disease, or severe degrees of malnutrition which could not be ameliorated by prolonged treatment with amino acids, whole blood, vitamins, and other means.

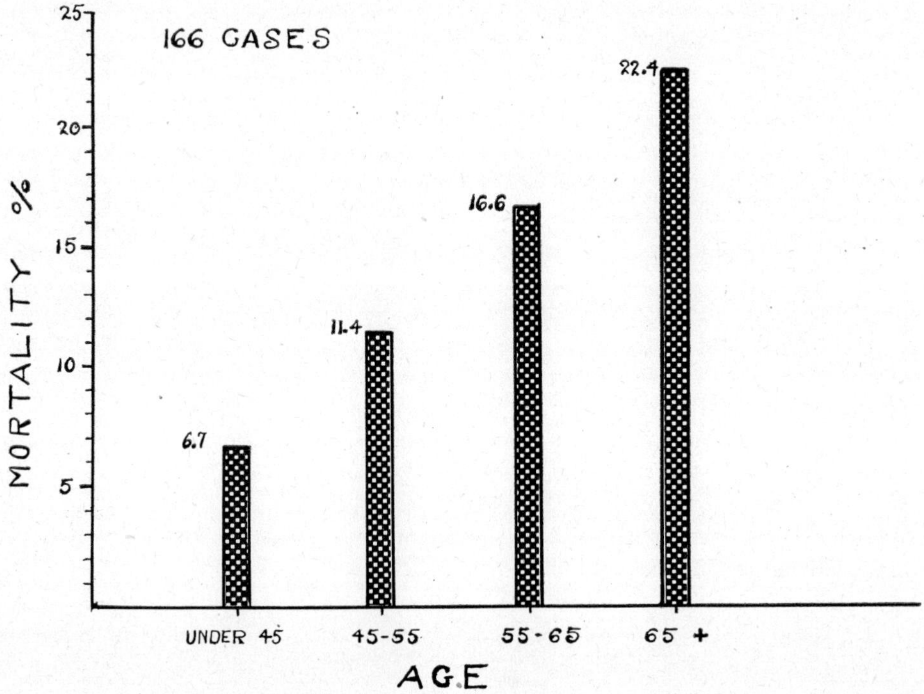

Chart 1.—Graph showing the relation of the operative mortality (per cent of patients who were treated by resection and anastomosis who died in the hospital) to the age of the patients in a series of 166 cases where the exact age was known.

In no case has the advanced age of the patient alone been allowed to militate against a decision to operate. It is well known that a large proportion of patients afflicted with carcinoma of the esophagus are elderly. Over 50 per cent of them are 65 years of age or older when seen for the first time by the surgeon. This policy with regard to the treatment of very old patients has been followed in spite of the realization that the mortality after esophagectomy is inevitably higher in the aged than in persons of younger years. Chart 1 illustrates the relationship between the age of the patient and the postoperative mortality rate.

It is based upon an analysis of 166 cases of carcinoma of the esophagus and cardia occurring in patients whose exact age was known. The steady rise from 6.7 per cent postoperative mortality in patients under 45 years of age to 22.4 per cent among those who were 65 or more years old is striking and significant. This fact, of course, tends to raise the average level of postoperative mortality for the series as a whole, but it would be inhumane to allow such a consideration to affect the decision to operate when the relief from suffering which the operation brings is usually so great.

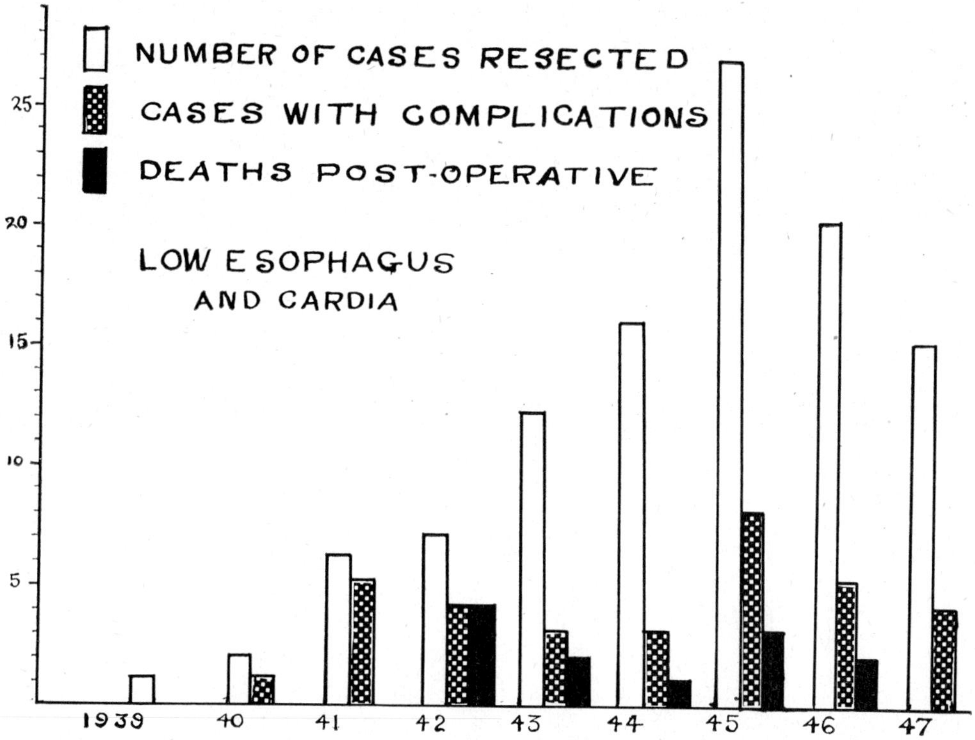

Chart 2.—Graph on carcinoma of the lower esophagus and cardia; the relationship between the number of patients operated upon by resection and anastomosis and the incidence of postoperative complications and deaths each year from 1939 through 1947.

An earnest effort is therefore made in every case of carcinoma of the esophagus or cardia to resect the growth if a primary anastomosis can be performed. In another place it was reported that as a result of following a radical policy regarding resection, the resectability for the entire series was in the vicinity of 65 per cent.[6]

The complications which have occurred and the causes of early postoperative death which have been observed were discussed recently in the communication just referred to and will not be described further here.[6] On the other hand, the relation between the number of patients operated upon each year and the occurrence of postoperative complications and death is of interest. These data are presented in Charts 2 and 3. Chart 2 deals with resections of carcinoma of the lower esophagus and cardia grouped together. The total number of cases of resection per year are shown and beside each column is a second column giving the number of cases of complicated recovery and a third column showing the number of cases resulting in death for each corresponding year. It is to be noted that although the relative number of cases of recovery with complications has remained essentially the same, the mortality rate in this group has shown a tendency to fall. Thus, in 1947, fifteen patients with carcinoma of the lower esophagus or cardia were operated upon by resection and esophagogastric anastomosis with no deaths.

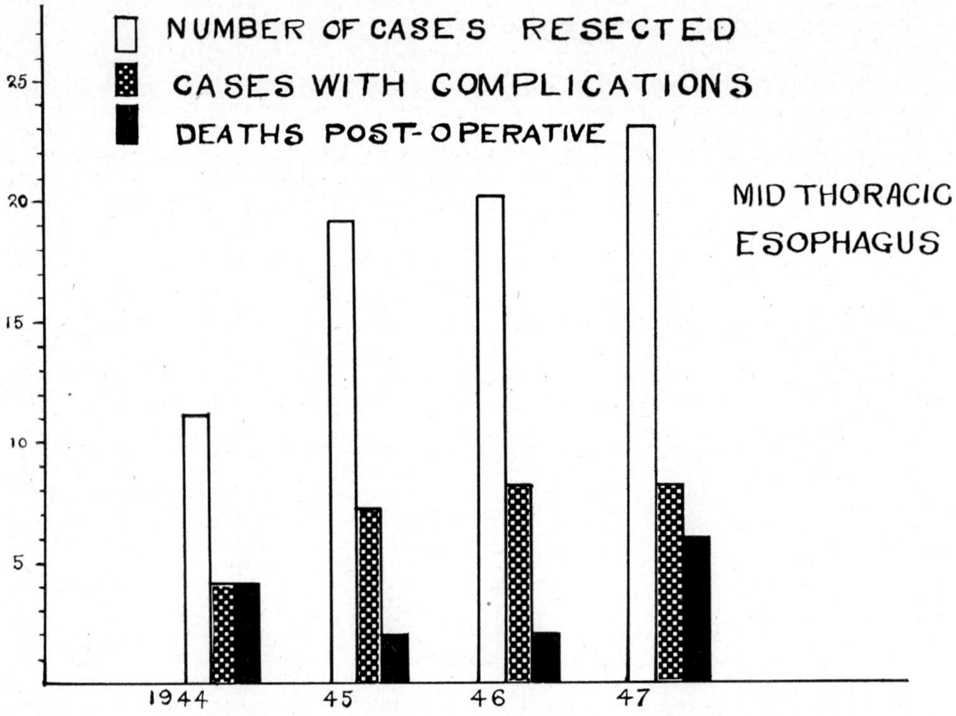

Chart 3.—Graph on carcinoma of the midthoracic segment of the esophagus; the relationship between the number of patients operated upon by resection and anastomosis and the incidence of postoperative complications and deaths each year from 1944 through 1947.

Chart 3 gives the same sort of information regarding the group of patients with carcinoma of the midthoracic region of the esophagus who were treated by resection and primary anastomosis. This procedure was not used in the treatment of such cases before the year 1944, but since then the number of cases has increased steadily from year to year. Here likewise the rate of occurrence of complications with recovery has not changed much. There was only a slight tendency to a decrease in the relative number of such complications. The death rate has fallen, however, with the exception of 1947, when three deaths from massive pulmonary embolism occurred. This unfortunate and unpredictable coincidence caused an unusually high postoperative death rate in that year.

End Results of Resection.—No detailed discussion of end results will be presented here. The last report in June, 1947,[6] suggested that carcinoma of the esophagus when treated by radical resection involving wide excision of the growth and concomitant removal of all possible regional lymph nodes will behave like carcinoma elsewhere in the body and that there will be enough cases of three- to 5-year survival to justify the use of the operation in the hope of effecting a cure. It should never be forgotten, however, that one of the major benefits of the operation in these cases is the palliation which the patient experiences from its use. The fact that many such patients live in relative comfort without any recurrence of dysphagia for as long as two or more years after operation serves to establish the value of radical resection as a palliative measure alone.

An encouraging beginning has been made in the treatment of carcinoma of the esophagus, and when we consider the progress which has already been made in the treatment of carcinoma of other organs, the future prospects of patients who have this dread disease are now, as compared with a few years ago, indeed hopeful.

REFERENCES

1. Adams, W. E., and Phemister, D. B.: Carcinoma of the Lower Thoracic Esophagus: Report of Successful Resection and Esophagogastrostomy, J. Thoracic Surg. **7:** 621, 1938.
2. Wookey, H.: The Surgical Treatment of Carcinoma of the Pharynx and Upper Esophagus, Surg. Gynec. & Obst. **75:** 499, 1942.
3. Sweet, R. H.: Carcinoma of the Superior Mediastinal Segment of the Esophagus; A Technic for Resection With Restoration of Continuity of the Alimentary Canal. (To be published.)
4. Sweet, R. H.: Carcinoma of the Midthoracic Esophagus; Its Treatment by Radical Resection and High Intrathoracic Esophagogastric Anastomosis, Ann. Surg. **124:** 653, 1946.
5. Sweet, R. H.: The Technic of Transthoracic Resection of the Stomach and Esophagus. Nelson's Loose-Leaf Surgery. (In Press.)
6. Sweet, R. H.: Carcinoma of the Esophagus and Cardiac End of the Stomach; Immediate and Late Results of Treatment by Resection and Primary Esophagogastric Anastomosis, J. A. M. A. **135:** 485, 1947.
7. Sweet, R. H.: Transthoracic Resection of the Esophagus and Stomach for Carcinoma; Analysis of the Postoperative Complications, Causes of Death, and Late Results of Operation, Ann. Surg. **121:** 272, 1945.
8. Sweet, R. H.: Surgical Management of Carcinoma of the Midthoracic esophagus, New England J. Med. **233:** 1, 1945.

SURGICAL TREATMENT OF CANCERS OF THE GASTRIC CARDIA

George T. Pack, M.D., and Gordon McNeer, M.D., New York, N. Y.
(From the Gastric Service, The Memorial Hospital for Cancer and Allied Diseases)

One hundred twenty-two cancers involving the gastric cardia have been resected on the gastric service of the Memorial Hospital. Sixty of these patients had total gastrectomy performed by the abdominal route with subdiaphragmatic esophagojejunostomy or esophagoduodenostomy; in these particular cases the gastric cancers although not necessarily originating in the cardiac region, involved so much of the proximal gastric segment as to necessitate total removal of the stomach. The indications, technique, and end results of total gastrectomy for cancer have been considered by us in detail in two previous publication.[55, 56] The present communication is limited to the study of our sixty-two patients who underwent transthoracic cardiectomy or the infrequently performed but feasible abdominal cardiectomy.

INCIDENCE

The contiguous parts of the stomach and esophagus, although anatomically different and harboring cancers of dissimilar histologic types, constitute from the therapeutic point of view a single surgical region. A study of the numerous tables compiled to show the incidence of gastric and esophageal cancers reveals the fact that about 12 to 16 per cent of all carcinomas of the stomach involve the proximal stomach and distal esophagus. If this ratio constantly obtains, 4,000 of the 25,000 Americans who die annually of malignant gastric neoplasms have cancers in the cardiac segment. Ten years ago all of these patients would have been declared inoperable and pronounced hopeless without even exploratory laparotomies. Today and with some assurance, we may offer these people a 33.3 per cent opportunity of five-year survival if they survive the operation. From 1931 (the date of reorganization of the gastric service) until May, 1940 (the date of the first transthoracic cardiectomy), 125 patients suffering from cancer of the gastric cardia were examined at the Memorial Hospital and all were classified as inoperable. With our present rate of resectability, 59 per cent of these patients would now have undergone the radical operation with hope for cure. In the Memorial Hospital series, 17 per cent of our patients with gastric cancer have the disease located in the proximal segment; these figures perhaps do not reflect the natural incidence because patients with cancer of this type are more inclined to gravitate to the cancer hospital than to general institutions.

Age and Sex Distribution.—The age of the average patient undergoing resection of the gastric cardia for cancer was 57.5 years. The proportion of males to females was 82 per cent to 18 per cent, a much greater disparity than exists for cancer of the stomach as a whole, which is 68.5 per cent males and 31.5 per cent females based on an analysis of 1200 patients (Table I).

Received for publication, May 4, 1948.

TABLE I. RESECTION OF THE GASTRIC CARDIA; AGE AND SEX DISTRIBUTION

	NUMBER	PER CENT	AVERAGE AGE (YEARS)	RANGE (YEARS)
Total	62		57.5	33-73
Males	51	82	57.2	39-72
Females	11	18	58.5	33-73

DIAGNOSIS OF TUMORS OF THE GASTRIC CARDIA

When obstruction of the distal esophagus has been produced at the cardiac orifice, a diagnosis of cancer is readily established and confirmed by clinical, radiographic, and endoscopic methods. Dysphagia and regurgitation of ingesta occur to a greater or lesser degree, depending on the extent of encroachment on the abdominal esophagus. Weight loss, emaciation, and dehydration are usually associated with such lesions. The resultant effect upon the human mechanism may be very profound, with hypoproteinemia and varying stages of avitaminosis the most prominent features, depending on the completeness of the obstruction and the elapsed time between its onset and the attempted correction.

The presence of dysphagia in a patient suspected of having cancer of the stomach is strong presumptive evidence that the disease involves the cardia. In our series of 1,117 patients with cancer of the stomach, analyzed as to symptomatology, without respect to the segmental location of the tumor, dysphagia was admitted by 20.4 per cent of patients and was the first symptom in 11.9 per cent. Of the patients with inoperable gastric cancers, 22.7 per cent experienced this discomfort and 17.8 per cent noted it as the initial symptom. Of the patients whose gastric cancers were resectable, only 11.5 per cent listed dysphagia as one of the complaints and only 8.3 per cent as the presenting symptom. The inference to be drawn from these data is that dysphagia should be considered, on the average, to be of serious prognostic import. Dysphagia was the first symptom in 40 per cent of the patients with cancer in the cardiac end of the stomach. There is both a qualitative and quantitative dysphagia, of which the first is the one most readily perceived. Sometimes the first observation by the patient has to do with the temperature of liquids and food ingested; cold liquids and edibles are usually provocative of the first evidence of discomfort. Apples, bread, leafy salads, and, later, meats are gradually abandoned and finally soft foods are replaced by liquids as the daily diet. The sense of discomfort or tightness on swallowing may be not only beneath the region of the xiphoid, but also referred to the base of the neck near the suprasternal space. The pain of dysphagia may actually simulate angina pectoris, with retrosternal discomfort radiating to the neck and down the left arm. Cardiologists have repeatedly stated that eating sometimes precipitates anginoid attacks, therefore, to have this erroneous diagnosis made is not to be wondered at.

The loss of weight and attendant metabolic changes become acute only as the obstruction nears completion. As a prognostic factor, the weight loss should be considered with due respect to (a) the rapidity with which it occurs, and (b) the relative weight loss when compared with the normal body weight. In our studies of the gastric acidity and anemia of patients with carcinoma of the stomach, we found no significant differences according to the segmental location of the cancers or their resectability.

Cancers of the gastric cardia not producing obstruction may offer many difficulties to the diagnostician, especially if the tumor is on the posterior wall of the stomach. The bony structure of the lower thorax prevents satisfactory palpation of this involved segment by both radiologist and surgeon. As motor activity is frequently not affected, symptoms peculiar to the gastrointestinal tract may not be produced. Most frequently an unexplained anemia, weight loss, and an appreciation of retarded bodily activity are the only clinical features of cancers in this silent portion of the stomach. Such tumors often attain enormous size before forcing the individual to realize that medical aid is imperative. Surprisingly enough, the surgical removal of such cancers frequently results in long-term survival.

Esophagoscopy and Gastroscopy.—Endoscopy should never be done without a preliminary barium swallowing and fluoroscopy or esophagograms. Such x-ray study furnishes information concerning the level and degree of obstruction and determines the choice of instruments, that is, the rigid esophagoscope or longer rigid gastroscope passed under direct visual guidance if the lesion obstructs the esophagus or cardia, and the flexible gastroscope passed blindly into the stomach if the proximal gastric segment is unobstructed. An immediate review or study of the x-ray films prior to endoscopy may lessen the hazard of accidental perforation by the examining instrument.

Esophagoscopy may be employed either to confirm the presence of a lesion of the cardia proved by roentgen examination or to discover (if possible) an early cancer that was not observed by x-ray study. Involvement of the abdominal esophagus is easily determined by use of the rigid esophagoscope or gastroscope, enabling the surgeon to choose whether the cardia should be approached by the abdominal, abdomino-thoracic, or transthoracic techniques. The removal of a biopsy specimen gives final support of the presumptive radiographic diagnosis, strengthening the hand of the surgeon in his management of the entire problem.

Routine gastroscopic examination is ill-advised because of the possibility of perforation or severe hemorrhage whenever the cancer encroaches on the cardiac orifice. If the x-ray films disclose no evidence of partial obstruction of the terminal esophagus, vertical gastroscopy with the flexible instrument may enable the examiner to visualize a lesion which cannot be demonstrated by other methods. In the procedure of vertical gastroscopy, the conscious patient sits on a low stool in moderate opisthotonos and the examiner stands on another stool, passing the instrument downward into the stomach. By this technique, the fundus and other portions of the proximal segment are better seen than in the usual lateral decubitus position[61] (Fig. 1).

Radiographic Diagnosis.—Stewart and Illick, in a classic summary of the cardinal x-ray signs of tumors of the cardia, emphasized the great importance of observing closely the very *first swallow* of barium as the stream enters the stomach. The normal manner in which the esophagus ejects the barium into the stomach by a characteristic spurt may be altered so that the fluid may flow in a constant stream without the transient hesitation. This phenomenon occurs when the cardia and esophagus are infiltrated by cancer, converting this channel into a rigid inelastic tube and with complete loss of its valvelike action. A too rapid emptying of the esophagus is, therefore, a sign of diagnostic importance. Instead of the barium stream dropping directly into the stomach,

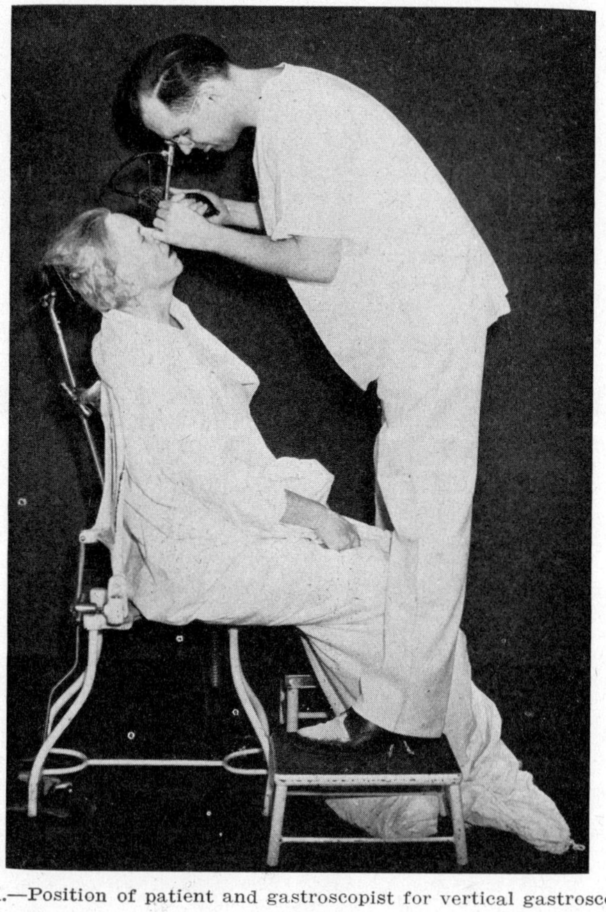

Fig. 1.—Position of patient and gastroscopist for vertical gastroscopy.

it may flow over the projecting cancer as if it were a precipice or in the so-called cascade effect; the barium stream may be visibly diverted. The cardiac sphincter may be obscured by the appearance of a long narrowed channel with irregular contour suggesting the encroachment of a cancer. The normal swaying or pendulum movements of the lower esophagus observed through the fluoroscope during the act of swallowing are frequently lost due to the rigidity and fixation of the esophageal wall. Any increase in the size of the esophageal lumen is cause for suspicion, especially if there is any tendency for retention

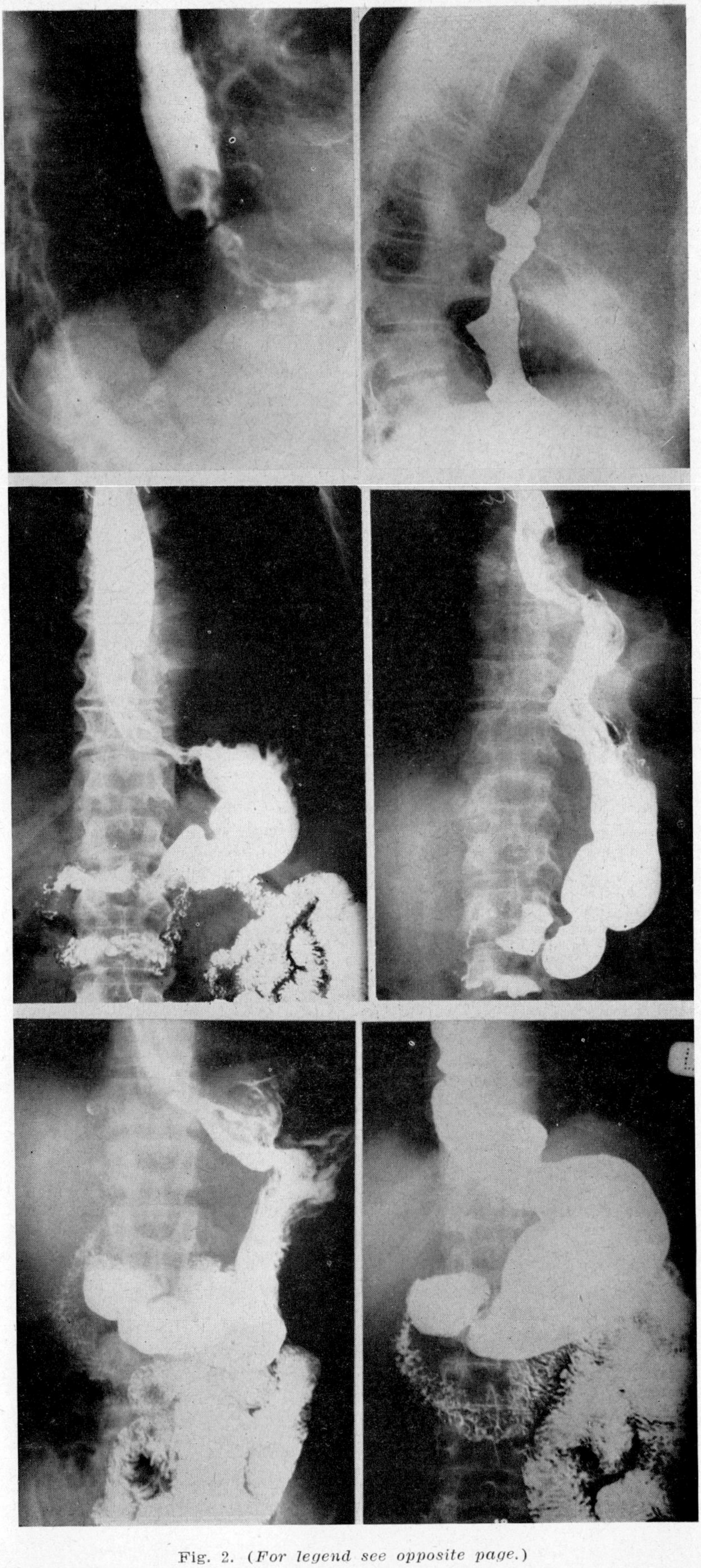

A.

B.

C.

D.

E.

F.

Fig. 2. (*For legend see opposite page.*)

of the barium in the esophagus. The caliber of the esophagus may be magnified two or three times the normal dimensions. The examination is repeated after heavy atropinization if the other signs of tumor are not strongly in evidence; a barium-filled capsule may be swallowed to test the patency of the cardiac orifice. Stewart and Illick have also called attention to the occurrence of antiperistalsis in the lower esophagus; one may see two or three antiperistaltic waves depending on the degree of obstruction. The mucosal pattern of the gastric rugae may be greatly altered by the cancer, and the size and configuration of the entire proximal gastric segment may be significantly changed so that the diagnosis of cancer is more easily made. The tumor mass can often be seen as an irregular density projecting into the hemispherical black shadow of the air bubble, or magenblase, in the fundus of the stomach. This ready aid to diagnosis can easily be obscured either by giving the patient too much barium or by unwisely placing him in the Trendelenburg position. The contrast of the tumor mass against the air bubble may be delineated more clearly in some instances by the use of Seidlitz powders or by inflating the stomach through a Levine tube under roentgenoscopic control as advocated by Wasch and Epstein (Fig. 2).

In our diagnostic study of more than 1,000 cases of gastric cancer at the Memorial Hospital, 292 gastroscopies and 1,022 gastrointestinal x-ray studies were completed. In summary, these two technical methods of diagnosis together were responsible for a diagnostic accuracy of 96.1 per cent, although 98.1 per cent of patients exhibited some abnormalities.

Differential Diagnosis.—Tumors of the esophagocardiac segment are not difficult to distinguish from such lesions as diaphragmatic hernia, diverticulum, varices, and extrinsic pressure. Cardiospasm may simulate cancer and is identified in the average case by its preponderance in females, constant location at or just above the diaphragm, funnel-shaped contour, smooth margins, greater dilatation of esophagus, longer duration of symptoms, esophagoscopic image, and biopsy negative for cancer.

Benign peptic ulcer may occur high on the lesser curvature and may involve the orifice. By contrast roentgenographic studies, it is sometimes possible to demonstrate converging mucosal rugae radiating around the ulcer, whereas with cancer the mucosal pattern is irregularly distorted. Gastric analysis is is not reliable as an important aid in differential diagnosis. If the law of averages is considered, the larger the ulcer crater, the greater likelihood exists that the defect is cancerous. If the ulcer completely and permanently disappears after conservative medical management, it may be assumed to be benign. We had a patient whose juxtacardiac ulcer healed and who gained weight under medical care; nine months later a total gastrectomy was done for an invasive

Fig. 2.—Transthoracic esophagogastrectomy. *A*, Preoperative roentgenogram of cancer of the cardia and esophagus; *B*, postoperative roentgenogram of intrathoracic anastomosis; *C*, preoperative roentgenogram of cancer of cardia and esophagus; *D*, postoperative roentgenogram of intrathoracic anastomosis; *E*, preoperative roentgenogram of cancer of cardia and esophagus; *F*, postoperative roentgenogram of intrathoracic anastomosis.

carcinoma. Malignant ulcers may show radiographic evidence of healing during a careful dietary regime. Apropos of this problem the following case history may be cited.

Case Report.—An elderly anemic woman, with kyphosis of such a degree as to prohibit endoscopic study, had a large obstructive ulcer involving the cardiac orifice. X-ray studies showed a soft tissue shadow just above the diaphragm, narrowing the esophageal lumen and assumed to be an upward extension of the cancer. She was too ill and emaciated to tolerate radical surgical treatment; a small laparotomy incision was done to construct a jejunostomy for feeding purposes. A palpating hand confirmed the presence of the large mass occupying the abdominal esophagocardiac segment. After six weeks of jejunostomy feedings, the patient had greatly improved, therefore a thoracotomy was performed with the intention of doing the routine esophagogastrectomy. The supradiaphragmatic shadow was due to a large lipoma which was easily enucleated; on severing the left diaphragmatic leaf the gastric lesion had entirely disappeared, the stomach had healed during the period of rest, and the proper diagnosis obviously should have been ulcer rather than cancer.

ANESTHESIA FOR THORACIC CARDIECTOMY*

The present-day success with the operation of transthoracic cardiectomy has been effected through the great advances in modern anesthesiology. Though ultimately bearing the responsibility of success or failure, the surgeon cannot have his attention withdrawn from the operative field and this radical and time-consuming operation in order to direct the management of the patient or combat the complications resulting from the anesthetic agent. The anesthetist has now assumed the application of methods to prevent and combat shock. Nowhere in the realm of surgery is close cooperation between surgical team, internist, and anesthetist more urgently required than in massive resections of the stomach and esophagus. In order safely to manage the patient through the operative experience, the anesthetist must have the knowledge of all the information about the patient's health discovered during the period of preoperative preparation. With these data at hand, an intelligent selection of the anesthetic agent and method best suited for the individual patient may be made.

The anesthetic agents most frequently used for the operation are cyclopropane or ether with a nitrous oxide-oxygen, ethylene, or cyclopropane induction. In our experience at the Memorial Hospital, intratracheal ether has been the anesthetic of choice.

During the period in which the pleural cavity is open it is frequently necessary to assist each involuntary inspiratory effort by the patient by gentle pressure on the rebreathing bag. This is done to secure adequate pulmonary ventilation in the presence of one open pleural cavity and the dependent position of the intact side of the thorax with consequent limitation of its expansion. In addition, the collapsed lung is reinflated by the application of positive pressure at periodic intervals every fifteen to thirty minutes during the operation as a precautionary measure to help prevent pulmonary edema during the operative period and atelectasis postoperatively.

---

*The anesthesias for these operations were under the management of Dr. Olga Schweizer, Director of Anesthesia in the Memorial Hospital.

The problem of secretions in the tracheobronchial tract is important; pulmonary diseases such as tuberculosis or bronchiectasis may be present concurrently with gastroesophageal cancer. In these cases collapse of the lung upon opening the pleura may force the abnormal secretions and exudates into the trachea and endotracheal tube. Preliminary preoperative measures ought to include postural drainage and vigorous coughing in an effort to bring up as much sputum as possible. Should flooding of the trachea occur during the operation, prompt aspiration is imperative to prevent an overflow into the dependent lung and to provide an absolutely free airway. In all cases of endotracheal intubation the tube must be sucked thoroughly before withdrawal at the end of the operation. The patient comes to the operating room with a Levine tube in residence within the stomach or terminal esophagus; this tube is constantly open for drainage and is intermittently aspirated by the anesthetist to avoid flooding the throat and trachea with the purulent and fermentative secretions from the stomach.

The technique of controlled respiration is frequently employed in inhalation anesthesia for transthoracic esophagocardiectomy because it permits the anesthetist to regulate the patient's respirations to the best advantage.

EVOLUTION OF THE OPERATION FOR CANCERS OF THE GASTRIC CARDIA

The radical surgical treatment of cancers of the gastric cardia was conceived early in the history of stomach surgery, but only sporadic application of this procedure was employed until the past decade. To the earliest period belong the researches of von Mikulicz, who established the fact that operative intervention may be done on the abdominal esophagus without causing tension pneumothorax. He was the first surgeon to report a gastric cardiectomy for cancer (1898); his patient died, as did the subsequent six patients operated on by other surgeons. Apparently the first successful cardiectomy in a human being was accomplished by Voelcker in 1908; in a communication to Parcelier he stated that the patient was alive three years postoperatively.

Von Mikulicz (1904) and later Sauerbruch (1906) had become the originators of transpleural thoracotomy by demonstrating the safety of opening the thorax under differential pressure. However, their patients subjected to cardiectomy failed to live, as was the outcome in the patient of Wendel (1907), likewise resected by the transthoracic route. Peritonitis was the usual cause of death in patients whose cancers of the gastric cardia were resected by the transperitoneal method, and shock was the cause of fatalities by the transpleural approach. With the exception of one of Zaaijer's patients (1913) operated on by a multiple stage transpleural technique with axillary esophagostomy, Brun (1916) and Bircher (1918) were the first to report operative survivals by any transpleural method of gastric cardiectomy.

Hörhammer in 1923 reported the survival of a patient for six and one-half years following a transabdominal cardiectomy for cancer of the proximal gastric segment. In 1925, Heuer, Andrus, and Bell, who were aware of the hazards of intrathoracic anastomosis of stomach and esophagus, designed an operation for transplanting the left leaf of the diaphragm high in the chest in order subsequently to perform an esophagogastrectomy with anastomosis below the diaphragm. The operation was successfully performed in dogs but led to a fatal outcome in the one human being on whom it was attempted.

Sauerbruch in 1925 was again unsuccessful but persisted in his belief that the transthoracic, transdiaphragmatic resection of the gastric cardia with immediate esophagogastrostomy was a feasible operative procedure. Marshall introduced this technique in the United States and accomplished the first successful transthoracic cardiectomy on July 31, 1937. His achievement was later repeated by Phemister on Jan. 26, 1938, and by Cattell on Aug. 27, 1938. However, Garlock in 1941 was apparently the first to appreciate the value and applicability of the transthoracic approach, because it was his perseverance and great experience which led to the popularization of the operation through the United States (Fig. 3).

Other historical details in the operation of cardiectomy for cancer:

1. Gregoire proposed rib resection followed by dissection of the pleura from the diaphragm with vertical division of the latter followed by resection and anastomosis. Rehn employed a somewhat similar principle, first mobilizing the left thorax through subperiosteal resection of the sixth to eleventh ribs. Subsequently posterior mediastinotomy with resection was performed. Clairmont and also Borches considered the best attack on the lower esophagus to be through the posterior mediastinum and by a retroperitoneal approach.

2. Radlinski described a technique for cardiectomy in which the esophagus was pulled down into the abdomen as far as possible. The stomach and esophagus were transsected and the tumor was removed. A permanent gastrostomy was constructed and the esophageal stump was at least temporarily disposed of by suturing a tube in it and bringing it to the skin as a fistula. Restoration of esophagogastric continuity appeared to be extremely problematical.

3. Jonas (1942) advised a preliminary jejunostomy for feeding, at the same time anchoring the upper gastric segment securely to a rib so that future tension on the suture line could be eliminated. Carter, Stevenson, and Abbott (1940) had previously recommended that the anastomosis be sutured to the chest wall in order to relieve tension at this site.

4. Schwers (1914) described a transpleural and transdiaphragmatic resection in two stages with rib resection. A U-shaped incision was made on the left edge of the sternum beginning at the base of the middle and lower thirds and proceeding over the costal arch. Extrapleural resection of the ninth to fifth ribs, inclusive, was done and the pleural cavity opened at the level of the fifth rib. The esophageal stump was isolated, followed by the isolation of the cardia with preservation of the vagi. A direct anastomosis was performed after resection of the cardia and esophagus.

5. Transpleural approach in the three- or four-stage operation of Zaaijer (1913). The first stage, laparotomy and gastrostomy. The second stage, subperiosteal resection of the left sixth to eighth ribs. The third stage, transpleural and transdiaphragmatic resection of the cardia, the esophageal stump being brought out through the lower axilla. The fourth stage, union of the two stomas with rubber tubing (Figs. 4 and 5).

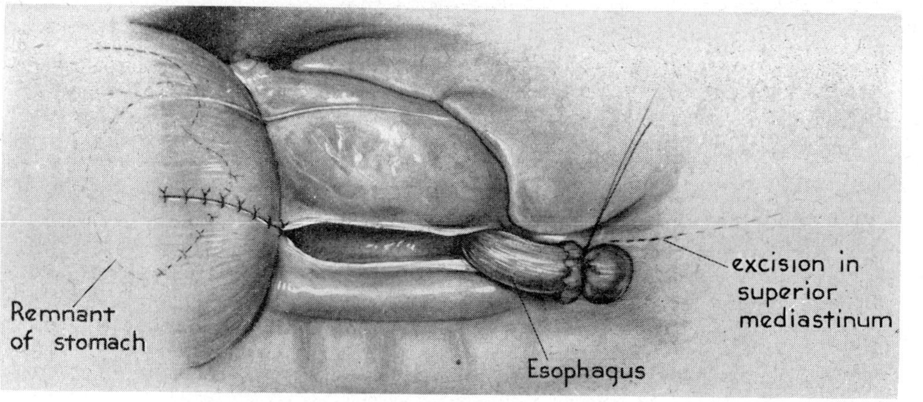

A.

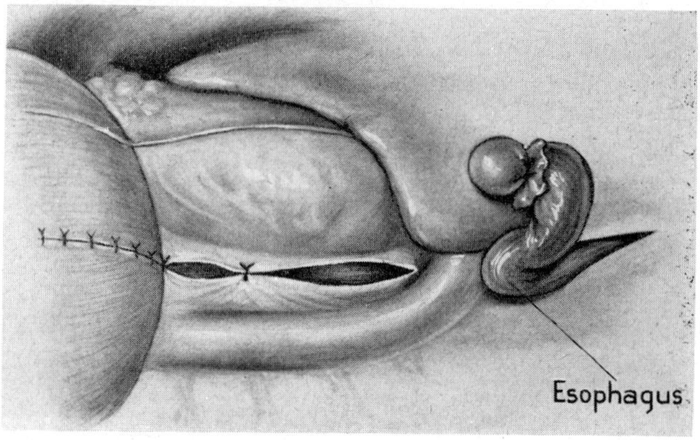

B.

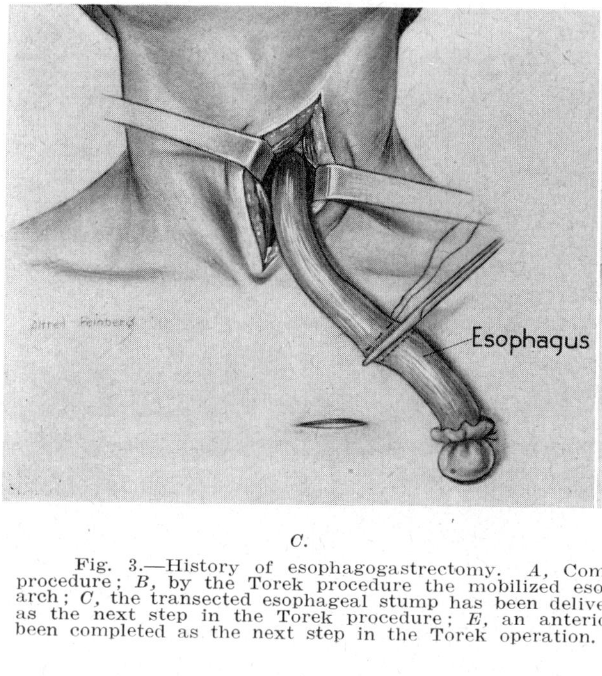

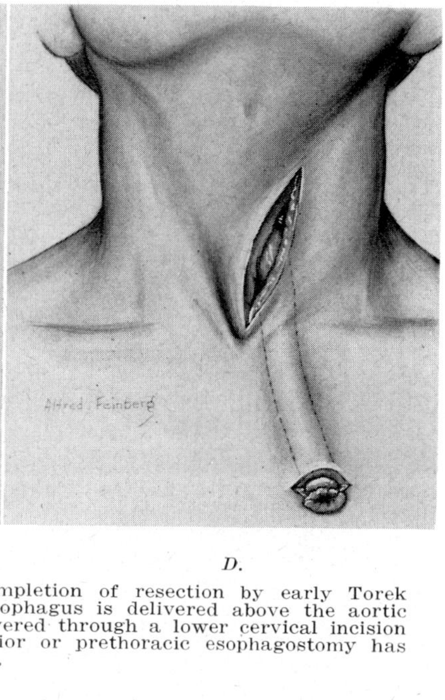

C. *D.*

Fig. 3.—History of esophagogastrectomy. *A*, Completion of resection by early Torek procedure; *B*, by the Torek procedure the mobilized esophagus is delivered above the aortic arch; *C*, the transected esophageal stump has been delivered through a lower cervical incision as the next step in the Torek procedure; *E*, an anterior or prethoracic esophagostomy has been completed as the next step in the Torek operation.

6. Technical features of the anastomosis. Miyagi (1927) stated categorically that no operator had ever succeeded in obtaining a good result by a direct suture of the esophagus to the stomach or jejunum. Clairmont asserted that if the defect after removal of the esophagus and cardia is longer than 8 cm., a direct anastomosis would not be possible. Ohsawa and Raven recommended that the anastomosis be covered with omentum to afford protection against leakage. Borches and Bircher attempted to cover the site with a peritoneal reflection freed from the diaphragm. Kümmell, Brun, Bircher, Küttner, and Clairmont completely divided the esophagus before starting the anastomosis, but Voelcker and Miyagi began the anastomosis before severance in order to eliminate the use of clamps on the delicate esophagus.

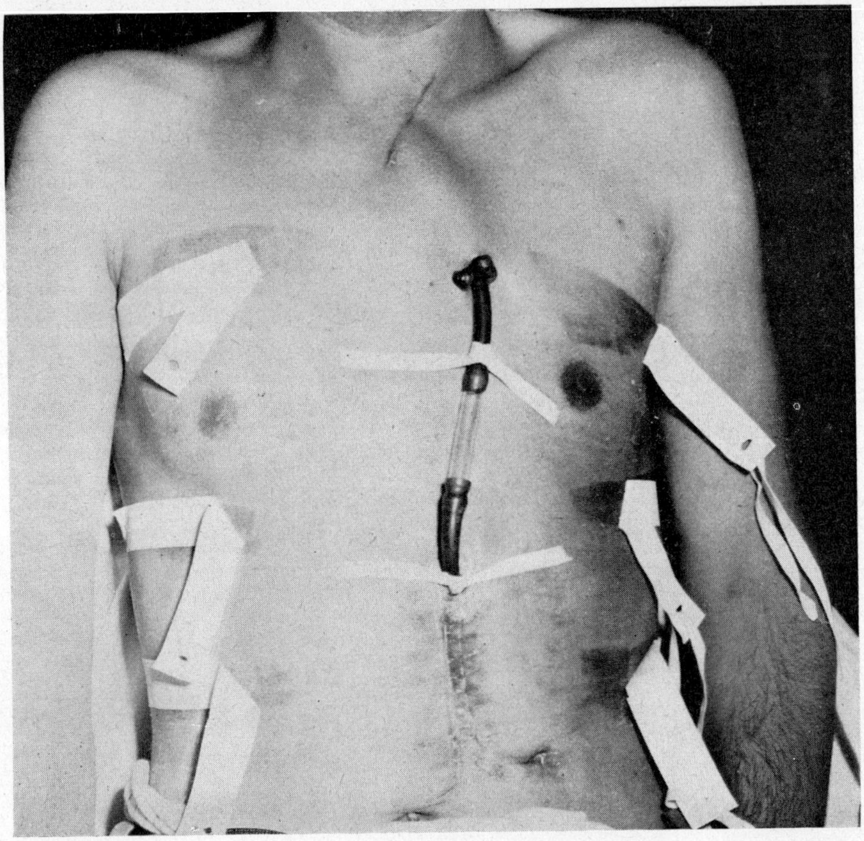

Fig. 4.—History of esophagogastrectomy. The completed Torek operation. In this patient the operation was done prior to the universal adoption of the intrathoracic type of anastomosis. The rubber feeding tube conjoins the prethoracic esophagostomy with a Janeway gastrostomy made with the remnant of stomach. This is an unsatisfactory mechanical arrangement, difficult to control.

7. Invagination method of anastomosis. The so-called invagination method has been described by Sauerbruch, Miyagi, Kader, Bircher, and Carter. This procedure involves the insertion of the distal esophageal stump into a carefully measured rent in the anterior wall of the gastric remnant, and traction downward by means of a clamp inserted into the gastric lumen distal to the site

of the anastomosis. It is then sutured in place. Of prime necessity is an adequate length of esophagus available for this technique. Sauerbruch employed this method in a one- or two-stage procedure with some variations. The chest was

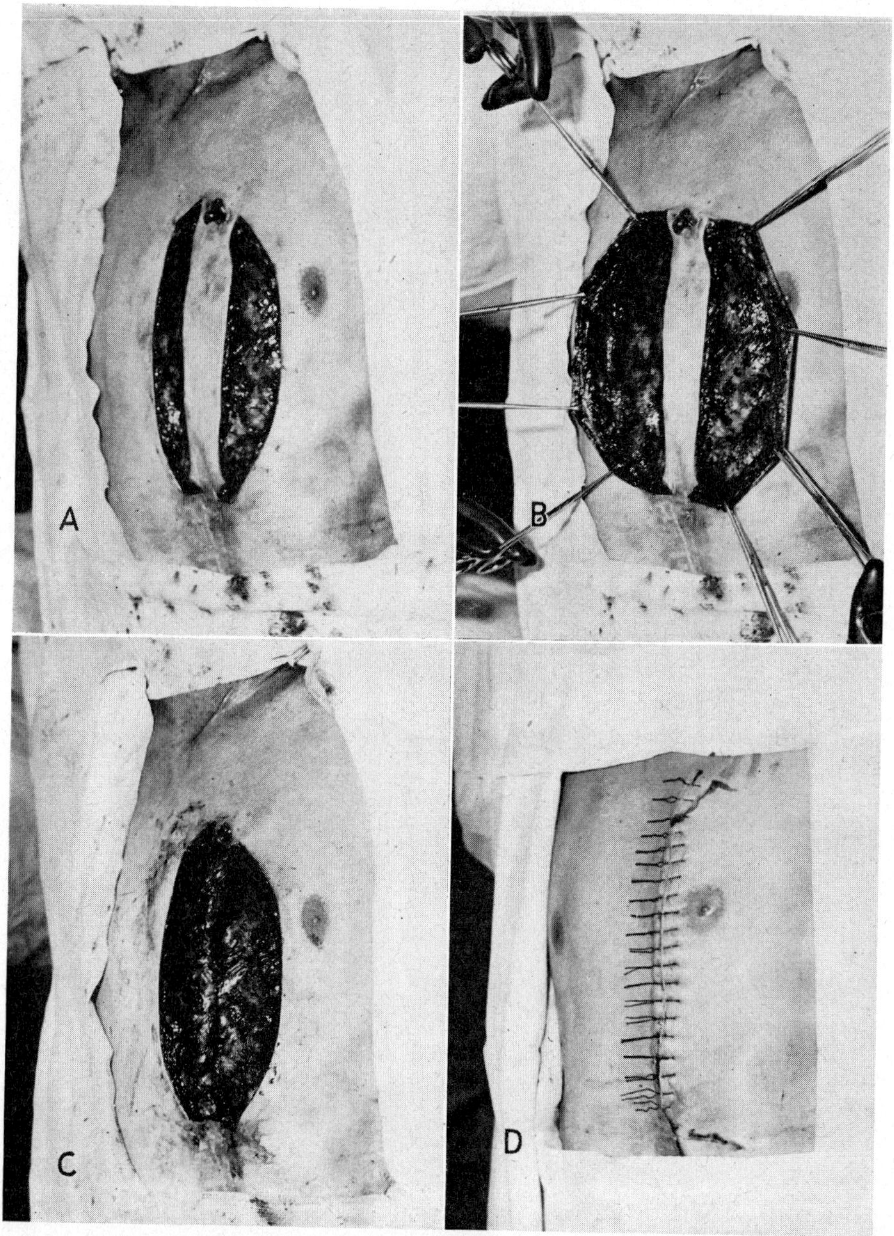

Fig. 5.—History of esophagogastrectomy. *A*, Early efforts to construct a prethoracic esophagus utilizing the skin of the chest wall; *B*, lateral skin flaps dissected widely back to permit approximation over the new rolled-in esophageal tube; *C*, the skin tube has been constructed by rolling in the tube; *D*, the new skin tube and the esophagostomy orifice have been covered by the lateral sliding skin flaps. The gastrostomy has not been connected. A jejunal loop should be used for the lower connection.

first explored and the resectability of the cancer determined, at which time the phrenic nerve was cut and the seventh to eleven ribs removed. Within two to three weeks the chest was again opened and adhesions divided. The involved cardiac segment was freed and the tumor-bearing portion actually invaginated deeply into the gastric lumen. The normal serosa of the stomach was sutured to the esophagus superior to the cancer. Some weeks later the necrotic tumor was removed through a gastrotomy incision. Sauerbruch employed this invagination technique on his first successful case; the patient lived for fourteen days and died of right-sided pneumonia. Kader used the invagination principle with excision of the cancer during the first operation. Both Ohsawa and Carter have tried the invagination technique and abandoned it because of the occurrence of postoperative stenosis. The sole advantage apparently is that it may have decreased the tendency to leakage of the line of sutures.

Types of Incisions for Cardiectomy.—The abdominal cavity has been opened in a great variety of ways by angle and transverse incisions. The costal arch incision, first suggested by Bozzi and later used by Hans Brun proceeded from the ensiform cartilage parallel to the costal margin up to the thirteenth rib. Marwedel made a curved incision two fingerbreadths below the costal arch and parallel to it, extending from the ensiform process to the tenth rib. In the medial angle of the wound the seventh rib and at the lateral angle the seventh, eighth, and ninth ribs were divided after bluntly stripping off the rectus and the external oblique muscles. The thoracic flap mobilized in this way could be conveniently closed above and offered a moderately satisfactory approach to the cardia and abdominal segment of the esophagus. Closure of this incision has been very tedious in our experience. The Baudet-Navarro exposure is somewhat similar; it permits the elevation of a costochondral flap which is later resutured into place. Voelcker (1908) opened the abdomen first by a median longitudinal incision from the ensiform process downward for 8 to 10 cm. and thus established the resectability of the cancer. Then the incision was continued at an angle and parallel to the costal arch up to the left anterior axillary line. The sixth and seventh ribs in their cartilaginous portion and the seventh, eighth, and ninth ribs were divided subperiosteally. This procedure is similar to that of Marwedel and offers a good approach to the gastric cardia.

CHOICE OF OPERATION PROCEDURES

Cancers of the gastric cardia may be removed by four different technical procedures, abdominal total gastrectomy, abdominal cardiectomy or proximal subtotal gastrectomy, laparothoracic resection or laparothoracotomy, and transthoracic or transdiaphragmatic esophagogastrectomy which may be subtotal or total. Among the factors influencing the surgeon to select one of these procedures as best suited for the individual case are the involvement or freedom of involvement of the esophagus, the regional localization of the cancer strictly to the cardia or fundus, the extension of the cancer for great distances along the lesser curvature, the presence of diffuse serosal invasion, peritoneal carcinosis of the lesser omental bursa, and adherence to and invasion of neighboring organs. The surgeon often cannot make this decision until the operative exploration has been done. The choice of procedures or modifications of these operations are sufficiently numerous to fit any surgical occasion, providing the cancer is not definitely inoperable. The specific indications and contraindications for these various technical procedures are given in detail elsewhere in this essay. Our own experience is adumbrated in Table II.

TABLE II. RESECTION OF THE GASTRIC CARDIA

PROCEDURES			NUMBER	PER CENT
Total cases (62 gastric cancers and 3 benign gastric ulcers)			65	100.0
I. Abdominal approach, total cases			10	15.4
Resection and esophagogastrostomy		9		
Resection and esophagogastrostomy plus partial pancreatectomy and partial hepatectomy		1		
II. Transthoracic approach, total cases			45	69.2
A. Multiple operations, total cases		6		
Jejunostomy; transthoracic resection and anterior thoracic esophagostomy; gastrostomy	1			
Jejunostomy; transthoracic resection and esophagogastrostomy	3			
Laparotomy; transthoracic resection and esophagogastrostomy	1			
Transthoracic resection and esophagogastrostomy; jejunostomy	1			
B. One-stage operations, total cases		39		
Transthoracic resection and esophagogastrostomy	36			
Transthoracic resection and esophagogastrostomy and splenectomy	1			
Transthoracic resection and esophagogastrostomy and partial pancreatectomy	1			
Transthoracic resection and esophagogastrostomy, splenectomy and partial pancreatectomy	1			
III. Abdominothoracic resection and esophagogastrostomy			6	9.2
IV. Transthoracic total resection, total cases			4	6.2
Total gastrectomy, esophagojejunostomy and jejunojejunostomy	3			
Total gastrectomy, esophagojejunostomy, jejunojejunostomy, and splenectomy	1			

THE TECHNIQUE OF TRANSTHORACIC ESOPHAGOGASTRECTOMY

The last barrier to the successful operative removal of all cancers of the stomach has been removed with the standardization of the operations involving resection of the terminal esophagus and gastric cardia. This dramatic change in the concept of the operability of gastric cancer has been effected in the past decade. Prior to this date, nearly all radiologists appended the word "inoperable" to most reports concerning cancers of the proximal gastric segment. At present no such tumor is so classified unless it is inseparably fixed to structures, the removal of which would result in the patient's death, or unless the presence of distant metastases can be demonstrated.

From our personal experience and study of the literature, the choice of a method can apply only to the individual case. Whereas the necessity for standardization of operative techniques forms the basis of sound surgical training, once these are mastered the ability to manage the problem at hand by any or a combination of methods is a requisite of the modern surgeon. Resection of the distal esophagus and gastric cardia by the transpleural, transdiaphragmatic approach has been so well standardized by now that the operation is routinely applied in all surgical clinics where gastric cancer is treated. Numerous surgeons employ a small preliminary laparotomy incision to determine the operability of the cancer. If resectability is decided upon, the thorax is opened through the left seven or eighth intercostal space. The patient lies in the right lateral decubitus position with the right thigh and knee flexed and the left arm suspended upward and forward by anchorage to a standard so as to elevate the scapula out of the way. Exploration and resection through a transthoracic incision alone have been widely employed in the greater number of instances. It is seldom necessary to resect a rib.

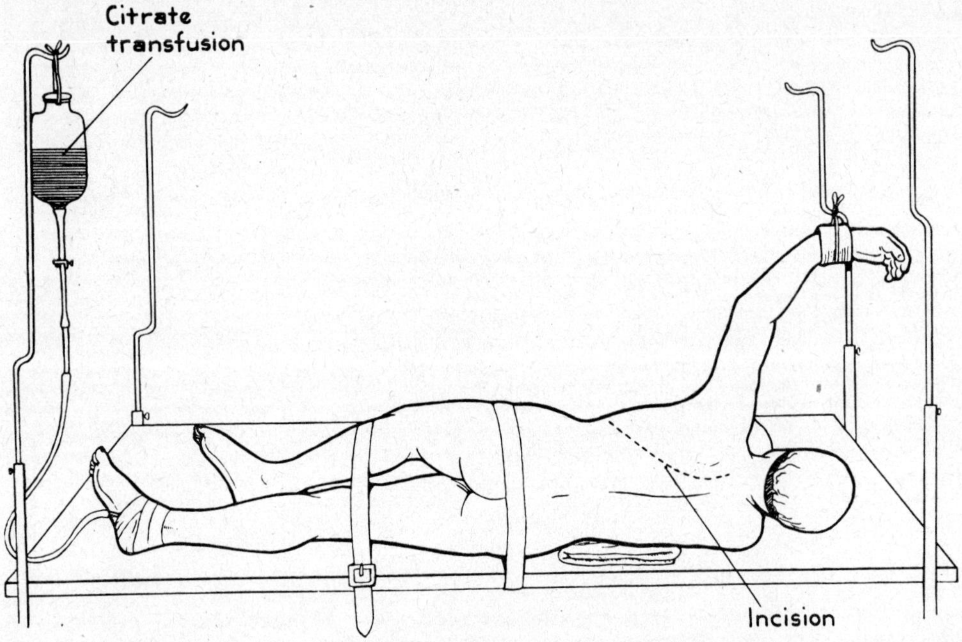

Fig. 6.—Position of patient for transthoracic transdiaphragmatic resection of esophagogastric cancer.

Recently the transabdominal, transthoracic incision originally advocated by Sauerbruch, Voelcker, Enderlein, and Wendel has been rediscovered in several surgical clinics. In fact, as previously stated, some surgeons, notably Garlock, have always advocated preliminary laparotomy to establish subdiaphragmatic operability. The incision may be vertical, as a left rectus muscle-splitting approach, a vertical paramedian epigastric approach, or a transverse upper abdominal approach, in each instance continuing the incision through the costochondral cartilages and along the ninth intercostal space if no contraindications to resection are discovered. Whenever the thoracotomy incision alone is to be used, the left side of the chest is uppermost at a ninety degree angle, but if the combined laparothoracotomy is to be done, the patient is rotated to the left (forty-five degree angle) to expose the abdominal wall (Fig. 6). The combined incision has the advantage of offering a complete abdominal exploration which cannot always be accomplished from above, and it affords an exposure which is superior to thoracotomy alone. The cul-de-sac, mesentery of the small and large

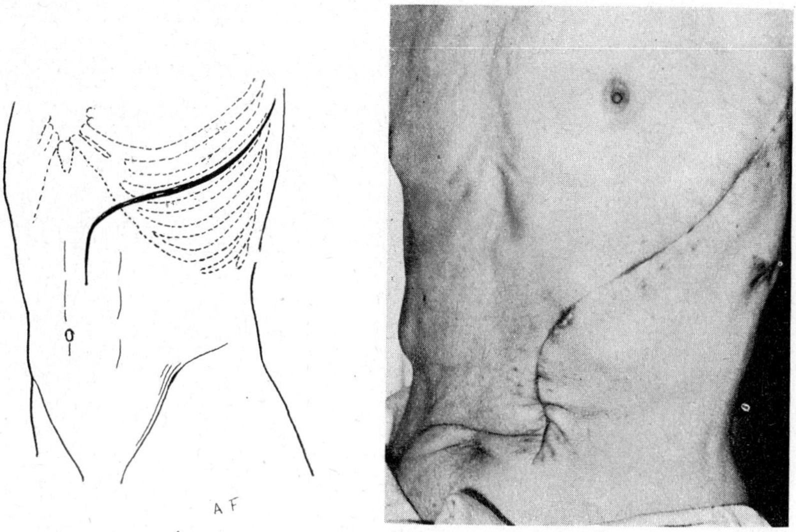

A. B.

Fig. 7.—*A*, Laparothoracotomy incision designed for preliminary abdominal exploration; *B*, scar of laparothoracotomy incision.

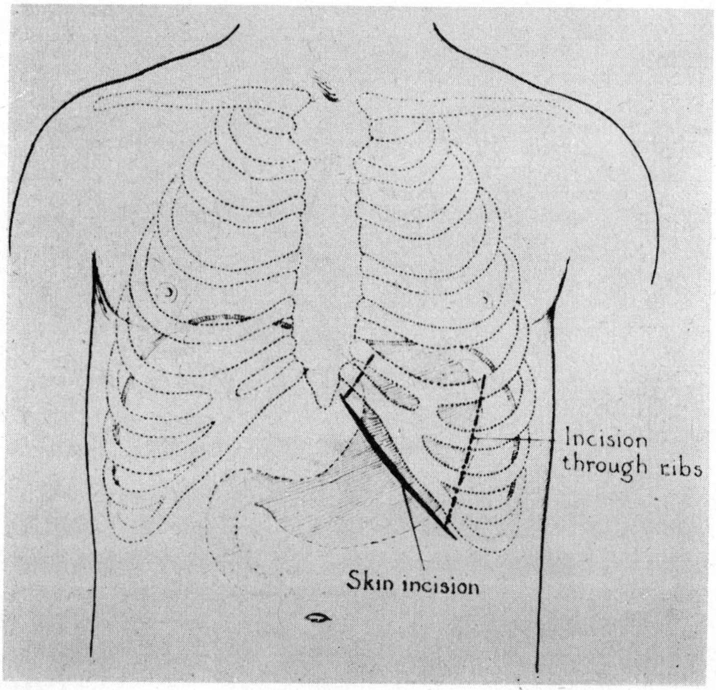

Fig. 8.—The Baudet-Navarro incision with rib flap for approach to the gastric cardia.

intestines, peritoneum, and all aspects of the liver are carefully examined for the presence of metastatic cancer before proceeding with the plan for resection. All the viscera which may be involved by an adherent or partially fixed cancer are directly beneath one's view. Resection of the spleen, pancreas, or left lobe of the liver is accomplished with relative ease and safety if the problem so requires. If, from the abdominal examination, the carcinoma is found to involve the entire abdominal esophagus, the thorax may be entered through a higher interspace or by rib resection (Figs. 7 and 8).

The left leaf of the diaphragm is severed in a radial direction down to and including the crural arch. The left phrenic nerve may be injected with Novocain solution where it is reflected from the pericardium onto the diaphragm. The presence or absence of intrathoracic metastases should be determined before the important blood supply of the organs about to be resected is compromised. Even small segments of the pericardium adherent to the cancer may be sacrificed. Insistence on the point of removing gastric cancers adherent to other organs has saved the lives of many patients who would have died of the disease in a relatively short time. In a recent study of our end results obtained in the treatment of all cancers of the stomach, about 33 per cent of the operative survivors of just such problems, that is, involvement of adjacent organs, lived for more than five years without recurrence.

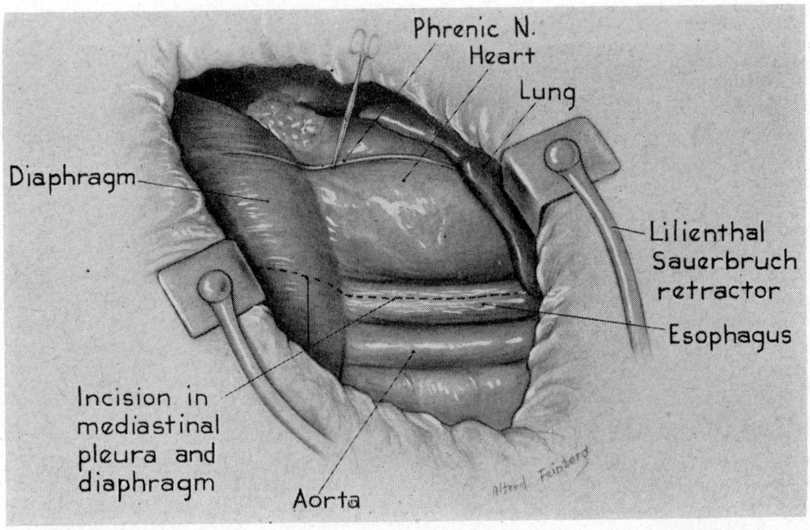

Fig. 9.—Transthoracic esophagogastrectomy. The ribs have been retracted. The esophagus, diaphragm, aorta, and phrenic nerve are in the operative field.

The pleural reflection of the lungs from the posterior mediastinum is released and the parietal pleura over the esophagus is incised. The lower esophagus is cautiously dissected free, care being taken not to enter the contralateral pleural space which is immediately adjacent (Fig. 9). The esophagus is palpated to determine the possible upper limits of the tumor; we have on numerous occasions found submucosal extension of the cancer well above the visible tumor. This fact is in keeping with the well-known tendency of both gastric and esophageal cancers to extend intramurally for surprisingly long distances up the esophagus. To avoid the embarrassment of being told by the pathologist that microscopic evidence of cancer was found at the line of transection of the esophagus, it is now our practice *not* to start the anastomosis until a frozen sec-

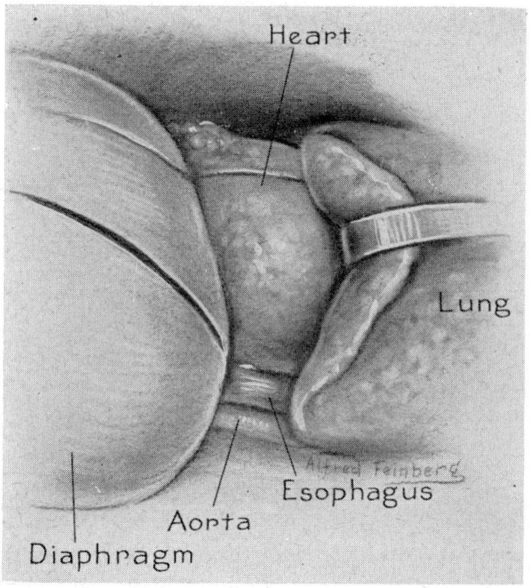

Fig. 10.—Transthoracic esophagogastrectomy. The left leaf of the diaphragm is severed in a radial direction from the rib margin to the crura.

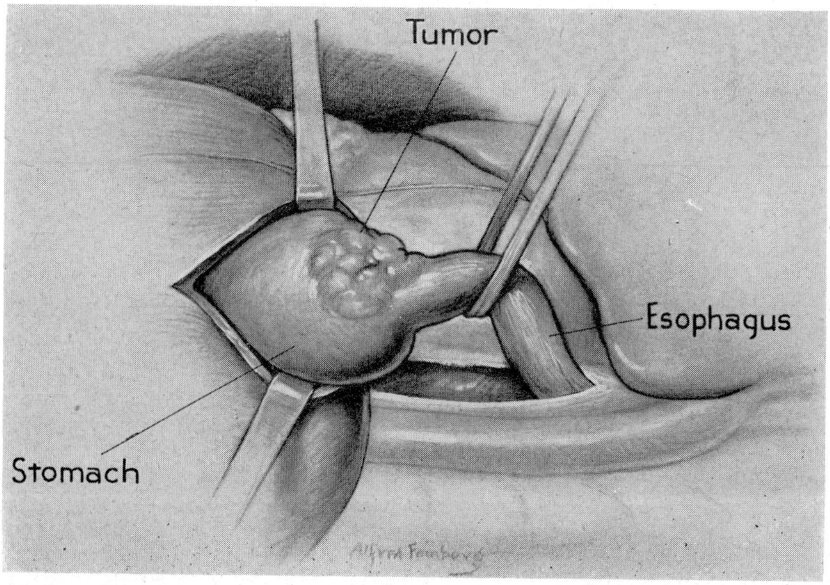

Fig. 11.—Transthoracic esophagogastrectomy. The lower thoracic esophagus has been elevated from the mediastinal bed and the mobilized proximal segment of the stomach appears in the diaphragmatic cleft.

tion specimen from the cut end of the esophagus has been studied microscopically and pronounced free of cancer by the pathologist.

The proximal gastric segment is then mobilized starting with complete severance of the diaphragmatic crura (Figs. 10 and 11). The coronary ligament containing the left gastric artery and vein is doubly clamped, severed, and ligated. The gastrohepatic ligament is similarly freed; in the resection of the cardia only, more of the lesser curvature is removed. The spleen constantly herniates into the chest through the rent in the diaphragm so that it is sometimes more convenient to remove it with the stomach whether or not the hilar nodes are involved. The great omentum is also removed but the right gastroepiploic vessels are carefully preserved. The line of transection of the stomach is chosen well below the inferior limits of the tumor (Fig. 12). The right

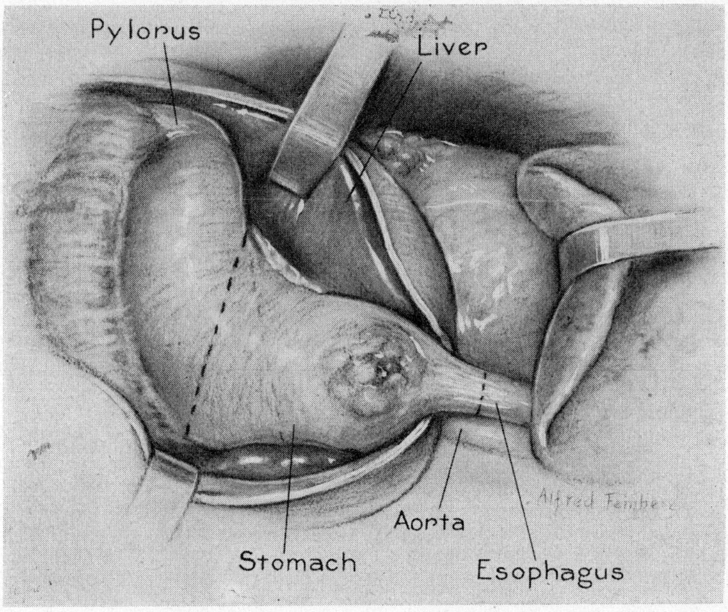

Fig. 12.—Transthoracic esophagogastrectomy. The lines of transection of esophagus and stomach are outlined. The resection includes a more liberal segment of the lesser curvature.

gastric artery is unmolested as every effort is made to ensure an abundant blood supply to the lower part of the stomach which will be used for the anastomosis. If the cancer invades the spleen, pancreas, left lobe of liver, or diaphragm, these organs should be included in the dissection. The de Petz clamp is applied across the stomach on a bias, sparing as much of the greater curvature as is compatible with an adequate resection for cancer, as it is the longer and more mobile greater curvature side which will be utilized for the anastomosis (Figs. 13 and 14). The distal gastric remnant is thereby converted into a tube, giving greatly added length with which to effect an anastomosis to the esophagus without tension. The cancer-bearing segment with attached structures such as mesentery, lymph nodes, spleen, and even the serosal lining of the lesser omental bursa is then ready for severance at the determined esophageal level.

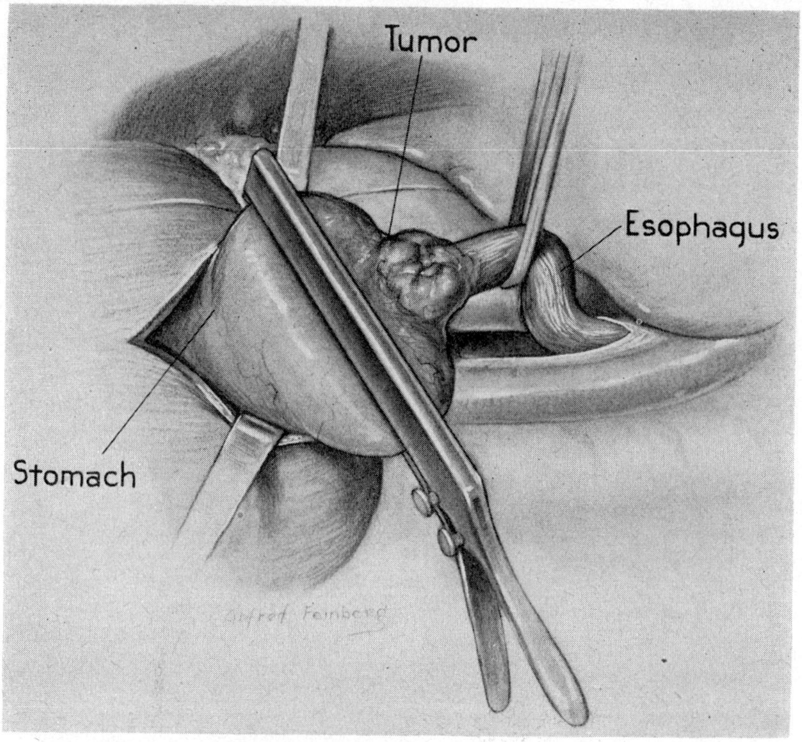

Fig. 13.—Transthoracic esophagogastrectomy. The de Petz sewing clamp has been applied distal to the gastric cancer.

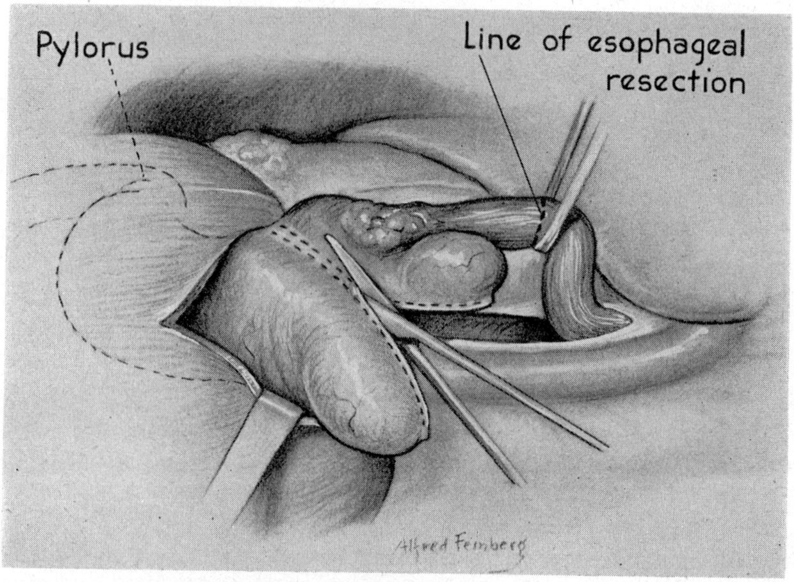

Fig. 14.—Transthoracic esophagogastrectomy. Resection of the cancer-bearing segment of stomach between two rows of de Petz metallic clips.

And end-to-end anastomosis is done by the open technique. The final level at which the esophagogastric anastomosis is done varies with the individual case. The anastomosis is always precarious because the esophagus unfortunately has no serosal coat and the longitudinal muscles of its wall do not permit the sutures to hold well. It is a well-established rule that the blood supply to the esophagus must be preserved and that the anastomosis should not be done at a distance greater than 2 cm. below one of its arterial vessels for fear of ischemia and perforation. In earlier years we employed an inner suture layer of continuous fine chromized catgut, but now we use interrupted silk sutures throughout, usually in two layers, sometimes in three. The initial posterior row of interrupted silk sutures is taken deeply and strongly. The completed anastomosis is invaginated after a fashion by pulling the seromuscular coat higher on the esophageal wall. In a few instances when we were dissatisfied about the possible integrity of the suture line we reinforced it by the application of a collar prepared by a free omental graft; it is difficult to evaluate the worth of this procedure, but it is a feasible thing to do, because in two patients coming to postmortem examination, the omental grafts were found to have taken completely.

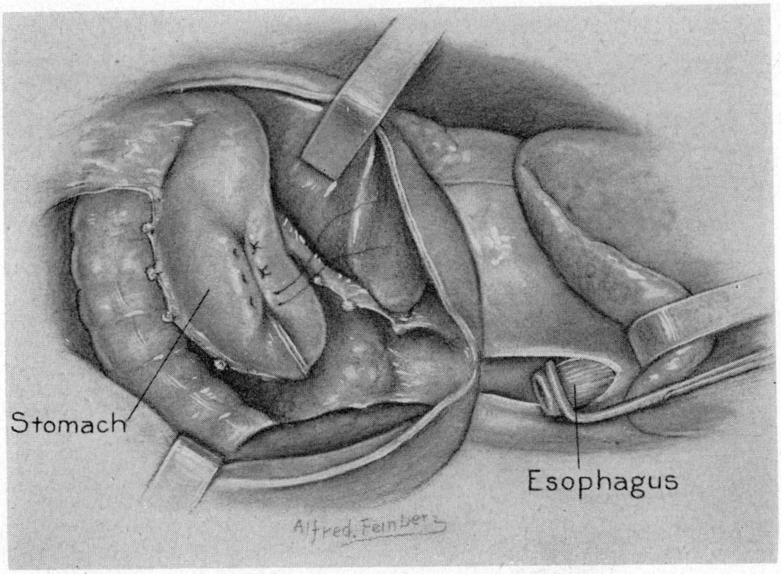

Fig. 15.—Transthoracic esophagogastrectomy. The gastric remnant is being constructed as a tube with which an anastomosis is to be effected with the esophagus.

The diaphragm is repaired by closure with two layers of interrupted silk sutures, leaving the newly constructed gastric tube within the thorax (Fig. 15). The new hiatus of the diaphragm is sutured to the wall of the stomach to aid in its suspension within the chest and further to seal off the two body cavities and prevent any possible herniation through the defect. The thoracic wall is closed in the usual manner employing underwater drainage, the intrapleural end of the tube lying fairly close to the anastomosis (Figs. 16, 17, 18 and 19).

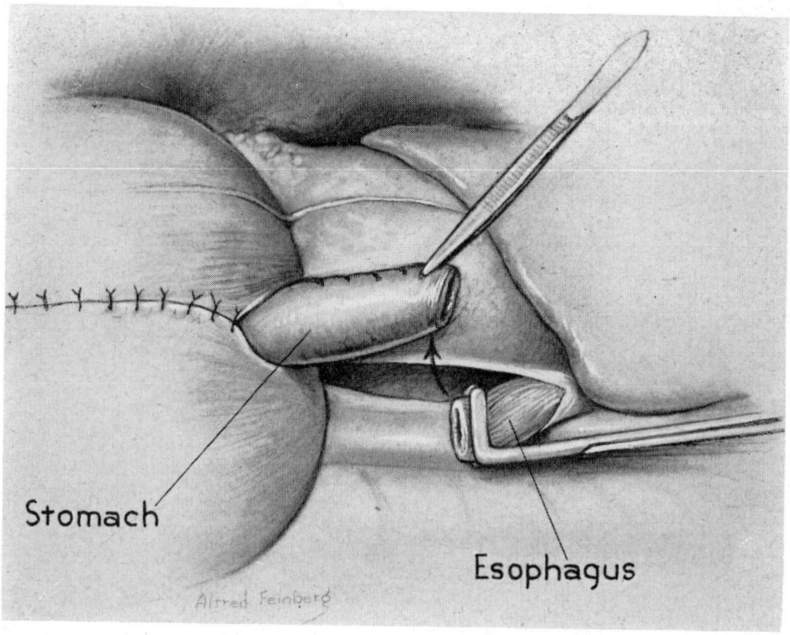

Fig. 16.—Transthoracic esophagogastrectomy. The distal segment of the stomach has been brought into its intrathoracic position, the diaphragm has been repaired, and an end-to-end anastomosis is to be done.

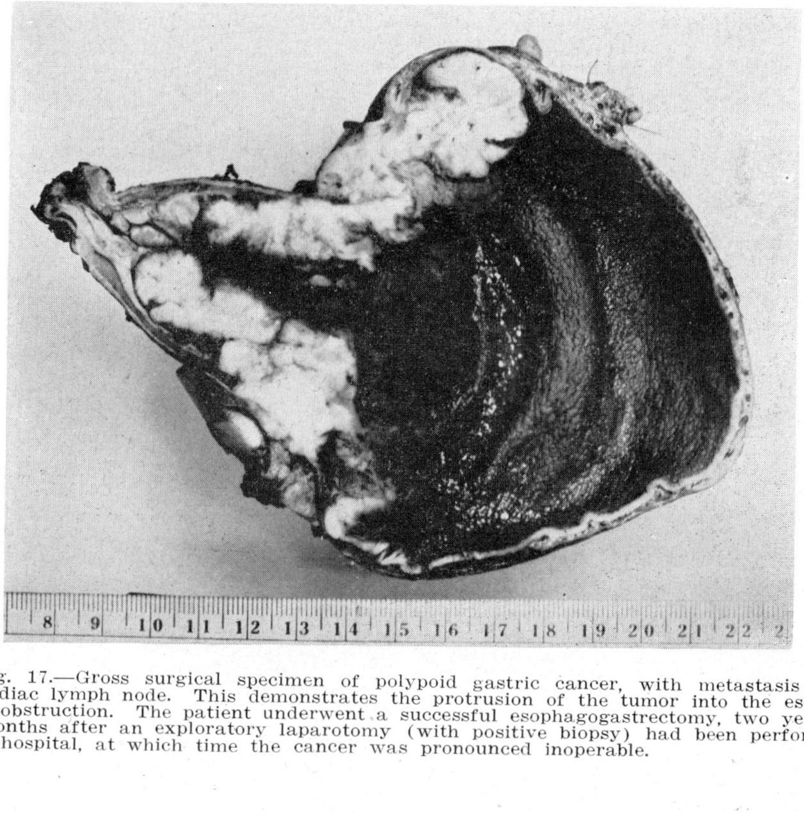

Fig. 17.—Gross surgical specimen of polypoid gastric cancer, with metastasis to one juxtacardiac lymph node. This demonstrates the protrusion of the tumor into the esophagus causing obstruction. The patient underwent a successful esophagogastrectomy, two years and three months after an exploratory laparotomy (with positive biopsy) had been performed at another hospital, at which time the cancer was pronounced inoperable.

A.

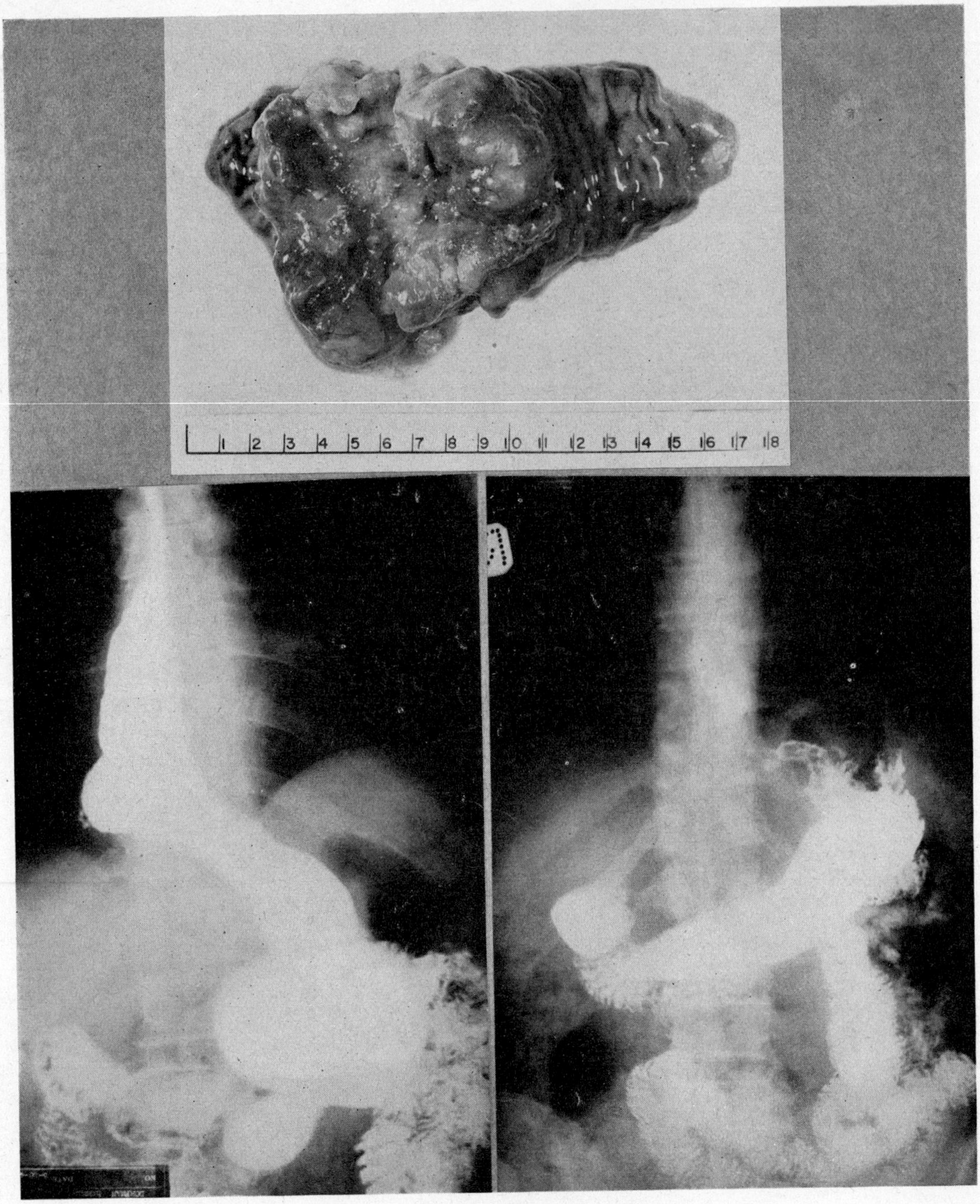

B. C.

Fig. 18—*A*, Gross specimen of resected cancer of cardioesophageal orifice. Pathology report was adenoma malignum, grade II, without metastatic involvement of regional lymph nodes. A 66-year-old man applied to the Memorial Hospital on Dec. 10, 1941, relating symptoms of seven months' duration, such as anorexia, weakness, dyspnea, loss of weight, and dysphagia. Roentgenograms showed a carcinoma of the cardiac end of the stomach with involvement of the abdominal esophagus. The lower esophagus and proximal half of the stomach were removed by the transthoracic, transdiaphragmatic route with an intrathoracic esophagogastric anastomosis. Convalescence was normal. A stricture subsequently developed and was successfully treated by peroral bouginage. The man was living and well six and one-half years following the operation. *B*, Preoperative x-ray film of cancer of cardioesophageal orifice; *C*, postoperative roentgenogram of intrathoracic esophagogastric anastomosis. Patient living and well more than six years.

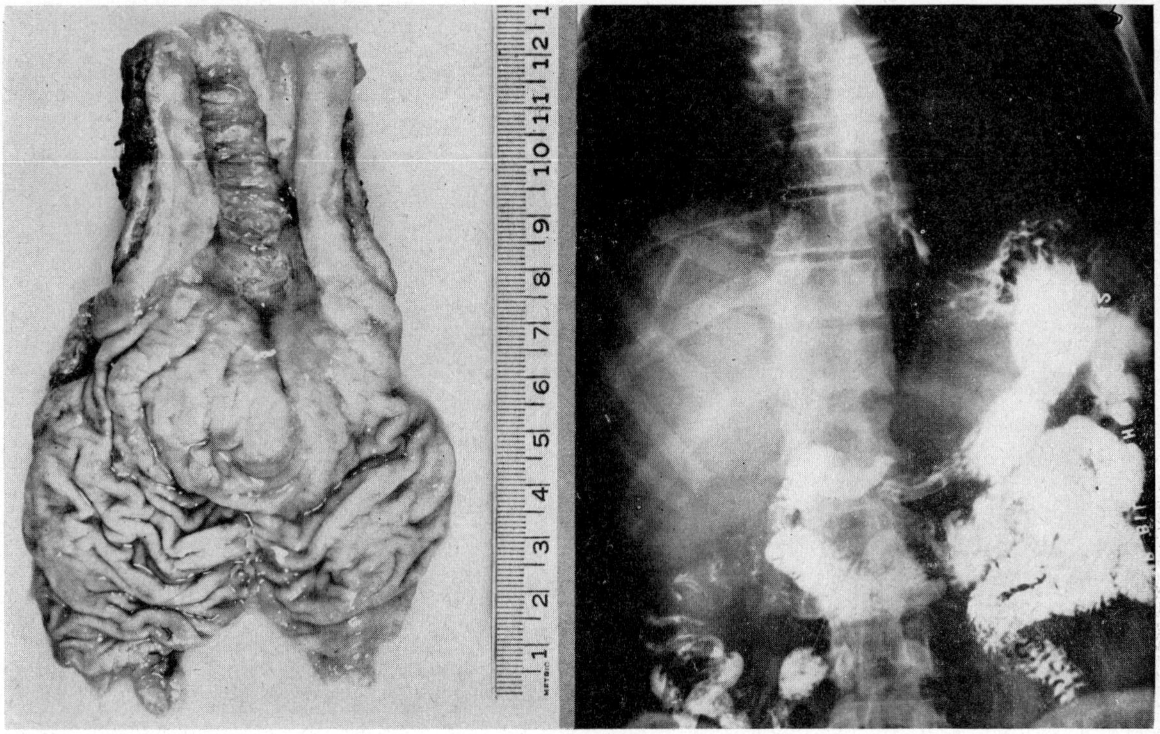

A. B.

Fig. 19.—*A*, Gross specimen of esophagogastric resection to show the location of the cancer involving the cardiac orifice and the lower esophagus. *B*, Preoperative roentgenogram to show the extent of gastric cancer in the esophagus.

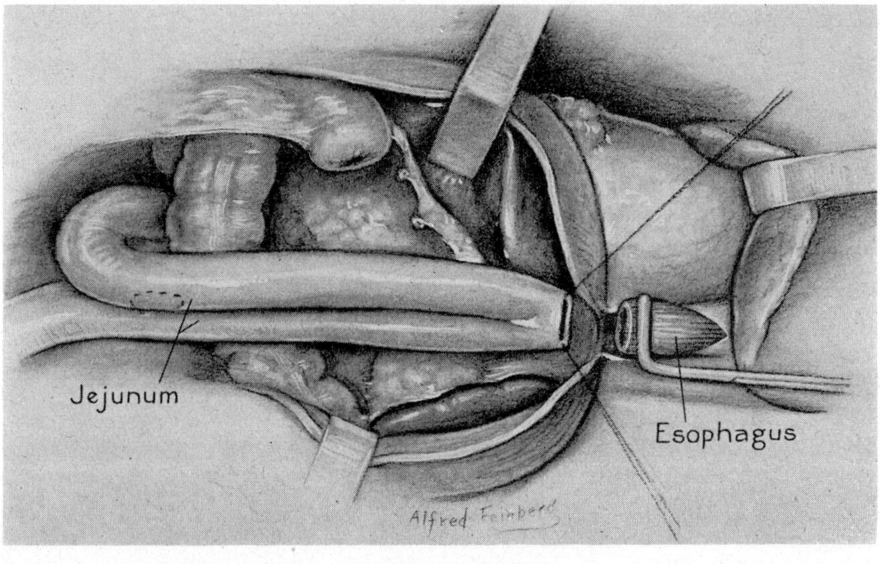

Fig. 20.—Transthoracic total gastrectomy. The entire stomach, great omentum, lesser omental bursa, and lower esophagus have been removed. The duodenal stump has been closed. A long jejunal loop has been brought up in the antecolic fashion for a terminolateral anastomosis with the esophagus. A supplementary enteroenterostomy (Braun anastomosis) has been done between the ascending and descending jejunal limbs.

Transthoracic Total Gastrectomy.—It is occasionally necessary to remove the entire stomach either by the transthoracic, transdiaphragmatic route or by the combined laparothoracotomy approach. The indications, of course, are the same as for total gastrectomy by the abdominal route, except that the esophagus too is implicated, thus requiring a supradiaphragmatic anastomosis. Involvement of the entire stomach, extension along the entire lesser curvature, diffuse invasion and nodularity of the gastric serosa, carcinosis of the lesser omental bursa, adherence to adjacent removable organs such as spleen, liver, tail of pancreas, etc., offer sufficient excuse and opportunity to remove the stomach in toto together with the necessary amount of esophagus (Fig. 20). The continuity of the alimentary tract is re-established by an intrathoracic esophagojejunostomy. The anastomosis is done either by a terminolateral (end-to-side)

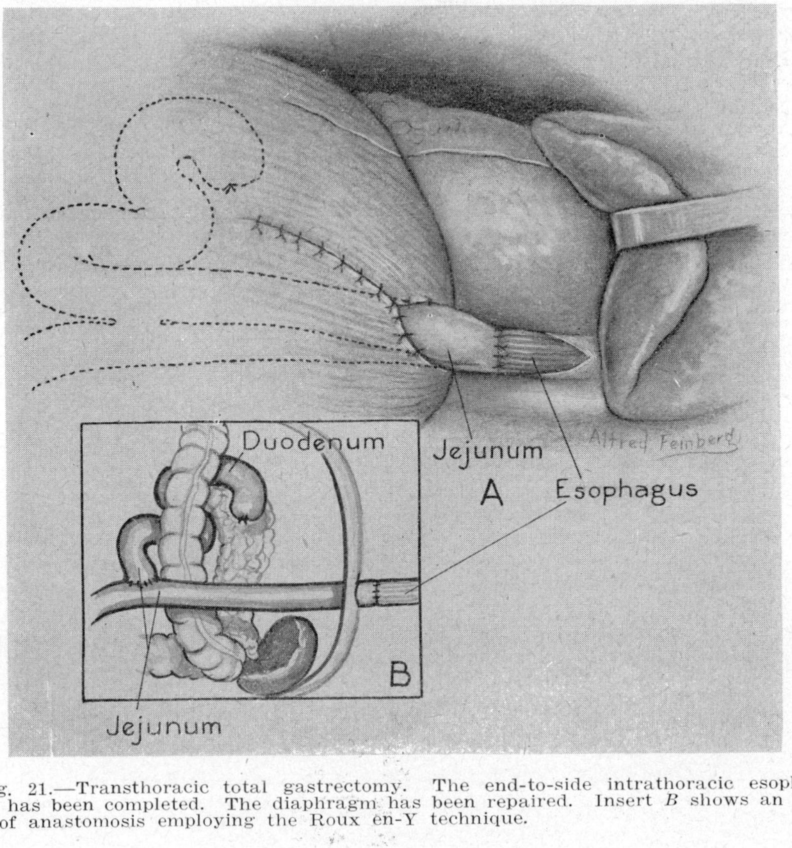

Fig. 21.—Transthoracic total gastrectomy. The end-to-side intrathoracic esophagojejunostomy has been completed. The diaphragm has been repaired. Insert *B* shows an alternate method of anastomosis employing the Roux en-Y technique.

union of the severed esophagus to a jejunal loop or by the Roux en-Y anastomosis, which is an end-to-end anastomosis of esophagus to the distal cut end of the jejunum, the proximal end of the severed jejunum being used to connect with the jejunum well below the diaphragm (Fig. 21). The jejunum may be elevated in the antecolic manner or retrocolic through a rent in the mesocolon. If the entire jejunal loop is long enough to be employed for this purpose, we usually perform an enteroenterostomy or Braun anastomosis between the ascending and descending jejunal limbs for the double purpose of permitting bile, pancreatic juice, and succus entericus to pass into the distal jejunum without regurgitation into the esophagus and also to facilitate the more direct passage of the food bolus regardless of whether it enters the ascending or descending jejunal limb.

TRANSTHORACIC RESECTION OF RECURRENT GELATINOUS CANCER AT INTRATHORACIC ANASTOMOTIC SITE OF ESOPHAGOJEJUNOSTOMY FOLLOWING TOTAL GASTRECTOMY

Case Report.—A 59-year-old man, whose mother had died of gastric cancer, applied to the gastric service of the Memorial Hospital, Nov. 3, 1947, complaining of lessened intake of food of one year's duration, severe dysphagia requiring a liquid diet of six weeks' duration, and loss of twenty pounds in weight (13.3 per cent of original body weight) in six months. Fluoroscopy and x-ray studies revealed a narrowing of the distal esophagus, a scalloping of the greater curvature of the fundus, a distortion of the mucosal pattern of the proximal gastric segment, and a cascade stomach without obstruction. An esophagoscopic biopsy taken at 40 cm. from the incisor teeth was positive for gelatinous adenocarcinoma.

On Dec. 2, 1947, a transthoracic, transdiaphragmatic total gastrectomy and splenectomy were done with an end-to-side intrathoracic esophagojejunostomy using a long jejunal loop united by a lateral enteroenterostomy. Convalescence was uneventful. The pathology report was signet-ring, gelatinous adenocarcinoma, grade II, with metastasis to omental lymph nodes. Although the esophagus was transected three fingerbreadths above the palpable upper margins of the tumor, the microscopic study showed submucosal extension of the cancer to a level only 0.8 cm. below the line of section.

Within three weeks after the operation, swallowing became progressively more difficult although the esophagogram was normal. Later the obstruction became complete as proved by the regurgitation of all food and liquids, by esophagoscopy, and fluoroscopy.

A second operation was done on Jan. 6, 1948, again by the transthoracic route. A firm, stenotic mass at the anastomotic site was considered to be recurrent or residual cancer. The previous anastomosis therefore was resected, one limb of the jejunal loop was closed, and a direct end-to-end anastomosis to the esophagus was effected with the other or distal jejunal limb. Again convalescence was uneventful. The pathological report on the second specimen was residual gelatinous carcinoma involving esophagus and jejunum. At the time of this communication the patient is in good health except for a slight benign stenosis of the anastomosis which is responding to peroral bouginage.

Epicrisis.—There are three valuable lessons to be learned from this surgical experience, namely: (1) the realization of the great tendency for cancers of this location to extend submucosally for long distances up the esophagus; (2) the wisdom of immediate frozen section microscopic study of the severed end of the esophagus before proceeding with the anastomosis, and (3) the feasibility of reoperating on such patients and resecting the locally recurrent cancer.

ABDOMINAL CARDIECTOMY

The repeatedly successful anastomosis of esophagus and stomach or esophagus and jejunum within the chest does not contradict the fact that the abdominal anastomosis is safer. In a group of more than sixty total gastrectomies done through the abdominal approach we have lost only one patient from the complication of leakage via the anastomosis, although we have had several patients with external fistulous tracts, whereas an intrathoracic leakage is of more serious import.

The questions may be asked, why not do a total gastrectomy instead of a subtotal resection of the proximal half of the stomach? Does the preservation of the distal and apparently normal half of the stomach add greatly to the risk of local recurrence? In answer to these queries, one may remark that surgeons are content to perform partial gastrectomies for cancers in the distal end of the stomach if they are assured by clinical inspection that the upper gastric segment is apparently normal. The partial removal of the upper half of the stomach in the transthoracic, transdiaphragmatic operations is considered the procedure of choice, yet by the abdominal route most surgeons believe they are compelled to sacrifice the entire stomach. In our own large group of patients treated by total gastrectomy, the chief indication for this operation was the regional location of the cancer in the proximal gastric segment. After total gastrectomy, a considerable number of patients experience postoperative abdominal discomfort; some have strictures and other mechanical disabilities; many have metabolic deficiencies such as anemia, steatorrhea, and inability to gain weight. These attendant sequels should be carefully considered in the elective choice of a total gastrectomy over partial gastrectomy (abdominal cardiectomy) for cancers of the proximal gastric segment.

The first and most essential criterion governing the suitability of any given case for abdominal cardiectomy is the confinement of the cancer strictly to the cardia without diffuse invasion of the esophagus or distal stomach. The localized polypoid tumors or ulcerocancers would seem to be the best suited for this operation of limited applicability. The notorious tendency of cancers to extend intramurally far up the esophageal wall beyond the palpable limits of the tumor must be taken into account in the preservation of sufficient abdominal esophagus to effect a subdiaphragmatic anastomosis. Mobilization of the esophagus by freeing it from the diaphragm (finger dissection) in order to increase its abdominal extension is easily done but there are limitations to this maneuver because of its precarious blood supply and fragility.

The incision for laparotomy may be either by the classical paramedian vertical approach or by the left Marwedel (paracostal) or Baudet-Navarro technique. The proximal gastric segment is mobilized by severing the gastrohepatic ligament, the coronary ligament with the left gastric artery and vein, the gastrosplenic and gastrophrenic attachments. The great omentum is removed, but the right gastroepiploic vessels and the right gastric vessels as well are preserved. If the nodes in the hilum of the spleen are involved or the cancer is adherent to the tail of the pancreas, these organs are removed en masse with the involved stomach. A peritoneal leaflet is elevated from the diaphragm and the left hepatic lobe is freed and retracted to the patient's right. The stomach is transected well below the cancer using the de Petz sewing clamp; the distal gastric tube is completed by inverting mattress sutures along the line of severance and is then ready to be joined to the esophagus. The cancerous proximal segment is elevated over the costal margin, exposing the posterior wall of the abdominal esophagus. The double posterior rows of sutures (interrupted silk) are inserted before the cancerous segment is cut away, after which the anterior rows of sutures are applied and the diaphragmatic leaflet is sewn onto the stomach below the level of the anastomosis, thereby adding greater safety and affording anchorage suspension for the otherwise unsupported remnant of stomach (Fig. 22).

The postoperative course has been good. There have been no operative fatalities in the group of ten patients on whom this operation has been done. In our first case, the patient was an obese male, weighing 285 pounds, with an anaplastic adenocarcinoma, grade IV, with metastases to three juxtacardiac lymph nodes. Postoperative pylorospasm has not been a complication, although both vagi nerves are routinely severed; in fact, the stomach has emptied with great facility (Fig. 23). There has been one exception.

PREOPERATIVE CARE

The profound effects of gastric cancer on the human mechanism are not well recognized nor understood. Conjoined studies from the Gastric Service and Laboratory for Clinical Investigation of the Memorial Hospital have demonstrated the frequent metabolic abnormalities associated with the presence of gastric cancer. The patients have usually undergone involuntary starvation for varying periods. Hepatic dysfunction as judged by a half dozen tests may be significantly impaired and yet return to normal limits after the offending cancer has been removed. Nitrogen imbalance, loss of protein stores, impaired protein synthesis, hypoproteinemia, hypoprothrombinemia, disturbed carbohydrate metabolism, and glycogen synthesis probably related to cortical adrenal dysfunction all are expressions of this metabolic disturbance and conspire to handicap the patient about to undergo radical gastric surgery. The slow but steady seepage of blood, the secondary anemia, and the absorption of toxic substances from grossly infected fungating cancers of the stomach produce circulatory changes of major importance. Imminent heart failure is frequently encountered. If partial or complete obstruction of the cardiac orifice has been produced, dehydration may have reached an alarming state of emergency. Whenever all these debilitating factors are working against an elderly individual, who from age alone is subject to various constitutional diseases, the surgeon realizes that considerable intelligent management is indicated before operative intervention is initiated.

The average patient requires about seven to ten days' time for careful preoperative preparation. The hazards of this operation are great enough without risking the patient's life by inadequate preparation. Three problems in this program are as follows: First, the fortification of the patient for the ordeal by the recognition and treatment of the incidental ailments such as heart disease, diabetes, kidney disease, etc.; second, the correction of the abnormalities attendant on the presence of the cancer such as anemia, dehydration, hypoproteinemia, inanition; and third, the preparation of the esophagus and stomach. The assignment of a medical consultant to assist in the preoperative management of these patients is one of the fundamental prerequisites of successful care. A careful estimate of the patient's general condition must be made. In addition

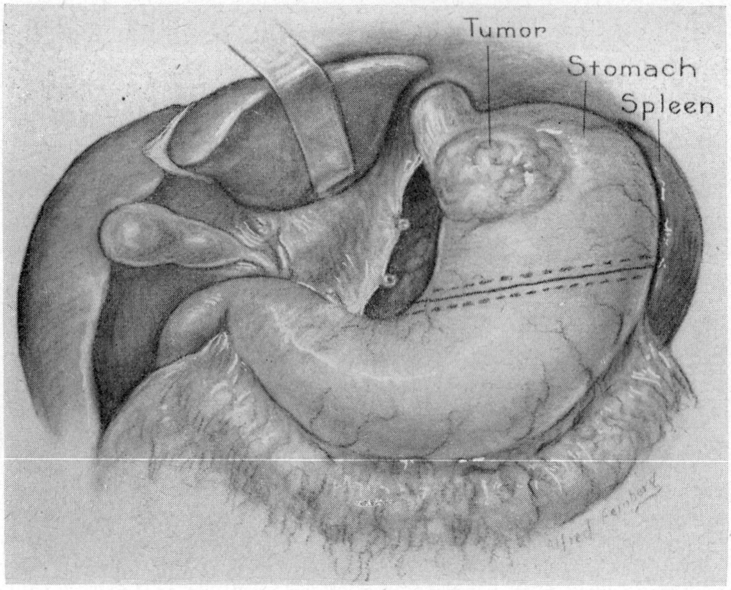

A.

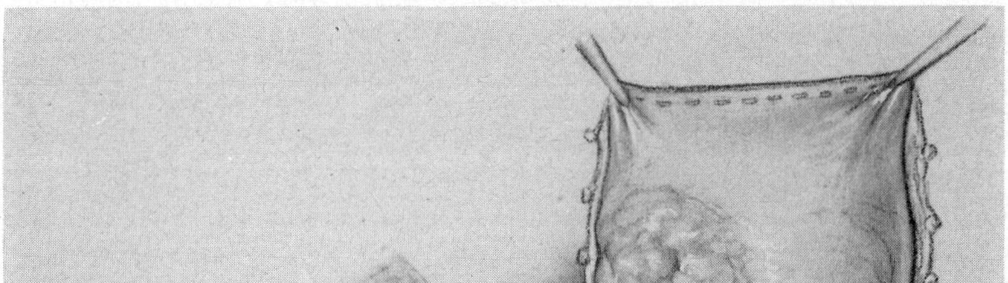

B.

Fig. 22.—Abdominal cardiectomy. *A*, Step one, mobilization of proximal gastric segment. The de Petz sutures have been applied preparatory to transection of the stomach below the cancer.

B, Step two, the cancerous proximal segment of the stomach is elevated by the Moynihan maneuver over the costal margin to expose the posterior wall of the abdominal esophagus. The distal stomach tube is being prepared by inverting the metallic clips with mattress sutures.

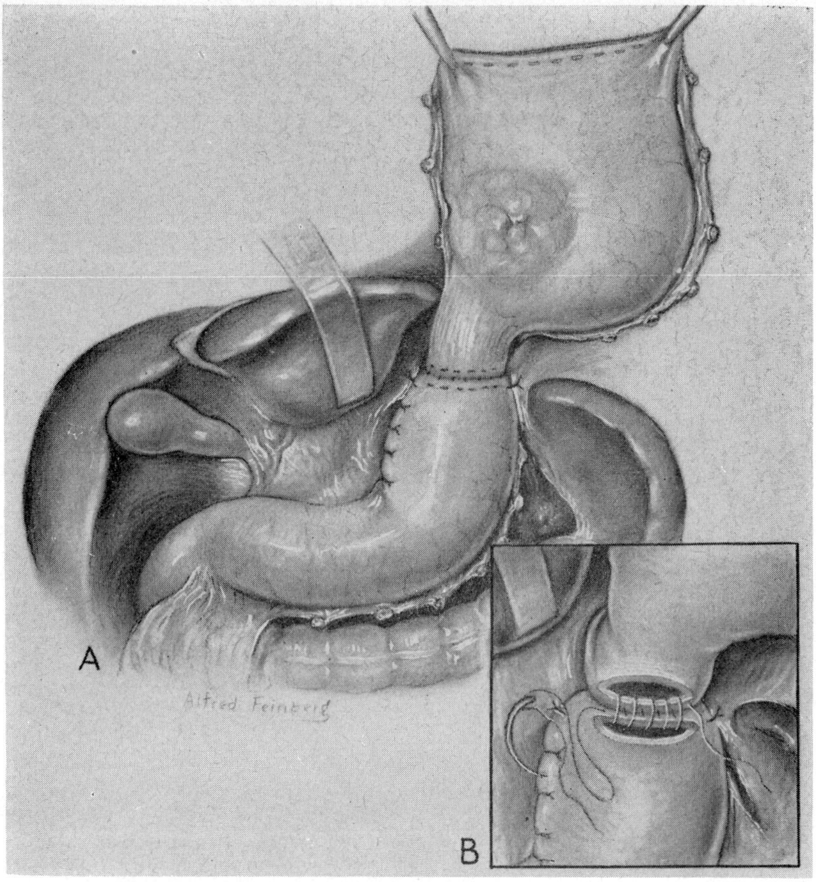

C.

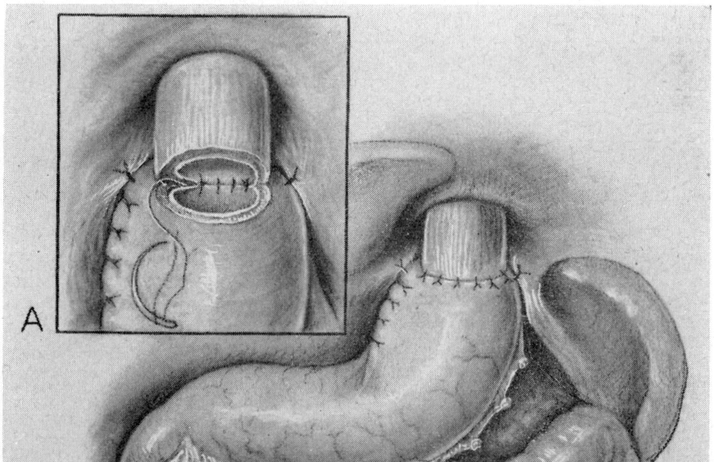

D.

Fig. 22.—*C*, Step three, the posterior rows of sutures are inserted for the esophagogastric anastomosis.

D, Step four, the completed subdiaphragmatic esophagogastric anastomosis following abdominal cardiectomy.

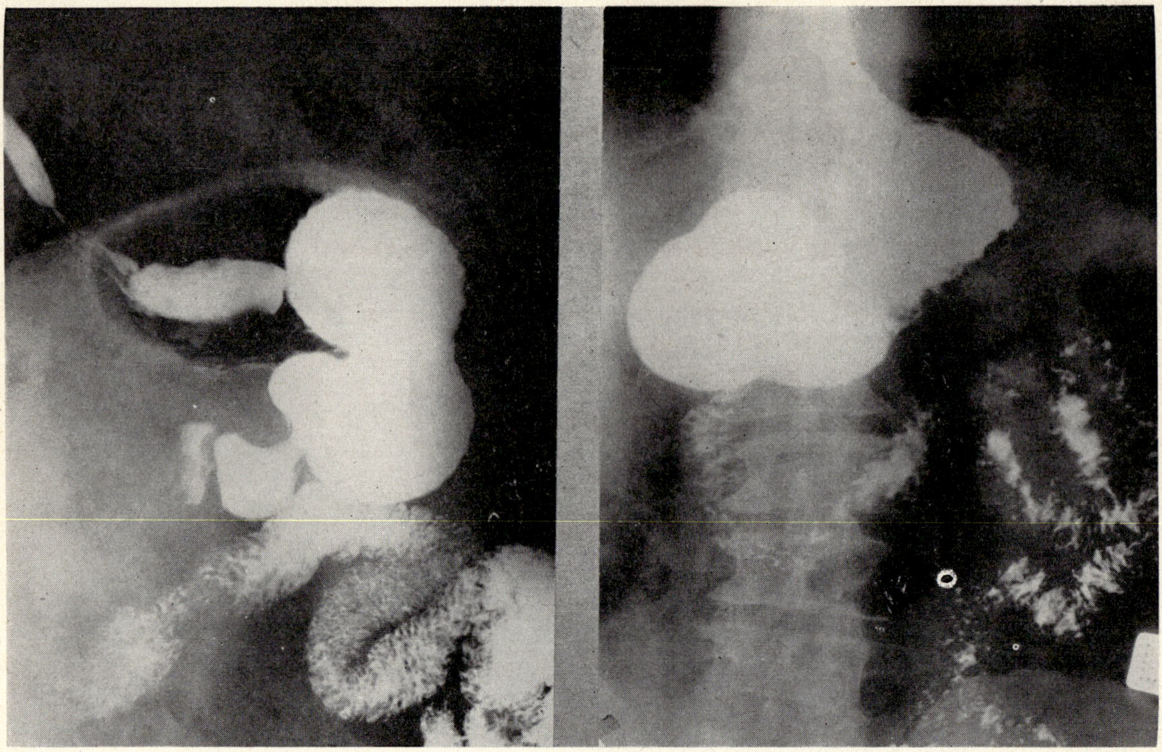

A. Fig. 23. *B.*

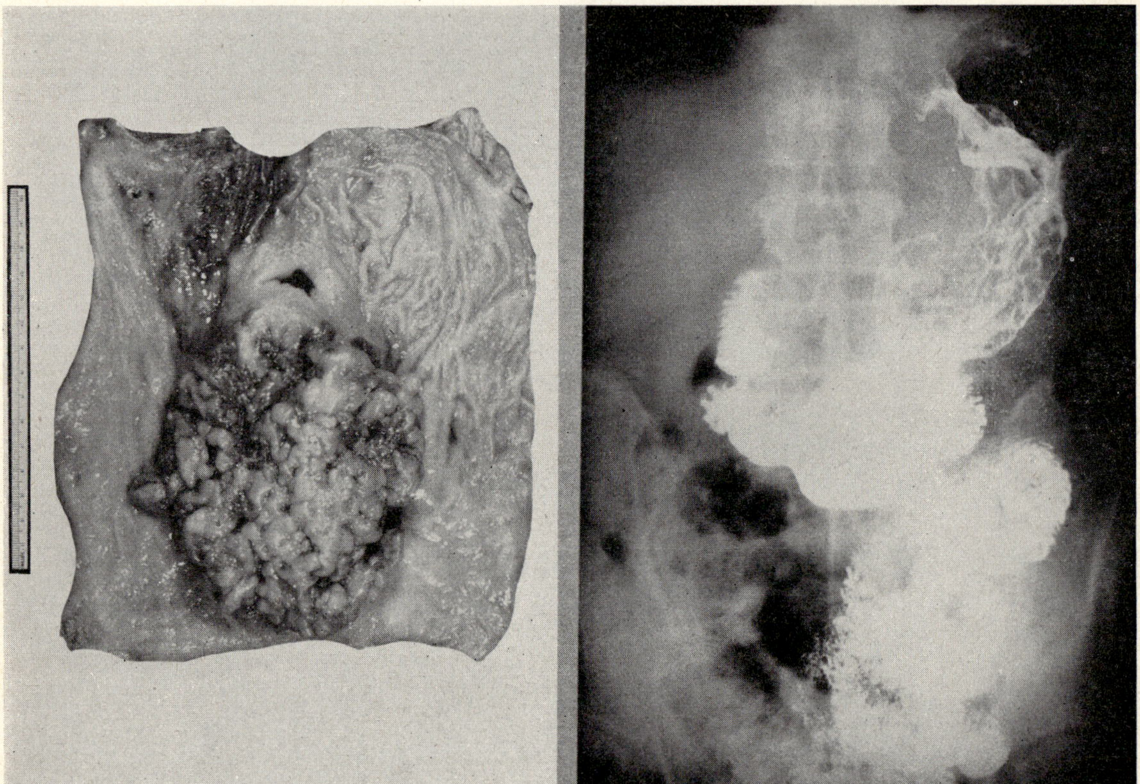

A. Fig. 24. *B.*

(For legends see opposite page.)

to the routine physical examination, special studies are done such as electrocardiography, survey films of the lungs, renal and hepatic tests of function.

Transfusions of whole blood in amounts necessary to combat anemia and increase the oxygen-carrying power are given daily. If these preliminary transfusions are only partly successful, it is wise to reserve at least 1000 c.c. of blood for the time of operation over and above the amount normally employed. In the preoperative treatment of hypoproteinemia we have employed the forced feedings of amino acids, protein hydrolysates, etc., but have observed that they

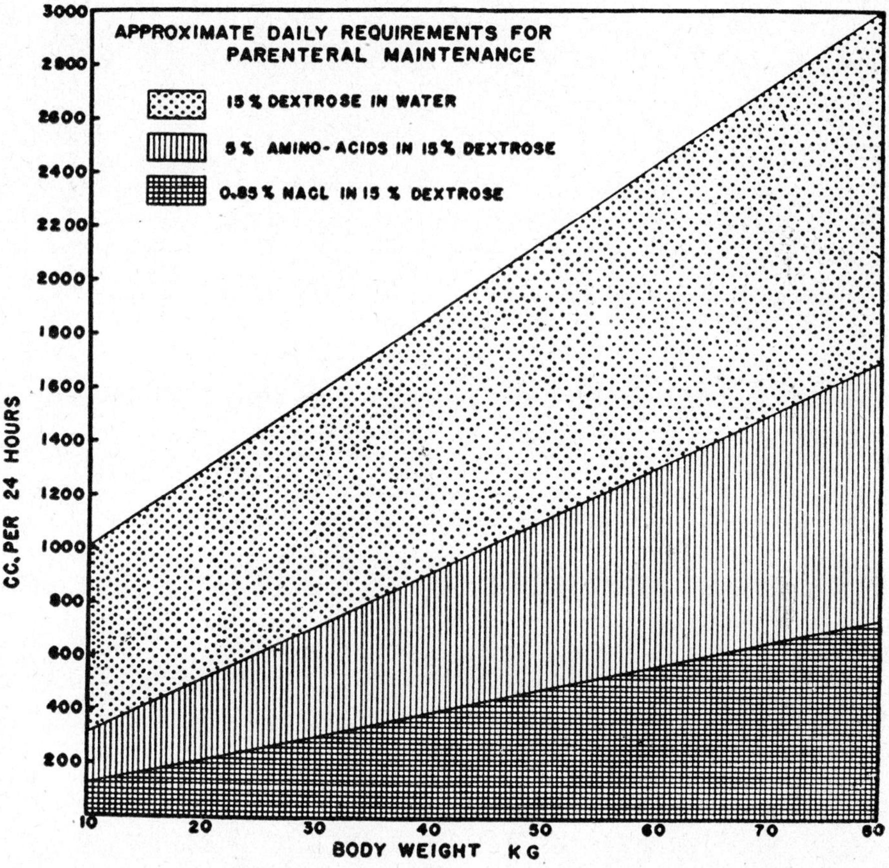

Fig. 25.—Approximate daily requirements of dextrose, amino acids, and sodium chloride for parenteral maintenance. (Courtesy of Butler, A. M., and Talbot, N. B., and the New England J. Med. 231: 585-590, 621-627, 1944.)

Fig. 23.—Abdominal cardiectomy. *A*, Roentgenogram of stomach made prior to operation. The tumor in the cardia may be seen outlined against the gas bubble. *B*, postoperative roentgenogram. The irregularity along the lesser curvature is due to the metallic suture clip. The gastric tube connecting the esophagus and pars media has been constructed from the greater curvature of the fundus.

Fig. 24.—*A*, Discrete, sessile, bulky, polypoid carcinoma in juxtacardiac position. The cardiac orifice is clearly seen. The operation performed was abdominal cardiectomy with subdiaphragmatic esophagogastrostomy. This patient was profoundly anemic and hypoproteinemic; the preoperative administration of many quarts of blood had little restorative effect. The red blood count and serum protein level became normal immediately after gastrectomy. *B*, Bulky defect in fundus of stomach produced by a huge polypoid carcinoma, as shown on roentgenogram, successfully treated by abdominal cardiectomy.

have not been as effectual as blood and plasma transfusions and the administration of human albumin. With severe anemia and severe hypoproteinemia, complete removal of the tumor is the only uniformly successful approach to the restoration of blood protein and blood counts to their normal levels. The addition of vitamin K is extremely important, because the prothrombin time is usually lower than normal, indicating liver damage. Some patients vomit uncontrollably prior to operation; intravenous fluids must be given to correct the dehydration, but it is important to remember too large and too frequent infusions of chlorides will affect adversely the ability of the plasma to regain a normal protein level and will otherwise disturb the electrolyte balance. The judicious use of glucose in distilled water may supplement the chloride infusions. The note inserted later in this paper by Homburger and the chart by Butler and Talbot (Fig. 25) may be consulted for greater detail.

POSTOPERATIVE MANAGEMENT

Resection of the gastric cardia with immediate esophagogastrostomy is of necessity a protracted operative procedure, requiring the surgeon to expose the pleural and peritoneal cavities. The main principle underlying the administration of fluids during the operation is the prevention rather than the treatment of shock. A slow infusion is started at the beginning of the operation and blood is added as soon as the preliminary exploratory procedures have been done and the cancer is considered operable. One transfusion of 600 c.c. of citrated blood is often sufficient, but if impending shock should become evident in spite of all precautions, it is treated with plasma or additional blood depending on the cause of the condition, trauma or hemorrhage.

Inasmuch as our postoperative care is directed at preventing or treating complications which may be fatal or seriously impede the patient's recovery, steps are taken in the operating room to institute this plan. The exposed lung is reinflated at frequent intervals during the operation. The anastomosis is reinforced, supported, and buttressed in every way in order to prevent leakage and subsequent empyema and/or mediastinitis. Tracheal suction is instituted by the anesthetist at the completion of the operation to free the bronchial tree of all thick secretions. Underwater tube drainage (a closed system) is established for the purpose of maintaining a negative pleural pressure, to permit the immediate escape of entrapped air and facilitate expansion of the lung, and to establish a fistulous tract for potential leakage, which seldom actually occurs. Before the chest cavity is closed, eucapin-in-oil is injected into the last five intercostal nerves for the purpose of anesthesia in the region of the operative incision. Spirometric readings after this technique of nerve blocking show a greatly improved vital capacity. The voluntary greater excursion of respiratory movements without pain is the result of the use of eucapin or similar long-lasting anesthetics in this manner. Furthermore, only minimal doses of morphine are required in the postoperative phase.

Even the application of the dressing is done with the idea of allowing full freedom of the thorax for respiration. The patient's bed is brought to the operating room and the patient transferred directly from the operating table. Just before leaving the operating room the lungs are inflated forcibly *not with oxygen* but *with ordinary air*. Because oxygen leaves the alveoli and enters the blood stream so rapidly, it may predispose to immediate atelectasis, therefore ordinary air is best for the final inflation of the lungs as the patient's respiratory movements are no longer controlled by outside influence. Before the patient is placed in an oxygen tent in his room, a portable x-ray film of the lungs is made in order to determine the degree of expansion of the lung and also the absence or unsuspected presence of air in the contralateral pleural space. Although this accident is occasionally encountered during the operative procedure, a small leak may not be observed. Aspiration of the air, preferably with the pneumothorax machine, must be immediately performed if its presence is detected, otherwise a tension pneumothorax might be set up very rapidly. No more serious complication may occur in this immediate phase. Subsequent radiographic studies of the chest are done as indicated.

The administration of oxygen either by bilateral nasal catheter or an oxygen tent is routine for the first few postoperative days in order to prevent any possible anoxia that might be a sequel to an operation involving the opening of the thoracic cavity. It is especially important in patients with heart disease. Very close observation of the underwater drainage system must be maintained at all times until the excursions become so limited, usually by the fourth or fifth day, that it may be discontinued.

One of the major dangers in the postoperative period is pulmonary atelectasis and its sequel, pneumonia. The atelectasis may be due to the presence of residual air in the chest cavity in spite of the procedure employed in the operating room to secure complete reinflation of the collapsed lung. Other factors such as a mucous plug or excess secretions may be present and active in producing this condition. Preventive measures are instituted as soon as the patient is returned to his room. He is turned at hourly intervals, lying alternately in the supine and lateral positions with the operative side down. Inhalations of pure carbon dioxide, administered by allowing the gas to flow from the tip of a tube held six inches above the patient's face, are given every half hour to every hour until consciousness is restored. The carbon dioxide serves the triple purpose of promoting deep respirations, permitting the expanded alveoli to fill with air which is reabsorbed very slowly, and aiding in the liquefaction and consequent easier expulsion of secretions. The carbon dioxide is continued after the patient regains consciousness if he is unwilling or unable voluntarily to perform deep breathing exercises every hour. These measures are carried out for the first forty-eight hours. The postoperative administration of morphine is reduced to the minimum necessary to control pain both with respect to the actual dose employed and the number of times it is given. In this way the respiratory and ciliary depressant effects of morphine are markedly decreased. If atelectasis does occur in spite of all precautions the treatment should be prompt and effective. The insertion of a small nasal catheter into the trachea and both major bronchi is readily accomplished and will induce coughing. The secretions dislodged by the cough can be aspirated by intermittent suction through the catheter. Should this method prove inadequate, suction bronchoscopy is indicated. Some degree of atelectasis, particularly of the left lower lobe, occurs in most instances in spite of these precautions. Pleural effusion is likewise a frequent complication requiring aspiration.

Early ambulation is practiced as soon as it is deemed advisable for the patient to leave the oxygen tent for even a short time. Every effort is made to encourage early and frequent movement in bed. Whenever possible the patient is encouraged to stand up or sit on the edge of the bed to urinate rather than to begin urethral catheterization too hurriedly. In forty-eight to seventy-two hours the patient is permitted to go to the bathroom for bowel movements and enemas.

Intravenous administration of normal salt solution is done in sparing amounts with full knowledge of the sodium and chloride balance. Once this requirement is met, we place more reliance on the use of glucose (5 and 10 per cent) in distilled water in quantities sufficient to produce a daily output of urine in the neighborhood of 1,200 c.c. Our recent experiences have caused us to recommend the employment of the subcutaneous rather than the intravenous route for the administration of parenteral fluids in many instances.

Patients may be fed high protein liquid nourishment by mouth, by jejunostomy, or by an indwelling tube which is passed through the nose, throat, and gullet, thence through the esophagojejunal or esophagogastric anastomosis. Orojejunal feedings through such a tube are started within twenty-four hours after the operation; the high protein, high caloric, and high vitamin diet given so early in the postoperative period speedily restores the nitrogen balance and is a decided advantage over the postoperative period of enforced starvation of earlier years. This tube has been left in place for eight days until the anastomosis is presumed to be safe, then oral feedings are resumed. This principle has been used in the case of ordinary partial gastrectomy for many years with no apparent serious complications, yet it is the opinion of one of us (G. McN.) that pulmonary complications occur more frequently with the use of such a tube and temporary jejunostomy has been used as a substitute. Some patients are intolerant of the tube passing through nose and throat and may complain bitterly.

Preoperative construction of a gastrostomy or jejunostomy for feeding purposes is not advised because of the interference with subsequent resection which these operative procedures might produce. Parenteral feeding has attained such a high degree of success that a preliminary jejunostomy is seldom necessary. Although we give our patients a high protein diet up to the very day of operation, soft or liquid foods are used depending upon the degree of obstruction at the cardia. Each evening the stomach or/and the esophagus are lavaged and emptied, using one-tenth normal hydrochloric acid for this purpose. Prophylactic penicillin is given prior to the operation and if the cancer is apparently badly infected with fever, etc., sulfonamides are added. Routine dental examination and treatment are part of the preparatory phase.

If the patient's general condition has been restored as close to normal as lies within our power, the surgeon must accept the risk of proceeding with the operation even in the face of certain systemic diseases which, in themselves, might well be definite contraindications.

Nutritional Management of Patients With Transthoracic-abdominal Resections of the Stomach

By F. Homburger, M.D.*

Nutritional Considerations in Regard to Operability.—It is my impression that any patient whose plasma proteins are lower than 6.0 Gm. per 100 ml. should not be subjected to this operation. High protein feedings may not be sufficient properly to prepare the patients, and transfusions of plasma will be necessary. In most patients with hypoproteinemia the use of large quantities of protein, perhaps protein hydrolysates and daily injections of plasma and preferably human albumin, will be necessary for longer periods than are now being used. One may encounter cases where the cardiovascular status of the patient does not permit plasma infusions. If such patients fail to respond to proper feedings and if their plasma protein values remain low, they may be considered unsuitable for the surgical procedure under discussion.

Nutritional Management in the Postoperative Phase.—In the postoperative phase, nutritional management depends upon the surgeon's decision as to whether or not a jejunal tube would be available. In my opinion the tube seems inevitably necessary whenever the patient's preoperative status suggests the possibility of cardiovascular complications in the postoperative phase. From the nutritionist's point of view, it does not matter whether the tube is orojejunal or through a jejunostomy. Regardless of the presence or absence of a feeding tube, the following measures should be observed:

1. Vitamin supplements: At least twice the average human requirement of all vitamins should be given parenterally. Thiamine is especially necessary for the oxidative processes in the postoperative phase and should be given at the rate of at least 20 to 40 mg. per day; riboflavin, about 20 to 40 mg. per day; pyridoxine 5 mg. (?); ascorbic acid, 500 to 1000 mg.; vitamin A, 15,000 U.; vitamin D, 1500 U. daily (?); nicotinic acid, 250 mg.; calcium pentothenate, 50 mg.

2. Maintenance of hemoglobin levels by adequate transfusion is necessary.

3. Maintenance of electrolyte balance. Reference is made to the papers by Butler and Talbot (Fig. 25).[16, 17] When patients are maintained on hydrolysate and sugar exclusively for more than one week, addition of mineral supplements may become necessary. The fact that more than the full sodium requirement is contained in the usual protein hydrolysates will have to be kept in mind.

*Homburger, in charge of the Laboratory for Clinical Investigation, has carried out fundamental studies on the metabolism of patients with cancer of the stomach in cooperation with the Gastric Service of the Memorial Hospital.

Nutritional management with tubes: The full protein and energy requirements can be covered by protein hydrolysate and dextrose for a few days. The fact that protein hydrolysate will be tolerated as soon as water can be taken cannot be overemphasized. Immediate feeding should be started instead of giving a large volume of water without nutrients. Diarrhea can be prevented by the use of Amphojel, Kaomagma, pectin, or certo and paregoric when necessary. It is important to use these substances at the first signs of diarrhea rather than to allow it to develop fully. After five or six days cream may be added to increase the caloric intake.

Nutritional management without intubation: Administration of adequate amounts of calories, proteins, and carbohydrates is possible by use of intravenous dextrose and intravenous hydrolysates (amigen) in quantities as indicated by Butler and Talbot. This may not suffice in patients with inoperable tumors and may have to be supplemented by plasma. The total fluid volumes necessary for proper nutrition may be excessive for the type of patient with whom we deal. Hydrolysate solutions by rectum are sometimes of help. The rectum should be cleaned with lukewarm water and a catheter inserted about twelve inches high. The rate of administration should be slow, controlled by Murphy drip, and the volume given at one time not to exceed 400 c.c. This may be repeated twice or three times and the total amount of hydrolysate to fill the patient's nitrogen requirement may be given in that manner in favorable cases.

It should be realized that no matter how well the nitrogen requirement may be covered, many patients will be unable to regenerate plasma protein and that in such cases plasma will have to be used in sufficient amounts to maintain a plasma protein of 6 Gm. per 100 ml.

LOCATION OF THE GASTRIC CANCER

The prime indication for the operation of cardiectomy or proximal gastrectomy is the localization of the cancer in the cardia, fundus, or upper half of the stomach. In 40 per cent of these resections, the esophagus was grossly involved by the cancer. If the abdominal esophagus is involved, the transthoracic approach should be used because of the well-known inclination of these cancers to extend submucosally high into the esophagus. In 30.7 per cent of the cancers resected, the lesion was confined to the cardia or cardia and lesser curvature without involvement of the abdominal esophagus; the decision to employ transthoracic esophagogastrectomy rather than total gastrectomy rests on numerous other factors, among which are the estimated technical ease of one approach over the other (Table III).

RESECTABILITY OF CANCERS OF THE GASTRIC CARDIA

Our rate of resectability for gastric cancers as a whole is 40 per cent. It would be higher were it not for the fact that the Memorial Hospital for Cancer, situated in a great metropolitan city, receives more than its quota of patients with advanced inoperable cancers deemed unsuitable for care in general institutions. Our rate of resectability for cancers of the gastric cardia, however, is 59.5 per cent, which is 50 per cent better than for gastric cancers as a whole.

TABLE III. RESECTION OF THE GASTRIC CARDIA; LOCATION OF GASTRIC CANCERS

LOCATION	NUMBER	PER CENT
Total cases	62	100.0
Cardia or cardia and lesser curvature	19	30.7
Cardia with involvement of esophagus	25	40.3
Extensive involvement of proximal segment	17	27.4
Multiple tumors:	1	1.6
Myosarcoma of the antrum and adenocarcinoma of the cardia		
LOCATION OF BENIGN GASTRIC ULCERS*		
Total cases (undergoing transthoracic esophagocardiectomy)		3
Cardia and lesser curvature		2
Multiple ulcers†		1

*These cases are not included in the statistical analyses except for Table II.

†In this patient, one large ulcer on the anterior wall at the cardia perforated the left lobe of the liver and diaphragm. Another huge ulcer of the posterior wall of the fundus was fixed to the pancreas and perforated into the spleen. The resection was a transabdominal, transdiaphragmatic esophagogastrectomy, splenectomy, partial pancreatectomy, and partial hepatectomy with esophagojejunostomy.

Therefore, it must be concluded that this regional localization is a favorable one for two reasons, namely, the earlier recognition of the cancers and the greater relative assurance of resectability. The advantages are somewhat neutralized by the higher operative mortality but this hazard is gradually lessening. Of the reasons for nonresectability, it may be seen that in only one instance was the condition of the patient a contraindication for the operation. Transthoracic esophagogastrectomy has been done in patients more than 70 years of age. Involvement of adjacent structures such as diaphragm, abdominal wall, spleen, left hepatic lobe, and pancreas has complicated the surgical problem but these structures have been removed if necessary and whenever possible; in thirteen patients this invasion and fixity was too great to be overcome by surgical attack. Distant metastases or peritoneal carcinosis determines the incurability of cancer and in twenty-six patients was the factor which influenced us in not attempting the operation, but in four patients with cancers of the gastric cardia admittedly incurable we performed palliative transthoracic esophagogastrectomies (Table IV).

TABLE IV. RESECTABILITY OF CANCERS OF THE GASTRIC CARDIA

CASES		NUMBER	PER CENT
Total cases, cancers of gastric cardia		104	
Total cases resected		62	59.5
Total cases nonresectable		42	40.5
Reasons for nonresectability			
1. Metastases to distant sites	26		
2. Involvement of/or fixation to neighboring organs	13		
3. Insuperable technical difficulties	2		
4. Condition of the patient	1		

NONFATAL COMPLICATIONS FOLLOWING RESECTION OF THE GASTRIC CARDIA

The great majority of the complications occurred in the days of our early experience in the performance of these operations. There have been fewer complications during the past eighteen months. The details of prevention of these complications are given in the sections dealing with pre- and postoperative care. The number of cardiovascular accidents has been lessened since we have had expert cardiologists prepare our patients with diseases of the heart and blood vessels and since we have lowered the incidence of phlebothrombosis by early ambulation and prevented hazardous and even fatal embolism by early, elective bilateral femoral and saphenous vein ligations. The pulmonary complications are prevented with greater ease than they are cured; these prophylactic measures are proper anesthesia, forceful aeration of lungs with ordinary air rather than oxygen at the completion of the operation, employment of the oxygen tent during the first few postoperative days, the prophylactic administration of penicillin and aerosal and the sulfonamides before and after the operation, and, most important of all, frequent aspirations of the trachea and bronchial tree by use of a suction catheter. The substitution of interrupted silk sutures throughout for two to three layers has been a definite improvement over the inner continuous catgut suture for the anastomosis as it has resulted in fewer leaks and fistulas and also in a lessened tendency for stricture formation. When external fistulas occur after abdominal total gastrectomy with subdiaphragmatic anastomoses, stenosis at the line of union has almost invariably developed, but on the contrary, external thoracic fistulas appearing after intrathoracic esophagogastric anastomoses have not resulted in strictures in our experience. Underwater drainage with the large fenestrated intrathoracic tube placed fairly close to the anastomosis has perhaps allowed the survival of some patients who developed leaks or ruptures of the anastomosis, as it led to temporary external fistula formation rather than fatal mediastinitis. The postoperative strictures are often amenable to dilatation by peroral bouginage. In one patient, a successful reoperation was done for resection of a cancer recurrent in an esophagojejunal anastomosis. In another instance the stricture was so renitent that a permanent jejunostomy for feeding was necessary. The information gleaned from the conjoined studies on the metabolism of patients with gastric cancer done by the Gastric Service and the Laboratory for Clinical Investigation of the Memorial Hospital (and previously published) has served in

TABLE V. NONFATAL COMPLICATIONS FOLLOWING RESECTION OF THE GASTRIC CARDIA FOR CARCINOMA

COMPLICATION	FREQUENCY
Number of operative survivals	41
Pulmonary Complications:	
Atelectasis	8
Pleural effusion	6
Pneumonia	14
Purulent bronchitis	1
Empyema	1
Subcutaneous emphysema	1
Abdominal Complications	
Ileus	1
Impaired motor function of gastric remnant	3
Anastomotic Complications:	
Fistula	4
Stenosis	4
Wound infection	1
Cardiovascular complications	8
Systemic complications (persistent hypoproteinemia, etc.)	3
Urinary complications (prostatic hypertrophy)	1
Patients having no complications*	12

*Of the twelve patients having no complications, eight were operated on in 1947 or later.

TABLE VI. END RESULTS FOLLOWING RESECTION OF THE GASTRIC CARDIA

Total cases of gastric cancer		62
Dead, total		42
Operative deaths	21	
Subsequent deaths	21	
Living, total		20
With disease	2	
Without disease	18	
Operative mortality	33 per cent	

There were no operative deaths following resection for ulcer (3 cases).

TABLE VII. CAUSE OF DEATH FOLLOWING RESECTION OF THE GASTRIC CARDIA

A. OPERATIVE DEATH

CAUSE OF DEATH	NUMBER
Number of operative deaths	21
Pulmonary and mediastinal complications	16
Cardiovascular complications	14
Anastomotic failure	4
Peritonitis	2
Esophagobronchial fistula	1
Subphrenic abscess	1
Rupture of intercostal artery	1

B. SUBSEQUENT DEATH

CAUSE OF DEATH	TOTAL CASES	METASTASIS TO REGIONAL LYMPH NODES	
		WITH	WITHOUT
Total	21	18	3
Metastasis	9	8	1
Recurrence	10	8	2
Suicide	1	1	
Undetermined	1	1	
Average postoperative duration	13.3 months	11.9 months	21.5 months

TABLE VIII. POSTOPERATIVE DURATION OF LIFE FOLLOWING RESECTION OF THE GASTRIC CARDIA FOR CANCER

POSTOPERATIVE DURATION OF LIFE	NUMBER SURVIVING OPERATION		WITH METASTASIS TO REGIONAL LYMPH NODES		WITHOUT METASTASIS TO REGIONAL LYMPH NODES	
	LIVING	DEAD	LIVING	DEAD	LIVING	DEAD
Total	20	21	10	18	10	3
With Disease	2	19		16	2	3
6 months or less		7		7		
7 to 12 months	2	5		4	2	1
13 to 24 months		5		4		1
25 to 36 months		2		1		1
Without Disease	18		10		8	
6 months or less	9		7		2	
7 to 12 months	1		1			
13 to 24 months	1				1	
25 to 36 months	4		1		3	
37 to 48 months	1		1			
49 to 60 months						
Over 60 months	2				2	
Undetermined		2		2		

good stead to lower the complications inherent in this source. Impaired motor function of the gastric remnant following cardiectomy has been observed three times, the pylorospasm with associated gastric atony no doubt being due to the vagotomy which is necessarily done if the operation is complete. This condition has been ameliorated by the use of urecholine, 5 to 10 mg., fifteen minutes before meals, three times daily. We have not been compelled to perform pyloroplasties or gastrojejunostomies on these patients. (Table V).

END RESULTS FOLLOWING RESECTION OF THE GASTRIC CARDIA

In our group of sixty-five cardiectomies (three for ulcer) the operative mortality was 32 per cent. This figure is distressingly and avoidably too high. The cases reported herein, however, include the entire experience of the department with all cases listed, done by junior members of the department and resident staff. Although the technical fallibilities of the operation have been largely eradicated, it must be realized that we are now extending the scope of the operation to include adjacent organs and these still more major procedures must be correspondingly more hazardous.

Twenty-one of these patients died as a result of the operation and twenty-one of the survivors ultimately succumbed due to continued growth and metastases of the cancers. The great majority of operative deaths was due to pulmonary and cardiovascular complications (see Table VI). By far the greater number of patients dying because of cardiopulmonary complications passed through a very uneven anesthetic experience. Surgical complications resulting from infections, trauma, faulty suture line, etc., and causing peritonitis, subphrenic abscess, anastomotic leakage, etc., accounted for only eight of the operative deaths. If one were positive that a sound anastomosis without tension had been effected and that no undue soiling had occurred, serious consideration would be given to the possibility of discontinuing the underwater drainage. Three of four patients who developed empyema of the pleural cavity after transthoracic esophagogastrectomy died of this complication (Tables VII and VIII).

Our first resection of the gastric cardia was performed on May 2, 1940. Only a few similar operations were done in the ensuing years; the yearly increment has been considerable and encouraging, but the number of cases available for the computation of five-year cures is not large enough to be conclusive or to ensure the accuracy of curability rates for this cancer. Of the nine patients on whom we operated more than five years ago, two are still living and well without evidence of recurrence, a five-year survival rate of 22 per cent. Twenty of the total number of patients are living, two with recurrent cancer and eighteen without evidence of this disease.

The authors wish to express their gratitude to Miss Mildred P. Ashley, their research associate and librarian for many years, for her invaluable aid in this work.

REFERENCES

1. Ach.: Beitrag zur Oesophagus Chirurgie, Verhandl. d. deutsch. Gesellsch. f. Chir. 42: 260-269, 1913.
2. Ayala Gonzales, Abraham, and Luna O., Antonio: Cáncer del esofago, Rev. de gastroenterol. de México 9: 55-89, 1944.

3. Beecher, H. K.: Shock and Anesthesia in Transthoracic Gastric Surgery, Surg., Gynec. & Obst. **76**: 331-336, 1943.
4. Bernstein, A.: Carcinoma of the Cardia, Rev. Gastroenterol. **8**: 234-238, 1941.
5. Biondi, D.: Esofago-gastrostomia sperimentale intrathoracica, Policlinico Suppl. **1**: 964, 1894-1895.
6. Bircher, E.: Operative Heilung eines Carcinoms am Übergang des Oesophagus in der Cardia, Correspondenzbl. f. Schweiz. Aertze. **48**: 467-478, 1918.
7. Bircher, E.: Die Technik der Magenchirurgie, Stuttgart, 1925, Ferdinand Enke, pp. 85-94.
8. Bird, C. E.: Recent Advances in Surgery of the Esophagus, SURGERY **6**: 772-801, 949, 1939.
9. Boit, H.: Die Radikaloperation des Karzinoms der Kardia und des abdominalen Oesophagus, Zentralbl. f. Chir. **41**: 846-849, 1914.
10. Borches, E.: Erfolgreiche Resektion der oberen Magenhälfte, Munchen. med. Wchnschr. **74**: 1454-1456, 1927.
11. Borches, E.: Die abdominale Resektion der oberen Magenhälfte (nach operationstechnichen Gesichtspunkten) Beitr. z. klin. Chir. **143**: 484-538, 1928.
12. Borelius, J.: Transpleural resektion av cardia och øesofagus, Hygiea (Stockholm) **77**: 1-8, 1915.
13. Bradshaw, H. H., and O'Neil, J. F.: Surgical Treatment of Some Lesions of the Upper Stomach, J. Thoracic Surg. **14**: 187-194, 1945.
14. Brun, H.: Zur Mobilisation und Verlagerung des Magens and Duodenums bei Operationen am Magen und unteren Abschnitt der Speiseröhre, Beitr. z. klin. Chir. **84**: 305-338, 1913.
15. Brun, H.: Ueber die Bedeutung und Unterbindung der Art. coronaria sin. bei Resektionen des Magens insbesondere der Kardia, Deutsche Ztschr. f. Chir. **135**: 81-100, 1916.
16. Butler, A. M., and Talbot, N. B.: Parenteral-fluid Therapy. I. Estimation and Provision of Daily Maintenance Requirements. New England J. Med. **231**: 585-590, 1944.
17. Butler, A. M., and Talbot, N. B.: Parenteral-fluid Therapy. II. The Estimation of Losses Incident to Starvation and Dehydration With Acidosis or Alkalosis and the Provision of Repair Therapy, New England J. Med. **231**: 621-627, 1944.
18. Carter, B. N., Stevenson, J., and Abbott, O. A.: Transpleural Esophagogastrostomy for Carcinoma of the Esophagus and for Carcinoma of the Cardiac Portion of the Stomach, SURGERY **8**: 587-603, 1940.
19. Cattell, R. B.: Resection of the Lower Esophagus for Carcinoma, S. Clin. North America **21**: 649-655, 1941.
20. Churchill, E. D., and Sweet, R. H.: Transthoracic Resection of Tumors of Stomach and Esophagus, Ann. Surg. **115**: 897-920, 1942.
21. Clagett, O. T., and Wiig, L. M.: Transthoracic Resection of the Esophagus and Stomach for Cancer, Proc. Staff Meet., Mayo Clin. **18**: 337-344, 1943.
22. Clagett, O. T., and Root, G. T.: Transthoracic Resection of the Cardia of the Stomach, Proc. Staff Meet., Mayo Clin. **19**: 187-191, 1944.
23. Clairmont, P.: Ueber die Extirpation des Kardiacarcinoms, Arch. f. klin. Chir. **140**: 343-377, 1926.
24. Fischer, H.: Surgical Treatment of the Esophagus, Arch. Surg. **6**: 256-273, 1923.
25. Garlock, J. H.: Problem of Carcinoma of Cardiac End of the Stomach, Surg., Gynec. & Obst. **73**: 244-256, 1941.
26. Garlock, J. H.: Combined Abdominothoracic Approach for Carcinoma of Cardia and Lower Esophagus, Surg., Gynec. & Obst. **83**: 737-741, 1946.
27. Garlock, J. H.: Technical Problems in Surgical Treatment of Carcinoma of the Esophagus and Upper Stomach, SURGERY **21**: 143, 1947.
28. Gosset, A.: De l'oesophago-gastrostomie transdiaphragmatique, Rev. de chir. **28**: 694-707, 1903.
29. Griswold, R. A.: Transthoracic Gastrectomy for Unusual Lesions of the Stomach, Ann. Surg. **121**: 600-619, 1945.
30. Von Hacker, V., and Lotheissen, G.: Resektion des Bauchstuckes und der Cardia, in Chirurgie der Speiseröhre, Stuttgart, 1926, Ferdinand Enke, pp. 447-460.
31. Hedblom, C. A.: Combined Transpleural and Transperitoneal Resection of the Thoracic Oesophagus and the Cardia for Carcinoma, Surg., Gynec. & Obst. **35**: 284-287, 1922.
32. Heuer, G. J., Andrus, W. DeW., and Bell, H. G.: The Experimental Transplantation of the Diaphragm as an Adjunct in the Treatment of Lesions of the Lower End of the Esophagus, Ann. Surg. **81**: 273-286, 1925.
33. Hörhammer, C.: Das Einmanschettierungsverfahren nach Goepel an den kardialen Magenpartien, mit besonderer Berücksichtigung der Einpflanzung des Osophagus Zentralbl. f. Chir. **50**: 633-636, 1923.
34. Homburger, F.: Use of Protein Hydrolysates by Mouth, Am. J. Med. **3**: 430-433, 1947.

35. Homburger, F., and Young, N. F.: Chemical Evolution and Labeling of Protein Hydrolysates for Human Consumption, Am. J. Med. 3: 427-429, 1947.
36. Homburger, F., and Young, N. F.: Studies on Hypoproteinemia. I. Hypoproteinemia in Patients With Gastric Cancer; its Persistence After Operation in the Presence of Body Tissue Repletion, Blood (In Press.)
37. Ingebrigtsen, R.: Resection du cardia cancéreux, Acta chir. Scandinav. **73**: 43-46, 1933.
38. Ingebrigtsen, R.: Om reseksjon av cardia og nedre ende av øesofagus (ved kancer), Norsk. mag. f. laegevidensk. **97**: 479-486, 1936.
39. Janeway, H. H., and Green, N. W.: Cancer of the Oesophagus and Cardia. A Description for Its Removal by the Transthoracic Route Under Conditions of Differential Pressure, Ann. Surg. **52**: 67-82, 1910.
40. Jonas, A. F., Jr.: Transpleural Esophago-gastrostomy, Arch. Surg. **44**: 556-569, 1942.
41. Kirschner, Theodore: Die Eingriffe in der Bauchhöle, in Chirurgische Operationslehre, 2 Bd. Spezieller Teil I, 1932, pp. 175-181.
42. Kümmell: Carcinom der Kardia, Verhandl. d. deutsch. Gesellsch. f. Chir. **39**: 96-97, 1910.
43. Lahey, F. H., and Marshall, S. F.: Some Unusual Gastro-enterological Surgical Problems, Am. J. Digest. Dis. **6**: 554-664, 1939.
44. Lotheissen, G.: Zur Radikaloperation des Speiseröhrenkrebses, Arch. f. klin. Chir. **131**: 200-225, 1924.
45. Marshall, S. F.: Carcinoma of the Esophagus, S. Clin. North America **18**: 643-648, 1938.
46. Meyer, H. W.: Intrathoracic Esophagojejunostomy for Total Gastrectomy With Lower Esophagectomy for Cancer, SURGERY **12**: 115-127, 1942.
47. Meyer, W.: Resection of the Cardia for Carcinoma, Ann. Surg. **62**: 693-709, 1915.
48. Von Mikulicz, J.: Beiträge zur Technik der Operation des Magencarcinoma, Verhandl. d. deutsch. Gesellsch. f. Chir. **27**: 252-260, 1898.
49. Von Mikulicz, J.: Chirurgische Erfahrungen über die Sauerbruch'sche Kammer Unter und Ueberdruck, Verhandl. d. deutsch. Gesellsch. f. Chir. **33**: 34-41, 1904.
50. Miyagi, J.: Unsere Erfahrungen mit der Resektion des Kardiakrebses, Arch. f. klin. Chir. **149**: 187-193, 1927.
51. Muir, E. G.: Resection of the Lower Oesophagus and Cardia, Lancet **2**: 75-77, 1936.
52. Nagel, G. W., and Menke, J. F.: Transthoracic Operations for Neoplasms of the Esophagus and Stomach, Surg., Gynec. & Obst. **83**: 657-666, 1946.
53. Ochsner, A., and DeBakey, M.: Surgical Aspects of Carcinoma of the Esophagus, J. Thoracic Surg. **10**: 401-445, 1941.
54. Pack, G. T., and Cameron, C. S.: Abdominal Cardiectomy or Subtotal Resection for Cancer of the Proximal Half of the Stomach, Am. J. Surg. **59**: 3-8, 1943.
55. Pack, G. T., and McNeer, G.: Total Gastrectomy for Cancer. A Collective Review of the Literature and an Original Report of Twenty Cases, Surg., Gynec. & Obst. **77**: 265-299, 1943.
56. Pack, G. T., McNeer, G., and Booher, R. J.: Principles Governing Total Gastrectomy, Arch. Surg. **55**: 457-485, 1947.
57. Pack, G. T., and Watson, W. L.: Transthoracic Subtotal Gastrectomy and Esophagectomy for Cancer, Arch. Surg. **46**: 930-938, 1943.
58. Parcelier, A.: Contribution à l'étude du cancer du cardia et en particulier de son traitement chirurgicale, Ann. internat. de chir. gastrointestinal **5**: 131-170, 1911; also in Arch. prov. de chir. **21**: 129-167, 1912.
59. Phemister, D. B.: Resection for Carcinoma of Esophagus (Editorial), Surg., Gynec. & Obst. **74**: 266-267, 1942.
60. Phemister, D. B.: Transthoracic Resection for Cancer of the Cardiac End of the Stomach, Arch. Surg. **46**: 915-929, 1943.
61. Pierson, J. C., and Pack, G. T.: Indications for Vertical Gastroscopy, Rev. Gastroenterol. **11**: 111-113, 1944.
62. Raven, R. W.: Thoracico-abdominal Gastrectomy for Carcinoma of the Thoracic Stomach, Brit. J. Surg. **29**: 39-46, 1941.
63. Rehn, Eduard: Osophagus-Chirurgie, Jena, 1914, Gustav Fischer, pp. 28-31; 86-90.
64. Sauerbruch, F.: Die Chirurgie des Brustteils der Spieseröhre, Beitr. z. klin. Chir. **46**: 405-494, 1905.
65. Sauerbruch, F.: Experimentelle Beiträge zur Oesophagus-chirurgie, Verhandl. d. deutsch. Gesellsch. f. Chir. **34**: 140-149, 1905.
66. Sauerbruch, F.: Ueber die Indikationen zur Resektion des Brustabschnittes der Speiseröhre, Deutsche Ztschr. f. Chir. **98**: 113-125, 1909.
67. Sauerbruch, F.: Bericht über die ersten in der pneumatischen Kammer der Breslauer Klinik ausgeführten Operationen, München. med. Wchnschr. **53**: 1-4, 1906.
68. Sauerbruch, F.: Die Kardiaresektion, in Chirurgie der Brustorgane, vol. II, Berlin, 1925, Julius Springer, pp. 639-650.
69. Schmieden, Victor: Die Resektion der Kardia und die Totalresektion des Magens, in Bier, Braun, Kümmell (Editors): Chirurgische Operationslehre, ed. 6, vol. III, Leipzig, 1933, Johann Ambrosius Barth, pp. 94-100.

70. Stewart, W. H., and Illick, H. E.: Roentgen Diagnosis of Carcinoma at the Cardia, Am. J. Roentgenol. **32**: 43-51, 1934.
71. Sweet, R. H.: Transthoracic Partial Gastrectomy for Carcinoma High in the Stomach, Rev. Gastroenterol. **9**: 264-269, 1942.
72. Sweet, R. H.: Transthoracic Resection of the Esophagus and Stomach for Cancer. Analysis of Postoperative Complications, Causes of Death and Late Results of Operation, Ann. Surg. **121**: 272-284, 1945.
73. Tiegel, M.: Zur Chirurgie des Oesophagus, Beitr. z. klin. Chir. **65**: 314-357, 1909.
74. Tiegel, M.: Die chirurgische Behandlung des Spieseröhrenkrebses, ihr gegenwärtiger Stand und ihre Aussichten für die Zukunft, München. med. Wchnschr. **57**: 896-899, 1910.
75. Voelcker: Ueber Extirpation der Cardia wegen Carcinom, Verhandl. d. deutsch. Gesellsch. f. Chir. **37**: 126-129, 1908.
76. Voelcker: Resektion der Kardia wegen Carcinom, Zentralbl. f. Chir. **41**: 333, 1914.
77. Wachtel, L.: Die operative Behandlung des Cardiacarcinoms, Inaug. Dissertation, Berlin, 1931.
78. Walters, W.: Transthoracic Resection of the Stomach and Esophagus for Carcinoma, Proc. Staff Meet., Mayo Clin. **17**: 241-247, 1942.
79. Wasch, M. G., and Epstein, B. S.: The Roentgen Visualization of Tumors of the Cardia, Am. J. Roentgenol. **51**: 564-571, 1944.
80. Wendel, W.: Beitrag zur endothorakalen Oesophagus-chirurgie, Arch. f. klin. Chir. **83**: 635-647, 1907.
81. Wendel, W.: Zur Chirurgie des Oesophagus, Verhandl. d. deutsch. Gesellsch. f. Chir. Pt. II, 588-606, 1910.
82. Wiener, J.: Osteoplastic Resection of the Costal Arch. Followed by Resection of Lesser Curvature of Stomach and Esophagus, and Esophagostomy, Ann. Surg. **48**: 530-540, 1908.
83. Woodsack, H.: Ueber die Resektion der Kardia, Beitr. z. klin Chir. **134**: 584-596, 1925.
84. Wu, Y. K., and Loucks, H. H.: Surgical Treatment of Carcinoma of the Esophagus, Chinese M. J. **60**: 1-33, 1941.
85. Zaaijer, J. H.: Erfolgreiche transpleurale Resektion eines Cardiacarcinoms, Beitr. z. klin. Chir. **83**: 419-430, 1913.
86. Zollinger, R.: Observations on the Use of Prolonged Anesthetic Agents in Upper Abdominal Incisions, SURGERY **10**: 27-36, 1941.

Book Reviews

Medical Education and the Changing Order. Raymond B. Allen, M.D., Ph.D. pp. 153. New York, 1946, Commonwealth Fund. $1.50.

This volume is one of the New York Academy of Medicine Series on Medicine and the Changing Order. The author, the executive dean of the Colleges of Dentistry, Medicine and Pharmacy of the University of Illinois and president-elect (now president) of the University of Washington, takes as his basic thesis the concept of "medicine . . . as a social science in the service of society." He examines the background of medical education and the recent trends, concluding that more stress has been given to the acquisition of scientific knowledge than to the development of a sound understanding of the social forces which affect the patient. He would not sacrifice the technical training through which modern medicine has made such advances, but would insist on the further development of a broad understanding of the social sciences. "The need is to bring the premedical and medical curricula up to date by recognizing the obvious fact that medicine has outgrown the limitations of the laboratory and the clinic and must add to itself *as required studies* pertinent phases of the disciplines of the social sciences and the humanities." He concludes with the very pointed statement that "it takes a man, not a machine, to understand mankind." This volume, highly objective in its analysis, frank in its expressions, and challenging in its ideas, should be read and reread by all who are interested in any phase of medical education. It will be equally interesting and valuable to all practitioners.

Announcement

The Society for Vascular Surgery will hold its second annual meeting, Sunday, June 20, 1948, at The Stevens hotel in Chicago. Arthur W. Allen will preside and deliver the presidential address; John Homans, Michael DeBakey and Alton Ochsner, Claude S. Beck, Geza de Takats, Herman E. Pearse, Daniel E. Elkin, J. Ross Veal, Frederick Coller, Reginald Smithwick, Louis G. Herman, Arthur H. Blakemore, Mims Gage, Norman E. Freeman, and Robert R. Linton will read papers, followed by short question periods.

The objects of this society are to promote the study and research in vascular diseases, to define more clearly the role of surgery in these diseases, to pool the experience and knowledge of its membership, to standardize nomenclature, to promote and encourage adequate teaching of these diseases to students, interns, and residents, to encourage hospitals to develop special sections in vascular surgery, and to provide special training for young surgeons interested in this field.

INDEX TO VOLUME 23

AUTHORS INDEX*

In this index following the author's name, the title of the subject is given as it appeared in the JOURNAL.

A

ACKERMAN, LAUREN V. Verrucous carcinoma of the oral cavity, 670
ALEXANDER, EBEN, JR. (*See* Ingraham, Matson, and Alexander, Jr.), 252
AMESTI, FELIX DE. (*See* De Amesti and Otaiza), 921
ANDRUS, WILLIAM DEWITT. George J. Heuer's contributions and his place in American surgery, 321

B

BAKER, JOEL W., AND DURHAM, MILTON W. Associated pancreatic necrosis and biliary disease, 301
BARNES, WILLIAM A. Unusual complications following resection of carcinoma of the cardiac end of the stomach, 522
BARONOFSKY, IVAN D. A cannula for pancreatic fistula, 665
BARRETO, H. (*See* Monteiro and Barreto), 178
BARSKY, ARTHUR J. Restoration of the thumb, 227
BELL, H. GLENN. The problem of gastric cancer in a university hospital, 351
BLACK, B. MARDEN. (*See* Evert, Black, and Dockerty), 185
BOSHER, LEWIS H., JR., AND WILLIAMS, CARRINGTON, JR. Herpes zoster and the surgical abdomen, 773
BOWERS, RALPH F. Observations of surgical training, 377
BRANE, CHARLES M. Penetrating wound of the chest with division of a bronchial artery, 476
BRUUSGAARD, CHRISTIAN. The operative treatment of chronic gastric and duodenal ulcer, 161
BURK, LLOYD B., JR. (*See* Buxton and Burk, JR.), 760
BURNETT, W. EMORY, AND CASWELL, H. TAYLOR. Lobectomy for pulmonary cysts in a fifteen-day-old infant with recovery, 84
BUXTON, ROBERT W. (*See* Cooper and Buxton), 821
—, AND BURK, LLOYD B., JR. Choledochotomy, 760

C

CARLQUIST, JOHN H. (*See* Hicken, Stevenson, and Carlquist), 682
CARTER, B. NOLAND. Twenty-five years of a graduate school of surgery founded by George J. Heuer, 326
CASWELL, H. TAYLOR. (*See* Burnett and Caswell), 84
CHENOWETH, ARTHUR I. (*See* Nickel, Jr., and Chenoweth), 480
CHILD, CHARLES G., III. (*See* Gill and Child, III), 571
—. Radical one-stage pancreaticoduodenectomy, 492
CLAGETT, O. THERON. (*See* Payne and Clagett), 912
—, AND SCHMIDT, HERBERT W. Surgical management of acquired stricture of the esophagus with esophagobronchial fistula and bronchiectasis of entire right lung, 221
CLIFFTON, EUGENE E. Tantalum foil cuffs in peripheral nerve surgery, 507
—. Unusual innervation of the intrinsic muscles of the hand by median and ulnar nerve, 12
CONWAY, HERBERT. (*See* Neumann and Conway), 584
—. Communication, 320
—. Evolution of treatment of capillary hemangiomas of the face with further observation on the value of camouflage by permanent pigment injection (tattooing), 389
COOPER, DONALD R., AND BUXTON, ROBERT W. Gastrostomy, 821
COOPER, WILLIAM A. End results in the treatment of peptic ulcer by posterior gastroenterostomy, 425
CORNELL, NELSON W. (*See* Maisel and Cornell), 591
CRUTCHER, RICHARD R., AND DANIEL, ROLLIN A., JR. Pulmonary embolism, 47
CURRY, G. J. A hip nail counterbore, 679

D

DANIEL, ROLLIN A., JR. (*See* Crutcher and Daniel, Jr.), 47
DE AMESTI, FELIX, AND OTAIZA, ELISEO. Cardioesophageal cancers treated via the transthoracic and transdiaphragmatic route, 921

*January, pp. 1-160; February, pp. 161-320; March, pp. 321-602; April, pp. 603-734; May, pp. 735-866; June, pp. 867-1934.

DEBAKEY, MICHAEL E., AND OCHSNER, ALTON. Subtotal esophagectomy and esophagogastrostomy for high intrathoracic esophageal lesions, 935
DILLER, THEODORE. (*See* Harris, Diller, and Marcus), 206
DINGWALL, JAMES A., LIN, DAVID T., AND LYON, JAMES A. The use of sodium tetradecyl sulfate in the sclerosing treatment of varicose veins, 599
DIVELEY, WALTER. (*See* McSwain and Diveley), 525
DOCKERTY, MALCOLM B. (*See* Evert, Black, and Dockerty), 185
DRAPER, JOHN W. Twenty-seven years of prostatic surgery at Bellevue hospital, 515
DURHAM, MILTON W. (*See* Baker and Durham), 301

E

ECKEL, JOHN H. Primary tumors of the jejunum and ileum, 467
EDWARDS, MONTE. Four metachronous malignant lesions of the colon, 808
EVERT, JOHN A., BLACK, B. MARDEN, AND DOCKERTY, MALCOLM B. Primary nonspecific ulcers of the small intestine, 185

F

FINDLEY, THOMAS. Indications for sympathectomy in the treatment of hypertension, 639
FINN, MINNIE. (*See* Friesen, State, Jasper, Finn, and Wangensteen), 167
FISHER, BERNARD. (*See* McClenahan and Fisher), 778
FOOT, N. CHANDLER, AND HUMPHREYS, GUSTAVUS A. The importance of accurate pathologic classification in the prognosis of renal tumors, 369
FRIESEN, STANLEY R., STATE, DAVID, JASPER, DONALD E., FINN, MINNIE, AND WANGENSTEEN, OWEN H. Production of allergic gastric and duodenal edema which predisposes to the histamine-provoked ulcer in dogs, 167

G

GAENSLER, EDWARD A., MCGOWAN, JOHN M., AND HENDERSON, FRANCIS F. A comparative study of the action of demerol and opium alkaloids in relation to biliary spasm, 211
GARDNER, CLARENCE E., JR. Foreign body localization in the soft parts, 275
GARLOCK, JOHN H. (*See* Sainburg and Garlock), 201
—. Progress in the surgical treatment of carcinoma of the esophagus and upper stomach, 906
GIANNESTRAS, N. J. The Magnuson-Stack procedure for recurrent dislocations of the shoulder, 794
GILL, DAN C., AND CHILD, CHARLES G., III. Esophagogastrostomy in the treatment of cardiospasm, 571
GLENN, FRANK. The surgical treatment of acute cholecystitis, 397
GROSS, ROBERT E. Treatment of short stricture of the esophagus by partial esophagectomy and end-to-end esophageal reconstruction, 735

H

HALPERT, BÉLA, AND YOUNG, MILLINGTON O. Carcinosarcoma of the mammary gland, 289
HAMILTON, ALFRED T. Subcutaneous rupture of the brachioradialis muscle, 806
HARRIS, FRANKLIN I., DILLER, THEODORE, AND MARCUS, SANFORD A. Hemorrhagic infarction of the greater omentum simulating acute appendicitis, 206
HEINBECKER, PETER. The pathogenesis of diastolic hypertension, 618
HENDERSON, FRANCIS F. (*See* Gaensler, Mc Gowan, and Henderson), 211
HENDRICKS, ROBERT. (*See* Moore and Hendricks), 442
HENRY, JAMES W. (*See* Vaughn, Lees, and Henry), 306
HICKEN, N. FREDERICK, STEVENSON, VERNON L., AND CARLQUIST, JOHN H. An unusually large myxosarcomatous tumor of the submaxillary gland, 682
HOLLENBERG, HENRY G. Amniotic hernia, 363
HOLMAN, CRANSTON W. Further observations on the treatment of bleeding peptic ulcer, 405
HOLZER, C. E., JR. Gunshot wounds involving the abdominal aorta, 645
HOMBURGER, F. Nutritional management of patients with transthoracic-abdominal resections of the stomach (in Pack and McNeer, Surgical treatment of cancers of the gastric cardia), 1011
HOWARD, RUTLEDGE W. (*See* Hufnagel, Walter, and Howard), 753
HUFNAGEL, CHARLES A., WALTER, CARL W., AND HOWARD, RUTLEDGE W. An in vivo method for evaluation of detergents and germicides, 753
HUMPHREYS, GUSTAVUS A. (*See* Foot and Humphreys), 369

I

INGRAHAM, FRANC D., MATSON, DONALD D., AND ALEXANDER, EBEN, JR. Experimental observations in the treatment of craniosynostosis, 252

J

JASPER, DONALD E. (*See* Friesen, State, Jasper, Finn, and Wangensteen), 167

JOHNSTON, J. HARVEY, JR. Fifty-ninth annual session of the Southern Surgical Association, 722

K

KASLOW, ARTHUR L. A new material and tube design in gastrointestinal intubation, 293

KENWORTHY, ROGER A., AND WELCH, C. STUART. Leiomyoma of the esophagus and cardia of the stomach, 745

KIRBY, CHARLES K. (*See* Royster, Kirby, and Wilbur), 248

KLEINSASSER, LEROY J. Intravenous clotting, 687

KLINE, EDITH. (*See* Puppel and Kline), 768

KNOX, GRAHAM. (*See* West and Knox), 450

KOSTRUBALA, JOSEPH G., AND WAGNER, ALBERT G. Electric lift, 298

KREMEN, ARNOLD J. The problem of parenteral nitrogen administration in surgical patients, 92

L

LASHER, EARL P., JR. The course of peptic ulceration in elderly persons, 501

LEES, WILLIAM M. (*See* Vaughn, Lees, and Henry), 306

LI, IRENE Y. Benign lymphoma of the rectum, 814

LIN, DAVID T. (*See* Dingwall, Lin, and Lyon), 599

LORD, JERE W., JR. Arterial and venous hypertensive states benefited by surgical intervention, 550

LYON, JAMES A. (*See* Dingwall, Lin, and Lyon), 599

M

MACQUIDDY, E. L., AND TOLLMAN, J. P. Observations on an absorbable powder to replace talc, 786

MAIER, HERBERT C. Preoperative, operative, and postoperative care in esophageal resections, 884

MAISEL, BERNARD, AND CORNELL, NELSON W. Conservative treatment of fractures of the tibial condyles, 591

MARCUS, SANFORD A. (*See* Harris, Diller, and Marcus), 206

MARSHALL, VICTOR F., AND SCHNITTMAN, MORRIS. Iliac lymphadenopathy as a cause of ureteral obstruction, 542

MATSON, DONALD D. (*See* Ingraham, Matson, and Alexander, Jr.), 252

MCCLENAHAN, J. E., AND FISHER, BERNARD. Mesenteric thrombosis, 778

MCCUNE, WILLIAM S. War wounds of the rectum and anal sphincter, 653

MCGOWAN, JOHN M. (*See* Gaensler, Mc Gowan, and Henderson), 211

MCNEER, GORDON. (*See* Pack and McNeer), 976

MCSWAIN, BARTON, AND DIVELEY, WALTER. Malignant tumors of the thyroid gland, 525

MONTEIRO, A., AND BARRETO, H. Aseptic gastric resection, Billroth I technique, 178

MOORE, S. W., AND HENDRICKS, ROBERT. Late results following perforated peptic ulcer, 442

MORRISON, DONALD R. The risk of surgery in heart disease, 561

N

NEUMANN, CHARLES G., AND CONWAY, HERBERT. Evaluation of skin grafting in the technique of radical mastectomy in relation to function of the arm, 584

NEWTON, FRANCIS C. In memoriam: Elliott Carr Cutler, 863

NICKEL, WILLIAM F., JR., AND CHENOWETH, ARTHUR I. Resection of the rectum with preservation of the anal sphincter, 480

O

OCHSNER, ALTON. (*See* DeBakey and Ochsner), 935

OPPENHEIMER, GORDON D. (*See* Rosenak and Oppenheimer), 832

OTAIZA, ELISEO. (*See* De Amesti and Otaiza), 921

P

PACK, GEORGE T. Introduction to symposium on cancer of the esophagus and gastric cardia, 867

—, AND MCNEER, GORDON. Surgical treatment of cancers of the gastric cardia, 976

PAYNE, JOHN H., AND CLAGETT, O. THERON. Transthoracic gastric resection for lesions of cardia of stomach and lower part of esophagus, 912

PEYTON, WILLIAM T., AND SIMMONS, DONALD R. Cyst formation at the operative site following cerebellar operations (pseudomeningocele), 269

POER, DAVID HENRY. Lymphosarcoma of the gastrointestinal tract, 354

POOL, JOHN L. (*See* Watson and Pool), 893

PUPPEL, I. DARIN, AND KLINE, EDITH. Myotonia acquisita due to chronic calculous cholecystitis and cured by cholecystectomy, 768

Q

QUIGLEY, THOMAS B. (*See* Urist, Ries, and Quigley), 801

R

RAVDIN, I. S. The changing status of surgical care, 603

RAY, BRONSON S., AND STEWART, HAROLD J. Role of the glossopharyngeal nerve in the carotid sinus reflex in man; relief of carotid sinus syndrome by intracranial section of the glossopharyngeal nerve, 411

RIES, LINCOLN. (*See* Urist, Ries, and Quigley), 801

ROBILLARD, GREGORY L. (*See* Shapiro and Robillard), 1

ROSENAK, STEPHAN S., AND OPPENHEIMER, GORDON D. An improved drain for peritoneal lavage, 832

ROYSTER, HENRY P., KIRBY, CHARLES K., AND WILBUR, ROBERT G. Typhoid osteomyelitis of the ribs treated with streptomycin and surgical excision, 248

S

SAINBURG, FRANK P., AND GARLOCK, JOHN H. Carcinoma of the gall bladder, 201

SCHMIDT, HERBERT W. (*See* Clagett and Schmidt), 221

SCHNITTMAN, MORRIS. (*See* Marshall and Schnittman), 542

SHAPIRO, ALFRED L., AND ROBILLARD, GREGORY L. The arterial blood supply of the common and hepatic bile ducts with reference to the problems of common duct injury and repair, 1

SHEINFELD, WILLIAM. Subcutaneous emphysema following chest trauma, 278

SHERMAN, ROBERT S. The roentgen diagnosis of cancer of the cardiac region of the stomach, 874

SIMMONS, DONALD R. (*See* Peyton and Simmons), 269

SINGLETON, A. O., JR. (*See* Singleton and Singleton, Jr.), 75

SINGLETON, A. O., AND SINGLETON, A. O., JR. Cerebral hemorrhage following repair of a common carotid-internal jugular arteriovenous fistula, 75

STATE, DAVID. (*See* Friesen, State, Jasper, Finn, and Wangensteen), 167

STEVENSON, VERNON J. (*See* Hicken, Stevenson, and Carlquist), 682

STEWART, HAROLD J. (*See* Ray and Stewart), 411

SWEET, RICHARD H. The treatment of carcinoma of the esophagus and cardiac end of the stomach by surgical extirpation, 952

T

THROCKMORTON, TOM DERCUM. Tantalum gauze in the repair of hernias complicated by tissue deficiency, 32

TOLLMAN, J. P. (*See* McQuiddy and Tollman), 786

TURELL, ROBERT. Tattooing with mercury sulfide for intractable anal pruritis, 63

U

URIST, MARSHALL R., RIES, LINCOLN, AND QUIGLEY, THOMAS B. A plaster traction splint for compound comminuted fractures of the tibia and fibula, 801

V

VAUGHN, ARKELL M., LEES, WILLIAM M., AND HENRY, JAMES W. Mesenteric cysts, 306

W

WAGNER, ALBERT G. (*See* Kostrubala and Wagner), 298

WALTER, CARL W. (*See* Hufnagel, Walter, and Howard), 753

WANGENSTEEN, OWEN H. (*See* Friesen, State, Jasper, Finn, and Wangensteen), 167

WATSON, WILLIAM L., AND POOL, JOHN L. Cancer of the cervical esophagus, 893

WELCH, C. STUART. (*See* Kenworthy and Welch), 745

WEST, JOHN P., AND KNOX, GRAHAM. Neurogenic tumors of the stomach, 450

WHITE, JAMES C. Progress in surgery of the autonomic nervous system, 1943-1946, 834

WILBUR, ROBERT G. (*See* Royster, Kirby, and Wilbur), 248

WILLIAMS, CARRINGTON, JR. (*See* Bosher, Jr., and Williams, Jr.), 773

Y

YOUNG, MILLINGTON O. (*See* Halpert and Young), 289

Z

ZINNINGER, M. M. Some experiences with anastomosis of the common bile duct to the duodenum, and repair of strictures of the common bile duct, 337

SUBJECT INDEX*

Book reviews are indicated by (*B. Rev.*)

A

Abdomen, surgical, herpes zoster and (Bosher, Jr., and Williams, Jr.), 773
Abdominal aorta, gunshot wounds involving (Holzer, Jr.), 645
cardiectomy; surgical treatment of cancers of gastric cardia (Pack and McNeer), 1001
Absorbable powder to replace talc, observations on (MacQuiddy and Tollman), 786
Administration, parenteral nitrogen, problem of, in surgical patients (Kremen), 92
Adrenals, diseases of, 158 (*B. Rev.*)
Alimentation, parenteral, in surgery, with reference to proteins and amino acids, 160 (*B. Rev.*)
Alkaloids, opium, and demerol, comparative study of action of, in relation to biliary spasm (Gaensler et al.), 211
Allergic gastric and duodenal edema, production of, which predisposes to histamine-provoked ulcer in dogs (Friesen et al.), 167
Ambulation, early, in surgical care (Ravdin), 615
Amino acids and proteins, with reference to parenteral alimentation in surgery, 160 (*B. Rev.*)
Amniotic hernia (Hollenberg), 363
Anal pruritus, intractable, tattooing with mercury sulfide for (Turell), 63
sphincter and rectum, war wounds of (McCune), 653
resection of rectum with preservation of (Nickel, Jr., and Chenoweth), 480
Anastomosis of common bile duct to duodenum, some experiences with, and repair of strictures of common bile duct (Zinninger), 337
Anatomic and clinical study of course of peptic ulceration in elderly persons (Lasher, Jr.), 501
Anesthesia in surgical care (Ravdin), 607
Announcements, 734, 1020
Aorta, abdominal, gunshot wounds involving (Holzer, Jr.), 645
Appendicitis, acute, hemorrhagic infarction of greater omentum simulating (Harris et al.), 206
Arm, function of, evaluation of skin grafting in technique of radical mastectomy in relation to (Neumann and Conway), 584
Army personnel at vascular centers, analysis of intravenous clotting in (Kleinsasser), 687
Arterial blood supply of common and hepatic bile ducts with reference to problems of common duct injury and repair (Shapiro and Robillard), 1
and venous hypertensive states benefited by surgical intervention (Lord, Jr.), 550
Arteriovenous fistula, common carotid-internal jugular, cerebral hemorrhage following repair of (Singleton and Singleton, Jr.), 75
Artery, bronchial, penetrating wound of chest with division of (Brane), 476
Aseptic gastric resection, Billroth I technique (Monteiro and Barreto), 178
Autonomic nervous system, progress in surgery of (White), 834
Autopsy and clinical studies on pulmonary embolism (Crutcher and Daniel, Jr.), 47

B

Balance, nitrogen, with problem of parenteral nitrogen administration in surgical patients (Kremen), 92
Benign lymphoma of rectum (Li), 814
Bile duct, common, some experiences with anastomosis of, to duodenum, and repair of strictures of common bile duct (Zinninger), 337
ducts, common and hepatic, arterial blood supply of, with reference to problems of common duct injury and repair (Shapiro and Robillard), 1
Biliary disease and associated pancreatic necrosis (Baker and Durham), 301
spasm, comparative study of action of demerol and opium alkaloids in relation to (Gaensler et al.), 211
Billroth I technique, aseptic gastric resection (Monteiro and Barreto), 178
Bleeding peptic ulcer, further observations on treatment of (Holman), 405
Blood supply, arterial, of common and hepatic bile ducts with reference to problems of common duct injury and repair (Shapiro and Robillard), 1
Book reviews, 154-160, 318-319, 1020
Brachioradialis muscle, subcutaneous rupture of (Hamilton), 806

*January, pp. 1-160; February, pp. 161-320; March, pp. 321-602; April, pp. 603-734; May, pp. 735-866; June, pp. 867-1034.

Bronchial artery, division of, penetrating wound of chest with (Brane), 476
Bronchiectasis of entire right lung and esophagobronchial fistula, surgical management of acquired stricture of esophagus with (Clagett and Schmidt), 221

C

Calcified cyst of mesentery; mesentery cysts (Vaughn et al.), 306
Calculous cholecystitis, chronic, myotonia acquisita due to, and cured by cholecystectomy (Puppel and Kline), 768
Camouflage by permanent pigment injection (tattooing), evolution of treatment of capillary hemangiomas of face with further observation on value of (Conway), 389
Cancer of cardiac region of stomach, roentgen diagnosis of (Sherman), 874
  cardioesophageal, treated via transthoracic and transdiaphragmatic route (De Amesti and Otaiza), 921
  of cervical esophagus (Watson and Pool), 893
  of esophagus and gastric cardia, introduction to symposium on (Pack), 867
    symposium on, 867-1019
  of gastric cardia, surgical treatment of (Pack and McNeer), 976
  gastric, problem of, in university hospital (Bell), 351
Cannula for pancreatic fistula (Baronofsky), 665
Capillary hemangiomas of face, evolution of treatment of, with further observation on value of camouflage by permanent pigment injection (tattooing) (Conway), 389
Carcinoma of cardiac end of stomach, resection of, unusual complications following (Barnes), 522
  of esophagus and cardiac end of stomach, treatment of, by surgical extirpation (Sweet), 952
    and upper stomach, progress in surgical treatment of (Garlock), 906
  of gall bladder (Sainburg and Garlock), 201
  verrucous, of oral cavity (Ackerman), 670
Carcinosarcoma of mammary gland (Halpert and Young), 289
Cardia, gastric, and esophagus, cancer of, introduction to symposium on (Pack), 867
    symposium on, 867-1019
  surgical treatment of cancers of (Pack and McNeer), 976
  of stomach and esophagus, leiomyoma of (Kenworthy and Welch), 745
    and lower part of esophagus, lesions of, transthoracic gastric resection for (Payne and Clagett), 912
Cardiac end of stomach and esophagus, treatment of carcinoma of, by surgical extirpation (Sweet), 952
    resection of carcinoma of, unusual complications following (Barnes), 522
  region of stomach, roentgen diagnosis of cancer of (Sherman), 874
Cardiectomy, abdominal; surgical treatment of cancers of gastric cardia (Pack and McNeer), 1001
  thoracic, anesthesia for; surgical treatment of cancers of gastric cardia (Pack and McNeer), 982
Cardioesophageal cancers treated via transthoracic and transdiaphragmatic route (De Amesti and Otaiza), 921
Cardiospasm, esophagogastrostomy in treatment of (Gill and Child, III), 571
Carotid sinus reflex in man, role of glossopharyngeal nerve in; relief of carotid sinus syndrome by intracranial section of glossopharyngeal nerve (Ray and Stewart), 411
Carotid-internal jugular arteriovenous fistula, common, cerebral hemorrhage following repair of (Singleton and Singleton, Jr.), 75
Cellulose gauze, oxidized, in craniosynostosis (Ingraham et al.), 257
Cerebellar operations, cyst formations at operative site following (pseudomeningocele) (Peyton and Simmons), 269
Cerebral hemorrhage following repair of common cartoid-internal jugular arteriovenous fistula (Singleton and Singleton, Jr.), 75
Cervical esophagus, cancer of (Watson and Pool), 893
Chemotherapy in surgical care (Ravdin), 610
Chest, penetrating wound of, with division of bronchial artery (Brane), 476
  principles in roentgen study of, 154 (*B. Rev.*)
  trauma, subcutaneous emphysema following (Sheinfeld), 278
Cholecystectomy, myotonia acquisita due to chronic calculous cholecystitis and cured by (Puppel and Kline), 768
Cholecystitis, acute, surgical treatment of (Glenn), 397
  chronic calculous, myotonia acquisita due to, and cured by cholecystectomy (Puppel and Kline), 768
Choledochotomy (Buxton and Burk, Jr.), 760
Classification, importance of accurate pathologic, in prognosis of renal tumors (Foot and Humphreys), 369
Clinical and anatomic study of course of peptic ulceration in elderly persons (Lasher, Jr.), 501
  and autopsy studies on pulmonary embolism (Crutcher and Daniel, Jr.), 47

Clotting, intravenous (Kleinsasser), 687
Colon, four metachronous malignant lesions of (Edwards), 808
Comminuted fractures, compound, of tibia and fibula, plaster traction splint for (Urist et al.), 801
Common bile duct, some experiences with anastomosis of, to duodenum, and repair of strictures of common bile duct (Zinninger), 337
carotid-internal jugular arteriovenous fistula, cerebral hemorrhage following repair of (Singleton and Singleton, Jr.), 75
and hepatic bile ducts, arterial blood supply of, with reference to problems of common duct injury and repair (Shapiro and Robillard), 1
Communication (Conway), 320
Compound comminuted fractures of tibia and fibula, plaster traction splint for (Urist et al.), 801
Condyles, tibial, fractures of, conservative treatment of (Maisel and Cornell), 591
Counterbore, hip nail (Curry), 679
Craniosynostosis, experimental observations in treatment of (Ingraham et al.), 252
Cuffs, tantalum foil, in peripheral nerve surgery (Cliffton), 507
Cutler, Elliott Carr. In memoriam (Newton), 863
Cyst formation at operative site following cerebellar operations (pseudomeningocele) (Peyton and Simmons), 269
mesenteric (Vaughn et al.), 306
pulmonary, lobectomy for, in fifteen-day-old infant with recovery (Burnett and Caswell), 84

D

Decubitus ulcers, aid in treatment of; electric lift (Kostrubala and Wagner), 298
Deficiency, tissue, tantalum gauze in repair of hernias complicated by (Throckmorton), 32
Demerol and opium alkaloids, comparative study of action of, in relation to biliary spasm (Gaensler et al.), 211
Desoxycorticosterone, epinephrine, and renin, sensitization to, in pathogenesis of diastolic hypertension (Heinbecker), 623
Detergents and germicides, in vivo method for evaluation of (Hufnagel et al.), 753
Device for permitting complete periodic experimental collection of pancreatic juice; cannula for pancreatic fistula (Baronofsky), 665
Diagnosis, roentgen, of cancer of cardiac region of stomach (Sherman), 874
Diagnosis—Cont'd
of tumors of gastric cardia; surgical treatment of cancers of gastric cardia (Pack and McNeer), 977
Diastolic hypertension, pathogenesis of (Heinbecker), 618
Diseases of adrenals, 158 (*B. Rev.*)
biliary, and associated pancreatic necrosis (Baker and Durham), 301
heart, risk of surgery in (Morrison), 561
Dislocations, recurrent, of shoulder, Magnuson-Stack procedure for (Giannestras), 794
Dogs, histamine-provoked ulcer in, production of allergic gastric and duodenal edema which predisposes to (Friesen et al.), 167
Drain, improved, for peritoneal lavage (Rosenak and Oppenheimer), 832
Duct, common bile, some experiences with anastomosis of, to duodenum, and repair of strictures of common bile duct (Zinninger), 337
common and hepatic bile, arterial blood supply of, with reference to problems of common duct injury and repair (Shapiro and Robillard), 1
Duodenal and gastric edema, allergic, production of, which predisposes to histamine-provoked ulcer in dogs (Friesen et al.), 167
ulcer, chronic, operative treatment of (Bruusgaard), 161
Duodenum, some experiences with anastomosis of common bile duct to, and repair of strictures of common bile duct (Zinninger), 337

E

Edema, allergic gastric and duodenal, production of, which predisposes to histamine-provoked ulcer in dogs (Friesen et al.), 167
Education, medical, and changing order, 1020 (*B. Rev.*)
Elderly persons, course of peptic ulceration in (Lasher, Jr.), 501
Electric lift (Kostrubala and Wagner), 298
Embolism, pulmonary (Crutcher and Daniel, Jr.), 47
Emphysema, subcutaneous, following chest trauma (Sheinfeld), 278
Epinephrine, renin, and desoxycorticosterone, sensitization to, in pathogenesis of diastolic hypertension (Heinbecker), 623
Esophageal lesions, high intrathoracic, subtotal esophagectomy and esophagogastrostomy for (DeBakey and Ochsner), 935
reconstruction, end-to-end, and partial esophagectomy, treatment of short stricture of esophagus by (Gross), 735
resections, preoperative, operative, and postoperative care in (Maier), 884

Esophagectomy, partial, and end-to-end esophageal reconstruction, treatment of short stricture of esophagus by (Gross), 735
subtotal, and esophagogastrostomy for high intrathoracic esophageal lesions (DeBakey and Ochsner), 935
Esophagogastrostomy and subtotal esophagectomy for high intrathoracic esophageal lesions (DeBakey and Ochsner), 935
in treament of cardiospasm (Gill and Child, III), 571
Esophagoscopy and gastroscopy in surgical treatment of cancers (Pack and McNeer), 978
Esophagus, acquired stricture of, with esophagobronchial fistula and bronchiectasis of entire right lung, surgical management of (Clagett and Schmidt), 221
and cardia of stomach, leiomyoma of (Kenworthy and Welch), 745
and cardiac end of stomach, treatment of carcinoma of, by surgical extirpation (Sweet), 952
cervical, cancer of (Watson and Pool), 893
and gastric cardia, cancer of, introduction to symposium on (Pack), 867
symposium on, 867-1019
lower part of, and cardia of stomach, lesions of, transthoracic gastric resection for (Payne and Clagett), 912
treatment of short stricture of, by partial esophagectomy and end-to-end esophageal reconstruction (Gross), 735
and upper stomach, carcinoma of, progress in surgical treatment of (Garlock), 906
Excision, surgical, and streptomycin, typhoid osteomyelitis of ribs treated with (Royster et al.), 248
Extirpation, surgical, treatment of carcinoma of esophagus and cardiac end of stomach by (Sweet), 952

F

Face, capillary hemangiomas of, evolution of treatment of, with further observation on value of camouflage by permanent pigment injection (tattooing) (Conway), 389
Fibrin film in craniosynostosis (Ingraham et al.), 255
Fibula and tibia, plaster traction splint for compound comminuted fractures of (Urist et al.), 801
Fistula, common carotid-internal jugular arteriovenous, cerebral hemorrhage following repair of (Singleton and Singleton, Jr.), 75
Fistula—Cont'd
esophagobronchial, and bronchiectasis of entire right lung, surgical management of acquired stricture of esophagus with (Clagett and Schmidt), 221
pancreatic, cannula for (Baronofsky), 665
Foil cuffs, tantalum, in peripheral nerve surgery (Cliffton), 507
Foreign body localization in soft parts (Gardner, Jr.), 275
Fractures, compound comminuted, of tibia and fibula, plaster traction splint for (Urist et al.), 801
handbook of, 318 (*B. Rev.*)
of tibial condyles, conservative treatment of (Maisel and Cornell), 591
Function of arm, evaluation of skin grafting in technique of radical mastectomy in relation to (Neumann and Conway), 584

G

Gall bladder, carcinoma of (Sainburg and Garlock), 201
Gastric cancer, problem of, in university hospital (Bell), 351
cardia and esophagus, cancer of, introduction to symposium on (Pack), 867
symposium on, 867-1019
surgical treatment of cancers of (Pack and McNeer), 976
and duodenal edema, allergic, production of, which predisposes to histamine-provoked ulcer in dogs (Friesen et al.), 167
ulcer, chronic, operative treatment of (Bruusgaard), 161
resection, aseptic, Billroth I technique (Monteiro and Barreto), 178
transthoracic, for lesions of cardia of stomach and lower part of esophagus (Payne and Clagett), 912
Gastroenterostomy, posterior, end results in treatment of peptic ulcer by (Cooper), 425
Gastrointestinal intubation, new material and tube design in (Kaslow), 293
in surgical care (Ravdin), 608
tract, lymphosarcoma of (Poer), 354
Gastroscopy and esophagoscopy in surgical treatment of cancers (Pack and McNeer), 978
Gastrostomy (Cooper and Buxton), 821
Gauze, tantalum, in repair of hernias complicated by tissue deficiency (Throckmorton), 32
Germicides and detergents, in vivo method for evaluation of (Hufnagel et al.), 753
Gland, mammary, carcinosarcoma of (Halpert and Young), 289
submaxillary, unusually large myxosarcomatous tumor of (Hicken et al.), 682
thyroid, malignant tumors of (McSwain and Diveley), 525

Glossopharyngeal nerve, role of, in carotid sinus reflex in man; relief of carotid sinus syndrome by intracranial section of glossopharyngeal nerve (Ray and Stewart), 411
Grafting, skin, evaluation of, in technique of radical mastectomy in relation to function of arm (Neumann and Conway), 584
Gunshot wounds involving abdominal aorta (Holzer, Jr.), 645
Gynecological and obstetrical pathology, 156 (*B. Rev.*)

H

Hand, intrinsic muscles of, unusual innervation of, by median and ulnar nerve (Cliffton), 12
Heart disease, risk of surgery in (Morrison), 561
Hemangiomas, capillary, of face, evolution of treatment of, with further observation on value of camouflage by permanent pigment injection (tattooing) (Conway), 389
Hemorrhage, cerebral, following repair of common carotid-internal jugular arteriovenous fistula (Singleton and Singleton, Jr.), 75
Hemorrhagic infarction of greater omentum simulating acute appendicitis (Harris et al.), 206
Hepatic and common bile ducts, arterial blood supply of, with reference to problems of common duct injury and repair (Shapiro and Robillard), 1
Hernia, amniotic (Hollenberg), 363
  tantalum gauze in repair of, complicated by tissue deficiency (Throckmorton), 32
Herniorrhaphy, tantalum gauze, technique of, in repair of hernias complicated by tissue deficiency (Throckmorton), 34
Herpes zoster and surgical abdomen (Bosher, Jr., and Williams, Jr.), 773
Heuer, George J., birthday volume, 321-602
  contributions and his place in American surgery (Andrus), 321
    twenty-five years of graduate school of surgery founded by (Carter), 326
  staff, photograph of members of, 602
Hip nail counterbore (Curry), 679
Histamine-provoked ulcer in dogs, production of allergic gastric and duodenal edema which predisposes to (Friesen et al.), 167
Hypertension, diastolic, pathogenesis of (Heinbecker), 618
  indications for sympathectomy in treatment of (Findley), 639
Hypertensive states, arterial and venous, benefited by surgical intervention (Lord, Jr.), 550
Hypophysis, neural, and control in pathogenesis of diastolic hypertension (Heinbecker), 619

I

Ileum and jejunum, primary tumors of (Eckel), 467
Iliac lymphadenopathy as cause of ureteral obstruction (Marshall and Schnittman), 542
In memoriam: Elliott Carr Cutler (Newton), 863
In vivo method for evaluation of detergents and germicides (Hufnagel et al.), 753
Infant, fifteen-day-old, lobectomy for pulmonary cysts in, with recovery (Burnett and Caswell), 84
Infarction, hemorrhagic, of greater omentum, simulating acute appendicitis (Harris et al.), 206
Injection, permanent pigment (tattooing), evolution of treatment of capillary hemangiomas of face with further observation on value of camouflage by (Conway), 389
Injury, common duct, and repair, arterial blood supply of common and hepatic bile ducts with reference to problems of (Shapiro and Robillard), 1
Innervation, unusual, of intrinsic muscles of hand by median and ulnar nerve (Cliffton), 12
Intervention, surgical, arterial and venous hypertensive states benefited by (Lord, Jr.), 550
Intestine, small, primary nonspecific ulcers of (Evert et al.), 185
Intracranial section of glossopharyngeal nerve, relief of carotid sinus syndrome by; role of glossopharyngeal nerve in carotid sinus reflex in man (Ray and Stewart), 411
Intrathoracic esophageal lesions, high, subtotal esophagectomy and esophagogastrostomy for (DeBakey and Ochsner), 935
Intravenous clotting (Kleinsasser), 687
Intrinsic muscles of hand, unusual innervation of, by median and ulnar nerve (Cliffton), 12
Intubation, gastrointestinal, new material and tube design in (Kaslow), 293

J

Jejunum and ileum, primary tumors of (Eckel), 467
Jugular arteriovenous fistula, common carotid-internal, cerebral hemorrhage following repair of (Singleton and Singleton, Jr.), 75

L

Lavage, peritoneal, improved drain for (Rosenak and Oppenheimer), 832
Leiomyoma of esophagus and cardia of stomach (Kenworthy and Welch), 745
Lesions of cardia of stomach and lower part of esophagus, transthoracic gastric resection for (Payne and Clagett), 912
four metachronous malignant, of colon (Edwards), 808
high intrathoracic esophageal, subtotal esophagectomy and esophagogastrostomy for (DeBakey and Ochsner), 935
Lift, electric (Kostrubala and Wagner), 298
Lobectomy for pulmonary cysts in fifteen-day-old infant with recovery (Burnett and Caswell), 84
Localization, foreign body, in soft parts (Gardner, Jr.), 275
Lung, entire right, bronchiectasis of, and esophagobronchial fistula, surgical management of acquired stricture of esophagus with (Clagett and Schmidt), 221
Lymphadenopathy, iliac, as cause of ureteral obstruction (Marshall and Schnittman), 542
Lymphoma, benign, of rectum (Li), 814
Lymphosarcoma of gastrointestinal tract (Poer), 354

M

Magnuson-Stack procedure for recurrent dislocations of shoulder (Giannestras), 794
Malignant lesions, four metachronous, of colon (Edwards), 808
tumors of thyroid gland (McSwain and Diveley), 525
Mammary gland, carcinosarcoma of (Halpert and Young), 289
Mastectomy, radical, evaluation of skin grafting in technique of, in relation to function of arm (Neumann and Conway), 584
Material and tube design, new, in gastrointestinal intubation (Kaslow), 293
Median and ulnar nerve, unusual innervation of intrinsic muscles of hand by (Cliffton), 12
Medical education and changing order, 1020 (*B. Rev.*)
Medicine in changing order, 158 (*B. Rev.*)
Meetings, review of recent, 722
Mercury sulfide, tattooing with, for intractable anal pruritus (Turell), 63
Mesenteric cysts (Vaughn et al.), 306
thrombosis (McClenahan and Fisher), 778
Metachronous malignant lesions of colon, four (Edwards), 808
Method, in vivo, for evaluation of detergents and germicides (Hufnagel et al.), 753
simple, requiring no especial training or equipment; foreign body localization in soft parts (Gardner, Jr.), 275
Methyl methacrylate in craniosynostosis (Ingraham et al.), 260
Mortality rates, study of comparative; twenty-seven years of prostatic surgery at Bellevue hospital (Draper), 515
Muscle, brachioradialis, subcutaneous rupture of (Hamilton), 806
intrinsic, of hand, unusual innervation of, by median and ulnar nerve (Cliffton), 12
Myotonia acquisita due to chronic calculous cholecystitis and cured by cholecystectomy (Puppel and Kline), 768
Myxosarcomatous tumor, unusually large, of submaxillary gland (Hicken et al.), 682

N

Nail, hip, counterbore (Curry), 679
Necrosis, associated pancreatic, and biliary disease (Baker and Durham), 301
Nerve, glossopharyngeal, role of, in carotid sinus reflex in man; relief of carotid sinus syndrome by intracranial section of glossopharyngeal nerve (Ray and Stewart), 411
median and ulnar, unusual innervation of intrinsic muscles of hand by (Cliffton), 12
spinal, outline of, 318 (*B. Rev.*)
surgery, peripheral, tantalum foil cuffs in (Cliffton), 507
Nervous system, autonomic, progress in surgery of (White), 834
surgical treatment of, 154 (*B. Rev.*)
Neurogenic tumors of stomach (West and Knox), 450
Neurology, penicillin in, 159 (*B. Rev.*)
psychiatry and neurosurgery, 1946 year book of, 157 (*B. Rev.*)
Neurosurgey, neurology, and psychiatry, 1946 year book of, 157 (*B. Rev.*)
Nitrogen administration, parenteral, problem of, in surgical patients (Kremen), 92
Nutrition in surgical care (Ravdin), 612
Nutritional management of patients with transthoracic-abdominal resections of stomach (Homburger), 1011

O

Obstetrical and gynecological pathology, 156 (*B. Rev.*)
Obstetrics, postgraduate, 159 (*B. Rev.*)
Obstruction, ureteral, iliac lymphadenopathy as cause of (Marshall and Schnittman), 542

Omentum, greater, hemorrhagic infarction of, simulating acute appendicitis (Harris et al.), 206
Operative, preoperative, and postoperative care in esophageal resections (Maier), 884
site, cyst formation at, following cerebellar operations (pseudomeningocele) (Peyton and Simmons), 269
treatment of chronic gastric and duodenal ulcer (Bruusgaard), 161
Opium alkaloids and demerol, comparative study of action of, in relation to biliary spasm (Gaensler et al.), 211
Oral cavity, verrucous carcinoma of (Ackerman), 670
Osteomyelitis, typhoid, of ribs treated with streptomycin and surgical excision (Royster et al.), 248

P

Pancreatic fistula, cannula for (Baronofsky), 665
necrosis, associated, and biliary disease (Baker and Durham), 301
Pancreaticoduodenectomy, radical one-stage (Child, III), 492
Parenteral alimentation in surgery, with reference to proteins and amino acids, 160 (*B. Rev.*)
nitrogen administration, problem of, in surgical patients (Kremen), 92
Pathogenesis of diastolic hypertension (Heinbecker), 618
Pathologic classification, importance of, in prognosis of renal tumors (Foot and Humphreys), 369
Patients, five million, 318 (*B. Rev.*)
surgical, problem of parenteral nitrogen administration in (Kremen), 92
Penetrating wound of chest with division of bronchial artery (Brane), 476
Penicillin in neurology, 159 (*B. Rev.*)
Peptic ulcer, bleeding, further observations on treatment of (Holman), 405
end results in treatment of, by posterior gastroenterostomy (Cooper), 425
perforated, late results following (Moore and Hendricks), 442
ulceration, course of, in elderly persons (Lasher, Jr.), 501
Perforated peptic ulcer, late results following (Moore and Hendricks), 442
Peripheral nerve surgery, tantalum foil cuffs in (Cliffton), 507
vascular collapse in surgical care (Ravdin), 608
Peritoneal lavage, improved drain for (Rosenak and Oppenheimer), 832
Pigment injection (tattooing), permanent, evolution of treatment of capillary hemangiomas of face with further observation on value of camouflage by (Conway), 389
Plaster traction splint for compound comminuted fractures of tibia and fibula (Urist et al.), 801
Plastic repair, transplantation, and prosthesis, restoration of thumb by (Barsky), 227
Polyethylene in craniosynostosis (Ingraham et al.), 262
Postoperative, operative, and preoperative care in esophageal resections (Maier), 884
Powder, absorbable, to replace talc, observations on (MacQuiddy and Tollman), 786
Preoperative, operative, and postoperative care in esophageal resections (Maier), 884
preparation and postoperative care in changing status of surgical care (Ravdin), 607
with problem of parenteral nitrogen administration in surgical patients (Kremen), 92
Preparation, preoperative, with problem of parenteral nitrogen administration in surgical patients (Kremen), 92
Procedure, Magnuson-Stack, for recurrent dislocations of shoulder (Giannestras), 794
Prognosis of renal tumors, importance of accurate pathologic classification in (Foot and Humphreys), 369
Prostatic surgery, twenty-seven years of, at Bellevue hospital (Draper), 515
Prosthesis, transplantation, and plastic repair, restoration of thumb by (Barsky), 227
Proteins and amino acids, parenteral alimentation in surgery, with reference to, 160 (*B. Rev.*)
metabolism with problem of parenteral nitrogen administration in surgical patients (Kremen), 93
Pruritus, intractable anal, tattooing with mercury sulfide for (Turell), 63
Pseudomeningocele; cyst formation at operative site following cerebellar operations (Peyton and Simmons), 269
Psychiatry, neurology, and neurosurgery, 1946 year book of, 157 (*B. Rev.*)
Pulmonary cysts, lobectomy for, in fifteen-day-old infant with recovery (Burnett and Caswell), 84
embolism (Crutcher and Daniel, Jr.), 47

R

Radical one-stage pancreaticoduodenectomy (Child, III), 492
mastectomy, evaluation of skin grafting in technique of, in relation to function of arm (Neumann and Conway), 584
Radiology for medical students, 156 (*B. Rev.*)

Reconstruction, end-to-end esophageal, and partial esophagectomy, treatment of short stricture of esophagus by (Gross), 735
Rectum and anal sphincter, war wounds of (McCune), 653
benign lymphoma of (Li), 814
resection of, with preservation of anal sphincter (Nickel, Jr., and Chenoweth), 480
Reflex, carotid sinus, in man, role of glossopharyngeal nerve in; relief of carotid sinus syndrome by intracranial section of glossopharyngeal nerve (Ray and Stewart), 411
Renal tumors, importance of accurate pathologic classification in prognosis of (Foot and Humphreys), 369
Renin, epinephrine, and desoxycorticosterone, sensitization to, in pathogenesis of diastolic hypertension (Heinbecker), 623
Repair of common carotid-internal jugular arteriovenous fistula, cerebral hemorrhage following (Singleton and Singleton, Jr.), 75
and common duct injury, arterial blood supply of common and hepatic bile ducts with reference to problems of (Shapiro and Robillard), 1
of hernias, tantalum gauze in, complicated by tissue deficiency (Throckmorton), 32
plastic, transplantation, and prosthesis, restoration of thumb by (Barsky), 227
Resection, aseptic gastric, Billroth I technique (Monteiro and Barreto), 178
of carcinoma of cardiac end of stomach, unusual complications following (Barnes), 522
esophageal, preoperative, operative, and postoperative care in (Maier), 884
of rectum with preservation of anal sphincter (Nickel, Jr., and Chenoweth), 480
of stomach, transthoracic-abdominal, nutritional management of patients with (Homburger), 1011
transthoracic gastric, for lesions of cardia of stomach and lower part of esophagus (Payne and Clagett), 912
Restoration of thumb (Barsky), 227
Review of recent meetings, 722
Ribs, typhoid osteomyelitis of, treated with streptomycin and surgical excision (Royster et al.), 248
Risk of surgery in heart disease (Morrison), 561
Roentgen diagnosis of cancer of cardiac region of stomach (Sherman), 874
study of chest, principles in, 154 (*B. Rev.*)
Rupture, subcutaneous, of brachioradialis muscle (Hamilton), 806

S

Sclerosing treatment of varicose veins, sodium tetradecyl sulfate in (Dingwall et al.), 599
Shoulder, recurrent dislocations of, Magnuson-Stack procedure for (Giannestras), 794
Sinus reflex, carotid, in man, role of glossopharyngeal nerve in; relief of carotid sinus syndrome by intracranial section of glossopharyngeal nerve (Ray and Stewart), 411
Skin grafting, evaluation of, in technique of radical mastectomy in relation to function of arm (Neumann and Conway), 584
Small intestine, primary nonspecific ulcers of (Evert et al.), 185
Sodium tetradecyl sulfate in sclerosing treatment of varicose veins (Dingwall et al.), 599
Southern Surgical Association, annual session of (Johnston, Jr.), 722
Spasm, biliary, comparative study of action of demerol and opium alkaloids in relation to (Gaensler et al.), 211
Sphincter, anal, and rectum, war wounds of (McCune), 653
resection of rectum with preservation of (Nickel, Jr., and Chenoweth), 480
Spinal nerves, outline of, 318 (*B. Rev.*)
Splint, plaster traction, for compound comminuted fractures of tibia and fibula (Urist et al.), 801
Stomach, carcinoma of cardiac end of, unusual complications following resection of (Barnes), 522
cardia of, and esophagus, leiomyoma of (Kenworthy and Welch), 745
and lower part of esophagus, lesions of, transthoracic gastric resection for (Payne and Clagett), 912
cardiac end of, and esophagus, treatment of carcinoma of, by surgical extirpation (Sweet), 952
region of, roentgen diagnosis of cancer of (Sherman), 874
neurogenic tumors of (West and Knox), 450
transthoracic-abdominal resections of, nutritional management of patients with (Homburger), 1011
upper, and esophagus, carcinoma of, progress in surgical treatment of (Garlock), 906
Streptomycin and surgical excision, typhoid osteomyelitis of ribs treated with (Royster et al.), 248
Stricture, acquired, of esophagus, surgical management of, with esophagobronchial fistula and bronchiectasis of entire right lung (Clagett and Schmidt), 221

Stricture—Cont'd
of common bile duct, repair of, some experiences with anastomosis of common bile duct to duodenum and (Zinninger), 337
short, of esophagus, treatment of, by partial esophagectomy and end-to-end esophageal reconstruction (Gross), 735
Students, medical, radiology for, 156 (*B. Rev.*)
Subcutaneous emphysema following chest trauma (Sheinfeld), 278
Submaxillary gland, unusually large myxosarcomatous tumor of (Hicken et al.), 682
Sulfate, sodium tetradecyl, in sclerosing treatment of varicose veins (Dingwall et al.), 599
Sulfide, mercury tattooing with, for intractable anal pruritus (Turell), 63
Supplies, medical and surgical, needed in war-devastated areas, 734
Surgery, American, George J. Heuer's contributions and his place in (Andrus), 321
of autonomic nervous system, progress in (White), 834
graduate school, twenty-five years of, founded by George J. Heuer (Carter), 326
peripheral nerve, tantalum foil cuffs in (Cliffton), 507
prostatic, twenty-seven years of, at Bellevue hospital (Draper), 515
risk of, in heart disease (Morrison), 561
Surgical abdomen and herpes zoster (Bosher, Jr., and Williams, Jr.), 773
Association, Southern, annual session of (Johnston, Jr.), 722
care, changing status of (Ravdin), 603
excision and streptomycin, typhoid osteomyelitis of ribs treated with (Royster et al.), 248
extirpation, treatment of carcinoma of esophagus and cardiac end of stomach by (Sweet), 952
intervention, arterial and venous hypertensive states benefited by (Lord, Jr.), 550
management of acquired stricture of esophagus with esophagobronchial fistula and bronchiectasis of entire right lung (Clagett and Schmidt), 221
patients, problem of parenteral nitrogen administration in (Kremen), 92
training, observations of (Bowers), 377
treatment of acute cholecystitis (Glenn), 397
of cancers of gastric cardia (Pack and McNeer), 976
of carcinoma of esophagus and upper stomach, progress in (Garlock), 906
of nervous ssytem, 154 (*B. Rev.*)
Sympathectomy, indications for, in treatment of hypertension (Findley), 639
Sympathectomy—Cont'd
in peripheral vascular disease; surgery of autonomic nervous system (White), 843
Symposium on cancer of esophagus and gastric cardia, 867-1019
Syndrome, carotid sinus, relief of, by intracranial section of glossopharyngeal nerve; role of glossopharyngeal nerve in carotid sinus reflex in man (Ray and Stewart), 411

T

Talc, observations on absorbable powder to replace (MacQuiddy and Tollman), 786
Tantalum in craniosynostosis (Ingraham et al.), 258
foil cuffs in peripheral nerve surgery (Cliffton), 507
gauze in repair of hernias complicated by tissue deficiency (Throckmorton), 32
Tattooing; evolution of treatment of capillary hemangiomas of face with further observation on value of camouflage by permanent pigment injection (Conway), 389
with mercury sulfide for intractable anal pruritus (Turell), 63
Technique, Billroth I, aseptic gastric resection (Monteiro and Barreto), 178
Tetradecyl sulfate, sodium, in sclerosing treatment of varicose veins (Dingwall et al.), 599
Thoracic cardiectomy, anesthesia for; surgical treatment of cancers of gastric cardia (Pack and McNeer), 982
Thrombosis and embolism in surgical care (Ravdin), 611
mesenteric (McClenahan and Fisher), 778
superior vena caval; intravenous clotting (Kleinsasser), 697
Thumb, restoration of (Barsky), 227
Thyroid gland, malignant tumors of (Mc Swain and Diveley), 525
Tibia and fibula, plaster traction splint for compound comminuted fractures of (Urist et al.), 801
Tibial condyles, fractures of, conservative treatment of (Maisel and Cornell), 591
Tissue deficiency, tantalum gauze in repair of hernias complicated by (Throckmorton), 32
Traction splint, plaster, for compound comminuted fractures of tibia and fibula (Urist et al.,), 801
Training, surgical, observations of (Bowers), 377
Transdiaphragmatic and transthoracic route, cardioesophageal cancers treated via (De Amesti and Otaiza), 921
Transplantation, plastic repair, and prosthesis, restoration of thumb by (Barsky), 227

Transthoracic gastric resection for lesions of cardia of stomach and lower part of esophagus (Payne and Clagett), 912
and transdiaphragmatic route, caridoesophageal cancers treated via (De Amesti and Otaiza), 921
Trauma, chest, subcutaneous emphysema following (Sheinfeld), 278
Treatment, conservative, of fractures of tibial condyles (Maisel and Cornell), 591
operative, of chronic gastric and duodenal ulcer (Bruusgaard), 161
sclerosing, of varicose veins, sodium tetradecyl sulfate in (Dingwall et al.), 599
surgical, of acute cholecystitis (Glenn), 397
of cancers of gastric cardia (Pack and McNeer), 976
of carcinoma of esophagus and upper stomach, progress in (Garlock), 906
Tube design and material, new, in gastrointestinal intubation (Kaslow), 293
Tumors, malignant, of thyroid gland (Mc Swain and Diveley), 525
myxosarcomatous, unusually large, of submaxillary gland (Hicken et al.), 682
neurogenic, of stomach (West and Knox), 450
primary, of jejunum and ileum (Eckel), 467
renal, importance of accurate pathologic classification in prognosis of (Foot and Humphreys), 369
Typhoid osteomyelitis of ribs treated with streptomycin and surgical excision (Royster et al.), 248

U

Ulcer, bleeding peptic, further observations on treatment of (Holman), 405
chronic gastric and duodenal, operative treatment of (Bruusgaard), 161
decubitus, aid in treatment of; electric lift (Kostrubala and Wagner), 298
histamine-provoked, in dogs, production of allergic gastric and duodenal edema which predisposes to (Friesen et al.), 167

Ulcer—Cont'd
peptic, end results in treatment of, by posterior gastroenterostomy (Cooper), 425
perforated peptic, late results following (Moore and Hendricks), 442
primary nonspecific, of small intestine (Evert et al.), 185
Ulceration, peptic, course of, in elderly persons (Lasher, Jr.), 501
Ulnar and median nerve, unusual innervation of intrinsic muscles of hand by (Cliffton), 12
Ureteral obstruction, iliac lymphadenopathy as cause of (Marshall and Schnittman), 542

V

Varicose veins, sodium tetradecyl sulfate in sclerosing treatment of (Dingwall et al.), 599
Vascular centers, Army personnel in, intravenous clotting observed in (Kleinsasser), 687
Surgery, society for, announcement, 1020
Veins, varicose, sodium tetradecyl sulfate in sclerosing treatment of (Dingwall et al.), 599
Venous and arterial hypertensive states benefited by surgical intervention (Lord, Jr.), 550
Verrucous carcinoma of oral cavity (Ackerman), 670
Visceromotor denervation; surgery of autonomic nervous system (White), 848
Viscerosensory denervation; surgery of autonomic nervous system (White), 852
Vulval pruritus, reference to, and evaluation of results; tattooing with mercury sulfide for intractable anal pruritus (Turell), 63

W

War wounds of rectum and anal sphincter (McCune), 653
War-devastated areas, medical and surgical supplies needed in, 734
Wounds, gunshot, involving abdominal aorta (Holzer, Jr.), 645
penetrating, of chest, with division of bronchial artery (Brane), 476
war, of rectum and anal sphincter (McCune), 653

A